Handbook of Drug Metabolism
Third Edition

DRUGS AND THE PHARMACEUTICAL SCIENCES
A Series of Textbooks and Monographs

Series Executive Editor
James Swarbrick
PharmaceuTech, Inc.
Pinehurst, North Carolina

Recent Titles in Series

Handbook of Drug Metabolism, Third Edition, *Paul G. Pearson and Larry C. Wienkers*

The Art and Science of Dermal Formulation Development, *Marc Brown and Adrian C. Williams*

Pharmaceutical Inhalation Aerosol Technology, Third Edition, *Anthony J. Hickey and Sandro R. da Rocha*

Good Manufacturing Practices for Pharmaceuticals, Seventh Edition, *Graham P. Bunn*

Pharmaceutical Extrusion Technology, Second Edition, *Isaac Ghebre-Sellassie, Charles E. Martin, Feng Zhang, and James Dinunzio*

Biosimilar Drug Product Development, *Laszlo Endrenyi, Paul Declerck, and Shein-Chung Chow*

High Throughput Screening in Drug Discovery, Amancio Carnero Generic Drug Product Development: International Regulatory Requirements for Bioequivalence, Second Edition, *Isadore Kanfer and Leon Shargel*

Aqueous Polymeric Coatings for Pharmaceutical Dosage Forms, Fourth Edition, *Linda A. Felton*

Good Design Practices for GMP Pharmaceutical Facilities, Second Edition, *Terry Jacobs and Andrew A. Signore*

Handbook of Bioequivalence Testing, Second Edition, *Sarfaraz K. Niazi*

Generic Drug Product Development: Solid Oral Dosage Forms, Second Edition, *edited by Leon Shargel and Isadore Kanfer*

A complete listing of all volumes in this series can be found at
www.crcpress.com

Handbook of Drug Metabolism

Third Edition

Edited by

Paul G. Pearson

Larry C. Wienkers

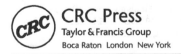

CRC Press

Taylor & Francis Group

Boca Raton London New York

CRC Press is an imprint of the
Taylor & Francis Group, an **informa** business

CRC Press
Taylor & Francis Group
6000 Broken Sound Parkway NW, Suite 300
Boca Raton, FL 33487-2742

First issued in paperback 2020

ISBN-13: 978-1-4822-6203-2 (hbk)
ISBN-13: 978-0-367-77976-4 (pbk)

Library of Congress Cataloging-in-Publication Data

Names: Pearson, Paul G. (Paul Gerard), 1960- editor. | Wienkers, Larry C., editor.
Title: Handbook of drug metabolism.
Description: Third edition / [edited by] Paul G. Pearson, Larry C. Wienkers. | Boca Raton, Florida : CRC Press, 2019. | Series: Drugs and the pharmaceutical sciences | Includes bibliographical references and index.
Identifiers: LCCN 2018057997| ISBN 9781482262032 (hardback : alk. paper) | ISBN 9780429190315 (ebook)
Subjects: LCSH: Drugs--Metabolism--Handbooks, manuals, etc.
Classification: LCC RM301.55 .H36 2019 | DDC 615.1--dc23
LC record available at https://lccn.loc.gov/2018057997

Visit the Taylor & Francis Web site at
http://www.taylorandfrancis.com

and the CRC Press Web site at
http://www.crcpress.com

This book is dedicated to Professors William F. Trager and Sidney D. Nelson

who trained and inspired a generation of drug metabolism scientists.

Contents

Section I   Fundamental Aspects of Drug Metabolism

Section II   Factors Which Affect Drug Metabolism

Section III Technologies to Study Drug Metabolism

Section IV Applications of Metabolism Studies in Drug Discovery and Development

Preface

It is almost a decade since the second edition of the *Handbook of Drug Metabolism* was published. Since its inception, the goal of the Handbook was to provide a comprehensive text to serve as a graduate course in Drug Metabolism, a useful reference for academic and industrial drug metabolism scientists, but also as an important reference tool for those pursuing a career in drug discovery and development. The third edition of the *Handbook of Drug Metabolism* has been markedly updated to capture a decade of advances in our understanding of factors that impact the pharmacokinetics and metabolism of therapeutic agents in humans. Moreover, we have sought to include new chapters that reflect significant advances that have occurred in major areas viz., the role transporters in drug disposition, active metabolites in drug development, predicting clinical pharmacokinetics, nonP450 biotransformation reactions, pharmacogenetics in drug metabolism and toxicity, drug interactions, and antibody drug conjugates.

The third edition of the *Handbook of Drug Metabolism* is organized into four sections. The first three sections capture scientific and experimental concepts around drug metabolism. Section I reviews fundamental aspects of drug metabolism, including a history of drug metabolism, a review of oxidative and non-oxidative biotransformation mechanisms, a review of liver structure, and function and pharmacokinetics of drugs metabolites. Section II details factors that impact drug metabolism, including pharmacogenetics, drug-drug interactions, and the role of extra-hepatic organs in drug biotransformation. Section III provides in depth insights into analytical technologies and methodologies to study drug metabolism at the molecular, subcellular, and cellular levels, and considerations of factors, viz. enzyme inhibition and induction that influence drug metabolism and therapeutic response. Section IV has been expanded substantially from the second edition to illustrate the highly integrated role of drug metabolism in drug discovery and drug development. In this regard, Section IV focuses on clinical and preclinical drug metabolism studies, safety considerations for drug metabolites (chemically-reactive and non-reactive metabolites) in the selection and development of promising therapeutic candidates and highlights the increased focus of regulatory agencies on safety considerations of drug metabolites.

The discipline of drug metabolism is now a highly integrated component of contemporary drug discovery and development programs—the results of these efforts have lead to only a small number of clinical development candidates that fail in clinical development for unacceptable pharmacokinetic and drug metabolism properties.

This book is dedicated to two groups of exceptional individuals. First, we thank the distinguished academic and industrial leaders (many of whom have contributed to this book) who have trained a generation, or more, of exceptional drug metabolism scientists. Second, we thank the many graduate students, post-doctoral fellows, and industrial colleagues who have challenged us and enriched our lives over the last two decades. We thank all of you for advancing the field of drug metabolism; your efforts have enabled our discipline to advance promising therapeutic agents with increased probability of success in finding medicines to treat serious illness.

Lastly, it has been a privilege to interact with this collection of expert authors, and we would like to express our sincere gratitude to them for their contributions to the third edition to the *Handbook of Drug Metabolism*.

Paul G. Pearson
Larry C. Wienkers

Editors

Paul G. Pearson is the president and CEO of Pearson Pharma Partners, Westlake Village, California, United States. Dr. Pearson received his PhD in Pharmaceutical Sciences from Aston University, Birmingham, UK. He has had an extensive and successful career in pharmaceutical science, previously serving as vice president of Pharmacokinetics and Drug Metabolism at Amgen, Inc. and executive director of Preclinical Drug Metabolism at Merck & Co, Inc. He is an active member of several international and national professional organizations. Dr. Pearson has contributed to numerous peer-reviewed publications and has been an honored invited lecturer at conferences, society meetings, and symposia on drug development, drug metabolism, and drug discovery. He is actively engaged in the discovery and development of new human therapeutics in the fields of oncology and neuroscience to make a dramatic difference to the lives of patients.

Larry C. Wienkers is a principal scientist, Wienkers Consulting, Bainbridge Island Washington, United States. Prior to consulting, Dr. Wienkers served as vice president of Pharmacokinetics and Drug Metabolism at Amgen, Inc. and senior director of Pharmacokinetics, Dynamics, and Metabolism at Pfizer. He obtained his PhD in Medicinal Chemistry from the University of Washington, Seattle, Washington, United States and in 2014 he was awarded the University of Washington, School of Pharmacy Distinguished Alumni Award in Pharmaceutical Science and Research. Larry is a member of several professional societies, where he has served as Chair of American Society of Pharmacology and Experimental Therapeutics Division of Drug Metabolism and in 2013 he was elected as a fellow in the American Association of Pharmaceutical Scientists. Dr. Wienkers has published over 80 peer-reviewed publications and book chapters, has been an invited lecturer at conferences and symposia on large- and small-molecule drug metabolism and drug discovery.

Contributors

Upendra A. Argikar
Pharmacokinetic Sciences Department
Novartis Institutes for BioMedical Research, Inc.
Cambridge, Massachusetts

Thomas A. Baillie
Department of Medicinal Chemistry
School of Pharmacy
University of Washington
Seattle, Washington

Sudheer Bobba
Department of Drug Metabolism and
    Pharmacokinetics
Genentech Inc.
South San Francisco, California

Yaofeng Cheng
Drug Metabolism
Gilead Sciences, Inc.
Foster City, California

Joshua G. Dekeyser
Department of Pharmacokinetics and Drug
    Metabolism
Amgen Inc.
One Amgen Center Drive
Thousand Oaks, California

Robert S. Foti
Department of Pharmacokinetics and Drug
    Metabolism
Amgen Inc.
Cambridge, Massachusetts

Enrico Garattini
Laboratory of Molecular Biology
IRCCS-Istituto di Ricerche Farmacologiche
    "Mario Negri"
Milano, Italy

F. Peter Guengerich
Department of Biochemistry
Vanderbilt University School of Medicine
Nashville, Tennessee

Kirk R. Henne
DMPK, Denali Therapeutics
South San Francisco, California

Emily J. Cox
Providence Medical Research Center
Providence Health & Services
Spokane, Washington

Amit S. Kalgutkar
Medicinal Sciences Department
Pfizer Worldwide Research and Development
Cambridge, Massachusetts

Sylvie E. Kandel
Department of Pharmacology, Toxicology and
    Therapeutics
The University of Kansas Medical Center
Kansas City, Kansas

S. Cyrus Khojasteh
Department of Drug Metabolism and
    Pharmacokinetics
Genentech Inc.
South San Francisco, California

Ken Korzekwa
Temple University School of Pharmacy
Philadelphia, Pennsylvania

Deanna L. Kroetz
Department of Bioengineering and
    Therapeutic Sciences
University of California
San Francisco, California

Sanjeev Kumar
Department of Drug Metabolism and
  Pharmacokinetics
Vertex Pharmaceuticals Incorporated
Boston, Massachusetts

Yurong Lai
Drug Metabolism
Gilead Sciences, Inc.
Foster City, California

John G. Lamb
Department of Pharmacology and Toxicology
College of Pharmacy
University of Utah
Salt Lake City, Utah

Jed N. Lampe
Department of Pharmacology, Toxicology and
  Therapeutics
The University of Kansas Medical Center
Kansas City, Kansas

Kimberly Lapham
Pharmacokinetics, Pharmacodynamics, and Drug
  Metabolism
Pfizer Global Research and Development
Groton, Connecticut

Lawrence H. Lash
Department of Pharmacology
Wayne State University School of Medicine
Detroit, Michigan

Jiunn H. Lin
Department of Drug Metabolism and
  Pharmacokinetics
Merck Research Laboratories
West Point, Pennsylvania

Shuguang Ma
Department of Drug Metabolism and
  Pharmacokinetics
Genentech Inc.
South San Francisco, California

Yong Ma
Department of Drug Metabolism and
  Pharmacokinetics
Genentech Inc.
South San Francisco, California

Kaushik Mitra
Department of Safety Assessment and Laboratory
  Animal Resources
Merck Research Laboratories (MRL)
Merck & Co., Inc.
West Point, Pennsylvania

Michael A. Mohutsy
Lilly Research Laboratories
Eli Lilly & Company
Indianapolis, Indiana

Patrick J. Murphy
Consultant, Drug Metabolism and Disposition
Carmel, Indiana

Swati Nagar
Temple University School of Pharmacy
Philadelphia, Pennsylvania

R. Scott Obach
Pharmacokinetics, Pharmacodynamics, and Drug
  Metabolism
Pfizer Global Research and Development
Groton, Connecticut

Paul R. Ortiz de Montellano
Department of Pharmaceutical Chemistry
School of Pharmacy
University of California
San Francisco, California

Mary F. Paine
Department of Pharmaceutical Sciences
College of Pharmacy and Pharmaceutical
  Sciences
Washington State University
Spokane, Washington

Cinthia Pastuskovas
Department of Pharmacokinetics and Drug
  Metabolism
Amgen Inc.
South San Francisco, California

Thomayant Prueksaritanont
Department of Drug Metabolism and
  Pharmacokinetics
Merck Research Laboratories
West Point, Pennsylvania

Christopher A. Reilly
Department of Pharmacology and Toxicology
College of Pharmacy
University of Utah
Salt Lake City, Utah

Brooke M. Rock
Department of Pharmacokinetics and Drug
    Metabolism
Amgen Inc.
South San Francisco, California

Dan Rock
Department of Pharmacokinetics and Drug
    Metabolism
Amgen Inc.
Seattle, Washington

Michael Schrag
Department of Drug Metabolism
Array BioPharma Inc.
Boulder, Colorado

Mark Seymour
Department of Metabolism, Covance
    Laboratories Ltd.,
Harrogate, United Kingdom

Raman Sharma
Pfizer, Inc.
Groton, Connecticut

Philip C. Smith
School of Pharmacy
University of North Carolina at Chapel Hill
Chapel Hill, North Carolina

Tore Bjerregaard Stage
Clinical Pharmacology and Pharmacy
Department of Public Health
University of Southern Denmark
Odense, Denmark

and

Department of Bioengineering and
    Therapeutic Sciences
University of California
San Francisco, California

Raju Subramanian
Department of Drug Metabolism and
    Pharmacokinetics
Gilead Sciences, Inc.
Foster City, California

Ryan H. Takahashi
Department of Drug Metabolism and
    Pharmacokinetics
Genentech Inc.
South San Francisco, California

Mineko Terao
Laboratory of Molecular Biology
IRCCS-Istituto di Ricerche Farmacologiche
    "Mario Negri"
Milano, Italy

Dan-Dan Tian
Department of Pharmaceutical Sciences
College of Pharmacy and Pharmaceutical
    Sciences
Washington State University
Spokane, Washington

George R. Tonn
DMPK, Denali Therapeutics
South San Francisco, California

Jan L. Wahlstrom
Department of Pharmacokinetics and Drug
    Metabolism
Amgen Inc.
One Amgen Center Drive
Thousand Oaks, California

Gregory S. Walker
Pfizer, Inc.
Groton, Connecticut

Shuai Wang
Department of Pharmacokinetics and Drug
    Metabolism
Amgen Inc.
Cambridge, Massachusetts

Nigel J. Waters
Nonclinical Development
Relay Therapeutics
Cambridge, Massachusetts

Bo Wen
Department of Drug Metabolism and
    Pharmacokinetics
GlaxoSmithKline
Collegeville, Pennsylvania

Larry C. Wienkers
Department of Pharmacokinetics and Drug
    Metabolism
Amgen Inc.
Seattle, Washington

Bradley K. Wong
Wong DMPK Consulting, LLC
Redwood City, California

Jiajie Yu
Department of Pharmacokinetics and Drug
    Metabolism
Amgen Inc.
South San Francisco, California

Donglu Zhang
Department of Drug Metabolism and
    Pharmacokinetics
Genentech Inc.
South San Francisco, California

Section I

Fundamental Aspects of Drug Metabolism

1

The Evolution of Drug Metabolism Research

Patrick J. Murphy

CONTENTS

Introduction

Drug metabolism research has grown from a desire to understand the workings of the human body in chemical terms to a major force in the effort to develop drugs tailored to the individual. This essay will trace the beginnings of what are now major branches of drug metabolism to provide some background to the current state of the art represented in the many chapters of this book.

Chemistry—Major Metabolic Routes

In 1828, the laboratory of Friedrich Woehler was abuzz with the synthesis of urea, the first "organic" synthetic achievement. Woehler then turned his attention to potential chemical transformations in the body. He had been interested in compounds found in urine since his undergraduate days, and when Liebig identified hippuric acid as a normal urinary product, Woehler suggested that it might be formed from benzoic acid and glycine in the body. His initial experiments in dogs, however, were inconclusive [1]. Alexander Ure, a physician seeking a cure for gout, heard about Woehler's idea and reasoned that if Woehler was correct then administration of benzoic acid to humans might lead to a diminished excretion of urea due to the use of nitrogen in the glycine conjugate. Ure took benzoic acid and isolated hippuric acid from his urine [2]. Woehler had his associate, Keller, repeat the experiment and confirmed that ingested benzoic acid was indeed excreted in the urine as hippuric acid [3].

These studies initiated a period lasting to the end of the nineteenth century when scientists and their collaborators subjected themselves to interesting molecules to "see what would happen." Many of the studies followed logical extensions of the earlier work.

Erdmann and Marchand administered cinnamic acid to volunteers and isolated a product tentatively identified as hippuric acid [4,5]. They proposed that the cinnamic acid was oxidized to benzoic acid and then conjugated with glycine. Woehler and Friederick Frerichs confirmed this transformation in dogs [6]. They also showed that benzaldehyde was converted to hippuric acid in dogs and rabbits.

The oxidation of benzene to phenol was discovered by the clinician, Bernhard Naunyn, during the course of experimental treatment of stomach "fermentation" with benzene. He was surprised to find that phenol was excreted following the administration of benzene. Naunyn then collaborated with the chemist, Schultzen, to study the fate of a number of hydrocarbons, including toluene, xylene, and larger molecules [7]. Aromatic hydroxylation, which had proven difficult for the chemists of the day, was readily accomplished in humans.

Studies on aromatic hydroxylation led Stadeler to discover conjugated phenols in human and animal urine [8]. Munk, after ingesting varying amounts of benzene, monitored the excretion of a "phenol-forming substance" in his urine by hydrolyzing the urine with acid and measuring the released phenol [9].

Baumann, using the color of indigo as his guide, purified an indigo-forming substance from urine and showed that upon hydrolysis both indigo and sulfate were released [10]. Baumann made many pioneering studies on sulfates formed from a variety of compounds, including catechol, bromobenzene, indole, and aniline.

The surprising ability of the body to methylate compounds was discovered by His in 1887 when he was able to isolate and identify *N*-methyl pyridinium hydroxide from the urine of dogs dosed with pyridine [11]. Over 60 years later, MacLagan and Wilkinson discovered the more significant *O*-methylation pathway using the phenol butyl-4-hydroxy 3,5-diiodobenzoate [12]. This is the pathway that led Axelrod to his Nobel Prize related to the methylation of catecholamines.

N-Acetylation was first described by Cohn in his studies on the fate of m-nitrobenzaldehyde. The oxidized, reduced compound is acetylated and conjugated with glycine to yield the hippurate of *N*-acetyl-m-aminobenzoic as a major metabolite [13].

Mercapturic acids were initially isolated in the laboratories of Baumann and Preuss studying the fate of bromobenzene and by Jaffe looking at chloro and iodobenzene [14,15]. The actual structure of these acetylcysteine conjugates was determined by Baumann in 1884 [16]. The nature of the cofactors in the conjugation reactions would not be known until the twentieth century.

A unique, primarily human, conjugation of glutamine with aryl acetic acids was discovered by Thierfelder and Sherwin in 1914 [17].

Active Metabolites

By the early part of the twentieth century, the major drug-metabolizing reactions had been identified. A unifying theory on the role of metabolism was developed by John Paxson Sherwin. Sherwin was one of the most prominent Americans in the field of metabolism [18]. A native of Bristol, Indiana, he was educated in Indiana and Illinois and then spent two years in Tubingen, Germany, before returning to the Midwest. He formulated the "chemical defense" theory elaborated in his reviews on drug metabolism in 1922, 1933, and 1935 [19–21]. The latter two reviews carried the title "Detoxication Mechanisms." This same title was used by R.T. Williams in his groundbreaking summaries of drug metabolism in 1947 and 1959 [22]. Although Williams was troubled with the general classification of all metabolic reactions as "detoxication," he accepted it as the most practical appellation. A mind-set that metabolism led to detoxication was so logical and had so many examples that when a compound was actually made more

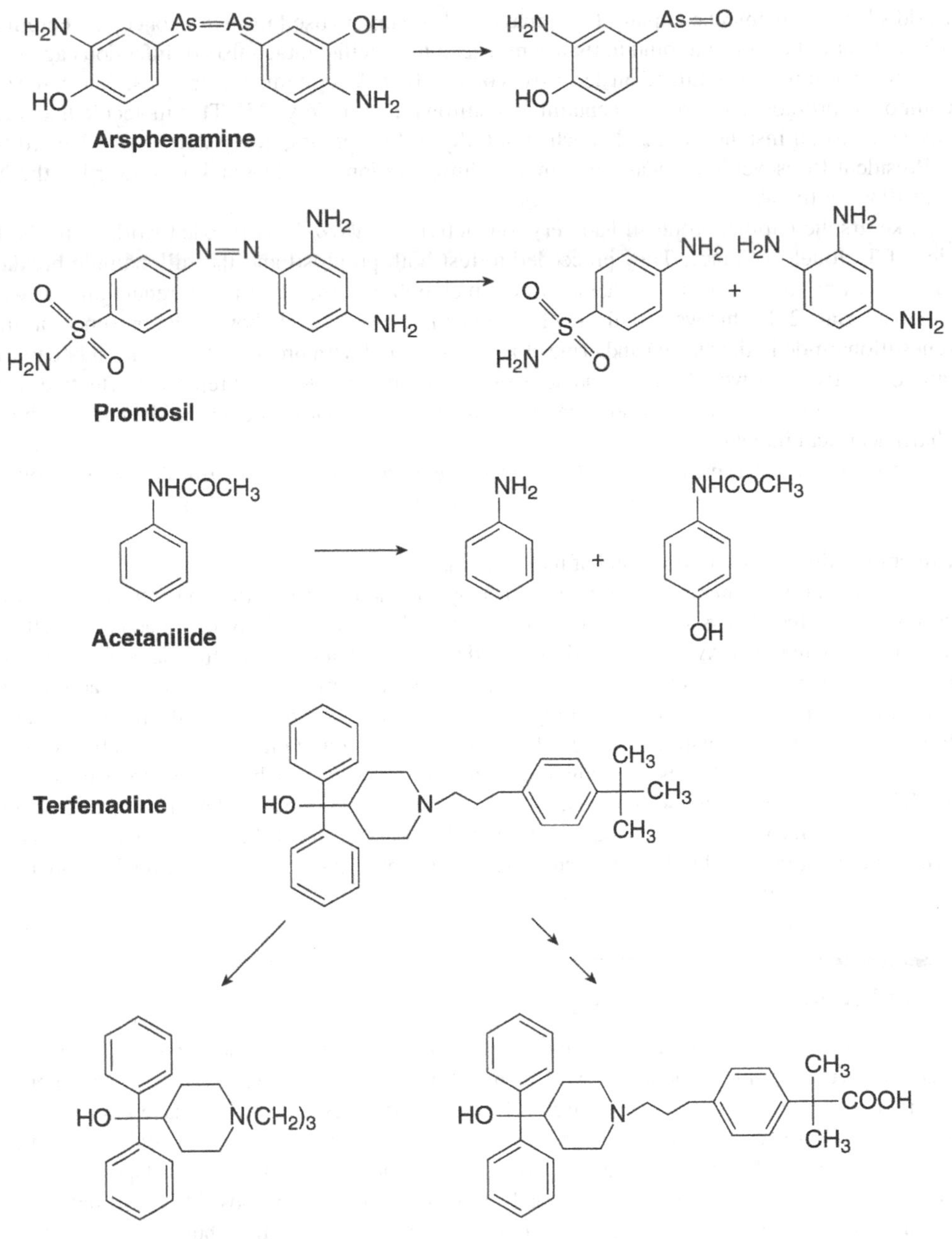

FIGURE 1.1 Examples of drug activation.

active, it engendered disbelief. But, even at this early stage of drug development, the examples of activation began to accumulate.

The world's first major drug, arsphenamine (Figure 1.1), an arsenical used for the treatment of syphilis, was ineffective *in vitro* [23]. Twelve years after its launch, studies showing that the drug worked through an oxidation product were published by Voegtlin and coworkers [24]. This compound, which evolved from the "magic bullet" concept of Ehrlich, set the stage for future worldwide "blockbusters."

A more dramatic impact of metabolism occurred with the launch of prontosil (Figure 1.1), the first major antibacterial agent. Prontosil was discovered in the early 1930s in the laboratories of I.G. Farben, the world's largest chemical company. G. Domagk and coworkers used Ehrlich's concept, wherein compounds that could be shown to bind to tissues may lead to specific antagonists of infectious agents. The early work, therefore, concentrated on derivatives of azo dyes. After numerous failures, they came across the compound prontosil, an azo dye containing a sulfonamide moiety [25]. This molecule had striking activity and was an instant success. Launched initially in Europe, it quickly stormed the United States when President Roosevelt's son was cured by its administration [26]. Domagk was awarded the Nobel Prize in 1939 for his work.

But, like arsphenamine, prontosil had very low activity *in vitro*. This puzzled workers in the laboratories of Trefouel in France. They proceeded to test both prontosil and the sulfonamide breakdown product and came to the conclusion that it was the metabolite formed by the azo reduction that was the true antibacterial [27]. This was confirmed by studies in England that showed the presence of aminobenzenesulfonamide in the plasma and urine of patients treated with prontosil [28]. Once it became clear that any derivative that would release the active sulfonamide *in vivo* could represent effective therapy, chemical companies around the world began making variations that would spawn the birth of the modern pharmaceutical industry.

Acetanilide (Figure 1.1) provides a bridge from active to toxic metabolites. Brodie and Axelrod found that acetanilide was converted to aniline, which explained the methemoglobinemia, which had been observed at high doses, and to acetaminophen, a superior analgesic [29]. This study launched the illustrious career of Julius Axelrod in the field of metabolism.

There are numerous examples of prodrugs, either by fortune or design, that must be activated for full pharmacological effect. Esters such as enalapril or clofibrate have to be hydrolyzed for activity. Methyldopa is decarboxylated and hydroxylated for activation, and cyclophosphamide is hydroxylated for activation.

There are also many other examples where the metabolites have some or all of the activity designated for the parent. One of the most striking and significant of these is the antihistamine terfenadine (Figure 1.1). The parent is oxidized to the active carboxylic acid and other metabolites by cytochrome P450 enzymes. When the P450s are inhibited, parent terfenadine reaches higher than normal levels [30,31]. This interaction led to cardiovascular problems in patients taking terfenadine and ketoconazole or erythromycin. Because of this interaction, terfenadine was taken off the market and new regulatory guidelines were put in place by the Food and Drug Administration (FDA) to alert drug developers of the need for interaction studies before approval.

Toxic and Reactive Metabolites

The products of metabolism are determined by the reaction mechanism of the enzymes involved and by the chemical structure of the reactant. Whether a metabolic product is more or less active is independent of these two interacting forces. Humans have evolved over the years, whereby we have a certain capacity to handle whatever the environment and our diets present. We learn to avoid certain toxins, which cannot be handled metabolically. The time frame of evolution does not permit the type of adaptation necessary to dispose of every new compound in a safe and beneficial manner. It is impossible to estimate what percentage of new molecular entities are converted to active or toxic metabolites, but it is clear that it has to be a higher percentage than we see just looking at marketed drugs. The fact is that if a toxic metabolite is produced during drug development, the candidate is usually eliminated from consideration. Therefore, the number of compounds actually activated by metabolism is necessarily higher than the overall documented occurrences. With any new compound, there is a significant chance that metabolism will yield pharmacologically active derivatives.

Reactive Intermediates

The formation of reactive intermediates is of particular concern in the development of new agents. Guroff and coworkers found that during the course of aromatic hydroxylation the hydrogen on the position to be hydroxylated could shift to the adjacent position [32]. This was termed the "NIH" shift and was subsequently explained by the formation of a reactive epoxide intermediate. The formation of "green pigments" during administration of 2-allyl-2-isopropylacetamide was shown by de Matteis to be due to destruction of P450 [33]. Ethylene and other olefins had similar destructive properties [34]. The most significant chemical moieties giving rise to reactive molecules and/or P450 inhibition have been reviewed [35]. Many of these compounds will react with glutathione in an inactivation step. Excretion of mercapturic acids is often taken as a sign of the formation of the reactive species. In the absence of adequate levels of glutathione or when the kinetics are favorable for protein binding, the formation of chemical-protein conjugates can lead to systemic toxicity.

The prototypical reactive intermediate is the quinone-imine formed from metabolism of acetaminophen. In a classic series of papers, Brodie and coworkers revealed the metabolic fate of acetaminophen and its potential tissue-binding metabolite [36–39]. While this compound is known to be hepatotoxic and readily binds to protein *in vitro*, it nonetheless remains a best-selling analgesic. Generally, at recommended doses, acetaminophen is efficiently removed by conjugation or, after oxidation, by glucuronidation and/or reaction with glutathione. At elevated doses or in conjunction with CYP2E1 induction, high levels of quinone-imine can lead to tissue damage [40].

Bioanalytical

The progress in drug metabolism is paralleled by, indeed dependent on, the advances in bioanalytical techniques. For most of the first century of drug metabolism research, identification of metabolites involved isolation, purification, and chemical manipulation leading to characterization. At the end of World War II, new technology developed during the war came into use in metabolism research. A study on the distribution of radioactivity in the mouse after administration of ^{14}C-dibenzanthracene set new standards for metabolic research [41]. The use of high-speed centrifuges to separate cellular components was another legacy of the Manhattan Project. The development of liquid-liquid partition chromatography by Martin and Synge [42] heralded the addition of new separation tools, including paper, thin layer, and gas chromatography. Spectrometry in biological media became routine with the Cary 14 spectrophotometer.

Mass spectrometry moved from the hands of specialists to the analytical laboratory with the launch of the LKB 9000 GC/MS. A crucial development for the eventual linking of mass spectrometry and liquid chromatography was the discovery of electrospray ionization by Fenn in 1980 [43]. LC/MS instruments from Sciex and Finnegan revolutionized the bioanalytical laboratories leading to increasingly more rapid and more efficient delineation of metabolic pathways. Newer analytical techniques permit the analysis of the chemical bound to protein and the characterization of the proteins involved. For example, Shin and coworkers recently identified binding of electrophiles to 263 proteins in human microsomal incubations [44]. Doss and Baillie [45] have suggested that drug developers use *in vitro* binding ability as a screen for potential reactive intermediates.

Enzymology—Mechanisms of Metabolism

Conjugation

The discovery of cofactor structures started with acetyl coA. This important cofactor, vital for intermediary metabolism, was identified using the acetylation of sulfanilamide as an assay. Lippman and coworkers painstakingly isolated and identified coenzyme A as the energy-containing component driving acetylation [46]. The principle of active cofactors led researchers to solving the structures of 3'-phosphoadenosine-5'-phosphosulfate (PAPS) [47], uridinediphosphoglucuronic acid (UDPGA) [48], and *S*-adenosylmethionine (SAM) [49]. Defining mercapturic acid formation took slightly longer because of the fact that the actual conjugating moiety was altered before elimination. The actual structure of mercapturic acids was solved when Baumann correctly identified the acetyl cysteine moiety [16]. Glutathione, originally isolated by M.J. de Rey Pailhade [50], was fully characterized by Hopkins in 1929 [51]. But it was not until 1959 when the relationship between glutathione conjugation and the formation of mercapturic acids was elucidated by Barnes and associates [52]. In 1961, Booth, Boyland, and Sims published data on the enzymatic formation of glutathione conjugates [53]. As a variation in the theme, it became clear that conjugation with amino acids such as glycine or glutamine involved initial activation of the substrate rather than the linking agent. The unique ability of humans and Old World monkeys to conjugate with glutamine was found to be due to the specificity of acyl transferase enzymes found in the mitochondria [54].

The structures of most of the human conjugating enzymes have now been elucidated, and in many cases, the enzymes have been cloned. Crystal structures have been slow to emerge for glucuronyl transferases because of the membrane-bound nature of these enzymes. There are 13 human sulfotransferases [55], 16 glucuronyl-transferases [56], multiple *N*-, *O*-, and *S* methyl transferases, 2 *N*-acetyl transferases [57], and 24 glutathione transferases [58]. The multiplicity of isozymes and overlapping specificities require extensive evaluation to understand which enzymes may be critical for a given drug.

Reduction

Some of the earliest *in vitro* experiments in metabolism dealt with enzymatic reduction. The importance of the azo derivatives of sulfanilamide led to initial experiments using neoprontosil as a model substrate. Bernheim reported the reduction of neoprontosil by liver homogenates [59]. Mueller and Miller studied the metabolism of the carcinogen dimethylaminoazobenzene (DAB) and found that in rat liver homogenates DAB was hydroxylated and demethylated and the azo linkage was reduced [60]. The reducing enzyme was shown to require reduced nicotinamide adenine dinucleotide phosphate (NADPH) and to reside in the particulate portion of the fragmented cells [61].

Oxidation

The incorporation of oxygen into drugs and endogenous molecules was found to occur directly from molecular oxygen using isotopically labeled oxygen [62,63]. This led to the definition of a new category of oxidases termed "monooxygenases" by Hayaishi and "mixed-function oxidases" by Mason. These oxidases required oxygen and a reductant, usually NADPH.

In Vitro Methodology/Enzymology

The unraveling of the secrets of the cell began with the development of the techniques of gently breaking the cell developed by Potter and Elvejham and then fractionating the fragments and components of the cell by differential centrifugation [64]. The first drug to be studied using these techniques was amphetamine. Axelrod examined the deamination of amphetamine and showed the activity to be dependent on oxygen and NADPH and to reside in the microsomal fraction of the cell [65]. Brodie's laboratory quickly examined a number of drug substrates and found them to be metabolized by the same microsomal system [66].

Further examination of microsomes by Klingenberg and Garfinkel revealed the presence of a pigment that had some of the properties of a cytochrome and a peak absorbance after reduction in the presence of CO at 450 nm [67,68]. The pigment was shown by Omura and Sato to be a cytochrome [69]. Estabrook Cooper and Rosenthal used light activation of the CO-inhibited system to prove that cytochrome P450 was the terminal oxidase in the oxidation of many classes of drug substrates [70]. The use of microsomes became standard practice in drug metabolism studies. However, the enzymes defied purification because of the fact that they were embedded in the membrane and solubilization inevitably led to denaturation.

Lu and Coon solved the problem of releasing the enzyme from the membrane using sodium deoxycholate in the presence of dithiothreitol and glycerol, rapidly expanding our knowledge of multiple

P450s [71]. Coon's laboratory, Wayne Levin and associates, and Fred Guengerich were among the pioneers in the separation and purification of P450s [72]. Nebert and coworkers developed a unifying nomenclature on the basis of the degree of similarity of the P450s, and the field began to blossom [73]. The culmination of the efforts to define human P450s came with the sequencing of the human genome. At that point, it was clear that there were 57 variants of human P450. The major ones involved in drug metabolism have been well characterized, while there are still some isozymes whose function is yet to be defined [72].

The physical characteristics of the enzymes are rapidly being defined. The first P450 to be crystallized and the first structure determined were from a pseudomonad, *Pseudomonas putida* [74]. This provided a blueprint for all the structures to come. Human P450s resisted crystallization until they were modified by shortening the amino terminus. It is this portion of the protein that binds the membrane, and by removing the amino terminal segment, it was possible to obtain a soluble, active P450 that could be crystallized and analyzed. The crystal structures of all of the major drug-metabolizing P450s now have been determined [75]. The knowledge of the crystal structures has helped in our understanding of the broad specificity of this class of enzymes, helped to determine the necessary properties of potential substrates, and led to the development of computer programs to predict whether a compound will be a substrate or not [76].

While the P450s have been the stars of drug metabolism, there are many other oxidative enzymes that can play a role, sometimes dominant, in the fate of new molecules. The flavin monooxygenases (FMOs), which are often involved in the metabolism of heterocyclic amines, sulfur, or phosphorous-containing compounds, have been characterized and five forms identified [77]. Aldehyde oxidase, a molybdenum-containing enzyme oxidizes nitrogen heterocycles and aldehydes [78], xanthine oxidase and xanthine dehydrogenase mainly involved in the production of uric acid [79], aldehyde dehydrogenase (3 classes, at least 17 genes [80], and alcohol dehydrogenase [23 distinct human forms]) [81] are among the enzymes most prominent in drug metabolism.

Genetic Characteristics of Drug-Metabolizing Enzymes

The drug-metabolizing enzymes showed early indications of genetic polymorphism on the basis of the individual variations in therapeutic effectiveness. The discovery of the utility of isoniazid in the treatment of tuberculosis was quickly followed by the realization that a significant portion of the patient population had elevated levels of isoniazid in the plasma. This was traced to a genetically determined deficiency in the *N*-acetyl transferase responsible for the inactivation of isoniazid [82]. Similarly, genetic variations in serum cholinesterase led to altered susceptibility to the effects of the muscle-relaxant succinyl choline [83]. A major breakthrough in the enzymes involved with drug oxidation came with the studies of Smith and coworkers on debrisoquine metabolism [84] and the work of Eichelbaum and coworkers on sparteine metabolism [85]. These discoveries led to a broad range of population studies on debrisoquine hydroxylase, later to be identified as CYP450 2D6. The variation in blood levels of these agents could be traced to whether patients had diminished levels of CYP2D6 or, in some cases, enhanced levels of CYP2D6.

As we learned more about the role of the isozymes of P450, genetic variations became a major topic of study. Significant polymorphic variations in CYP2C9, CYP 2C19, CYP2A6, and CYP2B6 must be taken into account for substrates of these enzymes [86]. Other oxidizing enzymes such as FMOs [87] and dihydropyrimidine dehydrogenase [88] also show genetic variation leading to drug toxicity. Conjugating enzymes such as thiopurine methyl transferase, *N*-acetyl transferase, and glucuronyl transferase have variants that have been shown to be important in altered response to drugs [89].

The message for drug development is clear. It is vital to know the enzymes involved in the breakdown of the administered drug. If a specific isozyme is responsible for either the majority of the inactivation or for the activation of an agent, then appropriate studies are required to determine the efficacy and/or toxicity of the drug over a spectrum of the population, including the genetic variants.

Induction-Control Mechanisms

One of the most striking features of drug-metabolizing enzymes is their ability to adapt to the substrate load. Early studies showed that ethanol administration to rats increased the ability of the kidney to metabolize ethanol [90], while borneol administration to dogs or menthol administration to mice led to increased β-glucuronidase activity in these species [91]. Conney et al. discovered enzyme induction by aromatic hydrocarbons [92], while Remmer and Merker reported phenobarbital induction of smooth endoplasmic reticulum in rabbits, rats, and dogs [93]. Studies on the induction phenomenon eventually led to discovery of the Ah receptor [94]. The mechanism of transcriptional regulation has been elucidated and forms the basis for our understanding of this superfamily of regulators [95]. Other receptors integral to the initiation of induction include peroxisome proliferator activated receptor (PPAR) [96], constitutive androstane receptor (CAR), and pregnane X receptor (PXR). Interactions between CAR and PXR have recently been reviewed [97]. The crystal structure of the human PXR ligand-binding domain in the presence and absence of ligands has been reported [98,99].

Inhibitors

Compounds that had broad specificity as inhibitors of P450 played a major role in the understanding of this class of enzymes. The discovery of SKF525a in the laboratories of SKF and its expanded use by Brodie and coworkers defined the microsomal oxidases before the discovery of P450 [100,101]. That one inhibitor could decrease the metabolism of so many diverse compounds argued for an enzyme with broad specificity or multiple enzymes with a common site of inhibition. Other inhibitors such as metyrapone, ketoconazole, and AIA were similarly employed. Attention was drawn to the role of inhibition in drug interactions when cimetidine, a popular proton pump inhibitor, was found to be a weak inhibitor of P450-catalyzed reactions [102]. The observation that grapefruit juice had inhibitory properties stimulated the studies of endogenous and environmental inhibitors resulting in adverse drug reactions [103]. Once the multiplicity of P450s was clear, specific inhibitors of individual isozymes were used to define activity [35]. These inhibitors included antibodies with unique specificities [104]. The field of specific inhibitors for targeted therapy is rapidly developing, as the roles of all 57 P450s are unraveled [105,106].

Transporters

The discovery of P-glycoprotein (P-gp or mdr1) in 1976 created an enhanced appreciation of the role of transporters in drug disposition [107]. In addition to playing an important role in drug penetration through the intestine, pgp plays a significant role in controlling the penetration of many drugs into the brain [108]. Umbenhauer and coworkers showed that a genetic deficiency in pgp correlated with the penetration of avermectin into the brain in mice [109,110]. Later studies showed a wide range of compounds controlled in a similar fashion. There are many other transporters that have yet to be characterized with regard to drug disposition. A total of 770 transporter proteins were predicted from analysis of the human genome. The ABC family, which contains pgp, consists of 47 members. The latest information and structural details on transporters can be found in the transporter protein analysis database [111]. The first crystal structure of an *S. aureus* ABC transporter was reported in 2007 [112]. In the drug development process, knowledge as to whether the candidate compounds are substrates for transporters is crucial to predicting bioavailability.

Drug Metabolism Research in Drug Development

The overall progression of drug metabolism from the determination of metabolic pathways to the current position in metabolic profiling is shown in Figure 1.2. The evolution of drug metabolism research has changed the role of the drug metabolism scientist in a most dramatic fashion. The modern day metabolism scientist must understand and evaluate not just the chemistry of metabolism but also the enzymatic, genetic, environmental, mechanistic, and interactive aspects of any new agent. The metabolism scientist must be able to develop a compound profile detailing all the nuances involved in proposed therapy. This profile, or metafile (Figure 1.3), must encompass a breadth of understanding enabling the design of clinical studies that facilitates the tailoring of the new agent to the most appropriate patient population.

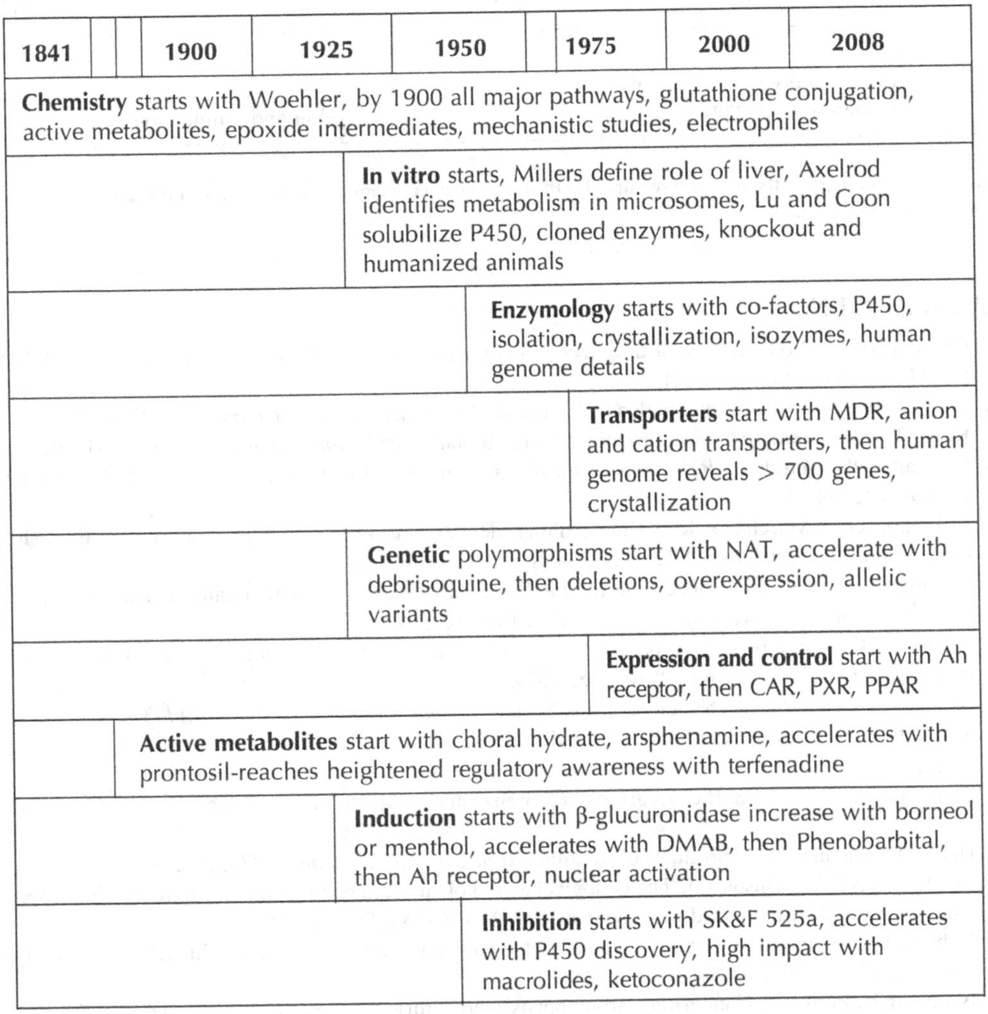

1841			1900	1925	1950	1975	2000	2008

Chemistry starts with Woehler, by 1900 all major pathways, glutathione conjugation, active metabolites, epoxide intermediates, mechanistic studies, electrophiles

In vitro starts, Millers define role of liver, Axelrod identifies metabolism in microsomes, Lu and Coon solubilize P450, cloned enzymes, knockout and humanized animals

Enzymology starts with co-factors, P450, isolation, crystallization, isozymes, human genome details

Transporters start with MDR, anion and cation transporters, then human genome reveals > 700 genes, crystallization

Genetic polymorphisms start with NAT, accelerate with debrisoquine, then deletions, overexpression, allelic variants

Expression and control start with Ah receptor, then CAR, PXR, PPAR

Active metabolites start with chloral hydrate, arsphenamine, accelerates with prontosil-reaches heightened regulatory awareness with terfenadine

Induction starts with β-glucuronidase increase with borneol or menthol, accelerates with DMAB, then Phenobarbital, then Ah receptor, nuclear activation

Inhibition starts with SK&F 525a, accelerates with P450 discovery, high impact with macrolides, ketoconazole

FIGURE 1.2 The evolution of drug metabolism research from the earliest days of discovery to the current broad-ranging research effort. Abbreviations: Peroxisome proliferator activated receptor, PPAR; constitutive androstane receptor, CAR; pregnane X receptor, PXR.

Metabolic Profile (Metafile)	

Transformation products
Identification
  -Human in vitro/in vivo
  -Animal in reference to efficacy
    models and toxicity models
Activity
  -Desirable
  -Extraneous, adverse
	Genetics
	  -Genotype for enzymes involved
	    in metabolism/disposition
	  -Phenotype for enzymes
	  -Impact of genetic polymorphisms
	  -species comparisons

Bioavailability
  -Methods of analysis
    parent/metabolites
  -Pharmacokinetics
	Interactions
	  -**Inhibition** by or of other drugs
	    Parent, metabolites
	  -**Induction** potentiality Parent,
	    metabolites

Enzymology
  -Enzymes involved in metabolism
  -Location of enzymes
	Transporters
	  -Transporters involved in
	    absorption and elimination

FIGURE 1.3 Summary of the research required for the creation of a compound profile. Many of these areas have greatly expanded in the last 25 years.

REFERENCES

1. Conti A, Bickel MH. History of drug metabolism: Discoveries of the major pathways in the 19th century. *Drug Metab Rev* 1977; 6:1–50.
2. Ure A. On gouty concretions; with a new method of treatment. *Pharm J Transact* 1841; 1:24.
3. Keller W. On the conversion of benzoic acid into hippuric acid. *Ann Chem Pharm* 1842; 43:108.
4. Erdmann OL, Marchand RF. Metabolism of cinnamic acid to hippuric acid in animals. *Ann Chem Pharm* 1842; 44:344.
5. Erdmann OL, Marchand RF. Umwandlung der Zimmtsa̋ure in Hippursa̋ure im thierishchen Organismus. *J Prakt Chem* 1842; 26:491–498.
6. Woehler F, Frerichs FT. Concerning the modifications which particular organic materials undergo in their transition to the urine. *Ann Chem Pharm* 1848; 63:335.
7. Schultzen O, Naunyn B. The behavior of benzene-derived hydrocarbons in the animal organism. *duBois-Reymond's Arch Anat Physiol* 1867:349.
8. Stadeler G. Ueber die flűchtigen Sa̋uren des Harns. *Ann Chem Liebigs* 1851; 77:17–37.
9. Munk I. Zur Kenntniss der phenolbildenden Substanz im Harn. *Arch Ges Physiol Pfluegers* 1876; 12:142–151.
10. Baumann E. Concerning the occurrence of Brenzcatechin in the urine. *Pfluger's Arch Physiol* 1876; 12:69.
11. His W. On the metabolic products of pyridine. *Arch Exp Path Pharmak* 1887; 22:253.
12. MacLagan NF, Wilkinson JH. The biological action of substances related to thyroxine. 7. The metabolism of butyl 4-hydroxy-3:5-diiodobenzoate. *Biochem J* 1954; 56:211–215.
13. Cohn R. Concerning the occurrence of acetylated conjugates following the administration of aldehydes. *Z Physiol Chem* 1893; 17:274.
14. Baumann E, Preuss C. Concerning Bromophenylmercapturic acid. *Ber Dtsch Chem Ges* 1879; 12:806.
15. Jaffe M. Ueber die nach einfuhrung von brombenzol und chlorbenzol im organismusentstehenden schwefelhaltigen sauren. *Ber Dtsch Chem Ges* 1879; 12:1092–1098.
16. Baumann E. Ueber cystin und cystein. *Z Physiol Chem* 1884; 8:299–305.
17. Thierfelder H, Sherwin CP. Phenylacetyl-glutamin, ein Stoffwechsel-Produkt des menschlichenKorpers nach Eingabe von Phenylessigsaure. *Ber Dtsch Chem Ges* 1914; 47:2630–2634.

18. Di Carlo FJ, Adams JD, Adams N. Carl Paxson Sherwin, American pioneer in drug metabolism. *Drug Metab Rev* 1992; 24:493–530.
19. Harrow B, Sherwin CP. Detoxication mechanisms. *Annu Rev Biochem* 1935; 4:263–278.
20. Ambrose AM, Sherwin CP. Detoxication mechanisms. *Annu Rev Biochem* 1933; 2:377–396.
21. Sherwin CP. The fate of foreign organic compounds in the animal body. *Physiol Rev* 1922;2:238–276.
22. Williams RT. *Detoxication Mechanisms*. 2nd ed. New York: John Wiley & Sons, 1959.
23. Ehrlich P, Hata S. *The Experimental Chemotherapy of Spirilloses*. English ed. New York: Rebman Company, 1911.
24. Voegtlin C, Smith HW. Quantitative studies in chemotherapy III. The oxidation of arsphenamine. *J Pharmacol Exp Ther* 1920; 16:199–217.
25. Domagk G. A report on the chemotherapy of bacterial infections. *Deut Med Woch* 1935; lxi:250.
26. Hager T. *The Demon Under the Microscope*. New York: Harmony Books, 2006.
27. Tréfouël J, Tréfouël J, Nitti F, Bovet D. Activity of p-aminophenylsulfamide in the experimental streptococcal infections of the mouse and rabbit. *C R Seances Soc Biol* 1935; 120:756.
28. Colebrook L, Kenny M. Treatment with prontosil of puerperal infections due to hemolyticstreptococci. *Lancet* 1936; 1:1319.
29. Brodie BB, Axelrod J. The fate of acetanilide in man. *J Pharmacol Exp Ther* 1948; 94:29–38.
30. Monahan BP, Ferguson CL, Killeavy ES, Lloyd BK, Troy J, Cantilena LR Jr, Torsades depointes occurring in association with terfenadine use. *JAMA* 1990; 264:2788–2790.
31. Jurima-Romet M, Crawford K, Cyr T, Inaba T. Terfenadine metabolism in human liver: *In Vitro* inhibition by macrolide antibiotics and azole antifungals. *Drug Metab Dispos* 1994; 22:849–856.
32. Guroff GDJ, Jerina DM, Renson J, Witkop B, Udenfriend S. Hydroxylation-induced migration: The NIH shift—Recent experiments reveal an unexpected and general result of enzymatic hydroxylation of aromatic compounds. *Science* 1967; 157:1524–1530.
33. De Matteis F. Loss of haem in rat liver caused by the porphyrogenic agent 2-allyl-2isopropylacetamide. *Biochem J* 1971; 124(4):767–777.
34. Ortiz de Montelano PR, Mico BA. Destruction of cytochrome P-450 by ethylene and other olefins. *Mol Pharm* 1980; 18:128–135.
35. Murray M, Reidy GF. Selectivity in the inhibition of mammalian cytochromes P-450 by chemical agents. *Pharmacol Rev* 1990; 42:85–101.
36. Jollow DJ, Mitchell JR, Potter WZ, Davis DC, Gillette JR, Brodie BB. Acetaminophen-induced hepatic necrosis. II. Role of covalent binding *in vivo*. *J Pharmacol Exp Ther* 1973; 187(1):195–202.
37. Mitchell JR, Jollow DJ, Potter WZ, Davis DC, Gillette JR, Brodie BB. Acetaminophen-induced hepatic necrosis. I. Role of drug metabolism. *J Pharmacol Exp Ther* 1973; 187(1):185–194.
38. Mitchell JR, Jollow DJ, Potter WZ, Gillette JR, Brodie BB. Acetaminophen-induced hepatic necrosis. IV. Protective role of glutathione. *J Pharmacol Exp Ther* 1973; 187(1):211–217.
39. Potter WZ, Davis DC, Mitchell JR, Jollow DJ, Gillette JR, Brodie BB. Acetaminophen-induced hepatic necrosis. III. Cytochrome P-450-mediated covalent binding *in vitro*. *J Pharmacol Exp Ther* 1973; 187(1):203–210.
40. Chen C, Krausz KW, Idle JR, Gonzalez FJ. Identification of novel toxicity-associated metabolites by metabolomics and mass isotopomer analysis of acetaminophen metabolism in wild-type and Cyp2e1-null mice. *J Biol Chem* 2008; 283:4543–4559.
41. Heidelberger C, Jones HB. The distribution of radioactivity in the mouse following administration of dibenzanthracene labeled in the 9 and 10 positions with carbon 14. *Cancer* 1948; 1:252–260.
42. Martin AJ, Synge RL. A new form of chromatogram employing two liquid phases: A theory of chromatography. 2. Application to the micro-determination of the higher monoamino-acids in proteins. *Biochem J* 1941; 35:1358–1368.
43. Fenn JB, Mann M, Meng CK, Wong SF, Whitehouse CM. Electrospray ionization for mass spectrometry of large biomolecules. *Science* 1989; 246:64–71.
44. Shin N, Liu Q, Stamer SL, Liebler DC. Protein targets of reactive electrophiles in human liver microsomes. *Chem Res Toxicol* 2007; 20:859–867.
45. Doss GA, Baillie TA. Addressing metabolic activation as an integral component of drug design. *Drug Metab Rev* 2006; 38:641–649.
46. Lipmann F. Acetylation of sulfanilamide by liver homogenates and extracts. *J Biol Chem* 1945; 160:173–190.

47. Robbins PW, Lipmann F. Isolation and identification of active sulfate. *J Biol Chem* 1957; 229:837–851.

48. Dutton GJ, Storey IDE. The isolation of a compound of uridine diphosphate and glucuronicacid from liver. *Biochem J* 1953; 53:37–38.

49. Cantoni GL. S-adenosylmethionine; a new intermediate formed enzymatically from l-methionine and adenosinetriphosphate. *J Biol Chem* 1953; 204:403–416.

50. De Rey-Pailhade J. Sur un corps d'origine organique hydrogenant le soufre a froid. (On a body of organic origin hydrogenated cold sulfur). *C R Hebd Seances Acad Sci* 1888;106:1683–1684 (in French).

51. Hopkins FG. On glutathione: A reinvestigation. *J Biol Chem* 1929; 84:269–320.

52. Barnes MM, James SP, Wood PB. The formation of mercapturic acids. 1. Formation of mercapturic acid and the levels of glutathione in tissues. *Biochem J* 1959; 71:680–690.

53. Booth J, Boyland E, Sims P. An enzyme from rat liver catalysing conjugations with glutathione. *Biochem J* 1961; 79:516–524.

54. Webster LT, Siddiqui, UA, Lucas, SV, Strong, JM, Mieyal, JJ. Identification of separateacyl-CoA: Glycine and acyl-CoA: L-glutamine N-acyltransferase activities in mitochondrial fractions from liver of rhesus monkey and man. *J Biol Chem* 1976; 251:3352–3358.

55. Allali-Hassani APP, Dombrovski L, Najmanovich R, Tempel W, Dong A, Loppnau P, Martin F et al. Structural and chemical profiling of the human cytosolic sulfotransferases. *PLoS Biol* 2007; 5:e97.

56. Tukey RH, Strassburg CP. Human UDP-glucuronosyltransferases: Metabolism, expression and disease. *Annu Rev Pharmacol Toxicol* 2000; 40:581–616.

57. Wu H, Dombrovsky L, Tempel W, Martin F, Loppnau P, Goodfellow GH, Grant DM, Plotnikov AN. Structural basis of substrate-binding specificity of human arylamine N-acetyltransferases. *J Biol Chem* 2007; 282:30189–30197.

58. Hayes JD, Flanagan JU, Jowsey IR. Glutathione transferases. *Annu Rev Pharmacol Toxicol* 2005; 45:51–88.

59. Bernheim F. The reduction of neoprontosil by tissues *in vitro*. *J Pharmacol Exp Ther* 1941;71:344–348.

60. Mueller GC, Miller JA. The metabolism of 4-dimethylaminoazobenzene by rat liverhomogenates. *J Biol Chem* 1948; 176:535–544.

61. Mueller GC, Miller JA. The reductive cleavage of 4-dimethylaminoazobenzene by rat liver: The intracellular distribution of the enzyme system and its requirement for triphosphopyridine nucleotide. *J Biol Chem* 1949; 180(3):1125–1136.

62. Hayaishi O, Katagiri M, Rothberg S. *J Am Chem Soc* 1955; 77:5450.

63. Mason HS, Fowlks WL, Peterson E. Oxygen transfer and electron transport by the phenolasecomplex. *J Am Chem Soc* 1955; 77(10):2914–2915.

64. De Duve C, Beaufay H. A short history of tissue fractionation. *J Cell Biol* 1981; 9:293s–299s.

65. Axelrod J. The enzymatic deamination of amphetamine (benzedrine). *J Biol Chem* 1955;214:753–763.

66. Brodie BB, Axelrod J, Cooper JR, Gaudette L, La Du B, Mitoma C, Udenfriend S. Detoxication of drugs and other foreign compounds by liver microsomes. *Science* 1955; 121:603–604.

67. Klingenberg M. Pigments of rat liver microsomes. *Arch Biochem Biophys* 1958; 75:376–386.

68. Garfinkel D. Studies on pig liver microsomes. I. Enzymic and pigment composition of different microsomal fractions. *Arch Biochem Biophys* 1958; 77:493–509.

69. Omura T, Sato R. A new cytochrome in liver microsomes. *J Biol Chem* 1962; 237:1375–1376.

70. Estabrook RW, Cooper DY, Rosenthal O. The light-reversible carbon monoxide inhibition of the steroid C-21 hydroxylation system of the adrenal cortex. *Biochem Z* 1963; 338:741–755.

71. Lu AYH, Coon MJ. Role of hemoprotein P450 in fatty acid o-hydroxylation in a soluble enzyme system from liver microsomes. *J Biol Chem* 1968; 243:1331–1332.

72. Guengerich FP. Human cytochrome P450 enzymes. In: Paul R Ortiz de Montellano, ed. *Cytochrome P450: Structure, Mechanism, and Biochemistry*. 3rd ed. New York: Kluwer Academic/Plenum Publishers, 2005:377–463.

73. Nebert DW, Adesnik M, Coon MJ, Estabrook RW, Gonzalez FJ, Guengerich FP, Gunsalus IC et al. The P450 gene superfamily: Recommended nomenclature. *DNA* 1987; 6:1–11.

74. Poulos TL, Finzel BC, Howard AJ. Crystal structure of substrate-free Pseudomonas putidacytochrome P-450. *Biochemistry* 1986; 25:5314–5322.

75. Rowland P, Blaney FE, Smyth MG, Jones JJ, Leydon VR, Oxbrow AK, Lewis CJ et al. Crystal structure of human cytochrome P450 2D6. *J Biol Chem* 2006; 281:7614–7622.

76. Yamashita F, Hashida M. In silico approaches for predicting ADME properties of drugs. *Drug Metab Pharmacokinet* 2004; 19:327–338.
77. Krueger SK, Williams DE. Mammalian flavin-containing monooxygenases: Structure/function, genetic polymorphisms and role in drug metabolism. *Pharmacol Ther* 2005; 106:357–387.
78. Garattini E, Mendel R, Romão MJ, Wright R, Terao M. Mammalian molybdo-flavoenzymes, an expanding family of proteins: Structure, genetics, regulation, function and pathophysiology. *Biochem J* 2003; 372(1):15–32.
79. Pacher P, Nivorozhkin A, Szabo´ C. Therapeutic effects of xanthine oxidase inhibitors: Renaissance half a century after the discovery of allopurinol. *Pharmacol Rev* 2006; 58:87–114.
80. Vasiliou V, Pappa A, Estey T. Role of human aldehyde dehydrogenases in enobiotic andxenobiotic metabolism. *Drug Metab Rev* 2004; 36:279–299.
81. Agarwal DP, Goedde HW. Pharmacogenetics of alcohol dehydrogenase. In: Kalow W, ed. *Pharmacogenetics of Drug Metabolism*. New York: Pergammon, 1992; 263–280.
82. Evans DA, Manley KA, McKusick VA. Genetic control of isoniazid metabolism in man. *Br Med J* 1960; 2:485–491.
83. Kalow W. Butyrylcholine esterase in the blood serum of man and animal. *Naunyn Schmiedebergs Arch Exp Pathol Pharmakol* 1952; 215:370–377.
84. Mahgoub A, Idle JR, Dring LG, Lancaster R, Smith RL. Polymorphic hydroxylation of debrisoquine in man. *Lancet* 1977; 2:584–586.
85. Eichelbaum M, Spannbrucker N, Dengler HJ. A probably genetic defect of the metabolism of sparteine. In: Gorrod JW, ed. *Biological Oxidation of Nitrogen*. Amsterdam, the Netherlands: Elsevier/NorthHoiland Biomedical Press, 1978:113–118.
86. Ingelman-Sundberg M, Sim SC, Gomez A, Rodriguez-Antona C. Influence of cytochrome P450 polymorphisms on drug therapies: Pharmacogenetic, pharmacoepigenetic and clinical aspects. *Pharmacol Ther* 2007; 116:496–526.
87. Koukouritaki SB, Poch MT, Henderson MC, Siddens LK, Krueger SK, VanDyke JE, Williams DE, Pajewski NM, Wang T, Hines RN. Identification and functional analysis of common human flavin-containing monooxygenase 3 genetic variants. *J Pharmacol Exp Ther* 2007; 320:266–273.
88. Harris BE, Carpenter JT, Diasio RB. Severe 5-fluorouracil toxicity secondary todihydropyrimidine dehydrogenase deficiency: A potentially more common pharmacogenetic syndrome. *Cancer* 1991; 68:499–501.
89. Gardiner SJ, Begg EJ. Pharmacogenetics, drug-metabolizing enzymes, and clinical practice. *Pharmacol Rev* 2006; 58:521–590.
90. Leloir LF, Mufioz JM. Ethyl alcohol metabolism in animal tissues. *Biochem J* 1938; 32:299–307.
91. Fishman WH. Studies on b-glucuronidase. III. The increase in b-glucuronidase activity of mammalian tissues induced by feeding glucuronidogenic substances. *J Biol Chem* 1940; 136:229–236.
92. Conney AH, Miller EC, Miller JA. The metabolism of methylated aminoazo dyes. V. Evidence for induction of enzyme synthesis in the rat by 3-methylcholanthrene. *Cancer Res* 1956; 16:450–459.
93. Remmer H, Merker HJ. Drug-induced changes in the liver endoplasmic reticulum: Association with drug-metabolizing enzymes. *Science* 1963; 142:1637–1638.
94. Poland A, Glover E, Kende AS. Stereospecific, high affinity binding of 2,3,7,8-tetrachlorodibenzo-p-dioxin by hepatic cytosol: Evidence that the binding species is receptor for induction of aryl hydrocarbon hydroxylase. *J Biol Chem* 1976; 251:4936–4946.
95. McMillan BJ, Bradfield CA. The aryl hydrocarbon receptor sans xenobiotics: Endogenous function in genetic model systems. *Mol Pharmacol* 2007; 72:487–498.
96. Michalik L, Auwerx J, Berger JP, Chatterjee VK, Glass CK, Gonzalez FJ, Grimaldi PA et al. International union of pharmacology. LXI. Peroxisome proliferator-activated receptors. *Pharmacol Rev* 2006; 58:726–741.
97. Moreau A, Vilarem MJ, Maurel Pl. Xenoreceptors CAR and PXR activation and consequences on lipid metabolism, glucose homeostasis, and inflammatory response. *Mol Pharm* 2008; 5:35–41.
98. Watkins RE, Wisely GB, Moore LB, Collins JL, Lambert MH, Williams SP, Willson TM, Kliewer SA, Redinbo MR. The human nuclear xenobiotic receptor PXR: Structural determinants of directed promiscuity. *Science* 2001; 292:2329–2333.
99. Xue Y, Moore LB, Orans J, Peng L, Bencharit S, Kliewer SA, Redinbo MR. Crystal structure of the pregnane X receptor-estradiol complex provides insights into endobiotic recognition. *Mol Endocrinol* 2007; 21:1028–1038.

100. Cooper JR, Axelrod J, Brodie BB. Inhibitory effects of b-diethylaminoethyldiphenylpropylacetate on a variety of drug metabolic pathways *in vitro. J Pharmacol Exp Ther* 1954; 112:55–63.
101. Axelrod J, Reichenthal J, Brodie BB. Mechanism of the potentiating action ofb-diethylaminoethyldiphenylpropylacetate. *J Pharmacol Exp Ther* 1954; 112:49–54.
102. Puurunen J, Pelkonen O. Cimetidine inhibits microsomal drug metabolism in the rat. *Eur J Pharmacol* 1979; 55:335–336.
103. Bailey DG, Spence JD, Munoz C, Arnold JM. Interaction of citrus juices with felodipine andnifedipine. *Lancet* 1991; 337:268–269.
104. Gelboin HV, Krausz K. Monoclonal antibodies and multifunctional cytochrome P450: Drug metabolism as paradigm. *J Clin Pharmacol* 2006; 46:353–372.
105. Haining RL, Nichols-Haining M. Cytochrome P450-catalyzed pathways in human brain: Metabolism meets pharmacology or old drugs with new mechanism of action? *Pharmacol Ther* 2007; 113:537–545.
106. Schuster I, Bernhardt R. Inhibition of cytochromes p450: Existing and new promising therapeutic targets. *Drug Metab Rev* 2007; 39:481–499.
107. Juliano RL, Ling V. A surface glycoprotein modulating drug permeability in Chinese hamster ovary cell mutants. *Biochim Biophys Acta* 1976; 455:152–162.
108. Schinkel AH, Smit JJ, van Tellingen O, Beijnen JH, Wagenaar E, van Deemter L et al. Disruption of the mouse mdr1a P-glycoprotein gene leads to a deficiency in the blood-brain barrier and to increased sensitivity to drugs. *Cell* 1994; 77:491–502.
109. Umbenhauer DR, Lankas GR, Pippert TR, Wise LD, Cartwright ME, Hall SJ, Beare CM. Identification of a p-glycoprotein-deficient subpopulation in the CF-1 mouse strain using a restriction fragment length polymorphism. *Toxicol Appl Pharmacol* 1997; 146:88–94.
110. Kwei GY, Alvaro RF, Chen Q, Jenkins HJ, Hop CE, Keohane CA et al. Disposition of ivermectin and cyclosporin A in CF-1 mice deficient in mdr1a P-glycoprotein. *Drug Metab Dispos* 1999; 27:581–587.
111. Ren Q, Chen K, Paulsen IT. Transport DB: A comprehensive database resource for cytoplasmic membrane transport systems and outer membrane channels. *Nucleic Acids Res* 2007;35: D274–D279.
112. Dawson RJ, Locher KP. Structure of the multidrug ABC transporter Sav1866 from Staphylococcus aureus in complex with AMP-PNP. *FEBS Lett* 2007; 581:935–938.

2

Pharmacokinetics of Drug Metabolites

Philip C. Smith

CONTENTS

Introduction

Drug metabolites and their disposition *in vivo* are well recognized by scientists, clinicians, and regulatory agencies to be important when evaluating a new drug entity. In the past several decades, increased attention has been placed on drug metabolism for several reasons. Firstly, the number of drugs with active metabolites, by design (i.e., prodrugs) or by chance, has increased (1–3). This is exemplified by the transition from terfenadine to its active metabolite fexofenadine (3) and interest in the contributions of morphine-6-glucuronide (M6G) toward the analgesic activity of the age-old drug, morphine, and potential development of this active metabolite (4). In addition, with the advent of methods to establish the metabolic genotype and characterize the phenotype of individual patients (5,6) and the identification of specific isoforms of enzymes of metabolism, there is an increased appreciation of how elimination of a drug by metabolism can influence drug bioavailability and clearance, and ultimately affect its efficacy and toxicity. These rapidly evolving methods can be translated to permit cost-effective individual optimization of drug therapy on the basis of a subject's metabolic capability (5,6), just as renal creatinine clearance has been used for years to assess renal function and permits individualized dose adjustment for drugs cleared by the kidney (7). Finally, the well accepted, though still poorly understood role of bioactivation in the potential toxicity of drugs and other xenobiotics (8,9) requires that metabolites continue to be evaluated and scrutinized for possible contributions to adverse effects observed *in vivo*. Though the importance of drug metabolism is seldom questioned, the interpretation and use of pharmacokinetic data on the disposition of metabolites is not well understood or fully implemented by some investigators. The objective of this chapter is to provide a basis for the interpretation and use of metabolite pharmacokinetic data from preclinical and clinical investigations.

A number of previous authors have reviewed methods and theory for the analysis of metabolite pharmacokinetics, with literature based upon simple models, as early as 1963 by Cummings and Martin (10). Thorough theoretical analyses and reviews have been published, notably by Houston (11,12), Pang (13), and Weiss (14). The topic of metabolite kinetics is not found in commonly employed textbooks on pharmacokinetics (15), though the topic is usually not presented or taught in an introductory course on pharmacokinetics. This chapter is not intended to present all aspects of basic pharmacokinetics that may be necessary for a thorough understanding of metabolite kinetics, and for this reason, motivated readers are recommended to consult other sources (15–19) if an introduction to basic pharmacokinetic principles is needed. This review will also not attempt to present or discuss all possible permutations of metabolite pharmacokinetics but will try to present and distinguish what can be assessed in humans and animals *in vivo* given commonly available experimental methods, which, in some cases, may be augmented by *in vitro* studies.

Metabolite Kinetics Following a Single Intravenous Dose of Parent Drug

General Considerations in Metabolite Disposition

Much of the theory presented here will be based upon primary metabolites, as shown in Scheme 2.1, which are formed directly from the parent drug or xenobiotic whose initial dose is known. In contrast, secondary or sequential metabolites, as indicated in Scheme 2.2, are formed from one or more primary

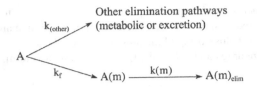

SCHEME 2.1 Drug metabolism to a primary metabolite followed by urinary or biliary excretion with parallel elimination pathways. The arrows indicate irreversible processes.

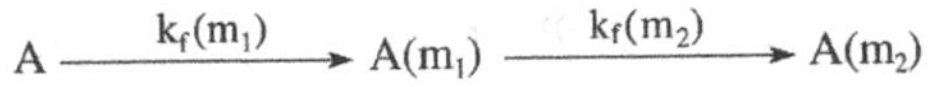

$$A \xrightarrow{k_f(m_1)} A(m_1) \xrightarrow{k_f(m_2)} A(m_2)$$

SCHEME 2.2 Sequential metabolism to a secondary metabolite, m_2, from a primary metabolite, m_1.

metabolites. The theory and resultant equations for the analysis of sequential metabolite kinetics are often more complex (see section "Sequential Metabolism") (13). Since most metabolites of interest are often primary metabolites, this review will focus on these, unless otherwise noted. Scheme 2.1 is the simplest model for one metabolite that can be measured *in vivo*, with other elimination pathways for the parent drug, either by metabolism or excretion (e.g., biliary or renal), represented as a combined first-order elimination term, k_{other}. Pharmacokinetic models will be presented here for conceptual reasons, but in the instances where model-independent or "non-compartmental" methods are appropriate, their applications will be discussed.

Here, A is the amount of drug or xenobiotic administered and $A(m)$ is the amount of a particular metabolite present in the body with time. When sequential metabolism is occurring, metabolites are distinguished with a subscript; $A(m_1)$ is the amount of primary metabolite present with time and $A(m_2)$ is the amount of secondary, or sequential, metabolite formed with time. $A(m)_{elim}$ is the amount of the primary metabolite of interest that is excreted (e.g., biliary or renal) and/or further metabolized. It is assumed that once metabolite is excreted in the urine or bile, it is not subject to reabsorption or cycling. The parameter k_f is the first-order formation rate constant for the metabolite and k_{other} represent a first-order rate constant for the sum of formation of other metabolites and elimination via other pathways. The constant $k(m)$ is the elimination rate constant for the metabolite, whereas the sum of k_f and k_{other} is k, the total first-order rate constant for the overall elimination of the parent drug. With this simple model, and derivations from this, the following assumptions will be employed unless otherwise noted:

1. The elimination and distribution processes are first order and thus linear; that is, they are not influenced by the concentration of drug or metabolite in the body. For example, saturation of enzyme and transport systems, co-substrate depletion, saturable plasma protein, or tissue binding does not occur.
2. All drug metabolism represents irreversible elimination of the parent drug; thus, there is no reversible metabolism, enterohepatic recycling, or bladder resorption.
3. For simplicity, a one-compartment model will be used, which assumes rapid distribution of parent drug and metabolite within the body.
4. There is no metabolism that results in metabolite being eliminated without first being presented to the systemic circulation.

From Scheme 2.1, the following equation is used to describe the rate of change in the amount of metabolite in the body at any time, which is equal to the rate of formation less the rate of elimination,

$$\frac{dA(m)}{dt} = k_f \cdot A - k(m) \cdot A(m) \tag{2.1}$$

This rate of input (i.e., formation) and output (i.e., elimination) is analogous to the form of the equation for first-order drug absorption and elimination (17). The amount of metabolite and parent drug present in the body upon initial intravenous bolus dosing of the drug is zero and the administered dose (D), respectively. The disposition of the parent drug can be described with an exponential term, as shown in Eq. 2.2,

$$A = D \cdot e^{-k \cdot t} \tag{2.2}$$

Substitution of A into Eq. 2.1 permits solving for $A(m)$ as a function of time (17),

$$A(m) = \frac{k_f \cdot D}{k(m) - k} \left[e^{-k \cdot t} - e^{-k(m) \cdot t} \right] \tag{2.3}$$

Since the amount of metabolite is often unknown, metabolite concentration, $C(m)$, is measured in plasma, which can be expressed by dividing both sides of Eq. 2.3 by the volume of distribution of the metabolite, $V(m)$, as follows,

$$C(m) = \frac{k_f \cdot D}{V(m) \cdot (k(m) - k)} \left[e^{-k \cdot t} - e^{-k(m) \cdot t} \right] \tag{2.4}$$

Equations 2.3 and 2.4 describe the amount and concentration, respectively, of a primary metabolite in the body over time after an intravenous bolus dose of the parent drug. Immediately after dosing there is no metabolite present, and the amount of metabolite will then reach a maximum when the rate of formation equals the rate of elimination of the metabolite. This peak occurs when $t_{m,peak} = \ln[k/k(m)]/[k - k(m)]$ (17). Here, k and $k(m)$ determine the shape of the drug and metabolite concentration versus time profiles, whereas k_f influences the fraction of the dose that is metabolized; thus, affecting the magnitude of the metabolite concentration. It is apparent that the relative magnitude or ratio of the two rate constants for the elimination of the parent drug and metabolite determines the overall profile of the metabolite relative to that of the parent drug, with two limiting cases described below.

Formation Rate-Limited Metabolism

In the first case, if $k(m) \gg k$, then the metabolite is eliminated by either excretion or further sequential metabolism much more rapidly than the rate at which the parent drug is eliminated. Since $k = k_f + k_{other}$, it also follows that $k(m) \gg k_f$. Under this condition, defined as formation rate-limited (FRL) metabolism, the exponential term describing metabolite elimination in Eqs. 2.3 and 2.4, $e^{-k(m) \cdot t}$, declines rapidly to zero relative to the exponential term describing parent drug elimination, $e^{-k \cdot t}$, and the term in the denominator, $[k(m) - k]$, approaches the value $k(m)$. Thus, shortly after an intravenous bolus dose of the parent drug, Eq. 2.3 simplifies to,

$$A(m) = \frac{k_f \cdot D}{k(m)} [e^{-k \cdot t}] \tag{2.5}$$

Equation 2.4 can be simplified similarly, and, if one takes the natural log (ln) of both sides of Eq. 2.5, then the amount of metabolite in the body can be described by a linear relationship with respect to time,

$$\ln A(m) = \ln\left(\frac{k_f \cdot D}{k(m)} \right) - k \cdot t \tag{2.6}$$

A similar relationship to Eq. 2.6 can be derived from Eq. 2.4 using concentrations rather than amounts when FRL metabolism applies. This log-linear relationship, common to first-order systems, indicates that when $k(m)$ k, the terminal half-life is measured for the metabolite amount or concentration versus time curves represent that of the parent drug, not that of the metabolite. This is shown below in Figures 2.1a and 2.2. Moreover, as $k(m)$ increases, the $t_{m,peak}$ for the metabolite approaches zero. In this case, the metabolite will reach peak concentrations very quickly after a bolus dose of the parent drug.

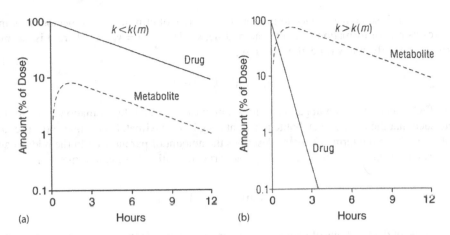

FIGURE 2.1 Drug and metabolite profiles simulated for the two common cases from Scheme 2.1. (a) Formation rate-limited metabolism where $k(m) > k$ [k_f, k_{other}, and $k(m)$ are 0.2, 0, and 2, respectively]. (b) Elimination rate-limited metabolism where $k(m) < k$ [k_f, k_{other}, and $k(m)$ are 2, 0, and 0.2, respectively]. Shown are amounts expressed as percentage of the dose; if converted to concentrations of parent drug and metabolite, the relative ratios of the curves may change as determined by V and $V(m)$, respectively. (From Rowland, M. and Tozer T.N., *Clinical Pharmacokinetics*, Lea and Febiger, Baltimore, MD, 1995.)

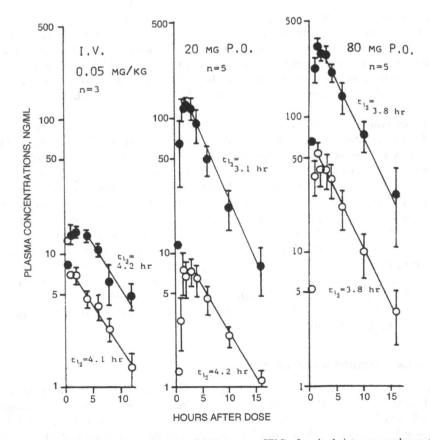

FIGURE 2.2 Plasma levels of NLA (●) and propranolol (o) (mean ± SEM) after single intravenous doses of propranolol in normal human subjects. NLA exhibits FRL metabolism with parallel half-lives and rapid attainment of peak levels. The higher ratios of NLA/propranolol at equilibrium are due to a much lower ratio of CL(m)/CL; however, $V(m)/V$ must be lower still (see Eq. 2.15) to provide $k(m)/k > 1$, characteristic of FRL metabolism. *Abbreviations:* NLA, naphthoxylacetic acid; FRL, formation rate limited. (From Walle, T. et al., *Clin. Pharmacol. Ther.*, 26, 548–554, 1979.)

Equation 2.5 can also be rearranged to indicate that the rate of elimination of metabolite, $k(m) \cdot A(m)$, approximates its rate of formation from the parent drug, $k_f \cdot D \cdot [e^{-k \cdot t}] = k_f \cdot A$, where A is the amount of parent drug in the body at any time after the dose,

$$k(m) \cdot A(m) = k_f \cdot D \cdot e^{-k \cdot t} \tag{2.7}$$

Thus, with FRL metabolism, an apparent equilibrium exists between the formation and elimination of metabolite such that the ratio of metabolite to parent drug is approximately constant soon after a dose of the parent drug. Since the term "$D \cdot e^{-k \cdot t}$" describes the amount of parent drug in the body at any time, shortly after an intravenous bolus dose of the parent drug, the ratio of amount of metabolite to drug is,

$$A(m) = \frac{k_f}{k(m)} \cdot A \tag{2.8}$$

Since the volume of distributions of parent drug (V) and metabolite [$V(m)$] are assumed constant, Eq. 2.8 can be rewritten by multiplying by volume terms to provide concentrations and clearance terms, where $CL_f = k_f V$ and $CL(m) = k(m) V(m)$ and the units of clearance are volume/time,

$$C(m) = \frac{k_f \cdot V}{k(m) \cdot V(m)} \cdot C = \frac{CL_f \cdot C}{CL(m)} \tag{2.9}$$

Though the metabolite concentration in the body, $C(m)$, at any time after a dose of parent drug can be determined by assay of plasma samples, in this case where $k(m) \gg k$, it is not possible to estimate $k(m)$ unambiguously. An estimate of $k(m)$ can only be determined by obtaining metabolite plasma concentration versus time data following an intravenous dose of the metabolite itself. These relationships do, however, indicate that the concentration ratio of metabolite versus parent drug will essentially be constant over time (Figure 2.1a). This ratio will be useful when relationships of concentration and clearance are discussed below.

With FRL metabolism, the observed apparent half-life of metabolite from concentration versus time curves is related to a first-order elimination rate constant of the parent drug, $t_{1/2} = \ln 2/k$, and the elimination half-life of the parent drug is longer than that of the metabolite if the metabolite were dosed independently. Since the metabolite is eliminated much faster than it is formed, its true half-life is not apparent, and the concentration versus time profile of the metabolite follows that of the parent drug as shown in Figures 2.1a and 2.2, where the log of the amount or plasma concentration are plotted on the ordinate. For naphthoxylacetic acid, a metabolite of propranolol (Figure 2.2), its plasma profile parallels that of propranolol whether the parent drug is given intravenously or orally (20). Even if the parent drug displayed more complex disposition characteristics with an initial distribution phase noted after an IV bolus dose (i.e., a two-compartment model) or perhaps secondary absorption peaks because of enterohepatic recycling, one would still expect to see a parallel profile for a metabolite subject to FRL metabolism. The observation of parallel metabolite and parent drug profiles after dosing the parent drug can also occur in cases of reversible metabolism; thus, this possibility should also be considered (see section "Reversible Metabolism").

Elimination Rate-Limited Metabolism

The second limiting case is when $k(m) \ll k$; that is, the elimination half-life of the metabolite is much longer than that of the parent drug. Here, the metabolite is eliminated by either excretion or sequential metabolism with a first-order rate constant that is much smaller than the rate constant for elimination of the parent drug ($k = k_f + k_{other}$), and this situation is defined as "elimination rate-limited" (ERL) metabolism. There is no requirement for the relative magnitude of $k(m)$ and k_f. Because of the differences between $k(m)$ and k, the exponential term $e^{-k \cdot t}$ in Eqs. 2.3 and 2.4 declines rapidly relative to the exponential term $e^{-k(m) \cdot t}$, and the term in the denominator, [$k(m) - k$], approaches the value of $-k$. Thus, when $k(m) \ll k$, after most of the parent drug has been eliminated, Eq. 2.3, which describes an IV bolus of parent drug, simplifies to

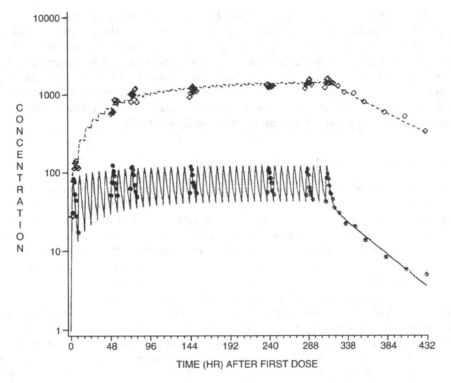

FIGURE 2.3 Plasma levels (ng/mL) of halazepam (⊙) and *N*-desalkylhalazepam (◇) after 40 mg halazepam every 8 hours for 14 days showing characteristics of elimination rate-limited metabolism. The estimated elimination half-lives for halazepam and *N*-desalkylhalazepam are 35 and 58 hours, respectively. Notable for the longer half-lives of the metabolite are a longer time to achieve steady-state than the parent drug, and smaller fluctuations between doses as seen in the simulated fit of the data. (From Chung, J.M. et al., *Clin. Pharmacol. Ther.*, 35, 838–842, 1984.)

$$A(\mathrm{m}) = \frac{k_f \cdot D}{k}[e^{-k(\mathrm{m})t}] \qquad (2.10)$$

With ERL metabolism, Eq. 2.4 also simplifies to express metabolite concentration versus time after an intravenous dose of the parent drug. This simplification indicates that with ERL metabolism, a log-linear plot of amount or concentration of metabolite versus time would have a terminal slope reflecting the true elimination half-life for the metabolite, i.e., $t_{1/2} = \ln 2/k(\mathrm{m})$. This is shown in Figure 2.1b, and an example of this type of metabolite profile is exemplified by the disposition of *N*-desalkylhalazepam, a metabolite of halazepam shown in Figure 2.3 (21). Under the condition of ERL metabolism, the elimination half-life of the metabolite is unambiguously and clearly resolved from that of the parent drug. Prodrugs are generally designed to follow ERL metabolism where the prodrug is rapidly metabolized to the active moiety that persists in the body for a much longer time than the parent prodrug, e.g., aspirin forming salicylate or mycophenolate mofetil forming mycophenolic acid. Considerations of possible accumulation of metabolite under ERL metabolism after the chronic dosing of the parent drug will be addressed below.

Rates of Metabolite Elimination Approximately Equal to Rates of Elimination of the Parent Drug

The above conditions of FRL and ERL metabolism permit simplification of the equations describing the disposition of the metabolite. However, in cases where $k(\mathrm{m})$ is close to the value of k, log-linear plots of metabolite concentration versus time do not, in theory, become apparently linear in the terminal phase of a concentration versus time profile because neither exponential term of Eq. 2.3 nor of Eq. 2.4 will become negligible and drop out as time progresses. Error in the analysis of plasma concentrations will also contribute to inability to discern a value for $k(m)$ from such a plot. Under these conditions, the use of log-linear plots to estimate $k(m)$, and subsequently the elimination half-life of the metabolite, will lead to an underestimation of $k(m)$ (12). Therefore, caution should be used when interpreting metabolite elimination rates and half-life data when clear distinction of $k(m)$ from k cannot be made. In practice, when $k(m) \cong k$, it is possible that noise in the data may make the terminal phase of the log concentration versus time plots appear reasonably log linear. A discussion of how to analyze data in instances where it appears that $k(m) \cong k$ is presented in the earlier review by Houston (12).

Clearance and Volume of Distribution for Metabolites

Most of the above discussion dealt with the amounts of drug and metabolite in the body and methods to simply distinguish FRL and ERL metabolism as well as to estimate $k(m)$ and half-life for a metabolite with ERL metabolism. However, in most instances, amounts are not known since concentrations of metabolite are determined in plasma or blood over time after dosing the parent drug. Since metabolites are seldom administered to humans (as an investigational new drug [IND] for the metabolite would require significant effort and expense), volume of distribution of the metabolite cannot be determined. Therefore, it is difficult for unambiguous conversion of observed metabolite concentrations to amount of metabolite in the body. It may be possible, given the availability of metabolite(s), to administer metabolite to animals to determine relevant pharmacokinetic parameters; however, extrapolation of pharmacokinetic values from animals to humans is complex and problematic. In general, volume terms more often extrapolate between species when scaling than do clearance estimates. If the preformed metabolite can be administered to humans, relevant pharmacokinetic parameters can be determined as commonly employed for the parent drug (16–19). However, one needs to consider the possibility that preformed metabolite dosed exogenously into the systemic circulation may behave differently than metabolite formed within specific tissues of the body, such as the liver or kidney, as summarized by Smith and Obach (9) and Prueksaritanont and Lin in this book (Chapter 25). Although a position paper addressing metabolites and drug safety stated that radiolabeled ADME (absorption, distribution, metabolism, and excretion) studies were adequate to address metabolite exposures (22), the Food and Drug Administration (FDA) issued a guidance on "major metabolites" that suggest to conduct animal studies of exogenously administered metabolites (23). Thus, there will likely be considerable information on metabolite distribution and pharmacokinetics in animals in the future. Much of the discussion here will focus on basic clearance of concepts that are applicable to metabolites, given limited knowledge of their disposition in humans, and may provide insight into the disposition of the metabolite if some assumptions are made.

The mass balance relationship in Eq. 2.1 can be modified by multiplying $k(m)$ by $V(m)$ and then dividing $A(m)$ by $V(m)$, which provide the values of metabolite clearance $CL(m)$ and $C(m)$, respectively. Similarly, multiplying and dividing the other terms in Eq. 2.1 by the volume of distribution of the parent drug V provides CL_f ($k_f \cdot V$) and C, respectively, where CL_f is the fractional clearance of the parent drug to form the metabolite and C is the concentration of the parent drug. CL_f can also be expressed as the product, $f_m \cdot CL$, where f_m is the fraction ($f_m = k_f / k = CL_f/CL$) of a systemically available dose of the parent drug that is converted irreversibly to the metabolite of interest. For the purpose of the discussion here, it will be assumed that any metabolite formed is systemically available and not subject to sequential metabolism or excretion without being presented to the systemic circulation. With this assumption and the above substitutions, Eq. 2.1 can be rewritten as

$$\frac{dA(m)}{dt} = CL_f \cdot C - CL(m) \cdot C(m) \qquad (2.11)$$

It is useful to consider the integration of Eq. 2.11 with respect to time from zero to infinity after an intravenous bolus of the parent drug. Since metabolite amounts in the body at times zero and infinity are zero and the terms of CL_f and $CL(m)$ are assumed to be constant, the integral of concentration versus time is the area under the concentration versus time curve (AUC). The following relationship is obtained,

$$CL_f \cdot AUC = CL(m) \cdot AUC(m) \tag{2.12}$$

where AUC(m) and AUC are the area under the plasma concentration versus time curve for the metabolite and parent drug, respectively. Since the product of a clearance and an AUC term is an amount, CL_f, AUC equals the amount of metabolite formed from the parent drug that reaches the systemic circulation, which for an intravenous dose equals f_m. The value of CL_f or f_m is usually not unambiguously known but may be estimated in some cases with some assumptions; for example, no sequential metabolism and all metabolite formed is excreted in the urine, or both urine and bile are collected in an animal model. Since CL_f is defined above as $f_m \cdot CL$, this can be substituted into Eq. 2.12 and then rearranged to provide,

$$\frac{f_m \cdot CL}{CL(m)} = \frac{AUC(m)}{AUC} \tag{2.13}$$

This relationship indicates that the relative AUCs of the metabolite versus parent drug will be dictated by the elimination clearances of metabolite and parent drug and the magnitude of the fraction of the dose that is directed toward the particular metabolite. For example, the AUC of morphine-3-glucuronide (M3G) is much greater than the AUC of morphine (ratio, ~7.8). Since the value of f_m cannot exceed unity, and a collection of urine long enough to estimate total recovery indicated that M3G averages 44% of the IV dose, it is apparent that the ratio of CL/CL(m) must be much greater than 1 (~17). It was reported that the half-lives of M3G and morphine were 3.9 and 1.7 hours (24), respectively; thus, M3G follows ERL metabolism, which is consistent with the much lower clearance of the metabolite contributing to its slow rate of elimination. With relative measures of clearance available from Eq. 2.13, one can also estimate the relative magnitude of the volume of distribution between metabolite and parent drug. Morphine, being basic, has a fairly large volume of distribution estimated to be 4 L/kg (24,25). In the case of ERL metabolism, where the relative values of k and $k(m)$ can be determined, one can substitute the relationship, $CL = k \cdot V$ into Eq. 2.13 and rearrange the equation to estimate relative values for the volumes of distribution,

$$\frac{V}{V(m)} = \frac{1}{f_m} \cdot \frac{k(m) \cdot AUC(m)}{k \cdot AUC} \tag{2.14}$$

Using the data presented in Figure 2.4 and associated data (20), Eq. 2.14 provides an estimate of $V(m)$ for M3G of about 0.5 L/kg, which is roughly one-seventh the value for V of morphine in adults. M3G has not been administered to humans, however, following an infusion of a diamorphine (a prodrug of morphine) to infants, the $V(m)$ of M3G was estimated to be 0.55 L/kg. Also, when its active analgetic isomer, M6G, was given to humans, it was determined to have a small volume of distribution of only 0.3 L/kg (26).

This example shows that the much larger AUC for M3G relative to morphine is due to a smaller clearance for the metabolite. The high peak M3G concentration is likely due to the rapid formation of the metabolite, which has a smaller volume of distribution because of its lower partitioning into tissues relative to the much more lipophilic parent drug, morphine.

The elimination rate constant, which is a parameter dependent on clearance and inversely dependent on the volume of distribution (i.e., $k = CL/V$), is lower for M3G because of $CL(m)$ being substantially smaller than CL. This relationship is summarized by the following equation,

$$\frac{k(m)}{k} = \frac{CL(m) \cdot V}{CL \cdot V(m)} \tag{2.15}$$

In cases where metabolism is FRL, the value of $k(m)$ cannot be estimated; thus, the relative volumes of distribution cannot be determined using Eq. 2.14, even when f_m is known. However, Eq. 2.13 is quite useful in estimating the important parameter, $CL(m)$, which can be used to predict average concentrations of the metabolite upon chronic administration, as will be discussed below. From Eq. 2.13 and the example of naphthoxylacetic acid/propranolol shown in Figure 2.2, where AUC(m)/AUC is much greater than 1,

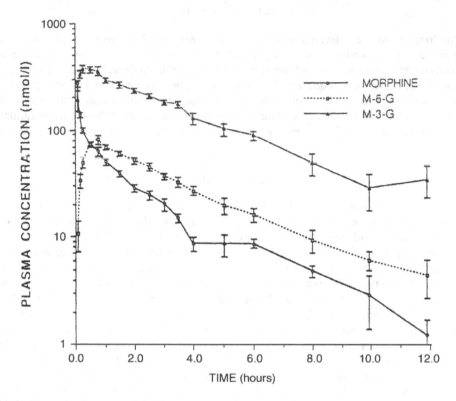

FIGURE 2.4 Plasma levels (mean ± SEM) for morphine, M6G and M3G in humans after a 5-mg intravenous bolus. The plot and associated data indicate that M3G has FRL metabolism, as its average half-life is more than twofold longer than that of morphine. *Abbreviations:* M6G, morphine-6-glucuronide; M3G, morphine-3-glucuronide; FRL, formation rate limited. (From Osborne, S. et al. *Clin. Pharmacol. Ther.* 47, 12–19, 1990.)

it is apparent that the clearance of naphthoxylacetic acid is much smaller than that of its parent drug [CL(m)/CL ≪ 1]; since the value of f_m cannot exceed unity, propranolol forms other known metabolites, and only 14% of the dose was excreted in urine as naphthoxylacetic acid. When Eq. 2.15 is considered and since $k(m)/k$ must exceed the value of 1 for FRL metabolism, it is apparent that the ratio of $V/V(m)$ must be large to compensate for the small ratio of CL(m)/CL for naphthoxylacetic acid/propranolol. Thus, $V(m)$ must be much smaller than V, which is also confirmed by the high concentrations of naphthoxyacetic acid relative to that of propranol shown in Figure 2.2 soon after the dose.

Consideration of the two primary pharmacokinetic parameters, clearance and volume, in Eq. 2.15 also provides an understanding of why FRL is more common than ERL metabolism, i.e., $k(m)/k$ is greater than 1 for a majority of metabolites. Most metabolites are more polar than the parent drug because of oxidation, hydrolysis, or conjugation; thus, they often distribute less extensively in the body [$V(m) < V$]. Exceptions to this may be metabolic products due to methylation or acetylation, which may be similar or more lipophilic than the respective parent drug. Most metabolites also have higher clearances than the parent drug, because of susceptibility to further phase II metabolism, enhanced biliary or renal secretion once a polar or charged functional group is added by biotransformation (e.g., oxidation to a carboxylic acid and conjugation with glucuronic acid, glycine, glutathione, or sulfate), or reduced protein binding, which may increase renal filtration clearance and increase clearance of metabolites with low extraction ratios. Together, these effects of a smaller volume and higher clearance, being the most commonly observed behavior for metabolites, result in FRL metabolism.

In the case of ERL metabolism, volume of distribution of a metabolite can be estimated using Eq. 2.14 if the parent drug can be administered as an intravenous dose to humans. As mentioned above, with FRL metabolism, $k(m)$ cannot often be unambiguously determined from plasma metabolite concentration versus time data in humans; therefore, $V(m)$ cannot be easily determined. However, volume of distribution for a metabolite in humans may be extrapolated from the values of $V(m)$ obtained in animals after intravenous dosing of the metabolite, if such data are available. Because volume is a parameter that is to a great extent dependent upon physicochemical properties of a compound and binding to tissues, this parameter, when corrected for differences in plasma, protein binding tends to be more amenable to interspecies scaling than is clearance (27–29). With a prediction of $V(m)$ in humans based on interspecies scaling, Eq. 2.15 may be used to estimate $k(m)$ for cases of FRL metabolism if f_m or $CL(m)$ is known.

Volume of distribution for a metabolite at steady-state $[V(m)_{ss}]$ can also be estimated from mean residence time (MRT) measurements as discussed below.

Mean Residence Time for Metabolites After an Intravenous Dose of the Parent Drug

MRT in the body is a measure of an average time that a molecule spends in the body after a dose and is a pharmacokinetic parameter that can be employed to describe metabolite disposition. MRT is considered a non-compartmental parameter on the basis of statistical moment theory (30); however, its use does assume that processes of metabolite formation and clearance are first order and linear (i.e., not dose or time dependent, the metabolite is formed irreversibly), and the metabolite is only eliminated from the sampling compartment (i.e., no peripheral tissues eliminate the metabolite by excretion or further metabolism). Hepatic and renal clearance are generally considered as part of the sampling compartment. There are more complex methods to estimate MRT that may accommodate reversible metabolism (31), though they are seldom employed or reported. MRT(m) is a time-average parameter, which is dependent on the disposition of the metabolite once formed. Thus, MRT(m) is of value in evaluating whether elimination and distribution of the metabolite have changed when the shape of the plasma metabolite concentration versus time curve is altered in response to changes in the disposition of the parent drug. Also, the relationship, $V(m)_{ss} = CL(m) \cdot MRT(m)_{m,iv}$, is useful to determine $V(m)_{ss}$, if $CL(m)$ can be determined (32).

When an intravenous bolus dose of preformed metabolite is administered, the $MRT(m)_{m,iv}$ is calculated as,

$$MRT(m)_{m,iv} = \frac{AUMC(m)_{m,iv}}{AUC(m)_{m,iv}} \tag{2.16}$$

where AUMC is the area under the first moment of the concentration versus time curve from the time of dosing, then estimated to infinity (17,30–33). The subscripts indicate the compound and route administered. A similar relationship describes the MRT of the parent drug if given as an intravenous bolus. $MRT(m)_{m,iv}$ measured after a rapid intravenous bolus of the metabolite reflects a mean time in the body for elimination and distribution of the metabolite. Measures of AUMC can be subject to substantially more error than AUC, primarily because of the need to extrapolate a larger portion of the first moment from the last sampling time to infinity (17,30).

When the metabolite is formed after intravenous dosing of the parent drug, the measured mean residence time reflects not only the mean time of metabolite in the body but also the time required for its formation from the parent drug. Therefore, the MRT(m) is corrected for this contribution by subtracting the MRT of the parent drug,

$$MRT(m)_{m,iv} = \frac{AUMC(m)_{p,iv}}{AUC(m)_{p,iv}} - \frac{AUMC_{p,iv}}{AUC_{p,iv}} \tag{2.17}$$

Here, the ratio $AUMC(m)_{p,iv}/AUC(m)_{p,iv}$ is sometimes referred to as the mean body residence time for the metabolite, MBRT(m), which reflects formation, distribution, and elimination processes, whereas the $MRT(m)_{m,iv}$ may be referred to as the mean disposition residence time, MDRT(m), reflecting only elimination and distribution (32). From Eq. 2.17, $MRT(m)_{m,iv}$ can be determined unambiguously from the plasma concentration versus time profiles of metabolite and parent drug after an intravenous dose of the parent drug, without the need for an intravenous dose of the metabolite (32,33). In a later section, $MRT(m)_{m,iv}$ will be derived following extravascular dosing of the parent drug.

Metabolite Kinetics After a Single Extravascular Dose of the Parent Drug

When a drug is not administered by an intravenous route, the rate of drug absorption from the site of extravascular administration, e.g., the gastrointestinal (GI) tract for peroral or the muscle for intramuscular, adds additional complexity to understanding the disposition of the metabolite. There are several confounding factors to be considered, the most obvious being both the extent of availability, F, of the parent drug and its rate of absorption, k_a, as defined by a rate constant. Here, for simplicity, a first-order rate of absorption will be employed, though drug inputs that approximate a zero-order process are also commonly found, especially with sustained or controlled release dosage forms. Additional considerations when extravascular administration is employed is estimating the fraction of the dose transformed into metabolite during absorption, which is referred to as "first-pass metabolite formation," and the fraction of metabolite that is formed during the absorption process reaching the plasma sampling site. These issues will be discussed later. It is instructive to first consider Scheme 2.3, which represents drugs with little or no first-pass metabolite formation, as commonly found for drugs with high oral availability. Again, for simplicity, it will be assumed that all metabolite formed after absorption of the parent compound reaches the systemic circulation prior to irreversible elimination, i.e., the availability of metabolite when formed *in vivo*, $F(m)$, is complete.

Metabolite Disposition After Extravascular Drug Administration with Limited Metabolite Formation During Absorption

Scheme 2.3 represents a drug where negligible metabolite forms during the absorption process. This scenario may be expected for drugs with high oral availability and low hepatic and gut wall metabolic clearance or drug administered by other extravascular administration routes where little or negligible metabolite may be formed during absorption, e.g., intramuscular administration. However, this scheme does not necessarily require high availability for the drug, but does assume that drug not reaching the systemic circulation is not because of biotransformation to the metabolite of interest, e.g., low availability may be due to poor dissolution, low GI membrane permeability, degradation at the site of absorption, or the formation of other metabolites. In this case, $F = f_a$, if no other first-pass metabolites are formed. Scheme 2.3 contains an absorption step, which was not present in Scheme 2.1. This catenary process with rate (k_a), drug elimination (k), and metabolite elimination $[k(m)]$ in series will influence metabolite disposition depending on the step that is rate-limiting.

For a drug with first-order absorption and elimination, the following bi-exponential equation describes the disposition of the parent drug (17),

$$C = \frac{k_a \cdot F \cdot D}{V \cdot (k_a - k)} \left[e^{-k \cdot t} - e^{-k_a \cdot t} \right] \tag{2.18}$$

This equation is mathematically analogous to Eqs. 2.3 and 2.4 (above) and, if multiplied by V, provides amounts rather than concentrations. If Eq. 2.18 is substituted into Eq. 2.1 and solved for the concentration

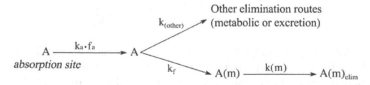

SCHEME 2.3 Absorption of drug and its metabolism to a primary metabolite, with no first-pass metabolism to the primary metabolite and parallel elimination pathways. Primary metabolite is eliminated by excretion or further metabolism.

of metabolite over time, one obtains a relationship with three exponentials, since there are two steps prior to the metabolite reaching the systemic circulation and one step influencing its elimination

$$C(m) = C_1 \cdot e^{-k \cdot t} + C_2 e^{-k(m) \cdot t} + C_3 \cdot e^{-k_a \cdot t} \qquad (2.19)$$

Here, the constants C_1, C_2, and C_3 are complex terms derived from the model in Scheme 2.3, which include the bioavailability of the parent drug, F, and dose, D, in their respective numerators, as well as the volume of distribution of the metabolite in the denominator. The values for these constants in Eq. 2.19 may be estimated by computer fitting of experimental data. Though the values of these constants have limited inherent utility themselves, the fitting process does provide a description of the time-dependent metabolite profile. Through the application of the superposition principle (17), the descriptive equation may be employed to estimate metabolite profiles at steady-state after chronic dosing or following irregular multiple dosing regimens of the parent drug.

Since Scheme 2.3 does not have any reversible processes, it is a catenary chain with simple constants for each exponential term in Eq. 2.19, which are easily conceptualized from the schematic model. These exponential terms indicate that any one of the processes of absorption, parent drug elimination, or metabolite elimination may be rate determining. The rate constant associated with the rate-limiting step (i.e., the slowest step) corresponds to the slope observed for the log-linear concentration versus time curve of the metabolite in plasma, assuming that one of the three rate constants is distinctly smaller. For drugs with FRL metabolism, either k or k_a will correspond to the terminal slope (and subsequently the observed half-life) and knowledge of the rates of absorption and elimination of the parent drug may be employed to discern which process or step may control the apparent terminal half-life of the metabolite concentration in plasma. For ERL metabolism, the elimination half-life of the metabolite is by definition longer than the elimination half-life of the parent drug. Therefore, if absorption is rate limiting, then the absorption rate may not only govern the observed terminal half-life of the parent drug but may also dictate the observed apparent terminal half-life of the metabolite. This is shown in Figure 2.5 where the rate of absorption of morphine is decreased after administration of a slow release buccal formulation such that the elimination rate for morphine cannot be distinguished from that of its metabolites (24). Without administration of an intravenous dose or an immediate release tablet of morphine (Figure 2.4), one could not discern from Figure 2.5 whether M3G follows ERL or FRL metabolism or whether the terminal half-life of Figure 2.5 is due to absorption.

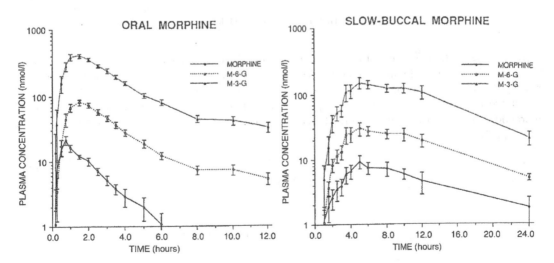

FIGURE 2.5 Comparison of immediate release oral (11.7 mg) versus slow-release buccal (14.2 mg) administration of morphine in humans on the profile of morphine, M6G and M3G. The common terminal half-life observed for parent drug and both metabolites shown for the slow-release buccal formulation are longer than obtained after the immediate release dosage form, suggestive of absorption being rate limiting. *Abbreviations:* M6G, morphine-6-glucuronide; M3G, morphine-3-glucuronide. (From Osborne, S. et al., *Clin. Pharmacol. Ther.*, 47, 12–19, 1990.)

Metabolite Disposition After Extravascular Drug Administration with Metabolite Formation During the Absorption Process

In numerous cases, as occurs for drugs with significant first-pass hepatic or gut wall metabolism, metabolite formed during absorption must be considered in characterizing the disposition of metabolite. Scheme 2.4 presents a model with one primary metabolite and other elimination pathways for the parent drug after absorption. Also introduced here is consideration of the availability of the metabolite once formed *in vivo* [$F(m)$].

Here the availability term, F, is the product of the fraction of dose of parent drug absorbed, f_a, and the fraction of dose reaching the liver that escapes biotransformation to metabolites (first-pass metabolism via the liver and/or GI tract) during first-pass absorption, F_H. As mentioned above, the term "f_a" includes drug not reaching the systemic circulation because of poor solubility, degradation, or low GI membrane permeability, and is often estimated by application of a mass balance approach after administration of radiolabeled drug. For example, if there is little radioactivity recovered in feces after an intravenous dose, then summation of the fraction of radiolabel in urine, tissues and expired breath after an oral dose of radiolabeled material would provide an estimate of f_a. The term "$1-F_H$" represents the fraction of drug absorbed that forms metabolites during the first-pass, which is also commonly defined as the extraction ratio across the organ, E. Also introduced here, is consideration of the availability of the metabolite, $F(m)$, which is the fraction of metabolite formed that is subsequently systemically available, e.g., not subject to sequential metabolism, intestinal efflux, or biliary excretion. In practice, $F(m)$ can only be determined unambiguously (assuming preformed metabolite behaves as does *in situ* generation of metabolite) after administration of the preformed metabolite by both the IV and extravascular routes, which is seldom possible in humans though may be feasible in animals (9). If other metabolites are also formed during absorption, then a fraction of the extraction ratio will represent the primary metabolite of interest (14). First-pass formation of metabolite via the gut wall is not considered separately here since the source of metabolite measured in the systemic circulation (either from the liver or GI wall) cannot be distinguished easily in human studies.

Assuming that there is no gut wall metabolism and that the fraction of metabolite formed during the first pass of drug through the liver is the same as subsequent passes (i.e., no saturable first-pass metabolism), then the amount of metabolite formed and presented to the systemic circulation is equal to the product of the AUC(m) and CL(m) (12),

$$f_a \cdot f_m \cdot F(m) \cdot D_{po} = CL(m) \cdot AUC(m)_{p,po} \tag{2.20}$$

where f_m is the fraction of dose that is converted to the metabolite of interest and the subscripts indicate that the parent drug was administered orally. A similar relationship exists for an intravenous dose of parent drug; however, f_a would be equal to unity. When the relationship of Eq. 2.20 is applied to both oral and intravenous doses of the parent drug (equal doses are used here; thus, doses cancel), the fraction of an oral dose of parent drug that is absorbed, f_a, can be estimated by measuring the metabolite exposure, AUC(m) (12),

$$f_a = \frac{AUC(m)_{p,po}}{AUC(m)_{p,iv}} \tag{2.21}$$

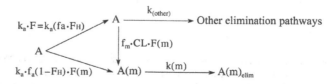

SCHEME 2.4 Absorption of drug and metabolism to a primary metabolite with first-pass formation of metabolite followed by excretion or metabolism.

With the assumption that first-pass loss of absorbed drug is only due to hepatic elimination, F_H can be estimated from the relationship, $F = f_a F_H$, where $F = \text{AUC}_{po}/\text{AUC}_{iv}$, if doses of parent drug are equal by both oral and intravenous routes. If the value of f_a as determined with Eq. 2.21 is greater than 1, this would suggest that GI wall metabolism is occurring. When the data of naphthoxylacetic acid/propranolol in Figure 2.2 is analyzed in this manner, f_a was estimated to be 0.98, which indicates that the absorption of propranolol is essentially complete and much of the formation of this metabolite is hepatic.

Estimating Fraction of Metabolite Formed and Formation Clearance

Commonly, values for f_m are reported for drugs administered to humans on the basis of collection of metabolite in urine after a dose of the parent drug. This, of course, assumes that all metabolite formed reaches the systemic circulation [i.e., $F(m) = 1$] and is then excreted into urine or that identification of sequential metabolites is accurate, and they are also efficiently excreted in urine. If metabolite can be administered independently, then additional calculations of f_m can be employed. Dosing preformed metabolite intravenously provides $\text{AUC}(m)_{m,iv}$, which can be compared to metabolite exposure from an intravenous dose of parent drug (34),

$$f_m \cdot F(m) = \frac{\text{AUC}(m)_{p,iv} \cdot M}{\left[\text{AUC}(m)_{m,iv} \cdot D\right]} \tag{2.22}$$

where M and D are molar doses of metabolite and parent drug, respectively. This relationship assumes that systemic clearance of the metabolite is independent of whether metabolite was dosed exogenously or formed from the parent drug *in vivo*. The term "$F(m)$" is present in Eq. 2.22 because availability of metabolite formed from intravenous parent drug may be less than complete. If the preformed metabolite was instead administered orally where it must also pass the liver before reaching the systemic circulation, then $F(m)$ cancels (12),

$$f_m = \frac{\text{AUC}(m)_{p,iv} \cdot M}{\left[\text{AUC}(m)_{m,po} \cdot D\right]} \tag{2.23}$$

The experimental approach of dosing the metabolite orally may be more easily performed, since it avoids the preparation and administration of an intravenous dose. However, use of Eq. 2.23 must now assume that the metabolite is well absorbed from the intestine, i.e., $f_a(m)$ is unity.

Once f_m is estimated, CL_f is simply the product of f_m and the total clearance of the parent drug, $CL_f = f_m CL$. An alternative approach to determine rate of metabolite formation and cumulative extent of formation is by the application of deconvolution analysis (35,36). With data from an intravenous dose of the metabolite, i.e., with a known input of the metabolite, the subsequent rate and extent of metabolite formation can be obtained by deconvolution (36) after any known input dose of the parent drug. This approach was applied to determine both metabolite formation rates and f_m for M6G after intravenous bolus and infusion doses of morphine, as shown in Figure 2.6 (26). The values of f_m when estimated by use of Eq. 2.22 [assuming $F(m) = 1$] and by deconvolution were 12 ± 2 (mean $\pm$ SD) and $9 \pm 1\%$ of the morphine dose, respectively, which is within anticipated experimental error (26). The advantage of the deconvolution approach is that it provides metabolite formation rates over time, which may be helpful in analyzing the system, and it has few assumptions for its application. A disadvantage of the method is that it requires an exogenous dose of the preformed metabolite and assumes that metabolite formed *in vivo* behaves similarly to that dosed as preformed metabolite.

MRT for Metabolite After an Extravascular Administration of Parent Drug

The $\text{MRT}(m)_{m,iv}$ can also be determined after an extravascular dose of the parent drug as long as the assumptions stated above in section "Mean Residence Time for Metabolites after an Intravenous Dose of Parent Drug" apply. The ability to obtain $\text{MRT}(m)_{m,iv}$ without an intravenous dose of the metabolite

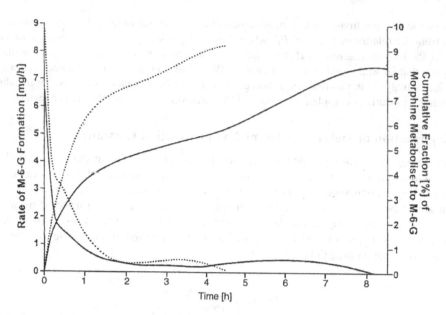

FIGURE 2.6 Deconvolution analysis of M6G/morphine to determine the rates of M6G formation (*left ordinate, descending lines*) and fraction of dose metabolized to M6G (*right ordinate, ascending lines*) after intravenous doses of morphine. Solid lines are data from a 0.13 mg/kg bolus followed by 0.005 mg/kg/hr infusion for 8 hours. Dotted lines are data from a 0.24 mg/kg bolus followed by 0.0069 mg/kg/hr infusion for 4 hours. *Abbreviation*: M6G, morphine-6-glucuronide. (From Lotsch, J. et al., *Clin. Pharmacol. Ther.* 60, 316–325, 1996.)

when there is no first-pass metabolism has been presented by several authors (32,33,37), and modifications to accommodate first-pass metabolite formation have been considered (38,39).

 If there is no first-pass formation of metabolite during the absorption process, then $MRT(m)_{m,iv}$ can be determined by correction of the MRT of metabolite in the body for contributions from the parent drug, which now include its absorption as well as distribution and elimination that were accounted for in Eq. 2.17,

$$MRT(m)_{m,iv} = \frac{AUMC(m)_{p,po}}{AUC(m)_{p,po}} - \frac{AUMC_{p,po}}{AUC_{p,po}} \tag{2.24}$$

The ratio $AUMC_{p,po}/AUC_{p,po}$ is defined as the MRT_{po} of the parent drug when given orally (or any other extravascular route) and is the sum of the MRT_{iv} and the mean absorption time (MAT) of the parent drug. Since the MRT_{po} is simply a ratio determined from observed plasma concentration profile of the parent drug after oral administration, $MRT(m)_{m,iv}$ can be estimated without intravenous administration of either parent drug or metabolite. As mentioned above in section "Mean Residence Time for Metabolites after an Intravenous Dose of Parent Drug," $MRT(m)_{m,iv}$ provides a parameter for the assessment of disposition (distribution and elimination) of the metabolite without consideration of its rate or time course of formation.

 If there is first-pass formation of metabolite, then Eq. 2.24 may introduce significant error in determining $MRT(m)_{m,iv}$ (38,39). To correct this error, the contribution of first-pass metabolism from an intravenous dose of the parent drug ($MRT_{p,iv} = AUMC/AUC$) and the fraction of the absorbed dose that escapes first-pass metabolism (F_H) need to be considered. Assuming that all metabolite formed from the first pass is due to a single metabolite,

$$MRT(m)_{m,iv} = \frac{AUMC(m)_{p,po}}{AUC(m)_{p,po}} - \frac{AUMC_{p,po}}{AUC_{p,po}} + (1 - F_H) \cdot MRT_{p,iv} \tag{2.25}$$

It is apparent that when first-pass metabolism is minimal, i.e., F_H is unity, then Eq. 2.25 collapses to Eq. 2.24. In addition, when $MRT_{p,iv}$ is small relative to the other terms as occurs with transient prodrugs such as aspirin, then the last term of Eq. 2.25 is again insignificant. However, when there is substantial first-pass metabolism, then use of Eq. 2.24 would provide a value that underestimates $MRT(m)_{m,iv}$. In practice, Eq. 2.24 may provide a value that is negative, indicating that there must be some first-pass metabolism occurring (39).

Metabolite Disposition After Chronic Administration of Parent Drug

Chronic administration of drugs by extravascular routes, multiple infusions, or continuous infusions is commonly employed in ambulatory and hospital settings. In these cases, active metabolites, toxic metabolites, or the impact of the metabolite on the disposition of the parent drug should be considered. Here, one needs to consider the accumulation of both the parent drug and metabolite to steady-state concentrations and the relationship between the steady-state characteristics of the parent drug relative to that of the metabolite, since these characteristics may differ from those observed after only a single dose of drug. The critical pharmacokinetic descriptors for the disposition of the metabolite on chronic drug administration are the time to achieve steady-state, peak, trough, and average concentrations at steady-state, the accumulation at steady-state relative to a single dose of parent drug, and metabolite clearance. Volume of distribution is a parameter that has little contribution in achieving steady-state levels but does impact the swings from peak to trough concentrations at steady-state because of its contribution in determining the half-life of parent drug and metabolite.

Time to Achieve Steady-State for a Metabolite

Following chronic extravascular administration or intravenous infusion for a sufficiently long time, parent drug and metabolite will eventually achieve steady-state concentrations where the input of the parent drug and metabolite (i.e., formation) into the systemic circulation on average equal their respective rates of elimination. The time to achieve such a steady-state is dependent on the half-life of the parent drug or metabolite and, if first-order elimination processes occur, generally it takes about 3.3 half-lives to reach 90% of the ultimate steady-state level, and after 5 half-lives, a compound would achieve about 97% of the theoretical steady-state level. In the case of a primary metabolite formed from the parent drug, it will be the slowest, rate-limiting process that governs when a metabolite reaches steady-state levels in the body. Therefore, for metabolites with FRL metabolism, the elimination half-life of the parent compound will control the time to achieve steady-state levels of the metabolite, whereas for ERL metabolism, the longer half-life of the metabolite will dictate the time needed for the metabolite to reach steady-state levels. ERL metabolism is shown in Figure 2.7, where the two metabolites of morphine take as much as 30 hours to accumulate to steady-state concentrations after bolus injection and continuous intravenous infusion of diamorphine (a prodrug of morphine) to infants, even though morphine rapidly attained steady-state (25). In this example, the mean elimination half-lives of the metabolites in 19 infants were estimated by the rate of attainment to steady-state (17) to be 11.1 and 18.2 hours for M3G and M6G, respectively (25), whereas these metabolites have reported half-lives estimated to be only several hours in adults (24,26).

On discontinuation of chronic or repetitive parent drug administration, the rate of decline in metabolite concentration will again be dependent upon whether FRL or ERL metabolism is operative. In the case of FRL metabolism, the rate of decline for the concentrations of the metabolite will simply follow that of the parent drug. In contrast, for ERL metabolism, metabolite levels will persist on the basis of their longer half-life as shown in Figure 2.8 for the metabolites of nitroglycerin (40).

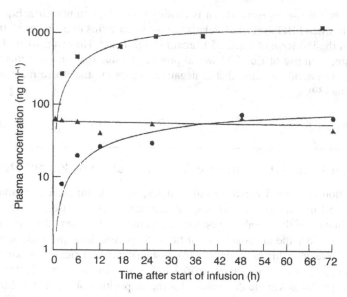

FIGURE 2.7 Disposition of morphine (▲), with the formation of M3G (■) and M6G (●), in a representative infant receiving diamorphine (prodrug of morphine) intravenous bolus followed by an infusion for 72 hours. The rate of attainment of steady-state for the metabolites is determined by the slowest rate constant, which provides estimated half-lives of 11 and 18 hours for M3G and M6G, respectively. *Abbreviations:* M6G, morphine-6-glucuronide; M3G, morphine-3-glucuronide. (From Barret, D.A. et al., *Br. J. Clin. Pharmacol.*, 41, 531–537, 1996.)

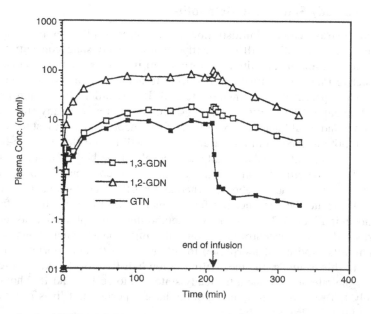

FIGURE 2.8 Plasma levels of GTN(■), 1,2-GDN (Δ), and 1,3-GDN (□) following an intravenous infusion of 0.070 mg/min GTN to a dog. The half-lives of the metabolites were much longer than the apparent half-life of approximately four minutes for GTN after the end of the infusion, and data suggest that the prolonged activity of GTN may be due to the metabolites. The prolonged residual GTN at very low concentrations is not understood nor is its slower than anticipated rise to steady-state. *Abbreviations:* GTN, glyceral trinitrate; GDN, glyceral dinitrate. (From Lee, F.W. et al., *J. Pharmacokinet. Biopharm.*, 21, 533–550, 1993.)

Metabolite Concentrations at Steady-State After Continuous Administration of Parent Drug

As mentioned above, at steady-state for the metabolite, the rate of formation equals the rate of elimination of the metabolite, i.e., $\Delta A(m)/\Delta t = 0$. Considering the fraction of metabolite formed from the parent drug, f_m, and the systemic bioavailability of the metabolite once formed, $F(m)$, from Eq. 2.11, the following relationship is defined at steady-state where the left term is the formation rate of metabolite that reaches the systemic circulation and the right term is its rate of elimination (11),

$$f_m \cdot F(m) \cdot CL \cdot C_{ss} = CL(m) \cdot C(m)_{ss} \tag{2.26}$$

Since at steady-state for the parent drug, CL C_{ss} is equal to the rate of infusion, R_o, this can be substituted into Eq. 2.26, which upon rearrangement provides the average concentration of metabolite at steady-state, $C(m)_{ss,ave}$.

$$C(m)_{ss,ave} = \frac{f_m \cdot F(m) \cdot R_o}{CL(m)} \tag{2.27}$$

This equation describes that $C(m)_{ss,ave}$ will be proportional to the infusion rate of the parent drug. However, the difficulties in obtaining estimates of the other terms of the equation without dosing of the metabolite limits the utility of Eq. 2.27. Alternatively, indirect approaches to estimate $C(m)_{ss,ave}$ from AUC data obtained after a single dose of the parent drug will be addressed below.

If, instead of intravenous infusions, drug input is via regular and repetitive extravascular administration, the rate of input R_o in Eq. 2.27 is modified to reflect an average drug administered at each dosing interval, D/τ. There is also a correction for the fraction of extravascular dose absorbed, f_a (11),

$$C(m)_{ss,ave} = \frac{f_m \cdot F(m) \cdot f_a \cdot D}{CL(m) \cdot \tau} \tag{2.28}$$

Here, the average rate of drug input is $f_a \cdot D/\tau$. The value of $C(m)_{ss,ave}$ obtained reflects the average level at steady-state but gives no information of relative fluctuations from peak to trough metabolite concentrations, $C(m)_{ss,max}/C(m)_{ss,min}$, at steady-state. The extent of this fluctuation for the metabolite levels will depend on whether FRL or ERL metabolism occurs. Assuming that absorption is not the rate-limiting process, for FRL metabolism, the metabolite rapidly equilibrates with the parent drug; thus, the peak to trough metabolite concentration ratio, $C(m)_{ss,max}/C(m)_{ss,min}$, will be similar to $C_{ss,max}/C_{ss,min}$ obtained for the parent drug. In contrast, for ERL metabolism, the longer elimination half-life of the metabolite will dampen its concentration swings at steady-state such that $C(m)_{s,max}/C(m)_{ss,min} < C_{ss,max}/C_{ss,min}$.

Estimating Metabolite Levels at Steady-State from a Single Dose

Superposition Principle to Estimate Metabolite Levels at Steady-State

When the metabolite and parent drug follow linear processes that are independent of dose and concentrations, i.e., no saturable processes occur, then prediction of metabolite concentrations after multiple doses or with a change of dose can be estimated if the route of drug administration does not change. Under these conditions, the time course of the metabolites as well as their average concentrations can be estimated by the principle of superposition (17). However, if the route of drug administration is different between the single dose administration and the chronic dosing without a change in bioavailability (e.g., single dose is an intravenous bolus, whereas the chronic administration is an intravenous infusion), the average concentration of the metabolite at steady-state can be predicted on the basis of relationships of clearance and AUC, as described below.

Superposition simply takes the plasma concentration versus time profile after a single dose and assumes that each successive dose would behave similarly, though the magnitude of concentration will vary proportionally with the dose administered. Thus, both the parent drug and metabolite profile can be summed over time. This can be done either by fitting the single dose data to appropriate mathematical functions as a sum of exponentials or polynomials and then summing this to infinity if the dosing regimen has a constant dosing interval (17). Alternatively, a more simple method, which is easily applied to even irregular dosing intervals, is to use a spreadsheet to sum the concentrations of metabolite from successive doses of the parent drug (15), making certain to have values or extrapolated metabolite concentrations for at least five elimination half-lives of metabolite or parent drug, whichever is longest.

Single Dose AUC Values to Predict Average Metabolite Levels at Steady-State

If an estimate of the average concentration of metabolite at steady-state is desired, then AUC(m) after a single dose can be employed effectively as shown by Lane and Levy (41).

This approach can also be used when the formulation of parent drug changed between single and chronic administration without altering availability of parent drug or fraction of metabolite formed (e.g., single dose is an oral suspension, whereas chronic administration is a sustained release capsule). From the relationship that the average rate of formation of metabolite is equal to its average rate of elimination at steady-state, as provided in Eq. 2.26 above, these authors then used the relationships of AUC and CL in Eq. 2.12 to derive the following from AUC data collected after a single dose of the parent drug,

$$\frac{C(m)_{ss,ave}}{C_{ss,ave}} = \frac{AUC(m)}{AUC} \tag{2.29}$$

This relationship assumes linearity (i.e., constant clearance) for the parent drug and metabolite with respect to changes in dose and time. Eq. 2.29 is applicable to any route of administration but does require that the route used for the single dose measurements of AUC be the same as that to be employed for steady-state measurements of concentrations. This requirement usually ensures that availabilities of the parent drug and metabolite formed are the same between single and chronic doses. This provides a means to estimate the average metabolite concentrations at steady-state from AUC(m)/AUC ratios from a single dose and knowledge of an estimated $C_{ss,ave}$ for the parent drug. Though initially derived from a one-compartment model, Eq. 2.29 was later extended with fewer restrictions by Weiss (14) using a noncompartmental approach.

When the route of administration changes, which may alter availability of the parent drug, the relationship of Eq. 2.29 must consider this change. If the initial single dose data were obtained from an intravenous dose, then the ratio of metabolite to parent drug concentrations at steady-state after oral dosing will be affected by fraction of parent drug systemically available (12,14). With an assumption that availability of the metabolite did not change with a change in the route of parent drug administration and there is no significant GI wall metabolism, the following relationship can be used,

$$\frac{C(m)_{ss,ave}}{C_{ss,ave}} = \frac{AUC(m)_{iv}}{AUC_{iv}} \left(\frac{1}{F_H} \right) \tag{2.30}$$

With regular doses and dosing intervals, τ, the AUC is equal to $C_{ss,ave} \cdot \tau$; therefore, Eq. 2.29 can be rearranged and written more simply as,

$$C(m)_{ss,ave} = \frac{AUC(m)}{\tau} \tag{2.31}$$

where AUC(m) is determined after a single dose of parent drug. Under these conditions of regular dosing to steady-state, data on the disposition of the parent drug are not necessarily required when estimating $C(m)_{ss,ave}$, though most often the parent drug data are available.

In cases where a single intravenous bolus dose of parent drug was used to obtain measurement of AUC(m), but then a continuous infusion of rate, R_0, is later employed, one can also derive $C(m)_{ss,ave}$ without complete knowledge of the disposition of parent drug. Since for continuous infusion, $C_{ss,ave} = R_0/CL$, and for a single IV bolus dose of parent drug, AUC = D/CL, substitution of these well-known relationships into Eq. 2.29 and rearrangement provides (41),

$$C(m)_{ss} = \frac{R_0 \cdot AUC(m)}{D} \qquad (2.32)$$

This relationship provides an actual level, since it is from an infusion where metabolite reaches a steady-state level. Only knowledge of the dose of drug employed for the single intravenous dose, D, and the resultant AUC(m) is needed.

Sequential Metabolism

A common scheme in drug metabolism is the concept of sequential metabolism where a parent drug is converted to one or more primary metabolites, which are then further converted to a secondary metabolite (Scheme 2.2, above). This process leads to two metabolites as shown in Figure 2.9, where

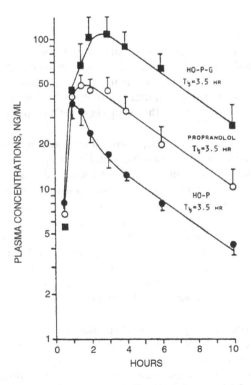

FIGURE 2.9 Disposition of propranol (o), its 4-OH metabolite (●), and sequential formation of its 4-OH-glucuronide metabolite (■) in humans after a single 80-mg oral dose. Data are mean ± SEM, N = 6. The initial rapid increase in 4-OH propranolol is followed by a later peak concentration of 4-OH-glucuronide due to sequential metabolism. The nonlinearity of the 4-OH metabolite immediately following its peak is likely due to significant formation of this metabolite during absorption, which takes time to distribute to tissues prior to equilibration with formation of the glucuronide. On the basis of urinary excretion data, most of the 4-OH propranolol is converted to propranolol glucuronide, and when Eq. 2.21 is applied to these two metabolites, the values of f_a are substantially greater than 1, suggestive of GI wall metabolism. (From Walle, T. et al., *Clin. Pharmacol. Ther.*, 27, 22–31, 1980.)

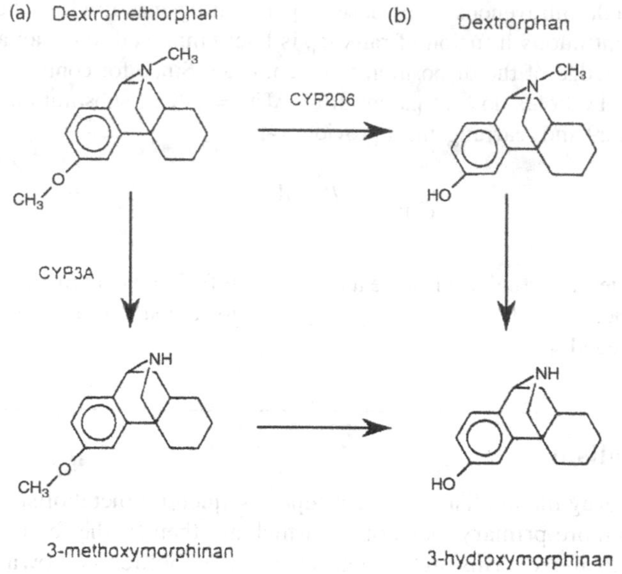

(a) Dextromethorphan   (b) Dextrorphan

CYP2D6

CYP3A

3-methoxymorphinan   3-hydroxymorphinan

SCHEME 2.5 Parallel metabolic pathways of dextromethorphan to a common metabolite (44).

propranolol is first oxidized to 4-hydroxy propranolol, which then undergoes sequential metabolism to 4-hydroxy propranolol glucuronide (42). Indeed, sequential metabolism formed the basis for the common nomenclature of phase I and phase II metabolism, coined by Williams (43). Another commonly observed sequence is that of parallel metabolism leading to a common metabolite as exemplified by the metabolism of dextromethorphan via CYP2D6 and CYP3A4 (44), as shown in Scheme 2.5.

For either of the two examples presented above, given that first-order processes apply, the equation that describes the disposition of the secondary metabolite would be complex polyexponential functions with the number of terms determined by the number of first-order processes leading to the penultimate metabolite of interest. Such processes may also include an absorption step (not shown in Scheme 2.5) if the parent compound is administered extravascularly. These processes can be dealt with by fitting the data with a polyexponential function or using other appropriate equations as presented by Eq. 2.19. A mathematical analysis of parallel and sequential systems has recently been developed (45). In the more simple, catenary chain represented by Scheme 2.2, the terminal apparent half-life of the secondary metabolite will be determined by the rate-limiting step, i.e., the step with the smallest rate constant among all steps describing the disposition of the metabolite. It is also possible in cases of sequential metabolism, depending on relative rates and competing pathways, that the primary metabolite (m_1 in Scheme 2.2) may not be observed at all, either in plasma or in urine.

Sequential metabolism is one of the primary reasons that the systemic availability F(m), of a primary metabolite once formed may be less than complete (46,47), as exemplified by 4-OH propranolol, which forms the glucuronide *in vivo* (Figure 2.9). Other factors impacting the systemic availability of a metabolite may include biliary and renal excretion of metabolites once formed in the liver and kidney, respectively, without access to the systemic circulation. Further complications arise when one considers the impact of sequential metabolism, intracellular access, and systemic availability of metabolites for evaluating the disposition of metabolite formed *in vivo* with that of preformed metabolite administered directly into the systemic circulation (41). To estimate actual pharmacokinetic parameters of metabolite, it is usually necessary to administer preformed metabolite, preferably by the intravenous route. However, inherent assumptions with such experiments are that the above-mentioned factors are independent of the route of metabolite administration.

Renal Clearance of Metabolites

Many metabolites are eliminated to a significant extent or almost exclusively into the urine. Collection and analysis of urine samples have some advantages—the primary one is that they are less invasive than blood sampling. Since urine production volume in a day, or during a dosing interval, is limited and usually a much smaller volume than V or $V(m)$, urine concentrations of metabolite or parent drug are often a great deal higher than those seen in plasma and thus more easily measured. Urine can also be collected incrementally, usually in intervals of one or more hours from humans, though this is often more difficult for small children, infants, and the elderly. For larger animals, catheterization can be performed to obtain continuous urine samples, but for smaller animals such as the rat, this becomes an invasive procedure that may alter renal function. When incremental urine samples cannot be collected, complete collections over four to five half-lives after a single dose or during one dosing interval at steady-state can be performed. Unfortunately, even though urine collection is noninvasive, urinary excretion data are all too often not included in clinical protocols, since these are considered as a secondary measure to plasma drug profiles. However, urinary metabolite excretion data can offer valuable information on the disposition of metabolites, especially when interpreting drug-drug interactions or the basis for altered pharmacokinetics in patient populations.

There are some assumptions that will be made in discussing renal clearance of metabolites that need to be considered. The first is that renal drug metabolism is not occurring, i.e., metabolite measured in plasma is what is filtered or transported into the renal tubule from the plasma, and parent drug does not convert to metabolite in the kidney. If renal drug metabolism does occur, the estimated renal clearance would be considered as an "apparent clearance," which is similar to estimating biliary clearance in a cannulated animal when hepatic metabolism of drug occurs without the metabolite being presented to the systemic circulation. Though the concept of drug metabolism in the liver prior to arrival of metabolite in the bile is well accepted, there appears to be a common, erroneous assumption that drug metabolism is unlikely to occur in the kidney. Another concern that is more easily tested is whether the metabolites are stable once excreted in the urine, since metabolites often reside in the bladder for periods of many hours prior to voiding. An example of this is the hydrolysis and acyl migration of ester glucuronides, which can be quite variable since it is a pH-dependent process (48,49). Finally, it is generally assumed that once a drug or metabolite arrives in the urinary bladder, it is irreversibly removed from the systemic circulation. However, studies have shown that resorption from the urinary bladder back into the systemic circulation can be significant for some compounds, and this phenomenon should be considered (50). For the purpose of discussion in this section, it will be assumed that these complicating factors are negligible, or if they are occurring, they are reproducible and permit calculations that provide estimates of apparent pharmacokinetic parameters.

Determination of Renal Clearance for Metabolites

Renal clearance is one pharmacokinetic parameter that can be determined for most metabolites as well as the parent drug regardless of the route of administration, dosing regimens, formulations, or availability. The data needed are urinary excretion rates and plasma concentrations. The following general equation applies to calculate renal clearance (CL_R) during a urine collection interval and is expressed for a metabolite (17),

$$CL_R(m) = \frac{\Delta A(m)_e / \Delta t}{C(m)_{ave}} \tag{2.33}$$

Here, $\Delta A(m)_e$ is the amount of metabolite excreted into the urine during the collection interval, Δt is the collection interval, and $C(m)_{ave}$ is the average plasma metabolite concentration over the interval. Intervals are typically at least two or several hours long for studies in humans due to the difficulty in voiding more frequently. If frequent, short incremental collections of urine are desired, it is common practice to provide oral fluids so that adequate (but not excessive) urine production rates are maintained.

The necessary collection interval makes the use of incremental renal clearance calculations difficult and less valuable for drugs with very short half-lives, such as less than an hour. The average plasma concentration is usually measured as the concentration at the midpoint of the collection interval or an average of the plasma concentrations at the beginning and end of a collection period.

An alternative calculation for incremental renal clearance is to rearrange Eq. 2.33, realizing that the product of the average plasma metabolite concentration and the time interval is the incremental AUC(m) for that collection period, i.e., $\Delta AUC(m) = C(m)_{ave} \cdot \Delta t$; thus,

$$CL_R(m) = \frac{\Delta A(m)_e}{\Delta AUC(m)} \tag{2.34}$$

Either of the above incremental renal clearance calculations can be applied to any collection interval, without consideration for the method of drug administration. These can also be applied to chronic multiple dose regimens where it is common to measure total urinary output over the dosing interval τ.

Incremental renal clearance calculations should result in values that are approximately constant if $CL_R(m)$ is constant across the periods collected, i.e., linear or concentration-independent pharmacokinetics (15,17–19). If they are not similar, a useful approach is to examine a plot of excretion rate, $\Delta A(m)_e/\Delta t$, as a function of metabolite plasma concentration, $C(m)_{ave}$. The slope of such a plot is $CL_R(m)$, and any nonlinearities may become apparent if renal clearance increases or decreases as concentrations of metabolite change over time or parent drug competes for active renal clearance process, i.e., active secretion or reabsorption.

Measuring incremental renal clearance is not routinely performed as it requires multiple urine collection over several intervals, which adds expense due to processing and analysis costs, or it may not be feasible for studies with children, small animals, or drugs with very short half-lives. Alternatively, a measure of average renal clearance can be determined following a single dose of parent drug using the following equation (17),

$$CL_R(m) = \frac{A_e(m)_{0-\infty}}{AUC(m)_{0-\infty}} \tag{2.35}$$

where $A_e(m)$ is the amount of metabolite excreted from initial time of dosing (time zero) to a later time, usually when almost all of the drug and metabolite have been eliminated from the body—4 or 5 elimination half-lives of parent or metabolite (whichever is rate limiting). AUC(m) is the area under the metabolite plasma concentration versus time curve for the same interval. For studies conducted with multiple doses to steady-state, the interval for collection of urine and measurement of AUC should be the dosing interval τ.

Use of Metabolite Excretion to Assess Disposition of Drug and Metabolite

Use of Metabolite Excretion Rate to Assess the Profile of Metabolite in Plasma

As mentioned above, metabolite concentrations are often more easily measured in urine than in plasma where concentrations may be below detection limits of the available assay. Assuming $CL_R(m)$ is constant, the excretion rate into urine should then parallel plasma concentrations of the metabolite as described by Eq. 2.33 (17). Since a fraction of the total systemic clearance of the metabolite, CL(m), may be due to renal excretion, $f_e(m) = CL_R(m)/CL(m)$, the rate of excretion can be expressed as,

$$\frac{\Delta A(m)_e}{\Delta t} = f_e(m) \cdot CL(m) \cdot C(m)_{ave} \tag{2.36}$$

Here, $C(m)_{ave}$ describes the average time course of plasma metabolite concentrations over time, whereas $f_e(m)$ and CL(m) are constant. Thus, urinary excretion data of metabolite when plotted versus time can characterize the profile of metabolite in plasma even when plasma concentrations of metabolite cannot be measured. This profile can be used to estimate the rates of initial increase in metabolite concentrations, the approximate time-to-peak metabolite levels in plasma, and the apparent elimination half-life of the metabolite.

Use of Metabolite Excretion Rates to Assess the Profile of the Parent Drug

For drugs exhibiting FRL metabolism, which is the most common situation, urinary excretion rates or fraction of dose excreted in the urine may be used to estimate the plasma profile of the parent drug. With FRL metabolism, the plasma profile of metabolite parallels that of the parent drug as shown in Eq. 2.9, which when substituted into Eq. 2.36 provides,

$$\frac{\Delta A(m)_e}{\Delta t} = f_e(m) \cdot CL_f \cdot C_{ave}$$

(2.37)

where C_{ave} is the average plasma concentration of parent drug over time. Thus, urinary excretion rate of the metabolite is directly proportional to the concentration of parent drug, which is expected under the conditions of FRL metabolism. Thus, a plot of metabolite excretion rates versus time provides a description of the parent drug profile and can be used to estimate the duration of the absorption phase, approximate time to peak concentration, and elimination half-life of the parent drug without the need to assay parent drug in plasma or urine. Also evident from Eq. 2.37 is that with FRL metabolism when values of $f_e(m)$ and $F(m)$ are both unity, then the excretion rate of metabolite equals its rate of formation from the parent drug.

Use of Metabolite Excretion Rates to Assess Formation Clearance of the Metabolite

Where drug concentrations can be measured in plasma, and f_e is known, under FRL metabolism, Eq. 2.38 can be rearranged to estimate formation clearance of the metabolite CL_f,

$$CL_f = \frac{\Delta A(m)_e / \Delta t}{f_e(m) \cdot C_{ave}}$$

(2.38)

where C_{ave} is the average concentration of drug during the period of urine collection. The use of Eq. 2.38 assumes that $F(m)$ of the metabolite is unity, i.e., all metabolite formed reaches the systemic circulation, though it does not require f_e to be equal to unity, though in practice this relationship has been applied to metabolites that are primarily excreted in the urine.

Alternatively, one could use amounts of metabolite and drug rather than concentrations using the same assumptions,

$$k_f = \frac{\Delta A(m)_e / \Delta t}{f_e(m) \cdot A_{ave}}$$

(2.39)

A classic example of the use of this approach is in Levy's studies of salicylate metabolism, which did not even require measurement of plasma salicylate concentrations (51). Salicylate has four major metabolites that are rapidly excreted in urine, so plasma concentrations of these metabolites were difficult to measure prior to the advent of modern liquid chromatography. Given that levels of metabolite in plasma were very low and urinary metabolites accounted for almost all of the salicylate dose, Levy estimated the amount of salicylate remaining in the body by using a mass balance approach where the amount remaining to be excreted at a given time interval represented A_{ave}. By evaluating urinary excretion rates versus A_{ave}, using a linear transformation of the Michaelis–Menton equation, the formation of the salicyluric acid and the phenol glucuronide metabolites were found to be saturable, and Michaelis–Menton constants, K_m and V_m, were determined, while the metabolism to gentisic acid and the acyl glucuronide were nonsaturable with constant k_f values over a large range of amounts of salicylate in the body.

When incremental collections of urine are not obtained, but the urine collection is for a sufficient number of elimination half-lives to approximate a complete collection of metabolite in the urine, then Eq. 2.37 can be rearranged and the integral of $C_{ave} \cdot \Delta t$ is the AUC for the parent drug,

$$CL_f = \frac{A(m)_e}{f_e(m) \times AUC} \tag{2.40}$$

The use of Eq. 2.40 is not dependent on rapid elimination of metabolite upon formation; thus, it is applicable to both conditions of FRL and ERL metabolism as long as urine is collected for a sufficient duration to account for all the metabolite formed after a single dose. The relationship is also applicable for the analysis of excretion data after chronic dosing to steady-state where amount of metabolite in urine and AUC is measured over the dosing interval τ. This equation, as written, does assume that $F(m)$ of the metabolite is unity for the CL_f value to be accurate, though use of an apparent CL_f may be adequate for comparative experiments if $F(m)$ is constant between experiments.

Assessment of Renal Metabolism

Using pharmacokinetic analysis to assess or quantify the extent of renal metabolism *in vivo* is difficult and not often employed. Renal and biliary clearance calculations employ the same equations and are both subject to errors if formation of metabolite occurs in the organ with subsequent excretion of metabolite without presentation of all metabolite to the systemic circulation. Biliary clearances of a metabolite can be determined by collection of bile in animals, but rarely in humans, and then are often referred to as *apparent* clearances because of the understanding that hepatic metabolism is likely occurring. In contrast, seldom are renal clearances of metabolites reported as *apparent* clearances; thus, there is an inherent assumption that none of the metabolite excreted in the urine is formed by the kidney and immediately excreted in the urine. Though there is little information to determine how often this assumption is valid, given the lower metabolic capability of the kidney relative to the liver for most substrates that have been examined, this assumption is usually accepted for renal clearance calculations. In contrast, such an assumption would probably be challenged if made for calculating biliary clearance of a metabolite.

If Eqs. 2.33 through 2.35 (above) are applied to metabolite excreted in the urine and the value of renal clearance based upon blood concentrations was very high, exceeding renal blood flow, then one may suspect that renal metabolism is occurring. This requires the use of clearance values on the basis of blood concentrations, which can be calculated from clearance in plasma and measurement of the blood/plasma concentration ratio, by the relationship, $CL\ C = CL_B\ C_B$, where the subscript B refers to blood. Therefore, ratios of metabolite concentration in blood relative to plasma need to be obtained and are easily determined *in vitro*. This phenomenon was reviewed by Vree et al. (52) in human studies. It is easy to conceptualize this phenomenon if one obtains extensive excretion of metabolite in urine when a very sensitive assay cannot even measure the metabolite in plasma. If the plasma concentration of metabolite is assigned a value of zero, then $CL_R(m)$ from the above equations is infinity, an unlikely event; therefore, renal metabolism should be considered. It would be more appropriate to conservatively assign the concentration of metabolite in plasma to a value just below the assay quantification limit rather than zero and then compare the clearance value on the basis of blood concentration to known renal blood flow.

An alternative, though more complex and invasive approach to assess renal metabolism was proposed and evaluated by Riegelman and coworkers (53,54), where parent drug and radiolabeled metabolite were infused simultaneously to estimate the renal clearance of the metabolite and formation rates. Contributions of hepatic metabolism to metabolite excreted in urine were determined with the assumption that the metabolism was FRL and $F(m)$ of metabolite formed in the liver was unity, i.e., these metabolites were not excreted in the bile or subject to sequential metabolism. The labeled dose of metabolite provides information supporting renal metabolism because the ratio of labeled to unlabeled metabolite in plasma versus urine will be different if parent drug is converted to metabolite when passing through the kidney. This approach revealed that 60%–70% of salicyluric acid metabolite produced from salicylate in a human subject was formed in the kidney (54). With the current availability of liquid chromatography-mass spectrometry, this method could be adapted to use stable isotope tracers of metabolites rather than radiolabeled material.

Biliary Clearance and Enterohepatic Recycling of Metabolites

Biliary clearance is an excretory route of elimination, in many ways similar to renal clearance discussed above. For some drugs, xenobiotics and metabolites, excretion into the bile can represent the major route for elimination. The mechanisms of bile formation, hepatobiliary transport, and excretion processes have been reviewed (55–57). Drugs can be eliminated in the bile by direct excretion without biotransformation; however, many drugs are excreted after metabolism to more polar, charged metabolites, often by conjugation with sulfate, glucuronic acid, or glutathione. Excretion via the bile can be an irreversible route of elimination for a drug if its metabolites have poor permeability (e.g., glucuronide or sulfate conjugates), the drug molecule is poorly absorbed, or the drug is subject to degradation or complexation in the intestinal contents. In contrast, there are numerous examples of conjugated (phase II) metabolites, which are excreted in the bile, cleaved to yield the parent drug, and then the parent drug is reabsorbed into the systemic circulation, i.e., enterohepatic recycling (EHC). The factors influencing EHC can be quite complex and have been reviewed (58).

Measurement of Biliary Clearance

Bile collection can occasionally be obtained from humans, such as in patients treated for biliary obstruction or post–liver transplant. Animal studies of biliary excretion are quite common, often conducted to provide insight into mechanistic processes of drug and metabolite disposition. When bile is collected after administration of the parent drug, *apparent* biliary clearance of metabolite can be determined using Eqs. 2.33 through 2.35 above, where the excretion rate of bile is substituted for that of urine. The term "*apparent*" is usually used because it is often the case that drug entering the hepatocyte is first metabolized and then the metabolite is excreted in the bile without subsequent access to the systemic circulation. If a preformed metabolite is administered directly, the same equations can be applied but may provide many different values for biliary clearance of the metabolite than the values determined when the parent drug is administered, since the metabolite need not be formed in the hepatocyte prior to excretion in the bile. Because of the potential rate-limiting steps involving active uptake or diffusion into the hepatocyte, metabolism in the hepatocyte and active transport from the hepatocyte into the bile, which may vary when parent drug versus metabolite is administered, the absolute value for metabolite biliary clearance using Eqs. 2.33 through 2.35 may not be that informative when preformed metabolite is administered directly.

More commonly employed when metabolite is formed in the hepatocyte and subsequently excreted in bile with negligible plasma levels is the measurement of the excretion rate of metabolite and/or parent drug in the bile as a function of parent drug concentration in plasma, which provides a measure of *apparent* biliary clearance,

$$\Delta A_{bile} / \Delta t = CL_{bile} \cdot C_{ave} \tag{2.41}$$

where ΔA_{bile} can include both parent drug and metabolite, though often metabolite(s) is (are) dominant, and C_{ave} refers to average plasma concentrations of the parent drug during the collection interval. If only metabolite is present in bile, but no metabolite is measurable in plasma, and metabolite once formed in the hepatocyte is not released into the systemic circulation, the term "CL_{bile}" represents an apparent formation clearance ($CL_{f,bile}$) for the metabolite in the liver. This relationship can be rewritten in terms of an AUC, either during an interval or until all the drug is eliminated after a single dose, where the subscript *bc* refers to the AUC obtained with an exteriorized bile cannula,

$$\Delta A_{bile} = CL_{bile} \cdot \Delta AUC_{bc} \tag{2.42}$$

Enterohepatic Recycling

EHC recycling via metabolites is considered a "futile cycle" because of the inefficiency of the metabolic process. The existence of EHC can be proven on the basis of several criteria as summarized by Duggan and Kwan (59). It can be proven unequivocally in animal studies by (i) linked experiments where the bile from a donor animal is infused into a recipient, (ii) a gradual establishment of a portal:systemic plasma concentration gradient after intravenous dosing of parent drug, and (iii) an increase in systemic clearance when there is irreversible bile diversion. In contrast, in most human studies, only suggestive evidence of EHC can be obtained. These include observations such as the presence of secondary peaks in plasma concentration versus time curves, often coincident with gallbladder discharge in response to a meal, or the presence of drug-derived material in the feces after administration via routes other than oral or rectal. It should be noted that secondary peaks due to EHC seen in humans would not initially be expected in the rat, which lacks a gallbladder. However, if reabsorption in the intestine is delayed because of regional distributions of β-glucuronidase or sulfatase, time-dependent hydrolysis of conjugates or site-specific permeability, secondary peaks may also be seen in the rat. Thus, secondary peaks in humans may be due to reasons other than EHC, such as delayed or irregular oral absorption.

When bile is diverted in animals, the AUC in plasma of parent drug will decrease relative to that obtained without diversion when enterohepatic recycling is operative. CL_{bile} determined with bile diversion using Eq. 2.43 can then be employed to estimate total biliary exposure or the total amount of drug/metabolite subject to EHC when cycling is operative without bile diversion (59),

$$\Sigma A_{bile} = CL_{bile} \cdot AUC \tag{2.43}$$

where AUC is the exposure to parent drug in plasma in an animal without biliary diversion and ΣA_{bile} is the estimated sum of all parent drug and metabolite that may be excreted in bile when EHC is operative, i.e., it is the cumulative drug exposure to the intestine. This measure of cumulative drug/metabolite exposure to the intestine due to EHC can result in an amount exceeding the intravenous dose when EHC is very extensive and efficient. For example, as shown in Table 2.1, indomethacin exposure in bile of the dog had an estimated 362% of the dose cycled, and the extent of cycling was inversely correlated with observed toxic doses across the species (59).

EHC can be very efficient, resulting in futile cycling. When this occurs, the metabolite formed and excreted in the bile does not represent an irreversible loss, instead the EHC process represents a distribution process with bile/intestine as a peripheral distribution compartment (58). One measure of the efficiency of EHC was provided by Tse et al. (60). From two experiments, conducted with and without bile collection, and AUC for the parent drug in plasma, which is measured in each treatment after a single intravenous dose, one can calculate the fraction of drug dose excreted in the bile as parent

TABLE 2.1

Species Differences in Indomethacin Biliary Exposure and Toxicity

Species	Clearance (mL/min/kg)			Area (µg·mL)		Plasma Gradient, $C_p^{port} dt / C_p^{ven}$	Total Exposure, $\Sigma_{bile}^{\%}$	Minimum Toxic Dosage (mg/kg/day)
	Plasma, $V_{cl,p}$	Urine, $V_{cl,r}$	Bile, $V_{cl,b}$	Venous, $\int_0^\infty C_p^{ven} dt$	Portal, $\int_0^\infty C_p^{port} dt$			
Dog	8.2	<0.1	13.3	122	310[a]	2.54[a]	362	0.5
Rat	0.32	0.01	0.39	3074	3535	1.15	134	0.75
Monkey	8.3	3.0	2.2	121	121	1.0	26	1.0
Guinea pig	6.25	1.85	1.20	158	181	1.15	21	6.0
Rabbit	3.62	1.09	0.40	278	334	1.20	13	20.0
Man	1.79	0.22	0.16[b]	592	592	1.0[c]	9.5	

Source: Duggan, D.E. and Kwan, K.C., *Drug Metab. Rev.*, 9, 21–41, 1979.

Portal/venous concentration ratios greatly exceeded 1 in the dog, and there was a strong inverse correlation between total biliary exposure and minimum toxic dosage.

Note: All disposition data for single intravenous dosage of 1 mg/kg, except man, for whom 25-mg total dosage normalized to 1 mg/kg.

[a] Based on complete 0- to 2-hr portal and systemic plasma profiles; for all other species, mean of more than five measurements at interval specified in text.

[b] Calculated from $f_{bile} = 0.09$ (H. B. Hucker, unpublished).

[c] Assumed.

drug and metabolites that are subject to possible cycling, F_b. From this information, and the definition that the amount of drug that is reabsorbed from the first cycle is $F_a \cdot F_b \cdot D$, together with the assumption that this fraction is constant with all subsequent cycles, the following relationship can be derived (60),

$$F_a = \left[1 - AUC_{bc} / AUC\right] / F_b \qquad (2.44)$$

where AUC_{bc} for the parent drug is measured with bile cannulation and drainage. The value of F_a obtained is a measure of the fraction of the sum of drug and metabolite excreted in the bile, which is then reabsorbed. When using this relationship, only metabolites that could be recycled (i.e., they are reversible to parent drug in the GI tract) would be included when estimating F_b. When F_b is a significant part of the dose, but AUC_{bc} is equivalent to AUC, it is apparent that bile diversion did not influence the amount of drug reaching the systemic circulation, and thus F_a is zero. In contrast, when a significant part of the dose is excreted in bile and AUC_{bc} is much less than AUC, then recycling is significant, and F_a can approach a value of 1.

Reversible Metabolism

Reversible metabolism occurs when a metabolite or biotransformation product and the parent drug undergo interconversion in both directions, as shown in Scheme 2.6. The scheme can also be written in terms of concentrations and clearance terms rather than amounts and rate constants, respectively, as shown in Scheme 2.6B using the common convention in the literature where the drug is considered in compartment 1 and the metabolite in compartment 2. These compartments are not to be confused with physiological spaces. Here, the "metabolite" may be the pharmacologically active species in the case of administration of a prodrug, an active metabolite, or an inactive metabolite. Generally, enzyme-catalyzed chiral inversion reactions are not reversible, such as the R to S conversion of ibuprofen (61,62), and these are not considered here. In contrast, chemical catalysis of the chiral inversion of thalidomide (63) would be expected to behave similarly to reversible metabolism, and the pharmacokinetic modeling would be the same.

Though reversible metabolism is less often addressed in reviews of drug metabolite kinetics (12), there are numerous examples occurring across a wide variety of compounds as noted in a recent review by Cheng and Jusko (64). These include phase I metabolic pathways for amines such as imipramine, alcohols such as corticosteroids and estradiol, lactones, and sulfides/sulfoxides such as captopril and sulindac. Examples for phase II metabolic pathways include carboxylic acids to their glucuronides, as in the case of ibuprofen, sulfation of phenols such as estrone, and acetylation of amines such as procainamide (64). Pharmacokinetic methods for the analysis of reversible metabolism are well described (64–67). More recently, considerations of statistical moment analysis as applied to reversible systems have also been addressed by Cheng (68,69).

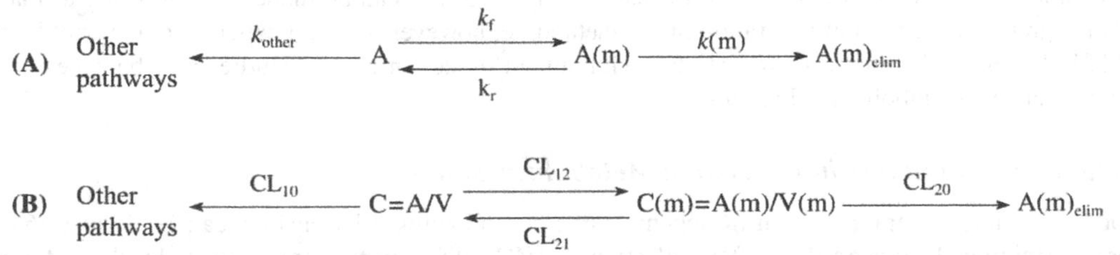

SCHEME 2.6 (a and b) Reversible conversion between metabolite and drug with parallel elimination pathways for the parent drug and metabolite.

Reversible metabolism is often ignored when analyzing the pharmacokinetic data of compounds that undergo metabolite interconversion. The pharmacokinetic parameter estimates obtained using methods or approaches that do not consider the reversible nature of the system are not true estimates of pharmacokinetic parameters and should be considered *apparent* parameter values. Indeed, regulatory agencies may not require rigorous evaluation of the true reversible metabolic parameters because the critical parameters of clearance, volume of distribution, and bioavailability can only be unambiguously obtained after direct administration of the preformed metabolite, which is usually not feasible in humans because of the need to secure an IND for the intravenous administration of the metabolite. Moreover, in many cases of reversible metabolism, the metabolite may only achieve low concentrations relative to the parent drug or is inactive; thus, a great deal of effort to fully elucidate its pharmacokinetics may be difficult or not justified on the basis of the considerable costs and efforts. There are, however, a number of common disease states, such as renal or hepatic impairment, which may dramatically alter the disposition of the metabolite; thus, significantly influencing the disposition of the parent drug, and these should be addressed. When a metabolite is active or of toxicological relevance, or when altered disposition of the metabolite substantially modifies the pharmacokinetic profile of the parent drug, efforts to more fully investigate reversible metabolism are warranted.

Determination of Primary Pharmacokinetic Parameters for Reversible Metabolic Systems

The primary pharmacokinetic parameters of clearance, volume, and availability, as well as commonly employed secondary parameters of half-life and MRT will be discussed here. Discussion of less commonly employed parameters can be found in other literature (64–69). However, difficulties in estimating parameters involving reversible metabolism, due to either the need to dose the metabolite directly or inherent errors in the complex equations employed, generally limit the utility of estimating some parameters. Other parameters unique to reversible metabolic systems are descriptors of the reversibility of the process that include the recycling numbers, recycled fraction, and exposure enhancement, which will be discussed below.

Half-Life in Reversible Metabolism Systems

As shown in Figure 2.10 for the interconversion of methylprednisone and methylprednisolone, which undergo the reversible metabolism of ketone/alcohol common with steroids, after the parent drug and metabolite reach equilibrium, the two compounds decline in parallel when either is administered intravenously (70). Because the terminal half-life reflects a hybrid of the clearance terms for the overall reversible system and the volumes of distribution of parent drug and metabolite, estimating changes in the half-life in response to an altered clearance or volume term is difficult. Although the use of "sojourn times" have been proposed as a measure of time a drug or metabolite is in the body before being eliminated or transformed in reversible systems (57), in practice, most often an *apparent* half-life is reported with the understanding that it may be subject to change in response to alterations of the disposition of parent drug or metabolite.

The fact that the terminal half-life of parent drug and metabolite are parallel when parent drug is administered could lead to an erroneous assumption that FRL metabolism is operative when in fact reversible metabolism is occurring. Confirmation of reversibility can be made by identifying formation of the parent drug after administration of the metabolite; however, such an experiment may not be feasible in humans. Therefore, *in vitro* studies with human tissues or animal studies may be necessary to infer reversible metabolism in humans.

Clearance Parameters in Reversible Metabolism Systems

For a reversible system as shown in Scheme 2.6B, the following relationships can be derived (64,65) for determining clearance values after collection of AUC data from an intravenous bolus dose of parent drug or metabolite on two separate occasions. These relationships assume that clearance and distribution processes are linear for both parent drug and metabolite, i.e., independent of concentration.

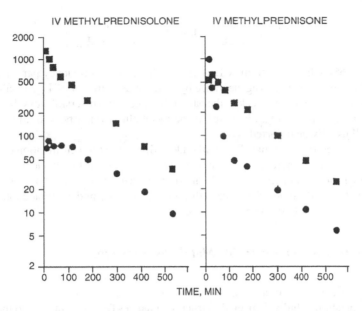

FIGURE 2.10 The reversible metabolism of methylprednisolone (■) and methylprednisone (●) when each is given on separate occasions as a 1.25 mg/kg intravenous bolus to a rabbit. The parallel profiles, constant concentration ratios at equilibrium, and formation of both compounds when either is administered, are characteristics of reversible metabolism. (From Ebling, W.F. et al., *Drug Metab. Dispos.*, 13, 296–301, 1985.)

$$CL_{10} = \frac{Dose^p \cdot AUC_m^m - Dose^m \cdot AUC_m^p}{AUC_p^p \cdot AUC_m^m - AUC_m^p \cdot AUC_p^m} \tag{2.45}$$

$$CL_{20} = \frac{Dose^m \cdot AUC_p^p - Dose^p \cdot AUC_p^m}{AUC_p^p \cdot AUC_m^m - AUC_m^p \cdot AUC_p^m} \tag{2.46}$$

$$CL_{21} = \frac{Dose^m \cdot AUC_m^p}{AUC_p^p \cdot AUC_m^m - AUC_m^p \cdot AUC_p^m} \tag{2.47}$$

$$CL_{21} = \frac{Dose^p \cdot AUC_p^m}{AUC_p^p \cdot AUC_m^m - AUC_m^p \cdot AUC_p^m} \tag{2.48}$$

Here, the superscript indicates the dose administered as being from the parent drug or metabolite, whereas the subscript refers to the compound that is measured in plasma. AUC is the total area under the plasma concentration versus time curve extrapolated to infinity. Similar equations can be derived when the compounds are infused to steady-state (67) where the values needed are infusion rates and steady-state concentrations. These relationships are not unique, as the model has also been applied to other two compartment pharmacokinetic systems with elimination occurring from each compartment, such as the reversible distribution and elimination from the maternal-fetal unit (71).

If apparent clearance terms are used for parent drug or metabolite, these will overestimate the true values for CL_{10} and CL_{20}, respectively. The magnitude of the error is a complex relationship of all the clearance terms as discussed by Ebling and Jusko (65) and is shown here for CL_{app} of the parent drug,

$$CL_{app} = \frac{D}{AUC} = CL_{10} + CL_{12}\left[\frac{CL_{20}}{CL_{21} + CL_{20}}\right] \tag{2.49}$$

Ebling and Jusko (65) defined the term "$CL_{20}/(CL_{21} + CL_{20})$" as an efficiency parameter because it is a fraction that defines the extent of drug clearance by metabolite formation (CL_{12}), resulting in metabolite that does not return or interconvert back to the parent drug, i.e., an irreversible loss. Similar relationships have been determined for $CL(m)_{app}$; however, if the metabolite cannot be administered, then only the term "CL_{app}" will usually be reported.

It is also evident from Eq. 2.49 that CL_{app} will underestimate the total elimination capacity for the parent drug, i.e., $CL_{10} + CL_{12}$, where CL_{12} is a measure of metabolite formation clearance, CL_f. Therefore, estimating the formation clearance of a metabolite from *in vivo* studies using $CL_f + CL_{app} - CL_{10}$ (where CL_{10} is determined from the other clearance pathways) may grossly underestimate total metabolic capability for the particular metabolic pathway *in vivo*.

Volume of Distribution in Reversible Metabolism Systems

Volume of distribution at steady-state for parent drug and metabolite in reversible metabolic systems are independent, but the equations to calculate the values necessitate consideration of the disposition of both parent drug and metabolite. Indeed, given the structural changes from parent drug to metabolites, as well as potential differences in protein binding and lipophilicity between the parent drug and metabolites, it is reasonable to expect that distribution in the body could be quite different, as previously mentioned for morphine and M6G. In the absence of interconversion, volume of distribution at steady-state $[V(m)_{ss,app}]$ is calculated with the following equation for the metabolite,

$$V(m)_{ss,app} = \frac{M \cdot AUMC_m^m}{\left(AUC_m^m\right)^2} \tag{2.50}$$

where AUMC(m) is the first moment of the plasma concentration versus time curve for the metabolite (17). This equation for apparent V_{ss} is in error if applied to reversible metabolism systems, since $V(m)_{ss,app}$ will overestimate the real $V(m)_{ss}$ because the parent drug reverts to the metabolite (65). Moreover, $V(m)_{ss,app}$ is not independent of clearance processes as is the true $V(m)_{ss}$; thus, changes in clearance terms of either parent drug or metabolite will modify the value of $V(m)_{ss,app}$ in reversible metabolism systems.

The relationship between the apparent and real parameter is described for the metabolite as follows (65),

$$V(m)_{ss,app} = V(m) + V_{ss}\left[\frac{CL_{12} \times CL_{21}}{\left(CL_{12} + CL_{10}\right)^2}\right] \tag{2.51}$$

The complexities of these relationships for volume and clearance combine, such that the following equation for $V(m)_{ss}$ is dependent on dose of metabolite and measured AUC and AUMC data (65),

$$V_{ss}(m) = \frac{M\left[\left(AUC_p^p\right)^2 \times AUMC_m^m - AUC_p^m \times AUC_m^p \times AUMC_p^p\right]}{\left(AUC_p^p \times AUC_m^m\right)^2 - \left(AUC_m^p \times AUC_p^m\right)^2} \tag{2.52}$$

Measures of AUMC used for Eqs. 2.50 and 2.52 are often criticized for the potential error that may be introduced when extrapolating the first-moment curve to infinity. Alternative equations derived for application of data obtained from infusions of metabolite and parent drug to steady-state may reduce some of the errors (67). Given the limited ability to dose preformed metabolite to humans and the potential error in determining V_{ss} for parent drug or metabolite within reversible systems, true values for the pharmacokinetic parameters in reversible metabolism systems have been determined in humans for very few compounds. Instead, it is more common to report $V_{ss,app}$ values, with an understanding that such values are inaccurate and subject to change if clearance is altered.

Bioavailability in Reversible Metabolism Systems

Interconversion of parent drug and metabolite also complicates the measures of bioavailability and consideration of this has led to the development of equations that assess absorption processes independent of clearance (64,72). However, the increased complexity of the relationships and the need to dose metabolite independently to assess the values have restricted their application. Thus, apparent bioavailability is often employed ignoring the contributions of reversible metabolism.

Measures of Reversibility in Drug Metabolism

Unique to reversible systems are measures defined as recycled fraction (RF), number of recyclings through the reversible process (R_I), as well as other terms (64,65). RF is a measure of the likelihood of a molecule going back and forth through the reversible system, i.e., being converted in both directions, and is a value between 0 and 1 determined from the relative values of clearance,

$$RF = \frac{CL_{12} \cdot CL_{21}}{CL_{11} \cdot CL_{22}} \tag{2.53}$$

where $CL_{11} = CL_{10} + CL_{12}$ and $CL_{22} = CL_{20} + CL_{21}$.

The number of recyclings, R_I, can exceed 1 and provides a measure of how exposure to parent or metabolite is enhanced by the interconversion process,

$$R_I = \frac{CL_{12} \cdot CL_{21}}{CL_{11} \cdot CL_{22} - CL_{12} \cdot CL_{21}} \tag{2.54}$$

Influence of Altered Metabolite Clearances on the Disposition of Parent Drug

Because metabolite and parent drug can interconvert, altered irreversible clearance of the metabolite (CL_{20}) can influence the disposition of the parent drug, causing changes in CL_{app}, i.e., Eq. 2.49. Examples of this include the non-steroidal anti-inflammatory drugs where renal clearance of labile ester glucuronide metabolite is reduced by renal dysfunction (73). For example, though diflunisal and other carboxylic acid-containing drugs are eliminated almost entirely by metabolism, simulation results shown in Table 2.2 show that when clearances that directly affect acyl glucuronides are altered, the AUC of both parent drug and metabolite can in some cases be significantly and seemingly unpredictably modified (74). This has potential clinical significance, since hepatobiliary or renal disease may alter clearance pathways of the metabolite and cause unanticipated alterations in the disposition of the parent drug, even though the parent drug itself is not eliminated directly into bile or into the urine.

TABLE 2.2

Relative Values of AUC for Acidic Drugs and Their Acyl Glucuronide Metabolites in Animals Obtained by Simulation Using the Model Shown When Individual Clearance Terms in the Scheme for Reversible Metabolism are Reduced to 10% of Their Initial Value

Clearance Terms Altered	Percentage of Normal AUC for Parent Compound (%)					
	DF	**S-ET**	**R-ET**	**VPA**	**S**	**Z**
Cl_{10}	241	380	242	477	791	850
Cl_{12}	146	119	146	112	103	102
Cl_{20}	144	117	141	111	103	102
Cl_{21}	75	99	99	96	83	100
Cl_{23}	93	89	79	96	100	94

Clearance Terms Altered	Percentage of Normal AUC for Acyl Glucuronide (%)					
	DFG	**S-ETG**	**R-ETG**	**VPAG**	**SG**	**ZG**
Cl_{10}	241	380	242	477	791	850
Cl_{12}	15	12	15	11	10	10
Cl_{20}	186	202	248	181	104	103
Cl_{21}	147	106	102	130	664	116
Cl_{23}	114	152	139	129	101	386

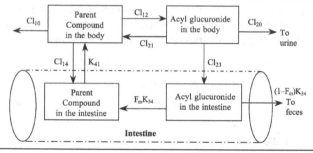

Source: Liu, J.H. and Smith, P.C., *Curr. Drug Metab.*, 7, 147–163, 2006.

The clearance terms are defined in the figure. Baseline value is 100. Data were obtained by Monte Carlo simulation using initial values obtained in animals.

Abbreviation: AUC, area under the curve.

Nonlinear Processes and Metabolite Disposition

Metabolite disposition is subject to the same sources of nonlinearity that can occur with the parent drug (17). These may include saturable enzymic metabolism, co-substrate depletion in phase II metabolism, saturable transport for biliary or renal excretion, saturable active uptake into hepatocytes, or saturable protein binding. In summary, metabolite disposition can be affected by nonlinearities involving both the rate of input (i.e., formation), rate of output (i.e., elimination), and distribution. Any nonlinearity in disposition of the parent drug, which is the precursor for the metabolite, will lead to increased complexities in predicting metabolite disposition; thus, the correlation between exposure to parent drug and exposure to the metabolite will not be predictable as dose is varied or may vary with time when dosing chronically. In this section, the most common source of nonlinearity will be considered and discussed, assuming that only one clearance parameter is nonlinear at a given time. However, one should realize that multiple nonlinearities may occur simultaneously, especially in animal toxicology studies where drug doses are intentionally pushed to levels much greater than those employed later in humans.

Michaelis–Menton Formation vs. Elimination of the Metabolite

The assumption that metabolite formation and elimination occur as first-order processes with constant CL_f and $CL(m)$ generally holds true for typical enzyme or active transport systems when concentrations of drug or metabolite, respectively, are below their K_m (Michaelis–Menton constant where the rate is half of the maximum velocity, V_m) (17) values. In cases where Michaelis–Menton kinetics apply for metabolite formation and elimination, with only a single pathway formation and elimination of metabolite, Eq. 2.11 can be rewritten as,

$$\frac{dA(m)}{dt} = \frac{V_{m,f} \cdot C}{K_{m,f} + C} - \frac{V_m(m) \cdot C(m)}{\left[K_m(m) + C(m) \right]} \tag{2.55}$$

It is apparent that $CL(m)$ and $k(m)$ are now functions of $K_m(m)$ and $V_m(m)$,

$$CL(m) = \frac{V_m(m)}{K_m(m) + C(m)} \tag{2.56}$$

$$k(m) = \frac{\dfrac{V_m(m)}{V(m)}}{\left[K_m(m) + C(m) \right]} \tag{2.57}$$

and similar relationships exist for CL_f and k_f. When $C \ll K_m$ and $C(m) \ll K_m(m)$, then both right-hand terms of Eq. 2.55 simplify, yielding first-order processes, since clearance of formation and the rate constant of elimination of the metabolite are essentially constant. However, if the elimination of the metabolite is saturable, i.e., when $C(m) > K_m(m)$, both $CL(m)$ and $k(m)$ become variable with $CL(m)$ and $k(m)$ decreasing as $C(m)$ increases; thus, the apparent half-life of the metabolite increases as $C(m)$ increases. When saturation of $CL(m)$ occurs, and CL_f is constant (i.e., formation of metabolite is not saturable in the concentration range of drug), then $C(m)/C$ and $AUC(m)/AUC$ will increase as the drug dose increases. Typically, plots of metabolite levels normalized to the drug dose should be superimposable, but with saturable elimination, the dose-normalized metabolite concentrations will increase with dose level. Even under conditions of FRL metabolism, saturation of metabolite elimination will increase these ratios as dose increases, though the metabolite concentration profile may still appear to be parallel to that of the parent drug profile. However, because the formation clearance (CL_f) of the metabolite did not change with dose, f_m would remain constant. Thus, for a metabolite that is primarily excreted in the urine, the percentage of the dose recovered in the urine as metabolite would be independent of dose.

For metabolites subject to ERL metabolism, saturable metabolite elimination may be noticeable from a profile of metabolite concentration versus time when parent drug is rapidly administered or absorbed. A semilog plot of metabolite concentrations versus time profile may show the classical concave shape at higher concentrations and then become loglinear at lower concentrations (15).

In contrast, if the metabolite formation clearance (CL_f) is saturable, while the elimination of metabolite is not, then $C(m)/C$ and $AUC(m)/AUC$ will decrease as drug dose increases. In this case, f_m will decline as the dose increases, assuming that there are other parallel pathways for drug elimination besides formation of the metabolite of interest. With FRL metabolism, the apparent half-life of the metabolite will increase if the saturable pathway of metabolism is a significant fraction of the overall elimination of parent drug, since the half-life of parent drug will increase. For ERL metabolism [$k(m) \ll k$], the profile of the metabolite after escalating single doses of parent drug may not be altered significantly, unless the elimination half-life of the parent drug increased significantly at higher doses such that value of k decreases to the extent that it approaches that of $k(m)$. In this case of saturable metabolite formation clearance, plotting metabolite concentration versus time profiles normalized to dose would show a decline in the AUC of the profiles as dose increased.

MRT concepts can also be applied to metabolites subject to Michaelis–Menton metabolism (31,69,75). Though there has been some debate about using MRT in nonlinear systems, a review addressed these concerns and with simulations showed that the values of MRT, V_{ss}, V_m, and K_m could be determined accurately (76). A potential advantage of MRT concepts for evaluating nonlinear systems is that they do not require multiple trials of various compartmental models normally employed when determining Michaelis–Menton parameters (76).

Conclusions

Even if some of the commonly employed mathematical relationships for performing pharmacokinetic analysis of the parent drug are also applicable to metabolites, because metabolites are formed *in vivo*, there are some unique methods applicable to describing metabolite disposition and an effort was made in this chapter to identify those methods. Many of the difficulties in analyzing metabolite pharmacokinetics stem from limited information about the rate and extent of their formation in the body, i.e., the input into the body is usually not known. Thus, many of the relationships described in this review are based upon derivations that do not require knowledge of the rate of metabolite input, but often make informed estimates of the extent of metabolite formation from the parent drug or assume that the extent of formation is constant between treatments or linear with dose. In many instances, especially when estimating levels after chronic administration of the parent drug, the extent of metabolite formed is more important than the rate at which it was formed. When possible, exogenous administration of preformed metabolite by a known input rate circumvents these limitations. However, due to the potential different behavior of preformed metabolite and that formed at tissue sites within the body (9,46,47), new assumptions arise that may be difficult to validate. One of the primary advantages of MRT approaches for describing metabolite pharmacokinetics is the fewer assumptions made for their application, but a lack of thorough understanding of their theory has limited their use by some investigators. Whatever approach is used, there is much to be gained from a better understanding of the pharmacokinetics of metabolites. Although data obtained in animals by administration of preformed metabolites will have to be interpreted with caution (9), the FDA guidance suggesting toxicology studies in animals with "major metabolites" (23) will in the future lead to substantially more data reported on metabolite disposition. Careful analysis of these data from exogenously administered metabolites relative to metabolites generated *in situ* from the parent drug should provide insight into whether such extraordinary efforts and cost can provide valuable information beyond that presently obtained by radiolabeled tracer studies.

This chapter did not present extensive derivations of some of the mathematical relationships provided. Earlier reviews on the pharmacokinetics of metabolites (12,14) or the primary literature cited should be consulted together with this chapter for further insight and understanding of the derivations and assumptions of the equations presented. In addition, some basic concepts in pharmacokinetics are needed for the full implementation of some of the relationships provided, and these can be found in textbooks on the topic (15–19). The pharmacokinetics and rates of metabolism are not necessarily limited by the metabolic step, and considerations of uptake and efflux transporters need to be considered when interpreting *in vivo* data. Topics such as reversible metabolism and MRT concepts are now better understood because of more recent work, and original literature should be consulted where appropriate. This review should provide a foundation for understanding how the complexities of metabolite formation and elimination may be analyzed. In conjunction with the other chapters in this text, this should assist scientists in the design of *in vitro* experiments, *in vivo* animal studies, and clinical trials to characterize the metabolism of drugs and other xenobiotics such that optimal information can be obtained about the disposition of metabolites in the body with as few assumptions as possible.

ACKNOWLEDGMENTS

The assistance and patience of Dr. Laurene Wang in reading, commenting, and editing this chapter is greatly appreciated.

REFERENCES

1. Atkinson AJ, Strong JM. Effect of active drug metabolites on plasma level response relationships. *J Pharmacokinet Biopharm* 1977; 5:95–109.
2. Sutfin TA, Jusko WJ. Compendium of active drug metabolites. In: Wilkinson GR, Rawlins MD, eds. *Drug Metabolism and Disposition: Considerations in Clinical Pharmacology.* Boston, MA: MTP Press, 1985:91–159.
3. Fura A. Role of pharmacologically active metabolites in drug discovery and development. *Drug Discov Today* 2006; 11:133–142.
4. Penson RT, Joel SP, Robert M, Gloyne A, Beckwith S, Slevin ML. The bioavailability and pharmacokinetics of subcutaneous, nebulized and oral morphine-6-glucuronide. *Br J Clin Pharmacol* 2002; 53:347–354.
5. Fuhr U, Jetter A, Kirchheiner J. Appropriate phenotyping procedures for drug metabolizing enzymes and transporters in humans and their simultaneous use in the "cocktail" approach. *Clin Pharmacol Ther* 2007; 81:270–283.
6. Relling MV, Giacomini KM. Pharmacogenomics. In: Burnton LL, Lazo JS, Parker KL, eds. *Goodman and Gillman's, The Pharmacological Basis of Therapeutics.* 11th ed. New York: McGraw-Hill, 2006:93–115.
7. Matzke GR, Comstock TJ. Influence of renal function and dialysis on drug disposition. In: Burton ME, Shaw LM, Schentag JJ, et al., eds. *Applied Pharmacokinetics and Pharmacodynamics.* 4th ed. New York: Lippincott Williams and Wilkins, 2006:187–212.
8. Uetrecht J. Idiosyncratic drug reactions: Past, present and future. *Chem Res Toxicol* 2008; 21:84–92.
9. Smith DA, Obach RS. Metabolites and safety: What are the concerns, and how should we address them? *Chem Res Toxicol* 2006; 19:1570–1579.
10. Cummings AJ, Martin BK. Excretion and accrual of drug metabolites. *Nature (London)* 1963; 200:1296–1297.
11. Houston JB, Taylor G. Drug metabolite concentration-time profiles: Influence of route of drug administration. *Br J Clin Pharmacol* 1984; 17:385–394.
12. Houston JB. Drug metabolite kinetics. *Pharmacol Ther* 1982; 15:521–552.
13. Pang KS. A review of metabolite kinetics. *J Pharmacokinet Biopharm* 1985; 13:632–662.
14. Weiss M. A general model of metabolite kinetics following intravenous and oral administration of the parent drug. *Biopharm Drug Dispos* 1988; 9:159–176.
15. Rowland M., Tozer TN. *Clinical Pharmacokinetics.* Baltimore, MD: Lea and Febiger, 1995.
16. Buxton ILO. Pharmacokinetics and pharmacodynamics: The dynamics of drug absorption, disposition, action and elimination. In: Burnton LL, Lazo JS, Parker KL, eds. *Goodman and Gillman's, The Pharmacological Basis of Therapeutics.* 11th ed. New York: McGraw-Hill, 2006:1–39.
17. Gibaldi M, Perrier D. *Pharmacokinetics.* 2nd ed. New York: Marcel Dekker, 1982.
18. Gibaldi M. *Biopharmaceutics and Clinical Pharmacokinetics,* 4th ed. Philadelphia, PA: Lea Febiger, 1991.
19. Shargel L, Wu-Pong S, Yu ABC. *Applied Biopharmaceutics and Pharmacokinetics.* 5th ed. New York: McGraw-Hill, 2005.
20. Walle T, Conradi EC, Walle UK, Fagan TC, Gaffrey TE. Naphthoxylacetic acid after single and long-term doses of propranolol. *Clin Pharmacol Ther* 1979; 26:548–554.
21. Chung JM, Hilbert RP, Gural E, Radwanski S, Symchowicz S, Zampaglione N. Multiple dose halazepam kinetics. *Clin Pharmacol Ther* 1984; 35:838–842.
22. Baillie TA, Cayen MN, Fouda H, Gerson RJ, Green JD, Grossman SJ. Klunk LJ, LeBlanc B, Perkins DG, Shipley LA. Drug metabolites in safety testing. *Toxicol Appl Pharmacol* 2002; 182:188–196.
23. Food and Drug Administration. Guidance for Industry: Safety testing of drug metabolites. Available at: www.fda.gov/cder/guidance/6897fnl.htm.
24. Osborne S, Joel D, Trew D, Slevin M. Morphine and metabolite behavior after different routes of morphine administration: Demonstration of the importance of the active metabolite morphine-6-glucuronide. *Clin Pharmacol Ther* 1990; 47:12–19.
25. Barret DA, Barker DP, Rutter N, Pawula M, Shaw PN. Morphine, morphine-6-glucuronide and morphine-3-glucuronide pharmacokinetics in newborn infants receiving diamorphine infusions. *Br J Clin Pharmacol* 1996; 41:531–537.

26. Lotsch J, Stockmann A, Kobal G, Brune K, Waibel R, Schmidt N, Geisslinger G. Pharmacokinetics of morphine and its glucuronides after intravenous infusion of morphine and morphine-6-glucuronide in healthy volunteers. *Clin Pharmacol Ther* 1996; 60:316–325.
27. Rowland M. Physiological pharmacokinetic models and interanimal species scaling. *Pharmacol Ther* 1985; 29:49–68.
28. Boxenbaum H. Interspecies scaling, allometry, physiological time, and the ground plan for pharmacokinetics. *J Pharmacokinet Biopharm* 1982; 10:201–227.
29. Mahmood I. Application of allometric principles for the prediction of pharmacokinetics inhuman and veterinary drug development. *Adv Drug Deliv Rev* 2007; 59:1177–1192.
30. Riegelman S, Collier P. The application of statistical moment theory to the evaluation of *in vivo* dissolution time and absorption time. *J Pharmacokinet Biopharm* 1980; 8:509.
31. Cheng H, Jusko WJ. Mean residence times and distribution volumes for drugs undergoing linear reversible metabolism and tissue distribution and linear or nonlinear elimination from the central compartment. *Pharm Res* 1991; 8:508–511.
32. Weiss M. Drug metabolite kinetics: Noncompartmental analysis. *Br J Clin Pharmacol* 1985; 19:855–856.
33. Veng SA-Pedersen, Gillespie WR. A method for evaluating the mean residence times of metabolites in the body, systemic circulation, and the peripheral tissue not requiring separate i.v. administration of the metabolite. *Biopharm Drug Dispos* 1987; 8:395–401.
34. Kaplan, Jack ML, Cotler S, Alexander K. Utilization of area under the curve to elucidate the disposition of an extensively biotransformed drug. *J Pharmacokinet Biopharm* 1973; 1:201–215.
35. Cutler DJ. Linear system analysis in pharmacokinetics. *J Pharmacokinet Biopharm* 1978; 6:265–282.
36. Karol MD, Goodrich S. Metabolite formation pharmacokinetics: Rate and extent determined by deconvolution. *Pharm Res* 1988; 5:347–351.
37. Murai Y, Nakagawa T, Yamaoka K, Uno T. High-performance liquid chromatographic determination and moment analysis of urinary excretion of flucloxacillin and its metabolites in man. *Int J Pharm* 1983; 15:309–320.
38. Weiss M. Metabolite residence time: Influence of the first-pass effect. *Br J Clin Pharmacol* 1986; 22:121–122.
39. Chan KKH, Gibaldi M. Effects of first-pass metabolisms and metabolite mean residence time determination after oral administration of parent drug. *Pharm Res* 1990; 7:59–63.
40. Lee FW, Salmonson T, Benet LZ. Pharmacokinetics and pharmacodynamics of nitroglycerin and its dinitrate metabolites in conscious dogs: Intravenous infusion studies. *J Pharmacokinet Biopharm* 1993; 21:533–550.
41. Lane EA, Levy RH. Prediction of steady-state behavior of metabolite from dosing of parent drug. *J Pharm Sci* 1980; 69:610–612.
42. Walle T, Conradi EC, Walle UK, Fagan TC, Gaffney TE. 4-Hydroxypropranolol and its glucuronide after single and long-term doses of propranolol. *Clin Pharmacol Ther* 1980; 27:22–31.
43. Williams RT. *Detoxification Mechanisms. The Metabolism of Drugs and Allied Organic Compounds.* New York: Wiley, 1947.
44. Jones D, Gorski C, Haehner BD, O'Mara EM, Hall SD. Determination of cytochrome P450 3A4/5 activity *in vivo* with dextromethorphan N-demethylation. *Clin Pharmacol Ther* 1996; 60:374–384.
45. Pang KS. Kinetics of sequential metabolism. *Drug Metab Dispos* 1995; 23:166–177.
46. Pang KS, Gillette JR. Sequential first-pass elimination of a metabolite derived from its precursor. *J Pharmacokinet Biopharm* 1979; 7:275–290.
47. Tirona RG, Pang KS. Sequestered endoplasma reticulum space for sequential metabolism of salicylamide: Coupling of hydroxylation and glucuronidation. *Drug Metab Dispos* 1996; 24:821–833.
48. Upton RA, Buskin JN, Williams RL, Holford NHG, Riegelman S. Negligible excretion of unchanged ketoprofen, naproxen and probenecid in urine. *J Pharm Sci* 1980; 69:1254–1257.
49. Smith PC, Hasegawa J, Langendijk PNJ, Benet LZ. Stability of acyl glucuronides in blood, plasma and urine: Studies with zomepirac. *Drug Metab Dispos* 1985; 13:110–112.
50. Dalton JT, Weintjes ME, Au JL. Effects of bladder reabsorption on pharmacokinetic data analysis. *J Pharmacokinet Biopharm* 1994; 22:183–205.
51. Levy G, Tsuchiya T, Amsel LP. Limited capacity for salicyl phenolic glucuronide formation and its effect on the kinetics of salicylate elimination in man. *Clin Pharmacol Ther* 1972; 13:258–268.
52. Vree TB, Hekster YA, Anderson PG. Contribution of the human kidney to the metabolic clearance of drugs. *Ann Pharmacother* 1992; 26:1421–1428.

53. Wan SH, Riegelman S. Renal contribution to overall metabolism of drugs I: Conversion of benzoic acid to hippuric acid. *J Pharm Sci* 1972; 61:1278–1284.
54. Lihmann BV, Wan SH, Riegelman S, Becker C. Renal contribution to overall metabolism of drugs IV: Biotransformation of salicylic acid to salicyluric acid in man. *J Pharm Sci* 1973; 62:1483–1486.
55. Bohan A, Boyer JL. Mechanisms of hepatic transport of drugs: Implications for cholestatic drug reactions. *Semin Liver Dis* 2002; 22:123–136.
56. Chandra P, Brouwer KL. The complexities of hepatic drug transport: Current knowledge and emerging concepts. *Pharm Res* 2004; 21:719–735.
57. Shitara Y, Sato H, Sugiyama Y. Evaluation of drug-drug interaction in the hepatobiliary and renal transport of drugs. *Annu Rev Pharmacol Toxicol* 2005; 45:689–723.
58. Roberts MS, Magnusson BM, Burczynski FJ, Weiss M. Enterohepatic circulation: Physiological, pharmacokinetic and clinical implications. *Clin Pharmacokinet* 2002; 41:751–790.
59. Duggan DE, Kwan KC. Enterohepatic recirculation of drugs as a determinant of therapeutic ratio. *Drug Metab Rev* 1979; 9:21–41.
60. Tse FLS, Ballard F, Skinn J. Estimating the fraction reabsorbed in drugs undergoing enterohepatic circulation. *J Pharmacokinet Biopharm* 1982; 10:455–461.
61. Hutt AJ, Caldwell J. The metabolic chiral inversion of 2-arylpropionic acids: A novel route with pharmacological consequences. *J Pharm Pharmacol* 1983; 35:693–704.
62. Baillie TA, Adams WJ, Kaiser DG, Olanoff LS, Halstead GW, Harpootlian H, Van Giessen GJ. Mechanistic studies of the metabolic chiral inversion of (R)-ibuprofen in humans. *J Pharmacol Exp Ther* 1989; 249:517–523.
63. Reist M, Carrupt PA, Francotte E, Testa B. Chiral inversion and hydrolysis of thalidomide: Mechanisms and catalysis by bases and serum albumin, and chiral stability of teratogenic metabolites. *Chem Res Toxicol* 1998; 11:1521–1528.
64. Cheng H, Jusko WJ. Pharmacokinetics of reversible metabolic systems. *Biopharm Drug Dispos* 1993; 14:721–766.
65. Ebling WF, Jusko WF. The determination of essential clearance, volume and residence time parameters of recirculating metabolic systems: The reversible metabolism of methylprednisolone and methylprednisone in rabbits. *J Pharmacokinet Biopharm* 1986; 14:557–599.
66. Wagner JG, DiSanto AR, Gillespie WR, Albert KS. Reversible metabolism and pharmacokinetics: Applications to prednisone-prednisolone. *Res Commun Chem Pathol Pharmacol* 1981; 32: 387–405.
67. Cheng H, Jusko WJ. Constant-rate intraneous infusion methods for estimating steady-state volumes of distribution and mean residence times in the body for drugs undergoing reversible metabolism. *Pharm Res* 1990; 7:628–632.
68. Cheng H. A method for calculating the mean transit times and distribution rate parameters of interconversion metabolites. *Biopharm Drug Dispos* 1993; 14:635–641.
69. Cheng H. Mean residence time of drugs administered non-instantaneously and undergoing linear tissue distribution and reversible metabolism and linear or non-linear elimination from the central compartment. *Biopharm Drug Dispos* 1995; 16:259–267.
70. Ebling WF, Szefler SJ, Jusko WJ. Methylprednisolone disposition in rabbits. Analysis, prodrug conversion, reversible metabolism. *Drug Metab Dispos* 1985; 13:296–301.
71. Wang LH, Rudolph AM, Benet LZ. Pharmacokinetic studies of the disposition of acetaminophen in the sheep maternal-fetal unit. *J Pharmacol Exp Ther* 1986; 238:198–205.
72. Hwang SS, Bayne WF. General method for assessing bioavailability of drugs undergoing reversible metabolism in a linear system. *J Pharm Sci* 1986; 75:820–821.
73. Faed EM. Decreased clearance of diflunisal in renal insufficiency: An alternative explanation. *Br J Clin Pharmacol* 1980; 10:185.
74. Liu JH, Smith PC. Predicting the pharmacokinetics of acyl glucuronides and their parent compounds in disease states. *Curr Drug Metab* 2006; 7:147–163.
75. Cheng H, Jusko WJ. Mean residence time for drugs showing simultaneous first-order and Michaelis-Menton elimination kinetics. *Pharm Res* 1989; 6:258–261.
76. Cheng H, Gillespie WR, Jusko WJ. Mean residence time concepts for nonlinear systems. *Biopharm Drug Dispos* 1995; 15:627–641.

3

The Cytochrome P450 Oxidative System

Paul R. Ortiz de Montellano

CONTENTS

Introduction to the Cytochrome P450 System

The cytochrome P450 (P450) enzymes are critically involved in the biosynthesis of sterols, eicosanoids, and other physiologically important substances. Conversely, they are also essential for the metabolism of endogenous lipophilic substrates, such as fatty acids, as well as most drugs and xenobiotics. Cytochrome P450 catalysis is uniquely suited to the introduction of hydroxyl groups and other polar functionalities into compounds as difficult to oxidize as saturated hydrocarbons. The introduction of such functionality is particularly critical for the metabolism and elimination of lipophilic compounds lacking functional groups suitable for conjugation reactions. On the dark side, the oxidative power of cytochrome P450 enzymes not infrequently transforms innocuous substrates into chemically reactive, toxic metabolites.

The P450 enzymes primarily involved in xenobiotic metabolism are widely distributed, with particularly high concentrations in the endoplasmic reticulum of the liver, kidney, lung, nasal passages, and gut, and significant concentrations in most other tissues.[1] In contrast, the sterol biosynthetic enzymes are concentrated in steroidogenic tissues such as the adrenals and testes. All the mammalian P450 enzymes are membrane bound, and the solubilization, purification, and reconstitution of the pure enzymes is technically challenging. However, all of the relevant enzymes can now be heterologously expressed in *Escherichia coli*, *Saccharomyces cerevisiae*, or in a baculovirus/insect cell system.

Each of these expression systems has advantages and disadvantages, but the bacterial and baculovirus systems are routinely used for the commercial production of mammalian P450 enzymes.

Cytochrome P450 Gene Family

Analysis of the human genome has identified a total of 57 human P450 enzymes, including many that were previously unknown and some of which have not yet been fully characterized (Table 3.1). The sequences of thousands of cytochrome P450 enzymes are now available and the number of additional sequences, particularly those of bacterial, insect, and plant origin, increases monthly (http://drnelson. utmem.edu/CytochromeP450.html). This flood of sequence information has led to a rational nomenclature based on the premise that the extent of sequence and functional identity decreases as a function of evolutionary distance from an ancestral precursor. In consequence, P450 enzymes are grouped in this nomenclature according to probable structural and functional similarity rather than, as in earlier days, on the basis of properties such as electrophoretic mobility, absorption spectrum, or substrate specificity. Although the cutoff lines are somewhat arbitrary, enzymes with more than 40% sequence identity are considered members of the same family and those with more than 55% identity are assigned to the same subfamily.[2,3] Thus, P450 enzymes are identified by a number denoting the family, a letter denoting the subfamily, and a number (and sometimes subsequent letters) identifying the specific member of the subfamily (Table 3.1). The identifying numbers can be associated with the term P450, as in P450 3A4, or more formally with the term CYP, as in CYP3A4. Thus, cytochrome P450 1A2 (CYP1A2) is the second member of subfamily A of family 1, and P450 3A4 is the fourth member of subfamily A of family 3. The trivial names of some substrate-specific enzymes continue to be used (e.g., aromatase for CYP19), but the P450 enzymes primarily involved in drug metabolism are now known by their systematic names.

Differences exist in the concentrations reported of the various drug metabolizing cytochrome P450 enzymes in human liver, but CYP3A4 is one of the most abundant isoforms (Figure 3.1). Other relatively abundant isoforms are CYP1A2, CYP2A6, CYP2C8, CYP2C9, CYP2D6, and CYP2E1.[1,4–6]

TABLE 3.1

The Human Complement of Cytochrome P450 Enzymes Grouped According to the Substrate Class that they Primarily Oxidize

Sterols	Xenobiotics	Fatty Acids	Eicosanoids	Vitamins	Unknown
1B1	1A1	2J2	4F2	2R1	2A7
7A1	1A2	2U1	4F3	24A1	2S1
7B1	2A6	4A11	4F8	26A1	2W1[a]
8B1	2A13	4B1	5A1	26B1	4A22
11A1	2B6	4F11	8A1	26C1	4F22
11B1	2C8	4F12		27B1	4X1
11B2	2C9	4V2		27C1	4Z1
17A1	2C18				20A1
19A1	2C19				
21A2	2D6				
27A1	2E1				
39A1	2F1				
46A1	3A4				
51A1	3A5				
	3A7				
	3A43				

Source: Guengerich, F.P., Human cytochrome P450 enzymes, in Ortiz de Montellano P.R., ed. *Cytochrome P450: Structure, Mechanism, and Biochemistry*, 4th ed., Springer, New York, 523–786, 2015.

[a] CYP2W1 has been shown to readily oxidize retinol and retinoic acid.[7] These compounds may be its natural substrates, but this remains to be clearly established.

(a)

(b)

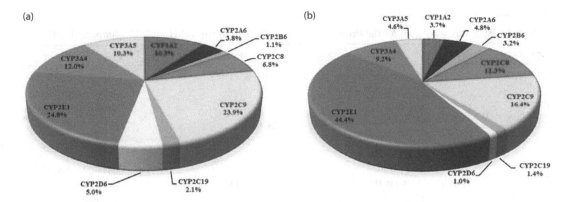

FIGURE 3.1 (a) The median amount of protein content for each P450 is shown as a percentage of the total median P450 protein content. (b) The median P450 mRNA expression level for each P450 is expressed as a percentage of the total median P450 mRNA expression. (From Zhang, H.-F. et al., *J. Pharmacol. Exp. Therap.*, 358, 83–93, 2016.)

The cytochrome P450-dependent metabolism of drugs and xenobiotics in humans is primarily mediated by enzymes of the CYP1, CYP2, and CYP3 families (Figure 3.2). The importance of the individual enzymes in drug metabolism depends on their abundance, their tissue localization, and the extent to which their substrate specificity coincides with the spectrum of drugs and xenobiotics to which the individual is exposed. CYP3A4, CYP2D6, and the CYP2C enzymes are responsible for the bulk of drug and xenobiotic metabolism, but other isoforms can be critical for the metabolism of specific substrates. In practice, CYP3A4/3A5 are thought to account for something between 20% and 30% of all P450-dependent drug metabolism, CYP2C9 and CYP2D6 for approximately 10% each, and the remaining enzymes, notably CYP2E1, CYP2C19, CYP2C8, CYP2B6, CYP2A6, CYP1B1, CYP1A2, and CYP1A1 for smaller percentages of the remaining total.[5,6] Furthermore, the relative importance of the different enzymes depends on the genetics of the individual and on the history of exposure to environmental factors, such as alcohol or drugs. Certain P450 enzymes, notably CYP2C19 and CYP2D6, are polymorphically distributed in the human population.[1,8] Thus, CYP2D6 levels are low in approximately 7% of the Caucasian population, and the ability of this subgroup to metabolize substrates such as debrisoquine is partially compromised.[9] CYP2C19 is in low titer in only 4% of the Caucasian population, but is low in 20% of the Asian population, as reflected by the relatively low ability of the latter subgroup to metabolize

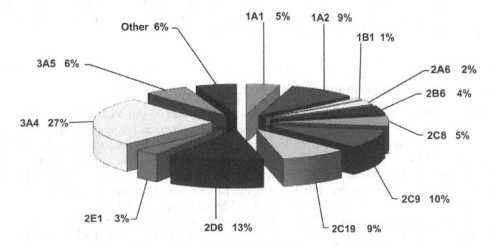

FIGURE 3.2 Extent to which individual human P450 enzymes contribute to the metabolism of drugs. A modestly different isoform distribution is observed for the metabolism of xenobiotics in general. (From Rendic, S. and Guengerich, F.P., *Chem. Res. Toxicol.*, 28, 38–42, 2015.)

TABLE 3.2

Selected List of the Substrates for the Primary Drug Metabolizing forms of Human Cytochrome P450

Enzyme	Substrates	Enzyme	Substrates
CYP1A1	Benzo[a]pyrene	CYP2E1	Caffeine
	Acetylaminofluorene		Chlorzoxazone
CYP1A2	Caffeine		N-nitrosodimethylamine
	Ethoxyresorufin		Acetaminophen
	2-acetylaminofluorene		Aflatoxin
	Acetaminophen		Aniline
	Phenacetin	CYP2F1	Naphthylamine
	Aflatoxin B1	CYP3A4	Aldrin
CYP2A6	Coumarin		Quinidine
	N-nitrosodiethylamine		Cyclosporin A
CYP2B6	7-ethoxycoumarin		Warfarin
CYP2C9	Benzphetamine		Erythromycin
	Aminopyrene		17β-estradiol
	Tienilic acid		Lidocaine
	Hexobarbital		Dapsone
	Tolbutamide		Sterigmatocystin
CYP2C19	Mephenytoin		Cortisol
CYP2D6	Bufuralol		Taxol
	Debrisoquine		Nifedipine
	Desipramine		Alfentanil
	Sparteine		Diltiazem
	Propranolol		Ethynylestradiol
	Dextromethorphan	CYP4A11	Arachidonic acid

Source: Guengerich, F.P., Human cytochrome P450 enzymes, in Ortiz de Montellano P.R., ed. *Cytochrome P450: Structure, Mechanism, and Biochemistry*, 4th ed., Springer, New York, 523–786, 2015.

substrates such as mephenytoin.[9,10] A number of criteria are required to unambiguously determine the role of a given P450 enzyme in the *in vivo* metabolism of a given agent. These include (a) demonstration that the purified enzyme has the required activity, (b) correlation of the activity in question in liver samples with the activities of the same samples toward substrates considered to be markers for the individual P450 enzymes, and (c) inhibition of the activity by isoform-selective or specific inhibitors, antibodies or, *in vivo*, by *si*RNA or gene silencing techniques (Table 3.2).

Structure of the Mammalian P450 Enzymes

The initial work on cytochrome P450 enzyme structure was carried out with the bacterial enzymes because they are generally soluble and relatively amenable to crystallization. Among the scores of bacterial P450 structures now available, are those of P450$_{cam}$ (CYP101),[11] P450BM-3 (CYP102),[12] P450$_{eryF}$ (CYP107A1),[13] and CYP119,[14] the structures on which much of our current understanding of P450 structure and mechanism is based. In contrast, the structures of the membrane-bound human P450 enzymes have only become available over the past decade. The first mammalian P450 structure, reported in 2000, was that of rabbit CYP2C5.[15] Since then, many human P450 structures have been determined in the presence and absence of ligands, including those of CYP1A1,[16] CYP1A2,[17] CYP1B1,[18] CYP2A6,[19,20] CYP2A13,[21,22] CYP2B4,[23] CYP2B6,[24] CYP2C8,[25,26] CYP2C9,[27,28] CYP2C19,[29] CYP2D6,[30,31] CYP2E1,[32] CYP2R1,[33] and CYP3A4.[34–36] The structures of several biosynthetic human P450 enzymes, including those of CYP7A1,[37] CYP11A1,[38] CYP17A1,[39] CYP21A2,[40] CYP24A1,[41] CYP46A1,[42] and CYP51[43] have also been determined. The human P450 structures generally confirm the mechanistic conclusions derived from the bacterial P450 enzymes but are naturally of much greater utility in helping to understand the substrate specificity and catalytic regiospecificity of the human P450 enzymes.

The cytochrome P450 enzymes are roughly triangular prisms in which 12 helical segments account for a large proportion of the amino acid residues.[15-43] The heme prosthetic group is generally anchored by at least three interactions: (a) the pincer action of two protein helices on the heme, (b) hydrogen bonds to the heme propionic acid groups, and (c) coordination of a cysteine thiolate ligand to the iron. A cysteine thiolate (Cys-S$^-$), rather than a protonated thiol (Cys-SH), is the proximal iron ligand in all active P450 enzymes. The active site cavity is generally lined with hydrophobic residues, as might be expected of an enzyme designed for the metabolism of lipophilic substrates. A few residues on the distal (substrate-binding) side of the heme are highly, but not universally, conserved throughout the P450 family. The most important of these is a catalytic threonine, Thr252 in P450$_{cam}$, which helps to stabilize the ferrous dioxy (Fe^{II}-OO$^-$) complex and to promote heterolysis of the dioxygen bond in the subsequent ferric peroxide (Fe^{III}-OOH) intermediate. The threonine is conserved in all the human P450 enzymes, but it is not absolutely essential because it is absent, for example, in the bacterial P450$_{eryF}$.[13] Nevertheless, it is important because its replacement by non-hydrogen bonding residues alters catalysis. Thus, mutation of Thr252 in P450$_{cam}$ greatly increases the degree of uncoupled turnover,[44,45] and mutation of the corresponding residue (Thr319) to an alanine in CYP1A2 suppresses the ability of the enzyme to oxidize benzphetamine but not 7-ethoxycoumarin.[46] In P450$_{eryF}$, the hydrogen-bonding role of the threonine is satisfied by a hydroxyl group on the substrate itself.[13]

Before mammalian P450 crystal structures were available, six domains of the primary sequences of P450 enzymes, known as Sequence Recognition Sequences (SRS), were proposed to be particularly important in determining substrate specificity.[47] These SRS were based on sequence alignments of the mammalian proteins with the sequences in the P450$_{cam}$ structure that interact with the substrate. The broad range of mammalian P450 crystal structures now available makes it possible to more precisely address the substrate specificity, hydroxylation regiochemistry and allosteric effects of cytochrome P450 enzymes. Extensive efforts to employ computational docking of potential ligands into P450 active sites to predict which compounds will be substrates for individual enzymes[48-53] have been undertaken in the hope of developing an *in silico* screen for potential drug-drug interactions. Such a screen would be highly useful if it could be applied at an early stage in the drug discovery process. Initially, these computational efforts were carried out with sequence-based homology models constructed by aligning the sequences of the human enzymes with those of crystallized bacterial P450 enzymes. However, these models are not sufficiently accurate for the analysis of substrate specificity. Furthermore, crystallographic, NMR, and other studies indicate that P450 enzymes undergo both minor and major conformational adjustments to accommodate the binding of specific ligands. For example, the crystal structure of CYP2C9 with warfarin bound in the active site places the substrate more than 10 Å away from the heme iron atom, whereas the structure of this enzyme with flurbiprofen positions the substrate close to the iron atom.[27,28] Substantial active site conformational differences are observed in the two crystal structures. A comparable conformational mobility has been found in the bacterial enzymes. For example, the binding of imidazole and 4-phenylimidazole to CYP119 causes a major internal rearrangement of an active site peptide.[14] NMR and crystallographic data show that addition of a 4-*para*-chloro substituent to the phenyl of 4-phenyimidazole engenders a third conformation.[54] The widespread observation of substrate-dependent active site conformational adjustments greatly complicates efforts to predict substrate specificity by computational docking.

As found originally for P450$_{cam}$,[11] the heme group and the substrate in P450 enzymes are buried deep within the protein. In the case of P450$_{cam}$, the camphor substrate is positioned ~4 Å above the heme iron atom by a hydrogen bond between the camphor ketone oxygen and a tyrosine residue (Tyr-96), as well as by contacts with a variety of other active site residues. A weakening of the interactions that position the substrate, either by mutation of the active site residues or alteration of the substrate itself, decreases the regiospecificity of the hydroxylation reaction and increases the extent to which catalytic turnover is coupled to camphor metabolite formation.[44,45] The binding of a substrate requires transient opening of a channel into the P450 active site. Indeed, DEER and crystallographic evidence indicates that the P450$_{cam}$ channel is open when the protein is in solution, but closes upon substrate binding.[55,56] NMR and crystallographic data suggest that CYP119 also has an open conformation in solution that closes upon the binding of some, but not all, ligands.[54] A crystal structure of the structure of unligated CYP2B4 reveals an open state of the entrance channel.[23] On complexation with 4-(4-chlorophenyl)imidazole, the protein closes by movement of a protein domain with intact secondary structure (i.e., essentially like a lid) to give a structure similar to that of the closed state of other P450 enzymes.[57] The structures of other complexes of this protein reveal a range of conformational states.[58–60] Analogous conformational changes have been observed in the crystal structures of several of the human P450 enzymes, including CYP2C8,[26] CYP2E1,[22] and CYP3A4.[61] Biophysical techniques, such as pressure perturbation EPR and FRET,[62,63] confirm the existence of multiple CYP3A4 conformational states in solution.

Spectroscopic Properties of Cytochrome P450 Enzymes

The cytochrome P450 chromophore provides information on the nature of the iron ligands, the iron oxidation state, and the nature of the heme environment.[64,65] The defining P450 spectrum is that of the ferrous-CO complex, which has an absorption maximum at 447–452 nm indicative of a thiolate-ligated hemoprotein. The thiolate ligand actually gives rise to a split Soret absorption with maxima at approximately 450 and 370 nm. Denaturation of the enzyme is associated with a shift of the absorption maximum of the ferrous-CO complex to ~420 nm, a value similar to that for the ferrous-CO complex of imidazole-ligated proteins such as myoglobin.[65] The enzyme with the 420 nm ferrous-CO absorbance maximum is inactive and formation of this 420 nm species is one of the earliest indicators of P450 denaturation.

The absorption spectrum of ferric cytochrome P450 depends on the ligation state of the iron.[64,65] The ferric low-spin state associated with the presence of two strong axial iron ligands has an absorption maximum at approximately 416–419 nm. The high-spin state in which one of the two coordination sites of the iron is either unoccupied or occupied by a weak ligand exhibits an absorption maximum at 390–416 nm. Cytochrome P450 enzymes commonly exist as an equilibrium mixture of the high- and low-spin states. In the P450 enzymes for which crystal structures are available, including the membrane-bound human enzymes, the ligand opposite to the cysteine thiolate, if one is present, is a water molecule.[11–43] The binding of a non-coordinating substrate, as illustrated by the binding of camphor to cytochrome P450$_{cam}$, is accompanied by extrusion of water from the active site, loss of the distal water ligand, and a general decrease in the active site polarity.[11] The loss of the distal ligand causes a shift from the hexacoordinated to a pentacoordinated iron state, which in turn results in a shift from the low- to the high-spin state. This transition is evidenced by a shift in the absorption maximum from 419 to 390 nm. The spectroscopic shift is usually determined from a difference spectrum in which the absorption of a solution containing everything except the compound of interest is subtracted from a similar sample that does contain the compound.[64] The binding of non-coordinating substrates to the ferric enzyme gives rise to what is known as a Type I difference spectrum with a maximum at 385–390 nm and a trough at approximately 420 nm. However, if the substrate can coordinate strongly to the iron atom, a Type II difference spectrum is observed with a maximum at approximately 425–435 nm and a trough at 390–405 nm. If the substrate only coordinates weakly to the iron, a variant of the Type II spectrum with a maximum at 420 nm and a trough at 388–390 nm is obtained. This latter spectrum is known as a Type III difference spectrum. Thus, substrate and inhibitor binding to P450 enzymes can be monitored spectroscopically. Some caution is required, however, because a Type II spectrum can be obtained with water as the distal iron ligand if it becomes a stronger ligand due to hydrogen bonding interactions with the substrate.[66] Furthermore, compounds are known that bind without significantly perturbing the spin state equilibrium and, therefore, do not give rise to a difference spectrum. An example of this is the binding of 2-isopropyl-4-pentenamide to microsomes from phenobarbital pretreated rats,[67] or the binding of non-coordinating ligands to CYP1A2, which unusually does not have a water coordinated to the heme iron in the ligand-free state.[17]

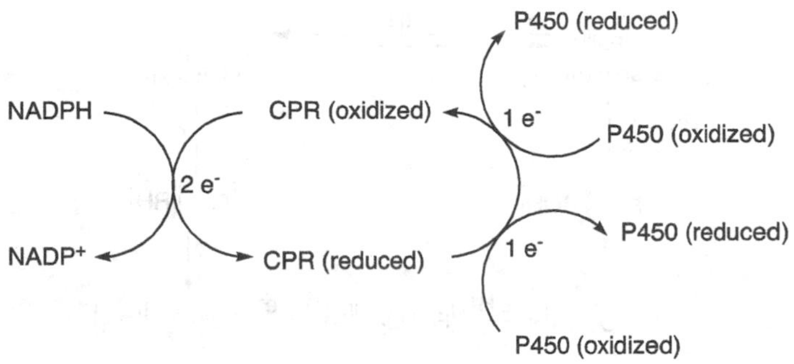

FIGURE 3.3 Cytochrome P450 reductase (CPR) transfers electrons from NADPH to cytochrome P450 enzymes in the mammalian endoplastic reticulum.

Cytochrome P450 Reductase and Cytochrome b_5

The catalytic turnover of most bacterial P450 enzymes and some human enzymes is supported by electrons provided by the coordinated action of a flavoprotein and an iron-sulfur protein. However, the electrons required for catalytic turnover of all the human xenobiotic-metabolizing cytochrome P450 enzymes are provided by NADPH-cytochrome P450 reductase (Figure 3.3).[68] This reductase is a 78 kDa protein that is anchored to the membrane by an N-terminal hydrophobic domain. Cytochrome P450 reductase binds one FMN and one FAD as prosthetic groups and is reduced by NADPH. NADPH transfers a hydride to the FAD group, which in turn uncouples the two associated electrons and transfers them to the heme via the FMN group. The reductase can be reduced by up to four electrons but under normal turnover conditions it cycles between the one- and three-electron reduced forms, both of which can transfer electrons to cytochrome P450. Limited tryptic digestion of liver microsomes releases a 72 kDa cytosolic reductase domain that binds NADPH and reduces cytochrome c but is no longer able to reduce cytochrome P450. The structure of the heterologously expressed cytochrome P450 reductase without the membrane-binding domain has been determined.[69,70]

In some instances, the catalytic turnover of mammalian cytochrome P450 enzymes can be synergistically increased or modified by cytochrome b_5.[71,72] Cytochrome b_5, which can be reduced by either NADH and cytochrome b_5 reductase or NADPH-cytochrome P450 reductase, with few exceptions is able to deliver the second but not the first electron required for catalytic turnover of cytochrome P450. The synergistic effect of cytochrome b_5 is due, at least in part, to an increase in the coupling of reduced pyridine nucleotide and oxygen utilization to product formation (i.e., to a decrease in uncoupled reduction of oxygen to give H_2O_2 or water rather than substrate oxidation). However, in some situations, cytochrome b_5 alters P450 catalysis by allosteric mechanisms independent of its ability to donate electrons. One example of this is the demonstration that apo cytochrome b_5 can stimulate the nifedipine oxidation and testosterone 6β-hydroxylation activities of CYP3A4.[71,73] Cytochrome b_5 also modulates the activities of steroid biosynthetic forms of cytochrome P450.[74]

Catalytic Cycle of Cytochrome P450

The catalytic cycle of cytochrome P450 has been most thoroughly defined for the bacterial cytochrome P450$_{cam}$,[75] but extensive work with the mammalian enzymes confirms that the same catalytic cycle, occasionally with minor variations, is in force (Figure 3.4). In P450$_{cam}$, the spin state change triggered by the binding of a non-coordinating substrate alters the redox potential of the heme and makes it possible for the electron-donor partner to transfer an electron to the iron. The redox potential shift from −300 to −170 mV on binding of camphor to P450$_{cam}$ enables its reduction by the iron-sulfur protein putidaredoxin ($E_{1/2}$ = −196 mV).[76] Catalytic turnover of the protein is thus initiated by substrate binding, a strategy that

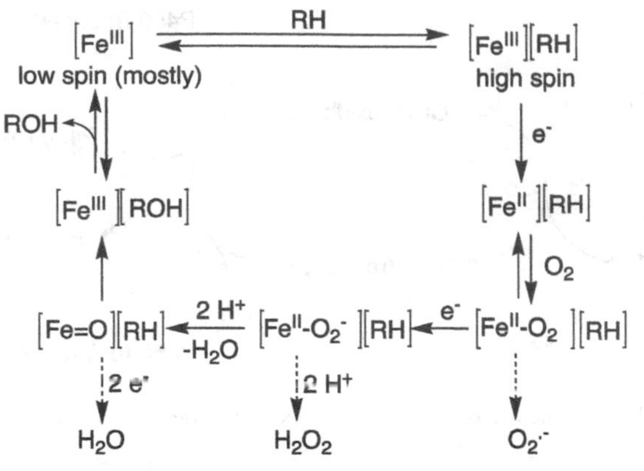

$$[Fe^{III}] \xrightleftharpoons{\text{RH}} [Fe^{III}][RH]$$

low spin (mostly)   high spin

ROH e^-

$$[Fe^{III}][ROH] \qquad [Fe^{II}][RH]$$

O_2

$$[Fe=O][RH] \xleftarrow[-H_2O]{2\,H^+} [Fe^{II}\text{-}O_2^-][RH] \xleftarrow{e^-} [Fe^{II}\text{-}O_2][RH]$$

$2\,e^-$ $2\,H^+$

$$H_2O \qquad H_2O_2 \qquad O_2^{\cdot-}$$

FIGURE 3.4 The cytochrome P450 catalytic cycle. The iron in brackets represent a cytochrome P450 prosthetic heme group and RH a substrate with an oxidizable C-H bond. The first electron is provided by CPR and the second by CPR or cytochrome b_5. The sites at which the catalytic cycle can be uncoupled to produce $O_2\cdot$-, H_2O_2, or H_2O rather than oxidized substrate (ROH) are indicated.

helps to minimize uncoupled turnover of the protein. Although studies of the mammalian enzymes in detergent and artificial lipid mixtures suggested that a similar spin-state-redox potential correlation did not hold with those proteins,[77] a study using a nanodisc environment that more closely resembles that in normal membranes has demonstrated that a similar correlation exists for at least CYP3A4.[78]

Reduction of the iron is followed by binding of oxygen to give the ferrous dioxy P450 complex, an intermediate that is unstable but has been observed under a variety of conditions. A further one-electron reduction of the ferrous dioxy complex produces the highly unstable ferric hydroperoxide (Fe^{III}-OOH) complex that has only been observed in cryogenic studies.[79] The formation of this intermediate is consistent with the finding that one of the products of uncoupled turnover of P450 is H_2O_2. It is also consistent with the fact that catalytic turnover of many P450 enzymes can be supported to some extent by exogenous H_2O_2 in the absence of cytochrome P450 reductase and NADPH. Heterolytic cleavage of the dioxygen bond in the ferric hydroperoxide complex concomitant with the uptake of two protons and the loss of a molecule of water produces the ferryl intermediate that is thought to be directly responsible for the oxidation most substrates.[75,80] The ferryl intermediate is two oxidation states above the ferric heme and is formally $Fe^V = O$, but it is more appropriately represented by an $Fe^{IV} = O$ coupled to a porphyrin radical cation. The ferryl species is the most transient of the catalytic intermediates, but it has been detected and characterized in the reactions of P450 enzymes with peroxides.[79–82] In most, but not all, instances the ferryl oxygen is transferred to the substrate to give an oxygenated metabolite. If the substrate is resistant to oxidation, the ferryl species can be reduced to a water molecule by further electrons from cytochrome P450 reductase or cytochrome b_5. To the extent that superoxide, H_2O_2, and water are produced at the expense of substrate oxidation during the catalytic turnover of cytochrome P450 the reaction is said to be uncoupled.

The possibility that substrate oxidation is mediated by intermediates in the oxygen activation cycle prior to the ferryl species has been explored. It is generally accepted that the ferric peroxy anion (Fe^{III}-OO$^-$) can add as a nucleophile to some carbonyl groups (and perhaps other highly electrophilic groups), resulting after homolytic cleavage of the dioxygen bond in carbon-carbon bond cleavage at the carbonyl carbon atom.[80] This reaction is thought to underlie the action of the biosynthetic P450 enzymes that catalyze lanosterol 14α-demethylation (CYP51) and removal of the progesterone side-chain to produce androstenedione (CYP17).[83] A similar mechanism has been widely accepted for the 19-demethylation and aromatization of testosterone that yields estradiol (CYP19), but recent work suggests that this reaction may be mediated by the normal ferryl intermediate.[84] More controversial is the proposal that the ferric hydroperoxide intermediate (Fe^{III}-OOH) can itself insert into CH bonds.[85] The evidence for this type of reactivity in normal P450 turnover is not compelling. If the ferric hydroperoxide plays any direct role in substrate oxidation, it is likely to be limited to the oxidation of electron-rich sulfur or nitrogen functionalities.

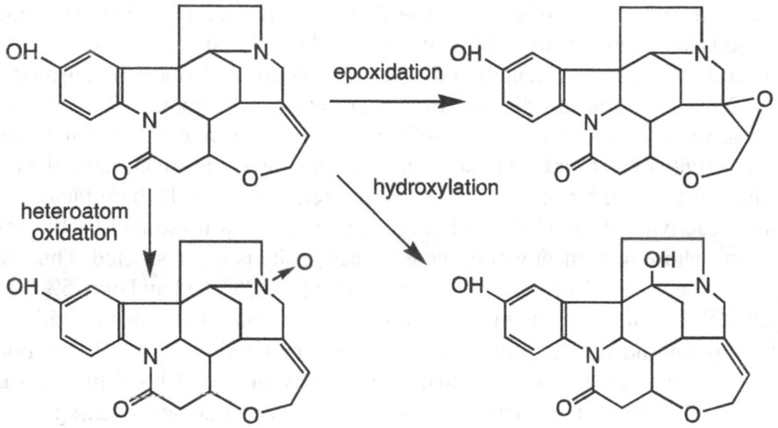

FIGURE 3.5 Hydroxylation, π-bond oxidation, and heteroatom oxidation, the three fundamental cytochrome P450-catalyzed reactions, are illustrated in the metabolism of strychnine. (From Oguri, K. et al., *Xenobiotica*, 19, 171–178, 1989.)

Cytochrome P450-Catalyzed Reactions

Cytochrome P450-catalyzed reactions produce a diversity of metabolites, many of which are formed by secondary, non-enzymatic decomposition of the initial products formed by the P450 reaction. Although the large list of reactions catalyzed by cytochrome P450 continues to expand, most of the reactions involve (a) insertion of an oxygen atom into the bond between a hydrogen and a carbon or other heavy atom (hydroxylation), (b) addition of an oxygen atom to a π-bond (epoxidation), or (c) addition of an oxygen atom to the electron pair on a heteroatom (heteroatom oxidation).[80] All three of these reactions are illustrated in the metabolism of strychnine (Figure 3.5).[86] Cytochrome P450 enzymes also catalyze reductive reactions under conditions of low oxygen tension. The oxidative catalytic process can be viewed as consisting of two stages: activation of molecular oxygen to the reactive (ferryl) oxidizing species followed by its reaction with the substrate. The cytochrome P450 catalytic machinery is primarily required for the first phase of this two-stage process. In contrast, the enzyme appears to contribute little to the reaction of the activated oxygen with the substrate beyond providing an appropriate environment for the reaction and, by only binding the substrate in certain orientations, limiting the sites on the substrate exposed to the activated oxygen. Therefore, the outcome of the catalytic process is largely determined by the position of the substrate within the active site, its mobility, and the relative reactivities of the functionalities on the substrate accessible to the activated oxygen in the enzyme-substrate complex.

Hydroxylation

Carbon Hydroxylation

The regio- and stereoselective hydroxylation of unactivated hydrocarbon functionalities is one of the most common but most difficult reactions catalyzed by cytochrome P450 enzymes. Isotope effects provide direct evidence that the reaction outcome depends on the reactivity of the accessible C-H bonds. Thus, hydroxylation of the undeuterated carbon is strongly favored in the oxidation of $[1,1\text{-}^2H_2]\text{-}1,3\text{-}$diphenylpropane (i.e., $C_6H_5CH_2CD_2C_6H_5$), a symmetric molecule in which the hydrogens are replaced by deuteriums on one of the two otherwise identical methylene groups. A large isotope effect ($k_H/k_D = 11$) is observed in the intramolecular preference for hydroxylation of the undeuterated methylene even though only a small kinetic isotope effect is observed on the overall rate of hydroxylated product formation.[87] The large intramolecular isotope effect indicates that the enzyme is sensitive to the different energies required to break C-H and C-D bonds, and is able to select between the two competing sites. Often only a relatively small kinetic isotope effect is observed on the rate of substrate consumption because the overall rate is determined by steps other than insertion of the oxygen into the C-H bond. However, the product distribution can be greatly altered by this "metabolic switching" process.[88,89]

The relationship between bond strength and susceptibility to oxidation is confirmed by the finding that the ease of P450-catalyzed insertion of an oxygen into hydrocarbon C-H bonds decreases in the order tertiary > secondary > primary,[90,91] a preference confirmed by computational studies.[49,92,93] The intrinsic higher reactivity of weaker C-H bonds can be masked by steric effects or by the protein-imposed orientation of the substrate with respect to the activated ferryl species. If these factors are minimized, then the intrinsic reactivity of the C-H bonds becomes evident, as illustrated by the hydroxylation of small hydrocarbons whose movement within the P450 active site is less restricted. Thus, the microsomal oxidation of *tert*-butane [CH(CH$_3$)$_3$] yields 95% *tert*-butanol [HOC(CH$_3$)$_3$] and only 5% 2-methylpropanol [CH$_3$CH(CH$_3$)CH$_2$OH].[90] The sterically-hindered, but weaker, tertiary C-H bond is oxidized in preference to the nine relatively unhindered but primary C-H bonds. The bond strengths of C-H bonds (Table 3.3) provide a good first approximation of the intrinsic reactivity of a C-H bond in a substrate molecule. Current efforts to predict substrate oxidation involve not only computational docking to crystallographic active sites, but also integration of this information with predictions of the relative reactivity of the various reaction sites on the substrate molecule.[91,94]

The relationship of bond-strength to enzymatic hydroxylation indicates that reactivity is related to the homolytic C-H bond scission energy, an inference consistent with a nonconcerted "oxygen-rebound" mechanism in which hydrogen abstraction by the activated oxygen is followed by recombination of the resulting radical species to give the hydroxylated product[80]:

$$[Fe^V = O] + R_3C\text{-}H \rightarrow [Fe^{IV}\text{-}OH] + R_3C\cdot \rightarrow [Fe^{III}] + R_3C\text{-}OH$$

As already noted, the $Fe^V = O$ in the above reaction sequence is likely to be an $Fe^{IV} = O$ coupled to a porphyrin radical cation. If a substrate radical is formed as a transient species, it should be possible to detect it in substrates in which the radical can undergo a sufficiently rapid rearrangement prior to recombination to give the hydroxylated product. Indeed, the hydroxylation of *exo*-tetradeuterated norbornane yields, among other products, the *endo*-deuterated alcohol metabolite.[95] This inversion of the deuterium stereochemistry requires the formation of either a radical or cationic intermediate in which the geometry of the tetrahedral carbon can be inverted. Numerous other examples are known of reactions that proceed with loss of stereo- or regiochemistry, including the allylic rearrangement that accompanies the CYP3A4-catalyzed hydroxylation of exemestane (Figure 3.6).[96]

Radical clock substrates have also been used to demonstrate the intervention of a substrate radical in hydrocarbon hydroxylation. A radical clock is a structure, commonly a cyclopropyl methylene group, which undergoes a radical rearrangement at a known rate. Despite some controversy,[97,98] the results confirm the radical nature of the reaction. Thus, β-thujone, a two-zone clock because the radical can be revealed by both a methyl group inversion and opening of the cyclopropyl ring (Figure 3.7), gives metabolites consistent with a radical intermediate.[99] Computation suggests that discrepancies in the results with radical clock substrates may be related to the existence of the ferryl species in multiple spin states.[93]

The cytochrome P450-catalyzed hydroxylation of hydrocarbon chains preferentially occurs at the carbon adjacent to the terminal (ω) carbon, i.e., at the ω-1 carbon, but hydroxylation can also occur

TABLE 3.3

Bond Strengths of Selected C-H Bonds

Bond	kcal/mol	Bond	kcal/mol
CH$_3$-H	104	HC≡CCH$_2$-H	88
Me$_2$CH-H	95	HOCH$_2$-H	94
Me$_3$C-H	92	H$_2$NCH$_2$-H	89
CH$_2$=CH$_2$CH$_2$-H	89	CH$_2$=CH-H	108
C$_6$H$_5$CH$_2$-H	85		

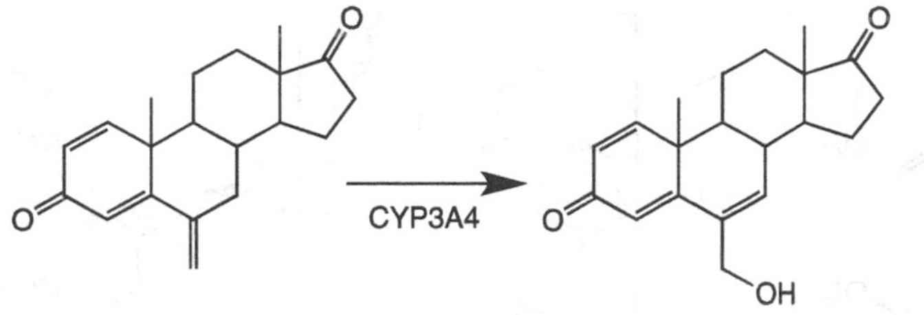

FIGURE 3.6 Rearrangement of the double bond accompanying the CYP3A4-catalyzed oxidation of exemestane. (From Kamdem, L.K. et al., *Drug Metab. Disp.*, 39, 98–105, 2011.)

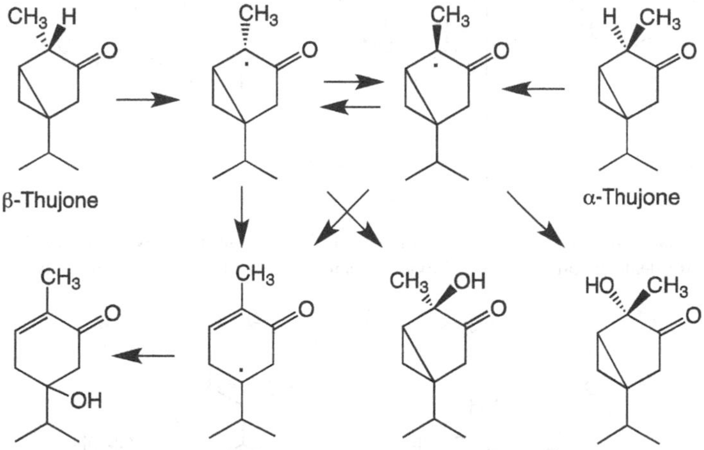

FIGURE 3.7 P450 oxidation of the radical clock substrates α- and β-thujone produces a C4 radical in which the methyl-substituted ring carbon can undergo both stereochemical inversion and cyclopropyl ring opening, two independent indicators of a radical intermediate. (From Jiang, Y. et al., *Biochemistry*, 45, 533–542, 2006.)

at the terminal carbon or at more internal sites in the hydrocarbon chain. ω-Hydroxylation is disfavored with respect to ω-1 hydroxylation by the higher strength of a primary than a secondary C-H bond (Table 3.3). Except for the CYP4 family of enzymes, which have evolved as specific fatty acid ω-hydroxylases, P450 enzymes preferentially catalyze the ω-1 hydroxylation of hydrocarbon chains. Of course, this reaction must compete with other favored reactions, such as allylic or benzylic hydroxylation. The hydroxylation of C-H bonds that are stronger than those of a terminal methyl group is essentially not observed. Thus, the direct oxidation of vinylic, acetylenic, or aromatic C-H bonds is negligible, although the π-bonds themselves are readily oxidized (see next section).

Carbon Hydroxylation Followed by Heteroatom Elimination

Hydroxylation adjacent to a heteroatom or a π-bond is highly favored by the weaker bond strength of C-H bonds adjacent to conjugating functionalities. In the case of sulfur, and particularly nitrogen, the availability of alternative mechanisms that lead to the same reaction outcome also enhances the reactivity at those positions. Allylic or benzylic hydroxylation normally produces a stable alcohol product, but hydroxylation adjacent to a heteroatom yields a product that readily eliminates the heteroatom to give two fragments, one containing a carbonyl group and the other retaining the heteroatom (Figure 3.8). Thus, oxidation adjacent to an oxygen normally results in O-dealkylation, adjacent to a nitrogen in N-dealkylation, adjacent to a sulfur in S-dealkylation, and adjacent to a halogen in oxidative dehalogenation (Figure 3.9).

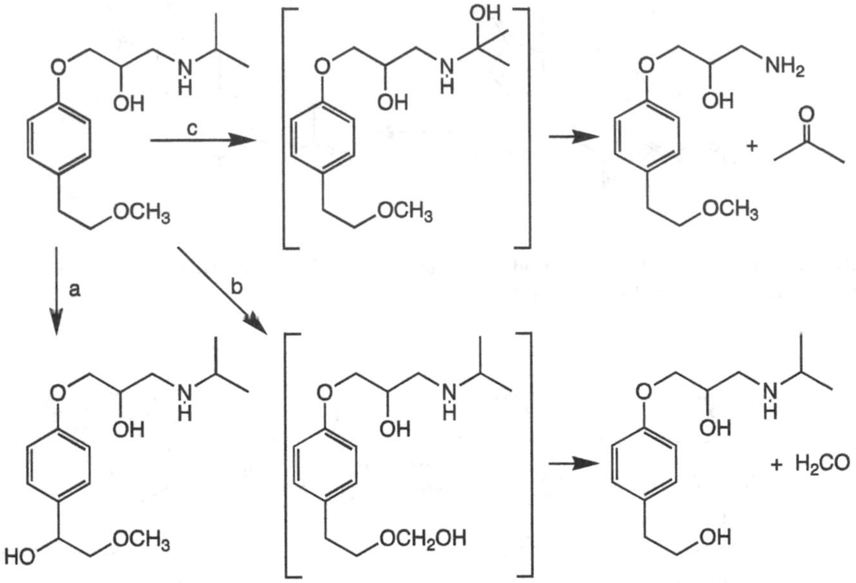

FIGURE 3.8   The oxidation of metoprolol illustrates (a) benzylic hydroxylation, (b) hydroxylation adjacent to an oxygen followed by elimination (O-dealkylation), and (c) hydroxylation adjacent to a nitrogen followed by elimination (N-dealkylation).

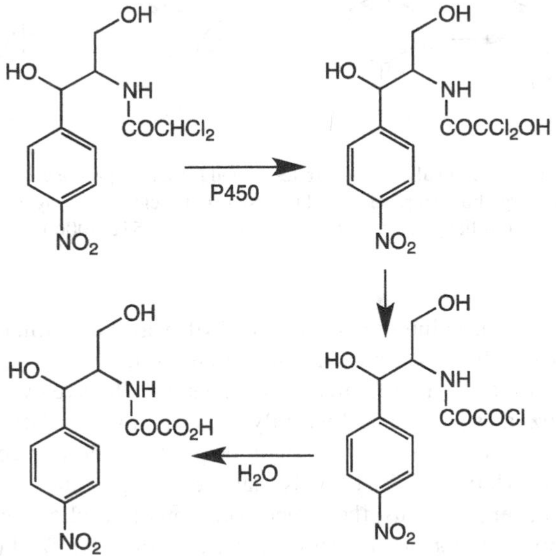

FIGURE 3.9   Hydroxylation adjacent to a halogen followed by elimination (oxidative dehalogenation), as illustrated by the oxidation of chloramphenicol. The acyl chloride produced from the dihalogenated carbon by the P450 reaction can react with water, as shown, or with other cellular nucleophiles.

Heteroatom Hydroxylation

The mechanism of cytochrome P450-catalyzed nitrogen hydroxylation is ambiguous because the reaction can proceed via insertion of an oxygen into the N-H bond or oxidation of the nitrogen to a nitroxide, followed by proton tautomerization to give the hydroxylamine. A similar ambiguity exists in the hydroxylation of sulfhydryl groups. N-hydroxylation via insertion into the N-H bond, as illustrated by the hydroxylation of p-chloroacetanilide, is favored in situations where the nitrogen electron pair is highly delocalized and, therefore, reacts poorly as an electron donor (Figure 3.10).[100]

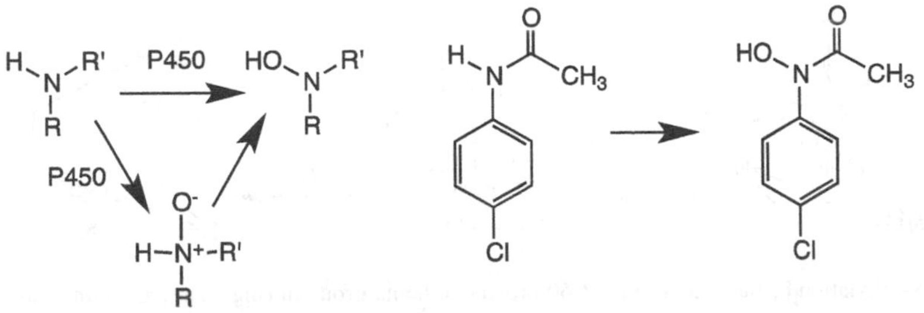

FIGURE 3.10 The "hydroxylation" of a nitrogen bearing a hydrogen atom can involve direct insertion into the N-H bond or transfer of the oxygen to the nitrogen followed by proton tautomerization. Insertion into the N-H bond is favored in amides. The hydroxylation of *p*-chloroacetanilide is shown as an example.

π-Bond Oxidation

Oxidation of Aliphatic π-Bonds

Cytochrome P450 enzymes normally oxidize double bonds to the corresponding epoxides (Figure 3.11). Retention of the olefin stereochemistry, as illustrated by the oxidation of *cis*-1-deuterated styrene (i.e., *cis* $C_6H_5CH=CHD$) to the epoxide without loss of stereochemistry,[101] suggests that the two carbon-oxygen bonds of the epoxide are formed without a discrete intermediate that allows rotation about the carbon-carbon bond. This strongly implies that both bonds are formed simultaneously, if not necessarily at the same rate. In general, the epoxidation of electron-rich double bonds is favored over that of electron-deficient double bonds because the ferryl P450 species is electron deficient. Although epoxides are usually the sole or dominant product of double bond oxidation, carbonyl products formed by migration of a hydrogen or halide from the carbon to which the oxygen is added to the adjacent carbon of the double bond are occasionally obtained. Two examples of this are the formation of trichloroacetaldehyde (CCl_3CHO) from 1,1,2-trichloroethylene ($CHCl=CCl_2$)[103] and the CYP7A1-catalyzed conversion of 7-dehydrocholesterol to 7-ketocholesterol (Figure 3.12).[104] The 1,2-migration of a hydrogen or halide indicates that a positive charge develops at the carbon towards which the

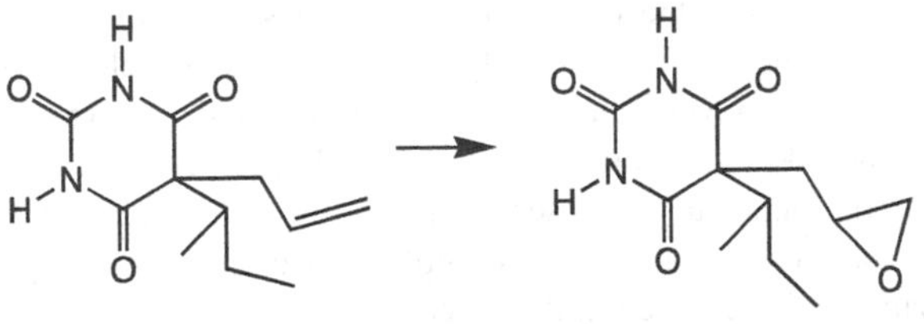

FIGURE 3.11 The cytochrome P450-catalyzed epoxidation of secobarbital. (From Harvey, D.J. et al., *Drug Metab. Dispos.*, 5, 527–546, 1977.)

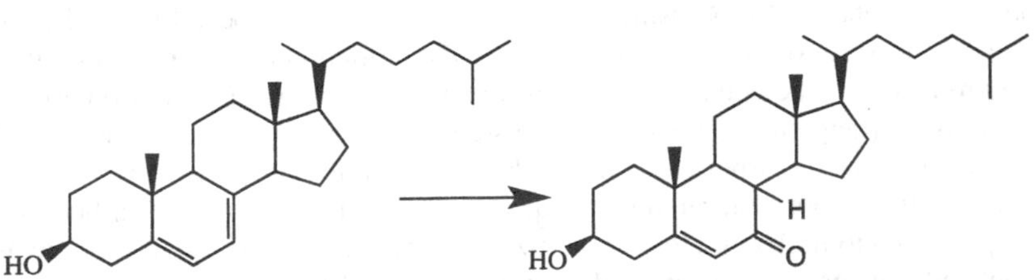

FIGURE 3.12 Oxidation of 7-dehydrocholesterol to 7-ketocholesterol by CYP7A1 does not involve formation of an epoxide intermediate.

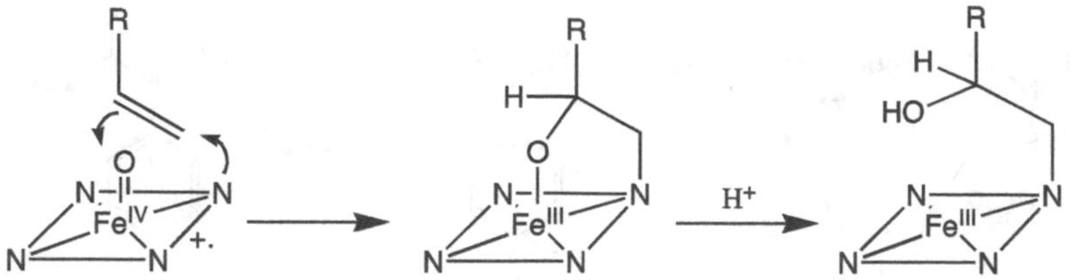

FIGURE 3.13 N-alkylation of the cytochrome P450 prosthetic heme group during terminal olefin oxidation. The P450 heme is represented by the square of nitrogen atoms surrounding an iron atom. The heme is shown in the proposed hypervalent activated state.

migration occurs. Thus, carbonyl products result from π-bond oxidations in which the two carbon-oxygen bonds are not simultaneously formed. Although this is a negligible reaction pathway for most olefinic substrates, it is an important reaction when the π-bond is part of an aromatic ring (see next section). Formation of epoxides by concerted oxygen insertion but carbonyl products by non-concerted oxygen transfer implies either that there are two independent reaction pathways or a single reaction manifold with a branchpoint leading to concerted (epoxide) versus non-concerted (carbonyl) products. Computational studies support the existence of a single pathway with a branchpoint determined by the spin state of the reactive species.[93]

The oxidation of terminal, unconjugated olefins results not only in olefin epoxidation but also frequently in inactivation of the cytochrome P450 enzyme.[105,106] In some instances, inactivation results from reaction of the epoxide metabolite with the protein, but in others inactivation involves alkylation of a nitrogen of the prosthetic heme group by a catalytically-activated form of the olefin (Figure 3.13). Characterization of the heme adducts shows that alkylation is initiated by oxygen transfer from the enzyme to the double bond but is not due to reaction with the actual epoxide metabolite. Thus, heme alkylation involves an asymmetric, non-concerted olefin oxidation pathway that may be part of the same manifold of reactions that produces the epoxide and carbonyl metabolites. In these heme alkylation reactions, the oxygen is added to the internal carbon of the double bond and the terminal carbon to the pyrrole nitrogen atom. Terminal acetylenes can participate in an analogous reaction in which ferryl oxygen transfer to the terminal carbon of the triple bond produces a ketene, which may react with the protein, whereas addition of the oxygen to the internal carbon leads to alkylation of a nitrogen of the heme.[106]

The reaction manifold that leads to the formation of epoxides, carbonyl products, and heme alkylation has not been definitively elucidated. It is likely that an initial complex involving some degree of charge-transfer between the ferryl oxygen and the π-bond decomposes by what appears to be (a) a concerted pathway leading to epoxide formation, (b) a free radical pathway that can lead to heme alkylation, and (c) a cationic pathway that leads to the observed 1,2-shifts of the olefin substituents (Figure 3.14). The computational studies suggest that the initial complex exists in different spin states, and that these states determine which pathway is followed in the reaction.[93]

Oxidation of Aromatic Rings

The cytochrome P450-catalyzed processing of aromatic systems is a special case of π-bond oxidation. In its simplest form, the oxidation is analogous to the oxidation of an isolated double bond and gives the same product, i.e., the epoxide. However, the epoxides derived from aromatic systems are unstable and readily rearrange to give phenols. The steps in this reaction are (a) heterolytic scission of one of the strained epoxide carbon-oxygen bonds, (b) migration of the hydrogen (or rarely some other substituent) on the carbon that retains the epoxide oxygen to the adjacent carbocation to give a ketone, and (c) proton tautomerization to rearomatize the structure, giving the phenol metabolite. The oxidation of fenbendazole provides an example of this reaction (Figure 3.15).[107] The net result is oxidation of an aromatic ring via an epoxide to the hydroxylated product that would formally result from insertion of oxygen into one of the aromatic C-H bonds. This aromatic "hydroxylation" mechanism

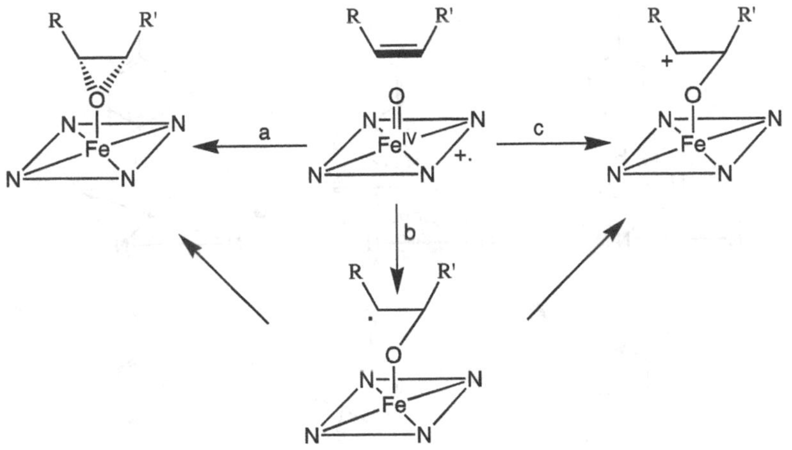

FIGURE 3.14 Reaction manifold in the cytochrome P450-catalyzed oxidation of olefins. Formation of a charge transfer complex may be followed by (a) apparently concerted epoxide formation, (b) non-concerted oxygen transfer to give a radical, or (c) non-concerted oxygen transfer to give a cation. The radical intermediate could give rise to both the epoxide and cation metabolites, but the retention of stereochemistry indicates it would have to be a very short-lived radical.

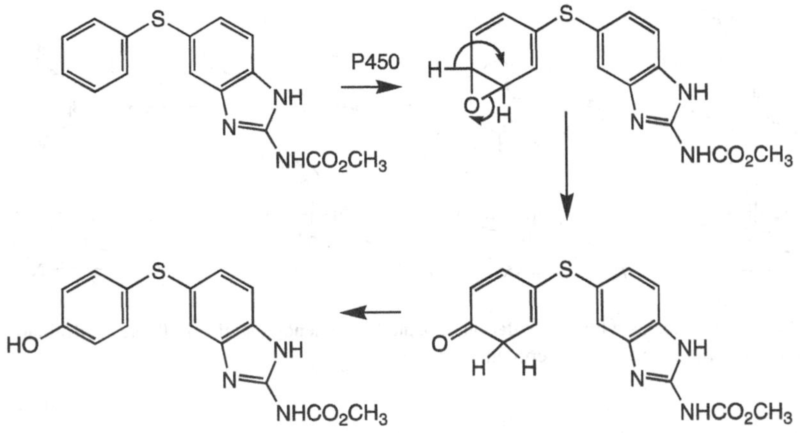

FIGURE 3.15 Cytochrome P450-catalyzed oxidation of fenbendazole illustrating the NIH shift mechanism for aromatic "hydroxylation". (From Barker, S.A. et al., *Biomed. Environ. Mass Spectrom.*, 14, 161–165, 1987.)

is known as the NIH shift because it was discovered at the National Institutes of Health.[108] The NIH shift of an epoxide can yield two different phenolic products, depending on which of the two epoxide carbon-oxygen bonds is broken. If the cation formed by breaking one of the bonds is significantly more stable than that obtained by breaking the other, the phenol produced by the lower energy pathway predominates. Substitution of an electron-donating group (e.g., alkoxy) promotes formation of the *ortho-* or *para*-hydroxy metabolite, whereas a strong electron withdrawing substituent (e.g., nitro) favors formation of the *meta*-hydroxy metabolite.

Aromatic π-bond oxidation is subject to mechanistic ambiguities comparable to those for the oxidation of simple olefins. Although the epoxides of some aromatic substrates have been isolated and shown to undergo the NIH shift, in other instances the epoxide is not a true intermediate in the reaction trajectory that produces the NIH shift. Asymmetric transfer of the ferryl oxygen to the aromatic π-bond may directly give a cation similar to that expected from cleavage of one of the epoxide carbon-oxygen bonds.

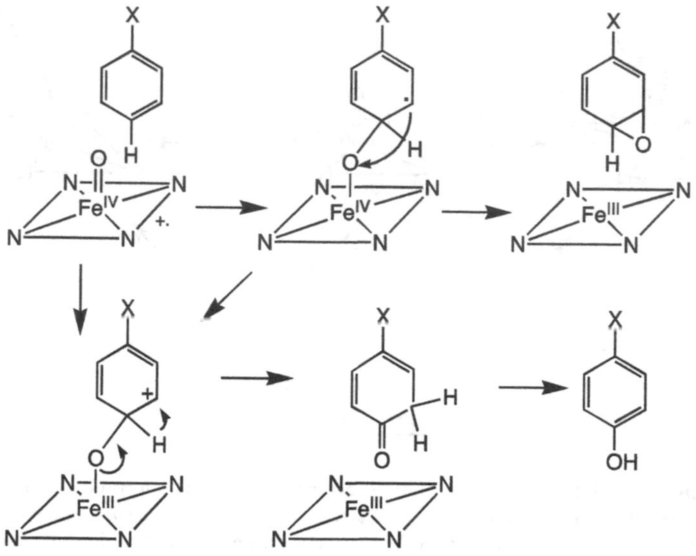

FIGURE 3.16 Hydroxylation of aromatic rings may occur without the formation of an epoxide intermediate. The putative cytochrome P450 heme reactive species is abbreviated as before.

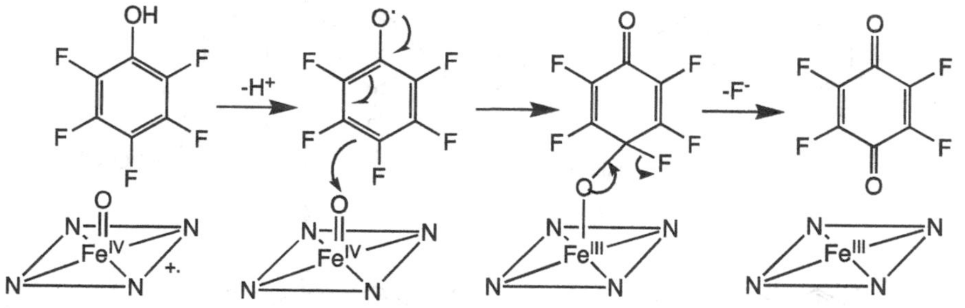

FIGURE 3.17 Proposed mechanism for the oxidation of pentafluorophenol resulting in fluoride elimination to give tetrafluoro *p*-quinone without the formation of an epoxide intermediate.

This intermediate then flows directly into the NIH shift (Figure 3.16). The reaction manifold can be diverted towards other reaction outcomes. An example of this is the oxidation of pentafluorophenol to 2,3,5,6- tetrafluoroquinone.[109] It appears that one-electron abstraction from the polyfluorinated phenol produces a phenoxy radical that combines with the ferryl oxygen at the carbon *para* to the oxygen. The resulting *para*-hydroxylated intermediate eliminates fluoride to give the quinone (Figure 3.17). As always, the reaction with the lowest energy barrier predominates!

Heteroatom Oxidation

The cytochrome P450 ferryl species is electron deficient and, therefore, has a propensity to react with the electron pairs on nitrogen and sulfur atoms. A similar reaction is not observed with oxygen electron pairs due to the much higher electronegativity of this atom. Halogen atoms, like oxygen, are highly electronegative and difficult to oxidize, but their oxidation can occur in special circumstances. One example is the oxidation of the chloride atom in 12-chlorododecanoic acid [i.e., $ClCH_2(CH_2)_{10}CO_2H$] by CYP4A1, an enzyme that normally oxidizes the terminal (ω) atom of a fatty acid chain.[110]

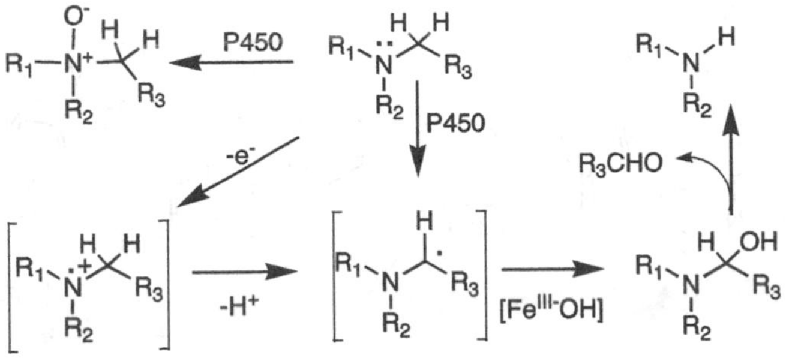

FIGURE 3.18 Cytochrome P450 can either oxidize a trisubstituted nitrogen to an N-oxide or introduce a hydroxyl adjacent to the nitrogen. The latter reaction can involve insertion of the oxygen into the adjacent C H bond or a reaction initiated by abstraction of an electron from the nitrogen followed by loss of a proton. [Fe^{III}-OH] represents the heme of P450 with a hydroxyl group on the ferric iron.

Nitrogen Oxidation

Tertiary amines can be oxidized to the corresponding N-oxides by both the cytochrome P450 enzymes and the flavin monooxygenases (Figure 3.18). In general, but not always,[111] cytochrome P450 enzymes preferentially catalyze the N-dealkylation of alkyl amines rather than formation of the N-oxide. The flavin monooxygenases only form the N-oxide. It is not possible to attribute the formation of an N-oxide to either the P450 or flavoprotein monooxygenase system without evidence that specifically implicates one or the other of these two enzyme systems.

The dealkylation of alkyl amines, ethers, thioethers, and other alkyl-substituted heteroatoms is catalyzed by cytochrome P450 but not by the flavin monooxygenase. As already described, this reaction can be viewed as proceeding via introduction of a hydroxyl group adjacent to the heteroatom followed by intramolecular elimination of the heteroatom (Figure 3.8). Therefore, the final products are an aldehyde or ketone and a heteroatom-containing substrate fragment. This conventional carbon hydroxylation mechanism operates in the case of ethers and halides. However, the lower electronegativity of nitrogen makes possible an alternative mechanism triggered by initial electron abstraction from the nitrogen atom by the ferryl species (Figure 3.18). Subsequent removal of a proton from the adjacent carbon by the partially reduced ferryl species, followed by recombination of the iron-bound hydroxyl group with the resulting radical, completes an indirect route to hydroxylation of the carbon adjacent to the nitrogen. Evidence is available for both reaction pathways and the pathway may be substrate-dependent.[80,112]

Sulfur Oxidation

The oxidation of thioethers to sulfoxides and the dealkylation of alkyl thioethers are subject to the same considerations as the metabolism of alkylamines. Sulfoxidation, as illustrated by the oxidation of ML3403 (Figure 3.19),[113] can be catalyzed by both the P450 enzymes and flavin monooxygenases. A thioether can be oxidized twice, first to the sulfoxide and then to the sulfone. The second oxidation is more difficult as the sulfur is more electron deficient after the first oxidation. S-dealkylation, like N- and O-dealkylations (Figure 3.8), is really a carbon hydroxylation reaction mediated by cytochrome P450 in which hydroxylation on the carbon adjacent to the sulfur is followed by extrusion of the heteroatom.

The P450-catalyzed oxidation of thiocarbonyl groups, as represented by the oxidation of thiopental (Figure 3.19) is unusual in that it leads to elimination of the sulfur to yield a simple carbonyl moiety. Transfer of the ferryl oxygen to the sulfur of the thiocarbonyl group produces an unsaturated sulfoxide that decomposes to the carbonyl product. The sulfur is eliminated, probably as HSOH, via a hydrolytic mechanism that may be assisted by glutathione.[114]

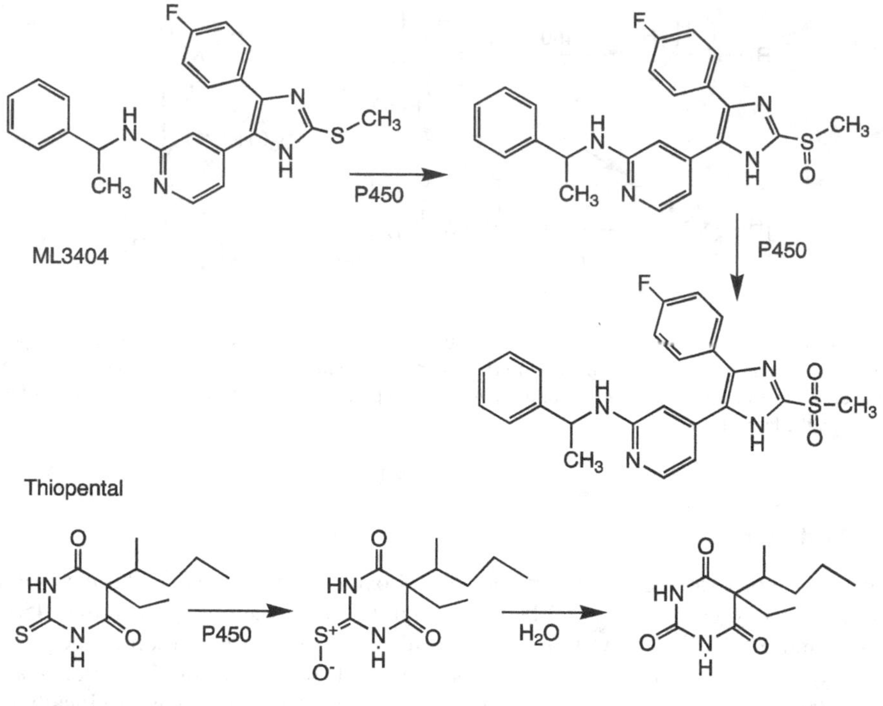

FIGURE 3.19 The P450-catalyzed oxidation of thioethers and thiocarbonyl groups as illustrated by the oxidations of ML3404 and thiopental. (From Kammerer, B. et al., *Drug Metab. Dispos.*, 35, 875–883, 2007.)

Unusual Oxidative Reactions

The range of reactions catalyzed by cytochrome P450 continues to grow, although some of the more novel reactions only occur in low yields, in special circumstances, or in substrate-specific plant or microbial P450 enzymes. One of these P450-catalyzed reactions is the desaturation of hydrocarbon functionalities. The most extensively characterized of these reactions is the desaturation of valproic acid to give the terminal olefin (Figure 3.20).[115] Isotope effect studies indicate that this reaction is initiated by hydrogen abstraction from the ω-1 position. This abstraction is followed either

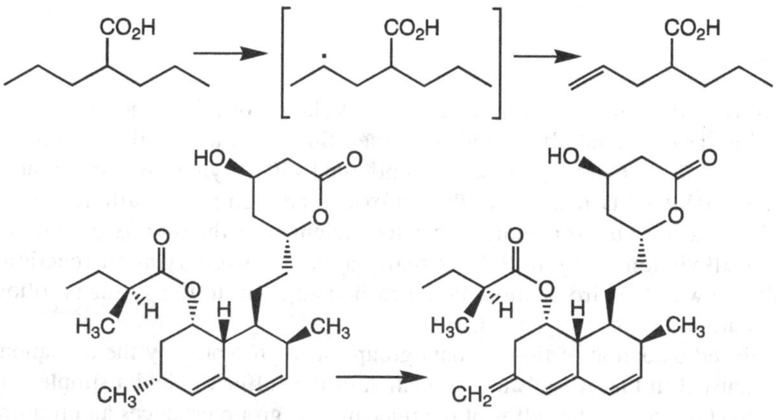

FIGURE 3.20 Cytochrome P450-catalyzed desaturation of valproic acid (above) and lovostatin (below). Isotope effects suggest that a radical intermediate, as shown for valproic acid, is involved in the reaction.

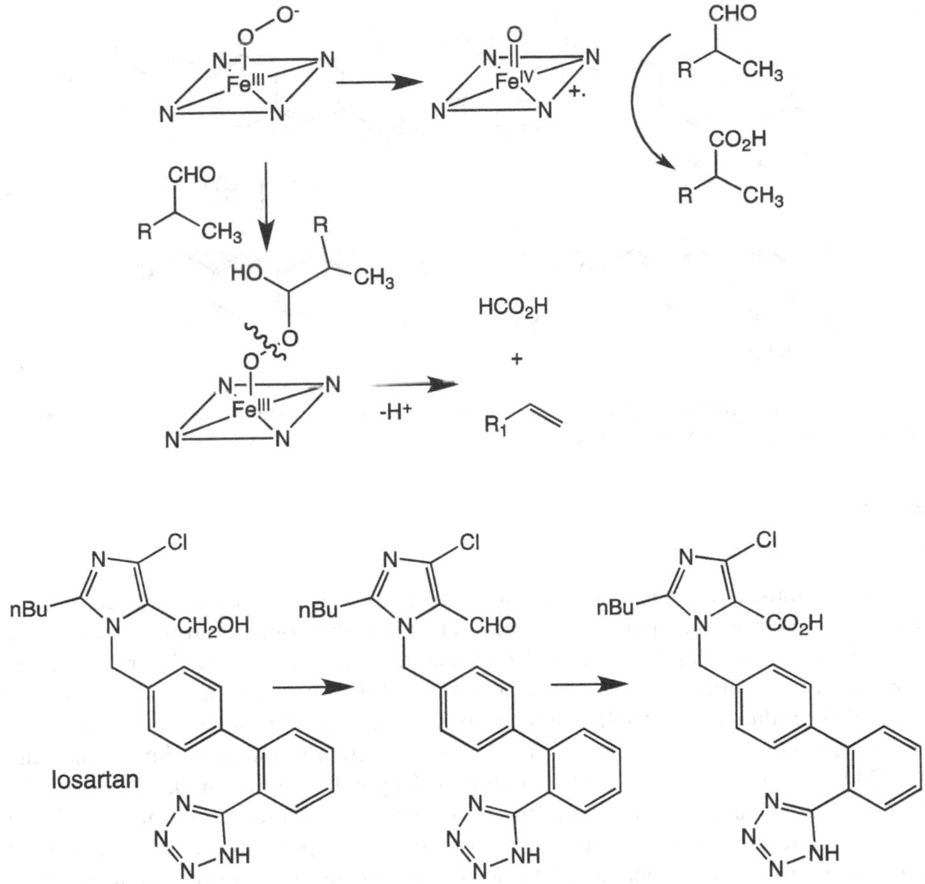

FIGURE 3.21 Aldehydes are generally oxidized by cytochrome P450 to the corresponding acids, but in some instances reaction of the aldehyde with the [Fe^{III}-OO-] intermediate results in loss of the aldehyde group as formic acid and formation of an unsaturated hydrocarbon.

by recombination to give the 4-hydroxy metabolite or, alternatively, by a second hydrogen atom abstraction from the terminal carbon to give the olefin. Other examples of desaturation reactions catalyzed by mammalian cytochrome P450 enzymes are the $\Delta^{6,7}$-desaturation of testosterone and the desaturation of lovastatin.[116,117]

The reaction of aldehydes with cytochrome P450 can follow one of two divergent pathways (Figure 3.21). The more common reaction is oxidation of the aldehyde to give a carboxylic acid, as illustrated by the metabolism of losartan (Figure 3.21).[118] The alternative pathway is a process that results in elimination of the aldehyde group as formic acid.[119] The carbon-carbon bond cleavage reaction finds strong precedent in the reactions catalyzed by biosynthetic P450 enzymes such as lanosterol demethylase. Cleavage of a carbon-carbon bond in the reaction catalyzed by this enzyme appears to involve the reaction of an aldehyde group on the substrate with the cytochrome P450 ferrous dioxy intermediate.[120] A similar mechanism is proposed for the reactions of some simple aldehydes with hepatic P450 enzymes, with the difference that the carbon-carbon bond cleavage process is the major or exclusive reaction in the biosynthetic enzymes but is often a minor reaction in the metabolism of xenobiotic aldehydes. Carbon-carbon bond cleavage reactions can also be observed with ketone substrates, particularly α-hydroxy ketones. The C^{17,20}-lyase reaction catalyzed by CYP17A1 is a classical example,[83] but a similar process occurs in the CYP1A2-catalyzed oxidation of the prodrug nabumetone to its truncated active form (Figure 3.22).[121] This reaction sequence also requires oxidation of the aldehyde intermediate that is first formed to the acid, the active drug.

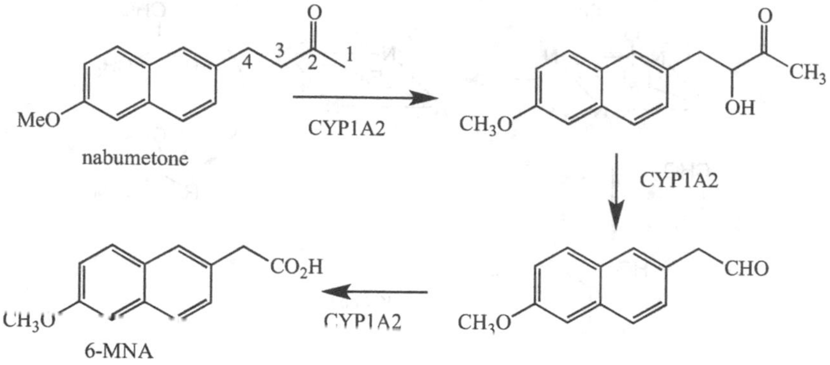

FIGURE 3.22 Oxidation of the prodrug nabumetone to the aldehyde via a C-C bond cleaving reaction, followed by oxidation of the aldehyde to the acid to give the active drug.

Reductive Reactions

In addition to oxidative reactions, cytochrome P450 is known to catalyze reductive reactions.[122] These reductive reactions are particularly relevant under anaerobic conditions but, under some aerobic conditions, can compete with oxidative reactions. A major reductive reaction catalyzed by cytochrome P450 is the dehalogenation of alkyl halides. Cytochrome P450, and sometimes cytochrome P450 reductase by itself, are also involved in reactions such as the reduction of azo and nitro compounds. Two examples of these reactions are the bioactivation of the anticancer prodrug AQ4N to the topoisomerase II inhibitor AQ4 by cytochrome P450,[123] and the bioactivation of the anticancer drug tirapazamine by electron transfer from cytochrome P450 reductase (Figure 3.23).[124] The important catalytic species in the P450-dependent reaction is presumably the ferrous deoxy intermediate in which the reduced iron has an open coordination position. Thus, reductive reactions compete with the binding and activation of oxygen, a fact that explains the oxygen sensitivity of the pathway.

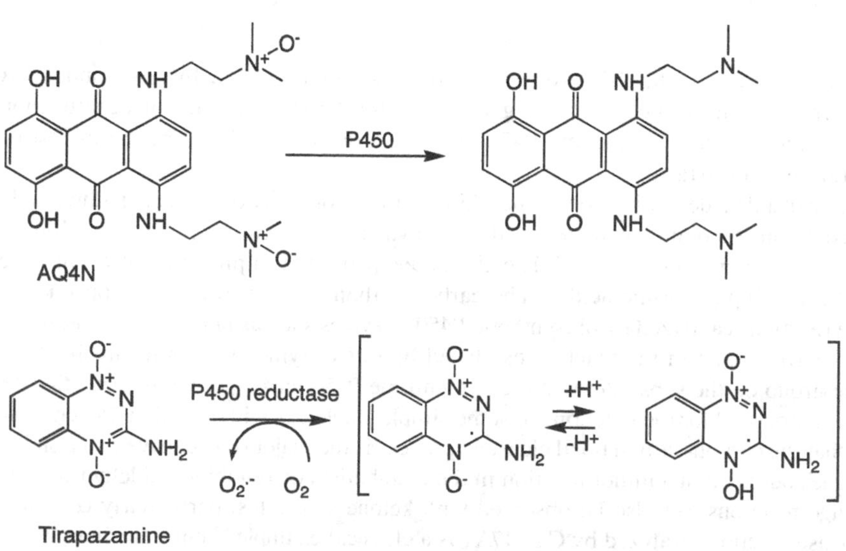

FIGURE 3.23 Reductive activation of the anticancer agents AQ4N and tirapazamine, the former by cytochrome P450 and the latter primarily by electron transfer from cytochrome P450 reductase.

REFERENCES

1. Guengerich, F.P. Human cytochrome P450 enzymes. In: Ortiz de Montellano P.R., ed. *Cytochrome P450: Structure, Mechanism, and Biochemistry*, 4th ed., (New York: Springer, 2015): 523–786.
2. Nelson, D., Koymans, L., Kamataki, T., et al. P450 superfamily: Update on new sequences, gene mapping, accession numbers and nomenclature. *Pharmacogenetics* 6 (1996): 1–42.
3. Nelson, D.R., Zeldin, D.C., Susan, M.G., et al. Comparison of cytochrome P450 (CYP) genes from the mouse and human genomes, including nomenclature recommendations for genes, pseudogenes and alternative splice variants. *Pharmacogenetics* 14 (2004): 1–18.
4. Michaels, S., and Wang, M.Z. The revised human liver cytochrome P450 "Pie". Absolute protein quantification of CYP4F and CYP3A4 enzymes using targeted quantitative proteomics. *Drug Metab. Dispos.* 42 (2014): 1241–1251.
5. Zhang, H.-F., Wang, H-H, Gao, N, et al. Physiological content and intrinsic activities of 10 cytochrome P450 isoforms in human normal liver microsomes. *J. Pharmacol. Exp. Therap.* 358 (2016): 83–93.
6. Rendic, S., and Guengerich, F.P. Survey of human oxidoreductases and cytochrome P450 enzymes involved in the metabolism of xenobiotic and natural chemicals. *Chem. Res. Toxicol.* 28 (2015): 38–42.
7. Zhao, Y., Wan, D., Yang, J., Hammock, B.D., and Ortiz de Montellano, P.R. Catalytic activities of tumor-specific human cytochrome P450 CYP2W1 towards endogenous substrates. *Drug Metab. Dispos.* 44 (2016): 771–780.
8. Evans, W.E., and Relling, M.V. Pharmacogenomics: Translating function genomics into rational therapeutics. *Science* 286 (1999): 487–491.
9. Nakamura, K., Goto, F., Ray, W.A., et al. Interethnic differences in genetic polymorphism of debrisoquine and mephenytoin hydroxylation between Japanese and Caucasian populations. *Clin. Pharmacol. Ther.* 38 (1987): 402–408.
10. Zanger, U.M., and Schwab, M. Cytochrome P450 enzymes in drug metabolism: Regulation of gene expression, enzyme activities, and impact of genetic variation. *Pharmacol. Therap.* 138 (2013): 103–141.
11. Poulos, T.L., Finzel, B.C., and Howard, A.J. High-resolution crystal structure of cytochrome P450$_{cam}$. *J. Mol. Biol.* 195 (1987): 687–700.
12. Ravichandran, K.G., Boddupalli, S.S., Hasemann, C.A., et al. Crystal structure of hemoprotein domain of P450BM-3, a prototype for microsomal P450s. *Science* 261 (1993): 731–736.
13. Cupp-Vickery, J.R., and Poulos, T.L. Structure of cytochrome P450eryF involved in erythromycin biosynthesis. *Struct. Biol.* 2 (1995): 144–153.
14. Yano, J.K., Koo, L.S., Schuller, D.J., Li, H., Ortiz de Montellano, P.R., and Poulos, T.L. Crystal structure of a thermophilic cytochrome P450 from the archaeon *Sulfolobus solfataricus*. *J. Biol. Chem.* 275 (2000): 31086–31092.
15. Williams, P.A., Cosme, J., Sridhar, V., et al. Mammalian microsomal cytochrome P450 monooxygenase: Structural adaptations for membrane binding and functional diversity. *Mol. Cell* 5 (2000): 121–131.
16. Walsh, A.A., Szklarz, G.D., and Scott, E.E. Human cytochrome P450 1A1 structure and utility in understanding drug and xenobiotic metabolism. *J. Biol. Chem.* 288 (2013): 2932–2943.
17. Sansen, S., Yano, J.K., Reynald, R.I., et al. Adaptations for the oxidation of polycyclic aromatic hydrocarbons exhibited by the structure of human P450 1A2. *J. Biol. Chem.* 282 (2007): 14348–14355.
18. Wang, A., Savas, U., Stout, C.D., and Johnson, E.F. Structural characterization of the complex between α-naphthoflavone and human cytochrome P450 1B1. *J. Biol. Chem.* 286 (2011): 5736–5743.
19. Yano, J.K., Hsu, M., Griffin, K.J., et al. Structures of human microsomal cytochrome P450 2A6 complexed with coumarin and methoxsalen. *Nature Struct. Molec. Biol.* 12 (2005): 822–823.
20. Yano, J.K., Denton, T.T., Cerny, M.A., Zhang, X., Johnson, E.F., and Cashman, J.R. Synthetic inhibitors of cytochrome P-450 2A6: Inhibitory activity, difference spectra, mechanism of inhibition, and protein co-crystallization. *J. Med. Chem.* 49 (2006): 6987–6901.
21. Smith, B.D., Sanders, J.L., Porubsky, P.R., et al. Structure of the human lung cytochrome P450 2A13. *J. Biol. Chem.* 282 (2007): 17306–17313.
22. DeVore, N.M., and Scott, E.E. Nicotine and 4-(methylnitrosamino)-1-(3-pridyl)-1-butanone binding and access channel in human cytochrome P450 2A6 and 2A13 enzymes. *J. Biol. Chem.* 287 (2012): 26576–26585.
23. Scott, E.E., He, Y.A., Wester, M.R., et al. An open conformation of mammalian cytochrome P450 2B4 at 1.6 Å-resolution. *Proc. Natl. Acad. Sci. U.S.A.* 100 (2003): 13196–13201.

24. Gay, S.C., Shah, M.B., Talakad, J.C., et al. Crystal structure of a cytochrome P450 2B6 genetic variant in complex with the inhibitor 4-(4-chlorophenyl)imidazole at 2.0-A resolution. *Mol. Pharmacol.* 77 (2010): 529–538.

25. Schoch, G.A., Yano, Y.K., Wester, M.R., et al. Structure of human microsomal cytochrome P450 2C8. Evidence for a peripheral fatty acid binding-site. *J. Biol. Chem.* 279 (2004): 9497–9503.

26. Schoch, G.A., Yano, J.K., Sansen, S., Dansette, P.M., Stout, C.D., and Johnson, E.F. Determinants of cytochrome P450 2C8 substrate binding: Structures of complexes with montelukast, troglitazone, felodipine or 9-*cis*-retinoic acid. *J. Biol. Chem.* 283 (2008): 17227–17237.

27. Williams, P.A., Cosme, J., Ward, A., et al. Crystal structure of human cytochrome P450 2C9 with bound warfarin. *Nature* 424 (2003): 464–468.

28. Wester, M.R., Yano, J.K., Schoch, G.A., et al. The structure of human cytochrome P450 2C9 complexed with flurbiprofen at 2.0-Å resolution. *J. Biol. Chem.* 279 (2004): 35630–35637.

29. Reynald, R.L., Sansen, S., Stout, C.D., and Johnson, E.F. Structural characterization of human cytochrome P450 2C19: Active site differences between P450s 2C8, 2C9, and 2C19. *J. Biol. Chem.* 53 (2012): 44581–44591.

30. Rowland, P., Blaney, F.E., Smyth, M.G., et al. Crystal structure of human cytochrome P450 2D6. *J. Biol. Chem.* 281 (2006): 7614–7622.

31. Wang, A., Savas, U., Hsu, M.H., Stout, C.D., and Johnson, E.F. Crystal structure of human cytochrome P450 2D6 with prinomastat bound. *J. Biol. Chem.* 287 (2012): 10834–10843.

32. Porubsky, P.R., Meneely, K.M., and Scott, E.E. Structures of human cytochrome P450 2E1: Insights into the binding of inhibitors and both small molecular weight and fatty acid substrates. *J. Biol. Chem.* 283 (2008): 33698–33707.

33. Strushkevich, N.V., Usanov, S.A., Plotnikov, A.N., Jones, G., and Park, H.W. Structural analysis of CYP2R1 with vitamin D3. *J. Mol. Biol.* 380 (2008): 95–106.

34. Williams, P.A., Cosme, J., Vincovic, V.M., et al. Crystal structures of human cytochrome P450 3A4 bound to metyrapone and progesterone. *Science* 305 (2004): 683–686.

35. Yano, J.K., Wester, M.R., Schoch, G.A., et al. The structure of human microsomal cytochrome P450 3A4 determined by X-ray crystallography to 2.05 Å resolution. *J. Biol. Chem.* 279 (2004): 38091–38094.

36. Sevrioukova, I.F., and Poulos, T.L. Structural and mechanistic insights into the interaction of cytochrome P4503A4 with bromoergocryptine, a type I ligand. *J. Biol. Chem.* 287 (2011): 3510–3517.

37. Tempel, W., Grabovec, I., MacKenzie, F., et al. Structural characterization of human cholesterol 7α-hydroxylase. *J. Lipid Res.* 55 (2014): 1925–1932.

38. Mast, N., Annalora, A.J., Lodowski, D.T., Palczewski, K., Stout, C.D., and Pikuleva, I.A. Structural basis for three-step sequential catalysis by the cholesterol side chain cleavage enzyme CYP11A1. *J. Biol. Chem.* 286 (2011): 5607–5613.

39. DeVore, N.M., and Scott, E.E.. Structures of cytochrome P450 17A1 with prostate cancer drugs abiraterone and TOK-001. *Nature* 482 (2012): 116–120.

40. Zhao, B., Lei, L., Kagawa, N., et al. A three-dimensional structure of steroid 21-hydroxylase (cytochrome P450 21A2) with two substrates reveals locations of disease-associated variants. *J. Biol. Chem.* 287 (2012): 10613–10622.

41. Annalora, A.J., Goodin, D.B., Hong, W.X., Zhang, Q., Johnson, E.F., and Stout, C.D. Crystal structure of CYP24A1, a mitochondrial cytochrome P450 involved in vitamin D metabolism. *J. Mol. Biol.* 396 (2010): 441–451.

42. Mast, N., White, M.A., Bjorkhem, I., Johnson, E.F., Stout, C.D., and Pikuleva, I.A. Crystal structures of substrate-bound and substrate-free cytochrome P450 46A1, the principal cholesterol hydroxylase in the brain. *Proc. Natl. Acad. Sci. U.S.A.* 105 (2008): 9546–9551.

43. Strushkevich, N., Usanov, S.A., and Park, H.W. Structural basis of human CYP51 inhibition by antifungal azoles. *J. Mol. Biol.* 397 (2010): 1067–1078.

44. Atkins, W.M., and Sligar, S.G. Molecular recognition in cytochrome P450: Alteration of regioselective alkane hydroxylation via protein engineering. *J. Am. Chem. Soc.* 111 (1989): 2715–2717.

45. Atkins, W.M., and Sligar, S.G. The roles of active site hydrogen bonding in cytochrome P-450$_{cam}$ as revealed by site-directed mutagenesis. *J. Biol. Chem.* 263 (1988): 18842–18849.

46. Furuya, H., Shimizu, T., Hirano, K., et al. Site-directed mutagenesis of rat liver cytochrome P-450d: Catalytic activities toward benzphetamine and 7-ethoxycoumarin. *Biochemistry* 28 (1989): 6848–6857.

47. Gotoh, O. Substrate recognition sites in cytochrome P450 family 2 (CYP2) proteins inferred from comparative analyses of amino acid and coding nucleotide sequences. *J. Biol. Chem.* 267 (1992): 83–90.
48. Cruciani, G., Carosati, E., De Boeck, B., et al. MetaSite: Understanding metabolism in human cytochromes from the perspective of the chemist. *J. Med. Chem.* 48 (2005): 6970–6979.
49. Afzelius, L., Arnby, C.H., Broo, A., et al. State-of-the-art tools for computational site of metabolism predictions: Comparative analysis, mechanistical insights, and future applications. *Drug Metab. Rev.* 39 (2007): 61–86.
50. Hritz, J., de Ruiter, A., and Oostenbrink, C. Impact of plasticity and flexibility on docking results for cytochrome P450 2D6: A combined approach of molecular dynamics and ligand docking. *J. Med. Chem.* 51 (2008): 7469–7477.
51. Moors, S.L.C., Vos, A.M., Cummings, M.D., Van Vlijmen, H., and Ceulemans, A. Structure-based site of metabolism prediction for cytochrome P450 2D6. *J. Med. Chem.* 54 (2011): 6098–6105.
52. Ford, K.A., Ryslik, G., Sodhi, J., et al. Computational predictions of the site of metabolism of cytochrome P450 2D6 substrates: Comparative analysis, molecular docking, bioactivation and toxicological implications. *Drug Metab. Rev.* 47 (2015): 291–319.
53. Hudelson, M.G., Ketkar, N.S., Holder, L.B., et al. High confidence predictions of drug-drug interactions: Predicting affinities for cytochrome P450 2C9 with multiple computational methods. *J. Med. Chem.* 51 (2008): 648–654.
54. Basudhar, D., Madrona, Y., Kandel, S., Lampe, J.N., Nishida, C.R., and Ortiz de Montellano, P.R. Analysis of cytochrome P450 CYP119 ligand-dependent conformational dynamics by two-dimensional NMR and x-ray crystallography. *J. Biol. Chem.* 290 (2015): 10000–10017.
55. Stoll, S., Lee, Y.T., Zhang, M., Wilson, R.F., Britt, R.D., and Goodin, D.B. Double electron-electron resonance shows cytochrome P450$_{cam}$ undergoes a conformational change in solution upon substrate binding. *Proc. Natl. Acad. Sci. U.S.A.* 109 (2012): 12888–12893.
56. Hollingsworth, S.A., Batabyal, D., Nguyen, B.D., and Poulos, T.L. Conformational selectivity in cytochrome P450 redox partner interactions. *Proc. Natl. Acad. Sci. U.S.A.* 113 (2016): 8723–8728.
57. Scott, E.E., White, M.A., He, Y.A., et al. Structure of mammalian cytochrome P450 2B4 complexed with 4-(4-chlorophenyl)imidazole at 1.9-Å resolution. *J. Biol. Chem.* 279 (2004): 27294–27301.
58. Zhao, Y., White, M.A., Muralidhara, B.K., Sun, L., Halpert, J.R., and Stout, C.D. Structure of microsomal cytochrome P450 2B4 complexed with the antifungal drug bifonazole. Insight into P450 conformational plasticity and membrane interaction. *J. Biol. Chem.* 281 (2006): 5973–5981.
59. Wilderman, P.R., Shah, M.B., Liu, T., et al. Plasticity of cytochrome P450 as investigated by hydrogen-deuterium exchange mass spectrometry and X-ray crystallography. *J. Biol. Chem.* 285 (2010): 38602–38611.
60. Shah, M.B., Kufareva, I., Pascual, J., Zhang, Q., Stout, C.D., and Halpert, J.R. A structural snapshot of CYP2B4 in complex with paroxetine provides insights into ligand binding and clusters of comformational states. *J. Pharmacol. Exp. Therap.* 346 (2013): 113–120.
61. Ekroos, M., and Sjögren, T. Structural basis for ligand promiscuity in cytochrome P450 3A4. *Proc. Natl. Acad. Sci. U.S.A.* 103 (2006): 13682–13687.
62. Davydov, D.R., Yang, Z., Davydova, N., Halpert, J.R., and Hubbell, W.L. Conformational mobility in cytochrome P450 3A4 explored by pressure-perturbation EPR spectroscopy. *Biophys. J.* 110 (2016): 1485–1498.
63. Davydov, D.R., Rumfeldt, J.A.O., Sineva, E.V., Fernando, H., Davydova, N.Y., and Halpert, J.R. Peripheral ligand binding site in cytochrome P450 3A4 located with fluorescence resonance energy transfer (FRET). *J. Biol. Chem.* 287 (2012): 6797–6809.
64. Schenkman, J.B., Sligar, S.G., and Cinti, D.L. Substrate interaction with cytochrome P450. In: Schenkman, J.B., Kupfer, D., eds. *Hepatic Cytochrome P-450 Monooxygenase System*, New York: Pergamon Press, (1982): 587–615.
65. Dawson, J.H., and Sono, M. Cytochrome P450 and chloroperoxidase: Thiolate-ligated heme enzymes. Spectroscopic determination of their active site structures and mechanistic implications of thiolate ligation. *Chem. Rev.* 87 (1987): 1255–1276.
66. Conner, K.P., Cruce, A.A., Krzyaniak, M.D., et al. Drug modulation of water-heme interactions in low-spin P450 complexes of CYP2C9d and CYP125A1. *Biochemistry* 54 (2015): 1198–1207.
67. Sweeney, G.D. and Rothwell, J.D. Spectroscopic evidence of interaction between 2-allyl-2-isopropylacetamide and cytochrome P-450 of rat liver microsomes. *Biochem. Biophys. Res. Commun.* 55 (1973): 798–804.

68. Waskell, L., and Kim, J.P. Electron transfer partners of cytochrome P450. In: Ortiz de Montellano PR, ed. *Cytochrome P450: Structure, Mechanism, and Biochemistry*, 4th ed. (New York: Springer, 2015): 33–68.

69. Wang, M., Roberts, D.L., Paschke, R., et al. Three-dimensional structure of NADPH-cytochrome P450 reductase: prototype for FMN- and FAD-containing enzymes. *Proc. Natl. Acad. Sci. U.S.A.* 94 (1997): 8411–8416.

70. Hamdane, D., Xia, C., Im, S.C., Zhang, H., Kim, J.P., and Waskell, L. Structure and function of an NADPH-cytochrome P450 oxidoreductase in an open conformation capable of reducing cytochrome P450. *J. Biol. Chem.* 284 (2009): 11374–11384.

71. Schenkman, J.B., and Jansson, I. The many roles of cytochrome b_5. *Pharmacol. Therap.* 97 (2003): 139–152.

72. Porter, T.D. The roles of cytochrome b_5 in cytochrome P450 reactions. *J. Biochem. Molec. Toxicol.* 16 (2002): 311–316.

73. Yamazaki, H., Johnson, W.W., Ueng, J.F., et al. Lack of electron transfer from cytochrome b_5 in stimulation of catalytic activities of cytochrome P450 3A4. Characterization of a reconstituted cytochrome P450 3A4/NADPH-cytochrome P450 reductase system and studies with apo-cytochrome b_5. *J. Biol. Chem.* 271 (1996): 27438–27444.

74. Storbeck, K.H., Swart, A.C., Fox, C.L., and Swart, P. Cytochrome b_5 modulates multiple reactions in steroidogenesis by diverse mechanisms. *J. Steroid Biochem. Molec. Biol.* 151 (2015): 66–73.

75. Denisov, I.G., and Sligar, S.G. Activation of molecular oxygen in cytochrome P450. In: Ortiz de Montellano PR, ed. *Cytochrome P450: Structure, Mechanism, and Biochemistry*, 4th ed. (New York: Springer, 2015): 69–109.

76. Sligar, S.G. Coupling of spin, substrate and redox equilibria in cytochrome P-450. *Biochemistry* 15 (1976): 5399-406.

77. Guengerich, F.P. Oxidation-reduction properties of rat liver cytochromes P-450 and NADPH-cytochrome P-450 reductase related to catalysis in reconstituted systems. *Biochemistry* 22 (1983): 2811–2820.

78. Das, A., Grinkova, Y.V., and Sligar, S.G. Redox potential control by drug binding to cytochrome P450 3A4. *J. Am. Chem. Soc.* 129 (2007): 13778–13779.

79. Schlichting, I., Berendzen, J., Chu, K., et al. The catalytic pathway of cytochrome P450$_{cam}$ at atomic resolution. *Science* 287 (2000): 1615–1622.

80. Ortiz de Montellano, P.R. Substrate oxidation by cytochrome P450 enzymes. In: Ortiz de Montellano, P.R., ed. *Cytochrome P450: Structure, Mechanism, and Biochemistry*, 4th ed., (New York: Springer, 2015): 111–176.

81. Rittle, J. and Green, M.T. Cytochrome P450 compound I: Capture, characterization, and C-H bond activation kinetics. *Science* 330 (2010): 933–937.

82. Wang, X., Peter, S., Kinne, M., Hofrichter, M., and Groves, J.T. Detection and kinetic characterization of a highly reactive heme-thiolate peroxygenase Compound I. *J. Am. Chem. Soc.* 134 (2012): 12897–12900.

83. Mak, P.J., Gregory, M.C., Denisov, I.G., Sligar, S.G., and Kincaid, J.R. Unveiling the crucial intermediates in androgen production. *Proc. Natl. Acad. Sci. U.S.A.* 112 (2015): 15856–15861.

84. Yoshimoto, F.K., and Guengerich, F.P. Mechanism of the third oxidative step in the conversion of androgens to estrogens by cytochrome P450 19A1 steroid aromatase. *J. Am. Chem. Soc.* 136 (2014): 15016–15025.

85. Sheng, X., Zhang, H., Hollenberg, P.F., and Newcomb, M. Kinetic isotope effects in hydroxylation reactions effected by cytochrome P450 Compounds I implicate multiple electrophilic oxidants for P450-catalyzed oxidations. *Biochemistry* 48 (2009): 1620–1627.

86. Oguri, K., Tanimoto, Y., and Yoshimura, H. Metabolite fate of strychnine in rats. *Xenobiotica* 19 (1989): 171–178.

87. Hjelmeland, L.M., Aronow, L., and Trudell, J.R. Intramolecular determination of primary kinetic isotope effects in hydroxylations catalyzed by cytochrome P-450. *Biochem. Biophys. Res. Commun.* 76 (1977): 541–549.

88. Foster, A.B. Deuterium isotope effects in the metabolism of drugs and xenobiotics: Implications for drug design. *Adv. Drug Res.* 14 (1985): 2–40.

89. Fisher, M.B., Henne, K.R., and Boer, J. The complexities inherent in attempts to decrease drug clearance by blocking sites of CYP-mediated metabolism. *Curr. Opin. Drug Disc. Develop.* 9 (2006): 101–109.

90. Frommer, U., Ullrich, V., and Staudinger, H. Hydroxylation of aliphatic compounds by liver microsomes. 1. The distribution of isomeric alcohols. *Hoppe-Seylers Z. Physiol. Chem.* 351 (1970): 903–912.

91. Sheridan, R.P., Korzekwa, K.R., Torres, R.A., and Walker, M.J. Empirical regioselectivity models for human cytochromes P450 3A4, 2D6, and 2C9. *J. Med. Chem.* 50 (2007): 3173–3184.

92. Shaik, S., Kumar, D., and de Visser, S.P. A valence bond modeling of trends in hydrogen abstraction barriers and transition states of hydroxylation reactions catalyzed by cytochrome P450 enzymes. *J. Am. Chem. Soc.* 130 (2008): 10128–10140.

93. Shaik, S., Cohen, S., Wang, Y., Chen, H., Kumar, D., and Thiel, W. P450 enzymes: Their structure, reactivity, and selectivity-modeled by QM/MM calculations. *Chem. Rev.* 110 (2010): 949–1017.

94. Kirchmair, J., Göller, A.H., Lang, D., et al. Predicting drug metabolism: Experiment and/or computation? *Nature Rev.* 14 (2015): 387–404.

95. Groves, J.T., McClusky, G.A., White, R.E., et al. Aliphatic hydroxylation by highly purified liver microsomal cytochrome P-450: Evidence for a carbon radical intermediate. *Biochem. Biophys. Res. Commun.* 81 (1978): 154–160.

96. Kamdem, L.K., Flockhart, D.A., and Desta, Z. *In vitro* cytochrome P450-mediated metabolism of exemestane. *Drug Metab. Disp.* 39 (2011): 98–105.

97. Auclair, K., Little, D.M., Ortiz de Montellano, P.R., and Groves, J.T. Revisiting the mechanism of P450 enzymes with the radical clocks norcarane and spiro[2,5]octane. *J. Am. Chem. Soc.* 124 (2002): 6020–6027.

98. Newcomb, M., Hollenberg, P.F., and Coon, M.J. Multiple mechanisms and multiple oxidants in P450-catalyzed hydroxylations. *Arch. Biochem. Biophys.* 409 (2003): 72–79.

99. Jiang, Y., He, X., and Ortiz de Montellano, P.R. Radical intermediates in the catalytic oxidation of hydrocarbons by bacterial and human cytochrome P450 enzymes. *Biochemistry* 45 (2006): 533–542.

100. Hinson, J.A., Mitchell, J.R., and Jollow, D.J. N-Hydroxylation of *p*-chloroacetanilide in hamsters. *Biochem. Pharmacol.* 25 (1975): 599–601.

101. Ortiz de Montellano, P.R., Mangold, B.L.K., Wheeler, C., et al. Stereochemistry of cytochrome P-450 catalyzed epoxidation and prosthetic heme alkylation. *J. Biol. Chem.* 258 (1983): 4208–4213.

102. Harvey, D.J., Glazener, L., Johnson, S.B., et al. Comparative metabolism of four allylic barbiturates and hexobarbital by rat and guinea pig. *Drug Metab. Dispos.* 5 (1977): 527–546.

103. Miller, R.E., and Guengerich, F.P. Oxidation of trichloroethylene by liver microsomal cytochrome P-450: Evidence for chlorine migration in a transition state not involving trichloroethylene oxide. *Biochemistry* 21 (1982): 1090–1097.

104. Shinkyo, R., Xu, L., Tallman, K.A., Cheng, Q., Porter, N.A., and Guengerich, F.P. Conversion of 7-dehydrocholesterol to 7-ketocholesterol is catalyzed by human cytochrome P450 7A1 and occurs by direct oxidation without an epoxide intermediate. *J. Biol. Chem.* 286 (2011): 33021–33028.

105. Correia, M.A., and Hollenberg, P.F. Inhibition of cytochrome P450 enzymes. In: Ortiz de Montellano, P.R., ed. *Cytochrome P450: Structure, Mechanism, and Biochemistry.* 4th ed. (New York: Springer, 2015): 177–259.

106. Kunze, K.L., Mangold, B.L.K., Wheeler, C., et al. The cytochrome P-450 active site. Regiospecificity of the prosthetic heme alkylation by olefins and acetylenes. *J. Biol. Chem.* 258 (1983): 4202–4207.

107. Barker, S.A., Hsieh, L.C., McDowell, T.R., et al. Short, qualitative and quantitative analysis of the anthelminthic febendazole and its metabolites in biological matrices by direct exposure probe mass spectrometry. *Biomed. Environ. Mass Spectrom.* 14 (1987): 161–165.

108. Jerina, D.M., and Daly, J.W. Arene oxides: A new aspect of drug metabolism. *Science* 185 (1974): 1573–1582.

109. Den Besten, C., van Bladeren, P.J., Duizer, E., et al. Cytochrome P450-mediated oxidation of pentafluorophenol to tetrafluorobenzoquinone as the primary reaction product. *Chem. Res. Toxicol.* 6 (1993): 674–680.

110. He, X., Cryle, M.J., De Voss, J.J., et al. Calibration of the channel that determines the ω-hydroxylation regiospecificity of cytochrome P4504A1. Catalytic oxidation of 12-halododecanoic acids. *J. Biol. Chem.* 280 (2005): 22697–22705.

111. Seto, Y., and Guengerich, F.P. Partitioning between N-dealkylation and N-oxygenation in the oxidation of N, N-dialkylarylamines catalyzed by cytochrome P450 2B1. *J. Biol. Chem.* 268 (1993): 9986–9997.

112. Karki, S.B., Dinnocenzo, J.P., Jones, J.P., et al. Mechanism of oxidative amine dealkylation of substituted N, N-dimethylanilines by cytochrome P-450: Application of isotope effect profiles. *J. Am. Chem. Soc.* 117 (1995): 3657–3664.
113. Kammerer, B., Scheible, H., Albrecht, W., et al. Pharmacokinetics of ML3403 ({4-[5-(4-fluorophenyl)-2-methylsulfanyl-3*H*-imidazol-4-yl]pyridine-2-yl}-(1-phenylethyl)-amine, a 4-pyridinylimidazole-type p38 mitogen-activated protein kinase inhibitor. *Drug Metab. Dispos.* 35 (2007): 875–883.
114. Madan, A., Williams, T.D., and Faiman, M.D. Glutathione- and glutathione-S-transferase-dependent oxidative desulfuration of the thione xenobiotic diethyldithiocarbamate methyl ester. Molec. *Pharmacol.* 46 (1994): 1217–1225.
115. Rettie, A.E., Boberg, M., Rettenmeier, A.W., et al. Cytochrome P-450-catalyzed desaturation of valproic acid *in vitro*: Species differences, induction effects, and mechanistic studies. *J. Biol. Chem.* 263 (1988): 13733–13738.
116. Korzekwa, K.R., Trager, W.F., Nagata, K., et al. Isotope effect studies on the mechanism of the cytochrome P450IIA1-catalyzed formation of Δ^6-testosterone from testosterone. *Drug Metab. Dispos.* 18 (1990): 974–979.
117. Vyas, K.P., Kari, P.H., Prakash, S.R., et al. Biotransformation of lovastatin. II. *In vitro* metabolism by rat and mouse liver microsomes and involvement of cytochrome P-450 in dehydrogenation of lovastatin. *Drug Metab. Dispos.* 18 (1990): 218–222.
118. Stearns, R.S., Chakravarty, P.K., Chen, R., et al. Biotransformation of losartan to its active carboxylic acid metabolite in human liver microsomes: Role of cytochrome P4502C and 3A subfamily members. *Drug Metab. Dispos.* 23 (1995): 207–215.
119. Roberts, E.S., Vaz, A.D., and Coon, M.J. Catalysis by cytochrome P-450 of an oxidative reaction in xenobiotic aldehyde metabolism: Deformylation with olefin formation. *Proc. Natl. Acad. Sci. U. S.A.* 88 (1991): 8963–8966.
120. Akhtar, M., Njar, V.C.O., and Wright, J.N. Mechanistic studies on aromatase and related C-C bond cleaving P-450 enzymes. *J. Steroid Biochem. Molec. Biol.* 44 (1993): 375–387.
121. Varfaj, F., Zulkifli, S.N.A., Park, H.-G., Challinor, V.L., De Voss, J.J., and Ortiz de Montellano P.R. Carbon-carbon bond cleavage in activation of the prodrug nabumetone. *Drug Metab. Dispos.* 42 (2014) 828–838.
122. Goeptar, A.R, Scheerens, H., and Vermeulen, N.P.E. Oxygen and xenobiotic reductase activities of cytochrome P450. *Crit. Rev. Toxicol.* 25 (1995): 25–65.
123. Patterson, L.H. Bioreductively activated antitumor N-oxides: The case of AQ4N, a unique approach to hypoxia-activated cancer chemotherapy. *Drug Metab. Rev.* 34 (2002): 581–592.
124. Saunders, M.P., Patterson, A.V., Chinje, E.C., et al. NADPH: Cytochrome c (P450) reductase activates tirapazamine (SR4233) to restore hypoxic and oxic cytotoxicity in anaerobic resistant derivative of the A549 lung cancer cell line. *Brit. J. Cancer* 82 (2000): 651–656.

4

Aldehyde Oxidases an Emerging Group of Enzymes Involved in Xenobiotic Metabolism: Evolution, Structure, and Function

Enrico Garattini and Mineko Terao

CONTENTS

Introduction

It is well established that phase I metabolism of clinically useful drugs is generally carried out by the family of cytochrome P450 mono-oxygenases (CYP450). These enzymes reside in the endoplasmic reticulum of the hepatocyte and oxidize various types of chemical functionalities with particular reference to aromatic rings, which are often the main structural components of different drugs. In spite of this, there is growing evidence for the involvement of a distinct enzyme, i.e. human aldehyde oxidase 1 (AOX1), in phase I metabolism (Garattini and Terao, 2011, 2012, 2013; Pryde et al., 2010). Human AOX1 (EC 1.2.3.1) is a cytosolic enzyme belonging to the family of molybdo-flavoproteins along with other mammalian AOX isoenzymes and the structurally related xanthine oxidoreductase (XOR) protein. AOXs and XOR are distributed throughout the animal kingdom and have been characterized in eukaryotic and prokaryotic organisms (Garattini et al., 2003; Hesberg et al., 2004; Mendel, 2007; Pritsos, 2000; Zhang and Gladyshev, 2008). While a single XOR form is known, up to four different AOXs have been described in insects (Marelja et al., 2014), plants (Kurosaki et al., 2013), and vertebrates (AOX1, AOX2; AOX3; AOX4) (Garattini et al., 2003, 2008; Kurosaki et al., 2013).

Mammalian XOR is the key enzyme in the catabolism of purines, catalyzing the oxidation of hypoxanthine into xanthine as well as xanthine into uric acid, whereas the physiological function of mammalian AOXs is still largely obscure.

The "aldehyde oxidase" denomination is due to the ability of these enzymes to oxidize aldehyde functionalities into the corresponding carboxylic acids. However, it must be stressed that the term is misleading, as aromatic and aliphatic aldehydes are not the major substrates of AOXs. In fact, aza-heterocycles and oxo-heterocycles are a much larger group of substrates that can be efficiently oxidized by AOXs. In the field of drug metabolism, this is the most relevant sub-group of substrates, as aza- and oxo-heterocycles are often present in the backbone of registered drugs and drug candidates. The broad substrate specificity of AOXs is at the basis of the recognized role played by these enzymes in phase I xenobiotic metabolism (Garattini et al., 2008, 2009; Garattini and Terao, 2011, 2012, 2013).

From a general point of view, AOXs are Mo-containing enzymes in which the molybdenum atom is coordinated to a molybdopterin cofactor (Hille, 1996) (Figure 4.1a). Enzymes dependent on this cofactor (Moco) are grouped into: (a) the xanthine oxidase family, (b) the dimethylsulfoxide (DMSO) reductase family, and (c) the sulfite oxidase family (Hille, 1996; Romao et al., 1997). Mammalian AOXs belong to the xanthine oxidase family of molybdoenzymes along with XOR. The primary structure of AOXs and XOR is very similar, and the catalytically active form of both types of enzymes is a homodimer consisting of two 150 kDa subunits (Figure 4.1a). The monomeric subunit of both AOXs and XDHs is divided into three distinct regions: an amino-terminal 25 kDa domain containing two non-identical 2Fe/2S redox centers, a central 40 kDa domain where the FAD-binding site is located, and a carboxy-terminal 85 kDa domain consisting of the Moco-binding site and the substrate pocket. In mammalian AOXs and XOR, the molybdenum atom is coordinated to one pyranopterin *via* two ene-dithiolate ligands, whereas, in the DMSO and sulfite oxidase families, the metal is coordinated into two pyranopterin molecules or one pyranopterin and a cysteine residue, respectively (Romao et al., 1997). The presence of Moco is fundamental for the catalytic activity of AOXs and XOR. Moco is not a dietary component and it is synthesized *de novo* by the living organism (Figure 4.2). Moco synthesis and assembly into AOX and XOR apo-proteins is a complex process, which is controlled by different enzymes. The first step of Moco bio-synthesis is radical-mediated cyclization of GTP to (8S)-3',8-cyclo-7,8-dihydroguanosine 5'-triphosphate (3',8-cH$_2$GTP), which is carried out by Moco Synthesis protein 1A (MOCS1A) in humans (Reiss et al., 1998, 1999). 3',8-cH$_2$GTP is subsequently biotransformed into cyclic pyranopterin monophosphate (cPMP) by MOCS1B (Hover et al., 2013, 2015a, 2015b). This is followed by the conversion of cPMP into molybdopterin (MPT) by MOCS2,

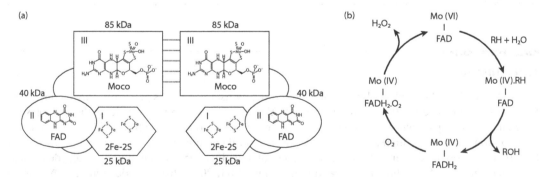

FIGURE 4.1 *Structure and catalytic activity of mammalian AOXs.* (a) All mammalian AOXs consist of two identical subunits divided in three distinct regions. The N-terminal domain containing the two iron-sulfur centers is connected to the FAD-containing intermediate domain *via* an unstructured and poorly conserved hinge region (black line). A second hinge region (black line) links the intermediate domain with the C-terminal Moco domain, which also contains the substrate pocket. (b) The catalytic cycle of AOXs is schematically represented. A generic type of substrate, RH, is oxidized into the corresponding product, ROH with concomitant reduction of Mo[VI] to Mo[IV]. Subsequently, the generated electrons are transferred to FAD with the production of FADH$_2$ and molecular O$_2$ that is the final electron acceptor producing H$_2$O$_2$.

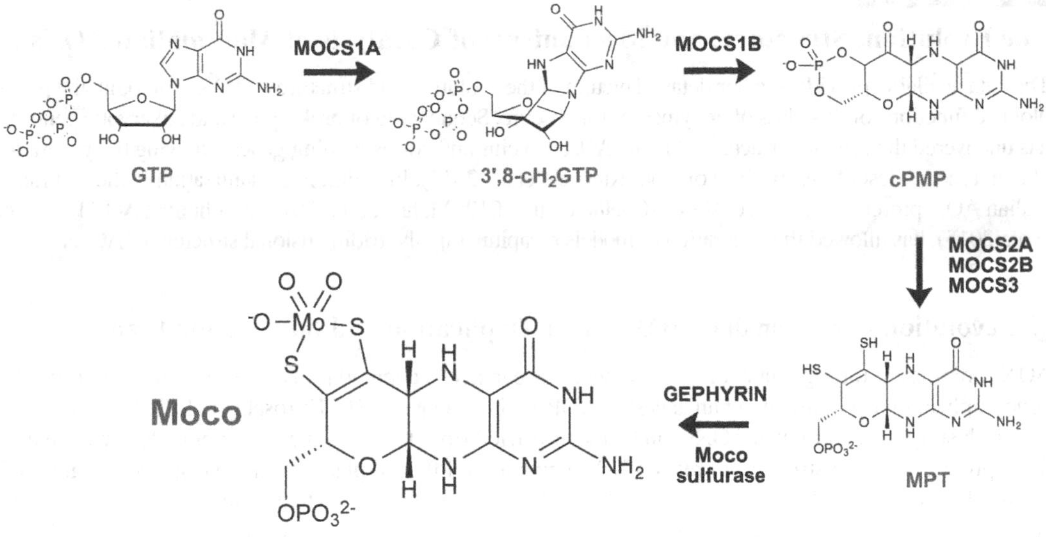

FIGURE 4.2 *Moco biosynthesis.* The figure illustrates the Moco bio-synthetic pathway in humans. GTP = guanosine triphosphate; cPMP = cyclic pyranopterin monophosphate; MPT = molybdopterin; Moco = moybdenum cofactor. The enzymes involved in the biosynthetic pathway are indicated: MOCS1A = molybdenum cofactor synthetase synthesis 1A; MOCS1B = molybdenum cofactor synthetase synthesis 1B; MOCS2A = molybdenum cofactor synthetase synthesis 2A; MOCS2B = molybdenum cofactor synthesis 2B; MOCS3 = molybdenum cofactor synthetase synthesis 3.

a heterodimeric protein consisting of MOCS2A, MOCS2B (Hahnewald et al., 2006; Reiss et al., 1999), and the adenylyltransferase, MOCS3 (Matthies et al., 2005). Finally, gephyrin catalyzes the insertion of molybdate into MPT to generate Moco (Stallmeyer et al., 1999). Given the complexity of the Moco biosynthetic pathway and the number of enzymes involved, it must be emphasized that expression of the AOX genes and corresponding apo-proteins in any given cell type does not guarantee synthesis of the catalytically active holoenzymes. In fact, assembly of the AOX holoezymes requires production of a sufficient amount of MoCo by the complex synthetic machinery, which is not necessarily present in every cell type.

As for the mechanisms of catalysis, XOR can use both NAD^+ and molecular oxygen as the final acceptors of the reducing equivalents generated during substrate oxidation depending on the enzyme being under the dehydrogenase (XDH) or oxidase (XO) form. Indeed, the enzyme can be reversibly or irreversibly converted from XDH to XO, which uses solely molecular oxygen as the electron acceptor. In contrast, the classic reactions catalyzed by AOXs produce electrons, which reduce only molecular oxygen and generate superoxide anions or hydrogen peroxide. The reactions catalyzed by AOXs generate reducing equivalents that lead to the concomitant reduction of molecular oxygen (O_2). O_2 reduction results in the generation of reactive oxygen species (ROS), like hydrogen peroxide and superoxide anions. A typical AOX catalytic cycle is represented in Figure 4.1b. The generic substrate, RH, is oxidized into its product, ROH, at the molybdenum center. The reducing equivalents generated biotransform FAD into $FADH_2$. Subsequently, $FADH_2$ is re-oxidized into FAD by molecular oxygen. The two 2Fe/2S redox centers present in the 25 kDa amino terminal region of AOXs mediate the transfer of electrons between Moco and FAD/$FADH_2$. Hence, they serve as electron sinks for the storage of the reducing equivalents generated during the catalytic cycle.

The objective of the book chapter is to provide an overview of the current knowledge on mammalian AOXs. We will provide information on the structure, evolution, and mechanisms of catalysis of mammalian AOXs. This will be followed by a discussion on the hypotheses regarding the physiological functions of mammalian AOXs. The emerging importance of human AOX1 and mammalian AOXs in xenobiotic metabolism will be covered in the last section, where emphasis will be given to the problems associated with the study of AOX-dependent drug and xenobiotic metabolism.

The Evolution, Structure, and Mechanisms of Catalysis of Mammalian AOXs

The data available provide a rather detailed picture of the evolution and structure of AOXs, although the physiological functions of this class of enzymes is still obscure. Sequencing of prokaryotic and eukaryotic genomes has uncovered the primary structure of many AOX proteins and corresponding genes, allowing the generation of a first model describing AOXs evolution (Kurosaki et al., 2013). In addition, crystallization of the first mammalian AOX protein, i.e., mouse AOX3 (Coelho et al., 2012; Mahro et al., 2011) and human AOX1 (Coelho et al., 2015), has allowed the generation of models recapitulating the tridimensional structure of AOXs.

The Evolution of Mammalian AOXs: Gene Duplication and Inactivation Events

AOXs are present throughout evolution and their appearance is deemed to have resulted from a primordial gene-duplication event involving an ancestral XOR-coding gene (*XDH*) (Kurosaki et al., 2013). The evolutionary history of mammalian AOXs can be reconstructed from the genomic sequencing data available for these proteins and the structurally related XOR enzyme in different plant and animal species (Figure 4.3) (Kurosaki et al., 2013). In vertebrates, a single *XDH* gene is present in practically all species, while the situation for the *AOX* genes is much more complex. Indeed, vertebrate genomes contain one or more *AOX* loci each coding for a distinct AOX isoenzyme, depending on the species considered. In particular, mammals present with a maximum of four *AOX* genes and the two extremes are represented by humans, which are characterized by a single active gene (*AOX1*), and rodents whose genomes contain four *AOX* loci coding for an equivalent number of proteins (AOX1; AOX2, also known as AOX3l1; AOX3; AOX4) (Figure 4.4). The *AOX* loci are structured in small gene clusters mapping to short regions of the same chromosome, namely Chromosome 1 in the case of mice (Kurosaki et al., 2013). The four mouse genes are located in close proximity in a head-to-tail configuration, according to the following order, *Aox1*, *Aox3*, *Aox4*, and *Aox2*.

Vertebrate AOXs and XORs are characterized not only by high levels of similarity in terms of their amino acid sequence, but also as far as the structure of the corresponding genes is concerned. In fact, the *AOX* and *XDH* genes consist of 35 and 36 exons, respectively, and the position of the 35 exon-intron junctions are highly conserved (Garattini et al., 2008; Kurosaki et al., 2013). These data support the idea that AOXs and XOR have the same evolutionary origin. We propose that the complement of vertebrate *AOX* loci results from independent gene-duplication and gene-deletion/inactivation events, which occurred during evolution (Garattini et al., 2008; Kurosaki et al., 2013; Rodriguez-Trelles et al., 2003; Terao et al., 2006). Prokaryotic AOXs are likely to have originated from a primordial gene-duplication event involving an ancestral *XDH* gene (Kurosaki et al., 2013). This was followed by the evolution of two distinct lines of AOXs, as indicated by the position by the two AOX clusters in the evolutionary dendrogram of Figure 4.3. On one hand, bacteria, algae, plant, and insects are characterized by a similar set of AOXs that are located on the right side of the tree whose central portion is occupied by XORs. On the other hand, vertebrate AOXs gather on the left side of the dendrogram, which is consistent with the idea that plant/insect and vertebrate *AOX* genes originated from distinct *XDH* gene-duplication events. Vertebrate AOXs evolution is characterized by a first phase consisting of a species-specific increase in the number of iso-enzymatic forms, which may reflect the necessity to acquire new physiological functions. The genome of the lamprey, the most ancient vertebrate for which sequencing data are available, is apparently devoid of *AOX* loci, although it contains a typical *XDH* gene. Ray-finned fishes are the first vertebrates endowed with *AOX* genes, as their genome is characterized by the presence of two such loci, i.e. *AOXα* and *AOXβ* (Garattini et al., 2008). *AOXα* is proposed to be the product of a first gene-duplication event from vertebrate *XDH*, while *AOXβ* must be the result of an independent and more recent duplication involving *AOXα* (Garattini et al., 2008; Kurosaki et al., 2013). The subsequent evolution of vertebrate *AOX* genes consists of at least two other duplication events, which must have occurred before the appearance of rodents. In mammals, a second evolutionary phase involving a progressive and species-specific deletion or pseudogenization of one or more *AOX* loci followed. In higher primates and humans, this process has resulted in the maintenance of a single active AOX gene, i.e. *AOX1*. In fact, human chromosome 2 presents with the vestiges of the mouse *AOX3* and *AOX2* orthologous genes, which underwent a process of pseudogenization and inactivation with the loss of several exons. No trace of sequences corresponding

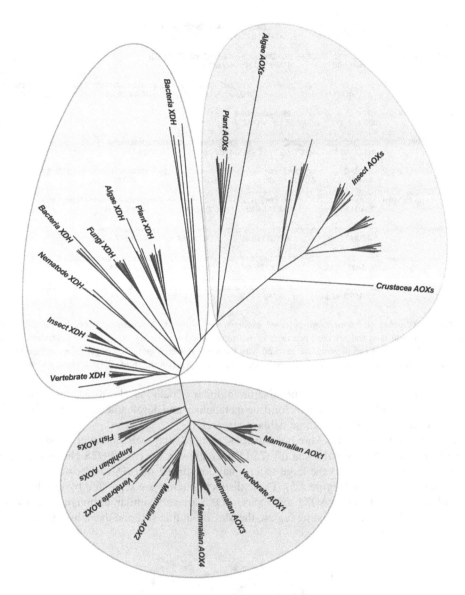

FIGURE 4.3   *Unrooted phylogenetic tree of AOXs and XDHs.* Phylogenesis of AOX isoenzymes and XOR (XDH) proteins in eukaryotes and prokaryotes. The phylogenetic tree is constructed aligning a large number of publicly available sequences using the CLUSTAL omega algorithm.

to the mouse *AOX4* ortholog are evident on chromosome 2 or in any other part of the human genome. In contrast, an active *AOX4* gene can be predicted in *Rhesus* monkeys, which is consistent with an *AOX4* deletion event during evolution from primates to humans. It is interesting to notice that the only active *AOX* gene is *AOX1*, which codes for the most ancient AOX isoform. The observation supports a nonredundant and common functional role of AOX1 in vertebrates.

Insights into the Structure of Mammalian AOXs from the Crystallization of Mouse AOX3 and Human AOX1

The first insights in the structural characteristics of mammalian AOXs derive from the data obtained after mouse liver AOX3 crystallization (Coelho et al., 2012; Mahro et al., 2011). Further information was gathered after crystallization of human AOX1, in its substrate-free form and complexed with the

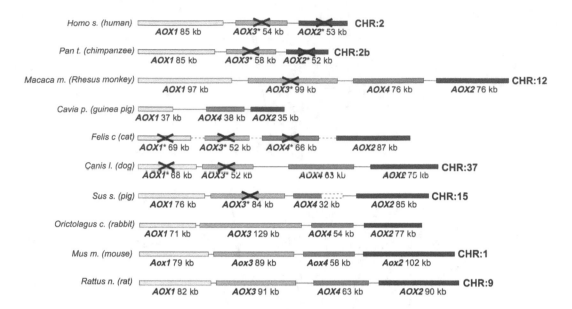

FIGURE 4.4 *AOX genes in humans and selected experimental animals.* A schematic representation of *AOX* genes and pseudogenes in humans and selected primates or mammals used for studies on drug and xenobiotic metabolism. Orthologous *AOX* genes and pseudogenes are marked with the same shade of grey. Pseudogenes are crossed and marked with an asterisk. When determined, the chromosomal location is indicated on the right: CHR = chromosome.

phthalazine substrate as well as the thioridazine inhibitor (Coelho et al., 2015). The resulting structural data have far-reaching implications for drug metabolism and development, given the importance of human AOX1 and mouse AOX3 in these fields of research.

Human AOX1 and mouse AOX3 are homodimeric proteins, and each monomer consists of three different domains: (a) an N-terminal domain I (25 kDa) containing the two 2Fe/2S clusters; (b) the FAD-binding domain II (40 kDa); (c) the large C-terminal domain III (85 kDa) harboring the MoCo- and substrate-interacting regions (Figure 4.5). These distinct domains are separated by two linker regions. The overall structures of human AOX1 and mouse AOX3 are very similar, although remarkable differences are observed in the FAD-binding region, the MoCo-binding site, and the substrate funnel. In both

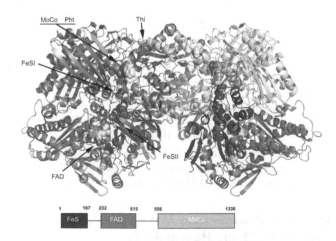

FIGURE 4.5 *Structure the human AOX1 protein.* Ribbon representation of the human AOX1 crystal structure. Monomer A is in gray on left of image and monomer B shows the three different protein domains on right of image: domain I = black (right center); domain II = dark gray (lower right); domain III = light gray (upper right). Domain III is separated from the FAD domain by linker 2. The protein cofactors (Moco, FeSI, FeSII and FAD) are indicated. Pht = phthalazine; Thi = thioridazine.

AOXs and XOR proteins, substrate access to the catalytic site is controlled by a wide and deep funnel. In human AOX1, many of the residues mapping to the entrance of the funnel are mobile and are part of two flexible loops influencing substrates entrance and products release. Thioridazine is an antipsychotic drug that inhibits liver AOX activity (Obach and Walsky, 2005; Rani Basu et al., 2005). Generation of human AOX1 crystals containing both phthalazine and thioridazine demonstrates the presence of distinct binding sites for the substrate and the inhibitor that are located at a remarkable distance from each other. The thioridazine-binding site is structurally conserved in other members of the molybdo-flavoprotein family, such as mouse AOXs and bovine XOR. Steady-state kinetic measurements show non-competitive inhibition of human AOX1 and mouse AOX3 by thioridazine, while bovine XOR is characterized by a mixed inhibition pattern. Finally, crystallization of the human AOX1 phthalazine/thioridazine complex provides information as to the modifications in the active site afforded by substrate/inhibitor binding (Terao et al., 2016).

Computational studies based on the crystal structure of human AOX1 and mouse AOX3 have resulted in the definition of some of the structural determinants modulating the substrate specificity and activity of the other mouse AOX isoforms, i.e. AOX1, AOX2, and AOX4 (Cerqueira et al., 2015). Major differences among mouse AOX1, AOX2, AOX3, and AOX4 are observed in the substrate-binding region. This is the basis of the differences in the catalytic activity and substrate/inhibitor specificities described for the different mouse AOX isoforms (Vila et al., 2004). Indeed, the substrate binding site is likely to consist of two different regions. The first region is common to all AOX isoforms and includes the active site consisting of a series of conserved amino acids (in mouse AOX3: Gln-772, Ala-807, Phe-909, and Phe-1014) as well as Lys-889 and Glu-1266, which are involved in the catalytic activity of these enzymes (Table 4.1, Figures 4.5 and 4.6). The second one is isoform-specific, and it is in the distal half of the catalytic tunnel. The conserved region is likely to control the correct alignment of the substrates into the active site of AOXs, while the variable and isoform-specific region may select the structure of the ligands specifically recognized by AOX1, AOX2, AOX3, and AOX4. Based on the available computational data, it is possible to predict that mouse AOX1 has an isoform-specific region that can accept substrates with variable shape, size, and nature. By converse, mouse AOX4 is predicted to bind only small and very hydrophobic substrates.

The Catalytic Activity of Mammalian AOXs

The development of efficient systems for the production and isolation of catalytically active mammalian AOX proteins is of fundamental importance to the study of the substrate specificity of this class of enzymes (Alfaro et al., 2009; Hartmann et al., 2012; Mahro et al., 2011). From a practical point of view, the availability of these tools would be of great help in the context of drug-development programs for identifying molecules that can be metabolized by AOXs.

Efficient expression of native and site-directed mutants of human and mouse AOX1 as well as mouse AOX3 in *E. coli* has provided new insights into the amino acid residues (Table 4.1) critical for the

TABLE 4.1

Comparison of the Relevant Amino Acid Residues of Human AOX1, Mouse AOX1, Mouse AOX2, Mouse AOX3, Mouse AOX4 and Bovine XOR

Human AOX1	Mouse AOX1	Mouse AOX2	Mouse AOX3	Mouse AOX4	Bovine XOR
Gln-776	Gln-771	Gln-782	Gln-772	Gln-774	Gln-767
Val-811	Val-806	Val-817	Ala-807	Val-809	Glu-802
Met-889	Met-884	Phe-895	Tyr-885	Phe-887	Arg-880
Lys-893	Lys-888	Lys-899	Lys-889	Lys-891	His-884
Phe-923	Phe-918	Phe-929	Phe-919	Phe-921	Phe-914
Leu-1018	Leu-1013	Phe-1024	Phe-1014	Val-1016	Phe-1009
Glu-1270	Glu-1265	Glu-1276	Glu-1266	Glu-1267	Glu-1261

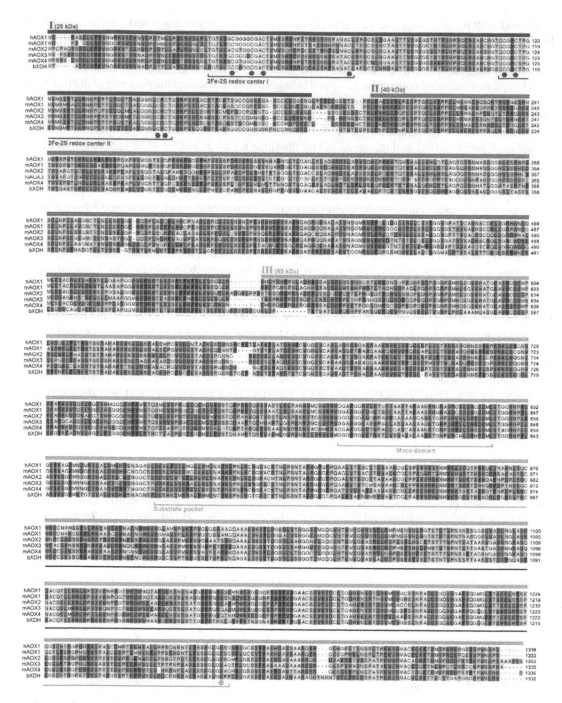

FIGURE 4.6 *Sequence alignment of human AOX1, mouse AOXs and bovine XDH.* The bovine XDH (bXDH) sequence is shown as a reference to highlight the sequence similarities between mammalian AOXs and XDH. The dark gray line above the sequences indicates the 25 kDa domain I containing the two 2Fe/2S redox centers whose eight cystein residues chelating the iron atoms are indicated by dark gray hexagon. The medium gray line indicates the 40 kDa domain II which contains the FAD binding site. The light gray line indicates the 85 kDa domain III which contains with the Moco binding site (Moco domain) and the substrate pocket as indicated. The Glu residue playing a fundamental role in the mechanisms of catalysis is marked by a light gray hexagon.

enzymatic activity of these proteins (Hartmann et al., 2012; Mahro et al., 2011; Schumann et al., 2009). As already observed in the case of XOR, the Glu residue present in the active site of AOXs (human AOX1 = Glu-1270; mouse AOX1 = Glu-1265; mouse AOX3 = Glu-1266) is essential for the catalytic activity of these enzymes. In fact, substitution of the amino acid with a Gln residue in mouse and human AOX1 inactivate the two enzymes (Mahro et al., 2013; Schumann et al., 2009). The situation is more complicated in the case of mouse AOX3, as the Glu-1266-Gln mutant maintains enzymatic activity with certain types of substrates, such as benzaldehyde, while it is inactive when challenged with N-heterocyclic compounds (Mahro et al., 2013).

The presence of highly conserved residues at the catalytic center (human AOX1: Glu-1270, Phe-923, Gln-776) (Table 4.1), suggests that the reaction mechanism of AOXs and XOR is similar, although the two types of enzymes have different substrate specificities (Cerqueira et al., 2015; Coelho et al., 2012; Mahro et al., 2013). One major difference between AOXs and XOR is represented by the Lys-893 residue (human AOX1 numbering). In fact, Lys-893 is a strictly conserved amino acid in AOXs, while it is substituted by an equally conserved His residue in XOR (bovine XOR: His-884). Lys-893 is located at a distance of approximately 10Å from the Mo center and 6Å from Glu-1270. Substrate docking into the active site causes the corresponding Lys residue of mouse AOX3 (Lys-889) to move from its original position, as indicated by molecular dynamics simulations (Coelho et al., 2012). The movement establishes new interactions with the mouse AOX3 residue equivalent to human Glu 1270 (Glu 1266) and/or the substrate itself.

The bovine XOR amino acids deemed to be involved in substrate binding, i.e. Glu-802 and Arg-880, are substituted by Val and Met, respectively, in human AOX1, as well as Ala and Tyr in mouse AOX3 (Schumann et al., 2009) (Table 4.1). In human XOR, substitution of these Glu and Arg residues with Val and Met, respectively, results in loss of activity towards purines as substrates and gain of activity towards aldehydes (Schumann et al., 2009; Yamaguchi et al., 2007). This indicates that the two residues contribute to substrate binding and determine substrate specificity. Specular substitutions of Val-806 with Glu and Met-884 with Arg in mouse AOX1 abolish catalytic activity when both purines and aldehydes are used as substrates (Schumann et al., 2009).

The influence exerted by two conserved residues (Ala-807 and Tyr-885) involved in substrate binding on the catalytic activity of mouse AOX3 has been investigated (Mahro et al., 2011). Mutation of Ala-807 into Val does not alter the kinetic constants when AOX3 is exposed to small substrates, like benzaldehyde or phthalazine. By converse, a slight decrease in the affinity for bulky substrates, such as phenanthridine, and a slight increase in catalytic efficiency are observed. As for the substitution of Tyr-885 with Met, the kinetic constants are also largely unaffected by small hydrophobic substrates, like benzaldehyde and phthalazine. In contrast, the Tyr-885-Met mutant converts bulkier substrates (phenanthridine) and charged substrates, such as N1-methylnicotinamide, more efficiently. Presumably, this is due to the greater flexibility of the Met side chain that facilitates binding of these substrates. All these effects are more evident if the double site-directed mutants of mouse AOX3 are considered.

Tissue Distribution, Regulation Endogenous Substrates, and Physiological Function of Mammalian AOXs

Although the role exerted by mammalian AOXs in drug and xenobiotic metabolism is ascertained, the physiological function(s) as well as the substrates and products of these enzymes are either unknown or just hypothesized. Another unclear aspect of AOX physiological function(s) is the reason as to why certain species of mammals are characterized multiple AOX isoenzymes, while the majority of primates as well as humans present with a single AOX protein. Since the decrease in the number of AOX isoenzymes from rodents to humans is the consequence of an evolutionary process involving the progressive deletion/inactivation of the relative genes, it can be hypothesized that the lost enzymes are not necessary for the homeostasis of the human organism. It can be also envisaged that the functional roles played by rodent AOX1, AOX2, AOX3, and AOX4 are concentrated in human AOX1. Indeed, it is possible that the evolutionary changes in the structure of human AOX1 broadened the range of substrates recognized by this enzyme to molecules originally specific to AOX2, AOX3, and AOX4. It can be equally hypothesized that mouse AOX2, AOX3, and AOX4 exert specialized functions in organs that have become dispensable in humans.

Tissue- and Cell-Specific Expression Profiles of Human AOX1 and Mouse AOXs

Comparison of the tissue- and cell distribution of human AOX1 and mouse AOX1, AOX2, AOX3, and AOX4 provides clues as to the role played by AOXs in physiological processes other than xenobiotic metabolism. In addition, the distribution data in humans and mouse gives hints on the relevance of mouse as a pre-clinical model to study the metabolism of drugs and xenobiotics, which are proved AOX substrates. A comparison between humans and mice is warranted because the mouse is a popular experimental animal and it is endowed with the maximum number of AOX isoenzymes observed in mammals.

The UNIGENE (UniGene Hs.406238) profile of human AOX1 mRNA tissue-specific expression (Figure 4.7) indicates that the transcript is detectable in various tissues. High levels of AOX1 mRNA are available in the adrenal gland, adipose tissue, and liver, followed by trachea, bone, kidney, and connective tissue. This is consistent with many of the results obtained at the protein level (Moriwaki et al., 2001). According to these last data, the richest source of human AOX1 is the liver, although significant amounts of the protein are present also in the respiratory, digestive, urogenital, and endocrine organs. High levels of the AOX1 protein are available in the tracheal and bronchial epithelium as well as the lung alveolar cells. Similarly, the epithelial component of the small and large intestine contains detectable amounts of human AOX1. Kidney tubules are endowed with significant levels of AOX1, while the glomeruli do not stain positive for the protein. The glandular epithelium of the prostate is also enriched in AOX1 protein. The large amounts of AOX1 protein present in the adrenal gland cortex are in line with role of the enzyme in steroid hormone synthesis. There is a single published study (Berger et al., 1995) on the expression of human AOX1 mRNA in the central nervous system (CNS) that demonstrates the presence of the transcript in the glial cells of the spinal cord.

Relative to human AOX1, the UNIGENE data indicate that the tissue-specific expression profile of the mouse orthologous mRNA (UNIGENE Mm.26787) is restricted (Figure 4.7). The richest sources of mouse AOX1 mRNA are the inner ear and the seminal vesicles followed by the liver and lung. Mouse AOX1 mRNA is also detectable in the CNS with particular reference to specific neuronal cells in the brain and the motoneuronal population of the spinal cord (Bendotti et al., 1997). This last observation is consistent with what reported for the human orthologue (Berger et al., 1995). Nevertheless, the highest levels of AOX1 mRNA are located in the epithelial layer of the choroid plexus, where the corresponding protein may be involved in cerebrospinal fluid absorption/secretion. It is worthwhile noting that the main sources of human and mouse AOX1 are not the same, with the exception of liver. The tissue-specific expression of mouse AOX3 mRNA (UNIGENE Mm.20108) is also restricted, being limited to the oviduct, liver, lung, and testis. Thus, mouse AOX3 and AOX1 seem to be co-expressed only in liver and lung. The tissue-distribution data for mouse AOX1 and AOX3 mRNAs levels are fully confirmed if the corresponding proteins are taken into consideration (Kurosaki et al., 1999; Terao et al., 2000). *In situ* hybridization experiments indicate that liver AOX1 and AOX3 mRNAs are synthesized by the hepatocyte, although it is unclear whether the same hepatocytic population is responsible for AOX1 and AOX3 synthesis. From a functional point of view, it would be important to understand why mouse and rat livers are endowed with AOX3 and AOX1, while the same organs in humans and other mammalian species contain only AOX1 (Vila et al., 2004). This is of particular interest in consideration of the fact that the mouse liver contains much higher levels of AOX3 than AOX1.

Large amounts of mouse AOX4 mRNA (UNIGENE Mm.244525) are observed in the fertilized ovum, the inner ear, and tongue (Figure 4.7). In the tongue, the AOX4 transcript is mainly expressed in the keratin-rich epithelial cells of the taste papillae (Terao et al., 2001). In the first part of the gastrointestinal tract, AOX4 mRNA expression extends to the keratinized epithelium lining the esophagus and the upper section of the stomach. Specific expression of the AOX4 mRNA and protein in keratinized epithelia is supported by the results obtained in the epidermal layer of the skin (Terao et al., 2009). However, the richest source of AOX4 is an organ present in most vertebrates, but not in humans and the majority of primates, i.e. the Harderian gland. The Harderian gland is an exocrine gland of the orbital cavity that secretes a lipid-rich fluid, which lubricates the eye surface and the fur (Buzzell, 1996; Hardeland et al., 2006; Payne, 1994). In furred animals, the fluid is a thermal isolator and contributes to the regulation of body temperature. Interestingly, skin sebaceous glands, which are related to and are also involved in fur lubrication and thermoregulation, are characterized by the same developmental origin as the Harderian gland and the same high levels of AOX4 (Terao et al., 2009).

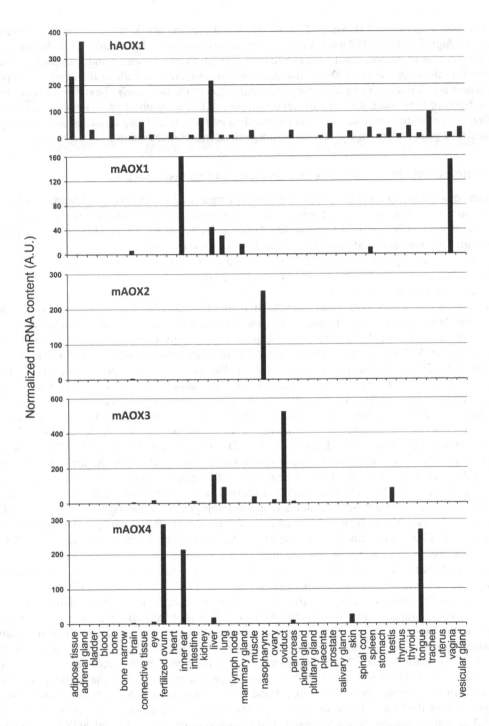

FIGURE 4.7 *Expression profiles of human AOX1 and mouse AOX1-AOX4.* The bar graphs indicate the normalized mRNA content of the indicated AOXs in the tissues considered. The results are based on the data contained in the UNIGENE section of the NCBI site: hAOX1 = human AOX1 (UniGene Hs.406238); mAOX1 = mouse AOX1 (UNIGENE Mm.26787); mAOX2 = mouse AOX2 (UNIGENE Mm.414292); mAOX3 = mouse AOX3 (UNIGENE Mm.20108); mAOX4 = mouse AOX4 (UNIGENE Mm.244525).

The mouse AOX2 mRNA (UNIGENE Mm.414292) is detectable only in the nasal cavity (Figure 4.7). In this site, high levels of AOX2 mRNA and protein are observed in the Bowman's gland, the major exocrine structure of the sub-mucosal layer (Terao et al., 2000). The Bowman's gland secretes the mucous fluid bathing the nasal cavity. AOX2 is also detectable in sustentacular cells of the nasal neuroepithelium, which are characterized by the same embryonal origin as the Bowman's gland (Huard et al., 1998). On the basis of these data, it can be hypothesized that AOX2 is involved in olfaction. The olfactory function is significantly more developed in rodents than humans, which may be the reason as to why the human *AOX2* gene underwent a process of pseudogenization and inactivation.

Regulation of Mammalian AOXs by Intrinsic and Extrinsic Factors

The number of studies on the factors and mechanisms regulating the expression of human AOX1 and other mammalian AOXs is limited. However, a discussion of the available data is of relevance for the role played by human AOX1 and other mammalian AOXs in drug metabolism. In addition, it may provide further hints as to the potential physiological functions of these enzymes.

Development and age control AOXs expression. Data on the influence exerted by the two factors on AOXs levels are available in humans and rodents. As for humans, young children (13 days to 4 months after birth) are known to express low levels of hepatic AOX1 enzymatic activity and protein. AOX1 activity and protein augment significantly in children after four months of age and reach adult levels by approximately two years of age (Tayama et al., 2012). These results are consistent with the data available on a larger cohort of children who were obtained with a non-invasive method based on the determination of the AOX1-dependent N(1)-methylnicotinamide metabolic product, pyridine, in the urine (Tayama et al., 2007a). As for rodents, limited data on the age-dependent expression of rat and mouse AOXs are available. In rat liver, AOX activity is barely detectable before 15 days from birth. From the second week of age, a rapid increase in AOX activity, which reaches a plateau at four weeks, is evident (Tayama et al., 2007b). However, these data do not take into account the fact that the AOX activity measured in rat liver is the sum of the enzymatic activities corresponding to AOX1 and AOX3. Thus, it would be important to know the developmental profile of expression of each single AOX isoenzyme. In fact, it is likely that the age-related expression profiles of liver AOX1 and AOX3 are distinct, as indicated by the data obtained in mice. In this rodent, liver AOX3 appears more precociously than the AOX1 isoenzyme (Terao et al., 2000). Mouse embryos are devoid of AOX3 and AOX1 mRNAs or proteins. The AOX3 protein is detectable in newborn animals and its levels plateau at five days. In contrast, the AOX1 counterpart is measurable only in adult animals. Currently, the effects exerted by aging on rodent liver AOX1 and AOX3 are unknown. By the same token, data on the developmental profiles of AOX2 and AOX4 in the tissues that express the two isozymes are not available.

A second factor influencing AOX expression is sex, which seems to control mouse liver AOX activity *via* the corresponding steroid hormones (Holmes, 1979; Ventura and Dachtler, 1980, 1981; Yoshihara and Tatsumi, 1997). In mice, liver AOX activity is higher in males than females. Castration of male mice or estrogen administration reduces liver AOX activity and administration of testosterone in castrated animals compensates this reduction. By converse, testosterone administration to female animals stimulates liver AOX activity. The results suggest that the androgen/estrogen ratio influences liver AOX enzymatic activity. The effects exerted by sex hormones on liver AOX activity are due to modulation of liver AOX1 and AOX3 mRNA as well as protein levels. In fact, the challenge of female animals with testosterone up-regulates AOX1 and AOX3 mRNAs, which results in a corresponding up-regulation of the encoded proteins and enzymatic activities (Kurosaki et al., 1999; Terao et al., 2000). The stimulating action of testosterone is not limited to mouse AOX1 and AOX3, as it extends to AOX4. In the Harderian gland, the levels of AOX4 are generally similar in adult male and female animals, although there is a restricted time-window in which the enzyme shows sexual dimorphism. At nine weeks of age, female Harderian glands contain significantly higher levels of AOX4 than the male counterparts (Terao et al., 2009). This is due to the suppressive action exerted by circulating testosterone on AOX4 expression. Thus, testosterone triggers an opposite effect on Harderian gland AOX4 and liver AOX1/AOX3 expression. In humans, the role played by gender and sex hormones on AOX1 expression is unclear, as a single study on the topic is available. In this study, the levels of

AOX1 protein were determined in the liver of few human donors using a mass-spectrometry assay. No significant difference was observed in female and male individuals (Fu et al., 2013).

Another intrinsic factor involved in the control of mammalian AOXs expression is circadian rhythm, as originally observed in guinea pig liver. In this animal, diurnal variations in AOX activity seem to be consequent to circadian variations in circulating melatonin (Beedham et al., 1989). Indeed, liver AOX enzymatic activity is increased by exposure to melatonin *via* undefined mechanisms. In mice, diurnal variations in liver AOX enzymatic activity are due to circadian oscillations in the levels of AOX1 and AOX3, which tend to be higher during the dark phase of the diurnal cycle (Terao et al., 2016). In this animal species, circadian variations in the expression levels are not a characteristic of AOX1 and AOX3, as they are observed also in the case of Harderian gland AOX4.

Knowledge on the extrinsic factors controlling AOX activity is of relevance to avoid toxic effects or a decrease in the therapeutic efficacy of drugs known to be metabolized by human AOX1. Specific components of the diet are among the extrinsic factors controlling AOXs activity and/or levels in humans and other mammals. Relative to appropriate control animals, diabetic rats show increased levels of AOX enzymatic activity in different tissues. In rats characterized by a streptozotocin-induced diabetic state, oral administration of vitamin E or sodium selenite reduces AOX activity in the liver, while it has no effect on the kidney or heart counterpart (Ghaffari et al., 2012). Consistent with this, selenium-deficient rats show an increase in the levels of liver AOX1 protein (Itoh et al., 2009). Tea consumption may also cause a decrease in AOX activity. In fact, exposure of human and rat liver cytosolic preparations to epicatechin or epicatechin gallate, two components of green tea, cause a significant inhibition of AOX enzymatic activity (Tayama et al., 2011).

Some environmental pollutants, toxic agents, and drugs modulate AOX levels or activity and may influence the therapeutic effects or toxicity of drugs that are AOX substrates. Phthalazine or 1-hydroxyphthalazine increases the enzymatic activity of rabbit liver AOX (Johnson et al., 1984), which is similar to what is observed in rats exposed to the alkylating agents, N-methyl-N'-nitro-N-nitrosoguanidine, N-methyl-N-nitrosourea, and methylmethansulfonate (Ohkubo et al., 1983a). Mouse AOX1 expression is induced by 2,3,7,8-tetrachlorodibenzo-p-dioxin (dioxin) in the *Hepa-1* hepatoma cell line and mouse liver because of the transcriptional effect triggered by the aryl-hydrocarbon-receptor (AHR) (Rivera et al., 2005). A transcriptional mechanism is also involved in the induction of mouse liver AOX1 mRNA following exposure to the chemopreventive agent, phenethyl isothiocyanate (Hu et al., 2006). In this case, the transcription factor that mediates AOX1 induction is NRF2, which seems to be a direct regulator of the corresponding gene. The rat and human *AOX1* orthologous genes are also direct targets of NRF2 (Maeda et al., 2012).

Predicted and Identified Endogenous Substrates of Mammalian AOXs

Clues as to the potential physiological function of human AOX1 and other mammalian AOXs may be gathered by the identification of endogenous substrates and products. Although direct evidence is not available, the KEGG database (http.//www.kegg.jp) implicates mammalian AOXs in several metabolic pathways. The involvement of AOXs in these pathways is generally speculative and based on indirect evidence indicating that selected endogenous molecules can be metabolized by AOX preparations of different origins. It must be emphasized that KEGG annotations are often based on the assumption that aliphatic or aromatic aldehydes are the sole substrates of AOXs, while AOXs hydroxylate many heterocyclic structures that are devoid of aldehyde functionalities. In addition, there is no *in vivo* evidence supporting the role of AOXs in any of the metabolic steps present in the KEGG database, with the exception of the few data obtained in the *Aox4* knock-out mouse (Terao et al., 2009). Finally, there is a virtual absence of data on the specificity of the proposed endogenous substrates for AOX1, AOX2, AOX3, or AOX4, which is a further problem for the mammalian species characterized by multiple AOX isoenzymatic forms. Despite these problems and biases, AOXs, including human AOX1, are deemed to be implicated in the following metabolic pathways: (a) *ec00280*: Valine, leucine and isoleucine degradation; (b) *ec00350*: Tyrosine metabolism; (c) *ec00380*: Tryptophan metabolism; (d) *ec00750*: vitamin B6 metabolism; (e) *ec00760*: nicotinate and nicotinamide metabolism; (f) *ec00830*: retinol metabolism.

In *ec00280*, human AOX1 is suggested to be involved into the oxidation of the L-valine catabolic product, (S)-methylmalonate semialdehyde, which results in the production of methylmalonate. In *ec00350*, the predicted AOX substrate is gentisate aldehyde that is transformed into gentisate. In the KEGG database, AOXs are predicted to be involved in tryptophan metabolism (*ec00380*), as they have the potential to oxidize 5-hydroxy indolacetaldehyde, a serotonin catabolite, into 5-hydroxy-indolacetic acid. Interestingly, recent metabolomics data obtained in the *Aox4* knock-out animal demonstrate that tryptophan and 5-hydroxy-indolacetic acid levels are much higher in the Harderian gland of these genetically engineered mice than in their wild-type counterparts (Terao et al., 2016). Further data generated with purified AOX4 and AOX3 proteins indicate that tryptophan and 5-hydroxy-indolacetic acid are also substrates of the two enzymes (Terao et al., 2016).

The inclusion of AOXs in the *ec00750* pathway is due to the fact that pyridoxal (vitamin B6) is a well-known AOX substrate (Schwartz and Kjeldgaard, 1951). AOXs metabolize pyridoxal into 4-pyridoxate, and the metabolic step is of physiological significance in insects (Cypher et al., 1982; Stanulovic and Chaykin, 1971). Interestingly, the isolated mouse AOX1 and AOX3 proteins recognize pyridoxal as a substrate, while the compound is not recognized by AOX4. Consistent with this, the phenotypes described in *Aox4* knock-out mice are not reconducible to alterations of vitamin B6 catabolism (Terao et al., 2009).

As for the role played in the *ec00760* pathway, human (Sugihara et al., 1997), monkey (Sugihara et al., 1997), rat (Ohkubo et al., 1983b), rabbit (Stoddart and Levine, 1992), and guinea pig (Yoshihara and Tatsumi, 1985) liver AOX(s) is capable of oxidizing N1-methyl-nicotinamide, a nicotinamide catabolic product, into N1-methyl-2-pyridone-5-carboxamide and N1-methyl-4-pyridone-5-carboxamide. N1-methyl-nicotinamide is the sole example of non-aldehydic AOX substrate included in the KEGG database. Human AOX1 is also hypothesized to oxidize nicotinamide riboside to 4-pyridone-3-carboxamide-1-β-d-ribonucleoside (PYR) (Pelikant-Malecka et al., 2015). Noticeably, PYR is an endothelial toxin that contributes to kidney insufficiency in uremic patients (Pelikant-Malecka et al., 2015).

The final KEGG pathway characterized by an AOX annotation is *ec00830*, which centers on vitamin A metabolism. Indeed, AOXs are implicated in the oxidation of 9-cis and all-trans retinal (RAL) to retinoic acid. All-trans retinoic acid (ATRA) is the active metabolite of vitamin A and it is a physiologically relevant molecule in the developing and adult organisms. Currently, RAL is the AOX candidate substrate for which the greatest amount of supporting evidence is available. Endogenous ATRA synthesis is a two-step process, involving a first step characterized by retinol oxidation into RAL *via* a reversible reaction catalyzed by various alcohol dehydrogenases (Molotkov et al., 2002). This is followed by an irreversible oxidative step resulting in the biotransformation of RAL into ATRA, which is purported to be predominantly carried out by the NAD-dependent aldehyde dehydrogenases, ALDH1A1, ALDH1A2, and ALDH1A3 (Niederreither et al., 1999). In mice and other mammals, AOXs are likely to catalyze the same metabolic step as ALDH1As. In fact, semi-purified rabbit liver AOX preparations are capable of oxidizing RAL into ATRA in a NAD-independent fashion (Huang and Ichikawa, 1994; Tomita et al., 1993; Tsujita et al., 1994). In addition, purified mouse AOX1 (Huang et al., 1999; Vila et al., 2004), AOX3 (Terao et al., 2001), AOX4 (Terao et al., 2009), and AOX2 (Kurosaki et al., 2004) recognize RAL as a substrate. AOXs are unlikely to oxidize RAL in mammalian embryos, as AOX enzymatic activity is detectable only after birth, at least in rodents. In adult mouse liver, AOX1 and AOX3 are equally unlikely to play a major role in ATRA synthesis given the low affinity of RAL for the two AOXs, the high levels of ALDH1A1, and cytosolic NAD-dependent RAL oxidizing activity (Terao et al., 2009). The same may be true for other mouse tissues characterized by co-expression of AOXs with ALDH1As. In contrast, mouse organs expressing AOX4, like the Harderian gland, tongue and skin, may represent rich sources of AOX-dependent ATRA synthesis (Terao et al., 2009). Indeed, *Aox4* knock-out mice show much lower levels of ATRA in the Harderian gland and skin relative to wild-type animals (Terao et al., 2009).

Clues on the Potential Physiological Function(s) of Mammalian AOXs

Although the number of relevant studies using direct approaches is very limited, the data available indicate that AOXs are involved in a varied array of physiological processes carried out by different tissues and cell types. In lung cells, human AOX1 contributes to the maintenance of the epithelial barrier integrity. In the 16HBE bronchial epithelial cell line, dexamethasone causes a marked increase in AOX1 expression, which is associated with a corresponding decrease in inter-cellular permeability. This recapitulates what is observed in asthmatic patients, where treatment with inhaled corticosteroids enhances the airway epithelial barrier integrity. In the same cell line, AOX1 knock-down blocks the decrease in inter-cellular permeability triggered by dexamethasone, suggesting a role for AOX1 in the control of cell-to-cell junctions (Shintani et al., 2015). Mouse AOX1 is implicated in the differentiation of myocytes along the myotube pathway, as the process is associated with AOX1 up-regulation and myotube fusion is blocked by AOX1 silencing (Kamli et al., 2014). Noticeably, myotube fusion involves an increase in inter-cellular contacts, which suggests that mouse and human AOX1 play a similar role in bronchial epithelial cells and developing myocytes, i.e. control of cell-cell interactions. The action exerted by AOX1 in bronchial and muscular cells may involve the production of H_2O_2 by the enzyme (Kamli et al., 2014).

Adipogenesis and liver fat storage are two other highly related processes mammalian AOXs contribute to. In pre-adipocytic mouse 3T3L1 cells, AOX1 is up-regulated in concomitance with adipocyte differentiation. In addition, fenofibrate, a hypocholesterolemic agent, down-regulates AOX1 in differentiated cells. AOX1 knock-down in preadipocytes, suppresses the storage of lipids and the secretion of adiponectin (a protein hormone stimulating fatty acid oxidation) subsequently activated in the differentiated adipocytes (Weigert et al., 2008). A role for AOXs in adipogenesis is further suggested by the high levels of AOX1 detected in human adipocytes (Weigert et al., 2008). As already alluded to, AOXs exert an action on lipid homeostasis not only in the adipose tissue, but also in the liver. In fact, AOX1 activity is increased during the process of steatosis triggered in rat liver by exposure to high-fat diets and administration of adiponectin or fenofibrate reduces the levels of hepatic AOX activity (Neumeier et al., 2006). The action of AOX1 on lipid homeostasis may be independent of its enzymatic activity. In contrast, it may be related to the interaction of AOX1 with the ABCA-1 lipid transporter, which is involved in the control of lipid efflux from the cell (Graessler and Fischer, 2007; Sigruener et al., 2007). AOX1 is not the only AOX isoenzyme involved in lipid homeostasis, as AOX4 seems to play a similar role in the process. Consistent with this, *AOX4* knock-out mice show resistance to obesity as well as hepatic steatosis upon exposure to high-fat diets. The two phenomena are accompanied by decreased fat deposition in visceral adipose tissue (Terao et al., 2016). The involvement of AOX4 in fat accumulation at the level of adipose tissue and liver is likely to be mediated by a systemic action of the enzyme. In fact, mouse adipocytes and hepatocytes do not synthesize detectable amounts of the AOX4 protein or mRNA. Interestingly, a similar resistance to obesity has been described in *Aldh1a1* knock-out mice exposed to high-fat diets (Ziouzenkova et al., 2007). Since both AOX4 and ALDH1a1 control the oxidation of RAL into ATRA, it is possible that the two retinoids are involved in fat deposition and resistance to obesity.

A last biological process for which there is direct evidence regarding the involvement of AOXs is nitric oxide synthesis, a process controlling local blood flow as well as the homeostasis of endothelial and other cell types under hypoxic conditions. During hypoxia, mammalian AOXs can reduce nitrite into nitric oxide (Li et al., 2008), and this enzymatic reaction has been shown to be particularly efficient in hepatocytes and human mammary epithelial cells grown under low oxygen tension (Maia et al., 2015).

The Role of Mammalian AOXs in Xenobiotic Metabolism

The role of human AOX1 in phase I metabolism of xenobiotics is well established, and the interest in this enzyme and other members of the AOX family is increasing given their emerging significance in drug-development programs (Garattini and Terao, 2011, 2012, 2013). In this last context, a major problem is represented by the animal models used during the preclinical phases of drug development aimed at evaluating the metabolism, pharmacokinetics, and pharmacodynamics of new therapeutic agents. Unlike humans, some of the most popular animal models are characterized by expression of other AOXs besides AOX1, as discussed in previous sections of the book chapter.

The Emerging Relevance of Mammalian AOXs in the Metabolism of Drugs

Mammalian AOXs are characterized by broad substrate specificity and recognize a variety of organic molecules regardless of the presence of an aldehyde function. These enzymes hydroxylate various aza-, oxo-, and sulfo-heterocycles and oxidize iminium functions to cyclic lactames. In certain conditions, such as hypoxia, AOXs act also as reductases, reducing N-oxides, sufoxides, nitro-compounds, and heterocycles (Dick et al., 2006; Kitamura and Tatsumi, 1984a, 1984b). All this along with the high levels of human AOX1 and mammalian AOX1 and/or AOX3 in liver is the basis for the role played by the two types of enzymes in drug and xenobiotic metabolism (Coelho et al., 2012; Sanoh et al., 2015; Zientek and Youdim, 2015). Indeed, the main function of AOXs and cytochrome P450 mono-oxygenases (CYP450s) in hepatic cells seems to be overlapping, as both types of enzymes are involved in the biotransformation/ inactivation of therapeutic agents and toxicants. While CYP450s are in the endoplasmic reticulum, the sub-cellular localization of AOX1 and AOX3 is the cytosol. Occasionally, AOXs and CYP450s act in concert, as exemplified by the SSRI (selective serotonin reuptake inhibitors), citalopram, whose tertiary amino group is oxidized to an aldehyde by CYP450 (Figure 4.8). Subsequently, AOX1 and/or AOX3 biotransform the aldehyde into the corresponding carboxylic acid. A variety of drugs are metabolized by AOXs, including anti-tumor, immunosuppressive, anti-malarial, and anti-viral agents as well as molecules acting in the central nervous system. As for the anti-tumor and immunosuppressive agents metabolized by AOXs, methotrexate and 6-mercaptopurine are two prominent examples. Methotrexate is oxidized into 7-hydroxy-methotrexate (Figure 4.8) by human AOX1 as well as rabbit, rat, mouse, and hamster AOXs (Chladek et al., 1997; Kitamura et al., 1999). AOX-dependent hydroxylation is fundamental for the pharmacokinetics and side effects of methotrexate, as 7-hydroxy-metotrexate is cytotoxic. In humans, methotrexate oxidation into 7-hydroxy-methotrexate is subject to inter-individual variability, and the biotransformation step is correlated to the levels of AOX1 enzymatic activity (Kitamura et al., 1999). 6-mercaptopurine, a major metabolite of the other immunosuppressant, azathioprine, is also a long-known AOX substrate (Beedham et al., 1987; Ding and Benet, 1979; Rooseboom et al., 2004). The imidazole ring of 6-mercaptopurine undergoes two successive hydroxylation steps, which are catalyzed by XOR and AOXs, respectively (Figure 4.8). AOX-dependent hydroxylation leads to metabolic inactivation and contributes to the pharmacokinetic profile of 6-mercaptopurine in humans and experimental animals. A last example of an immunosuppressant for which some of the toxic metabolites are generated by AOX1 is thiopurine (Chouchana et al., 2012).

Other well-known drugs for which there is evidence of AOX-dependent metabolism are certain anti-malarial and anti-viral agents. For instance, the anti-malarial cryptolepine (Figure 4.8) is oxidized to cryptolepine-11-one by rabbit liver AOX activity (Stell et al., 2012). Quinine is a further example of anti-malarial drug whose bio-disposition is dependent on AOX activity, which generates the 2-quinone derivative (Beedham et al., 1992). Dog and rat livers contain undetectable and low levels of cytosolic quinine oxidase activity, respectively. The first observation is consistent with the absence of AOX1 and AOX3 proteins (Terao et al., 2006) in dog liver due to pseudogenization/inactivation of the corresponding genes (Kurosaki et al., 2013). In contrast, the observation made in rats suggests that quinine is a much better substrate of AOX3 than AOX1. The hypothesis is supported by the results obtained in baboon liver, which contains high levels of quinine oxidizing activity despite pseudogenization/inactivation of the *AOX3* gene (Kurosaki et al., 2013). Further support is provided by the observation that guinea pig and marmoset livers, which are also characterized by deletion and pseudogenization of the *AOX3* gene (Kurosaki et al., 2013), oxidize quinine into 2-quinone at the same extent as the human counterpart.

There are at least three issues that should be considered in discussing the role played by human AOX1 and other mammalian AOXs in drug metabolism. First, AOX-dependent metabolic inactivation of drugs does not simply involve oxidation, as these AOXs are also capable of reducing appropriate substrates, as already mentioned. With respect to this, a relevant example is ziprasidone, which is used for the treatment of different psychiatric disorders. In humans, ziprasidone is reduced by AOX1 and subsequently methylated by thiol-methyl-transferase (Obach et al., 2012). Second, AOX-dependent oxidation of drugs does not necessarily cause metabolic inactivation. In fact, metabolic activation of prodrugs by human AOX1 has been exploited to avoid pharmacokinetic problems. A relevant example of this strategy is represented by the clinical development of the 5-iodo-2-deoxyuridine precursor, 5-iodo-2-pyrimidinone-2-deoxyribose

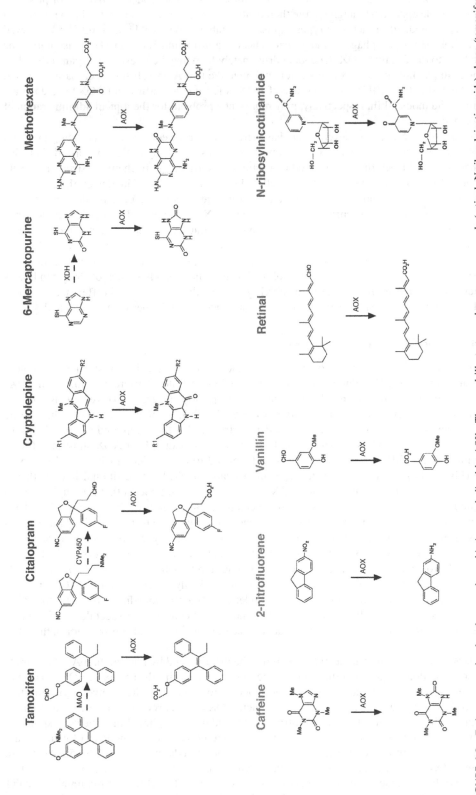

FIGURE 4.8 *Endogenous molecules, drugs and xenobiotics metabolized by AOXs.* The panel illustrates endogenous compounds (retinal, N-ribosylnicotinamide), drugs (tamoxifen, citalopram, cryptolepin, 6-mercaptopurine, methotrexate), xenobiotics of toxicological interest (caffeine, 2-nitrofluorene, vanillin) and AOX-dependent metabolites. When AOXs act on metabolic intermediates of the parental drug, the enzymes involved in the primary metabolic step are also indicated: MAO = monoamine oxidase; CYP450 = cytochrome P450 dependent mono-oxygenase; XDH = xanthine dehydrogenase.

(Kinsella et al., 1994, 1998, 2000). In the near future, human AOX1-dependent activation of prodrugs may represent a viable approach to augment the therapeutic index of anti-tumor agents via an increase in tumor selectivity. Indeed, different tumor types express detectable amounts of human AOX1, as observed in the case of glioblastoma, esophageal, and gastric cancer (Garattini and Terao, 2011). A last point to be mentioned relates to the fact that AOX-dependent drug metabolism may be relevant in organs other than the liver. For example, human skin explants can metabolize the two AOX substrates, carbarazepan and zoniporide (Manevski et al., 2014). The presence of AOX1 (Terao et al., 2016) and AOX4 (Terao et al., 2009) in human and mouse skin, respectively, may represent a problem for the topical administration of drugs and cosmetics.

The importance of AOXs in drug development has increased over the course of the last few years with the synthesis of an ever increasing number of organic molecules specifically designed to avoid CYP450-dependent metabolism. In fact, this has resulted in a significant enrichment in chemical structures likely to be metabolized by human AOX1 (Barr et al., 2014; Fratelli et al., 2013; Hutzler et al., 2013). The problem has led to new medicinal chemistry approaches aimed at avoiding AOX-dependent metabolism (Pryde et al., 2012). In addition, the enrichment in potential AOX substrates underscores the importance of the availability of appropriate *in vitro* screening assays to validate AOX-dependent metabolism. Such assays are likely to become fundamental tools in any drug development program (Garattini and Terao, 2011, 2013). A further problematic issue in drug development is represented by the selection of the most appropriate *in vivo* model to study the pharmacokinetics and pharmacodynamics of drug candidates with the potential to be metabolized by human AOX1, given the already discussed differences between humans and many mammalian species in the complement of active *AOX* genes (Figures 4.4 and 4.7).

AOX Substrates of Toxicological Interest

AOXs metabolize not only drugs, but also various molecules of toxicological interest, such as phthalazines, which are environmental pollutants and are typical AOX substrates. Different mammalian AOXs oxidize phthalazine into 1-hydroxy-phthalazine, which, subsequently, undergoes irreversible isomerization into 1-phthalazinone (Beedham et al., 1990; Coelho et al., 2015; Stubley et al., 1979). Phthalazine administration increases rabbit liver AOX activity, demonstrating that the compound is not only a substrate, but it is also an AOX inducer (Johnson et al., 1984). Another example of AOX substrate of toxicological significance is caffeine, which is rapidly metabolized to an oxo-derivative by AOXs (Castro et al., 2001) (Figure 4.8). Vanillin, a sweetener, is an aromatic aldehyde of nutritional interest that is oxidized into a carboxylic acid by mammalian AOXs (Figure 4.8). A last toxicant that is thought to be an AOX substrate is acetaldehyde, the primary ethanol metabolite. Based on this observation, AOXs have been implicated in the liver toxicity associated with alcohol consumption. The hypothesized mechanism underlying AOX-dependent liver toxicity is the production of reactive oxygen species during acetaldehyde oxidation (Shaw and Jayatilleke, 1990). However, the results obtained in the liver of AOX deficient *DBA/2* and AOX proficient *CD1* mice are not consistent with the hypothesis. In fact, *CD1* and *DBA/2* mice, whose livers contain undetectable levels of AOX3 and markedly lower amounts of AOX1 relative to *CD1* animals, show the same amounts of liver acetaldehyde after ethanol administration (Vila et al., 2004). This supports the concept that neither liver AOX1 nor AOX3 contributes to acetaldehyde metabolism in mice. The finding is also in line with the fact that acetaldehyde is a bad substrate for both AOX1 and AOX3.

Another class of toxic agents that has the potential to be metabolized by mammalian AOXs consists of nitro compounds. Molecules containing a nitro functionality exemplify the ability of AOXs to act not only as oxidases, but also as reductases in the presence of electron donors, such as 2-hydroxypyrimidine (Tatsumi et al., 1986; Ueda et al., 2003, 2005). In fact, AOXs can carry out the nitro-reduction of the widespread pollutants, 2-nitrofluorene, 1-nitro-pyrene, and 4-nitrobiphenyl into the corresponding amines. Interestingly, AOX-dependent nitro-reduction is observed not only in the liver (Tatsumi et al., 1986), but also in the skin of experimental animals, like mice (Ueda et al., 2003, 2005). As mouse liver expresses AOX1 and AOX3, while the main enzyme expressed in mouse skin is AOX4, nitro-reduction may not be a characteristic of a specific AOX isoenzyme. The ability of mammalian AOX1 to carry out nitro-reduction and the presence of AOXs in the skin has far-reaching implications for the human situation. In fact, human skin contains AOX1 enzymatic activity (Manevski et al., 2014), and AOX-dependent reduction of environmental nitro-compounds may represent a defense reaction in man and various other mammalian species. A further example of AOX-dependent nitro-reductive metabolism is represented by the neonicotinoid, imidacloprid. Neonicotinoids are insecticides whose nitroimino functionality is reduced by AOXs *in vitro*. The relative contribution of liver AOXs and CYP450s in the metabolism of the neonicotinoid, imidacloprid, was recently assessed *in vivo* (Swenson and Casida, 2013). Addition of the AOX inhibitors, tungsten or hydralazine, in the drinking water of C57BL/6J mice causes a selective reduction in the levels of liver AOX activity and no change in CYP450 activity. In tungsten and hydralazine treated mice, CYP450-dependent imidacloprid metabolism is unaffected, whereas the AOX-generated nitrosoguanidine metabolite is significantly decreased. The study provides direct *in vivo* evidence that mouse liver AOX1 and AOX3 play a major role in the reduction of imidacloprid.

Single Nucleotide Polymorphisms Affecting Human AOX1 Activity

The ever-increasing significance of human AOX1 in drug and xenobiotic metabolism has spurred interest in the identification of single nucleotide polymorphisms (SNPs), which may affect the expression or the catalytic activity of the enzyme. Identification of this type of SNPs in the human population is likely to allow the definition of fast and slow metabolizers as for known or predicted AOX1 substrates. Indeed, SNPs mapping to the coding region of the human *AOX1* gene are likely to represent a major source of inter-individual variability as to AOX1 activity. Various *AOX1* SNPs are listed in the NCBI database (http://www.ncbi.nlm.nih.gov/snp). The allelic frequency of some of these SNPs was determined in 180 Northern Italian volunteers (Hartmann et al., 2012), which led to the identification of one non-sense, one synonymous, and five non-synonymous polymorphisms. *R1297K* is the most frequent non-synonymous polymorphism followed by the *L1271S* and *N1135S* AOX1 variants. The amino acid substitutions, *R802C* and *R921H* are characterized by a much lower frequency. The recombinant *R802C* and *R921H* AOX1 proteins have reduced catalytic activity upon challenge with a number of classic substrates, while the *N1135S* and *H1297R* variants are endowed with increased enzymatic activity. Thus, individuals characterized by the presence of the *R802C* or *R921H* and the *N1135S* or *H1297R* variants, respectively, are predicted to be poor and extensive metabolizers of drugs biotransformed by human AOX1. A similar situation is observed in certain strains of rats, where non-synonymous polymorphisms affect the catalytic activity of certain AOXs (Adachi et al., 2007; Hartmann et al., 2012).

Conclusion

Thanks to the recent crystallization of mouse AOX3 (Coelho et al., 2012; Mahro et al., 2011) and human AOX1 (Coelho et al., 2015), fundamental insights into the tridimensional structure of mammalian AOXs are now available. In addition, the development of efficient methods for the purification of recombinant mammalian AOXs has provided an ever-increasing amount of data on the mechanisms underlying the catalytic activity of these enzymes. Despite this, we are still far away from the solution of a fundamental problem in mammalian AOXs biology. In fact, it remains to be established why a single AOX isoform is present in humans, while multiple enzyme isoforms have been described in other mammalian species. An answer to this specific issue may come from the identification of common and specific substrates for human AOX1 and the other mouse AOX isoforms.

The sequencing data available for a series of prokaryotic and eukaryotic genomes has allowed the determination of the primary structure of many AOX proteins (Kurosaki et al., 2013) as well as the prediction of the complement of active and inactive *AOX* genes in a significant number of vertebrate species. This type of information is of major interest from a basic and an applied point of view. At the basic level, it has permitted the reconstruction of AOXs evolution. At the applied level, with particular reference to the realms of pharmacology and toxicology, the data available have permitted the identification of the AOX isoforms expressed in animal models used for the pre-clinical studies of new drug candidates.

In the drug-development field, AOX-dependent metabolism is becoming a serious problem (Garattini and Terao, 2012, 2013). In fact, an ever-increasing number of new drug candidates are based on chemical structures, which are designed to avoid CYP450-dependent metabolism and inactivation. Unfortunately, this organic synthesis strategy has resulted in an enrichment for chemical structures recognized by human AOX1 (Pryde et al., 2012). As common models, like mice and rats, do not recapitulate the human situation in terms of AOX-dependent metabolism, pre-clinical pharmacokinetics and pharmacodynamics studies performed in these animal species on potential AOX-substrates are unlikely to provide clinically useful results. This has been proposed as the basis of the possible failures of drugs metabolized by human AOX1 in clinical trials (Choughule et al., 2013, 2015; Dalvie et al., 2013; Diamond et al., 2010). The available genomic data indicate that the best animal models for the study of drugs predicted to be human AOX1 targets are the chimpanzee, followed by the guinea pig and the pig, since the corresponding livers express only the human AOX1 orthologous protein (Figure 4.4). However, it should be noted that guinea pigs and pigs are likely to express AOX2 and AOX4 in tissues other than the liver, which may represent a serious confounding factor. The problem represented by a good and cost-effective experimental model may be solved with the development of a genetically engineered animal expressing human AOX1 in the context of an AOX-null mouse or rat. Another important issue in the fields of drug development and environmental toxicology, which has been touched upon in this chapter, is the development of simple *in vitro* paradigms to be used for the prediction of human AOX1-dependent metabolism. Cellular models genetically engineered for the efficient expression of human AOX1 and the availability of an *E. coli* system for the production of the human AOX1 recombinant protein are likely to address this issue.

A last point that should be stressed in the current discussion on mammalian AOXs is the primary physiological role of this class of enzymes, which is unlikely to be xenobiotic metabolism. In fact, multiple human tissues, some of which are characterized by very specialized functions, express significant amounts AOX1. In addition, the expression of rodent AOX1, AOX2, AOX3, and AOX4 is tissue-specific. The data obtained on the *Aox4* knock-out mouse demonstrate an involvement of AOX4 in the systemic control of circadian rhythms, locomotor activity, and adipogenesis (Terao et al., 2016). In particular, AOX4 inactivation causes resistance to obesity due to reduced fat deposition in the adipose tissue. With respect to this, it is interesting to notice that human AOX1 is likely to exert a similar action in the adipocyte (Sigruener et al., 2007; Weigert et al., 2008). This finding is of potential interest in the field of medicinal chemistry, since human AOX1 may represent a new and viable target for the development of specific inhibitors as potential anti-obesity drugs.

REFERENCES

Adachi, M., Itoh, K., Masubuchi, A., Watanabe, N., and Tanaka, Y. (2007). Construction and expression of mutant cDNAs responsible for genetic polymorphism in aldehyde oxidase in Donryu strain rats. *J Biochem Mol Biol 40*, 1021–1027.

Alfaro, J.F., Joswig-Jones, C.A., Ouyang, W., Nichols, J., Crouch, G.J., and Jones, J.P. (2009). Purification and mechanism of human aldehyde oxidase expressed in Escherichia coli. *Drug Metab Dispos 37*, 2393–2398.

Barr, J.T., Choughule, K., and Jones, J.P. (2014). Enzyme kinetics, inhibition, and regioselectivity of aldehyde oxidase. *Methods Mol Biol 1113*, 167–186.

Beedham, C., al-Tayib, Y., and Smith, J.A. (1992). Role of guinea pig and rabbit hepatic aldehyde oxidase in oxidative in vitro metabolism of cinchona antimalarials. *Drug Metab Dispos 20*, 889–895.

Beedham, C., Bruce, S.E., Critchley, D.J., al-Tayib, Y., and Rance, D.J. (1987). Species variation in hepatic aldehyde oxidase activity. *Eur J Drug Metab Pharmacokinet 12*, 307–310.

Beedham, C., Bruce, S.E., Critchley, D.J., and Rance, D.J. (1990). 1-substituted phthalazines as probes of the substrate-binding site of mammalian molybdenum hydroxylases. *Biochem Pharmacol 39*, 1213–1221.

Beedham, C., Padwick, D.J., al-Tayib, Y., and Smith, J.A. (1989). Diurnal variation and melatonin induction of hepatic molybdenum hydroxylase activity in the guinea-pig. *Biochem Pharmacol 38*, 1459–1464.

Bendotti, C., Prosperini, E., Kurosaki, M., Garattini, E., and Terao, M. (1997). Selective localization of mouse aldehyde oxidase mRNA in the choroid plexus and motor neurons. *Neuroreport 8*, 2343–2349.

Berger, R., Mezey, E., Clancy, K.P., Harta, G., Wright, R.M., Repine, J.E., Brown, R.H., Brownstein, M., and Patterson, D. (1995). Analysis of aldehyde oxidase and xanthine dehydrogenase/oxidase as possible candidate genes for autosomal recessive familial amyotrophic lateral sclerosis. *Somat Cell Mol Genet 21*, 121–131.

Buzzell, G.R. (1996). The Harderian gland: Perspectives. *Microsc Res Tech 34*, 2–5.

Castro, G.D., Delgado de Layno, A.M., Costantini, M.H., and Castro, J.A. (2001). Cytosolic xanthine oxido-reductase mediated bioactivation of ethanol to acetaldehyde and free radicals in rat breast tissue. Its potential role in alcohol-promoted mammary cancer. *Toxicology 160*, 11–18.

Cerqueira, N.M., Coelho, C., Bras, N.F., Fernandes, P.A., Garattini, E., Terao, M., Romao, M.J., and Ramos, M.J. (2015). Insights into the structural determinants of substrate specificity and activity in mouse aldehyde oxidases. *J Biol Inorg Chem 20*, 209–217.

Chladek, J., Martinkova, J., and Sispera, L. (1997). An in vitro study on methotrexate hydroxylation in rat and human liver. *Physiol Res 46*, 371–379.

Chouchana, L., Narjoz, C., Beaune, P., Loriot, M.A., and Roblin, X. (2012). Review article: The benefits of pharmacogenetics for improving thiopurine therapy in inflammatory bowel disease. *Aliment Pharmacol Ther 35*, 15–36.

Choughule, K.V., Barr, J.T., and Jones, J.P. (2013). Evaluation of rhesus monkey and guinea pig hepatic cytosol fractions as models for human aldehyde oxidase. *Drug Metab Dispos 41*, 1852–1858.

Choughule, K.V., Joswig-Jones, C.A., and Jones, J.P. (2015). Interspecies differences in the metabolism of methotrexate: An insight into the active site differences between human and rabbit aldehyde oxidase. *Biochem Pharmacol 96*, 288–295.

Coelho, C., Foti, A., Hartmann, T., Santos-Silva, T., Leimkuhler, S., and Romao, M.J. (2015). Structural insights into xenobiotic and inhibitor binding to human aldehyde oxidase. *Nat Chem Biol 11*, 779–783.

Coelho, C., Mahro, M., Trincao, J., Carvalho, A.T., Ramos, M.J., Terao, M., Garattini, E., Leimkuhler, S., and Romao, M.J. (2012). The first mammalian aldehyde oxidase crystal structure: Insights into substrate specificity. *J Biol Chem 287*, 40690–40702.

Cypher, J.J., Tedesco, J.L., Courtright, J.B., and Kumaran, A.K. (1982). Tissue-specific and substrate-specific detection of aldehyde and pyridoxal oxidase in larval and imaginal tissues of Drosophila melanogaster. *Biochem Genet 20*, 315–332.

Dalvie, D., Xiang, C., Kang, P., and Zhou, S. (2013). Interspecies variation in the metabolism of zoniporide by aldehyde oxidase. *Xenobiotica 43*, 399–408.

Diamond, S., Boer, J., Maduskuie, T.P., Jr., Falahatpisheh, N., Li, Y., and Yeleswaram, S. (2010). Species-specific metabolism of SGX523 by aldehyde oxidase and the toxicological implications. *Drug Metab Dispos 38*, 1277–1285.

Dick, R.A., Kanne, D.B., and Casida, J.E. (2006). Substrate specificity of rabbit aldehyde oxidase for nitrogua-nidine and nitromethylene neonicotinoid insecticides. *Chem Res Toxicol 19*, 38–43.

Ding, T.L. and Benet, L.Z. (1979). Comparative bioavailability and pharmacokinetic studies of azathioprine and 6-mercaptopurine in the rhesus monkey. *Drug Metab Dispos 7*, 373–377.

Fratelli, M., Fisher, J.N., Paroni, G., Di Francesco, A.M., Pierri, F., Pisano, C., Godl, K., Marx, S., Tebbe, A., Valli, C. et al. (2013). New insights into the molecular mechanisms underlying sensitivity/resistance to the atypical retinoid ST1926 in acute myeloid leukaemia cells: The role of histone H2A.Z, cAMP-dependent protein kinase A and the proteasome. *Eur J Cancer 49*, 1491–1500.

Fu, C., Di, L., Han, X., Soderstrom, C., Snyder, M., Troutman, M.D., Obach, R.S., and Zhang, H. (2013). Aldehyde oxidase 1 (AOX1) in human liver cytosols: Quantitative characterization of AOX1 expression level and activity relationship. *Drug Metab Dispos 41*, 1797–1804.

Garattini, E., Fratelli, M., and Terao, M. (2008). Mammalian aldehyde oxidases: Genetics, evolution and bio-chemistry. *Cell Mol Life Sci 65*, 1019–1048.

Garattini, E., Fratelli, M., and Terao, M. (2009). The mammalian aldehyde oxidase gene family. *Hum Genomics 4*, 119–130.

Garattini, E., Mendel, R., Romao, M.J., Wright, R., and Terao, M. (2003). Mammalian molybdo-flavoenzymes, an expanding family of proteins: Structure, genetics, regulation, function and pathophysiology. *Biochem J 372*, 15–32.

Garattini, E. and Terao, M. (2011). Increasing recognition of the importance of aldehyde oxidase in drug development and discovery. *Drug Metab Rev 43*, 374–386.

Garattini, E. and Terao, M. (2012). The role of aldehyde oxidase in drug metabolism. *Expert Opin Drug Metab Toxicol 8*, 487–503.

Garattini, E. and Terao, M. (2013). Aldehyde oxidase and its importance in novel drug discovery: Present and future challenges. *Expert Opin Drug Discov 8*, 641–654.

Ghaffari, T., Nouri, M., Saei, A.A., and Rashidi, M.R. (2012). Aldehyde and xanthine oxidase activities in tissues of streptozotocin-induced diabetic rats: Effects of vitamin E and selenium supplementation. *Biol Trace Elem Res 147*, 217–225.

Graessler, J. and Fischer, S. (2007). The dual substrate specificity of aldehyde oxidase 1 for retinal and acetaldehyde and its role in ABCA1 mediated efflux. *Horm Metab Res 39*, 775–776.

Hahnewald, R., Leimkuhler, S., Vilaseca, A., Acquaviva-Bourdain, C., Lenz, U., and Reiss, J. (2006). A novel MOCS2 mutation reveals coordinated expression of the small and large subunit of molybdopterin synthase. *Mol Genet Metab 89*, 210–213.

Hardeland, R., Pandi-Perumal, S.R., and Cardinali, D.P. (2006). Melatonin. *Int J Biochem Cell Biol 38*, 313–316.

Hartmann, T., Terao, M., Garattini, E., Teutloff, C., Alfaro, J.F., Jones, J.P., and Leimkuhler, S. (2012). The impact of single nucleotide polymorphisms on human aldehyde oxidase. *Drug Metab Dispos 40*, 856–864.

Hesberg, C., Hansch, R., Mendel, R.R., and Bittner, F. (2004). Tandem orientation of duplicated xanthine dehydrogenase genes from Arabidopsis thaliana: Differential gene expression and enzyme activities. *J Biol Chem 279*, 13547–13554.

Hille, R. (1996). The mononuclear molybdenum enzymes. *Chem Rev 96*, 2757–2816.

Holmes, R.S. (1979). Genetics, ontogeny, and testosterone inducibility of aldehyde oxidase isozymes in the mouse: Evidence for two genetic loci (Aox-1 and Aox-2) closely linked on chromosome 1. *Biochem Genet 17*, 517–527.

Hover, B.M., Lilla, E.A., and Yokoyama, K. (2015a). Mechanistic investigation of cPMP synthase in molybdenum cofactor biosynthesis using an uncleavable substrate analogue. *Biochemistry 54*, 7229–7236.

Hover, B.M., Loksztejn, A., Ribeiro, A.A., and Yokoyama, K. (2013). Identification of a cyclic nucleotide as a cryptic intermediate in molybdenum cofactor biosynthesis. *J Am Chem Soc 135*, 7019–7032.

Hover, B.M., Tonthat, N.K., Schumacher, M.A., and Yokoyama, K. (2015b). Mechanism of pyranopterin ring formation in molybdenum cofactor biosynthesis. *Proc Natl Acad Sci USA 112*, 6347–6352.

Hu, R., Xu, C., Shen, G., Jain, M.R., Khor, T.O., Gopalkrishnan, A., Lin, W., Reddy, B., Chan, J.Y., and Kong, A.N. (2006). Identification of Nrf2-regulated genes induced by chemopreventive isothiocyanate PEITC by oligonucleotide microarray. *Life Sci 79*, 1944–1955.

Huang, D.Y., Furukawa, A., and Ichikawa, Y. (1999). Molecular cloning of retinal oxidase/aldehyde oxidase cDNAs from rabbit and mouse livers and functional expression of recombinant mouse retinal oxidase cDNA in Escherichia coli. *Arch Biochem Biophys 364*, 264–272.

Huang, D.Y. and Ichikawa, Y. (1994). Two different enzymes are primarily responsible for retinoic acid synthesis in rabbit liver cytosol. *Biochem Biophys Res Commun 205*, 1278–1283.

Huard, J.M., Youngentob, S.L., Goldstein, B.J., Luskin, M.B., and Schwob, J.E. (1998). Adult olfactory epithelium contains multipotent progenitors that give rise to neurons and non-neural cells. *J Comp Neurol 400*, 469–486.

Hutzler, J.M., Obach, R.S., Dalvie, D., and Zientek, M.A. (2013). Strategies for a comprehensive understanding of metabolism by aldehyde oxidase. *Expert Opin Drug Metab Toxicol 9*, 153–168.

Itoh, K., Adachi, M., Sato, J., Shouji, K., Fukiya, K., Fujii, K., and Tanaka, Y. (2009). Effects of selenium deficiency on aldehyde oxidase 1 in rats. *Biol Pharm Bull 32*, 190–194.

Johnson, C., Stubley-Beedham, C., and Stell, J.G. (1984). Elevation of molybdenum hydroxylase levels in rabbit liver after ingestion of phthalazine or its hydroxylated metabolite. *Biochem Pharmacol 33*, 3699–3705.

Kamli, M.R., Kim, J., Pokharel, S., Jan, A.T., Lee, E.J., and Choi, I. (2014). Expressional studies of the aldehyde oxidase (AOX1) gene during myogenic differentiation in C2C12 cells. *Biochem Biophys Res Commun 450*, 1291–1296.

Kinsella, T.J., Kunugi, K.A., Vielhuber, K.A., McCulloch, W., Liu, S.H., and Cheng, Y.C. (1994). An in vivo comparison of oral 5-iodo-2′-deoxyuridine and 5-iodo-2-pyrimidinone-2′-deoxyribose toxicity, pharmacokinetics, and DNA incorporation in athymic mouse tissues and the human colon cancer xenograft, HCT-116. *Cancer Res 54*, 2695–2700.

Kinsella, T.J., Kunugi, K.A., Vielhuber, K.A., Potter, D.M., Fitzsimmons, M.E., and Collins, J.M. (1998). Preclinical evaluation of 5-iodo-2-pyrimidinone-2′-deoxyribose as a prodrug for 5-iodo-2′-deoxyuridine-mediated radiosensitization in mouse and human tissues. *Clin Cancer Res 4*, 99–109.

Kinsella, T.J., Schupp, J.E., Davis, T.W., Berry, S.E., Hwang, H.S., Warren, K., Balis, F., Barnett, J., and Sands, H. (2000). Preclinical study of the systemic toxicity and pharmacokinetics of 5-iodo-2-deoxypyrimidinone-2′-deoxyribose as a radiosensitizing prodrug in two, non-rodent animal species: implications for phase I study design. *Clin Cancer Res 6*, 3670–3679.

Kitamura, S., Sugihara, K., Nakatani, K., Ohta, S., Ohhara, T., Ninomiya, S., Green, C.E., and Tyson, C.A. (1999). Variation of hepatic methotrexate 7-hydroxylase activity in animals and humans. *IUBMB Life 48*, 607–611.

Kitamura, S. and Tatsumi, K. (1984a). Involvement of liver aldehyde oxidase in the reduction of nicotinamide N-oxide. *Biochem Biophys Res Commun 120*, 602–606.

Kitamura, S. and Tatsumi, K. (1984b). Reduction of tertiary amine N-oxides by liver preparations: Function of aldehyde oxidase as a major N-oxide reductase. *Biochem Biophys Res Commun 121*, 749–754.

Kurosaki, M., Bolis, M., Fratelli, M., Barzago, M.M., Pattini, L., Perretta, G., Terao, M., and Garattini, E. (2013). Structure and evolution of vertebrate aldehyde oxidases: From gene duplication to gene suppression. *Cell Mol Life Sci 70*, 1807–1830.

Kurosaki, M., Demontis, S., Barzago, M.M., Garattini, E., and Terao, M. (1999). Molecular cloning of the cDNA coding for mouse aldehyde oxidase: Tissue distribution and regulation in vivo by testosterone. *Biochem J 341 (Pt 1)*, 71–80.

Kurosaki, M., Terao, M., Barzago, M.M., Bastone, A., Bernardinello, D., Salmona, M., and Garattini, E. (2004). The aldehyde oxidase gene cluster in mice and rats. Aldehyde oxidase homologue 3, a novel member of the molybdo-flavoenzyme family with selective expression in the olfactory mucosa. *J Biol Chem 279*, 50482–50498.

Li, H., Cui, H., Kundu, T.K., Alzawahra, W., and Zweier, J.L. (2008). Nitric oxide production from nitrite occurs primarily in tissues not in the blood: Critical role of xanthine oxidase and aldehyde oxidase. *J Biol Chem 283*, 17855–17863.

Maeda, K., Ohno, T., Igarashi, S., Yoshimura, T., Yamashiro, K., and Sakai, M. (2012). Aldehyde oxidase 1 gene is regulated by Nrf2 pathway. *Gene 505*, 374–378.

Mahro, M., Bras, N.F., Cerqueira, N.M., Teutloff, C., Coelho, C., Romao, M.J., and Leimkuhler, S. (2013). Identification of crucial amino acids in mouse aldehyde oxidase 3 that determine substrate specificity. *PLoS One 8*, e82285.

Mahro, M., Coelho, C., Trincao, J., Rodrigues, D., Terao, M., Garattini, E., Saggu, M., Lendzian, F., Hildebrandt, P., Romao, M.J., et al. (2011). Characterization and crystallization of mouse aldehyde oxidase 3: From mouse liver to Escherichia coli heterologous protein expression. *Drug Metab Dispos 39*, 1939–1945.

Maia, L.B., Pereira, V., Mira, L., and Moura, J.J. (2015). Nitrite reductase activity of rat and human xanthine oxidase, xanthine dehydrogenase, and aldehyde oxidase: Evaluation of their contribution to NO formation in vivo. *Biochemistry 54*, 685–710.

Manevski, N., Balavenkatraman, K.K., Bertschi, B., Swart, P., Walles, M., Camenisch, G., Schiller, H., Kretz, O., Ling, B., Wettstein, R., et al. (2014). Aldehyde oxidase activity in fresh human skin. *Drug Metab Dispos 42*, 2049–2057.

Marelja, Z., Dambowsky, M., Bolis, M., Georgiou, M.L., Garattini, E., Missirlis, F., and Leimkuhler, S. (2014). The four aldehyde oxidases of Drosophila melanogaster have different gene expression patterns and enzyme substrate specificities. *J Exp Biol 217*, 2201–2211.

Matthies, A., Nimtz, M., and Leimkuhler, S. (2005). Molybdenum cofactor biosynthesis in humans: Identification of a persulfide group in the rhodanese-like domain of MOCS3 by mass spectrometry. *Biochemistry 44*, 7912–7920.

Mendel, R.R. (2007). Biology of the molybdenum cofactor. *J Exp Bot 58*, 2289–2296.

Molotkov, A., Fan, X., Deltour, L., Foglio, M.H., Martras, S., Farres, J., Pares, X., and Duester, G. (2002). Stimulation of retinoic acid production and growth by ubiquitously expressed alcohol dehydrogenase Adh3. *Proc Natl Acad Sci USA 99*, 5337–5342.

Moriwaki, Y., Yamamoto, T., Takahashi, S., Tsutsumi, Z., and Hada, T. (2001). Widespread cellular distribution of aldehyde oxidase in human tissues found by immunohistochemistry staining. *Histol Histopathol 16*, 745–753.

Neumeier, M., Hellerbrand, C., Gabele, E., Buettner, R., Bollheimer, C., Weigert, J., Schaffler, A., Weiss, T.S., Lichtenauer, M., Scholmerich, J., et al. (2006). Adiponectin and its receptors in rodent models of fatty liver disease and liver cirrhosis. *World J Gastroenterol 12*, 5490–5494.

Niederreither, K., Subbarayan, V., Dolle, P., and Chambon, P. (1999). Embryonic retinoic acid synthesis is essential for early mouse post-implantation development. *Nat Genet 21*, 444–448.

Obach, R.S., Prakash, C., and Kamel, A.M. (2012). Reduction and methylation of ziprasidone by glutathione, aldehyde oxidase, and thiol S-methyltransferase in humans: An in vitro study. *Xenobiotica 42*, 1049–1057.

Obach, R.S. and Walsky, R.L. (2005). Drugs that inhibit oxidation reactions catalyzed by aldehyde oxidase do not inhibit the reductive metabolism of ziprasidone to its major metabolite, S-methyldihydroziprasidone: An in vitro study. *J Clin Psychopharmacol 25*, 605–608.

Ohkubo, M., Sakiyama, S., and Fujimura, S. (1983a). Increase of nicotinamide methyltransferase and N1-methyl-nicotinamide oxidase activities in the livers of the rats administered alkylating agents. *Cancer Lett 21*, 175–181.

Ohkubo, M., Sakiyama, S., and Fujimura, S. (1983b). Purification and characterization of N1-methylnicotinamide oxidases I and II separated from rat liver. *Arch Biochem Biophys 221*, 534–542.

Payne, A.P. (1994). The harderian gland: A tercentennial review. *J Anat 185 (Pt 1)*, 1–49.

Pelikant-Malecka, I., Sielicka, A., Kaniewska, E., Smolenski, R.T., and Slominska, E.M. (2015). Endothelial toxicity of unusual nucleotide metabolites. *Pharmacol Rep 67*, 818–822.

Pritsos, C.A. (2000). Cellular distribution, metabolism and regulation of the xanthine oxidoreductase enzyme system. *Chem Biol Interact 129*, 195–208.

Pryde, D.C., Dalvie, D., Hu, Q., Jones, P., Obach, R.S., and Tran, T.D. (2010). Aldehyde oxidase: An enzyme of emerging importance in drug discovery. *J Med Chem 53*, 8441–8460.

Pryde, D.C., Tran, T.D., Jones, P., Duckworth, J., Howard, M., Gardner, I., Hyland, R., Webster, R., Wenham, T., Bagal, S., et al. (2012). Medicinal chemistry approaches to avoid aldehyde oxidase metabolism. *Bioorg Med Chem Lett 22*, 2856–2860.

Rani Basu, L., Mazumdar, K., Dutta, N.K., Karak, P., and Dastidar, S.G. (2005). Antibacterial property of the antipsychotic agent prochlorperazine, and its synergism with methdilazine. *Microbiol Res 160*, 95–100.

Reiss, J., Cohen, N., Dorche, C., Mandel, H., Mendel, R.R., Stallmeyer, B., Zabot, M.T., and Dierks, T. (1998). Mutations in a polycistronic nuclear gene associated with molybdenum cofactor deficiency. *Nat Genet 20*, 51–53.

Reiss, J., Dorche, C., Stallmeyer, B., Mendel, R.R., Cohen, N., and Zabot, M.T. (1999). Human molybdopterin synthase gene: Genomic structure and mutations in molybdenum cofactor deficiency type B. *Am J Hum Genet 64*, 706–711.

Rivera, S.P., Choi, H.H., Chapman, B., Whitekus, M.J., Terao, M., Garattini, E., and Hankinson, O. (2005). Identification of aldehyde oxidase 1 and aldehyde oxidase homologue 1 as dioxin-inducible genes. *Toxicology 207*, 401–409.

Rodriguez-Trelles, F., Tarrio, R., and Ayala, F.J. (2003). Convergent neofunctionalization by positive Darwinian selection after ancient recurrent duplications of the xanthine dehydrogenase gene. *Proc Natl Acad Sci USA 100*, 13413–13417.

Romao, M.J., Knablein, J., Huber, R., and Moura, J.J. (1997). Structure and function of molybdopterin containing enzymes. *Prog Biophys Mol Biol 68*, 121–144.

Rooseboom, M., Commandeur, J.N., and Vermeulen, N.P. (2004). Enzyme-catalyzed activation of anticancer prodrugs. *Pharmacol Rev 56*, 53–102.

Sanoh, S., Tayama, Y., Sugihara, K., Kitamura, S., and Ohta, S. (2015). Significance of aldehyde oxidase during drug development: Effects on drug metabolism, pharmacokinetics, toxicity, and efficacy. *Drug Metab Pharmacokinet 30*, 52–63.

Schumann, S., Terao, M., Garattini, E., Saggu, M., Lendzian, F., Hildebrandt, P., and Leimkuhler, S. (2009). Site directed mutagenesis of amino acid residues at the active site of mouse aldehyde oxidase AOX1. *PLoS One 4*, e5348.

Schwartz, R. and Kjeldgaard, N.O. (1951). The enzymic oxidation of pyridoxal by liver aldehyde oxidase. *Biochem J 48*, 333–337.

Shaw, S. and Jayatilleke, E. (1990). The role of aldehyde oxidase in ethanol-induced hepatic lipid peroxidation in the rat. *Biochem J 268*, 579–583.

Shintani, Y., Maruoka, S., Gon, Y., Koyama, D., Yoshida, A., Kozu, Y., Kuroda, K., Takeshita, I., Tsuboi, E., Soda, K., et al. (2015). Nuclear factor erythroid 2-related factor 2 (Nrf2) regulates airway epithelial barrier integrity. *Allergol Int 64 Suppl*, S54–S63.

Sigruener, A., Buechler, C., Orso, E., Hartmann, A., Wild, P.J., Terracciano, L., Roncalli, M., Bornstein, S.R., and Schmitz, G. (2007). Human aldehyde oxidase 1 interacts with ATP-binding cassette transporter-1 and modulates its activity in hepatocytes. *Horm Metab Res 39*, 781–789.

Stallmeyer, B., Drugeon, G., Reiss, J., Haenni, A.L., and Mendel, R.R. (1999). Human molybdopterin synthase gene: Identification of a bicistronic transcript with overlapping reading frames. *Am J Hum Genet 64*, 698–705.

Stanulovic, M. and Chaykin, S. (1971). Aldehyde oxidase: Catalysis of the oxidation of N 1 -methylnicotinamide and pyridoxal. *Arch Biochem Biophys 145*, 27–34.

Stell, J.G., Wheelhouse, R.T., and Wright, C.W. (2012). Metabolism of cryptolepine and 2-fluorocryptolepine by aldehyde oxidase. *J Pharm Pharmacol 64*, 237–243.

Stoddart, A.M. and Levine, W.G. (1992). Azoreductase activity by purified rabbit liver aldehyde oxidase. *Biochem Pharmacol 43*, 2227–2235.

Stubley, C., Stell, J.G., and Mathieson, D.W. (1979). The oxidation of azaheterocycles with mammalian liver aldehyde oxidase. *Xenobiotica 9*, 475–484.

Sugihara, K., Kitamura, S., Tatsumi, K., Asahara, T., and Dohi, K. (1997). Differences in aldehyde oxidase activity in cytosolic preparations of human and monkey liver. *Biochem Mol Biol Int 41*, 1153–1160.

Swenson, T.L. and Casida, J.E. (2013). Aldehyde oxidase importance in vivo in xenobiotic metabolism: Imidacloprid nitroreduction in mice. *Toxicol Sci 133*, 22–28.

Tatsumi, K., Kitamura, S., and Narai, N. (1986). Reductive metabolism of aromatic nitro compounds including carcinogens by rabbit liver preparations. *Cancer Res 46*, 1089–1093.

Tayama, Y., Miyake, K., Sugihara, K., Kitamura, S., Kobayashi, M., Morita, S., Ohta, S., and Kihira, K. (2007a). Developmental changes of aldehyde oxidase activity in young Japanese children. *Clin Pharmacol Ther 81*, 567–572.

Tayama, Y., Moriyasu, A., Sugihara, K., Ohta, S., and Kitamura, S. (2007b). Developmental changes of aldehyde oxidase in postnatal rat liver. *Drug Metab Pharmacokinet 22*, 119–124.

Tayama, Y., Sugihara, K., Sanoh, S., Miyake, K., Kitamura, S., and Ohta, S. (2012). Developmental changes of aldehyde oxidase activity and protein expression in human liver cytosol. *Drug Metab Pharmacokinet 27*, 543–547.

Tayama, Y., Sugihara, K., Sanoh, S., Miyake, K., Morita, S., Kitamura, S., and Ohta, S. (2011). Effect of tea beverages on aldehyde oxidase activity. *Drug Metab Pharmacokinet 26*, 94–101.

Terao, M., Barzago, M.M., Kurosaki, M., Fratelli, M., Bolis, M., Borsotti, A., Bigini, P., Micotti, E., Carli, M., Invernizzi, R.W., et al. (2016). Mouse aldehyde-oxidase-4 controls diurnal rhythms, fat deposition and locomotor activity. *Sci Rep 6*, 30343.

Terao, M., Kurosaki, M., Barzago, M.M., Fratelli, M., Bagnati, R., Bastone, A., Giudice, C., Scanziani, E., Mancuso, A., Tiveron, C., et al. (2009). Role of the molybdoflavoenzyme aldehyde oxidase homolog 2 in the biosynthesis of retinoic acid: Generation and characterization of a knockout mouse. *Mol Cell Biol 29*, 357–377.

Terao, M., Kurosaki, M., Barzago, M.M., Varasano, E., Boldetti, A., Bastone, A., Fratelli, M., and Garattini, E. (2006). Avian and canine aldehyde oxidases: Novel insights into the biology and evolution of molybdoflavoenzymes. *J Biol Chem 281*, 19748–19761.

Terao, M., Kurosaki, M., Marini, M., Vanoni, M.A., Saltini, G., Bonetto, V., Bastone, A., Federico, C., Saccone, S., Fanelli, R., et al. (2001). Purification of the aldehyde oxidase homolog 1 (AOH1) protein and cloning of the AOH1 and aldehyde oxidase homolog 2 (AOH2) genes: Identification of a novel molybdo-flavoprotein gene cluster on mouse chromosome 1. *J Biol Chem 276*, 46347–46363.

Terao, M., Kurosaki, M., Saltini, G., Demontis, S., Marini, M., Salmona, M., and Garattini, E. (2000). Cloning of the cDNAs coding for two novel molybdo-flavoproteins showing high similarity with aldehyde oxidase and xanthine oxidoreductase. *J Biol Chem 275*, 30690–30700.

Tomita, S., Tsujita, M., and Ichikawa, Y. (1993). Retinal oxidase is identical to aldehyde oxidase. *FEBS Lett 336*, 272–274.

Tsujita, M., Tomita, S., Miura, S., and Ichikawa, Y. (1994). Characteristic properties of retinal oxidase (retinoic acid synthase) from rabbit hepatocytes. *Biochim Biophys Acta 1204*, 108–116.

Ueda, O., Kitamura, S., Ohashi, K., Sugihara, K., and Ohta, S. (2003). Xanthine oxidase-catalyzed metabolism of 2-nitrofluorene, a carcinogenic air pollutant, in rat skin. *Drug Metab Dispos 31*, 367–372.

Ueda, O., Sugihara, K., Ohta, S., and Kitamura, S. (2005). Involvement of molybdenum hydroxylases in reductive metabolism of nitro polycyclic aromatic hydrocarbons in mammalian skin. *Drug Metab Dispos 33*, 1312–1318.

Ventura, S.M. and Dachtler, S.L. (1980). Development and maturation of aldehyde oxidase levels in fetal hepatic tissue of C57BL/6J mice. *Enzyme 25*, 213–219.

Ventura, S.M. and Dachtler, S.L. (1981). Effects of sex hormones on hepatic aldehyde oxidase activity in C57BL/6J mice. *Horm Res 14*, 250–259.

Vila, R., Kurosaki, M., Barzago, M.M., Kolek, M., Bastone, A., Colombo, L., Salmona, M., Terao, M., and Garattini, E. (2004). Regulation and biochemistry of mouse molybdo-flavoenzymes: The DBA/2 mouse is selectively deficient in the expression of aldehyde oxidase homologues 1 and 2 and represents a unique source for the purification and characterization of aldehyde oxidase. *J Biol Chem 279*, 8668–8683.

Weigert, J., Neumeier, M., Bauer, S., Mages, W., Schnitzbauer, A.A., Obed, A., Groschl, B., Hartmann, A., Schaffler, A., Aslanidis, C., et al. (2008). Small-interference RNA-mediated knock-down of aldehyde oxidase 1 in 3T3-L1 cells impairs adipogenesis and adiponectin release. *FEBS Lett 582*, 2965–2972.

Yamaguchi, Y., Matsumura, T., Ichida, K., Okamoto, K., and Nishino, T. (2007). Human xanthine oxidase changes its substrate specificity to aldehyde oxidase type upon mutation of amino acid residues in the active site: Roles of active site residues in binding and activation of purine substrate. *J Biochem 141*, 513–524.

Yoshihara, S. and Tatsumi, K. (1985). Guinea pig liver aldehyde oxidase as a sulfoxide reductase: Its purification and characterization. *Arch Biochem Biophys 242*, 213–224.

Yoshihara, S. and Tatsumi, K. (1997). Purification and characterization of hepatic aldehyde oxidase in male and female mice. *Arch Biochem Biophys 338*, 29–34.

Zhang, Y. and Gladyshev, V.N. (2008). Molybdoproteomes and evolution of molybdenum utilization. *J Mol Biol 379*, 881–899.

Zientek, M.A. and Youdim, K. (2015). Reaction phenotyping: Advances in the experimental strategies used to characterize the contribution of drug-metabolizing enzymes. *Drug Metab Dispos 43*, 163–181.

Ziouzenkova, O., Orasanu, G., Sharlach, M., Akiyama, T.E., Berger, J.P., Viereck, J., Hamilton, J.A., Tang, G., Dolnikowski, G.G., Vogel, S., et al. (2007). Retinaldehyde represses adipogenesis and diet-induced obesity. *Nat Med 13*, 695–702.

5

UDP-Glucuronosyltransferases

Robert S. Foti and Upendra A. Argikar

CONTENTS

Introduction

The uridine diphosphate glucuronosyltransferases (UGTs) represent a super-family of Phase II membrane-bound drug metabolizing enzymes (MW = 50–60 kDa) that are responsible for the transfer of glucuronic acid from the cofactor uridine diphosphoglucuronic acid (UDPGA), to a nucleophilic acceptor substrate (Dutton 1980, 1997, Mackenzie et al. 1997, King et al. 2000, Tephly and Green 2000, Tukey and Strassburg 2000, Rowland et al. 2013). The resulting glucuronide conjugates are more water soluble than the parent drug molecule (aglycone), thus rendering them subject to facile excretion. UGT-catalyzed glucuronidation is generally accepted to be the second most prevalent metabolic pathway, with only cytochrome P450 oxidation contributing to a greater percentage of drugs cleared by metabolism (Williams et al. 2004). To date, more than 20 individual UGT isoforms have been identified in humans, with the majority of xenobiotic metabolism being catalyzed by isoforms in the UGT1A and UGT2B subfamilies. UGTs are also capable of catalyzing the addition of other sugar moieties such as glucose or xylose to an aglycone acceptor molecule (Mackenzie et al. 2008, 2011, Meech et al. 2015). Well-documented structural moieties that can serve as nucleophilic acceptors for glucuronidation, include alcohols (aromatic or aliphatic), carboxylic acids (resulting in the formation of acyl glucuronides), thiols, amines, and nucleophilic carbon atoms (Figure 5.1) (Richter et al. 1975, Sorich et al. 2006). This chapter will cover basic UGT enzymology, as well as the important role that UGTs play in drug metabolism, drug interactions and drug efficacy, and safety. UGT ontogeny, *in vitro-in vivo* extrapolation (IVIVE) for UGT substrates, analytical challenges with glucuronide metabolites and general experimental considerations with the UGTs will also be reviewed.

General Enzymology, Reaction Mechanism, and Atypical Kinetics

UGT enzymes are widely expressed throughout the body with the liver having the highest expression levels of the enzymes (Tukey and Strassburg 2000, Nakamura et al. 2008, Izukawa et al. 2009, Ohno and Nakajin 2009, Court et al. 2012, Vildhede et al. 2015). Additional sites of expression include

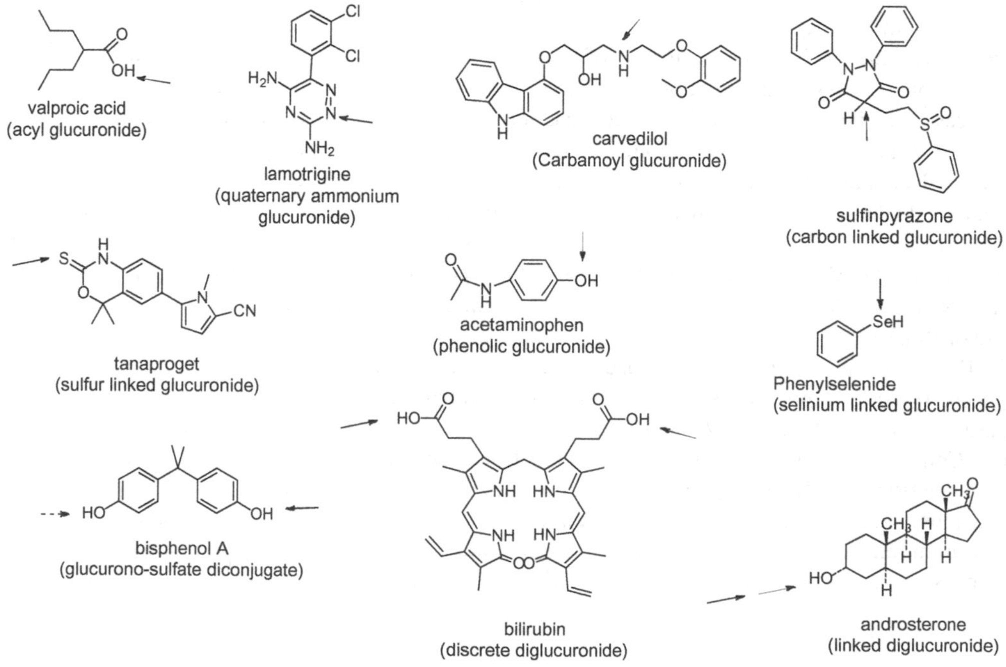

FIGURE 5.1 Examples of glucuronides. The site of conjugation is indicated by an arrow for each substrate.

the intestine, kidneys, colon, lungs, testis, ovaries, rectum, and prostate (Radominska-Pandya et al. 1998, Turgeon et al. 2001, Nakamura et al. 2008, Margaillan et al. 2015, Wijayakumara et al. 2015, Asher et al. 2016). Many of the UGT isoforms display tissue-dependent expression patterns, such as UGT1A8 and UGT1A10, which are primarily expressed in the intestine, or UGT2B17, which is has its highest expression levels in prostate (Cheng et al. 1998, Mojarrabi and Mackenzie 1998, Barbier et al. 2000b, Mizuma 2009). Within cells, UGTs are transmembrane proteins that are primarily found in the smooth endoplasmic reticulum (Radominska-Pandya et al. 1999, Bock and Kohle 2009, Magdalou et al. 2010). A hypothetical structure of UGTs is illustrated in Figure 5.2. The substrate binding domain is located on the luminal side of the membrane, a fact that often renders the use of pore-forming reagents, such as alamethicin, necessary when conducting glucuronidation reactions in vitro (Fisher et al. 2000). As such, it has been demonstrated that the N-terminal domain, which resides on the luminal side of the membrane, plays a key role in the substrate recognition properties of the enzymes (Radominska-Pandya et al. 1999, 2005, Coffman et al. 2001, 2003, Lewis et al. 2007, Kerdpin et al. 2009, Dong et al. 2012). Conversely, the cofactor binding domain is oriented near the C-terminus of the protein, which is also located on the luminal side of the endoplasmic reticulum (ER) membrane (Radominska-Pandya et al. 1999, 2005, 2010, Banerjee et al. 2008,

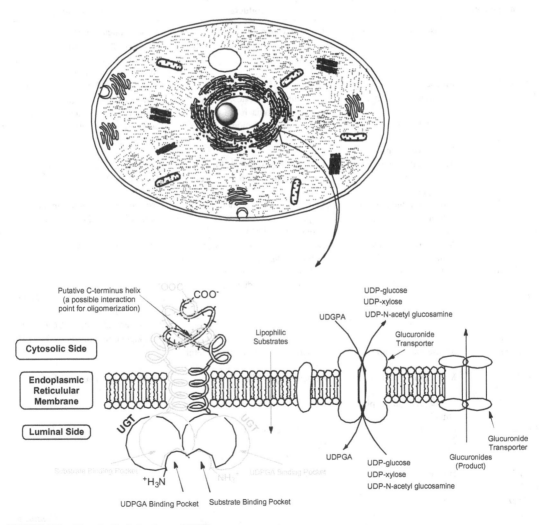

FIGURE 5.2 Hypothetical structure of UGTs.

Xiong et al. 2008, Meech et al. 2012, Nair et al. 2015). Because of the charged nature of sugars such as UDP-glucuronic acid and the resulting glucuronic acid metabolites, active transporters have been postulated to facilitate the transfer of these molecules across the membrane of the endoplasmic reticulum *in vivo* (Bossuyt and Blanckaert 1997, Meech and Mackenzie 1997a, Radominska-Pandya et al. 1999, Kobayashi et al. 2006, Rowland et al. 2015).

Pharmacogenetics

Over 20 human UGT isoforms have been identified and are divided into the UGT1, UGT2, UGT3 and UGT4 subfamilies based on protein and substrate similarity (Table 5.1, Figure 5.3). Many of the UGT genes have been widely studied for polymorphic variants, with UGT1A1 being the most well

TABLE 5.1

A Simplified Snapshot of Genes from UGT Superfamily

UGT Gene (nomenclature shown for human genes)	Species	Tissue Based Expression of Products	Comments
UGT1A1	Mouse, rat, cat, human	Liver, intestine, bile duct, stomach, colon, mammary gland	Disease states implication: defective gene – Crigler-Najjar syndrome and reduced expression in Gilbert's syndrome.
UGT1A2	Mouse, rat, cat, monkey		Pseudogene in humans (*UGT1A2P*)
UGT1A3	Rat, monkey, human	Liver, intestine, testes, prostate, bile duct, stomach, colon	Pseudogene in mice (*ugt1a3-ps*) and mRNA undetectable in rat
UGT1A4	Rabbit, human	Liver, bile duct, colon	Pseudogene in mouse and rat (*ugt1a4-ps*)
UGT1A5	Mouse, rat, human		
UGT1A6	Mouse, rat, dog, monkey, human, rabbit, cow, sheep, ferret	Liver, kidney, intestine, brain, ovary, testes, bile duct, spleen, skin	Pseudogene in cat, leopard (*UGT1A6P*)
UGT1A7	Mouse, rat, human, rabbit, sheep, guinea pig	Stomach (gastric epithelium), esophagus	Two other pseudogenes in mouse (*ugt1a7a-ps* and *ugt1a7b-ps*)
UGT1A8	Monkey, human	Esophagus, intestine	
UGT1A9	Mouse, rat, monkey, human	Liver, kidney ovary, testes, spleen, skin, esophagus	Pseudogene in rat (*ugt1a9-ps*)
UGT1A10	Mouse, rat, human	Intestine, lung, stomach, esophagus, bile duct	
UGT1A11			Pseudogene in mouse (*ugt1a11-ps*) and human (*UGT1A11P*)
UGT1A12			Pseudogene in human (*UGT1A12P*)
UGT1A13			Pseudogene in human (*UGT1A13P*)
UGT2A1	Mouse, rat, human	Olfactory epithelium, brain, fetal lung	
UGT2A2	Mouse, rat, rabbit, human	Olfactory epithelium	Rabbit *UGT2C1* renamed as *UGT2A2*
UGT2A3	Mouse, rat, guinea pig, human	Olfactory epithelium	
UGT2B1	Mouse, rat	Liver, kidney, intestine, testes	
UGT2B2	Rat	Liver	
UGT2B3	Rat		
UGT2B4	Human	Liver	
UGT2B5	Mouse		
UGT2B6	Rat		

(Continued)

TABLE 5.1 (*Continued*)

A Simplified Snapshot of Genes from UGT Superfamily

UGT Gene (nomenclature shown for human genes)	Species	Tissue Based Expression of Products	Comments
UGT2B7	Human	Liver, kidney, esophagus, intestine, brain, kidney, pancreas	
UGT2B8	Rat	Liver	
UGT2B9	Monkey	Liver	
UGT2B10	Human	Liver, adrenals, prostate, mammary gland, esophagus	
UGT2B11	Human	Liver, kidney, mammary gland, prostate, skin, adipose, adrenal gland, lung, and adipose	
UGT2B12	Rat	Liver, kidney, intestine	
UGT2B13	Rabbit	Liver (adult)	
UGT2B14	Rabbit	Liver (adult)	
UGT2B15	Human	Liver, prostate, testes, esophagus	
UGT2B16	Rabbit		
UGT2B17	Human	Liver, kidney, prostate, testes, uterus, placenta, mammary glands, adrenals, skin	
UGT2B18	Monkey		
UGT2B19	Monkey		
UGT2B20	Monkey		
UGT2B21	Guinea pig		
UGT2B22	Guinea pig		
UGT2B23	Monkey		
UGT2B24			Pseudogene in human (UGT1B24P)
UGT2B25			Pseudogene in human (UGT1B25P)
UGT2B26			Pseudogene in human (UGT1B26P)
UGT2B27			Pseudogene in human (UGT1B27P)
UGT2B28	Human		
UGT2B29			Pseudogene in human (UGT1B29P)
UGT2B30	Monkey		
UGT2B31	Dog, pig		
UGT2B32	Guinea pig		
UGT2B33	Monkey		
UGT2B34	Mouse, rat		
UGT2B35	Mouse		
UGT2B36	Mouse		
UGT2B37	Mouse		
UGT2B38	Mouse		
UGT3A1	Mouse, human		
UGT3A2	Mouse, human		
UGT8A1	Mouse, rat, monkey, human, cow		

The genes in human and other mammalian species are exemplified. The genes are denoted in all caps (as opposed to denoting rodent genes in uncapitalized letters) for simplicity. Additional information can be obtained at https://www.flinders.edu.au/medicine/sites/clinical-pharmacology/current-nomenclature.cfm (date accessed September 15, 2016). Site maintained by Karli Goodwin. Last modified date: September 15, 2016.

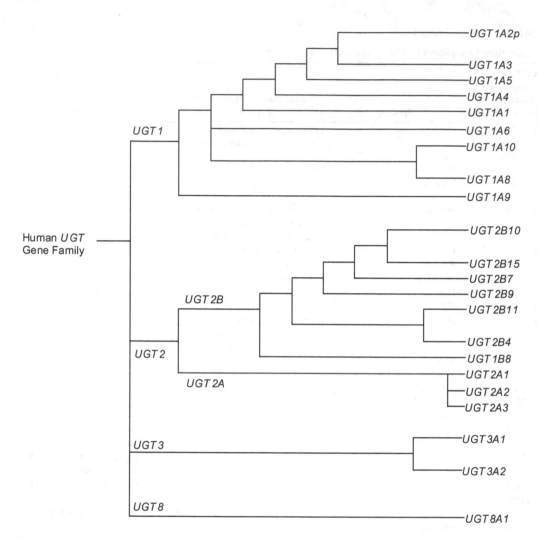

FIGURE 5.3 Human UGT gene family.

characterized. A number of comprehensive compilations of UGT pharmacogenetics (Guillemette 2003) and their relevance to cancer (Nagar and Remmel 2006b) along with the tools to evaluate UGT polymorphisms can be found in the literature (Argikar et al. 2008). Further, a detailed discussion on the allelic variants, their resulting protein product and the effect on functional activity from a drug interaction perspective can be found in a book chapter on UGTs by Remmel and coworkers (Remmel et al. 2008). The section below attempts to summarize some of the key findings to date with a focus on UGT pharmacogenetics and disease states.

UGT1A1

UGT1A1 gene polymorphisms have been comprehensively studied. These manifest in a rare inborn error of bilirubin metabolism, resulting in Crigler-Najjar syndrome (Types I and II). Type I Crigler-Najjar syndrome requires liver transplantation, whereas Type II is treatable with *UGT1A1* inducers such as phenobarbital. Decreased expression of UGT1A1 is observed in Gilbert's patients (asymptomatic unconjugated hyperbilirubinemia), which has been linked to the presence of a seventh (TA) repeat in addition to generally observed six (TA) repeats (*UGT1A1*28*) (Monaghan et al. 1996, Guillemette 2003), resulting in approximately a 70% decrease in UGT1A1 enzyme expression in the liver of homozygous subjects. *UGT1A1*6* and other mutations in the *UGT1A1* gene besides the (TA)$_7$TAA genotype also contribute to unconjugated hyperbilirubinemia (Akaba et al. 1998, Urawa et al. 2006). A mutation in phenobarbital-response element, resulting in a regulatory defect is also linked with Gilbert's syndrome, and is shown to be in linkage disequilibrium with *UGT1A1*28* (Guillemette 2003, Kitagawa et al. 2005, Costa 2006, Ferraris et al. 2006).

The HIV protease inhibitors atazanavir and indinavir are known to increase unconjugated bilirubin levels by inhibiting UGT1A1, especially in patients with Gilbert's syndrome (Rotger et al. 2005, Lankisch et al. 2006). The role of the *UGT1A1*28* polymorphism in toxicity of the anticancer prodrug irinotecan has been well documented (Ando et al. 1998, Iyer et al. 1998, Innocenti and Ratain 2006). Irinotecan is rapidly converted by esterases to an active phenolic compound, SN-38, which is metabolically inactivated by UGT1A1 via glucuronidation. Patients with the *UGT1A1*28* allele are at a significantly higher risk for neutropenia; therefore, FDA has recommended that patients should be genotyped prior to use of irinotecan.

UGT1A3 and UGT1A4

UGT1A3 and UGT1A4 are often implicated in the formation of quaternary ammonium glucuronide metabolites, as well as being capable of glucuronidating other substrates. Iwai et al. identified four non-synonymous single nucleotide polymorphisms (SNPs) in the *UGT1A3* sequence (Iwai et al. 2004). The presence of the *UGT1A3*2* allele resulted in an altered protein sequence (W11R, V47A) that showed an increase in the efficiency of estrone glucuronidation. The variants also showed increased activity toward glucuronidation of a variety of flavonoids in general (Chen et al. 2006), but the R45W variant resulted in decreased estrone glucuronidation (Iwai et al. 2004). Two variants in the *UGT1A4* gene have also been identified, but the effect on activity appears to vary depending upon the substrate. The P24T SNP resulting from *UGT1A4*2* variant showed decreased intrinsic clearance for the anticonvulsant drug lamotrigine, a probe substrate documented to show a fivefold variation in intrinsic clearance values across human liver microsomal bank (Argikar and Remmel 2009b). The L48V mutant resulting from *UGT1A4*3* has been shown to either not retain catalytic activity toward dihydrotestosterone glucuronidation (Ehmer et al. 2004) or, in contrast, has shown higher activity (Zhou et al. 2011). It has also been shown to be more efficient for 4-(methylnitrosamino)-1-(3-pyridyl)-1-butanol (NNAL) (Wiener et al. 2004) and clozapine (Mori et al. 2005) or less efficient for substrates such as trans-Androsterone and lamotrigine (Mori et al. 2005, Zhou et al. 2011). In vitro findings for lamotrigine were validated *in vivo* in a clinical study (Gulcebi et al. 2011).

UGT1A6

UGT1A6 plays a primary role in the metabolism of analgesic drugs such as acetaminophen, as well as the neurotransmitters serotonin and 5-hydroxytryptophol. Krishnaswamy and coworkers identified several variants of the *UGT1A6* gene, with polymorphisms in the regulatory region as well as exon 1 (Krishnaswamy et al. 2005a). The *UGT1A6*2* variant resulted in a protein that showed altered Km values for numerous substrates, including serotonin (Krishnaswamy et al. 2005b). Interestingly, beta-thalassemia/hemoglobin E patients with an *UGT1A6*2* variant and no *UGT1A1*28* polymorphism showed a remarkably lower AUC of acetaminophen (substrate UGTs 1A1, 1A6 and 1A9) and its metabolites (Tankanitlert et al. 2007).

UGT1A8 and UGT1A10

UGT1A8 and UGT1A10 are extrahepatic UGT isoforms with broad substrate specificity. One silent mutation and three other variants have been detected for UGT1A8. The proteins resulting from *UGT1A8*1* and *UGT1A8*2* did not show any change in in vitro activity toward numerous substrates; however, the protein from the *UGT1A8*3* variant showed little to no activity toward any substrate studied (Huang et al. 2002b, Thibaudeau et al. 2006). Variants in *UGT1A10* gene that result in lower catalytic activity have been reported. One variant, *UGT1A10*2*, results in a corresponding protein that has significantly lower activity for phenolic compounds (Elahi et al. 2003). Polymorphic enzymes resulting from coding region SNPs showed reduced catalytic efficiency toward estradiol glucuronidation (Saeki et al. 2002, Jinno, Saeki, Tanaka-Kagawa et al. 2003).

UGT1A9

UGT1A9 is primarily expressed in the kidneys and is often associated with the metabolism of the anesthetic propofol. *UGT1A9* coding region mutants are observed at low allele frequencies, whereas regulatory region mutations are more common and may result in increased expression of UGT1A9. Girard and coworkers showed that the functionally expressed UGT1A9.3 enzyme, resulting from a coding region mutation, had reduced SN-38 glucuronidation (Girard et al. 2004). Jinno and coworkers reported similar findings for a genetic variant 766G>A, resulting in a non-synonymous mutation of D256N, a protein with 20-fold lower intrinsic clearance as compared to the wild-type (Jinno, Saeki, Saito et al. 2003). While moderate to no change has been reported in the oral clearance of mycophenolic acid, a linkage disequilibrium between the two regulatory mutations of *UGT1A9* and mutation of *UGT1A1* has been reported (Innocenti et al. 2005). The *UGT1A9*22* mutation possesses an $AT_{10}AT$ repeat instead of the more common AT_9AT repeat (Yamanaka et al. 2004), possibly resulting in higher expression levels of UGT1A9.22 (Innocenti et al. 2005).

UGT2B4 and UGT2B7

UGT2B4 and UGT2B7 are primarily hepatic isoforms and are capable of metabolizing many of the same substrates such as codeine and various bile acids. *UGT2B4*2* has been identified as a polymorphic variant of *UGT2B4* (Lampe et al. 2000, Saeki et al. 2004). A common variant of *UGT2B7* observed across a diverse population, namely *UGT2B7*2*, has been shown to produce an enzyme with altered activity towards select substrates (Bhasker et al. 2000, Court et al. 2003, Girard et al. 2004) and can result in activity toward substrates not typically glucuronidated by the wild type enzyme (Coffman et al. 1998). *UGT2B7*2* was identified to be present in linkage disequilibrium with a regulatory region mutation of *UGT2B7*, possibly explaining the lower glucuronidation of morphine in subjects with *UGT2B7*2* (Holthe et al. 2002, Sawyer et al. 2003).

UGT2B15 and UGTB17

UGT2B15 and UGT2B17 are major UGTs in human prostate and are responsible for inactivation of androgens by glucuronidation (Belanger et al. 2003, Court et al. 2004, Chouinard et al. 2007). Court and coworkers showed that *UGT2B15*2* results in approximately 50% lower activity for S-oxazepam but increased activity for androgens in genotyped microsomes (Court et al. 2004). The UGT2B15.2 variant (D85Y) was observed to a greater extent in Asian population than Caucasians (Lampe et al. 2000). UGT2B15.4 variant enzyme showed no change in activity, whereas a rare variant, UGT2B15.6, showed increased enzymatic activity. *UGT2B15*1* homozygous subjects have been shown to be at increased risk of prostate cancer (Park et al. 2004).

   A deletion of an approximately 170kB stretch of DNA encompassing the entire *UGT2B17* locus has been reported by Wilson and coworkers, resulting in *UGT2B17*2* (Wilson et al. 2004). Intrinsic clearance for dihydroexemestane glucuronidation in microsomes that were genotyped as *UGT2B17*2/*2* was dramatically lower as compared to wild-type (Sun et al. 2010). Similarly, urinary ratios of testosterone glucuronide to epitestosterone glucuronide are widely used for testing of testosterone abuse, especially in athletes. Ratios greater than 4 are normally considered to be indicative of testosterone overuse. Interestingly, Schulze and coworkers reported that administration of testosterone to persons with the *UGT2B17* deletion genotype, results in the majority of the ratios being 20-fold lower on average, suggesting that such individuals may not test positive for testosterone if evaluated using the ratio test, even during testosterone abuse (Schulze et al. 2008, 2011).

Ontogeny

Understanding the ontogeny of drug metabolizing enzymes is critical to ensuring the safe administration of drugs across pediatric, adult, and geriatric populations. The developmental aspects of UGT expression came to light in the mid-twentieth century with the attribution of grey baby syndrome due to the lack of UGT-catalyzed chloramphenicol metabolism (Sutherland 1959, Weiss et al. 1960, Laferriere and Marks 1982, Pineiro-Carrero and Pineiro 2004). Further, the onset of jaundice in newborns was shown to be due to low activity of UGT1A1 and the resulting inability of the newborn to metabolize and eliminate bilirubin (Maruo et al. 1999, Huang et al. 2002a, Bartlett and Gourley 2011, Zaja et al. 2014). Subsequently, many in vitro and *in vivo* studies evaluating the mRNA or protein expression, enzyme activity or *in vivo* hepatic clearance have been undertaken to understand the expression levels and activity of UGT isoforms from the developing fetus to pediatric subjects and on through adulthood. Though the quantitation of UGT protein levels has been hampered by the availability of selective antibodies, recent advancements in mass spectrometry-based proteomics may shed new light on expression levels for individual isoforms at various life stages (Fallon et al. 2013a, 2013b). The propensity for UGTs to undergo post-translational modifications or interact with other proteins in order to achieve their active states has further complicated ontogeny studies with this family of enzymes (Barbier et al. 2000a, Luquita et al. 2001, Riches and Collier 2015).

In general, it appears that fetal expression of UGTs is low relative to adults, with the majority of fetal UGT expression being comprised of UGT2B isoforms as shown by the example in Figure 5.4 (de Wildt et al. 1999, Strassburg et al. 2002, Krekels et al. 2012, Coughtrie 2015). After birth, a rapid increase in expression levels is observed, with UGT expression reaching adult levels during childhood development, though the exact maturation period can be isoform dependent. UGT1A1, for example, has been reported to reach adult expression levels between 4 and 24 months of age, while UGT2B7 expression achieves adult expressions levels at approximately 7–24 months or 12–17 years, depending on the study (Onishi et al. 1979, Strassburg et al. 2002, Zaya et al. 2006, Miyagi and Collier 2011). In vitro studies with the non-selective UGT substrate 4-methylumbelliferone suggest maximal aggregate UGT activity is reached at between 8 and 20 months post-birth (Miyagi and Collier 2011).

The ontogeny of UGT enzyme expression and activity may also differ from the observed ability of the enzymes to contribute to the hepatic clearance of a drug. The hepatic clearance capacities of UGT1A1 and UGT1A6, for example, are comparable to adult capacities at approximately 2 years post birth, while UGT1A9 clearance does not reach maturity until approximately 18 years post birth (Miyagi and Collier 2011, Miyagi et al. 2012). Similarly, allometric scaling techniques suggest the intrinsic hepatic clearance

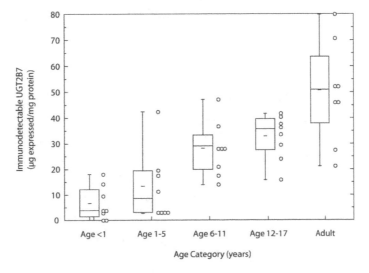

FIGURE 5.4 UGT ontogeny as exemplified by the increase in UGT2B7 protein expression observed from birth through adulthood. (Reproduced with permission from Zaya, M.J. et al., *Drug Metab. Dispos.*, 34, 2097–2101, 2006.)

of trifluoperazine, a UGT1A4 substrate, reaches adult levels between 18 and 20 years of age, though the isoform is thought to reach adult levels of expression and activity in early childhood (Miyagi and Collier 2007). Adult levels of hepatic clearance for UGT2B7 have been reported to be achieved within the first 3 months to 2.5 years post-birth, using glucuronidation of morphine as a selective *in vivo* marker of UGT2B7 activity (McRorie et al. 1992, Lynn et al. 1998, 2000, Bouwmeester et al. 2004). Increases in observed UGT activity have also been shown to be dependent upon overall gestation period, with the time needed to reach adult levels of UGT clearance being shorter for those infants carried to full term, as opposed to those born prematurely (Mirochnick et al. 1999, Knibbe et al. 2009).

Reaction Mechanism

The transfer of glucuronic acid from UDPGA to the aglycone involves an acid-base mechanism that begins with a deprotonation of the aglycone by a conserved histidine or proline residue in the UGT active site (Figure 5.5). The protonated histidine is rendered stable through interactions with a neighboring

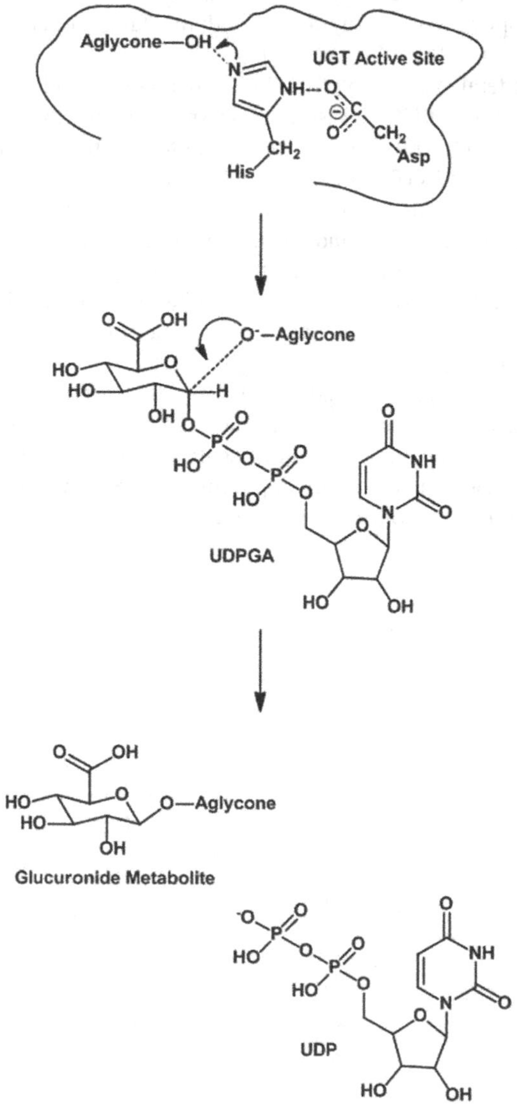

FIGURE 5.5 UGT reaction mechanism.

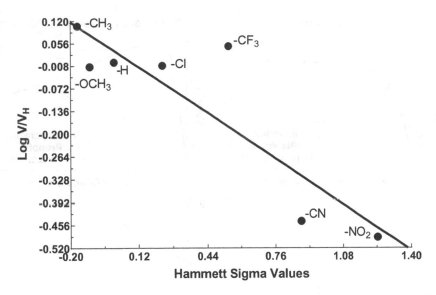

FIGURE 5.6 Effect of substituents on maximal rate of phenol glucuronidation as evidence that glucuronidation occurs via an S_N2 mechanism (Reproduced with permission from Yin, H. et al., *Chem. Biol. Interact.*, 90, 47–58, 1994.)

aspartic acid residue, which is also thought to be conserved across the UGTs (Li et al. 2007, Miley et al. 2007). Subsequently, the putative glucuronide metabolite is formed through an S_N2 nucleophilic attack by the aglycone at the C1-carbon of UDPGA, with the C1-carbon undergoing an inversion in stereochemistry from the β-configuration in UDPGA to the β-configuration in the glucuronide metabolite (Johnson and Fenselau 1978). The proposed S_N2 reaction mechanism has been supported by seminal work demonstrating that increasing the nucleophilicity of the aglycone directly increases the rate of the glucuronidation reaction (Figure 5.6), while further mechanistic evaluations have made use of the unique properties of the anomeric proton present on the C1-carbon atom (Yin et al. 1994, Walker et al. 2007, Malik and Black 2012). In addition to the nucleophilicity of the aglycone, the lipophilicity of a molecule has also been shown to be a key factor in determining its susceptibility to glucuronidation, with a log P of approximately 2 appearing to favor binding within the active sites of UGTs (Kim 1991, Smith et al. 2003).

Remarkably, literature reports document that infrequently, glucuronides are also formed upon N-carbamoylation of primary and secondary amines, at carbon atoms, and at selenium atoms. In addition to mono-glucuronides, two types of diglucuronide conjugates have also been documented. These can be classified into two distinct types: "discrete diglucuronides," which are formed when glucuronidation occurs at two different functional groups on the same aglycone; and "linked diglucuronides," which are formed whenever the second glucuronidation occurs on a hydroxyl group of the first glucuronide's sugar moiety (glycone) rather than directly on the parent molecule (Argikar 2012).

Atypical Kinetics

The bi-substrate S_N2 glucuronidation reaction can be described by multiple kinetic models, including Michaelis-Menten, sigmoidal (activation), bi-phasic, and substrate or product inhibition (Figure 5.7) (Zhou and Miners 2014). The mechanism itself has been reported to be a compulsory-ordered bi bi mechanism, whereby UDP-glucuronic acid binds first followed by binding of the aglycone, though other mechanisms have been proposed (Potrepka and Spratt 1972, Vessey and Zakim 1972, Sanchez and Tephly 1975, Rao et al. 1976, Koster and Noordhoek 1983, Falany et al. 1987, Yin et al. 1994, Luukkanen et al. 2005). In general, under saturating concentrations of UDP-glucuronic acid (>> Km),

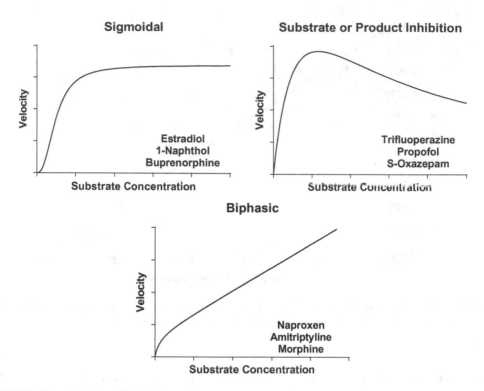

FIGURE 5.7 Examples of atypical kinetic profiles often demonstrated by UGT substrates.

the observed kinetics will appear to be Michaelis-Menten and are often defined as such. However, more mechanistic evaluations of glucuronidation kinetics have revealed the ability of UGTs to bind multiple aglycones, either simultaneously or sequentially, resulting in the aforementioned atypical kinetic profiles (Rios and Tephly 2002, Stone et al. 2003, Iwuchukwu and Nagar 2008, Uchaipichat et al. 2008, Zhou et al. 2010).

Substrates and Inhibitors

The pursuit of selective substrates and inhibitors for UGT isoforms remains a key area of research owing to the overlap of ligand pharmacophores among the various UGTs. Similar to many of the known probe substrates of the cytochrome P450 enzymes, probe substrates for UGTs can be useful in reaction phenotyping and *in vitro* drug interaction studies, as well as in more mechanistic experiments. Both endogenous and xenobiotic compounds have been evaluated and suggested as useful probe substrates or inhibitors of UGTs and a comprehensive table is shown in Table 5.2. Well-characterized endogenous substrates include bilirubin and estradiol (UGT1A1), serotonin (UGT1A6), testosterone (UGT2B15 and UGT2B17), and other estrogens, androgens, or arachidonic acid metabolites (multiple UGTs). Many xenobiotics have been characterized in regard to UGT specificity, with compounds such as trifluoperazine (UGT1A4), propofol (UGT1A9), morphine (UGT2B7), and S-oxazepam (UGT2B15), in addition to others, being proposed as selective substrates (Oda et al. 2015). It is important to note that in certain cases, the selectivity of a substrate is also dependent upon the organ-specific expression patterns of a given UGT isoform, as is the case with propofol, which is glucuronidated solely by UGT1A9 in the liver but is also a substrate of multiple extrahepatic UGTs (Court 2005). Selective UGT inhibitors include atazanavir and erlotinib (UGT1A1), hecogenin (UGT1A4), fluconazole (UGT2B7), and S-nicotine (UGT2B10).

TABLE 5.2

A List of Endogenous and Exogenous Substrates, Inducers and Inhibitors of Major Human UGTs

Iso-enzyme	Trivial Names	Endogenous Substrates	Drug or Xenobiotic Substrates	Inducers	Inhibitors
UGT1A1	Rat B1 HP3 HUG$_{Br-1}$ UGTBr1	*Bilirubin, estradiol* (3-hydroxy), 2-hydroxyestrone, 2-hydroxyestradiol trans-retinoic acid, Catechol estrogens (2- & 4-hydroxy), thyroxine	*Ethinyl estradiol, morphine* (3-hydroxy), buprenorphine, Ferulic acid, genistein Naltrexone (low), naloxone (low), SN-38 (active metabolite of irinotecan) alizarin, quinalizarin, raltegravir, muraglitazar (3–8 µM km), 6-hydroxy warfarin, glycerrhetinic acid	Bilirubin, chlorophenoxypropionic acid, chrysin, clofibrate 3-methylcholanthrene, phenylpropionic acid, phenobarbital, etc. pregnenolone-16α-nitrile & dexamethasone, clotrimazole, rifampin, and St. John's wort.	Atazanavir, erlotinib, indinavir
UGT1A3	Rat B3 H 1c	Bile acids (carboxyl functional group), catechol estrogens (2-OH >4-OH), 2-OH-estrone, 2-hydroxyestradiol, decanoic acid, dodecanoic acid, bilirubin (low), thyroxine	*Cyproheptadine, alizarin, buprenorphine*, norbuprenorphine, bropirimine, diphenylamine, diprenorphine, emodin, esculetin, eugenol, ezetimibe, fisetin, genestein, desacetylcinobufagin (16-OH) 3-hydroxydesloratadine, 7-hydroxyflavone, hydromorphone, 4-methylumbelliferone, morphine, nalorphine, naloxone, naltrexone, *naringenin*, quercehtin, scopoletin, thymol, umbelliferone. Carboxyl group: clofibrate, ciprofibrate, etodolac, fenoprofen, ibuprofen, ketoprofen, naproxen (racemic > S), valproic acid, formation of simvastatin & atorvastatin lactones via an intermediate acyl glucuronide, fenofibric acid, glycerrhetininc acid (highest activity by UGT1A3), muraglitazar (3–7 µM Km),	β-Naphthoflavone, Rifampin (?)	
UGT1A4	HUG$_{Br-2}$	Estrogens: 2-hydroxy-estrone and 2-hydroxy estradiol, 4-hydroxy	Tertiary amines: amitriptyline, chlorpheniramine, chlorpromazine,	Phenobarbital, phenytoin, and carbamazepine	Hecogenin

(Continued)

TABLE 5.2 (*Continued*)

A List of Endogenous and Exogenous Substrates, Inducers and Inhibitors of Major Human UGTs

Iso-enzyme	Trivial Names	Endogenous Substrates	Drug or Xenobiotic Substrates	Inducers	Inhibitors
		catechol estrogens(low), estriol, Progestins: 5α-pregnan-3α,20α-diol, 16α-hydroxy pregnenolone, 19-hydroxy and 21-hydroxy pregnenolone, pregnenelone, androsterone, epiandrosterone, etiocholanone Androgens: dehydroepiandro- sterone, dihydrotestosterone, epitestosterone, testosterone, 5α-androstan-3α, 17β-diol, 5β-androstan-3α,11α, 17β-triol; bilirubin (very low), F_6-1α,23S,25 (OH)$_3$D$_3$–a hexafluorinated Vit D$_3$ analog	clozapine, cyproheptadine, desacetylcinobufagin (3-OH), diphenylamine, doxepin, *imipramine*, ketotifen, loxapine, promethazine, tripellenamine, *trifluoperazine* Aromatic heterocyclic amines: croconazole, lamotrigine, nicotine (30X velocity than UGT1A3), 1-phenylimidazole, posaconazole, retigabine Primary & secondary amines: 2- & 4-aminobiphenyl, diphenylamine, desmethylclozapine Alcoholic & phenolic substrates: borneol, carveol, carvacrol diosgenin, *hecogenin*, isomenthol, menthol, neomenthol, 1- and 2-naphthol (low), p-nitrophenol (low), nopol, tigogenin, medetomide, midazolam (N-glucuronide on N of imidazole), glycerrhetinic acid, senecionine		
UGT1A6	HP1 HlugP1 UGT1-6 Rat4NP	*Serotonin*, 3-hydroxy methyl DOPA	Phenols: acetaminophen, 2-amino-5-nitro-4- trifluoromethylphenol (flutamide metabolite), BHA, BHT, 7-hydroxy coumarin, 4-hydroxy- coumarin (low), dobutamine, 4-ethylphenol, 3-ethylphenol, 4-fluorocatechol, 2-hydroxybiphenyl, 4-iodophenol, 4-isopropylphenol (low), 4-methylcatechol, 4-methylphenol, methylsalicylate, 4-methylumbelliferone, 4-nitrophenol, 4-nitrocatechol, octylgallate, phenol, 4-propylphenol (low), cis-resveratrol, salicylate, 4-tert-butylphenol (low), tetrachlorocatechol, vanillin	TCDD, β-naphtoflavone, 3-methyl chloranthrene	α-napthol, 4-t-butyl phenol, 4-methylumbelliferone, 7-hydroxy coumarin

(Continued)

TABLE 5.2 (*Continued*)

A List of Endogenous and Exogenous Substrates, Inducers and Inhibitors of Major Human UGTs

Iso-enzyme	Trivial Names	Endogenous Substrates	Drug or Xenobiotic Substrates	Inducers	Inhibitors
			Amines: 4-aminobiphenyl, 1-naphthylamine>2-naphthylamine, N-OH-2-naphthylamine. Drugs: acetaminophen, beta blocking adrenergic agents (low activity) such as atenolol, labetolol, metoprolol, pindolol, propranolol. naproxen (R>>S for rat 1A6), salicylate, valproic acid. Flavonoids: chrysin, 7-hydroxy flavone, naringenin, gaboxadol (minor), fenofibric acid Others: Protocatechic aldehyde, daphetin		
UGT1A7	Rat A2 H 1g	estriol, 2-OH-estradiol, 4-OH-estrone	Benzo(a)pyrene phenols (7-OH>>9-OH>3-OH), Benzo(a)pyrene-t-7,8-dihydrodiol (7R-glucuronide, low affinity), 2-OH-biphenyl, 4-methylumbelliferone, 1- and 2-naphthol, 4-nitrophenol, octylgallate, vanillin, gaboxadol (minor)	TCDD	magnolol
UGT1A8/9[a]	HP4 Hlug P4	2-hydroxy estrone, 4-hydroxy estrone, 2-hydroxy estradiol, 4-hydroxy estradiol, estrone, dihydrotestosterone, trans-retinoic acid, 4-hydroxy retinoic acid, hyocholic acid, hyodeoxyc holic, testosterone, leukotriene B4	Alizarin, anthraflavic acid, apigenin, Benzo(a) pyrene-t-7,8-dihydrodiol (7R- and 8S-glucuronides), emodin, fisetin, flavoperidol, genistein, naringenin, quercetin, quinalizarin, 4-methylumbelliferone, scopoletin, carvacrol, eugenol, 1-naphthol, p-nitrophenol, 4-aminobiphenyl, 2-hydroxy, 3-hydroxy, and 4-hydroxy biphenyl, buprenorphine (low), morphine (low), naloxone, naltrexone, ciprofibrate, diflunisal, diphenylamine, furosemide, mycophenolic acid (high), phenolphthalein, propofol, valproic acid,	3-Methyl cloranthrene	

(*Continued*)

TABLE 5.2 (*Continued*)

A List of Endogenous and Exogenous Substrates, Inducers and Inhibitors of Major Human UGTs

Iso-enzyme	Trivial Names	Endogenous Substrates	Drug or Xenobiotic Substrates	Inducers	Inhibitors
			nandrolone, 1-methyl-5α-androst-1-en-17b-ol-3-one (metabolite of metenolone), 5α-androstane-3α,17b-diol (metabolite of testosterone), (−)-epigallocatechin gallate (tea phenol), SN-38 (low)[metabolite of irinotecan], troglitazone (moderate), raloxifene (both 6b- and 4'-b-glucuronides), quercetin, luteolin, gaboxadol (minor), indomethacin,		
UGT1A9/8[a]	H 1h	Retinoic acid, thyroxine (T4), tri-iodothyronine (T3; minor), 4-hydroxyestrone, 4-hydroxyestradiol (major)	Planar Phenols: Phenol, acetaminophen, 2-hydroxybiphenyl, 4-iodophenol, 4-propylphenol, 4-isopropylphenol (low), 4-ethylphenol, 3-ethylphenol, 4-methylphenol, 4-nitrophenol, 4-tert-butylphenol (low), methylsalicylate, salicylate, mono(ethylhexyl) salicylate, mono(ethylhexyl) phthalate, BHA, BHT, vanillin, 7-hydroxycoumarin, 4-hydroxycoumarin (low), 4-methylumbelliferone Bulky Phenols: phenol red, phenolphthalein, fluorescein Simple Catechols: *octyl gallate, propyl gallate* Primary Amines: 4-aminobiphenyl Xenobiotics: acetaminophen, p-HPPH (phenytoin metabolite), retigabine fenofibric acid, gemfibrozil, ciprofibric acid, clofibric acid, troglitazone (10-fold lower activity than fibrates),	TCDD, tetrabutyl hydroquinone, clofibric acid	High concentrations of propofol, niflumic acid (ki ~100 nM), magnolol

(Continued)

TABLE 5.2 (Continued)

A List of Endogenous and Exogenous Substrates, Inducers and Inhibitors of Major Human UGTs

Iso-enzyme	Trivial Names	Endogenous Substrates	Drug or Xenobiotic Substrates	Inducers	Inhibitors
			SN-38 (active metabolite of irinotecan), mycophenolic acid, *propfol*, atenolol, labetolol, metoprolol, pindolol, propranolol, diflunisal, fenoprofen, ibuprofen, ketoprofen, mefenamic acid, naproxen (low activity against all NSAIDs), bumetanide, furosemide, (dapsone), ethi'nyl estradiol -minor), dobutamine, dopamine, levodopa, carbidopa, entacapone, R –oxazepam, emodin, chrysin, 7-Hydroxyflavone, galangin, naringenin, quercetin carveol, nopol, citronellol, 6-hydroxychrysene, gaboxadol (major), muraglitazar (2.1 uM Km), valproic acid, daphnetin,		
UGT1A10	H 1j	2-OH-estrone (low), 4-OH estrone (low), dihydrotestosterone, testosterone	Alizarin, anthraflavic acid, apigenin, Benzo(a) pyrene-t-7,8-dihydrodiol (7R- and 8S-glucuronides, high affinity), emodin, fisetin, genistein, naringenin, quercetin, quinalizarin, 4-methylumbelliferone, scopoletin, carvacrol, eugenol, mycophenolic acid, 17β-methyl-5β-– androst-4-ene-3α,17α-diol (metabolite of metadienone), nandrolone, 1-methyl-5α- androst-1-en-17β–ol-3-one (metabolite of metenolone), 5α-androstane-3α,17β-diol (metabo lite of testosterone), SN-38 (minor), raloxifene (4'-β-glucuronide only), dopamine (low affinity, high specificity), Hydrozyimidazoacridones (C-1311, C-1305)		
UGT2A1			Etiocholanolone (low affinity), epitestosterone, testosterone		

(Continued)

TABLE 5.2 (Continued)

A List of Endogenous and Exogenous Substrates, Inducers and Inhibitors of Major Human UGTs

Iso-enzyme	Trivial Names	Endogenous Substrates	Drug or Xenobiotic Substrates	Inducers	Inhibitors
UGT2B4	Hlug 25, h-1, h-20	6α-hydroxy bile acids, 3α-hydroxy pregnanes, 3α-, 16α-, 17β-androgens. metabolites of poly unsaturated fatty acids (PUFA), arachidonic and linoleic acids, estriol, 2-hydroxy estriol, 4-hydroxy estrone, HDCA, 17-epiestriol	Phenols: Eugenol, 4-nitrophenol, 2-aminophenol, 4-methyl umbelliferone, morphine	Fenofibric acid, chenodeoxycholic acid-activated FXR	
UGT2B7	h-2, Hlug6	Arachidonic acid metabolites: Leukotriene B4 (LTB4), 5-hydroxyeicosatetraenoic acid (HETE), 12-HETE, 15-HETE, and 13-hydroxyoctadecadienoic acid (HODE) Bile acids: hyodexycholic acid Estrogens: Estriol, estradiol (17β-hydroxy), 4-hydroxy estrone (high), 2-hydroxy estrone, 2-hydroxy estriol, 17-epiestriol, epitestosterone Pregnanes: 3α-hydroxy pregnanes, Androgens: 3α-, 16α-, 17β-androgens, Others: 5α- and 5β-dihydroaldosterone, trans-retinoic acid,	*R-oxazepam*, naproxen, menthol, *AZT (zidovudine)*, abacavir, acetaminophen, almokalant, carvedilol, chloramphenicol, epirubicin, 1′-hydroxy estragole, 5-hydroxy rofecoxib, lorazepam, menthol, 4-methylumbelliferone, 1-naphthol (low), 4-nitrophenol, octylgallate, propranolol, temazepam, finofibric acid (high Clint >> UGTs 1A3, 1A6, 1A9), efavirenz, indomethacin, glycerrhetinic acid, 2,2-bis(bromomethyl)-1,3-propandiol, PR-104A, carbinol (metabolite of letrozole) Carboxylic acid-containing drugs: benoxaprofen, ciprofibrate, clofibric acid, diflunisal, dimethylxanthenone-4-acetic acid (DMXAA), fenoprofen, ibuprofen, indomethacin, ketoprofen, naproxen, pitavastatin, simvastatin acid, tiaprofenic acid, valproic acid, zaltoprofen, zomepirac. Opioids: morphine 3OH>6OH, buprenorphine, nalorphine, naltrexone, codeine (low) and naloxone.	Rifampin, Phenobarbital, HNF1α	R-oxazepam and zidovudine (competitive), Flunitrazepam relatively potent (Ki ~50–90 µM), but also inhibits UGT1A3 (Ki = 20–30 µM for 2-hydroxy estrogens) and UGT1A1 (Ki > 200 µM). Diclofenac, Etonitazenyl, genistein, herbimycin A, amytryptalline (Low concentrations)?.

(Continued)

TABLE 5.2 (*Continued*)

A List of Endogenous and Exogenous Substrates, Inducers and Inhibitors of Major Human UGTs

Iso-enzyme	Trivial Names	Endogenous Substrates	Drug or Xenobiotic Substrates	Inducers	Inhibitors
					diclofenac (58 uM IC50), diflunisal (37 uM IC50), indomethacin (88uM IC50), fluconazole (529 uM IC50),
UGT2B10	h-46	No known substrates	Medetomine (levo and dextro), amitryptalline, imipramine, clomipramine, trimipramine, senecionine		S-nicotine
UGT2B11		No known substrates			
UGT2B15	h-3	*Testosterone*, dihydrotestosterone			
UGT2B17	Hlug 4	*Testosterone*, androsterone, epitestosterone			
UGT2B28		Steroids, bile acids		Eugenol	
UGT3A1		Ursodeoxycholic acid, 17-β-estradiol,	4-nitrophenol		
UGT3A2					
UGT8A1		No known substrates			

aUGT1A8 and UGT1A9 were previously mislabeled. The old UGT1A8 is now UGT1A9 and vice versa.

AhR activators in humans (Aromatic hydrocarbon Receptor)—Tetrachlorodibenzodioxin (TCDD), α-Naphthoflavone, 3-Methylcloranthrene.

PXR (Pregnenolone-16-α-nitrile-X-Receptor) activators in rodents—pregnenolone-16α-nitrile (PCN), dexamethasone.

PXR (Pregnenolone-16-α-nitrile-X-Receptor) activators in humans—clotrimazole, rifampin, and St. John's wort.

CAR (Constitutive Androstane Receptor) activators in humans—3-methylcholanthrene, phenylpropionic acid, Phenobarbital, Phenytoin, carbamazepine.

PPAR α (Peroxisome Proliferated-Activated Receptor-α) activator in humans—clofibric acid, fenobibric acid, pirinixic acid.

PPAR α (Peroxisome Proliferated-Activated Receptor-α) activator in humans—rosiglitazone.

FXR (Farnesoid-X-Receptor) activators in humans—chenodeoxycholic acid.

LXR (Liver-X-Receptor).

RXR (Retinod-X-Receptor).

Underlined substrates denote the most commonly used probes for enzymatic activity.

UGT Drug and Protein Interactions

Traditionally, the potential for clinically relevant drug interactions involving the UGTs to occur was considered to be low based on the relatively low affinities of UGT substrates and inhibitors as well as the overlapping specificities of most UGT ligands (Williams et al. 2004). *In vitro* studies have shown the UGTs to be susceptible to both inhibition and induction, though the observed alteration of enzymatic activity does not necessarily translate into the clinic (Goon et al. 2016). Further, cases where clinically relevant UGT drug interactions appear to be occurring can be complicated by concomitant interactions with transporters or pharmacodynamic targets (Burckhardt and Burckhardt 2003). Specific topics related to UGT drug interactions are discussed below, and have been covered in full detail in previous chapters on UGTs (Remmel et al. 2008).

Acyl Glucuronides

Formation of acyl glucuronides, their subsequent chemical and biochemical reactivity, and hepatic disposition have been extensively documented and have been the subject matter of many reviews over multiple decades (Faed 1984, Sallustio et al. 2000, Bailey and Dickinson 2003, Skonberg et al. 2008, Regan et al. 2010, Dickinson 2011, Stachulski 2011). All glucuronides that are formed are beta-glucuronides due to the nature of the biochemical reaction described earlier. Acyl glucuronides can be quickly confirmed by a quick derivatization reaction with 55% hydroxyl amine solution to their corresponding hydroxamic acids (Vaz et al. 2010). Once the acyl 1-beta-glucuronides are formed, the glucuronides may undergo acyl migration, a phenomenon where the acyl group of the drug migrates to the 2-, 3-, or 4- beta isomers. These 2-, 3-, and 4-beta forms may undergo anomerization to the corresponding 2,3,4 alpha isomers, respectively. Once formed, the alpha isomers cannot be cleaved by physiological beta-glucuronidases that are present in blood and tissues. Anomerization has been documented to be predominant at lower pHs, whereas transacylation is shown to be promoted at higher pHs. It should be noted that Amadori rearrangement can only occur with 3-beta and 4-beta positional isomers and possibly by 3-alpha and 4-alpha anomers (Hodge 1955). The reaction is driven by the open form aldose intermediate, which reacts with the nucleophilic amino groups of a protein or peptide. The molecular rearrangement is driven by formation of a stable 1-amino-1-deoxy-2-ketose form, and as such, the 1-beta isomer cannot form the aldose intermediate and 2-positional isomers cannot undergo Amadori rearrangement. Acyl-SG pathways are thought to be bioactivation pathways eventually promoting protein adducts similar to transacylation (Boelsterli 2002, Grillo 2011) and can be reasoned to occur with any and all reactive positional isomers of acyl glucuronides. From a chemical reactivity stand point, thio-acyl GSH conjugates are more reactive than acyl glucuronides, as was demonstrated by reaction of diclofenac acyl glucuronide and diclofenac-S-acyl GSH respectively with N-acetyl cysteine (Grillo 2011). Reactive drug-acyl glucuronides as well as drug-thio-acyl GSH conjugates are thought to play a substantial role in the toxicokinetics of non-steroidal anti-inflammatory drugs but not via biochemical reactivity. Acyl glucuronides are actively taken up in the gut and cleaved intracellularly via beta-glucuronidases or due to higher pH to release the aglycone. This is thought to result in high local concentrations of the parent drug, potentially leading to damaging effects (Boelsterli 2011). Figure 5.8 illustrates general reactivity of acyl glucuronides.

Due to the potential risk of acyl glucuronide reactivity, many experiments have been designed over the years with the aim of potentially screening out reactive/toxic acyl glucuronides in early discovery or with the objective of characterizing the risk assessment of potential clinical candidates in development. Stability of acyl glucuronides has been studied in buffers, plasma, and human serum albumin solutions, with buffer at pH 7.4 showing potential for categorization of potential compounds into "safe," "withdrawn," or "warning" categories (Sawamura et al. 2010). Similarly, reaction with peptides is acknowledged as a reasonable surrogate for biochemical reactivity of acyl glucuronides (Wang et al. 2004). Walker et al. have reported an NMR-based methodology to evaluate reactivity of acyl glucuronides (Walker et al. 2007). This method relies on the disappearance of the anomeric resonance of 1-beta-acyl glucuronide as a marker of degradation or rearrangement kinetics and ultimately the stability of acyl glucuronides. Some of the assays employed for risk assessment in the industry are of a "reconstitution"

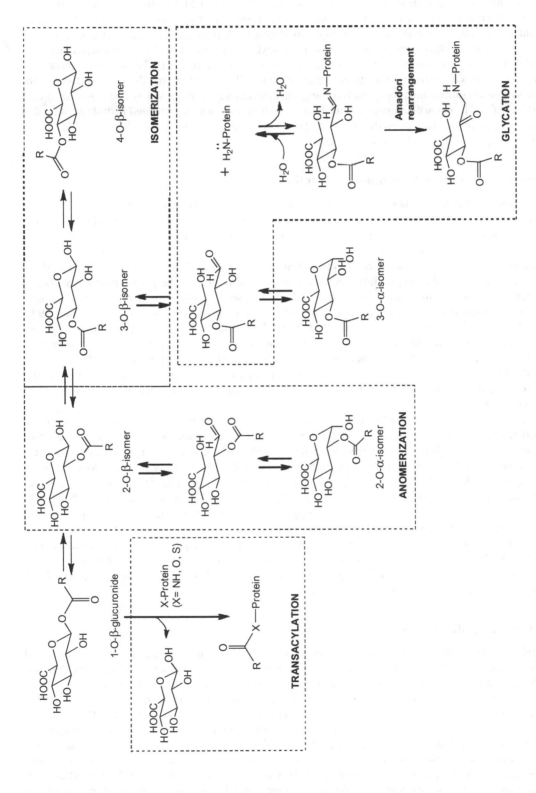

FIGURE 5.8 Transacylation, glycation, anomerization and regio-isomerization of acyl glucuronides.

nature, where the need for synthesis of an acyl glucuronide has been eliminated by utilizing lyophilized extracts from an *in vitro* incubation as a surrogate (Zhong et al. 2015). Finally, a recent experimental report by Iwamura and coworkers, points toward two additional dimensions in the reactivity of acyl glucuronides. The authors describe immunostimulation in human peripheral blood mononuclear cells by acyl glucuronides of withdrawn drugs, such as zomepirac acyl glucuronide, and also point toward induction of mRNA of five genes assessed via DNA microarrays (Iwamura et al. 2015). An *in silico* approach for predicting the reactivity of acyl glucuronides that can be readily applied in early discovery without needing to synthesize glucuronide compounds or carry out kinetic assays is proposed by Potter and coworkers (Potter et al. 2011). For six commercially available NSAIDS, the authors correlated hydrolysis of methyl esters of acyl chemicals with predicted ^{13}C-NMR chemical shifts of the carbonyl carbons along with steric descriptors in a partial least square model.

Cytochrome P450—Glucuronide Interactions

The inhibition of drug metabolizing enzymes by metabolites is a well-recognized occurrence and can result in the inhibition of the enzyme involved in the formation of the metabolite (product inhibition) or in the inhibition of other drug metabolizing enzymes. Glucuronide metabolites are no exception to this rule, with multiple examples of inhibition of UGT or cytochrome P450 (CYP) enzymes by glucuronides having been described in recent years (Backman et al. 2016, Sane et al. 2016, Tornio et al. 2016). Perhaps one of the most studied examples involves the inhibition of CYP2C8 by the glucuronide metabolite of gemfibrozil. While gemfibrozil is an inhibitor of CYP2C9 *in vitro*, its glucuronide metabolite is a potent and mechanism-based inactivator of CYP2C8, both *in vitro* and *in vivo* (Sallustio and Foster 1995, Wen et al. 2001, Wang et al. 2002, Shitara et al. 2004). Interestingly, though glucuronidation of gemfibrozil by UGT2B7 results in the formation of an acyl glucuronide, rearrangement of the acyl glucuronide is not the mechanism of CYP2C8 inactivation by gemfibrozil glucuronide. Rather, NADPH-dependent oxidation of the dimethylphenoxy moiety by CYP2C8 results in the formation of a radical intermediate and subsequent alkylation of the heme prosthetic group (Figure 5.9, top panel) (Ogilvie et al. 2006, Baer et al. 2009).

The metabolism of glucuronide conjugates by cytochrome P450 enzymes has been described for other glucuronides as well. For example, CYP2C8 has been shown to catalyze the formation of 2-hydroxyestradiol-17β-glucuronide from estradiol 17β-glucuronide and of 4-hydroxydiclofenac acyl glucuronide from diclofenac acyl glucuronide (Kumar et al. 2002, Delaforge et al. 2005). More recently, the respective roles of CYP2C8 and UGT2B10 in the formation of 3-hydroxydesloratadine were evaluated. The proposed reaction mechanism involves the glucuronidation of desloratadine by UGT2B10 followed by oxidation at the 3-position of the pyridine ring and subsequent deconjugation to form 3-hydroxydesloratadine (Kazmi et al. 2015). No oxidation at the 3-position was detected in the absence of glucuronidation, suggesting that an initial conjugation step was a requirement for subsequent oxidation by CYP2C8 (Figure 5.9, bottom panel). CYP2C8 has also been implicated in the dealkylation of the anti-diabetic agent sipoglitazar through a glucuronide intermediate, with no direct dealkylation of sipoglitazar being observed (Nishihara et al. 2012).

UGT Protein Interactions

Beginning with research on rat UGT isoforms in the early 1980s, the formation of UGT homo- and hetero-oligomers and the resulting impact on UGT activity has been the focus of many mechanistic studies and reviews (Ikushiro et al. 1997, Taura et al. 2000, Kurkela et al. 2003, Fremont et al. 2005, Ishii et al. 2005, 2010, Takeda et al. 2005, Iyanagi 2007, Nakajima et al. 2007, Operana and Tukey 2007, Finel and Kurkela 2008, Bock and Kohle 2009, Lewis et al. 2011, Konopnicki et al. 2013). The oligomers exist as either dimers or tetramers, as have been observed in the formation of diglucuronide metabolites (Peters and Jansen 1986, Gschaidmeier et al. 1995). The mechanism of UGT oligomer formation has been attributed to multiple protein domains that govern the protein interactions, many of which also confer the membrane binding properties of the UGTs (Ghosh et al. 2001, Lewis et al. 2011, Rouleau et al. 2013). Most studies have implicated the N-terminal domain of UGT isoforms as the primary contributor

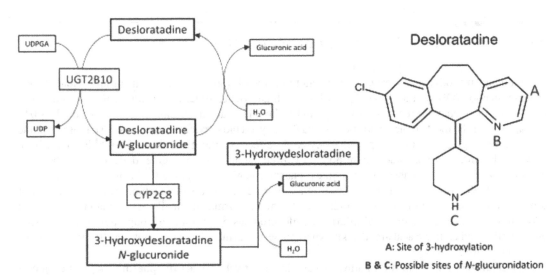

FIGURE 5.9 Examples of P450—glucuronide interactions as represented by the heme alkylation and subsequent inactivation of CYP2C8 by gemfibrozil 1-O-β-glucuronide (top panel) and the required formation of desloratadine N-glucuronide in the CYP2C8-catalyzed formation of 3-hydroxydesloratadine (bottom panel). (Reproduced with permission from Baer, B.R. et al., *Chem. Res. Toxicol.*, 22, 1298–1309, 2009 and Kazmi, F. et al., *Drug Metab. Dispos.*, 43, 1294–1302, 2015.)

to oligomerization, though a role for the C-terminal domain has also been suggested, and the potential for disulfide bond formation between UGTs remains a possibility (Meech and Mackenzie 1997b, Ghosh et al. 2001, Kurkela et al. 2007, Olson et al. 2009, Yuan et al. 2015). Based on the formation of UGT1A dimers after co-expression in Sf9 cells and the lack thereof after the simple mixing of lysates, the oligomerization of UGTs most likely requires regulated cellular synthesis as opposed to simple binding interactions (Operana and Tukey 2007, Yuan et al. 2015, Liu et al. 2016). The resulting oligomers affect both the activity and conformation of UGTs, and it has been suggested that protein interactions may also affect the thermal stability of UGT isoforms (Fujiwara et al. 2007, 2010, Fujiwara and Itoh 2014). The occurrence of protein oligomers is not limited to interactions among the UGTs, but has been observed between UGTs and cytochrome P450 isozymes as well (Fremont et al. 2005, Ishii et al. 2010).

Common techniques that have been used to characterize UGT protein interactions include co-immunoprecipitation, fluorescence resonance energy transfer (FRET), and two-hybrid screening protocols in transfected cell lines (Ghosh et al. 2001, Kurkela et al. 2003, Operana and Tukey 2007, Liu et al. 2016). Without exception, all of the aforementioned techniques have successfully identified oligomerizations between UGT isoforms as well as between UGT and other drug metabolizing enzymes such as the cytochrome P450s. Specific examples include interactions between a soluble form of UGT1A9 and UGT1A4, resulting in changes to the glucuronidation rates of entacapone and scoleptin, as well as interactions between UGT2B7 and CYP3A4, which affected both the kinetics as well as the regioselectivity of UGT2B7-mediated morphine glucuronidation (Kurkela et al. 2004, Takeda et al. 2005, 2009). Elegant studies using a FRET-based approach and fluorescently-labeled UGT1A isoforms further confirmed that the formation of homo-and hetero-dimers occurs readily among UGT1A family members, albeit in an isoform-dependent manner (Operana and Tukey 2007).

More recently, studies conducted in more physiologically relevant *in vitro* systems, such as human hepatocytes, have utilized siRNA down-regulation of UGT expression to study potential protein interactions (Konopnicki et al. 2013). Upon selective down regulation of UGT2B7, a decrease in UGT1A9 activity was also observed, confirming earlier observations made in doubly-transfected HEK293 cells and implying functional protein interactions between UGT1A9 and UGT2B7 (Fujiwara et al. 2010, Konopnicki et al. 2013). The results further emphasize the importance in the choice of *in vitro* systems when evaluating glucuronidation reactions, given the potential (or lack thereof) for protein interactions to occur within a given system, depending on the enzymes present.

Pharmacodynamic and Toxicological Role of UGTs

In addition to their role as prominent drug metabolizing enzymes, the UGTs can play a role in the observed pharmacodynamics, efficacy, and safety profile of a given drug, often through bioactivation or detoxification (Olson et al. 1992, Spahn-Langguth and Benet 1992, Ritter 2000). Research has also shown that the metabolic function of UGTs can be altered in various disease states (Wells et al. 2004). Perhaps one of the most studied examples of UGT-catalyzed bioactivation is the conversion of morphine to morphine-6-glucuronide. The pharmacodynamic effects of the glucuronide metabolite have been shown to be orders of magnitude more potent than the parent drug morphine, depending on the route of administration and contribute to the clinical pharmacology of morphine (Osborne et al. 1988, 1992, Paul et al. 1989, Portenoy et al. 1991, Loser et al. 1996). In an analogous fashion, the glucuronides of some retinoids, such as retinyl glucuronide, are also more pharmacologically active than their parental aglycones (Prabhala et al. 1989). Similarly, the glucuronides of gemfibrozil, buprenorphine or norbuprenorphine, and clofibric acid are also known to possess pharmacological activity (Sallustio et al. 1997, Brown et al. 2011).

UGT-catalyzed glucuronidation pathways can also negatively impact the pharmacological profile of a drug through rapid elimination of the drug or through the onset of drug resistance (Mazerska et al. 2016). Lamotrigine (epilepsy; UGT1A4), efavirenz (HIV; UGT1A1/2B7) and telmisartan (hypertension; UGT1A3) are all examples where increased UGT activity due to either polymorphic expression or enzyme induction have been shown or suggested to decrease the effectiveness of the drugs in patients (Kwara et al. 2009, Habtewold et al. 2011, Ieiri et al. 2011, Yamada et al. 2011, Ghosh et al. 2013, Chang et al. 2014, Metzger et al. 2014). UGT-mediated drug resistance has also received attention in oncology settings where alterations to UGT expression levels in tumors can affect the therapeutic outcome. For example, UGT expression has been shown to be lower in tumor-derived tissue from breast cancer patients as opposed to healthy tissue, while in biopsies from colon, pancreatic, or stomach tumors, a higher level of UGT activity relative to healthy tissue was reported (Starlard-Davenport et al. 2008, Jones and Lazarus 2014, Cengiz et al. 2015, Dates et al. 2015, Lu et al. 2015, Yilmaz et al. 2015). As such, drugs such as tamoxifen, belinostat, and etoposide are all subject to changes in their pharmacodynamics based upon the UGT expression levels in patients and, more specifically, in the tumor tissue itself (Poon et al. 1993, Watanabe et al. 2003, Zheng et al. 2007, Ahern et al. 2011, Wang et al. 2013, Goey and Figg 2016). Regarding safety profiles, the impact of glucuronidation on irinotecan-mediated toxicity has been well characterized, with intestinal glucuronidation thought to play a key role in diminishing the toxicological effects of irinotecan (Takahashi et al. 1997, Iyer et al. 2002, Han et al. 2006, Nagar and Blanchard 2006a, Toffoli et al. 2006, Tallman et al. 2007, Fujita and Sparreboom 2010, Di Paolo et al. 2011, Chen et al. 2013, Wang et al. 2014, Etienne-Grimaldi et al. 2015).

Alterations of UGT expression or activity can also affect the metabolism of endogenous compounds and result in the onset of various disease states. Bilirubin, formed by the breakdown of erythrocytic heme and other heme containing enzymes, undergoes multifaceted disposition. Primarily formed in blood, unconjugated bilirubin is transported to the liver by binding to albumin, where it's taken up by OATP1B1 and OATP1B3 into hepatocytes. Bilirubin undergoes glucuronidation to mono- and di-glucuronides, a reaction catalyzed only by UGT1A1. MPR2 is responsible for the active efflux of bilirubin to its conjugated form into bile, where it may be unconjugated or reduced by gut bacteria to form urobilinogen and excreted. Inhibition of the uptake transporters or UGT1A1 may lead to unconjugated hyperbilirubinemia. Similarly, polymorphic variants of UGT1A1 can result in individuals with reduced expression or dysfunctional enzyme who cannot metabolize bilirubin efficiently and display unconjugated hyperbilirubinemia. Deconvoluting hyperbilirubinemia is extremely challenging due the complex interplay of glucuronidation and transport mechanisms, and a couple case examples that show case methodologies and caveats are recommended for further reading (Templeton et al. 2014).

Estimation of *In Vivo* Glucuronidation Parameters

There are numerous *in vitro* and *in vivo* challenges associated with UGTs and glucuronidation. As previously mentioned, glucuronidation as a metabolic pathway is dependent on a substrate's entry into the cell and may be rate limiting to a substrate's exit out of the cell. Thus, kinetics in microsomes may not always translate to hepatocytes. Furthermore, the active site of UGTs faces the inner lumen of the ER membrane and, therefore, faces inward in microsomes. *In vitro* incubations need to utilize pore-forming agents in appropriate amounts for reproducible kinetics. IVIVE is further complicated when the UGT substrate is also a substrate for one or more uptake and efflux transporters. Many of these difficulties result in inaccurate clearance prediction of UGT substrates, even when glucuronidation is the major route of elimination. In addition, challenges related to *in vitro* kinetic models and *in vivo* preclinical studies are an added complicating aspect and are discussed herein. Broadly these can be classified into the categories below.

Sources of Variability in UGT-Catalyzed Reactions

A number of sources of variability exist when assessing glucuronidation reactions *in vitro*, many of which stem from the propensity of the UGTs to be involved in protein-protein interactions as well as from the localization of the UGT active sites on the luminal side of the ER membrane. As such, the choice of *in vitro* systems (i.e., recombinantly expressed single enzyme systems, sub-cellular fractions, or hepatocytes) can quantitatively and qualitatively impact the observed results, and caveats exist when using any *in vitro* approach (Radominska-Pandya et al. 1999). For example, single enzymes systems such as transfected cell lines or recombinantly expressed UGTs have the advantage of being able to mechanistically assess the contributions of an individual isoform to a glucuronidation reaction, though are limited in that oligomerization with other drug metabolizing enzymes is unable to occur (Konopnicki et al. 2013). UGT enzymes are often over-expressed in recombinant systems, and as such, the observed kinetics in recombinant systems cannot be directly translated to microsomes or hepatocytes. Elucidation of atypical kinetics in recombinant systems is also difficult. For example, a general UGT substrate, 4-methyl umbelliferone, shows Michaelis-Menten kinetics in HLM; however, atypical kinetics are observed in recombinant enzyme systems: hyperbolic kinetics are observed with UGT1A1, substrate inhibition is observed with UGT1A3, and homotropic cooperativity is seen in incubations with UGT2B7 (Miners et al. 2004, Argikar et al. 2011).

Sub-cellular fractions such as microsomes or S9 fractions are preferred from the standpoint of protein-protein interactions as well as in the flexibility to separate glucuronidation reactions from their oxidative counterparts through the addition (or omission) of individual cofactors such as NADPH or UDPGA (Fisher et al. 2002, Kilford et al. 2009). A caveat to the use of subcellular fractions is the need to overcome the UGT-latency often observed in these systems through the means of artificial pore-forming approaches such as alamethicin, detergents, or sonication (Lueders and Kuff 1967, Little et al. 1997, Fisher et al. 2000, Kurkela et al. 2003, Soars et al. 2003, Mazur et al. 2010, Walsky et al. 2012, Ladd et al. 2016). Finally, from the standpoint of physiological relevance, assessing glucuronidation reactions in hepatocytes represents the *in vitro* approach most likely to correlate with *in vivo* results, though the contributions of oxidation, conjugation, hydrolysis, and transport to the metabolic fate of the agly-cone can make interpreting the overall role of glucuronidation somewhat complex (Miners et al. 2006, Naritomi et al. 2015).

Beyond the choice of *in vitro* systems, additional factors can affect glucuronidation reactions and can often have a significant impact on the translatability of *in vitro* results to their clinical outcomes. For example, numerous studies have shown that, in general, an under-prediction of *in vivo* clearance occurs when using intrinsic clearance values obtained from liver microsomal systems (Boase and Miners 2002, Soars et al. 2002, Engtrakul et al. 2005, Miners et al. 2010, Naritomi et al. 2015). A key factor histori-cally implicated in the under-prediction has been the effect of endogenous fatty acids on UGT activ-ity *in vitro*. Microsomal fatty acids are released during *in vitro* incubations in various concentrations. Fatty acids from caprylic acid (C8) to nervonic acid (C24) have been reported to be liberated from rat, monkey, and human liver microsomes during incubations in a time-dependent manner. The concentra-tions of the acids are also known to be varied across liver microsomes from rat, monkey, and human in a species-dependent fashion (Bushee et al. 2014). Careful consideration needs to be given to which of these fatty acids are important depending on the species of interest and the substrate/inhibitor under investigation, while performing detailed kinetic studies. The fatty acids outcompete the substrates; thus, yielding artificially high Km values (high µM to low mM). The competitive inhibition of various UGT isoforms by unsaturated fatty acids is well documented, with the addition of albumin (generally bovine serum albumin, fatty acid-free human serum albumin, or intestinal fatty acid binding protein) having been shown to bind endogenous fatty acids; thus, improving the IVIVE by attenuating the observed UGT inhibition (Rowland et al. 2007, 2008, Manevski et al. 2011, Gill et al. 2012, Sekimoto et al. 2016). Although these have been shown to help the IVIVE of UGT1A9 and UGT2B7 substrates, Km parameters remain unaltered for substrates of UGTs 1A4, 1A1, and 1A6 (low µM) (Tsoutsikos et al. 2004, Rowland et al. 2007, 2008).

The type of buffer system and other reagents used for *in vitro* glucuronidation reactions can also affect the resulting kinetics, as has been shown for cytochrome P450 catalyzed reactions. For example, altera-tions to the observed UGT kinetics for 3′-azido-3′-deoxythymidine were noted when carbonate buffer was used as opposed to the more commonly used potassium phosphate or Tris buffer systems (Engtrakul et al. 2005). Similarly, in HLM, UGT1A4, and UGT1A9 showed up to 2× higher activity in Tris-HCl buffer, than phosphate buffer. The use of β-glucuronidase inhibitors is a further source of variation among *in vitro* UGT protocols. The enzyme is readily expressed in most mammalian tissues including the major organs involved in drug metabolism and is responsible for the hydrolysis of glucuronide metabolites back to their respective aglycones (Marsh et al. 1952, Levvy and Marsh 1959). While the inclusion of β-glucuronidase inhibitors such as D-saccharic acid 1,4-lactone may have limited physiological rel-evance, their inclusion in *in vitro* assays has been shown to improve IVIVE from microsomal data and may provide additional mechanistic insights into a given glucuronidation pathway (Oleson and Court 2008, Walsky et al. 2012). It is believed that increased glucuronidation activity in the presence of saccha-rolactone may actually be due to a decrease in pH and not necessarily inhibition of beta-glucuronidases.

Further differences in incubation conditions can arise from pore forming reagents, choice and concentra-tion of organic solvent, and methods of glucuronide quantitation, all of which can lead to variations in Km and Vmax across laboratories. In general, alamethicin is recommended over surfactants such as Triton-X and Brij58. It has been reported optimal concentrations of the pore forming reagent are 50 µg alamethicin / mg of protein (if the protein concentration is greater than 0.17 mg/mL) or 10 µg alamethicin / mL of incuba-tion (Fisher et al. 2000, Soars et al. 2003, Walsky et al. 2012). Organic solvents utilized in incubations also lead to observable differences in enzyme kinetics for a given substrate. In general, organic solvents are rec-ommended to be less than 1% in an *in vitro* incubation. It should be noted that UGT1A9 and UGT2B17 are not as well tolerant of DMSO as other UGTs (Chauret et al. 1998, Uchaipichat et al. 2004). Finally, accurate kinetic studies for formation of glucuronides are performed by either using a synthetic reference standard for the glucuronide or by the use of ^{14}C-UDPGA to form the glucuronide. Neither technique is time and cost effective. Synthesis of glucuronides as reference standards is demanding, and formation kinetics of gluc-uronides is resource intensive. Thus, there exists a general dependency on substrate depletion kinetics even in the presence of competing metabolic pathways. Absolute quantification of the glucuronide metabolite in circulation is challenging due to this and other analytical challenges.

Effect of Enterohepatic Recirculation

Due to constant recycling of the parent drug and or its glucuronide metabolite, this phenomenon presents a remarkable challenge in estimating the fraction of the drug (dose) that is metabolized via glucuronidation. Enterohepatic recirculation of glucuronides begins with the uptake of the glucuronide metabolite from the blood compartment into hepatocytes, subsequent biliary excretion, and reabsorption in the intestine (Vasilyeva et al. 2015). Interconversion between the glucuronide metabolite and the parent offers an additional complicating factor. The molecular weight, chemical structure, and polarity of the glucuronide in conjunction with co-administered medications, disease state, age, and gender can all affect the rate and extent of enterohepatic recirculation (Malik et al. 2016). Recirculation has been noted for glucuronides of drugs such as sorafenib, retigabine, lorazepam and acetaminophen. While information on entero-hepatic recirculation of a new chemical entity may not be readily available in early discovery, it is recommended that preclinical models in drug-development phases undergo iterative refinement as additional details on entero-hepatic recirculation are revealed.

Species-Dependent Glucuronidation

Expression of UGT isoforms in preclinical species and human is different, often leading to a poor translation of the rate or extent of glucuronidation from preclinical models to human. Species differences in expression of UGTs are known, but are not well understood. Moreover, the expression of UGT isoforms is tissue-specific in preclinical species and human. Further, a role for extrahepatic glucuronidation as a metabolic component has recently been gaining attention in more complex attempts to accurately estimate glucuronidation clearance. Species differences in extra-hepatic expression and function of UGTs are even less well-understood, and genetic polymorphisms and disease states are a further complicating factor (Cappiello et al. 1991, Burchell et al. 1998, Tukey and Strassburg 2000, Burchell 2003, Mackenzie et al. 2005).

Analytical Challenges with Glucuronide Metabolites

Advancements in mass spectrometry have resulted in highly sensitive instruments with softer ionization techniques and robust precursor and fragment ion detection (Bushee and Argikar 2011). This has resulted in qualitative and quantitative assessments of metabolites that were previously below limits of quantification or detection by HPLC-UV methods. Despite this, glucuronides as metabolites can be complicated to quantify by modern day analytical techniques. Some of the difficulties with respect to sample preparation and analysis are discussed below. Active tissue beta glucuronidases will cleave the glucuronides to form the parent drug. Similarly, some acyl glucuronides may be unstable at high or low pHs, as is the case with clopidogrel acyl glucuronide at pH values below 5.5. Where acidification is a commonly utilized strategy to prevent rearrangement when quantifying acyl glucuronides and use of 0.1% formic acid is generally a default mobile phase, a pH dependent sample work-up should be used with caution for glucuronides of new chemical entities. Extra precaution is recommended where re-analysis, incurred sample analysis, or multiple freeze thaw cycles of samples are involved. Concerns connected with acyl glucuronide reactivity are discussed separately in this chapter. In general, chromatographic separation of glucuronides and their parent compounds is a must to avoid over-estimation of the parent molecule by in-source fragmentation of the glucuronide. Most glucuronides elute very close to the solvent front in reverse-phase HPLC conditions, but due attention is needed while running shorter gradients, especially LC methods that run over a few minutes, or high-throughput, high capacity non-LC-based MS techniques. Further, glucuronides such as valproic acid glucuronide are unstable at high temperatures (Argikar and Remmel 2009a). In general, inaccurate estimation of glucuronides or parent molecules leads to overestimation of PK, TK and skewed PK-PD relationships. Unusual glucuronides need to be accounted for during metabolite identification studies. These glucuronides may not add up to the usual m/z values or neutral losses in a mass list. Finally, the importance of an authentic, pure reference standard for quantification cannot be stressed more and has been discussed in a separate section in this chapter.

In Vivo Estimation of Glucuronidation Kinetics from *In Vitro* Data

The above challenges can all translate to poor IVIVE, and glucuronidation rates, in general, tend to be underpredicted (Miners et al. 2006, Gill et al. 2012, Naritomi et al. 2015). A few valuable approaches exist that may be utilized in research and early development to aid IVIVE of UGT substrates (Argikar et al. 2016). These are listed below along with their strengths and weaknesses.

Quantitative IVIVE: Prediction of Human *In Vivo* Hepatic Clearance Using Human Liver Microsomes or Hepatocytes

This is a widely utilized, simple technique for the extrapolation of microsomal or hepatocellular *in vitro* data to predict *in vivo* hepatic clearance (Soars et al. 2002, Miners et al. 2006, Naritomi et al. 2015). It calculates intrinsic clearance from either substrate disappearance or product formation assays in microsomes or hepatocytes. This value is then corrected for fraction unbound, and the scaled *in vivo* hepatic CL is calculated using the well-stirred equations shown below based on whether the data was generated in microsomes (top equation) or hepatocytes (bottom equation).

$$CLint = \frac{0.693}{\text{in vitro t1}/2} \times \frac{\text{mL incubation}}{\text{mg microsomes}} \times \frac{40 \text{ mg microsomes}}{\text{g Liver}} \times \frac{21.4 \text{ g Liver}}{\text{kg body weight}}$$

$$CLint = \frac{0.693}{\text{in vitro t1}/2} \times \frac{\text{mL incubation}}{\text{million cells}} \times \frac{99 \text{ million cells}}{\text{g Liver}} \times \frac{21.4 \text{ g Liver}}{\text{kg body weight}}$$

$$CLH = \frac{QH \times fu \times CLint}{QH + (fu \times CLint)}$$

Hepatocytes have been shown to result in more accurate predictions of *in vivo* clearance parameters for UGT substrates, as discussed earlier. A few of the major limitations of this method are that it discounts extrahepatic metabolism and hepatocellular assay cannot be reliably applied to compounds with poor passive permeability and little to no active uptake.

Use of Relative Activity Factors (RAFs)

This approach works very well when authentic glucuronide reference standards are available for estimation of intrinsic clearance or when glucuronidation is the predominant pathway, ideally with one glucuronide metabolite (Gibson et al. 2013). RAFs are calculated by measuring the intrinsic clearance of a specific UGT substrate in microsomes and purified, recombinant enzyme as depicted in the equation below. This is semi-mechanistic in nature and can be a powerful tool when cross-checked with UGT protein concentrations. It can also be applied when interspecies differences in rate and/or extent of glucuronidation are observed. In addition, it can be applied to other organs to estimate clearance, when extra-hepatic glucuronidation is observed. A benefit is that large animal PK data are not needed, but UGT phenotyping data are required. A potential drawback is that some UGTs such as UGT1A9 and UGT2B7 are shown to work better in the presence of BSA. The absence of specific UGT substrates for calculation of RAFs is an additional complicating factor (i.e., estimation of relative activities may include contribution of other hepatic UGTs as well). For example, estradiol, which is used for UGT1A1, is also a UGT1A3 substrate; chenodeoxy cholic acid can be used for UGT1A3 RAF estimation but is also a UGT1A1 and UGT2B7 substrate; AZT, although historically used for calculation of RAF for UGT2B7, is metabolized by UGT2B4 and UGT2B17 (Court et al. 2003).

$$RAF = \frac{CLint, u(HLM)}{CLint, u(rUGT)}$$

CL Delta: fmCYP and fmUGT Approach

This method is another semi-mechanistic approach, which is applicable when interspecies differences in rate and/or extent of glucuronidation are observed (Cubitt et al. 2009, 2011, Kilford et al. 2009, Gill et al. 2012). It relies on calculating metabolic contributions by CYPs and UGTs to a given compounds overall metabolism. f_{mCYP} and f_{mUGT} are calculated from incubations containing UDPGA, NADPH, and both cofactors, as per the equations below. Like the RAF approach, it can be applied to other organs for clearance estimation (e.g. kidney [UGT1A9], intestine [UGT1A8, UGT1A10]). While neither UGT phenotyping nor large animal PK data are necessary, this method is laborious, especially if fraction unbound (f_u), and intrinsic CL with and without BSA are estimated. This is a useful tool to utilize *in vitro* high-throughput ADME/metabolism data from human liver microsomes, but sequential and concurrent metabolism in hepatocytes can act as limiting factors for broader application.

$$fm,\ UGT = \frac{CLint,\ UGT}{\left(CLint,\ UGT + CLint,\ CYP\right)}$$

$$fm,\ CYP = \frac{CLint,\ CYP}{\left(CLint,\ UGT + CLint,\ CYP\right)}$$

As mentioned previously, some UGTs are extrahepatic and are known to be expressed in either a tissue-specific or tissue predominant manner (Burchell et al. 1998, Tukey and Strassburg 2000). Intestine (Radominska-Pandya et al. 1998, Strassburg et al. 1999), kidney (McGurk et al. 1998), placenta (Collier et al. 2002, 2015), lung, eye, spleen, and others, have been shown to express UGTs (Table 5.1), and glucuronidation pathways of several endobiotics and xenobiotics have been characterized in drug metabolism models derived from these organs. Therefore, inclusion of a glucuronidation component from such organs in clearance estimations, especially intestine and kidney, has enabled improved prediction of total clearance for substrates of such UGTs (Cubitt et al. 2009, 2011, Gill et al. 2012, Naritomi et al. 2015). In many similar instances, whole body physiologically-based pharmacokinetic (PBPK) modeling approaches may be worth investigating and may be a more appropriate method than static modeling, due to the model's ability to integrate individual organ contributions to clearance (Galetin 2014).

Allometry-Based Approaches to Predicting *In Vivo* Glucuronidation: Single-Species Scaling Based on Monkey Pharmacokinetics

Single-species scaling of human pharmacokinetics from monkey pharmacokinetics have been described in much detail (Deguchi et al. 2011, Lombardo et al. 2013a, 2013b). This approach is by far the simplest scaling approach based on *in vivo* data and has been shown to be reliable for a large data set of compounds. Neither extensive modeling and data generation nor a synthetic reference standard of the glucuronide metabolite are needed, and the methodology can be applied for a broad range of UGT substrates regardless of their chemical properties. As with all allometric approaches, it is non-mechanistic in nature and agnostic to potential differences between species at the enzyme level. The foundation of this approach is based on relative differences in physiological attributes underlying drug disposition between monkey and human (e.g., liver weight, hepatic blood flow, glomerular filtration rate). Coefficients derived for each species represent an undefined amalgam of such constants and are represented in the equation below:

$$CL_{human} = CL_{monkey} \times (Wt_{human}/Wt_{monkey})^{0.75}$$

where CL represents clearance, Wt represents body weight in the respective species, and 0.75 is a fixed exponent.

Special Considerations with Regard to Glucuronidation Reactions

The following key points detailing known intricacies with regard to conducting glucuronidation studies and using the data to extrapolate to humans are worthy of careful consideration while investigating UGT-catalyzed metabolic pathways.

1. Uridine diphosphate (UDP) has not been shown to be a reliable pan-inhibitor of glucuronidation reactions. Inhibition by UDP has been documented for UGTs 1A1 and 1A4 in liver microsomes, but the same data was not substantiated in recombinantly expressed single enzyme systems. Similarly, while this method was successfully applied to UGT1A9 in sf9 cell lysate supernatants, these findings were not confirmed in either recombinant systems or microsomes (Fujiwara et al. 2008, Manevski et al. 2011). Thus, to date, there is no confirmation that this is a valid method of inhibiting hepatic and/or extra-hepatic UGTs in any of the commonly used cellular or subcellular models of drug metabolism. Furthermore, different *in vitro* systems inherently bring in additional complications such as differences in protein expression, lipid compositions, and functional activity. Although based on the sequential bi bi nature of the glucuronidation reactions, one may be tempted to apply UDP inhibition to estimate UGT activity, especially in the absence of specific inhibitors, and many more experiments are needed before this method can be considered a general or reliable approach to determine contribution of glucuronidation towards clearance.

2. Whenever fatty acid quenching proteins such as BSA, has, or IFABP are utilized in UGT incubations for UGTs, such as UGT2B7, it is imperative to use unbound substrate concentrations and not total substrate concentrations. This is discussed in detail in the earlier section on clearance prediction. Unbound fraction determinations should be made under the same experimental conditions used in the *in vitro* clearance assay.

3. Micheals-Menten kinetics are not to be assumed for any glucuronidation reaction and the dataset needs to be carefully examined for presence of atypical kinetics such as homotropic/heterotropic activation. This is discussed in detail in the earlier section on UGT reaction mechanisms.

4. Estimation of kinetic rates (i.e., Vmax) without an authentic reference standard of the glucuronide is incorrect and should not be undertaken in any event (Argikar and Nagar 2014). Firstly, such an approach assumes that ionization of the parent and the glucuronide metabolite are equivalent in the mass spectrometer (MS), but this assumption is fundamentally wrong. It is well established that ionization of parent and the metabolite by MS is dramatically different (Dahal et al. 2011). The scenario is even worse when one compares metabolites like glucuronides or sulfates, because addition of polar bulky groups like glucuronic acid dramatically impacts MS ionization due to changes in the liquid gas phase properties for LC-MS/MS analyses (Figure 5.10). Furthermore, the MS responses are a function of the constituents and pH of the mobile phase, the flow rates and the MS source parameters. Many techniques such as low flow or calculation of ionization properties tend to negate the variability in MS response, but these techniques are far from generating equimolar responses for analytes such as parent and glucuronide metabolites. Secondly, calculation of metabolite formation kinetics on relative peak areas in the absence of a reference standard is also incorrect. It is understood that Michaelis-Menten kinetics describe a process at steady-state. As we know, Km represents the substrate concentration at half-maximal velocity, i.e., concentration at Vmax/2 and has units of concentration. As we know, Vmax is a rate, and therefore, it has units of concentration per unit time (normalized to concentration of enzyme used in the experiment). To obtain Vmax, reaction velocity (v) is plotted versus substrate concentration [S] (Seibert and Tracy 2014). A true Vmax cannot be obtained by plotting relative peak areas of metabolites to parent. Saturation (Vmax type effect) observed in such a plot can be an artifact due to MS detector saturation, i.e., a plateau in detector response when the analyte concentration is beyond the detector's dynamic range. Therefore, the MS measurements and the subsequent kinetic analysis are fundamentally incorrect.

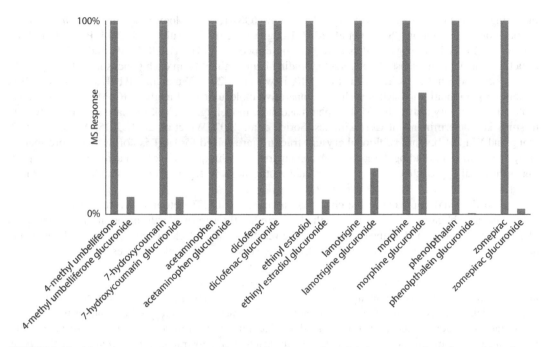

FIGURE 5.10 Mass spectrometric responses observed for compounds and their corresponding glucuronides after an equal volume injection at 1 μM in Orbitrap-XL in either ESI positive ionization in acidic mobile phase or ESI negative ionization in neutral mobile phase at a flow rate of 250 μL/min. The mass spectrometric responses for metabolites are shown as a percentage of their respective parent drug's response. The data illustrates that mass spectrometric responses are multifactorial even at equimolar concentrations and peak areas of glucuronide metabolites are not recommended to be utilized as a reliable estimate for quantification in the absence of an authentic reference standard.

Future Directions and Technologies

Though the study of UGTs and glucuronidation mechanisms is a decades old endeavor, the technologies available to aid in these enzymatic studies continue to evolve. As mentioned previously, hepatocytes represent one of the most physiologically relevant *in vitro* systems in which to study drug metabolism, especially in regard to phase II drug metabolism and transporter-mediated processes. However, under many typical *in vitro* protocols, hepatocyte incubations can have challenges in maintaining their morphology and viability over prolonged periods of time or when being used to assess the metabolism of low clearance compounds (Di et al. 2012, 2013, Ramaiahgari et al. 2014, Vivares et al. 2015). To this end, there has been an increased interest in evaluating *in vitro* systems, such as bioreactors, microfluidic platforms, spheroids, and other three-dimensional cellular models, which allow for a more robust determination of the drug metabolism and toxicology properties of a given compound (Novik et al. 2010, Nakamura et al. 2011, Fey and Wrzesinski 2012, LeCluyse et al. 2012, Godoy et al. 2013, Gomez-Lechon et al. 2014, Esch et al. 2015). Assessments of UGT activity in these systems have been promising, with UGT substrates such as hydrocortisone, morphine, lamotrigine, and diclofenac, in addition to others, being profiled to support the utility of these systems in evaluating conjugative metabolism (Wang et al. 2010, Kampe et al. 2014, Ohkura et al. 2014, Sarkar et al. 2015).

Beyond *in vitro* technologies, the use of *in silico* approaches to predict and characterize UGT-mediated reactions also remains a current area of research. Owing to the general lack of UGT crystal structures and related structural knowledge of the substrate binding domain of many UGT isoforms, mechanistic studies to study UGT substrate binding remain challenging. To indirectly begin to explore substrate binding interactions and UGT substrate specificity, multiple computational approaches have been described, including quantitative structure activity relationships (QSAR), homology modeling, and *in silico* site of metabolism predictions (Sorich et al. 2008, Dong et al. 2012, Tripathi et al. 2013, Peng et al. 2014, Nair et al. 2015). Homology models have been described for UGT1A1, UGT1A9, and UGT2B7, with structural insights into substrate or cofactor binding being gained from each (Locuson and Tracy 2007, Laakkonen and Finel 2010, Takaoka et al. 2010, Lewis et al. 2011, Wu et al. 2011, Tripathi et al. 2013). Other computational approaches such as comparative molecular field analysis (CoMFA), comparative molecular similarity indices (CoMSIA), pharmacophore modeling, and VolSurf have been recently used to study key determinants of UGT kinetics (Sorich et al. 2002, Wu et al. 2011, 2015, Ako et al. 2012, Dong and Wu 2012). Until additional crystal structures are solved for UGT isoforms, and more specifically, their substrate binding domains, such computational techniques will continue to be key in supporting orthogonal approaches such as site-directed mutagenesis in regard to understanding UGT protein structure.

As an orthogonal approach to the characterization of the UGT protein structures, there have been a number of publications on *in silico* methods to predict the site of glucuronidation, the contribution of glucuronidation as a clearance pathway, or the reactivity of acyl glucuronides. Peng and coworkers applied a bioinformatics approach with the help of local and global molecular descriptors that defined physicochemical properties, such as chemical reactivity, bond strength, and molecular volume, for a training set of 300+ compounds. Their predictions for sites of glucuronidation correlated to experimental data with 84% success rate using a test set of over 50 molecules (Peng et al. 2014). Non-training set based models such as Metasite® depend on molecular interaction fields to predict a site of metabolism. A limitation of such models is that, in general, they assume a given molecule to be a substrate and the model itself is unable to differentiate between substrates, non-substrates, and inhibitors. Furthermore, the model cannot distinguish between various types of binding modes or types of kinetic reactions such as atypical kinetics versus Michealis-Menten kinetics. Most importantly, such models cannot provide a distinction between multiple possible sites of conjugative metabolism for substrates with multiple unmasked nucleophilic groups (polyfunctional substrates), and use of these models to estimate the contribution of glucuronidation to the overall clearance of a molecule should be approached with caution. Conversely, the application of predictive models toward *in silico* UGT reaction phenotyping and estimation of kinetic parameters may provide an alternative to predict the role of glucuronidation in the clearance of a drug. Varying degrees of success with UGTs 1A1 and 1A4 based on 2D- and 3D-QSAR approaches and QSMR data have been reported for a set of compounds (Miners et al. 2004), but routine use of these models toward a new chemical entity will require additional research efforts.

A number of *in vivo* models have been developed with the aim of studying induction, regulation, and polymorphisms of UGTs in preclinical species (Chen et al. 2005). Such models with knocked-out mouse gene(s) in conjunction with knocked-in human genes have been instrumental in deciphering the role of specific nuclear receptors, such as CAR, PXR, and PPARs, signaling pathways such as nrf2-keap1, in the regulation of UGT isoforms, and their effect on UGT substrates (Verreault et al. 2006, Bonzo et al. 2007, Senekeo-Effenberger et al. 2007, Yueh and Tukey 2007, Argikar et al. 2009). These models employ mouse nuclear receptor elements, unless the knock-in/knock-out sequence has been performed for a specific nuclear receptor. An alternative animal model, such as the chimeric mice, where greater than 70% of the mouse hepatocytes have been replaced by human hepatocytes, constitute a method to test human-specific nuclear receptors UGTs in mice (Strom et al. 2010, Nishimura et al. 2013, Bateman et al. 2014, Sanoh and Ohta 2014).

Finally, focused research efforts into identifying additional selective substrates and inhibitors for UGT isoforms, the enzymology of UGTs in preclinical species, and the role of UGT pharmacogenetics in personalized medicine will most likely continue to be of interest in the near future. While UGTs are known to share overlapping substrate specificities, recent efforts have begun to identify isoform selective substrates and inhibitors, tools that will continue to expand the UGT drug interaction and reaction phenotyping resources (Miners et al. 2010, Fedejko-Kap et al. 2012, Lee et al. 2015, Pattanawongsa et al. 2016). Towards the role of glucuronidation in preclinical species, the knowledge surrounding the enzymology of UGTs in these species lags behind that of the cytochromes P450, with recent efforts seeking to expand that knowledge base in species commonly used in safety studies, such as dogs and rodents (Soars et al. 2001, Kaivosaari et al. 2011, Furukawa et al. 2014, Troberg et al. 2015).

Similarly, building on the well documented role of UGT polymorphisms in determine absorption, distribution, metabolism, excretion and toxicity (ADMET) properties, efforts are underway to identify more rapid and precise screening methods to characterize UGT polymorphisms within individuals with a focus on ensuring optimal safety and efficacy in each patient (Minucci et al. 2014, Gammal et al. 2016, Shahandeh et al. 2016).

Conclusions

The aim of this chapter was to provide a basic overview of UGT enzymology, pharmacogenetics, ontogeny, drug interactions, and *in vivo* predictions. Detailed information is available in the many exceptional reviews, book chapters, and research papers referenced herein, which have been published on UGT-related topics over the years. While much of the enzymatic phenomena surrounding UGTs has been investigated in detail through highly mechanistic studies, a great deal of research remains, with areas such as UGT protein structure, isoform-specific inhibitors, protein-protein interactions, engineered *in vitro* systems and in silico models still receiving a great deal of interest. Transgenic and humanized models can serve as an important translational tools of tissue specific human UGT enzymes. Modulation of function and capacity of UGTs in disease states is an exciting avenue, and developments in this arena will serve as a foundation for personalized medicine. As our UGT knowledge base continues to expand, so will our ability to rapidly and confidently provide pharmacokinetic, safety, and efficacy data for UGT substrates across the discovery and development continuum.

ABBREVIATIONS

UGT   UDP-Glucuronosyltransferase
UDPGA   uridine diphosphoglucuronic acid UDP, uridine diphosphate
IVIVE   *in vitro–in vivo* extrapolation
RAF   relative activity factor
MS   mass spectrometer

REFERENCES

Ahern, T. P., M. Christensen, D. P. Cronin-Fenton, K. L. Lunetta, H. Soiland, J. Gjerde, J. P. Garne et al. 2011. "Functional polymorphisms in UDP-glucuronosyl transferases and recurrence in tamoxifen-treated breast cancer survivors." *Cancer Epidemiol Biomarkers Prev* no. 20 (9):1937–1943. doi:10.1158/1055-9965.EPI-11-0419.

Akaba, K., T. Kimura, A. Sasaki, S. Tanabe, T. Ikegami, M. Hashimoto, H. Umeda et al. 1998. "Neonatal hyperbilirubinemia and mutation of the bilirubin uridine diphosphate-glucuronosyltransferase gene: A common missense mutation among Japanese, Koreans and Chinese." *Biochem Mol Biol Int* no. 46 (1):21–26.

Ako, R., D. Dong, and B. Wu. 2012. "3D-QSAR studies on UDP-glucuronosyltransferase 2B7 substrates using the pharmacophore and VolSurf approaches." *Xenobiotica* no. 42 (9):891–900. doi:10.3109/00498254.2012.675094.

Ando, Y., H. Saka, G. Asai, S. Sugiura, K. Shimokata, and T. Kamataki. 1998. "UGT1A1 genotypes and glucuronidation of SN-38, the active metabolite of irinotecan." *Ann Oncol* no. 9 (8):845–847.

Argikar, U. A. 2012. "Unusual glucuronides." *Drug Metab Dispos* no. 40 (7):1239–1251. doi:10.1124/dmd.112.045096.

Argikar, U. A., O. F. Iwuchukwu, and S. Nagar. 2008. "Update on tools for evaluation of uridine diphosphoglucuronosyltransferase polymorphisms." *Expert Opin Drug Metab Toxicol* no. 4 (7):879–894. doi:10.1517/17425255.4.7.879.

Argikar, U. A., G. Liang, J. L. Bushee, V. P. Hosagrahara, and W. Lee. 2011. "Evaluation of pharmaceutical excipients as cosolvents in 4-methyl umbelliferone glucuronidation in human liver microsomes: Applications for compounds with low solubility." *Drug Metab Pharmacokinet* no. 26 (1):102–106.

Argikar, U. A. and S. Nagar. 2014. "Case study 2. Practical analytical considerations for conducting in vitro enzyme kinetic studies." *Methods Mol Biol* no. 1113:431–439. doi:10.1007/978-1-62703-758-7_19.

Argikar, U. A., P. M. Potter, J. M. Hutzler, and P. H. Marathe. 2016. "Challenges and opportunities with non-CYP enzymes aldehyde oxidase, carboxylesterase, and UDP-glucuronosyltransferase: Focus on reaction phenotyping and prediction of human clearance." *AAPS J.* doi:10.1208/s12248-016-9962-6.

Argikar, U. A. and R. P. Remmel. 2009a. "Effect of aging on glucuronidation of valproic acid in human liver microsomes and the role of UDP-glucuronosyltransferase UGT1A4, UGT1A8, and UGT1A10." *Drug Metab Dispos* no. 37 (1):229–236.

Argikar, U. A. and R. P. Remmel. 2009b. "Variation in glucuronidation of lamotrigine in human liver microsomes." *Xenobiotica* no. 39 (5):355–363.

Argikar, U. A., K. Senekeo-Effenberger, E. E. Larson, R. H. Tukey, and R. P. Remmel. 2009. "Studies on induction of lamotrigine metabolism in transgenic UGT1 mice." *Xenobiotica* no. 39 (11):826–835.

Asher, G. N., J. K. Fallon, and P. C. Smith. 2016. "UGT concentrations in human rectal tissue after multidose, oral curcumin." *Pharmacol Res Perspect* no. 4 (2):e00222. doi:10.1002/prp2.222.

Backman, J. T., A. M. Filppula, M. Niemi, and P. J. Neuvonen. 2016. "Role of cytochrome P450 2C8 in drug metabolism and interactions." *Pharmacol Rev* no. 68 (1):168–241. doi:10.1124/pr.115.011411.

Baer, B. R., R. K. DeLisle, and A. Allen. 2009. "Benzylic oxidation of gemfibrozil-1-O-beta-glucuronide by P450 2C8 leads to heme alkylation and irreversible inhibition." *Chem Res Toxicol* no. 22 (7):1298–1309.

Bailey, M. J. and R. G. Dickinson. 2003. "Acyl glucuronide reactivity in perspective: Biological consequences." *Chem Biol Interact* no. 145 (2):117–137.

Banerjee, R., M. W. Pennington, A. Garza, and I. S. Owens. 2008. "Mapping the UDP-glucuronic acid binding site in UDP-glucuronosyltransferase-1A10 by homology-based modeling: Confirmation with biochemical evidence." *Biochemistry* no. 47 (28):7385–7392. doi:10.1021/bi8006127.

Barbier, O., C. Girard, R. Breton, A. Belanger, and D. W. Hum. 2000a. "N-glycosylation and residue 96 are involved in the functional properties of UDP-glucuronosyltransferase enzymes." *Biochemistry* no. 39 (38):11540–11552.

Barbier, O., H. Lapointe, M. El Alfy, D. W. Hum, and A. Belanger. 2000b. "Cellular localization of uridine diphosphoglucuronosyltransferase 2B enzymes in the human prostate by in situ hybridization and immunohistochemistry." *J Clin Endocrinol Metab* no. 85 (12):4819–4826. doi:10.1210/jcem.85.12.7019.

Bartlett, M. G. and G. R. Gourley. 2011. "Assessment of UGT polymorphisms and neonatal jaundice." *Semin Perinatol* no. 35 (3):127–133. doi:10.1053/j.semperi.2011.02.006.

Bateman, T. J., V. G. Reddy, M. Kakuni, Y. Morikawa, and S. Kumar. 2014. "Application of chimeric mice with humanized liver for study of human-specific drug metabolism." *Drug Metab Dispos* no. 42 (6):1055–1065. doi:10.1124/dmd.114.056978.

Belanger, A., G. Pelletier, F. Labrie, O. Barbier, and S. Chouinard. 2003. "Inactivation of androgens by UDP-glucuronosyltransferase enzymes in humans." *Trends Endocrinol Metab* no. 14 (10):473–479.

Bhasker, C. R., W. McKinnon, A. Stone, A. C. Lo, T. Kubota, T. Ishizaki, and J. O. Miners. 2000. "Genetic polymorphism of UDP-glucuronosyltransferase 2B7 (UGT2B7) at amino acid 268: Ethnic diversity of alleles and potential clinical significance." *Pharmacogenetics* no. 10 (8):679–685.

Boase, S. and J. O. Miners. 2002. "In vitro-in vivo correlations for drugs eliminated by glucuronidation: Investigations with the model substrate zidovudine." *Br J Clin Pharmacol* no. 54 (5):493–503.

Bock, K. W. and C. Kohle. 2009. "Topological aspects of oligomeric UDP-glucuronosyltransferases in endoplasmic reticulum membranes: Advances and open questions." *Biochem Pharmacol* no. 77 (9):1458–1465. doi:S0006-2952(08)00891-5 [pii].

Boelsterli, U. A. 2002. "Xenobiotic acyl glucuronides and acyl CoA thioesters as protein-reactive metabolites with the potential to cause idiosyncratic drug reactions." *Curr Drug Metab* no. 3 (4):439–450.

Boelsterli, U. A. 2011. "Acyl glucuronides: Mechanistic role in drug toxicity?" *Curr Drug Metab* no. 12 (3):213–214.

Bonzo, J. A., A. Belanger, and R. H. Tukey. 2007. "The role of chrysin and the ah receptor in induction of the human UGT1A1 gene in vitro and in transgenic UGT1 mice." *Hepatology* no. 45 (2):349–360.

Bossuyt, X. and N. Blanckaert. 1997. "Carrier-mediated transport of uridine diphosphoglucuronic acid across the endoplasmic reticulum membrane is a prerequisite for UDP-glucuronosyltransferase activity in rat liver." *Biochem J* no. 323 (Pt 3):645–648.

Bouwmeester, N. J., B. J. Anderson, D. Tibboel, and N. H. Holford. 2004. "Developmental pharmacokinetics of morphine and its metabolites in neonates, infants and young children." *Br J Anaesth* no. 92 (2):208–217.

Brown, S. M., M. Holtzman, T. Kim, and E. D. Kharasch. 2011. "Buprenorphine metabolites, buprenorphine-3-glucuronide and norbuprenorphine-3-glucuronide, are biologically active." *Anesthesiology* no. 115 (6):1251–1260. doi:10.1097/ALN.0b013e318238fea0.

Burchell, B. 2003. "Genetic variation of human UDP-glucuronosyltransferase: Implications in disease and drug glucuronidation." *Am J Pharmacogenomics* no. 3 (1):37–52.

Burchell, B., C. H. Brierley, G. Monaghan, and D. J. Clarke. 1998. "The structure and function of the UDP-glucuronosyltransferase gene family." *Adv Pharmacol* no. 42:335–338.

Burckhardt, B. C. and G. Burckhardt. 2003. "Transport of organic anions across the basolateral membrane of proximal tubule cells." *Rev Physiol Biochem Pharmacol* no. 146:95–158. doi:10.1007/s10254-002-0003-8.

Bushee, J. L. and U. A. Argikar. 2011. "An experimental approach to enhance precursor ion fragmentation for metabolite identification studies: Application of dual collision cells in an orbital trap." *Rapid Commun Mass Spectrom* no. 25 (10):1356–1362.

Bushee, J. L., G. Liang, C. E. Dunne, S. P. Harriman, and U. A. Argikar. 2014. "Identification of saturated and unsaturated fatty acids released during microsomal incubations." *Xenobiotica* no. 44 (8):687–695. doi:10.3109/00498254.2014.884253.

Cappiello, M., L. Giuliani, and G. M. Pacifici. 1991. "Distribution of UDP-glucuronosyltransferase and its endogenous substrate uridine 5′-diphosphoglucuronic acid in human tissues." *Eur J Clin Pharmacol* no. 41 (4):345–350.

Cengiz, B., O. Yumrutas, E. Bozgeyik, E. Borazan, Y. Z. Igci, I. Bozgeyik, and S. Oztuzcu. 2015. "Differential expression of the UGT1A family of genes in stomach cancer tissues." *Tumour Biol* no. 36 (8):5831–5837. doi:10.1007/s13277-015-3253-1.

Chang, Y., L. Y. Yang, M. C. Zhang, and S. Y. Liu. 2014. "Correlation of the UGT1A4 gene polymorphism with serum concentration and therapeutic efficacy of lamotrigine in Han Chinese of Northern China." *Eur J Clin Pharmacol* no. 70 (8):941–946. doi:10.1007/s00228-014-1690-1.

Chauret, N., A. Gauthier, and D. A. Nicoll-Griffith. 1998. "Effect of common organic solvents on in vitro cytochrome P450-mediated metabolic activities in human liver microsomes." *Drug Metab Dispos* no. 26 (1):1–4.

Chen, S., D. Beaton, N. Nguyen, K. Senekeo-Effenberger, E. Brace-Sinnokrak, U. Argikar, R. P. Remmel, J. Trottier, O. Barbier, J. K. Ritter, and R. H. Tukey. 2005. "Tissue-specific, inducible, and hormonal control of the human UDP-glucuronosyltransferase-1 (UGT1) locus." *J Biol Chem* no. 280 (45):37547–37557.

Chen, S., M. F. Yueh, C. Bigo, O. Barbier, K. Wang, M. Karin, N. Nguyen, and R. H. Tukey. 2013. "Intestinal glucuronidation protects against chemotherapy-induced toxicity by irinotecan (CPT-11)." *Proc Natl Acad Sci USA* no. 110 (47):19143–19148. doi:10.1073/pnas.1319123110.

Chen, Y., S. Chen, X. Li, X. Wang, and S. Zeng. 2006. "Genetic variants of human UGT1A3: Functional characterization and frequency distribution in a Chinese Han population." *Drug Metab Dispos* no. 34 (9):1462–1467.

Cheng, Z., A. Radominska-Pandya, and T. R. Tephly. 1998. "Cloning and expression of human UDP-glucuronosyltransferase (UGT) 1A8." *Arch Biochem Biophys* no. 356 (2):301–305. doi:10.1006/abbi.1998.0781.

Chouinard, S., O. Barbier, and A. Belanger. 2007. "UDP-glucuronosyltransferase 2B15 (UGT2B15) and UGT2B17 enzymes are major determinants of the androgen response in prostate cancer LNCaP cells." *J Biol Chem* no. 282 (46):33466–33474.

Coffman, B. L., W. R. Kearney, S. Goldsmith, B. M. Knosp, and T. R. Tephly. 2003. "Opioids bind to the amino acids 84 to 118 of UDP-glucuronosyltransferase UGT2B7." *Mol Pharmacol* no. 63 (2):283–288.

Coffman, B. L., W. R. Kearney, M. D. Green, R. G. Lowery, and T. R. Tephly. 2001. "Analysis of opioid binding to UDP-glucuronosyltransferase 2B7 fusion proteins using nuclear magnetic resonance spectroscopy." *Mol Pharmacol* no. 59 (6):1464–1469.

Coffman, B. L., C. D. King, G. R. Rios, and T. R. Tephly. 1998. "The glucuronidation of opioids, other xenobiotics, and androgens by human UGT2B7Y(268) and UGT2B7H(268)." *Drug Metab Dispos* no. 26 (1):73–77.

Collier, A. C., N. A. Ganley, M. D. Tingle, M. Blumenstein, K. W. Marvin, J. W. Paxton, M. D. Mitchell, and J. A. Keelan. 2002. "UDP-glucuronosyltransferase activity, expression and cellular localization in human placenta at term." *Biochem Pharmacol* no. 63 (3):409–419.

Collier, A. C., A. D. Thevenon, W. Goh, M. Hiraoka, and C. E. Kendal-Wright. 2015. "Placental profiling of UGT1A enzyme expression and activity and interactions with preeclampsia at term." *Eur J Drug Metab Pharmacokinet* no. 40 (4):471–480. doi:10.1007/s13318-014-0243-4.

Costa, E. 2006. "Hematologically important mutations: Bilirubin UDP-glucuronosyltransferase gene mutations in Gilbert and Crigler-Najjar syndromes." *Blood Cells Mol Dis* no. 36 (1):77–80.

Coughtrie, M. W. 2015. "Ontogeny of human conjugating enzymes." *Drug Metab Lett* no. 9 (2):99–108.

Court, M. H. 2005. "Isoform-selective probe substrates for in vitro studies of human UDP-glucuronosyltransferases." *Methods Enzymol* no. 400:104–116. doi:10.1016/S0076-6879(05)00007-8.

Court, M. H., Q. Hao, S. Krishnaswamy, T. Bekaii-Saab, A. Al-Rohaimi, L. L. von Moltke, and D. J. Greenblatt. 2004. "UDP-glucuronosyltransferase (UGT) 2B15 pharmacogenetics: UGT2B15 D85Y genotype and gender are major determinants of oxazepam glucuronidation by human liver." *J Pharmacol Exp Ther* no. 310 (2):656–665.

Court, M. H., S. Krishnaswamy, Q. Hao, S. X. Duan, C. J. Patten, L. L. Von Moltke, and D. J. Greenblatt. 2003. "Evaluation of 3'-azido-3'-deoxythymidine, morphine, and codeine as probe substrates for UDP-glucuronosyltransferase 2B7 (UGT2B7) in human liver microsomes: Specificity and influence of the UGT2B7*2 polymorphism." *Drug Metab Dispos* no. 31 (9):1125–1133.

Court, M. H., X. Zhang, X. Ding, K. K. Yee, L. M. Hesse, and M. Finel. 2012. "Quantitative distribution of mRNAs encoding the 19 human UDP-glucuronosyltransferase enzymes in 26 adult and 3 fetal tissues." *Xenobiotica* no. 42 (3):266–277. doi:10.3109/00498254.2011.618954.

Cubitt, H. E., J. B. Houston, and A. Galetin. 2009. "Relative importance of intestinal and hepatic glucuronidation-impact on the prediction of drug clearance." *Pharm Res* no. 26 (5):1073–1083. doi:10.1007/s11095-008-9823-9.

Cubitt, H. E., J. B. Houston, and A. Galetin. 2011. "Prediction of human drug clearance by multiple metabolic pathways: Integration of hepatic and intestinal microsomal and cytosolic data." *Drug Metab Dispos* no. 39 (5):864–873. doi:10.1124/dmd.110.036566.

Dahal, U. P., J. P. Jones, J. A. Davis, and D. A. Rock. 2011. "Small molecule quantification by liquid chromatography-mass spectrometry for metabolites of drugs and drug candidates." *Drug Metab Dispos* no. 39 (12):2355–2360. doi:10.1124/dmd.111.040865.

Dates, C. R., T. Fahmi, S. J. Pyrek, A. Yao-Borengasser, B. Borowa-Mazgaj, S. M. Bratton, S. A. Kadlubar, P. I. Mackenzie, R. S. Haun, and A. Radominska-Pandya. 2015. "Human UDP-glucuronosyltransferases: Effects of altered expression in breast and pancreatic cancer cell lines." *Cancer Biol Ther* no. 16 (5):714–723. doi:10.1080/15384047.2015.1026480.

de Wildt, S. N., G. L. Kearns, J. S. Leeder, and J. N. van den Anker. 1999. "Glucuronidation in humans: Pharmacogenetic and developmental aspects." *Clin Pharmacokinet* no. 36 (6):439–452. doi:10.2165/00003088-199936060-00005.

Deguchi, T., N. Watanabe, A. Kurihara, K. Igeta, H. Ikenaga, K. Fusegawa, N. Suzuki et al. 2011. "Human pharmacokinetic prediction of UDP-glucuronosyltransferase substrates with an animal scale-up approach." *Drug Metab Dispos* no. 39 (5):820–829. doi:10.1124/dmd.110.037457.

Delaforge, M., A. Pruvost, L. Perrin, and F. Andre. 2005. "Cytochrome P450-mediated oxidation of glucuronide derivatives: Example of estradiol-17beta-glucuronide oxidation to 2-hydroxy-estradiol-17beta-glucuronide by CYP 2C8." *Drug Metab Dispos* no. 33 (3):466–473. doi:10.1124/dmd.104.002097.

Di, L., K. Atkinson, C. C. Orozco, C. Funk, H. Zhang, T. S. McDonald, B. Tan, J. Lin, C. Chang, and R. S. Obach. 2013. "In vitro-in vivo correlation for low-clearance compounds using hepatocyte relay method." *Drug Metab Dispos* no. 41 (12):2018–2023. doi:10.1124/dmd.113.053322.

Di, L., P. Trapa, R. S. Obach, K. Atkinson, Y. A. Bi, A. C. Wolford, B. Tan, T. S. McDonald, Y. Lai, and L. M. Tremaine. 2012. "A novel relay method for determining low-clearance values." *Drug Metab Dispos* no. 40 (9):1860–1865. doi:10.1124/dmd.112.046425.

Di Paolo, A., G. Bocci, M. Polillo, M. Del Re, T. Di Desidero, M. Lastella, and R. Danesi. 2011. "Pharmacokinetic and pharmacogenetic predictive markers of irinotecan activity and toxicity." *Curr Drug Metab* no. 12 (10):932–943.

Dickinson, R. G. 2011. "Iso-glucuronides." *Curr Drug Metab* no. 12 (3):222–228.

Dong, D., R. Ako, M. Hu, and B. Wu. 2012. "Understanding substrate selectivity of human UDP-glucuronosyltransferases through QSAR modeling and analysis of homologous enzymes." *Xenobiotica* no. 42 (8):808–820. doi:10.3109/00498254.2012.663515.

Dong, D. and B. Wu. 2012. "In silico modeling of UDP-glucuronosyltransferase 1A10 substrates using the VolSurf approach." *J Pharm Sci* no. 101 (9):3531–3539. doi:10.1002/jps.23100.

Dutton, G. J. 1997. "Raising the colors: Personal reflections on the glucuronidation revolution 1950–1970." *Drug Metab Rev* no. 29 (4):997–1024. doi:10.3109/03602539709002241.

Dutton, G. J. 1980. "Structures and properties of glucuronides." In *Glucuronidation of Drugs and Other Compounds*. Boca Raton, FL: CRC Press.

Ehmer, U., A. Vogel, J. K. Schutte, B. Krone, M. P. Manns, and C. P. Strassburg. 2004. "Variation of hepatic glucuronidation: Novel functional polymorphisms of the UDP-glucuronosyltransferase UGT1A4." *Hepatology* no. 39 (4):970–977.

Elahi, A., J. Bendaly, Z. Zheng, J. E. Muscat, J. P. Richie, Jr., S. P. Schantz, and P. Lazarus. 2003. "Detection of UGT1A10 polymorphisms and their association with orolaryngeal carcinoma risk." *Cancer* no. 98 (4):872–880.

Engtrakul, J. J., R. S. Foti, T. J. Strelevitz, and M. B. Fisher. 2005. "Altered AZT (3'-azido-3'-deoxythymidine) glucuronidation kinetics in liver microsomes as an explanation for underprediction of in vivo clearance: Comparison to hepatocytes and effect of incubation environment." *Drug Metab Dispos* no. 33 (11):1621–1627. doi:10.1124/dmd.105.005058.

Esch, E. W., A. Bahinski, and D. Huh. 2015. "Organs-on-chips at the frontiers of drug discovery." *Nat Rev Drug Discov* no. 14 (4):248–260. doi:10.1038/nrd4539.

Etienne-Grimaldi, M. C., J. C. Boyer, F. Thomas, S. Quaranta, N. Picard, M. A. Loriot, C. Narjoz et al. 2015. "UGT1A1 genotype and irinotecan therapy: General review and implementation in routine practice." *Fundam Clin Pharmacol* no. 29 (3):219–237. doi:10.1111/fcp.12117.

Faed, E. M. 1984. "Properties of acyl glucuronides: Implications for studies of the pharmacokinetics and metabolism of acidic drugs." *Drug Metab Rev* no. 15 (5–6):1213–1249. doi:10.3109/03602538409033562.

Falany, C. N., M. D. Green, and T. R. Tephly. 1987. "The enzymatic mechanism of glucuronidation catalyzed by two purified rat liver steroid UDP-glucuronosyltransferases." *J Biol Chem* no. 262 (3):1218–1222.

Fallon, J. K., H. Neubert, T. C. Goosen, and P. C. Smith. 2013a. "Targeted precise quantification of 12 human recombinant uridine-diphosphate glucuronosyl transferase 1A and 2B isoforms using nano-ultra-high-performance liquid chromatography/tandem mass spectrometry with selected reaction monitoring." *Drug Metab Dispos* no. 41 (12):2076–2080. doi:10.1124/dmd.113.053801.

Fallon, J. K., H. Neubert, R. Hyland, T. C. Goosen, and P. C. Smith. 2013b. "Targeted quantitative proteomics for the analysis of 14 UGT1As and -2Bs in human liver using NanoUPLC-MS/MS with selected reaction monitoring." *J Proteome Res* no. 12 (10):4402–4413. doi:10.1021/pr4004213.

Fedejko-Kap, B., S. M. Bratton, M. Finel, A. Radominska-Pandya, and Z. Mazerska. 2012. "Role of human UDP-glucuronosyltransferases in the biotransformation of the triazoloacridinone and imidazoacridinone antitumor agents C-1305 and C-1311: Highly selective substrates for UGT1A10." *Drug Metab Dispos* no. 40 (9):1736–1743. doi:10.1124/dmd.112.045401.

Ferraris, A., G. D'Amato, V. Nobili, B. Torres, M. Marcellini, and B. Dallapiccola. 2006. "Combined test for UGT1A1 -3279T-->G and A(TA)nTAA polymorphisms best predicts Gilbert's syndrome in Italian pediatric patients." *Genet Test* no. 10 (2):121–125.

Fey, S. J. and K. Wrzesinski. 2012. "Determination of drug toxicity using 3D spheroids constructed from an immortal human hepatocyte cell line." *Toxicol Sci* no. 127 (2):403–411. doi:10.1093/toxsci/kfs122.

Finel, M. and M. Kurkela. 2008. "The UDP-glucuronosyltransferases as oligomeric enzymes." *Curr Drug Metab* no. 9 (1):70–76.

Fisher, M. B., K. Campanale, B. L. Ackermann, M. VandenBranden, and S. A. Wrighton. 2000. "In vitro glucuronidation using human liver microsomes and the pore-forming peptide alamethicin." *Drug Metab Dispos* no. 28 (5):560–566.

Fisher, M. B., D. Jackson, A. Kaerner, S. A. Wrighton, and A. G. Borel. 2002. "Characterization by liquid chromatography-nuclear magnetic resonance spectroscopy and liquid chromatography-mass spectrometry of two coupled oxidative-conjugative metabolic pathways for 7-ethoxycoumarin in human liver microsomes treated with alamethicin." *Drug Metab Dispos* no. 30 (3):270–275.

Fremont, J. J., R. W. Wang, and C. D. King. 2005. "Coimmunoprecipitation of UDP-glucuronosyltransferase isoforms and cytochrome P450 3A4." *Mol Pharmacol* no. 67 (1):260–262. doi:10.1124/mol.104.006361.

Fujita, K. and A. Sparreboom. 2010. "Pharmacogenetics of irinotecan disposition and toxicity: A review." *Curr Clin Pharmacol* no. 5 (3):209–217.

Fujiwara, R. and T. Itoh. 2014. "Extensive protein-protein interactions involving UDP-glucuronosyltransferase (UGT) 2B7 in human liver microsomes." *Drug Metab Pharmacokinet* no. 29 (3):259–265.

Fujiwara, R., M. Nakajima, S. Oda, H. Yamanaka, S. Ikushiro, T. Sakaki, and T. Yokoi. 2010. "Interactions between human UDP-glucuronosyltransferase (UGT) 2B7 and UGT1A enzymes." *J Pharm Sci* no. 99 (1):442–454. doi:10.1002/jps.21830.

Fujiwara, R., M. Nakajima, H. Yamanaka, M. Katoh, and T. Yokoi. 2008. "Product inhibition of UDP-glucuronosyltransferase (UGT) enzymes by UDP obfuscates the inhibitory effects of UGT substrates." *Drug Metab Dispos* no. 36 (2):361–367. doi:dmd.107.018705 [pii].

Fujiwara, R., M. Nakajima, H. Yamanaka, A. Nakamura, M. Katoh, S. Ikushiro, T. Sakaki, and T. Yokoi. 2007. "Effects of coexpression of UGT1A9 on enzymatic activities of human UGT1A isoforms." *Drug Metab Dispos* no. 35 (5):747–757. doi:10.1124/dmd.106.014191.

Furukawa, T., Y. Naritomi, K. Tetsuka, F. Nakamori, H. Moriguchi, K. Yamano, S. Terashita, K. Tabata, and T. Teramura. 2014. "Species differences in intestinal glucuronidation activities between humans, rats, dogs and monkeys." *Xenobiotica* no. 44 (3):205–216. doi:10.3109/00498254.2013.828362.

Galetin, A. 2014. "Rationalizing underprediction of drug clearance from enzyme and transporter kinetic data: From in vitro tools to mechanistic modeling." *Methods Mol Biol* no. 1113:255–288. doi:10.1007/978-1-62703-758-7_13.

Gammal, R. S., M. H. Court, C. E. Haidar, O. F. Iwuchukwu, A. H. Gaur, M. Alvarellos, C. Guillemette et al. 2016. "Clinical Pharmacogenetics Implementation Consortium (CPIC) Guideline for UGT1A1 and Atazanavir Prescribing." *Clin Pharmacol Ther* no. 99 (4):363–369. doi:10.1002/cpt.269.

Ghosh, C., M. Hossain, V. Puvenna, J. Martinez-Gonzalez, A. Alexopolous, D. Janigro, and N. Marchi. 2013. "Expression and functional relevance of UGT1A4 in a cohort of human drug-resistant epileptic brains." *Epilepsia* no. 54 (9):1562–1570. doi:10.1111/epi.12318.

Ghosh, S. S., B. S. Sappal, G. V. Kalpana, S. W. Lee, J. R. Chowdhury, and N. R. Chowdhury. 2001. "Homodimerization of human bilirubin-uridine-diphosphoglucuronate glucuronosyltransferase-1 (UGT1A1) and its functional implications." *J Biol Chem* no. 276 (45):42108–42115. doi:10.1074/jbc. M106742200.

Gibson, C. R., P. Lu, C. Maciolek, C. Wudarski, Z. Barter, K. Rowland-Yeo, M. Stroh, E. Lai, and D. A. Nicoll-Griffith. 2013. "Using human recombinant UDP-glucuronosyltransferase isoforms and a relative activity factor approach to model total body clearance of laropiprant (MK-0524) in humans." *Xenobiotica* no. 43 (12):1027–1036. doi:10.3109/00498254.2013.791761.

Gill, K. L., J. B. Houston, and A. Galetin. 2012. "Characterization of in vitro glucuronidation clearance of a range of drugs in human kidney microsomes: Comparison with liver and intestinal glucuronidation and impact of albumin." *Drug Metab Dispos* no. 40 (4):825–835. doi:10.1124/dmd.111.043984.

Girard, H., M. H. Court, O. Bernard, L. C. Fortier, L. Villeneuve, Q. Hao, D. J. Greenblatt, L. L. von Moltke, L. Perussed, and C. Guillemette. 2004. "Identification of common polymorphisms in the promoter of the UGT1A9 gene: Evidence that UGT1A9 protein and activity levels are strongly genetically controlled in the liver." *Pharmacogenetics* no. 14 (8):501–515.

Godoy, P., N. J. Hewitt, U. Albrecht, M. E. Andersen, N. Ansari, S. Bhattacharya, J. G. Bode et al. 2013. "Recent advances in 2D and 3D in vitro systems using primary hepatocytes, alternative hepatocyte sources and non-parenchymal liver cells and their use in investigating mechanisms of hepatotoxicity, cell signaling and ADME." *Arch Toxicol* no. 87 (8):1315–1530. doi:10.1007/s00204-013-1078-5.

Goey, A. K. and W. D. Figg. 2016. "UGT genotyping in belinostat dosing." *Pharmacol Res* no. 105:22–27. doi:10.1016/j.phrs.2016.01.002.

Gomez-Lechon, M. J., L. Tolosa, I. Conde, and M. T. Donato. 2014. "Competency of different cell models to predict human hepatotoxic drugs." *Expert Opin Drug Metab Toxicol* no. 10 (11):1553–1568. doi:10.1517/17425255.2014.967680.

Goon, C. P., L. Z. Wang, F. C. Wong, W. L. Thuya, P. C. Ho, and B. C. Goh. 2016. "UGT1A1 mediated drug interactions and its clinical relevance." *Curr Drug Metab* no. 17 (2):100–106.

Grillo, M. P. 2011. "Drug-S-acyl-glutathione thioesters: Synthesis, bioanalytical properties, chemical reactivity, biological formation and degradation." *Curr Drug Metab* no. 12 (3):229–244.

Gschaidmeier, H., A. Seidel, B. Burchell, and K. W. Bock. 1995. "Formation of mono- and diglucuronides and other glycosides of benzo(a)pyrene-3,6-quinol by V79 cell-expressed human phenol UDP-glucuronosyltransferases of the UGT1 gene complex." *Biochem Pharmacol* no. 49 (11):1601–1606.

Guillemette, C. 2003. "Pharmacogenomics of human UDP-glucuronosyltransferase enzymes." *Pharmacogenomics J* no. 3 (3):136–158.

Gulcebi, M. I., A. Ozkaynakci, M. Z. Goren, R. G. Aker, C. Ozkara, and F. Y. Onat. 2011. "The relationship between UGT1A4 polymorphism and serum concentration of lamotrigine in patients with epilepsy." *Epilepsy Res* no. 95 (1–2):1–8. doi:10.1016/j.eplepsyres.2011.01.016.

Habtewold, A., W. Amogne, E. Makonnen, G. Yimer, K. D. Riedel, N. Ueda, A. Worku et al. 2011. "Long-term effect of efavirenz autoinduction on plasma/peripheral blood mononuclear cell drug exposure and CD4 count is influenced by UGT2B7 and CYP2B6 genotypes among HIV patients." *J Antimicrob Chemother* no. 66 (10):2350–2361. doi:10.1093/jac/dkr304.

Han, J. Y., H. S. Lim, E. S. Shin, Y. K. Yoo, Y. H. Park, J. E. Lee, I. J. Jang, D. H. Lee, and J. S. Lee. 2006. "Comprehensive analysis of UGT1A polymorphisms predictive for pharmacokinetics and treatment outcome in patients with non-small-cell lung cancer treated with irinotecan and cisplatin." *J Clin Oncol* no. 24 (15):2237–2244. doi:10.1200/JCO.2005.03.0239.

Hodge, J. E. 1955. "The amadori rearrangement." *Adv Carbohydr Chem* no. 10:169–205.

Holthe, M., P. Klepstad, K. Zahlsen, P. C. Borchgrevink, L. Hagen, O. Dale, S. Kaasa, H. E. Krokan, and F. Skorpen. 2002. "Morphine glucuronide-to-morphine plasma ratios are unaffected by the UGT2B7 H268Y and UGT1A1*28 polymorphisms in cancer patients on chronic morphine therapy." *Eur J Clin Pharmacol* no. 58 (5):353–356.

Huang, C. S., P. F. Chang, M. J. Huang, E. S. Chen, K. L. Hung, and K. I. Tsou. 2002a. "Relationship between bilirubin UDP-glucuronosyl transferase 1A1 gene and neonatal hyperbilirubinemia." *Pediatr Res* no. 52 (4):601–605. doi:10.1203/00006450-200210000-00022.

Huang, Y. H., A. Galijatovic, N. Nguyen, D. Geske, D. Beaton, J. Green, M. Green, W. H. Peters, and R. H. Tukey. 2002b. "Identification and functional characterization of UDP-glucuronosyltransferases UGT1A8*1, UGT1A8*2 and UGT1A8*3." *Pharmacogenetics* no. 12 (4):287–297.

Ieiri, I., C. Nishimura, K. Maeda, T. Sasaki, M. Kimura, T. Chiyoda, T. Hirota et al. 2011. "Pharmacokinetic and pharmacogenomic profiles of telmisartan after the oral microdose and therapeutic dose." *Pharmacogenet Genomics* no. 21 (8):495–505. doi:10.1097/FPC.0b013e3283489ce2.

Ikushiro, S., Y. Emi, and T. Iyanagi. 1997. "Protein-protein interactions between UDP-glucuronosyltransferase isozymes in rat hepatic microsomes." *Biochemistry* no. 36 (23):7154–7161. doi:10.1021/bi9702344.

Innocenti, F., W. Liu, P. Chen, A. A. Desai, S. Das, and M. J. Ratain. 2005. "Haplotypes of variants in the UDP-glucuronosyltransferase1A9 and 1A1 genes." *Pharmacogenet Genomics* no. 15 (5):295–301.

Innocenti, F. and M. J. Ratain. 2006. "Pharmacogenetics of irinotecan: Clinical perspectives on the utility of genotyping." *Pharmacogenomics* no. 7 (8):1211–1221.

Ishii, Y., S. Takeda, and H. Yamada. 2010. "Modulation of UDP-glucuronosyltransferase activity by protein-protein association." *Drug Metab Rev* no. 42 (1):145–158. doi:10.3109/03602530903208579.

Ishii, Y., S. Takeda, H. Yamada, and K. Oguri. 2005. "Functional protein-protein interaction of drug metabolizing enzymes." *Front Biosci* no. 10:887–895.

Iwai, M., Y. Maruo, M. Ito, K. Yamamoto, H. Sato, and Y. Takeuchi. 2004. "Six novel UDP-glucuronosyltransferase (UGT1A3) polymorphisms with varying activity." *J Hum Genet* no. 49 (3):123–128.

Iwamura, A., M. Ito, H. Mitsui, J. Hasegawa, K. Kosaka, I. Kino, M. Tsuda, M. Nakajima, T. Yokoi, and T. Kume. 2015. "Toxicological evaluation of acyl glucuronides utilizing half-lives, peptide adducts, and immunostimulation assays." *Toxicol In Vitro* no. 30 (1 Pt B):241–249. doi:10.1016/j.tiv.2015.10.013.

Iwuchukwu, O. F. and S. Nagar. 2008. "Resveratrol (trans-resveratrol, 3,5,4′-trihydroxy-trans-stilbene) glucuronidation exhibits atypical enzyme kinetics in various protein sources." *Drug Metab Dispos* no. 36 (2):322–330. doi:10.1124/dmd.107.018788.

Iyanagi, T. 2007. "Molecular mechanism of phase I and phase II drug-metabolizing enzymes: Implications for detoxification." *Int Rev Cytol* no. 260:35–112. doi:10.1016/S0074-7696(06)60002-8.

Iyer, L., S. Das, L. Janisch, M. Wen, J. Ramirez, T. Karrison, G. F. Fleming, E. E. Vokes, R. L. Schilsky, and M. J. Ratain. 2002. "UGT1A1*28 polymorphism as a determinant of irinotecan disposition and toxicity." *Pharmacogenomics J* no. 2 (1):43–47.

Iyer, L., C. D. King, P. F. Whitington, M. D. Green, S. K. Roy, T. R. Tephly, B. L. Coffman, and M. J. Ratain. 1998. "Genetic predisposition to the metabolism of irinotecan (CPT-11). Role of uridine diphosphate glucuronosyltransferase isoform 1A1 in the glucuronidation of its active metabolite (SN-38) in human liver microsomes." *J Clin Invest* no. 101 (4):847–854.

Izukawa, T., M. Nakajima, R. Fujiwara, H. Yamanaka, T. Fukami, M. Takamiya, Y. Aoki, S. Ikushiro, T. Sakaki, and T. Yokoi. 2009. "Quantitative analysis of UDP-glucuronosyltransferase (UGT) 1A and UGT2B expression levels in human livers." *Drug Metab Dispos* no. 37 (8):1759–1768. doi:10.1124/dmd.109.027227.

Jinno, H., M. Saeki, Y. Saito, T. Tanaka-Kagawa, N. Hanioka, K. Sai, N. Kaniwa et al. 2003. "Functional characterization of human UDP-glucuronosyltransferase 1A9 variant, D256N, found in Japanese cancer patients." *J Pharmacol Exp Ther* no. 306 (2):688–693.

Jinno, H., M. Saeki, T. Tanaka-Kagawa, N. Hanioka, Y. Saito, S. Ozawa, M. Ando et al. 2003. "Functional characterization of wild-type and variant (T202I and M59I) human UDP-glucuronosyltransferase 1A10." *Drug Metab Dispos* no. 31 (5):528–532.

Johnson, L. P. and C. Fenselau. 1978. "Enzymatic conjugation and hydrolysis of [18O]isoborneol glucuronide." *Drug Metab Dispos* no. 6 (6):677–679.

Jones, N. R. and P. Lazarus. 2014. "UGT2B gene expression analysis in multiple tobacco carcinogen-targeted tissues." *Drug Metab Dispos* no. 42 (4):529–536. doi:10.1124/dmd.113.054718.

Kaivosaari, S., M. Finel, and M. Koskinen. 2011. "N-glucuronidation of drugs and other xenobiotics by human and animal UDP-glucuronosyltransferases." *Xenobiotica* no. 41 (8):652–669. doi:10.3109/00498254.2011.563327.

Kampe, T., A. Konig, H. Schroeder, J. G. Hengstler, and C. M. Niemeyer. 2014. "Modular microfluidic system for emulation of human phase I/phase II metabolism." *Anal Chem* no. 86 (6):3068–3074. doi:10.1021/ac404128k.

Kazmi, F., P. Yerino, J. E. Barbara, and A. Parkinson. 2015. "Further characterization of the metabolism of desloratadine and its cytochrome P450 and UDP-glucuronosyltransferase Inhibition Potential: Identification of Desloratadine as a Relatively Selective UGT2B10 Inhibitor." *Drug Metab Dispos* no. 43 (9):1294–1302. doi:10.1124/dmd.115.065011.

Kerdpin, O., P. I. Mackenzie, K. Bowalgaha, M. Finel, and J. O. Miners. 2009. "Influence of N-terminal domain histidine and proline residues on the substrate selectivities of human UDP-glucuronosyltransferase 1A1, 1A6, 1A9, 2B7, and 2B10." *Drug Metab Dispos* no. 37 (9):1948–1955. doi:10.1124/dmd.109.028225.

Kilford, P. J., R. Stringer, B. Sohal, J. B. Houston, and A. Galetin. 2009. "Prediction of drug clearance by glucuronidation from in vitro data: Use of combined cytochrome P450 and UDP-glucuronosyltransferase cofactors in alamethicin-activated human liver microsomes." *Drug Metab Dispos* no. 37 (1):82–89. doi:10.1124/dmd.108.023853.

Kim, K. H. 1991. "Quantitative structure-activity relationships of the metabolism of drugs by uridine diphosphate glucuronosyltransferase." *J Pharm Sci* no. 80 (10):966–970.

King, C. D., G. R. Rios, M. D. Green, and T. R. Tephly. 2000. "UDP-glucuronosyltransferases." *Curr Drug Metab* no. 1 (2):143–161.

Kitagawa, C., M. Ando, Y. Ando, Y. Sekido, K. Wakai, K. Imaizumi, K. Shimokata, and Y. Hasegawa. 2005. "Genetic polymorphism in the phenobarbital-responsive enhancer module of the UDP-glucuronosyltransferase 1A1 gene and irinotecan toxicity." *Pharmacogenet Genomics* no. 15 (1):35–41.

Knibbe, C. A., E. H. Krekels, J. N. van den Anker, J. DeJongh, G. W. Santen, M. van Dijk, S. H. Simons et al. 2009. "Morphine glucuronidation in preterm neonates, infants and children younger than 3 years." *Clin Pharmacokinet* no. 48 (6):371–385. doi:10.2165/00003088-200948060-00003.

Kobayashi, T., J. E. Sleeman, M. W. Coughtrie, and B. Burchell. 2006. "Molecular and functional characterization of microsomal UDP-glucuronic acid uptake by members of the nucleotide sugar transporter (NST) family." *Biochem J* no. 400 (2):281–289. doi:10.1042/BJ20060429.

Konopnicki, C. M., L. J. Dickmann, J. M. Tracy, R. H. Tukey, L. C. Wienkers, and R. S. Foti. 2013. "Evaluation of UGT protein interactions in human hepatocytes: Effect of siRNA down regulation of UGT1A9 and UGT2B7 on propofol glucuronidation in human hepatocytes." *Arch Biochem Biophys* no. 535 (2):143–149. doi:10.1016/j.abb.2013.03.012.

Koster, A. S. and J. Noordhoek. 1983. "Kinetic properties of the rat intestinal microsomal 1-naphthol: UDP-glucuronosyl transferase. Inhibition by UDP and UDP-N-acetylglucosamine." *Biochim Biophys Acta* no. 761 (1):76–85.

Krekels, E. H., M. Danhof, D. Tibboel, and C. A. Knibbe. 2012. "Ontogeny of hepatic glucuronidation; methods and results." *Curr Drug Metab* no. 13 (6):728–743.

Krishnaswamy, S., Q. Hao, A. Al-Rohaimi, L. M. Hesse, L. L. von Moltke, D. J. Greenblatt, and M. H. Court. 2005a. "UDP glucuronosyltransferase (UGT) 1A6 pharmacogenetics: I. Identification of polymorphisms in the 5′-regulatory and exon 1 regions, and association with human liver UGT1A6 gene expression and glucuronidation." *J Pharmacol Exp Ther* no. 313 (3):1331–1339.

Krishnaswamy, S., Q. Hao, A. Al-Rohaimi, L. M. Hesse, L. L. von Moltke, D. J. Greenblatt, and M. H. Court. 2005b. "UDP glucuronosyltransferase (UGT) 1A6 pharmacogenetics: II. Functional impact of the three most common nonsynonymous UGT1A6 polymorphisms (S7A, T181A, and R184S)." *J Pharmacol Exp Ther* no. 313 (3):1340–1346.

Kumar, S., K. Samuel, R. Subramanian, M. P. Braun, R. A. Stearns, S. H. Chiu, D. C. Evans, and T. A. Baillie. 2002. "Extrapolation of diclofenac clearance from in vitro microsomal metabolism data: Role of acyl glucuronidation and sequential oxidative metabolism of the acyl glucuronide." *J Pharmacol Exp Ther* no. 303 (3):969–978. doi:10.1124/jpet.102.038992.

Kurkela, M., J. A. Garcia-Horsman, L. Luukkanen, S. Morsky, J. Taskinen, M. Baumann, R. Kostiainen, J. Hirvonen, and M. Finel. 2003. "Expression and characterization of recombinant human UDP-glucuronosyltransferases (UGTs): UGT1A9 is more resistant to detergent inhibition than other UGTs and was purified as an active dimeric enzyme." *J Biol Chem* no. 278 (6):3536–3544. doi:10.1074/jbc. M206136200.

Kurkela, M., J. Hirvonen, R. Kostiainen, and M. Finel. 2004. "The interactions between the N-terminal and C-terminal domains of the human UDP-glucuronosyltransferases are partly isoform-specific, and may involve both monomers." *Biochem Pharmacol* no. 68 (12):2443–2450. doi:10.1016/j.bcp.2004.08.019.

Kurkela, M., A. S. Patana, P. I. Mackenzie, M. H. Court, C. G. Tate, J. Hirvonen, A. Goldman, and M. Finel. 2007. "Interactions with other human UDP-glucuronosyltransferases attenuate the consequences of the Y485D mutation on the activity and substrate affinity of UGT1A6." *Pharmacogenet Genomics* no. 17 (2):115–126. doi:10.1097/FPC.0b013e328011b598.

Kwara, A., M. Lartey, K. W. Sagoe, E. Kenu, and M. H. Court. 2009. "CYP2B6, CYP2A6 and UGT2B7 genetic polymorphisms are predictors of efavirenz mid-dose concentration in HIV-infected patients." *AIDS* no. 23 (16):2101–2106. doi:10.1097/QAD.0b013e3283319908.

Laakkonen, L. and M. Finel. 2010. "A molecular model of the human UDP-glucuronosyltransferase 1A1, its membrane orientation, and the interactions between different parts of the enzyme." *Mol Pharmacol* no. 77 (6):931–939. doi:10.1124/mol.109.063289.

Ladd, M. A., P. N. Fitzsimmons, and J. W. Nichols. 2016. "Optimization of a UDP-glucuronosyltransferase assay for trout liver S9 fractions: Activity enhancement by alamethicin, a pore-forming peptide." *Xenobiotica*:1–10. doi:10.3109/00498254.2016.1149634.

Laferriere, C. I. and M. I. Marks. 1982. "Chloramphenicol: Properties and clinical use." *Pediatr Infect Dis* no. 1 (4):257–264.

Lampe, J. W., J. Bigler, A. C. Bush, and J. D. Potter. 2000. "Prevalence of polymorphisms in the human UDP-glucuronosyltransferase 2B family: UGT2B4(D458E), UGT2B7(H268Y), and UGT2B15(D85Y)." *Cancer Epidemiol Biomarkers Prev* no. 9 (3):329–333.

Lankisch, T. O., U. Moebius, M. Wehmeier, G. Behrens, M. P. Manns, R. E. Schmidt, and C. P. Strassburg. 2006. "Gilbert's disease and atazanavir: From phenotype to UDP-glucuronosyltransferase haplotype." *Hepatology* no. 44 (5):1324–1332.

LeCluyse, E. L., R. P. Witek, M. E. Andersen, and M. J. Powers. 2012. "Organotypic liver culture models: Meeting current challenges in toxicity testing." *Crit Rev Toxicol* no. 42 (6):501–548. doi:10.3109/10408 444.2012.682115.

Lee, S. J., J. B. Park, D. Kim, S. H. Bae, Y. W. Chin, E. Oh, and S. K. Bae. 2015. "In vitro selective inhibition of human UDP-glucuronosyltransferase (UGT) 1A4 by finasteride, and prediction of in vivo drug-drug interactions." *Toxicol Lett* no. 232 (2):458–465. doi:10.1016/j.toxlet.2014.11.018.

Levvy, G. A. and C. A. Marsh. 1959. "Preparation and properties of beta-glucuronidase." *Adv Carbohydr Chem* no. 14:381–428.

Lewis, B. C., P. I. Mackenzie, D. J. Elliot, B. Burchell, C. R. Bhasker, and J. O. Miners. 2007. "Amino terminal domains of human UDP-glucuronosyltransferases (UGT) 2B7 and 2B15 associated with substrate selectivity and autoactivation." *Biochem Pharmacol* no. 73 (9):1463–1473. doi:10.1016/j.bcp.2006.12.021.

Lewis, B. C., P. I. Mackenzie, and J. O. Miners. 2011. "Homodimerization of UDP-glucuronosyltransferase 2B7 (UGT2B7) and identification of a putative dimerization domain by protein homology modeling." *Biochem Pharmacol* no. 82 (12):2016–2023. doi:10.1016/j.bcp.2011.09.007.

Li, D., S. Fournel-Gigleux, L. Barre, G. Mulliert, P. Netter, J. Magdalou, and M. Ouzzine. 2007. "Identification of aspartic acid and histidine residues mediating the reaction mechanism and the substrate specificity of the human UDP-glucuronosyltransferases 1A." *J Biol Chem* no. 282 (50):36514–36524. doi:10.1074/jbc. M703107200.

Little, J. M., P. A. Lehman, S. Nowell, V. Samokyszyn, and A. Radominska. 1997. "Glucuronidation of all-trans-retinoic acid and 5,6-epoxy-all-trans-retinoic acid. Activation of rat liver microsomal UDP-glucuronosyltransferase activity by alamethicin." *Drug Metab Dispos* no. 25 (1):5–11.

Liu, Y. Q., L. M. Yuan, Z. Z. Gao, Y. S. Xiao, H. Y. Sun, L. S. Yu, and S. Zeng. 2016. "Dimerization of human uridine diphosphate glucuronosyltransferase allozymes 1A1 and 1A9 alters their quercetin glucuronidation activities." *Sci Rep* no. 6:23763. doi:10.1038/srep23763.

Locuson, C. W. and T. S. Tracy. 2007. "Comparative modelling of the human UDP-glucuronosyltransferases: Insights into structure and mechanism." *Xenobiotica* no. 37 (2):155–168. doi:10.1080/00498250601129109.

Lombardo, F., N. J. Waters, U. A. Argikar, M. K. Dennehy, J. Zhan, M. Gunduz, S. P. Harriman, G. Berellini, I. L. Rajlic, and R. S. Obach. 2013a. "Comprehensive assessment of human pharmacokinetic prediction based on in vivo animal pharmacokinetic data, part 2: Clearance." *J Clin Pharmacol* no. 53 (2):178–191. doi:10.1177/0091270012440282.

Lombardo, F., N. J. Waters, U. A. Argikar, M. K. Dennehy, J. Zhan, M. Gunduz, S. P. Harriman, G. Berellini, I. L. Rajlic, and R. S. Obach. 2013b. "Comprehensive assessment of human pharmacokinetic prediction based on in vivo animal pharmacokinetic data, part 1: Volume of distribution at steady state." *J Clin Pharmacol* no. 53 (2):167–177. doi:10.1177/0091270012440281.

Loser, S. V., J. Meyer, S. Freudenthaler, M. Sattler, C. Desel, I. Meineke, and U. Gundert-Remy. 1996. "Morphine-6-O-beta-D-glucuronide but not morphine-3-O-beta-D-glucuronide binds to mu-, delta- and kappa- specific opioid binding sites in cerebral membranes." *Naunyn Schmiedebergs Arch Pharmacol* no. 354 (2):192–197.

Lu, L., J. Zhou, J. Shi, X. J. Peng, X. X. Qi, Y. Wang, F. Y. Li, F. Y. Zhou, L. Liu, and Z. Q. Liu. 2015. "Drug-metabolizing activity, protein and gene expression of UDP-glucuronosyltransferases are significantly altered in hepatocellular carcinoma patients." *PLoS One* no. 10 (5):e0127524. doi:10.1371/journal.pone.0127524.

Lueders, K. K. and E. L. Kuff. 1967. "Spontaneous and detergent activation of a glucuronyltransferase in vitro." *Arch Biochem Biophys* no. 120 (1):198–203.

Luquita, M. G., V. A. Catania, E. J. Pozzi, L. M. Veggi, T. Hoffman, J. M. Pellegrino, S. Ikushiro et al. 2001. "Molecular basis of perinatal changes in UDP-glucuronosyltransferase activity in maternal rat liver." *J Pharmacol Exp Ther* no. 298 (1):49–56.

Luukkanen, L., J. Taskinen, M. Kurkela, R. Kostiainen, J. Hirvonen, and M. Finel. 2005. "Kinetic characterization of the 1A subfamily of recombinant human UDP-glucuronosyltransferases." *Drug Metab Dispos* no. 33 (7):1017–1026. doi:10.1124/dmd.105.004093.

Lynn, A. M., M. K. Nespeca, S. L. Bratton, and D. D. Shen. 2000. "Intravenous morphine in postoperative infants: Intermittent bolus dosing versus targeted continuous infusions." *Pain* no. 88 (1):89–95.

Lynn, A., M., M. K. Nespeca, S. L. Bratton, S. G. Strauss, and D. D. Shen. 1998. "Clearance of morphine in postoperative infants during intravenous infusion: The influence of age and surgery." *Anesth Analg* no. 86 (5):958–963.

Mackenzie, P. I., K. W. Bock, B. Burchell, C. Guillemette, S. Ikushiro, T. Iyanagi, J. O. Miners, I. S. Owens, and D. W. Nebert. 2005. "Nomenclature update for the mammalian UDP glycosyltransferase (UGT) gene superfamily." *Pharmacogenet Genomics* no. 15 (10):677–685.

Mackenzie, P. I., I. S. Owens, B. Burchell, K. W. Bock, A. Bairoch, A. Belanger, S. Fournel-Gigleux et al. 1997. "The UDP glycosyltransferase gene superfamily: Recommended nomenclature update based on evolutionary divergence." *Pharmacogenetics* no. 7 (4):255–269.

MacKenzie, P. I., A. Rogers, D. J. Elliot, N. Chau, J. A. Hulin, J. O. Miners, and R. Meech. 2011. "The novel UDP glycosyltransferase 3A2: Cloning, catalytic properties, and tissue distribution." *Mol Pharmacol* no. 79 (3):472–478. doi:10.1124/mol.110.069336.

Mackenzie, P. I., A. Rogers, J. Treloar, B. R. Jorgensen, J. O. Miners, and R. Meech. 2008. "Identification of UDP glycosyltransferase 3A1 as a UDP N-acetylglucosaminyltransferase." *J Biol Chem* no. 283 (52):36205–36210. doi:10.1074/jbc. M807961200.

Magdalou, J., S. Fournel-Gigleux, and M. Ouzzine. 2010. "Insights on membrane topology and structure/function of UDP-glucuronosyltransferases." *Drug Metab Rev* no. 42 (1):159–166. doi:10.3109/03602530903209270.

Malik, M. Y., S. Jaiswal, A. Sharma, M. Shukla, and J. Lal. 2016. "Role of enterohepatic recirculation in drug disposition: Cooperation and complications." *Drug Metab Rev* no. 48 (2):281–327. doi:10.3109/036025 32.2016.1157600.

Malik, V. and G. W. Black. 2012. "Structural, functional, and mutagenesis studies of UDP-glycosyltransferases." *Adv Protein Chem Struct Biol* no. 87:87–115. doi:10.1016/B978-0-12-398312-1.00004-4.

Manevski, N., P. S. Moreolo, J. Yli-Kauhaluoma, and M. Finel. 2011. "Bovine serum albumin decreases Km values of human UDP-glucuronosyltransferases 1A9 and 2B7 and increases Vmax values of UGT1A9." *Drug Metab Dispos* no. 39 (11):2117–2129. doi:10.1124/dmd.111.041418.

Margaillan, G., M. Rouleau, J. K. Fallon, P. Caron, L. Villeneuve, V. Turcotte, P. C. Smith, M. S. Joy, and C. Guillemette. 2015. "Quantitative profiling of human renal UDP-glucuronosyltransferases and glucuronidation activity: A comparison of normal and tumoral kidney tissues." *Drug Metab Dispos* no. 43 (4):611–619. doi:10.1124/dmd.114.062877.

Marsh, C. A., F. Alexander, and G. A. Levvy. 1952. "Glucuronide decomposition in the digestive tract." *Nature* no. 170 (4317):163–164.

Maruo, Y., K. Nishizawa, H. Sato, Y. Doida, and M. Shimada. 1999. "Association of neonatal hyperbilirubinemia with bilirubin UDP-glucuronosyltransferase polymorphism." *Pediatrics* no. 103 (6 Pt 1):1224–1227.

Mazerska, Z., A. Mroz, M. Pawlowska, and E. Augustin. 2016. "The role of glucuronidation in drug resistance." *Pharmacol Ther* no. 159:35–55. doi:10.1016/j.pharmthera.2016.01.009.

Mazur, C. S., J. F. Kenneke, J. K. Hess-Wilson, and J. C. Lipscomb. 2010. "Differences between human and rat intestinal and hepatic bisphenol a glucuronidation and the influence of alamethicin on in vitro kinetic measurements." *Drug Metab Dispos* no. 38 (12):2232–2238. doi:10.1124/dmd.110.034819.

McGurk, K. A., C. H. Brierley, and B. Burchell. 1998. "Drug glucuronidation by human renal UDP-glucuronosyltransferases." *Biochem Pharmacol* no. 55 (7):1005–1012.

McRorie, T. I., A. M. Lynn, M. K. Nespeca, K. E. Opheim, and J. T. Slattery. 1992. "The maturation of morphine clearance and metabolism." *Am J Dis Child* no. 146 (8):972–976.

Meech, R. and P. I. Mackenzie. 1997a. "Structure and function of uridine diphosphate glucuronosyltransferases." *Clin Exp Pharmacol Physiol* no. 24 (12):907–915.

Meech, R. and P. I. Mackenzie. 1997b. "UDP-glucuronosyltransferase, the role of the amino terminus in dimerization." *J Biol Chem* no. 272 (43):26913–26917.

Meech, R., N. Mubarokah, A. Shivasami, A. Rogers, P. C. Nair, D. G. Hu, R. A. McKinnon, and P. I. Mackenzie. 2015. "A novel function for UDP glycosyltransferase 8: Galactosidation of bile acids." *Mol Pharmacol* no. 87 (3):442–450. doi:10.1124/mol.114.093823.

Meech, R., A. Rogers, L. Zhuang, B. C. Lewis, J. O. Miners, and P. I. Mackenzie. 2012. "Identification of residues that confer sugar selectivity to UDP-glycosyltransferase 3A (UGT3A) enzymes." *J Biol Chem* no. 287 (29):24122–24130. doi:10.1074/jbc.M112.343608.

Metzger, I. F., T. C. Quigg, N. Epstein, A. O. Aregbe, N. Thong, J. T. Callaghan, D. A. Flockhart et al. 2014. "Substantial effect of efavirenz monotherapy on bilirubin levels in healthy volunteers." *Curr Ther Res Clin Exp* no. 76:64–69. doi:10.1016/j.curtheres.2014.05.002.

Miley, M. J., A. K. Zielinska, J. E. Keenan, S. M. Bratton, A. Radominska-Pandya, and M. R. Redinbo. 2007. "Crystal structure of the cofactor-binding domain of the human phase II drug-metabolism enzyme UDP-glucuronosyltransferase 2B7." *J Mol Biol* no. 369 (2):498–511. doi:10.1016/j.jmb.2007.03.066.

Miners, J. O., K. M. Knights, J. B. Houston, and P. I. Mackenzie. 2006. "In vitro-in vivo correlation for drugs and other compounds eliminated by glucuronidation in humans: Pitfalls and promises." *Biochem Pharmacol* no. 71 (11):1531–1539. doi:10.1016/j.bcp.2005.12.019.

Miners, J. O., P. I. Mackenzie, and K. M. Knights. 2010. "The prediction of drug-glucuronidation parameters in humans: UDP-glucuronosyltransferase enzyme-selective substrate and inhibitor probes for reaction phenotyping and in vitro-in vivo extrapolation of drug clearance and drug-drug interaction potential." *Drug Metab Rev* no. 42 (1):196–208. doi:10.3109/03602530903210716.

Miners, J. O., P. A. Smith, M. J. Sorich, R. A. McKinnon, and P. I. Mackenzie. 2004. "Predicting human drug glucuronidation parameters: Application of in vitro and in silico modeling approaches." *Annu Rev Pharmacol Toxicol* no. 44:1–25. doi:10.1146/annurev.pharmtox.44.101802.121546.

Minucci, A., G. Canu, M. De Bonis, E. Delibato, and E. Capoluongo. 2014. "Is capillary electrophoresis on microchip devices able to genotype uridine diphosphate glucuronosyltransferase 1A1 TATA-box polymorphisms?" *J Sep Sci* no. 37 (12):1521–1523. doi:10.1002/jssc.201400235.

Mirochnick, M., E. Capparelli, and J. Connor. 1999. "Pharmacokinetics of zidovudine in infants: A population analysis across studies." *Clin Pharmacol Ther* no. 66 (1):16–24. doi:10.1016/S0009-9236(99)70049-4.

Miyagi, S. J. and A. C. Collier. 2007. "Pediatric development of glucuronidation: The ontogeny of hepatic UGT1A4." *Drug Metab Dispos* no. 35 (9):1587–1592. doi:10.1124/dmd.107.015214.

Miyagi, S. J. and A. C. Collier. 2011. "The development of UDP-glucuronosyltransferases 1A1 and 1A6 in the pediatric liver." *Drug Metab Dispos* no. 39 (5):912–919. doi:10.1124/dmd.110.037192.

Miyagi, S. J., A. M. Milne, M. W. Coughtrie, and A. C. Collier. 2012. "Neonatal development of hepatic UGT1A9: Implications of pediatric pharmacokinetics." *Drug Metab Dispos* no. 40 (7):1321–1327. doi:10.1124/dmd.111.043752.

Mizuma, T. 2009. "Intestinal glucuronidation metabolism may have a greater impact on oral bioavailability than hepatic glucuronidation metabolism in humans: A study with raloxifene, substrate for UGT1A1, 1A8, 1A9, and 1A10." *Int J Pharm* no. 378 (1–2):140–141. doi:10.1016/j.ijpharm.2009.05.044.

Mojarrabi, B. and P. I. Mackenzie. 1998. "Characterization of two UDP glucuronosyltransferases that are predominantly expressed in human colon." *Biochem Biophys Res Commun* no. 247 (3):704–709. doi:10.1006/bbrc.1998.8843.

Monaghan, G., M. Ryan, R. Seddon, R. Hume, and B. Burchell. 1996. "Genetic variation in bilirubin UPD-glucuronosyltransferase gene promoter and Gilbert's syndrome." *Lancet* no. 347 (9001):578–581.

Mori, A., Y. Maruo, M. Iwai, H. Sato, and Y. Takeuchi. 2005. "UDP-glucuronosyltransferase 1A4 polymorphisms in a Japanese population and kinetics of clozapine glucuronidation." *Drug Metab Dispos* no. 33 (5):672–675.

Nagar, S. and R. L. Blanchard. 2006a. "Pharmacogenetics of uridine diphosphoglucuronosyltransferase (UGT) 1A family members and its role in patient response to irinotecan." *Drug Metab Rev* no. 38 (3):393–409. doi:10.1080/03602530600739835.

Nagar, S. and R. P. Remmel. 2006b. "Uridine diphosphoglucuronosyltransferase pharmacogenetics and cancer." *Oncogene* no. 25 (11):1659–1672. doi:1209375 [pii].

Nair, P. C., R. Meech, P. I. Mackenzie, R. A. McKinnon, and J. O. Miners. 2015. "Insights into the UDP-sugar selectivities of human UDP-glycosyltransferases (UGT): A molecular modeling perspective." *Drug Metab Rev* no. 47 (3):335–345. doi:10.3109/03602532.2015.1071835.

Nakajima, M., H. Yamanaka, R. Fujiwara, M. Katoh, and T. Yokoi. 2007. "Stereoselective glucuronidation of 5-(4'-hydroxyphenyl)-5-phenylhydantoin by human UDP-glucuronosyltransferase (UGT) 1A1, UGT1A9, and UGT2B15: Effects of UGT-UGT interactions." *Drug Metab Dispos* no. 35 (9):1679–1686. doi:10.1124/dmd.107.015909.

Nakamura, A., M. Nakajima, H. Yamanaka, R. Fujiwara, and T. Yokoi. 2008. "Expression of UGT1A and UGT2B mRNA in human normal tissues and various cell lines." *Drug Metab Dispos* no. 36 (8):1461–1464. doi:10.1124/dmd.108.021428.

Nakamura, K., R. Mizutani, A. Sanbe, S. Enosawa, M. Kasahara, A. Nakagawa, Y. Ejiri et al. 2011. "Evaluation of drug toxicity with hepatocytes cultured in a micro-space cell culture system." *J Biosci Bioeng* no. 111 (1):78–84. doi:10.1016/j.jbiosc.2010.08.008.

Naritomi, Y., F. Nakamori, T. Furukawa, and K. Tabata. 2015. "Prediction of hepatic and intestinal glucuronidation using in vitro-in vivo extrapolation." *Drug Metab Pharmacokinet* no. 30 (1):21–29. doi:10.1016/j.dmpk.2014.10.001.

Nishihara, M., M. Sudo, N. Kawaguchi, J. Takahashi, Y. Kiyota, T. Kondo, and S. Asahi. 2012. "An unusual metabolic pathway of sipoglitazar, a novel antidiabetic agent: Cytochrome P450-catalyzed oxidation of sipoglitazar acyl glucuronide." *Drug Metab Dispos* no. 40 (2):249–258. doi:10.1124/dmd.111.040105.

Nishimura, T., Y. Hu, M. Wu, E. Pham, H. Suemizu, M. Elazar, M. Liu et al. 2013. "Using chimeric mice with humanized livers to predict human drug metabolism and a drug-drug interaction." *J Pharmacol Exp Ther* no. 344 (2):388–396. doi:10.1124/jpet.112.198697.

Novik, E., T. J. Maguire, P. Chao, K. C. Cheng, and M. L. Yarmush. 2010. "A microfluidic hepatic coculture platform for cell-based drug metabolism studies." *Biochem Pharmacol* no. 79 (7):1036–1044. doi:10.1016/j.bcp.2009.11.010.

Oda, S., T. Fukami, T. Yokoi, and M. Nakajima. 2015. "A comprehensive review of UDP-glucuronosyltransferase and esterases for drug development." *Drug Metab Pharmacokinet* no. 30 (1):30–51. doi:10.1016/j.dmpk.2014.12.001.

Ogilvie, B. W., D. Zhang, W. Li, A. D. Rodrigues, A. E. Gipson, J. Holsapple, P. Toren, and A. Parkinson. 2006. "Glucuronidation converts gemfibrozil to a potent, metabolism-dependent inhibitor of CYP2C8: Implications for drug-drug interactions." *Drug Metab Dispos* no. 34 (1):191–197. doi:10.1124/dmd.105.007633.

Ohkura, T., K. Ohta, T. Nagao, K. Kusumoto, A. Koeda, T. Ueda, T. Jomura et al. 2014. "Evaluation of human hepatocytes cultured by three-dimensional spheroid systems for drug metabolism." *Drug Metab Pharmacokinet* no. 29 (5):373–378.

Ohno, S. and S. Nakajin. 2009. "Determination of mRNA expression of human UDP-glucuronosyltransferases and application for localization in various human tissues by real-time reverse transcriptase-polymerase chain reaction." *Drug Metab Dispos* no. 37 (1):32–40. doi:10.1124/dmd.108.023598.

Oleson, L. and M. H. Court. 2008. "Effect of the beta-glucuronidase inhibitor saccharolactone on glucuronidation by human tissue microsomes and recombinant UDP-glucuronosyltransferases." *J Pharm Pharmacol* no. 60 (9):1175–1182. doi:10.1211/jpp.60.9.0009.

Olson, J. A., R. C. Moon, M. W. Anders, C. Fenselau, and B. Shane. 1992. "Enhancement of biological activity by conjugation reactions." *J Nutr* no. 122 (3 Suppl):615–624.

Olson, K. C., R. W. Dellinger, Q. Zhong, D. Sun, S. Amin, T. E. Spratt, and P. Lazarus. 2009. "Functional characterization of low-prevalence missense polymorphisms in the UDP-glucuronosyltransferase 1A9 gene." *Drug Metab Dispos* no. 37 (10):1999–2007. doi:10.1124/dmd.108.024596.

Onishi, S., N. Kawade, S. Itoh, K. Isobe, and S. Sugiyama. 1979. "Postnatal development of uridine diphosphate glucuronyltransferase activity towards bilirubin and 2-aminophenol in human liver." *Biochem J* no. 184 (3):705–707.

Operana, T. N. and R. H. Tukey. 2007. "Oligomerization of the UDP-glucuronosyltransferase 1A proteins: Homo- and heterodimerization analysis by fluorescence resonance energy transfer and co-immunoprecipitation." *J Biol Chem* no. 282 (7):4821–4829. doi:10.1074/jbc. M609417200.

Osborne, R., S. Joel, D. Trew, and M. Slevin. 1988. "Analgesic activity of morphine-6-glucuronide." *Lancet* no. 1 (8589):828.

Osborne, R., P. Thompson, S. Joel, D. Trew, N. Patel, and M. Slevin. 1992. "The analgesic activity of morphine-6-glucuronide." *Br J Clin Pharmacol* no. 34 (2):130–138.

Park, J., L. Chen, K. Shade, P. Lazarus, J. Seigne, S. Patterson, M. Helal, and J. Pow-Sang. 2004. "Asp85tyr polymorphism in the udp-glucuronosyltransferase (UGT) 2B15 gene and the risk of prostate cancer." *J Urol* no. 171 (6 Pt 1):2484–2488.

Pattanawongsa, A., P. C. Nair, A. Rowland, and J. O. Miners. 2016. "Human UDP-glucuronosyltransferase (UGT) 2B10: Validation of cotinine as a selective probe substrate, inhibition by UGT enzyme-selective inhibitors and antidepressant and antipsychotic drugs, and structural determinants of enzyme inhibition." *Drug Metab Dispos* no. 44 (3):378–388. doi:10.1124/dmd.115.068213.

Paul, D., K. M. Standifer, C. E. Inturrisi, and G. W. Pasternak. 1989. "Pharmacological characterization of morphine-6 beta-glucuronide, a very potent morphine metabolite." *J Pharmacol Exp Ther* no. 251 (2):477–483.

Peng, J., J. Lu, Q. Shen, M. Zheng, X. Luo, W. Zhu, H. Jiang, and K. Chen. 2014. "In silico site of metabolism prediction for human UGT-catalyzed reactions." *Bioinformatics* no. 30 (3):398–405. doi:10.1093/bioinformatics/btt681.

Peters, W. H. and P. L. Jansen. 1986. "Microsomal UDP-glucuronyltransferase-catalyzed bilirubin diglucuronide formation in human liver." *J Hepatol* no. 2 (2):182–194.

Pineiro-Carrero, V. M. and E. O. Pineiro. 2004. "Liver." *Pediatrics* no. 113 (4 Suppl):1097–1106.

Poon, G. K., Y. C. Chui, R. McCague, P. E. Llnning, R. Feng, M. G. Rowlands, and M. Jarman. 1993. "Analysis of phase I and phase II metabolites of tamoxifen in breast cancer patients." *Drug Metab Dispos* no. 21 (6):1119–1124.

Portenoy, R. K., E. Khan, M. Layman, J. Lapin, M. G. Malkin, K. M. Foley, H. T. Thaler, D. J. Cerbone, and C. E. Inturrisi. 1991. "Chronic morphine therapy for cancer pain: plasma and cerebrospinal fluid morphine and morphine-6-glucuronide concentrations." *Neurology* no. 41 (9):1457–1461.

Potrepka, R. F. and J. L. Spratt. 1972. "A study on the enzymatic mechanism of guinea-pig hepatic-microsomal bilirubin glucuronyl transferase." *Eur J Biochem* no. 29 (3):433–439.

Potter, T., R. Lewis, T. Luker, R. Bonnert, M. A. Bernstein, T. N. Birkinshaw, S. Thom, M. Wenlock, and S. Paine. 2011. "In silico prediction of acyl glucuronide reactivity." *J Comput Aided Mol Des* no. 25 (11):997–1005. doi:10.1007/s10822-011-9479-0.

Prabhala, R. H., V. Maxey, M. J. Hicks, and R. R. Watson. 1989. "Enhancement of the expression of activation markers on human peripheral blood mononuclear cells by in vitro culture with retinoids and carotenoids." *J Leukoc Biol* no. 45 (3):249–254.

Radominska-Pandya, A., S. M. Bratton, M. R. Redinbo, and M. J. Miley. 2010. "The crystal structure of human UDP-glucuronosyltransferase 2B7 C-terminal end is the first mammalian UGT target to be revealed: The significance for human UGTs from both the 1A and 2B families." *Drug Metab Rev* no. 42 (1):133–144. doi:10.3109/03602530903209049.

Radominska-Pandya, A., P. J. Czernik, J. M. Little, E. Battaglia, and P. I. Mackenzie. 1999. "Structural and functional studies of UDP-glucuronosyltransferases." *Drug Metab Rev* no. 31 (4):817–899.

Radominska-Pandya, A., J. M. Little, J. T. Pandya, T. R. Tephly, C. D. King, G. W. Barone, and J. P. Raufman. 1998. "UDP-glucuronosyltransferases in human intestinal mucosa." *Biochim Biophys Acta* no. 1394 (2–3):199–208.

Radominska-Pandya, A., M. Ouzzine, S. Fournel-Gigleux, and J. Magdalou. 2005. "Structure of UDP-glucuronosyltransferases in membranes." *Methods Enzymol* no. 400:116–147. doi:10.1016/S0076-6879(05)00008-X.

Ramaiahgari, S. C., M. W. den Braver, B. Herpers, V. Terpstra, J. N. Commandeur, B. van de Water, and L. S. Price. 2014. "A 3D in vitro model of differentiated HepG2 cell spheroids with improved liver-like properties for repeated dose high-throughput toxicity studies." *Arch Toxicol* no. 88 (5):1083–1095. doi:10.1007/s00204-014-1215-9.

Rao, M. L., G. S. Rao, and H. Breuer. 1976. "Investigations on the kinetic properties of estrone glucuronyl-transferase from pig kidney." *Biochim Biophys Acta* no. 452 (1):89–100.

Regan, S. L., J. L. Maggs, T. G. Hammond, C. Lambert, D. P. Williams, and B. K. Park. 2010. "Acyl glucuro-nides: The good, the bad and the ugly." *Biopharm Drug Dispos* no. 31 (7):367–395. doi:10.1002/bdd.720.

Remmel, R. P., J. Zhou, and U. A. Argikar. 2008. "UDP-glucuronosyl transferases." In *Drug-Drug Interactions*, edited by D.A. Rodrigues, 744. New York: Informa Health Care.

Riches, Z. and A. C. Collier. 2015. "Posttranscriptional regulation of uridine diphosphate glucuronosyltrans-ferases." *Expert Opin Drug Metab Toxicol* no. 11 (6):949–965. doi:10.1517/17425255.2015.1028355.

Richter, W. J., K. O. Alt, W. Dieterle, J. W. Faigle, H. P. Kriemler, H. Mory, and T. Winkler. 1975. "C-glucuronides, a novel type of drug metabolites." *Helv Chim Acta* no. 58 (8):2512–2517. doi:10.1002/hlca.19750580833.

Rios, G. R. and T. R. Tephly. 2002. "Inhibition and active sites of UDP-glucuronosyltransferases 2B7 and 1A1." *Drug Metab Dispos* no. 30 (12):1364–1367.

Ritter, J. K. 2000. "Roles of glucuronidation and UDP-glucuronosyltransferases in xenobiotic bioactivation reactions." *Chem Biol Interact* no. 129 (1–2):171–193.

Rotger, M., P. Taffe, G. Bleiber, H. F. Gunthard, H. Furrer, P. Vernazza, H. Drechsler, E. Bernasconi, M. Rickenbach, and A. Telenti. 2005. "Gilbert syndrome and the development of antiretroviral therapy-associated hyperbilirubinemia." *J Infect Dis* no. 192 (8):1381–1386.

Rouleau, M., P. Collin, J. Bellemare, M. Harvey, and C. Guillemette. 2013. "Protein-protein interactions between the bilirubin-conjugating UDP-glucuronosyltransferase UGT1A1 and its shorter isoform 2 regulatory partner derived from alternative splicing." *Biochem J* no. 450 (1):107–114. doi:10.1042/BJ20121594.

Rowland, A., P. Gaganis, D. J. Elliot, P. I. Mackenzie, K. M. Knights, and J. O. Miners. 2007. "Binding of inhibitory fatty acids is responsible for the enhancement of UDP-glucuronosyltransferase 2B7 activity by albumin: Implications for in vitro-in vivo extrapolation." *J Pharmacol Exp Ther* no. 321 (1):137–147. doi:10.1124/jpet.106.118216.

Rowland, A., K. M. Knights, P. I. Mackenzie, and J. O. Miners. 2008. "The 'albumin effect' and drug gluc-uronidation: Bovine serum albumin and fatty acid-free human serum albumin enhance the glucuronida-tion of UDP-glucuronosyltransferase (UGT) 1A9 substrates but not UGT1A1 and UGT1A6 activities." *Drug Metab Dispos* no. 36 (6):1056–1062. doi:10.1124/dmd.108.021105.

Rowland, A., P. I. Mackenzie, and J. O. Miners. 2015. "Transporter-mediated uptake of UDP-glucuronic acid by human liver microsomes: Assay conditions, kinetics, and inhibition." *Drug Metab Dispos* no. 43 (1):147–153. doi:10.1124/dmd.114.060509.

Rowland, A., J. O. Miners, and P. I. Mackenzie. 2013. "The UDP-glucuronosyltransferases: Their role in drug metabolism and detoxification." *Int J Biochem Cell Biol* no. 45 (6):1121–1132. doi:10.1016/j.biocel.2013.02.019.

Saeki, M., S. Ozawa, Y. Saito, H. Jinno, T. Hamaguchi, H. Nokihara, Y. Shimada et al. 2002. "Three novel single nucleotide polymorphisms in UGT1A10." *Drug Metab Pharmacokinet* no. 17 (5):488–490.

Saeki, M., Y. Saito, H. Jinno, T. Tanaka-Kagawa, A. Ohno, S. Ozawa, K. Ueno et al. 2004. "Single nucleotide polymorphisms and haplotype frequencies of UGT2B4 and UGT2B7 in a Japanese population." *Drug Metab Dispos* no. 32 (9):1048–1054.

Sallustio, B. C. and D. J. Foster. 1995. "Reactivity of gemfibrozil 1-o-beta-acyl glucuronide. Pharmacokinetics of covalently bound gemfibrozil-protein adducts in rats." *Drug Metab Dispos* no. 23 (9):892–899.

Sallustio, B. C., L. A. Harkin, M. C. Mann, S. J. Krivickas, and P. C. Burcham. 1997. "Genotoxicity of acyl glucuronide metabolites formed from clofibric acid and gemfibrozil: A novel role for phase-II-mediated bioactivation in the hepatocarcinogenicity of the parent aglycones?" *Toxicol Appl Pharmacol* no. 147 (2):459–464. doi:10.1006/taap.1997.8322.

Sallustio, B. C., L. Sabordo, A. M. Evans, and R. L. Nation. 2000. "Hepatic disposition of electrophilic acyl glucuronide conjugates." *Curr Drug Metab* no. 1 (2):163–180.

Sanchez, E. and T. R. Tephly. 1975. "Morphine metabolism. IV. Studies on the mechanism of morphine: Uridine diphosphoglucuronyltransferase and its activation by bilirubin." *Mol Pharmacol* no. 11 (5):613–620.

Sane, R. S., D. Ramsden, J. P. Sabo, C. Cooper, L. Rowland, N. Ting, A. Whitcher-Johnstone, and D. J. Tweedie. 2016. "Contribution of major metabolites toward complex drug-drug interactions of deleobuvir: In vitro predictions and in vivo outcomes." *Drug Metab Dispos* no. 44 (3):466–475. doi:10.1124/dmd.115.066985.

Sanoh, S. and S. Ohta. 2014. "Chimeric mice transplanted with human hepatocytes as a model for prediction of human drug metabolism and pharmacokinetics." *Biopharm Drug Dispos* no. 35 (2):71–86. doi:10.1002/bdd.1864.

Sarkar, U., D. Rivera-Burgos, E. M. Large, D. J. Hughes, K. C. Ravindra, R. L. Dyer, M. R. Ebrahimkhani, J. S. Wishnok, L. G. Griffith, and S. R. Tannenbaum. 2015. "Metabolite profiling and pharmacokinetic evaluation of hydrocortisone in a perfused three-dimensional human liver bioreactor." *Drug Metab Dispos* no. 43 (7):1091–1099. doi:10.1124/dmd.115.063495.

Sawamura, R., N. Okudaira, K. Watanabe, T. Murai, Y. Kobayashi, M. Tachibana, T. Ohnuki et al. 2010. "Predictability of idiosyncratic drug toxicity risk for carboxylic acid-containing drugs based on the chemical stability of acyl glucuronide." *Drug Metab Dispos* no. 38 (10):1857–1864. doi:10.1124/dmd.110.034173.

Sawyer, M. B., F. Innocenti, S. Das, C. Cheng, J. Ramirez, F. H. Pantle-Fisher, C. Wright et al. 2003. "A pharmacogenetic study of uridine diphosphate-glucuronosyltransferase 2B7 in patients receiving morphine." *Clin Pharmacol Ther* no. 73 (6):566–574.

Schulze, J. J., J. Lundmark, M. Garle, I. Skilving, L. Ekstrom, and A. Rane. 2008. "Doping test results dependent on genotype of uridine diphospho-glucuronosyl transferase 2B17, the major enzyme for testosterone glucuronidation." *J Clin Endocrinol Metab* no. 93 (7):2500–2506. doi:10.1210/jc.2008-0218.

Schulze, J. J., J. O. Thorngren, M. Garle, L. Ekstrom, and A. Rane. 2011. "Androgen sulfation in healthy UDP-glucuronosyl transferase 2B17 enzyme-deficient men." *J Clin Endocrinol Metab* no. 96 (11):3440–3447. doi:10.1210/jc.2011-0521.

Seibert, E. and T. S. Tracy. 2014. "Fundamentals of enzyme kinetics." *Methods Mol Biol* no. 1113:9–22. doi:10.1007/978-1-62703-758-7_2.

Sekimoto, M., T. Takamori, S. Nakamura, and M. Taguchi. 2016. "In vitro enhancement of carvedilol glucuronidation by amiodarone-mediated altered protein binding in incubation mixture of human liver microsomes with bovine serum albumin." *Biol Pharm Bull* no. 39 (8):1359–1363. doi:10.1248/bpb.b16-00360.

Senekeo-Effenberger, K., S. Chen, E. Brace-Sinnokrak, J. A. Bonzo, M. F. Yueh, U. Argikar, J. Kaeding et al. 2007. "Expression of the human UGT1 locus in transgenic mice by 4-chloro-6-(2,3-xylidino)-2-pyrimidinylthioacetic acid (WY-14643) and implications on drug metabolism through peroxisome proliferator-activated receptor alpha activation." *Drug Metab Dispos* no. 35 (3):419–427.

Shahandeh, A., D. M. Johnstone, J. R. Atkins, J. M. Sontag, M. Heidari, N. Daneshi, E. Freeman-Acquah, and E. A. Milward. 2016. "Advantages of array-based technologies for pre-emptive pharmacogenomics testing." *Microarrays (Basel)* no. 5 (2). doi:10.3390/microarrays5020012.

Shitara, Y., M. Hirano, H. Sato, and Y. Sugiyama. 2004. "Gemfibrozil and its glucuronide inhibit the organic anion transporting polypeptide 2 (OATP2/OATP1B1:SLC21A6)-mediated hepatic uptake and CYP2C8-mediated metabolism of cerivastatin: Analysis of the mechanism of the clinically relevant drug-drug interaction between cerivastatin and gemfibrozil." *J Pharmacol Exp Ther* no. 311 (1):228–236. doi:10.1124/jpet.104.068536.

Skonberg, C., J. Olsen, K. G. Madsen, S. H. Hansen, and M. P. Grillo. 2008. "Metabolic activation of carboxylic acids." *Expert Opin Drug Metab Toxicol* no. 4 (4):425–438. doi:10.1517/17425255.4.4.425.

Smith, P. A., M. J. Sorich, R. A. McKinnon, and J. O. Miners. 2003. "In silico insights: Chemical and structural characteristics associated with uridine diphosphate-glucuronosyltransferase substrate selectivity." *Clin Exp Pharmacol Physiol* no. 30 (11):836–840.

Soars, M. G., B. Burchell, and R. J. Riley. 2002. "In vitro analysis of human drug glucuronidation and prediction of in vivo metabolic clearance." *J Pharmacol Exp Ther* no. 301 (1):382–390.

Soars, M. G., B. J. Ring, and S. A. Wrighton. 2003. "The effect of incubation conditions on the enzyme kinetics of udp-glucuronosyltransferases." *Drug Metab Dispos* no. 31 (6):762–767.

Soars, M. G., D. J. Smith, R. J. Riley, and B. Burchell. 2001. "Cloning and characterization of a canine UDP-glucuronosyltransferase." *Arch Biochem Biophys* no. 391 (2):218–224. doi:10.1006/abbi.2001.2383.

Sorich, M. J., R. A. McKinnon, J. O. Miners, and P. A. Smith. 2006. "The importance of local chemical structure for chemical metabolism by human uridine 5'-diphosphate-glucuronosyltransferase." *J Chem Inf Model* no. 46 (6):2692–2697. doi:10.1021/ci600248e.

Sorich, M. J., P. A. Smith, R. A. McKinnon, and J. O. Miners. 2002. "Pharmacophore and quantitative structure activity relationship modelling of UDP-glucuronosyltransferase 1A1 (UGT1A1) substrates." *Pharmacogenetics* no. 12 (8):635–645.

Sorich, M. J., P. A. Smith, J. O. Miners, P. I. Mackenzie, and R. A. McKinnon. 2008. "Recent advances in the in silico modelling of UDP glucuronosyltransferase substrates." *Curr Drug Metab* no. 9 (1):60–69.

Spahn-Langguth, H. and L. Z. Benet. 1992. "Acyl glucuronides revisited: Is the glucuronidation process a toxification as well as a detoxification mechanism?" *Drug Metab Rev* no. 24 (1):5–47. doi:10.3109/03602539208996289.

Stachulski, A. V. 2011. "Chemistry and reactivity of acyl glucuronides." *Curr Drug Metab* no. 12 (3):215–221.

Starlard-Davenport, A., B. Lyn-Cook, and A. Radominska-Pandya. 2008. "Identification of UDP-glucuronosyltransferase 1A10 in non-malignant and malignant human breast tissues." *Steroids* no. 73 (6):611–620. doi:10.1016/j.steroids.2008.01.019.

Stone, A. N., P. I. Mackenzie, A. Galetin, J. B. Houston, and J. O. Miners. 2003. "Isoform selectivity and kinetics of morphine 3- and 6-glucuronidation by human udp-glucuronosyltransferases: Evidence for atypical glucuronidation kinetics by UGT2B7." *Drug Metab Dispos* no. 31 (9):1086–1089.

Strassburg, C. P., N. Nguyen, M. P. Manns, and R. H. Tukey. 1999. "UDP-glucuronosyltransferase activity in human liver and colon." *Gastroenterology* no. 116 (1):149–160.

Strassburg, C. P., A. Strassburg, S. Kneip, A. Barut, R. H. Tukey, B. Rodeck, and M. P. Manns. 2002. "Developmental aspects of human hepatic drug glucuronidation in young children and adults." *Gut* no. 50 (2):259–265.

Strom, S. C., J. Davila, and M. Grompe. 2010. "Chimeric mice with humanized liver: Tools for the study of drug metabolism, excretion, and toxicity." *Methods Mol Biol* no. 640:491–509. doi:10.1007/978-1-60761-688-7_27.

Sun, D., G. Chen, R. W. Dellinger, A. K. Sharma, and P. Lazarus. 2010. "Characterization of 17-dihydroexemestane glucuronidation: Potential role of the UGT2B17 deletion in exemestane pharmacogenetics." *Pharmacogenet Genomics* no. 20 (10):575–585. doi:10.1097/FPC.0b013e32833b04af.

Sutherland, J. M. 1959. "Fatal cardiovascular collapse of infants receiving large amounts of chloramphenicol." *AMA J Dis Child* no. 97 (6):761–767.

Takahashi, T., Y. Fujiwara, M. Yamakido, O. Katoh, H. Watanabe, and P. I. Mackenzie. 1997. "The role of glucuronidation in 7-ethyl-10-hydroxycamptothecin resistance in vitro." *Jpn J Cancer Res* no. 88 (12):1211–1217.

Takaoka, Y., M. Ohta, A. Takeuchi, K. Miura, M. Matsuo, T. Sakaeda, A. Sugano, and H. Nishio. 2010. "Ligand orientation governs conjugation capacity of UDP-glucuronosyltransferase 1A1." *J Biochem* no. 148 (1):25–28. doi:10.1093/jb/mvq048.

Takeda, S., Y. Ishii, M. Iwanaga, P. I. Mackenzie, K. Nagata, Y. Yamazoe, K. Oguri, and H. Yamada. 2005. "Modulation of UDP-glucuronosyltransferase function by cytochrome P450: Evidence for the alteration of UGT2B7-catalyzed glucuronidation of morphine by CYP3A4." *Mol Pharmacol* no. 67 (3):665–672. doi:10.1124/mol.104.007641.

Takeda, S., Y. Ishii, M. Iwanaga, A. Nurrochmad, Y. Ito, P. I. Mackenzie, K. Nagata, Y. Yamazoe, K. Oguri, and H. Yamada. 2009. "Interaction of cytochrome P450 3A4 and UDP-glucuronosyltransferase 2B7: Evidence for protein-protein association and possible involvement of CYP3A4 J-helix in the interaction." *Mol Pharmacol* no. 75 (4):956–964. doi:10.1124/mol.108.052001.

Tallman, M. N., K. K. Miles, F. K. Kessler, J. N. Nielsen, X. Tian, J. K. Ritter, and P. C. Smith. 2007. "The contribution of intestinal UDP-glucuronosyltransferases in modulating 7-ethyl-10-hydroxy-camptothecin (SN-38)-induced gastrointestinal toxicity in rats." *J Pharmacol Exp Ther* no. 320 (1):29–37. doi:10.1124/jpet.106.110924.

Tankanitlert, J., N. P. Morales, T. A. Howard, P. Fucharoen, R. E. Ware, S. Fucharoen, and U. Chantharaksri. 2007. "Effects of combined UDP-Glucuronosyltransferase (UGT) 1A1*28 and 1A6*2 on paracetamol pharmacokinetics in beta-thalassemia/HbE." *Pharmacology* no. 79 (2):97–103.

Taura, K. I., H. Yamada, Y. Hagino, Y. Ishii, M. A. Mori, and K. Oguri. 2000. "Interaction between cytochrome P450 and other drug-metabolizing enzymes: Evidence for an association of CYP1A1 with microsomal epoxide hydrolase and UDP-glucuronosyltransferase." *Biochem Biophys Res Commun* no. 273 (3):1048–1052. doi:10.1006/bbrc.2000.3076.

Templeton, I., G. Eichenbaum, R. Sane, and J. Zhou. 2014. "Case study 5. Deconvoluting hyperbilirubinemia: Differentiating between hepatotoxicity and reversible inhibition of UGT1A1, MRP2, or OATP1B1 in drug development." *Methods Mol Biol* no. 1113:471–483. doi:10.1007/978-1-62703-758-7_22.

Tephly, T. and M.D. Green. 2000. "UDP-glucuronosyltransferases." In *Metabolic Drug Interactions*, edited by R. H. Levy, K.E. Thummel, W.F. Trager, P.D. Hansten and M. Eichelbaum, 160–173. Philadelphia, Pennsylvania: Lippincott Williams and Wilkins.

Thibaudeau, J., J. Lepine, J. Tojcic, Y. Duguay, G. Pelletier, M. Plante, J. Brisson et al. 2006. "Characterization of common UGT1A8, UGT1A9, and UGT2B7 variants with different capacities to inactivate mutagenic 4-hydroxylated metabolites of estradiol and estrone." *Cancer Res* no. 66 (1):125–133.

Toffoli, G., E. Cecchin, G. Corona, A. Russo, A. Buonadonna, M. D'Andrea, L. M. Pasetto et al. 2006. "The role of UGT1A1*28 polymorphism in the pharmacodynamics and pharmacokinetics of irinotecan in patients with metastatic colorectal cancer." *J Clin Oncol* no. 24 (19):3061–3068. doi:10.1200/JCO.2005.05.5400.

Tornio, A., P. J. Neuvonen, M. Niemi, and J. T. Backman. 2016. "Role of gemfibrozil as an inhibitor of CYP2C8 and membrane transporters." *Expert Opin Drug Metab Toxicol* 1–13. doi:10.1080/17425255.2016.1227791.

Tripathi, S. P., A. Bhadauriya, A. Patil, and A. T. Sangamwar. 2013. "Substrate selectivity of human intestinal UDP-glucuronosyltransferases (UGTs): In silico and in vitro insights." *Drug Metab Rev* no. 45 (2):231–252. doi:10.3109/03602532.2013.767345.

Troberg, J., E. Jarvinen, M. Muniz, N. Sneitz, J. Mosorin, M. Hagstrom, and M. Finel. 2015. "Dog UDP-glucuronosyltransferase enzymes of subfamily 1A: Cloning, expression, and activity." *Drug Metab Dispos* no. 43 (1):107–118. doi:10.1124/dmd.114.059303.

Tsoutsikos, P., J. O. Miners, A. Stapleton, A. Thomas, B. C. Sallustio, and K. M. Knights. 2004. "Evidence that unsaturated fatty acids are potent inhibitors of renal UDP-glucuronosyltransferases (UGT): Kinetic studies using human kidney cortical microsomes and recombinant UGT1A9 and UGT2B7." *Biochem Pharmacol* no. 67 (1):191–199.

Tukey, R. H. and C. P. Strassburg. 2000. "Human UDP-glucuronosyltransferases: Metabolism, expression, and disease." *Annu Rev Pharmacol Toxicol* no. 40:581–616.

Turgeon, D., J. S. Carrier, E. Levesque, D. W. Hum, and A. Belanger. 2001. "Relative enzymatic activity, protein stability, and tissue distribution of human steroid-metabolizing UGT2B subfamily members." *Endocrinology* no. 142 (2):778–787. doi:10.1210/endo.142.2.7958.

Uchaipichat, V., A. Galetin, J. B. Houston, P. I. Mackenzie, J. A. Williams, and J. O. Miners. 2008. "Kinetic modeling of the interactions between 4-methylumbelliferone, 1-naphthol, and zidovudine glucuronidation by udp-glucuronosyltransferase 2B7 (UGT2B7) provides evidence for multiple substrate binding and effector sites." *Mol Pharmacol* no. 74 (4):1152–1162. doi:10.1124/mol.108.048645.

Uchaipichat, V., P. I. Mackenzie, X. H. Guo, D. Gardner-Stephen, A. Galetin, J. B. Houston, and J. O. Miners. 2004. "Human udp-glucuronosyltransferases: Isoform selectivity and kinetics of 4-methylumbelliferone and 1-naphthol glucuronidation, effects of organic solvents, and inhibition by diclofenac and probenecid." *Drug Metab Dispos* no. 32 (4):413–423. doi:10.1124/dmd.32.4.413.

Urawa, N., Y. Kobayashi, J. Araki, R. Sugimoto, M. Iwasa, M. Kaito, and Y. Adachi. 2006. "Linkage disequilibrium of UGT1A1*6 and UGT1A1*28 in relation to UGT1A6 and UGT1A7 polymorphisms." *Oncol Rep* no. 16 (4):801–806.

Vasilyeva, A., S. Durmus, L. Li, E. Wagenaar, S. Hu, A. A. Gibson, J. C. Panetta et al. 2015. "Hepatocellular shuttling and recirculation of sorafenib-glucuronide is dependent on Abcc2, Abcc3, and Oatp1a/1b." *Cancer Res* no. 75 (13):2729–2736. doi:10.1158/0008-5472.CAN-15-0280.

Vaz, A. D., W. W. Wang, A. J. Bessire, R. Sharma, and A. E. Hagen. 2010. "A rapid and specific derivatization procedure to identify acyl-glucuronides by mass spectrometry." *Rapid Commun Mass Spectrom* no. 24 (14):2109–2121. doi:10.1002/rcm.4621.

Verreault, M., K. Senekeo-Effenberger, J. Trottier, J. A. Bonzo, J. Belanger, J. Kaeding, B. Staels, P. Caron, R. H. Tukey, and O. Barbier. 2006. "The liver X-receptor alpha controls hepatic expression of the human bile acid-glucuronidating UGT1A3 enzyme in human cells and transgenic mice." *Hepatology* no. 44 (2):368–378.

Vessey, D. A. and D. Zakim. 1972. "Regulation of microsomal enzymes by phospholipids. V. Kinetic studies of hepatic uridine diphosphate-glucuronyltransferase." *J Biol Chem* no. 247 (10):3023–3028.

Vildhede, A., J. R. Wisniewski, A. Noren, M. Karlgren, and P. Artursson. 2015. "Comparative proteomic analysis of human liver tissue and isolated hepatocytes with a focus on proteins determining drug exposure." *J Proteome Res* no. 14 (8):3305–3314. doi:10.1021/acs.jproteome.5b00334.

Vivares, A., S. Salle-Lefort, C. Arabeyre-Fabre, R. Ngo, G. Penarier, M. Bremond, P. Moliner, J. F. Gallas, G. Fabre, and S. Klieber. 2015. "Morphological behaviour and metabolic capacity of cryopreserved human primary hepatocytes cultivated in a perfused multiwell device." *Xenobiotica* no. 45 (1):29–44. doi:10.3109/00498254.2014.944612.

Walker, G. S., J. Atherton, J. Bauman, C. Kohl, W. Lam, M. Reily, Z. Lou, and A. Mutlib. 2007. "Determination of degradation pathways and kinetics of acyl glucuronides by NMR spectroscopy." *Chem Res Toxicol* no. 20 (6):876–886. doi:10.1021/tx600297u.

Walsky, R. L., J. N. Bauman, K. Bourcier, G. Giddens, K. Lapham, A. Negahban, T. F. Ryder, R. S. Obach, R. Hyland, and T. C. Goosen. 2012. "Optimized assays for human UDP-glucuronosyltransferase (UGT) activities: Altered alamethicin concentration and utility to screen for UGT inhibitors." *Drug Metab Dispos* no. 40 (5):1051–1065. doi:10.1124/dmd.111.043117.

Wang, H., T. Bian, T. Jin, Y. Chen, A. Lin, and C. Chen. 2014. "Association analysis of UGT1A genotype and haplotype with SN-38 glucuronidation in human livers." *Pharmacogenomics* no. 15 (6):785–798. doi:10.2217/pgs.14.29.

Wang, J., M. Davis, F. Li, F. Azam, J. Scatina, and R. Talaat. 2004. "A novel approach for predicting acyl glucuronide reactivity via Schiff base formation: Development of rapidly formed peptide adducts for LC/MS/MS measurements." *Chem Res Toxicol* no. 17 (9):1206–1216. doi:10.1021/tx049900+.

Wang, J. S., M. Neuvonen, X. Wen, J. T. Backman, and P. J. Neuvonen. 2002. "Gemfibrozil inhibits CYP2C8-mediated cerivastatin metabolism in human liver microsomes." *Drug Metab Dispos* no. 30 (12):1352–1356.

Wang, L. Z., J. Ramirez, W. Yeo, M. Y. Chan, W. L. Thuya, J. Y. Lau, S. C. Wan et al. 2013. "Glucuronidation by UGT1A1 is the dominant pathway of the metabolic disposition of belinostat in liver cancer patients." *PLoS One* no. 8 (1):e54522. doi:10.1371/journal.pone.0054522.

Wang, W. W., S. R. Khetani, S. Krzyzewski, D. B. Duignan, and R. S. Obach. 2010. "Assessment of a micropatterned hepatocyte coculture system to generate major human excretory and circulating drug metabolites." *Drug Metab Dispos* no. 38 (10):1900–1905. doi:10.1124/dmd.110.034876.

Watanabe, Y., M. Nakajima, N. Ohashi, T. Kume, and T. Yokoi. 2003. "Glucuronidation of etoposide in human liver microsomes is specifically catalyzed by UDP-glucuronosyltransferase 1A1." *Drug Metab Dispos* no. 31 (5):589–595.

Weiss, C. F., A. J. Glazko, and J. K. Weston. 1960. "Chloramphenicol in the newborn infant. A physiologic explanation of its toxicity when given in excessive doses." *N Engl J Med* no. 262:787–794. doi:10.1056/NEJM196004212621601.

Wells, P. G., P. I. Mackenzie, J. R. Chowdhury, C. Guillemette, P. A. Gregory, Y. Ishii, A. J. Hansen et al. 2004. "Glucuronidation and the UDP-glucuronosyltransferases in health and disease." *Drug Metab Dispos* no. 32 (3):281–290. doi:10.1124/dmd.32.3.281.

Wen, X., J. S. Wang, J. T. Backman, K. T. Kivisto, and P. J. Neuvonen. 2001. "Gemfibrozil is a potent inhibitor of human cytochrome P450 2C9." *Drug Metab Dispos* no. 29 (11):1359–1361.

Wiener, D., D. R. Doerge, J. L. Fang, P. Upadhyaya, and P. Lazarus. 2004. "Characterization of N-glucuronidation of the lung carcinogen 4-(methylnitrosamino)-1-(3-pyridyl)-1-butanol (NNAL) in human liver: Importance of UDP-glucuronosyltransferase 1A4." *Drug Metab Dispos* no. 32 (1):72–79.

Wijayakumara, D. D., D. G. Hu, R. Meech, R. A. McKinnon, and P. I. Mackenzie. 2015. "Regulation of human UGT2B15 and UGT2B17 by miR-376c in prostate cancer cell lines." *J Pharmacol Exp Ther* no. 354 (3):417–425. doi:10.1124/jpet.115.226118.

Williams, J. A., R. Hyland, B. C. Jones, D. A. Smith, S. Hurst, T. C. Goosen, V. Peterkin, J. R. Koup, and S. E. Ball. 2004. "Drug-drug interactions for UDP-glucuronosyltransferase substrates: A pharmacokinetic explanation for typically observed low exposure (AUCi/AUC) ratios." *Drug Metab Dispos* no. 32 (11):1201–1208. doi:10.1124/dmd.104.000794.

Wilson, W., 3rd, F. Pardo-Manuel de Villena, B. D. Lyn-Cook, P. K. Chatterjee, T. A. Bell, D. A. Detwiler, R. C. Gilmore et al. 2004. "Characterization of a common deletion polymorphism of the UGT2B17 gene linked to UGT2B15." *Genomics* no. 84 (4):707–714.

Wu, B., J. K. Morrow, R. Singh, S. Zhang, and M. Hu. 2011. "Three-dimensional quantitative structure-activity relationship studies on UGT1A9-mediated 3-O-glucuronidation of natural flavonols using a pharmacophore-based comparative molecular field analysis model." *J Pharmacol Exp Ther* no. 336 (2):403–413. doi:10.1124/jpet.110.175356.

Wu, Z., X. Zhang, Z. Ma, and B. Wu. 2015. "Establishment of pharmacophore and VolSurf models to predict the substrates of UDP-glucuronosyltransferase1A3." *Xenobiotica* no. 45 (8):653–662. doi:10.3109/0049 8254.2015.1016136.

Xiong, Y., A. S. Patana, M. J. Miley, A. K. Zielinska, S. M. Bratton, G. P. Miller, A. Goldman, M. Finel, M. R. Redinbo, and A. Radominska-Pandya. 2008. "The first aspartic acid of the DQxD motif for human UDP-glucuronosyltransferase 1A10 interacts with UDP-glucuronic acid during catalysis." *Drug Metab Dispos* no. 36 (3):517–522. doi:10.1124/dmd.107.016469.

Yamada, A., K. Maeda, N. Ishiguro, Y. Tsuda, T. Igarashi, T. Ebner, W. Roth, S. Ikushiro, and Y. Sugiyama. 2011. "The impact of pharmacogenetics of metabolic enzymes and transporters on the pharmacokinetics of telmisartan in healthy volunteers." *Pharmacogenet Genomics* no. 21 (9):523–530. doi:10.1097/ FPC.0b013e3283482502.

Yamanaka, H., M. Nakajima, M. Katoh, Y. Hara, O. Tachibana, J. Yamashita, H. L. McLeod, and T. Yokoi. 2004. "A novel polymorphism in the promoter region of human UGT1A9 gene (UGT1A9*22) and its effects on the transcriptional activity." *Pharmacogenetics* no. 14 (5):329–332.

Yilmaz, L., E. Borazan, T. Aytekin, I. Baskonus, A. Aytekin, S. Oztuzcu, Z. Bozdag, and A. Balik. 2015. "Increased UGT1A3 and UGT1A7 expression is associated with pancreatic cancer." *Asian Pac J Cancer Prev* no. 16 (4):1651–1655.

Yin, H., G. Bennett, and J. P. Jones. 1994. "Mechanistic studies of uridine diphosphate glucuronosyltransferase." *Chem Biol Interact* no. 90 (1):47–58.

Yuan, L., S. Qian, Y. Xiao, H. Sun, and S. Zeng. 2015. "Homo- and hetero-dimerization of human UDP-glucuronosyltransferase 2B7 (UGT2B7) wild type and its allelic variants affect zidovudine glucuronidation activity." *Biochem Pharmacol* no. 95 (1):58–70. doi:10.1016/j.bcp.2015.03.002.

Yueh, M. F. and R. H. Tukey. 2007. "Nrf2-Keap1 signaling pathway regulates human UGT1A1 expression in vitro and in transgenic UGT1 mice." *J Biol Chem* no. 282 (12):8749–8758.

Zaja, O., M. K. Tiljak, M. Stefanovic, J. Tumbri, and Z. Jurcic. 2014. "Correlation of UGT1A1 TATA-box polymorphism and jaundice in breastfed newborns-early presentation of Gilbert's syndrome." *J Matern Fetal Neonatal Med* no. 27 (8):844–850. doi:10.3109/14767058.2013.837879.

Zaya, M. J., R. N. Hines, and J. C. Stevens. 2006. "Epirubicin glucuronidation and UGT2B7 developmental expression." *Drug Metab Dispos* no. 34 (12):2097–2101. doi:10.1124/dmd.106.011387.

Zheng, Y., D. Sun, A. K. Sharma, G. Chen, S. Amin, and P. Lazarus. 2007. "Elimination of antiestrogenic effects of active tamoxifen metabolites by glucuronidation." *Drug Metab Dispos* no. 35 (10):1942–1948. doi:10.1124/dmd.107.016279.

Zhong, S., R. Jones, W. Lu, S. Schadt, and G. Ottaviani. 2015. "A new rapid in vitro assay for assessing reactivity of acyl glucuronides." *Drug Metab Dispos* no. 43 (11):1711–1717. doi:10.1124/dmd.115.066159.

Zhou, J., U. A. Argikar, and R. P. Remmel. 2011. "Functional analysis of UGT1A4(P24T) and UGT1A4(L48V) variant enzymes." *Pharmacogenomics* no. 12 (12):1671–1679.

Zhou, J. and J. O. Miners. 2014. "Enzyme kinetics of uridine diphosphate glucuronosyltransferases (UGTs)." *Methods Mol Biol* no. 1113:203–228. doi:10.1007/978-1-62703-758-7_11.

Zhou, J., T. S. Tracy, and R. P. Remmel. 2010. "Glucuronidation of dihydrotestosterone and trans-androsterone by recombinant UDP-glucuronosyltransferase (UGT) 1A4: Evidence for multiple UGT1A4 aglycone binding sites." *Drug Metab Dispos* no. 38 (3):431–440. doi:10.1124/dmd.109.028712.Danis quas sitendi

Section II

Factors Which Affect Drug Metabolism

6

Non-CYP Drug Metabolizing
Enzymes and Their Reactions

Shuguang Ma, Ryan H. Takahashi, Yong Ma, Sudheer Bobba,
Donglu Zhang, and S. Cyrus Khojasteh

CONTENTS

Introduction

Metabolism is the major elimination pathway of a drug from the body initiated by drug metabolizing enzymes (DMEs). DMEs are present mainly in the liver, intestine, and blood and facilitate the excretion of xenobiotics from the body by converting lipophilic drugs into hydrophilic compounds. Cytochrome P450 enzymes (CYPs) are responsible for the clearance of a majority of drugs on the market, and, accordingly, much emphasis has been placed on understanding the role of CYPs in metabolism, clearance, drug-drug interactions, and oral bioavailability [1].

The widespread use of metabolic stability screening using microsomal fractions or hepatocytes for oxidative and glucuronic acid conjugative metabolism at the early discovery stage has greatly increased the number of drug candidates with a high level of metabolic stability. This screening strategy, however, has forced new chemical entities (NCEs) into chemical spaces that rely on non-CYP enzymes for clearance, and therefore, the importance of non-CYP enzymes in the elimination of drugs has been increasingly recognized in drug discovery and development [2–4]. In a recent survey of a set of 125 small molecule drugs approved by the United States Food and Drug Administration (FDA) from 2006 to 2015, approximately 30% of the metabolism of these drugs is carried out by non-CYP enzymes [5]. These non-CYP enzymes can also modulate efficacy, contribute to detoxification, or produce therapeutically active or reactive/toxic metabolites [6,7]. Here, we discuss the non-CYP enzymes involved in drug metabolism reactions (except for enzymes discussed in Chapters 4 and 5) and their subcellular locations, organ distributions, mechanisms of reactions, and typical substrates and inhibitors.

Flavin-Containing Monooxygenases

The flavin-containing monooxygenase (FMO) (EC 1.14.13.8) enzymes are NADPH-dependent, membrane bound to the endoplasmic reticulum (ER), and have molecular weights of approximately 60 kDa. FMOs metabolize a wide range of substrates by oxidizing nitrogen, sulfur, phosphorous, and selenium atoms. The source of the added oxygen atom is molecular O_2.

The role of FMO is often underestimated in the calculation of total clearance because several of the reactions they carry out are similar to those mediated by CYPs. In addition, CYPs use the same cofactor and are also located on the ER [8]. FMO-mediated reactions can be distinguished from those mediated by CYPs by the following observations:

1. FMO activity is optimal at a pH of >9 while CYP activity is optimal at a pH of 7.4.
2. All FMOs, except for FMO2, are thermally unstable when pre-incubated in the absence of NADPH.
3. 1-Aminobenzotriazole (ABT) inactivates CYP enzymes in a time-dependent manner but does not inhibit FMOs.
4. Inhibitory antibodies to cytochrome P450 reductase will impact CYP-dependent processes, but not those that are FMO-dependent.
5. Detergents (such as Triton-X 100) inhibit CYP enzymes but have little effect on FMO activity.
6. Recombinant enzymes can be used to distinguish between FMO- and CYP-catalyzed reactions.
7. FMOs are rarely induced, but many CYPs are inducible.

Subcellular Location and Organ Distribution

FMOs are distributed differently in organs throughout the body depending on the isoform (Table 6.1) [9]. In humans, the five functional forms of FMO (FMO1 through FMO5) share 50%–55% sequence identity. Even though FMO1 is the major form in many animals, in humans, this isoform is found only in fetal livers and is absent in adults [9]. FMO1 has a shallow substrate binding channel and, therefore, broad substrate specificity. The highest concentration of FMO2 is in lung tissue, followed by the kidney where the concentration is 7-fold less. FMO3 is the major isoform in human liver at a concentration of 46 pmol/mg [10] but is present at much lower amounts in the lung and kidney (<5%). FMO3 has a deep substrate binding channel (8–10 Å) and, therefore, a narrower substrate specificity than FMO1. FMO4 and FMO5 play minor roles in drug metabolism.

In humans, trimethylamine, a foul-smelling chemical derived from dietary sources, such as choline and carnitine, is metabolized by FMO3 to an odorless *N*-oxide metabolite. FMO3 deficiency leads to trimethylaminuria ("fish-like odor syndrome") [11].

TABLE 6.1

FMO Distribution in Different Species

Form	Mouse	Rat	Monkey	Human
FMO1	Kidney	Liver, kidney	Kidney	Kidney >> lung, small intestine >> liver
FMO2	Lung	Lung	Lung	Lung >> kidney > liver, small intestine
FMO3	Liver, kidney	Kidney	Liver, kidney	Liver >> lung > kidney >> small intestine

Multiplicity and Species Differences

Pronounced differences in FMO expression exist amongst preclinical species [12–13]. The flavin adenine dinucleotide (FAD) and NADPH binding domains, with 4–32 and 186–213 residues, respectively, are the conserved regions across species.

Young female mice have very high expressions of FMO3 and FMO5, which most closely resembles FMO expression in the adult human liver. The FMO3 activity in young female rats is 5–10 fold higher than that in male rats. Adult rats have relatively low FMO3 and FMO5 expressions and a similar FMO1 expression to humans.

Catalytic Mechanism

The overall reaction of FMO-mediated metabolism involves the use of FAD as a prosthetic group to initiate a two-electron oxidation (Figure 6.1). The steps of this reaction are described below:

1. At resting state, the enzyme is present as a 4α-hydroperoxyflavin (FAD-OOH). The distal oxygen is electrophilic.
2. A nucleophilic substrate (X:) attacks the distal oxygen of FAD-OOH and results in formation of an oxygenated product (O-X) and 4α-hydroxyflavin (FAD-OH).
3. The metabolite is released, and FAD-OH loses a water molecule to form FAD. This is thought to be the rate-limiting step of the reaction.
4. FAD receives an electron from NADPH to form $FADH_2$ (not shown). This is further oxidized by O_2 to form FAD-OOH. This step returns FMO to its resting state.

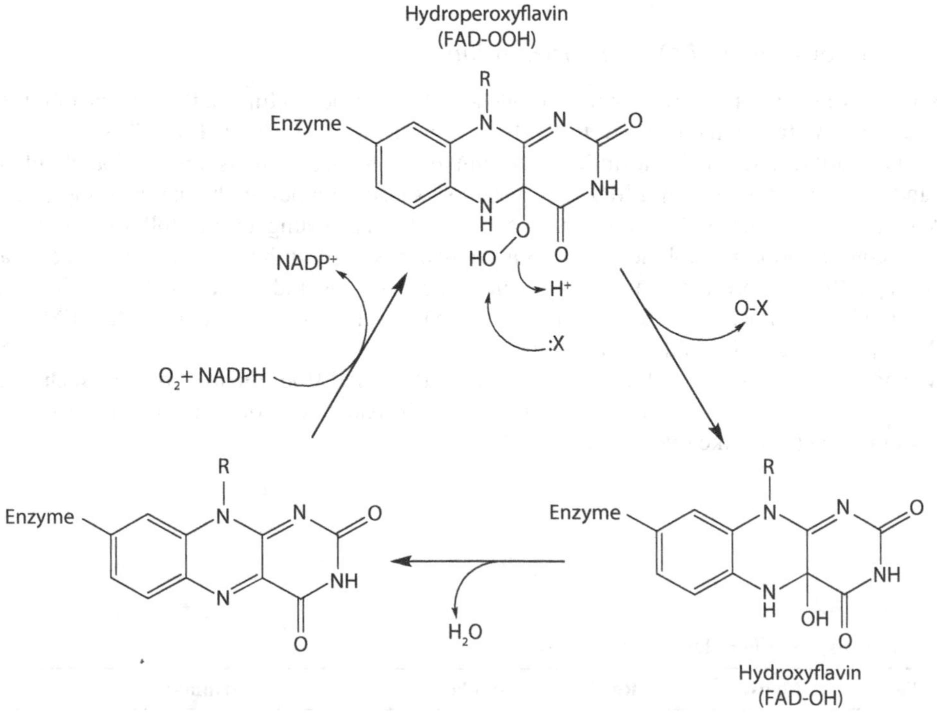

FIGURE 6.1   Reaction mechanism for oxidation by flavin-containing monooxygenases.

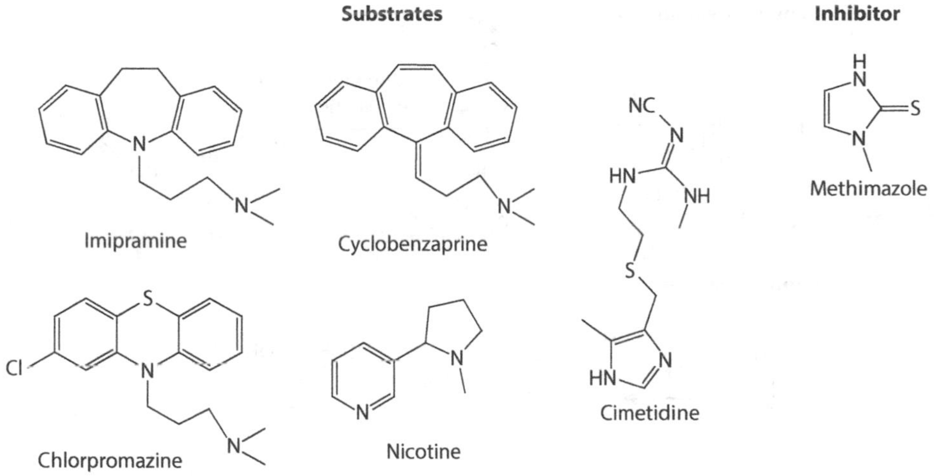

FIGURE 6.2 Examples of substrates and inhibitors of flavin-containing monooxygenase.

Substrates and Inhibitors

FMOs catalyze the *N*-oxidation of substrates that contain a nitrogen atom with sp³ centers (Figure 6.2). Such substrates include benzydamine, chlorpromazine, clozapine, cyclobenzaprine, ephedrine, imipramine (FMO1 isoform), itopride, *N*-methylamphetamine, nicotine (FMO3 isoform), norcocaine, phenothiazine, and trimethylamine. FMOs can also mediate the *S*-oxidation of thioethers to sulfoxides, and rarely, the further oxidation of these sulfoxides to sulfones. Examples are cimetidine, sulindac, and tazarotenic acid.

Methimazole, n-octylamine, and thiourea are FMO inhibitors. Note that n-octylamine is also an inactivator of FMO. Caution needs to be taken when using methimazole since the compound also inhibits several CYP isoforms. No inhibitory antibodies are commercially available, but antibodies are available for Western blot studies.

Reactions and Relevance to Human Drug Metabolism

FMOs contribute to the clearance of several drugs through *N*- or *S*-oxidation. For example, FMO1 in renal tissue is involved in the oxidative metabolism of lorcaserin at the nitrogen atom [14]. In addition to the oxidation of heteroatoms, FMOs have been implicated in several less common, yet important, reactions (Figure 6.3). These include Cope-type elimination driven by the loss of a side chain after *N*-oxide formation. Oxime formation can also occur following consecutive oxidation by FMOs. Finally, even though carbon oxidation by FMOs is uncommon, it can occur, as is the case with 4-fluoroaniline.

Monoamine Oxidases

Monoamine oxidase (MAO) (EC 1.4.3.4) enzymes are bound to the outer membrane of mitochondria, and although they are widely distributed in many tissues, their activity in the brain has been a focus of therapeutic research. MAOs oxidize primary, secondary, and tertiary amines to aldehydes, while the endogenous substrates of MAOs are primary amines, such as histamine. The key feature of MAO substrates is that the amine is neighboring a carbon with a hydrogen atom.

Subcellular Location and Organ Distribution

MAOs are expressed in most tissues and are present in two isoforms, MAO-A and MAO-B, which share a 70% sequence identity. Most tissues express both isoforms in the same cell, with the exception of

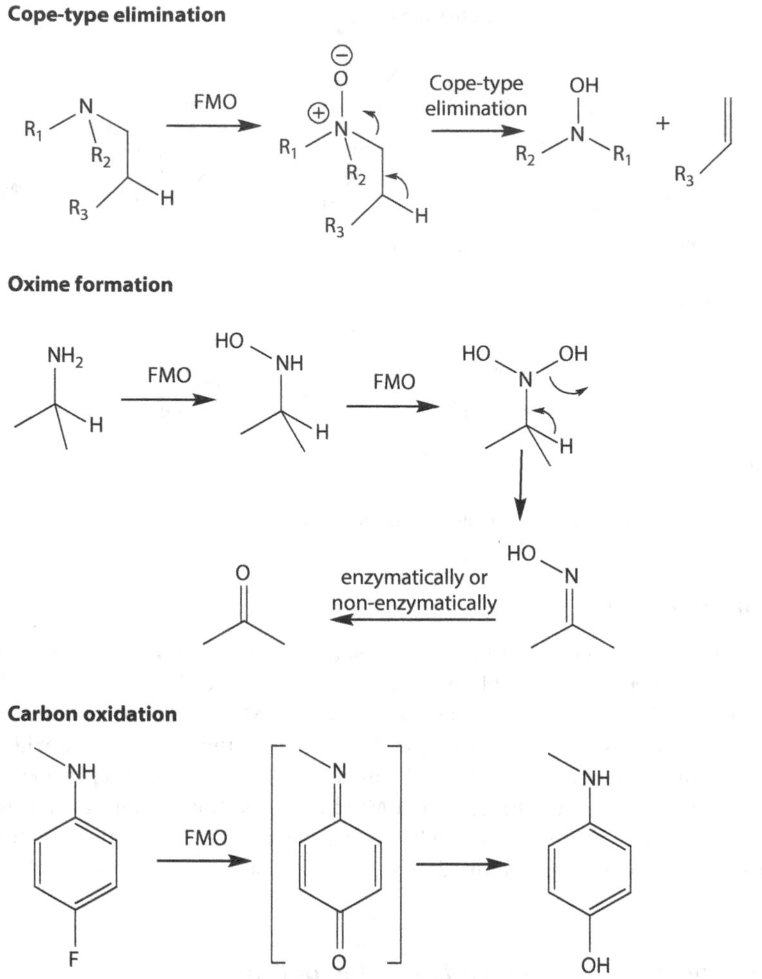

Cope-type elimination

Oxime formation

Carbon oxidation

FIGURE 6.3   Uncommon oxidation reactions mediated by flavin-containing monooxygenases (FMOs).

platelets that express only MAO-B. The highest expression of MAOs is in the liver and placenta while the lowest concentration is in the spleen. In the brain, MAO-A is distributed mainly in dopaminergic neurons versus MAO-B, which is localized in serotonergic neurons.

Catalytic Mechanism

The prosthetic group in MAO is FAD. Multiple mechanisms have been proposed for MAO-catalyzed metabolism, but one of the most accepted involves a single electron transfer to form radical intermediates. In the first step, FAD abstracts a single electron from the nitrogen atom (amine) to form an amine radical cation (Step 1). The nitrogen radical cation then facilitates the abstraction of a hydrogen atom from the neighboring carbon atom (Step 2). An imine is formed by loss of a second electron, while FAD is reduced to $FADH_2$ (Step 3). $FADH_2$ oxidizes molecular O_2, leading to formation of the resting state of the enzyme (FAD) and hydrogen peroxide (Step 4), while the imine is converted into an aldehyde and ammonia (Step 5).

1. $FAD + RCH_2NH_2$ (substrate) $\rightarrow FAD^- + RCH_2(H_2)N^{+\cdot}$
2. $RCH_2(H_2)N^{+\cdot} \rightarrow R(H)C^{+\cdot}(H_2)N:$

3. $FAD^- + R(H)C^{\cdot+}(H_2)N: \rightarrow FADH_2 + RCH=NH$
4. $FADH_2 + O_2 \rightarrow FAD + H_2O_2$
5. $RCH=NH + H_2O \rightarrow RCH=O + NH_3$

The aldehyde product is often further oxidized to an acid or reduced to an alcohol by other enzymes.

Substrates and Inhibitors

Dopamine and tryptamine are metabolized by both MAO isoforms. Substrates of MAO-A include almotriptan, biogenic amines, 5-hydroxytryptamine (5-HT or serotonin), melatonin, norepinephrine (catechol-containing), rizatriptan, sumatriptan, tyramine, and zolmitriptan (Figure 6.4). The substrates of MAO-B include 2-phenylethylamine (PEA), benzylamine (non-catechol-containing), and tertiary amines.

Pargyline is a mechanism-based inactivator of both MAO isoforms, and it binds to N5 of FAD (Figure 6.4). Selective inhibitors of MAO-A, such as clorgyline and moclobemide, are typically used in the treatment of depression [15]. MAO-B inhibitors, such as (*R*)-deprenyl (selegiline; irreversible inhibition) and desmethoxyyangonin (reversible inhibition), are typically used in the treatment of Parkinson's disease [16].

Reactions and Relevance to Human Drug Metabolism

1-Methyl-4-phenyl-1,2,3,6-tetrahydropyridine (MPTP) is a neurotoxin that causes permanent brain damage and Parkinsonism. The mechanism of toxicity is conversion to MPP$^+$ by MAO-B in glial cells in the brain (Figure 6.5). This metabolite kills dopamine-producing neurons in the substantia nigra and, hence, induces the effects of Parkinson's disease [17].

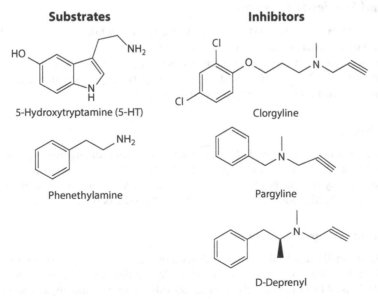

FIGURE 6.4 Substrates and inhibitors of monoamine oxidases.

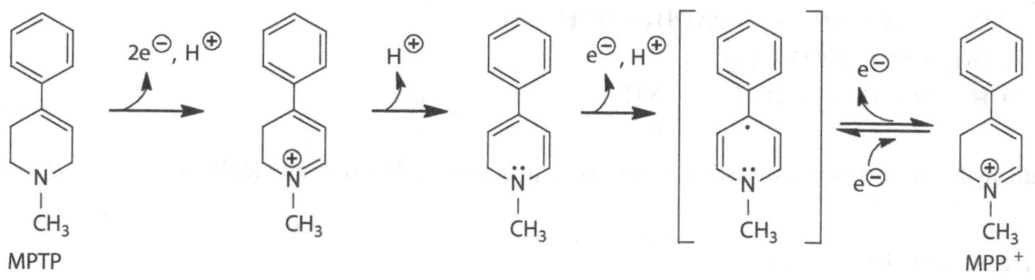

FIGURE 6.5 Bioactivation of *N*-methyl-4-phenyl-1,2,3,6-tetrahydropyridine (MPTP) to form the neurotoxin, *N*-methyl-4-phenylpyridinium (MPP+), mediated by MAO-B.

Alcohol Dehydrogenases

Alcohol dehydrogenases (ADHs) (EC 1.1.1.1) are a group of zinc-containing enzymes that facilitate the inter-conversion between alcohols and aldehydes or ketones by converting the cofactor nicotinamide adenine dinucleotide (NAD+) to its reduced form (NADH). The overall reaction is:

$$R\text{-}CH_2\text{-}OH + NAD^+ \rightarrow R\text{-}CHO + NADH + H^+$$

ADHs comprise a complex enzyme system that are grouped into six classes (ADH1 to ADH6), of which the first five have been identified in humans [18]. The major human ADHs are ADH1 and ADH5, both of which are dimeric proteins consisting of two 40 kDa subunits.

Subcellular Location and Organ Distribution

ADHs are located almost exclusively in cytosol and blood. They are widely distributed in various organs [19]. ADH1 is abundant in the liver, with lower levels in the gastrointestinal tract, kidneys, and lungs. ADH2 is found only in the liver. ADH3 exists in most tissues. ADH4 is expressed mainly in the stomach and esophagus, although it is also present in much lower levels in liver, skin, and cornea. ADH5 is found in gastric epithelium, and ADH6 is expressed principally in the liver of rats.

Multiplicity and Species Differences

Humans have three ADH1(ADH1A, ADH1B and ADH1C) genes, while mouse and rat have only one. ADH5 is present only in humans and ADH6 is present only in rats.

ADH enzymes show marked genetic variation. Allelic variants occur at *ADH1B* to give *ADH1B1*, −2 and −3, and at *ADH1C* to give *ADH1C1* and −2. All these polymorphic subunits can combine to form homodimers or heterodimers, leading to extensive multiplicity [6].

Catalytic Mechanism

In the oxidation mechanism (Figure 6.6), ADH uses zinc to position the hydroxyl group of the alcohol in a conformation that allows for oxidation to occur. NAD+ acts as a co-substrate and performs the oxidation. While the enzyme attaches to the two substrates (NAD+ and alcohol), the hydrogen is formally transferred from the alcohol to NAD+, resulting in the products NADH and a ketone or aldehyde.

Substrates, Inhibitors, and Inducers

Human ADH1 is primarily involved in the metabolism of ethanol and other small aliphatic alcohols. ADH2 shows a high K_m value for ethanol and preferentially oxidizes aromatic or medium to long chain alkyl aliphatic alcohols. ADH3 is relatively inactive towards ethanol oxidation, and its major activity is as a glutathione-dependent formaldehyde dehydrogenase. ADH4 is highly active towards alcohol and

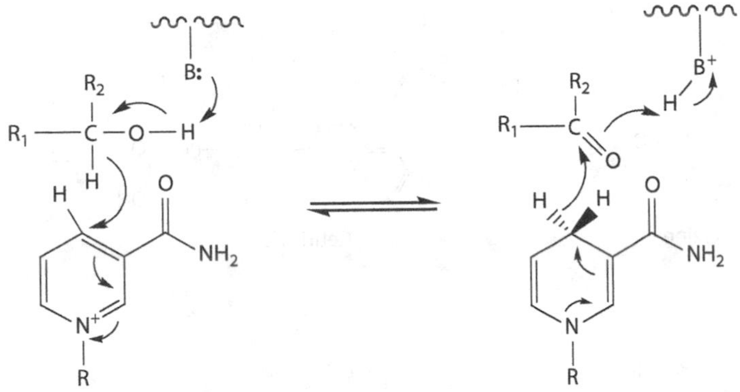

FIGURE 6.6 Catalytic mechanism of alcohol dehydrogenase.

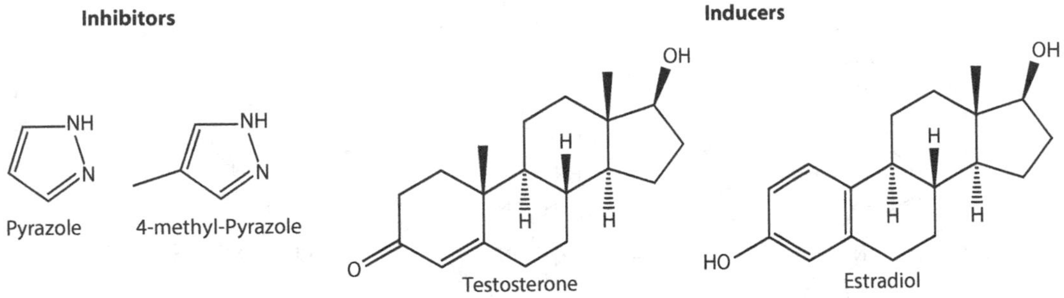

FIGURE 6.7 Inhibitors and inducers of alcohol dehydrogenase.

retinoids. ADH5 is a fetal alcohol dehydrogenase, which has been less studied and, therefore, little is known about its substrates and characteristics.

Pyrazole and its 4-alkyl-substituted derivatives (e.g., 4-methylpyrazole) are potent, although not selective, inhibitors for ADH1s. ADH enzymes are also inducible. Induction of ADH in mouse and/or rat by androgen (e.g., testosterone) and estradiol has been demonstrated (Figure 6.7) [20–21].

Reactions and Relevance to Human Drug Metabolism

ADH is involved in the metabolism of a number of drugs (Figure 6.8). Hydroxyzine is a first-generation antihistamine for the treatment of allergic conditions and is extensively metabolized in the liver to cetirizine through oxidation of the alcohol moiety to a carboxylic acid mediated by ADH. It is also involved in the metabolism of celecoxib, a selective cyclooxygenase-2 inhibitor. Following methyl hydroxylation by CYP2C9, ADH1, and ADH2 subsequently oxidizes the alcohol to carboxycelecoxib [22].

Abacavir is a reverse transcriptase inhibitor approved for treatment of HIV/AIDS as a single agent or as part of a two-drug or three-drug pill combination. Abacavir is a prodrug that is converted to the active metabolite, carbovir triphosphate, which is responsible for the inhibition of viral replication. In humans, abacavir is extensively metabolized in the liver to form an inactive glucuronide metabolite and a carboxylic acid metabolite catalyzed by ADH1A [23].

ADH might be also involved in the metabolic pathway of felbamate that leads to its toxicity. Felbamate is a broad-spectrum antiepileptic drug for the treatment of several forms of epilepsy. After its introduction, cases of aplastic anemia and hepatotoxicity associated with its use were reported. The observed toxicity might be related to the formation of a reactive atropaldehyde metabolite by ADH-mediated oxidation of the felbamate monocarbamate metabolite, followed by spontaneous loses of carbon dioxide and ammonia [24].

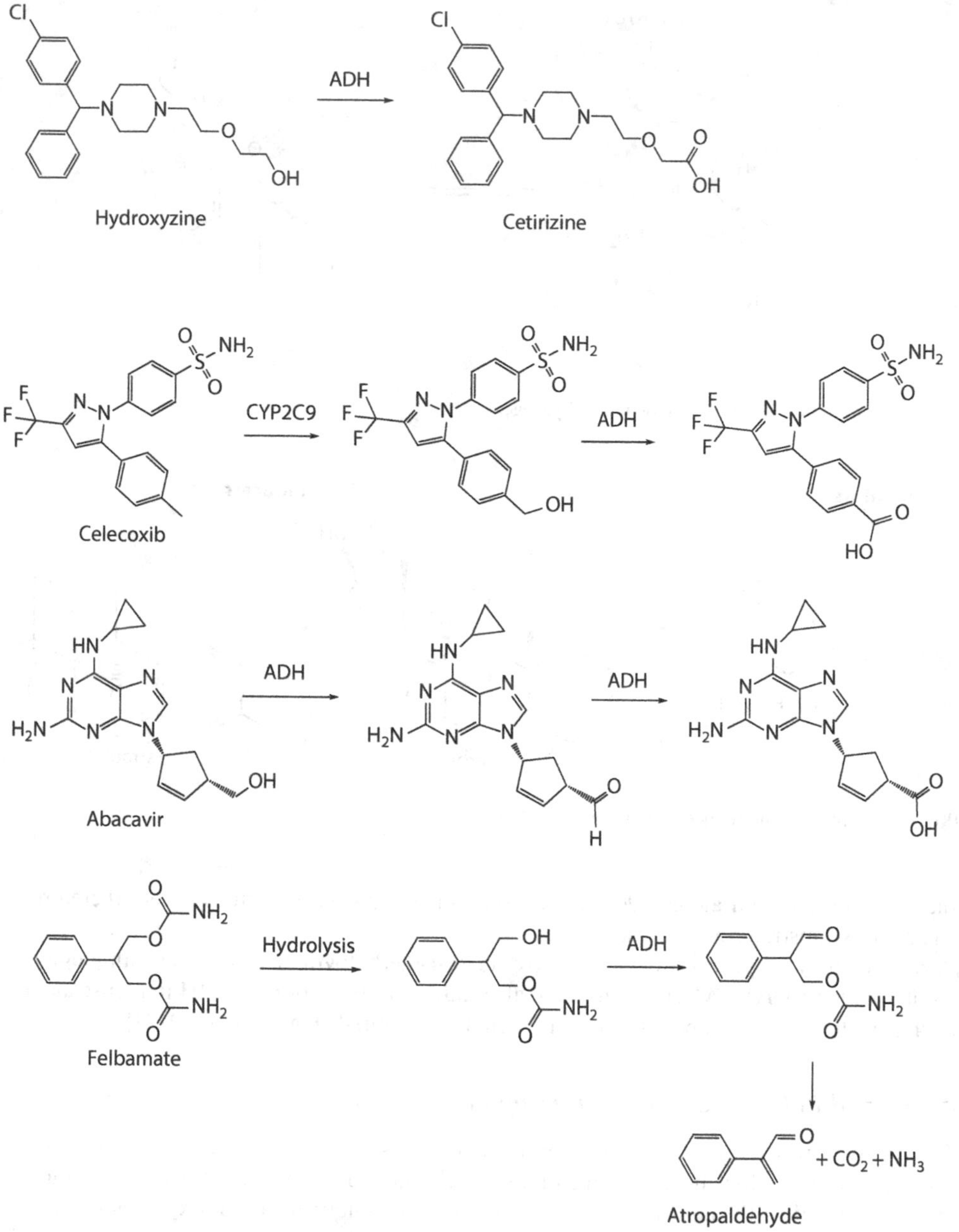

FIGURE 6.8 Metabolic reactions catalyzed by alcohol dehydrogenase (ADH).

Aldehyde Dehydrogenases

Aldehyde dehydrogenases (ALDHs) (EC 1.2.1.3) are a group of enzymes that irreversibly catalyze the oxidation of aldehydes to carboxylic acids.

$$RCHO + NAD^+ + H_2O \rightarrow RCOOH + NADH + H^+$$

Some ALDH enzymes also show esterase activity.

The human genome contains 19 genes that are members of the ALDH superfamily [25], which are classified as class (1) (low K_m, cytosolic), class (2) (low K_m, mitochondrial), and class (3) (high K_m)

based on their kinetic properties and sequence similarities. The ALDH enzymes differ in their primary amino acid sequences and in the quaternary structures. For example, ALDH3 is a dimer of two 85 kDa subunits, whereas ALDH1 and ALDH2 are homo-tetramers of 54 kDa subunits. ALDH enzymes consist of three domains: a substrate-binding (catalytic) domain, a cofactor $(NAD(P)^+)$ binding domain, and a dimerization/tetramerization domain.

Subcellular Location and Organ Distribution

ALDHs are found in all subcellular regions including the cytosol, mitochondria, endoplasmic reticulum, and nucleus. Most ALDHs have a wide tissue distribution, with the highest level in the liver, followed by kidney, uterus, and brain. The name, subcellular location, tissue distribution, and major substrate for each ALDH enzyme are summarized in Table 6.2 [25].

TABLE 6.2

Human ALDH Enzymes and Their Location, Tissue Distribution, and Substrates

ALDH Isoform	Subcellular Location	Tissue Distribution	Major Substrate
ALDH1A1	Cytosol	Testis, brain, eye lens, liver, kidney, lung, and retina	Retinal
ALDH1A2	Cytosol	Intestine, testis, liver, kidney, lung, brain, and retina	Retinal
ALDH1A3	Cytosol	Salivary gland, stomach, breast, kidney, and fetal nasal mucosa	Retinal
ALDH1B1	Mitochondria	Liver, testis, kidney, skeletal, muscle, heart, placenta, brain, and lung	Acetaldehyde
ALDH1L1	Cytosol	Liver, kidney, pancreas, lung, prostate, brain, skeletal muscle, heart, ovary, thymus, and testis	10-Formyltetrahydrofolate
ALDH1L2	Unknown	Spleen and corpus callosum	Unknown
ALDH2	Mitochondria	Liver, kidney, lung, heart, and brain	Acetaldehyde
ALDH3A1	Cytosol, nucleus	Cornea, stomach, esophagus, and lung	Aromatic, aliphatic aldehyde
ALDH3A2	Microsomes, peroxisomes	Liver, kidney, intestine, stomach, skeletal, muscles, skin, lung, pancreas, placenta, heart, and brain	Fatty aldehydes
ALDH3B1	Cytosol	Kidney, liver, lung, and brain	Unknown
ALDH3B2	Unknown	Salivary gland	Unknown
ALDH4A1	Mitochondria	Liver, skeletal muscle and kidney	Glutamate γ-semialdehyde
ALDH5A1	Mitochondria	Liver. kidney, skeletal muscle, and brain	Succinate semialdehyde
ALDH6A1	Mitochondria	Liver, kidney, heart, muscle, and brain	Malonate semialdehyde
ALDH7A1	Cytosol, nucleus, mitochondria	Cochlea, eye, ovary, heart, kidney, liver, spleen, muscle, lung, and brain	α-Aminoadipic semialdehyde
ALDH8A1	Cytosol	liver, kidney, brain, spinal cord, mammary gland, thymus, adrenal, testis, prostate, and gastrointestinal tract	Retinal
ALDH9A1	Cytosol	Liver, skeletal muscle, kidney, and brain	γ-Aminobutyraldehyde
ALDH16A1	Unknown	Bone marrow, heart, kidney, and lung	Unknown
ALDH18A1	Mitochondria	Pancreas, ovary, testis, and kidney	Unknown

Multiplicity and Species Differences

The genetic polymorphism of ALDH2 occurs in about 50% of the Asian population. The alcohol flushing syndrome observed in this population is caused by acetaldehyde accumulation as a result of reduced ALDH2 activity associated with the expression of ALDH2 * 2 in this population. Mutation and genetic deficiencies in other ALDHs impair the metabolism of other aldehydes, which is the underlying cause of certain types of diseases. ALDH4A1 deficiency disturbs proline metabolism, resulting in type II hyperprolinemia. Genetic polymorphism that results in diminished activity of the fatty aldehyde dehydrogenase gene (ALDH3A2) is associated with Sjogren-Larsson syndrome.

Catalytic Mechanism

ALDH enzymes share a number of highly conserved residues necessary for catalysis and cofactor binding. Catalysis occurs in six steps (Figure 6.9) [26]: (i) activation of the catalytic Cys243 (numbering based on the mature human ALDH3 protein) via a water-mediated proton abstraction by Glu333 and consequent nucleophilic attack on the electrophilic aldehyde by the thiolate group of Cys243, (ii) formation of a tetrahedral thiohemiacetal intermediate with concomitant hydride transfer to the pyridine ring of NAD$^+$, (iii) formation of a thioester intermediate, (iv) formation of a second tetrahedral intermediate, (v) formation of the product acid, which may re-protonate the thiolate, and (vi) dissociation of the reduced cofactor and subsequent regeneration of the enzyme by NAD$^+$ binding.

Substrates, Inhibitors, and Inducers

The ALDH enzymes catalyze oxidation reaction of a wide range of endogenous and exogenous aldehyde substrates. Even though ALDHs display distinct substrate specificities [27], they also show an overlapping spectrum of substrates. The ALDH1A subfamily enzymes, comprising ALDH 1A1, 1A2, and 1A3, synthesize retinoic acid from retinal and have a high substrate affinity (K_m in the low μM range).

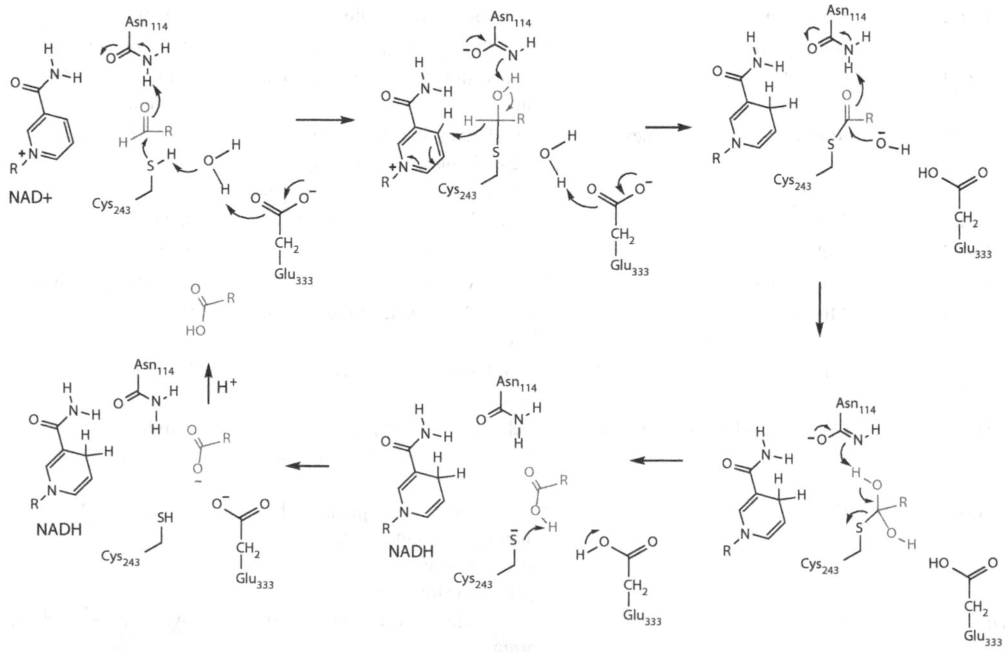

FIGURE 6.9 Proposed mechanism of aldehyde oxidation to carboxylic acid by class 3 aldehyde dehydrogenase (substrate is depicted as OHC-R in center of top left reaction scheme).

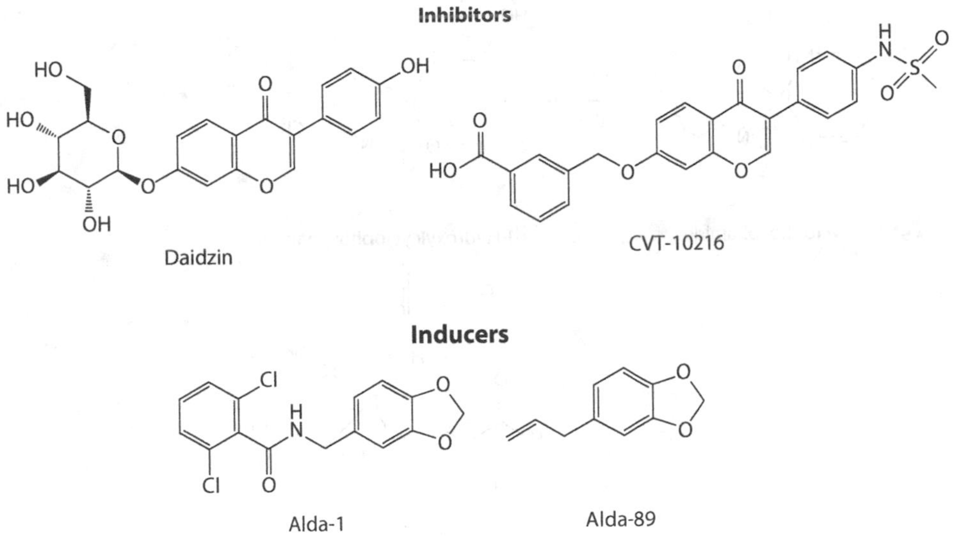

Inhibitors

Daidzin

CVT-10216

Inducers

Alda-1

Alda-89

FIGURE 6.10 Inhibitors and inducers of aldehyde dehydrogenase.

ALDH2 has a high substrate affinity and is predominantly associated with acetaldehyde oxidation in the second step of alcohol metabolism ($K_m < 5$ μM). Major substrates for other ALDH enzymes are listed in Table 6.2.

Pharmacological inhibitors have been developed for only 3 of the 19 ALDH isozymes: ALDH2, ALDH1A1, and ALDH3A1 [28]. Daidzin and its structural analog (CVT-10216, Figure 6.10) are among the very few highly potent inhibitors of the ALDH2 isozyme (IC_{50}, 80 and 29 nM, respectively). Alda-1 and Alda-89 are small-molecule inducers of ALDH. Alda-1 increases acetaldehyde metabolism of ALDH2 by 2-fold with an EC_{50} of about 6 μM. Alda-89 increases acetaldehyde metabolism of ALDH3A1 by 5-fold with an EC_{50} of about 20 μM [29].

Reactions and Relevance to Human Drug Metabolism

ALDHs play a pivotal role in the metabolism of endogenous and exogenous aldehydes. Generally considered to be detoxification enzymes, ALDHs serve to protect cells by eliminating the reactive aldehydes derived from lipid peroxidation by oxidizing them to their respective carboxylic acids. This is evident from several studies in which an ALDH has been shown to protect against aldehyde-induced cytotoxicity.

Cyclophosphamide is an alkylation agent of the nitrogen mustard type used for the treatment of cancers, autoimmune diseases and amyloid light-chain amyloidosis. It is a prodrug that requires activation by CYP to convert it to 4-hydroxycyclophosphamide, which exists in equilibrium with the ring-opened aldophosphamide. Under anaerobic conditions in tumor cells, aldophosphamide undergoes β-elimination to produce acrolein and phosphoramide mustard, the active metabolite that ultimately forms DNA cross-links resulting cell apoptosis. ALDH plays a pivotal role in the detoxification of cyclophosphamide. Aldophosphamide is oxidized to an inactive metabolite, carboxyphosphamide, in target and healthy cells by ALDH1 or tumor-specific ALDH3 (Figure 6.11). On the other hand, elevated levels of ALDH in tumor cells can lead to an acquired resistance to cyclophosphamide.

Peroxidases

Peroxidases (EC 1.11.1.X) are enzymes that catalyze the oxidation of substrates via peroxide. Peroxidases are widely distributed in almost all living organisms in nature. In humans, peroxidases play an important role in the metabolism of a variety of endogenous substances, xenobiotics, and drugs [30]. The major peroxidases in humans include glutathione peroxidase (GPx), catalase (CAT), myeloperoxidase (MPO),

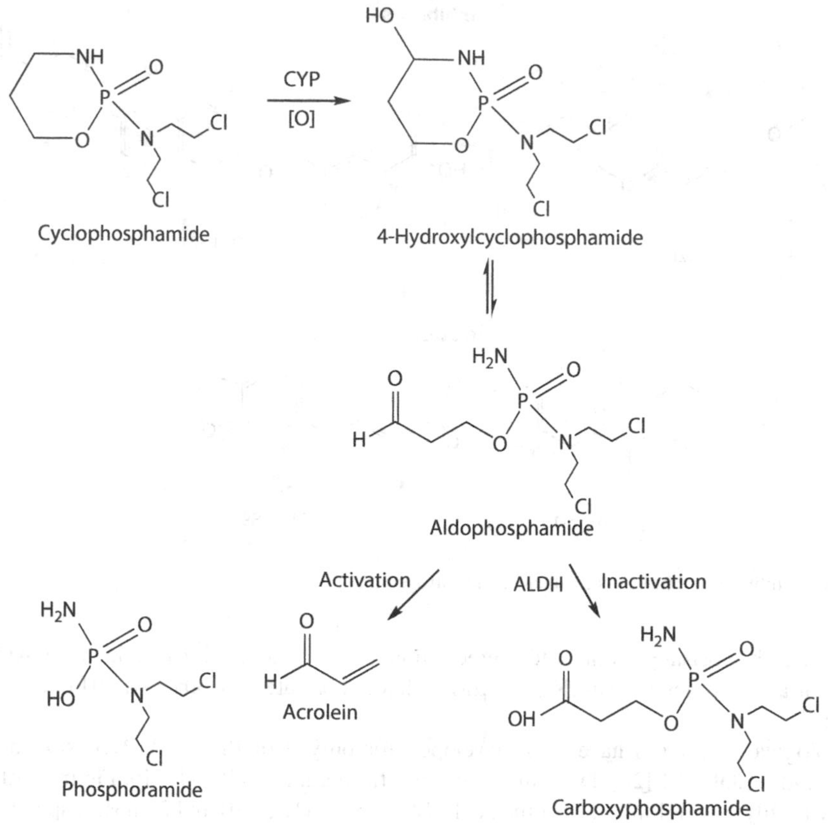

FIGURE 6.11 Activation and inactivation of cyclophosphamide.

eosinophil peroxidase (EPO), lactoperoxidase (LPO), thyroid peroxidase (TPO), and prostaglandin-endoperoxide synthases (PTGSs) [31]. GPx is a family of non-heme peroxidases with an oxidizable selenocysteine residue in the active center, and their function is to eliminate hydrogen peroxide and lipid hydroperoxides from the human body using endogenous glutathione as the electron donor [32]. All the other major peroxidases listed here are heme peroxidases. The information regarding the distribution, subcellular location, molecular weight, gene locus, substrates, and inhibitors of the major human heme peroxidases are summarized in Table 6.3.

Catalytic Mechanism

In most of the human heme peroxidases that are relevant to drug metabolism, the heme Fe(III) is bound to four pyrrole nitrogen atoms of ferriprotoporphyrin IX. The Fe(III) is also coordinated by an axial histidyl imidazole, leaving the other side of heme vacant and available for substrate binding. The catalyzing cycle of peroxidase can be described by the following Equations 6.1 through 6.3:

$$\text{Peroxidase} + \text{ROOH} \rightarrow \text{Compound I} + \text{ROH} \tag{6.1}$$

$$\text{Compound I} + \text{AH}_2 \rightarrow \text{Compound II} + \text{AH}^\bullet \tag{6.2}$$

$$\text{Compound II} + \text{AH}_2 \rightarrow \text{Peroxidase} + \text{AH}^\bullet + \text{H}_2\text{O} \tag{6.3}$$

or

$$\text{Compound II} + \text{AH}^\bullet \rightarrow \text{Peroxidase} + \text{A} + \text{H}_2\text{O} \tag{6.3}$$

TABLE 6.3

The Properties of Human Heme Peroxidases

Name	Distribution	Subcellular Location	MW (kD)	Gene Locus	Substrates	Inhibitors	References
CAT	Universal, particularly in liver	Peroxisomes	240 (tetramer)	11p13	H_2O_2, chlorpromazine, phenylhydrazine, ethylhydrazine	CN^-, azides, hydroxylamines, 3-amino-1,2,4-triazole, mercaptoethanol, vitamin C	[30]
MPO	Neutrophils	Lysosomes	150 (dimer)	17p13	Cl^-, Br^-, I^-, SCN^-, phenylbutazone, dapsone, sulphonamides, procainamide, clozapine, amodiaquine, vesnarinone, 5-aminosalicylic acid, aminopyrine, propylthiouracil, etoposide, carbamazepine, phenytoin, glafenine, ellipticine	4-amino-benzoic acid hydrazide, AZD3241, AZD5904, PF-1355, dapsone, salicylhydroxamic acid, paracetamol, isoniazid, 2-thioxanthines	[31,36]
EPO	Eosinophils	Lysosomes	70	17q22	Cl^-, Br^-, I^-, SCN^-, thiocyanates	Dapsone, melatonin	[31,37]
LPO	Secreted from the secretory cells in the exocrine glands	Extracellular milk, saliva, tears	80	17p13	Cl^-, Br^-, I^-, SCN^-, 3-amino-1,2,4-triazole, indomethacin, tamoxifen, thiocyanates, thiol drugs (e.g., cysteamine, *N*-acetylcysteine, penicillamine, and captopril)	3-amino-1,2,4-triazole, salicylhydroxamic acid, benzohydroxamic acid, ketamine and bupivacaine, propofol, sulphanilimide, melatonin, serotonin, vitamin C, vitamin K3, folic acid	[31,38]
TPO	Secreted from thyroid follicular cells	Extracellular (thyroid follicle)	105	2p25	I^-, 3-amino-1,2,4-triazole, resorcinol, flavonoids, minocycline, anti-thyroid thioamides (e.g., methimazole and propylthiouracil)	3-amino-1,2,4-triazole, resorcinol, flavoncids, minocycline, anti-thyroid thioamides (e.g., methimazole and propylthiouracil)	[31,39]
PTGS-1	Universal	Endoplasmic reticulum	140 (dimer)	9q32	Prostaglandin G_2, etoposide, felodipine, phenytoin, acetaminophen, paracetamol, tamoxifen, ellipticine	Non-steroidal anti-inflammatory drugs (e.g., indomethacin, ibuprofen, aspirin, and piroxicam)	[31,40]
PTGS-2	Inflammatory tissues and cancer cells	Endoplasmic reticulum; nuclear envelope	140 (dimer)	1q25.2		Non-steroidal anti-inflammatory drugs (e.g., indomethacin, ibuprofen, aspirin and piroxicam); selective inhibitors (e.g., clecoxib and rofecoxib)	[31,40]

where Compound I is a highly reactive intermediate comprising Fe(IV) = O coupled with a porphyrin or tyrosyl radical cation in the active center, and compound II is a Fe(IV) = O species following one electron transfer from the substrate [30–31]. Thus, the overall reaction cycle catalyzed by peroxidases can be summarized as:

$$AH_2 + ROOH \rightarrow A + H_2O + ROH \text{ or } 2AH_2 + ROOH \rightarrow 2AH^{\cdot} + H_2O + ROH \tag{6.4}$$

Peroxidases can use peroxide to oxidize electron-rich substrates and generate either stable or reactive metabolites.

Reactions and Relevance to Human Drug Metabolism

Peroxidases can participate in the metabolism of a number of drugs, although in most cases they are not considered to be the major drug metabolizing enzymes. However, the reactive drug metabolites generated by peroxidases can be of interest because they may be involved in the adverse effects and metabolism-induced toxicities of drugs [7]. For example, the use of the antipsychotic agent clozapine in patients is associated with a high incidence of agranulocytosis. Clozapine and its stable metabolites generated by CYPs do not lead to this adverse effect; however, MPO mediates the oxidation of clozapine in activated neutrophils to form a reactive nitrenium ion. This reactive intermediate can irreversibly bind to neutrophils, increasing the level of intracellular oxidative stress and the potential of agranulocytosis (Figure 6.12a) [7,33]. The anti-seizure agent phenytoin can be oxidized by PTGS, TPO, or MPO to produce multiple highly reactive metabolites that covalently bind to proteins and neutrophils, leading to idiosyncratic drug reactions (Figure 6.12b) [7,30]. Sometimes, oxidation by peroxidase helps to convert an inactive prodrug to the active species and, thus, enhances drug efficacy. For example, the antineoplastic agent ellipticine can be oxidized by PTGS or other peroxidases in cancer cells to form a carbon radical that can alkylate DNA, which leads to its anti-tumor activities in animal models (Figure 6.12c) [7,34].

Stable drug metabolites can also be generated from the reactions catalyzed by peroxidases. 1,4-Dihydropyridine calcium channel blockers (e.g., felodipine and nifedipine) are a class of antihypertensive drugs that undergo oxidation by PTGS peroxidase. The peroxidase catalyzes the transformation of the 1,4-dihydropyridine moiety of felodipine to an aromatic pyridine (Figure 6.12d) [7,35].

Aldo-keto Reductases

Aldo-keto reductases (AKRs) are a superfamily of proteins that catalyze the NAD(P)H-dependent reduction of carbonyl-containing compounds to their respective alcohol metabolites [41]. They may also mediate the corresponding reverse oxidative reactions. AKRs are generally monomeric proteins comprised of approximately 320 amino acids and are found in mammals, amphibians, plants, yeast, protozoa, and bacteria.

The general AKR protein structure is an $(\alpha/\beta)_8$ barrel with eight repeated units of alpha helixes and beta sheets, with the beta sheets forming the sides of the barrel that lead to a conserved active site for catalysis [42,43]. The nomenclature system for this superfamily distinguishes between protein isoforms on the basis of unique amino acid sequences. The designation "AKR" identifies the protein as a member of the superfamily; a numeric figure designates family, defined by 40% shared sequence identity; a letter designates subfamily, defined by 60% shared sequence identity; and another numeric figure designates a unique protein sequence. Proteins that share 95% or greater sequence identity must demonstrate distinct functions to be considered unique; otherwise, they are considered to be variant alleles of a single isoform.

Currently, 115 members of the AKR superfamily have been identified and are grouped into 15 families (http://www.med.upenn.edu/akr/). In humans, 13 AKR proteins have been identified, belonging to the AKR1, 6, and 7 subfamilies. The AKR1 proteins are the human homologs of reductases that are expressed across many species and include aldose reductases, aldehyde reductase, hydroxysteroid

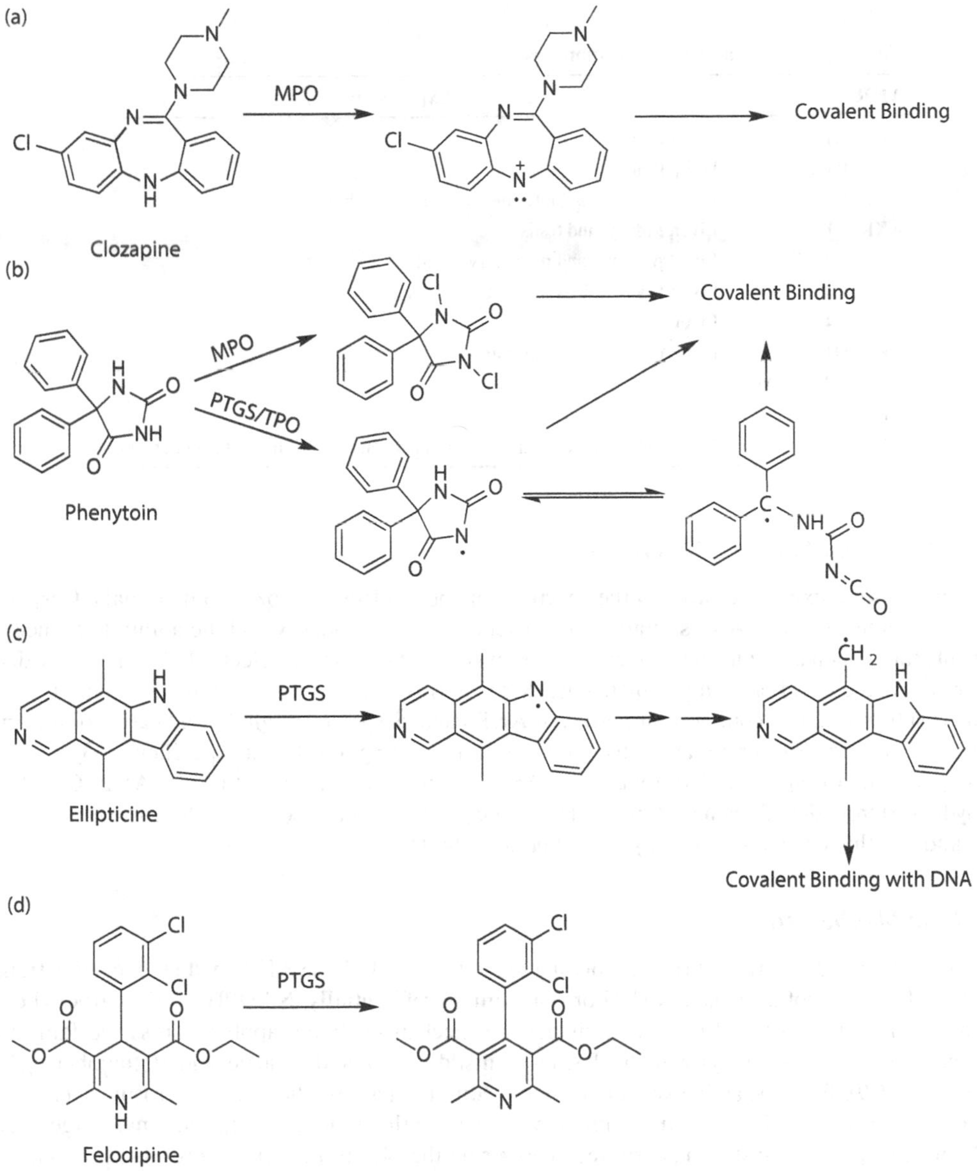

FIGURE 6.12 Metabolic reactions catalyzed by peroxidases. (a) Formation of nitrenium ion of clozapine by myeloperoxidase (MPO). (b) Formation of reactive metabolites of phenytoin by MPO and prostaglandin-endoperoxide synthases (PTGS), and thyroid peroxidase (TPO). (c) Formation of a carbon radical of ellipticine by PTGS. (d) Formation of pyridine by PTGS.

reductases, and steroid 5′-reductase. The AKR6 and AKR7 proteins have vastly different functions and are human homologs of potassium channel subunits and aflatoxin aldehyde reductase, respectively.

Subcellular Location and Organ Distribution

AKRs are widely expressed throughout the human body, and the distributions differ for various isoforms. A summary of the expression patterns of human AKRs is presented in Table 6.4 [44–46].

High expression levels of AKRs have been associated with some cancer cell lines and tumor types, suggesting a possible link to carcinogenesis. In addition, AKRs can have protective (e.g., by reducing acute toxic effects of polycyclic aromatic hydrocarbon metabolites) or procarcinogenic (e.g., by dysregulation of regulators of cell migration or proliferation) roles.

TABLE 6.4

The Expression Patterns of Human AKRs

AKR	Expression
AKR1A1	Ubiquitous
AKR1B1	Ubiquitous
AKR1B10	Liver, colon, small intestine, thymus, and adrenal gland
AKR1C1	Liver, kidney, and testis
AKR1C2	Liver, prostate, and mammary gland
AKR1C3	Liver, brain, kidney, placenta, and testis
AKR1C4	Liver
AKR1D1	Liver, colon, brain, and testis
AKR6A3, A5, A9	Heart and brain
AKR7A2	Ubiquitous
AKR7A3	Liver, kidney, colon, pancreas, stomach, endometrium, and adenocarcinoma

Multiplicity and Species Differences

AKR proteins are expressed through the spectrum of species from protozoa to mammals. Despite vast species differences, many AKRs retain a high level of sequence identity and the ability to reduce common substrates such as 4-nitrobenzaldehyde. However, in other cases, a select AKR can display distinct substrate specificities. For example, different AKR isoforms exhibit a high level of selectivity for steroid or sugar substrates. The common properties of AKRs across species might be indicative of a common multifunctional ancestor protein that diverged over time, leading to substrate specificity [43].

An example of species differences in AKR expression and function is AKR1C2 (human 3α-hydroxysteroid dehydrogenase type 3). The single gene in humans corresponds to five or six genes in mice and rats that encode structurally related proteins [47].

Catalytic Mechanism

In the reduction of carbonyl to its corresponding secondary alcohol, the AKR-mediated reaction transfers a hydride from the cofactor (i.e., NADH or, sometimes preferentially, NADPH) to the carbonyl carbon and a proton to the carbonyl oxygen. This general mechanism likely applies across the family [42]. A tetrad of residues, namely tyrosine-55, lysine-84, histidine-117, and aspartic acid-50 (numbering based on rat AKR1C9), form the active site and is highly conserved across the family. Tyrosine acts as a general acid in 3-ketosteroid reduction and provides the proton that is added to the carbonyl oxygen. Lysine facilitates this proton transfer to substrates by lowering the pKa of the tyrosine residue through proton donation. Both residues are critical to protein function. The histidine and aspartic acid participate in proton donation or removal by the essential tyrosine.

Substrates and Inhibitors

AKRs catalyze reduction reactions of highly diverse endogenous and xenobiotic substrates. These enzymes are involved in the biotransformation of aldehydes resulting from lipid peroxidation, prostaglandins, steroids, neurotransmitters, and sugars, suggesting that AKRs act as regulators of key biological processes. Xenobiotics such as aflatoxin B1, the tobacco product nicotine-derived nitrosamine ketone (NNK), and a wide range of pharmaceuticals (e.g., NSAIDs, anthracyclines, naloxone) are also substrates for AKRs (Figure 6.13).

Chemical inhibition of AKRs has been investigated as a possible therapeutic strategy for cancer treatment, with AKR1B10 and AKR1C3 currently considered plausible targets [48,49]. A challenge in *in vitro* drug metabolism studies has been to identify and validate AKR isoform-selective chemical inhibitors. This is further complicated by the often incomplete inhibition of reductase activities, as

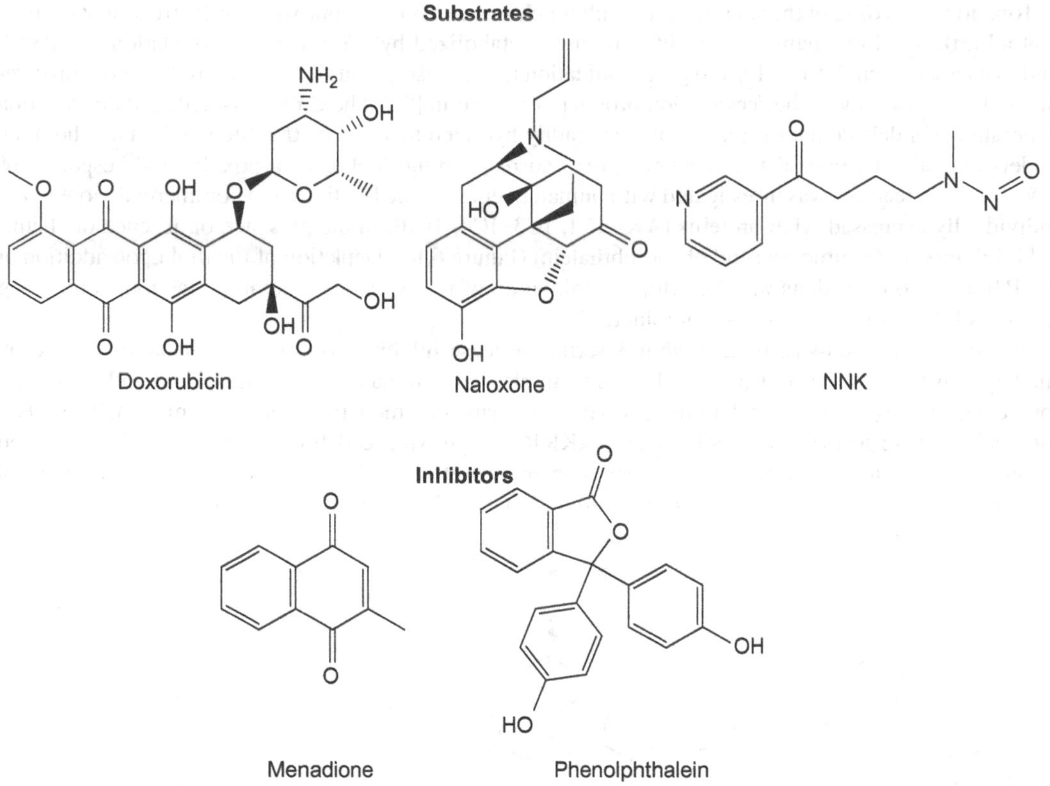

FIGURE 6.13 Substrates and inhibitors of aldo-keto reductases.

well as the overlapping inhibitor sensitivities of closely related enzymes such as alcohol dehydrogenases, short chain dehydrogenases/reductases (i.e., carbonyl reductases (CBRs) and 11β-hydroxysteroid dehydrogenase), and quinone reductases. Chemical inhibitors that have demonstrated some selectivity for AKRs are menadione, ethacrynic acid, mefenamic acid, phenolphthalein, flufenamic acid, and medroxyprogesterone.

Reactions and Relevance to Human Drug Metabolism

Warfarin is a highly effective anticoagulant normally used to prevent the formation of blood clots in blood vessels. It was first approved for use as a medication in 1954 and remains an important medicine; it is the most widely prescribed oral anticoagulant drug in North America. The reduction product, (*SR*)-warfarin alcohol, is the major human metabolite. Since warfarin is administered as a racemic mixture and reduction at the side chain carbonyl group to its corresponding secondary alcohol creates a second stereocenter, four warfarin alcohol enantiomers may be formed. Malatkova et al. characterized the cytosolic enzymes that mediate warfarin reduction in humans [50]. By use of recombinant and purified reductases (AKR1A1, 1B1, 1B10, 1C1, 1C2, 1C3, 1C4, and CBR1 and 3), AKR1C3 showed the greatest reductive activities for warfarin with a V_{max} of 19 nmol/mg protein/min, which was more than 100-fold higher than the next most active reductase, CBR1. The observed affinities (K_m) were 288 and 183 μM for AKR1C3 and CBR1, respectively. AKR1C3 showed stereoselective reduction forming predominantly the (*RS/SR*) warfarin-alcohol(s), whereas CBR1 formed a mixture of (*RS/SR*) and (*RR/SS*)-warfarin alcohols. Assuming comparable expression for AKR1C3 and CBR1, these results indicate that AKR1C3 is the primary reductase that forms the major human warfarin metabolite.

Tofacitinib is a drug of the janus kinase inhibitor class that has been approved for the treatment of rheumatoid arthritis. In humans, tofacitinib is mainly metabolized by CYP-mediated oxidation (CYP3A4, and to a lesser extent CYP2C19) and glucuronidation [51]. Investigations by Le et al. indicate the involvement of AKR to convert the decyanation product of tofacitinib [52]. The CYP3A4-mediated decyanation generated an aldehyde intermediate that was readily hydrated to a diol metabolite (MX). This diol then underwent reductive or oxidative conversion to its corresponding alcohol or carboxylic acid, respectively. The reductive reaction was investigated with human liver cytosolic fractions and commercially obtained, individually expressed AKR proteins (AKR1C1, 1C3, 1C4, 1B10) in the presence or absence of chemical inhibitors (flufenamic acid and phenolphthalein) (Figure 6.14). Depletion of the diol upon addition of AKR1C1 was observed, as was the effective inhibition of the AKR1C1-mediated reaction, confirming the role of AKR in the metabolism of tofactinib.

Boceprevir is a non-structural protein 3 serine protease inhibitor used to treat hepatitis caused by the hepatitis C virus (HCV) genotype 1. In human plasma, two major metabolites, M28 and M31, with molecular masses 2 Da higher than boceprevir were formed by reductive biotransformation. These two metabolites were formed in AKR1C2- and AKR1C3-expressing cell lines, and these AKRs showed stereoselectivity for boceprevir or its diastereomer to preferentially form the corresponding alcohol metabolite (Figure 6.14). The results of this inhibition experiment support the involvement of AKRs in the formation of boceprevir reduction products [53].

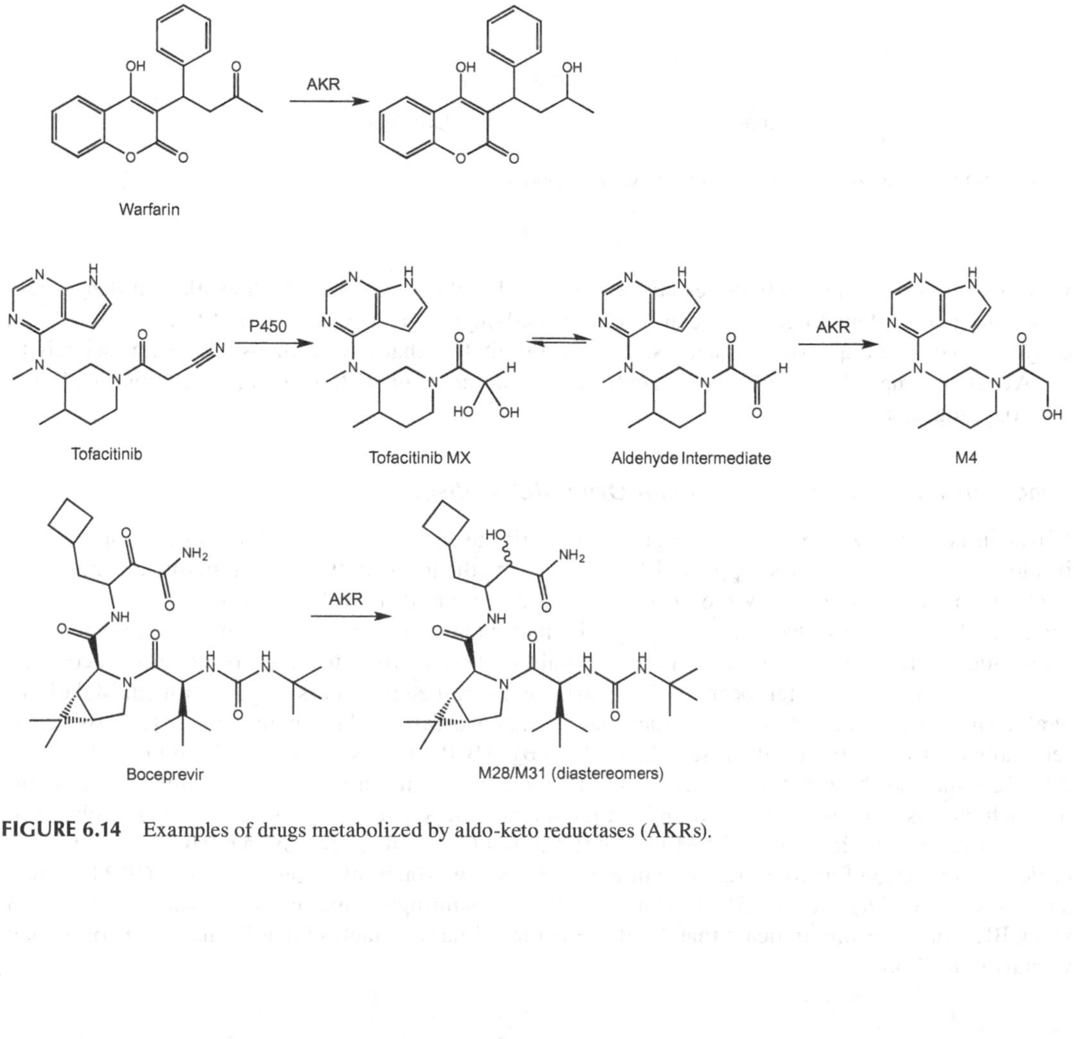

FIGURE 6.14 Examples of drugs metabolized by aldo-keto reductases (AKRs).

Epoxide Hydrolases

Epoxide hydrolases (EC 3.3.2.9) are a ubiquitous and important class of enzymes that play a prominent role in the detoxification of xenobiotics as well as in the control of physiological signaling molecules. Five distinct forms of epoxide hydrolase are present in mammals: cholesterol epoxide hydrolase, hepoxilin hydrolase, leukotriene A4 hydrolase, soluble epoxide hydrolase (sEH), microsomal epoxide hydrolase (mEH). The latter two enzymes, sEH and mEH, are involved in xenobiotic biotransformations.

Epoxide hydrolases are members of the α/β-hydrolase superfamily. The epoxide hydrolase shares the α/β-hydrolase fold domain with a number of other hydrolytic enzymes of widely differing phylogenetic origins and catalytic functions such as esterases, lipases, and hydrolases.

As the name suggests, epoxide hydrolases catalyze the hydrolysis of an epoxide by the addition of H_2O. Simple epoxides are hydrated to their corresponding vicinal dihydrodiols, and arene oxides are converted to a trans-dihydrodiol [54]. Epoxide hydrolases have broad substrate specificity and display a surprisingly high apparent affinity to structurally divergent substrates. While the hydrolysis of these substrates to the corresponding dihydrodiol usually results in termination of chemical reactivity, the dihydrodiol product can be a precursor to reactive metabolites of genotoxic potential. One well known example of this involves the bay region dihydrodiol epoxides of polycyclic aromatic compounds, such as benzo[a]pyrene-7,8-dihydrodiol-9,10-epoxide [55]. Many epoxides are sufficiently reactive as a result of their strained ring structures and can react with electron-rich structures in proteins and nucleic acids, leading to the formation of protein or DNA adducts [56].

Subcellular Location and Organ Distribution

Although levels vary, epoxide hydrolases are present in every tissue, with the highest concentration of mEH and sEH found in the endoplasmic reticulum and cytosol, respectively, of liver. Among the five epoxide hydrolases, mEH and sEH have been extensively characterized because of their potential clinical value and involvement in the metabolism of xenobiotics [57].

Multiplicity and Species Differences

mEH and sEH are present in all mammalian species including mouse, rat, dog, monkey, and humans. Sex and species differences in hepatic epoxide hydrolase activities towards cis- and *trans*-stilbene oxide were studied. Although some similarities in the specificity across different animal strains were observed, overall these seems to be no good laboratory animal model that compares well with humans in terms of the hydrolase activity [58]. The specific activity with *cis*-stilbene oxide as a substrate was highest in the microsomal fraction. The lowest activities were found in mice, while rat and monkey liver microsomes demonstrated several fold higher specific activities [59].

Catalytic Mechanism

The catalytic site of epoxide hydrolase comprises three amino acid residues that form a catalytic triad (Figure 6.15) [60]. In mEH, Asp226 functions as the nucleophile, His431 the base, and Glu404 as the acid. mEH catalyzes the addition of water to epoxides through a general base catalysis. This reaction can be described with the two-carbon cyclic ether substrate oxirane. The catalytic activity is initiated by the attack of the nucleophile Asp226 on the carbon of the oxirane ring leading to the formation of an acyl-enzyme intermediate, with the negative charge developing on the oxygen stabilized by a putative oxyanion hole. The His431 residue activates a water molecule by abstracting a proton, which then attacks the carbon atom of Asp226, resulting in the hydrolysis of the ester bond in the acyl-enzyme intermediate, thus restoring the active enzyme and formation of a vicinal diol [57].

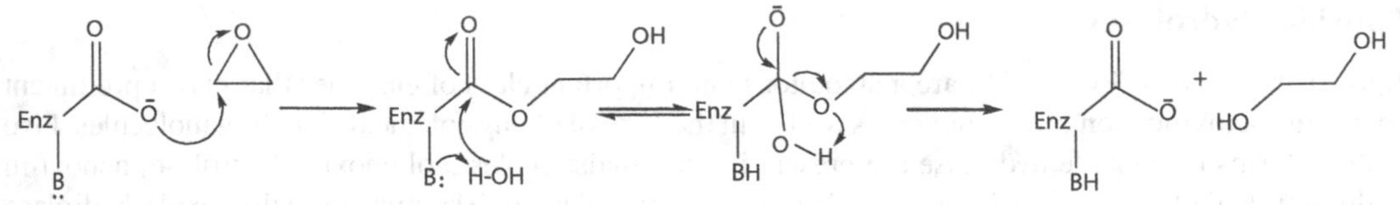

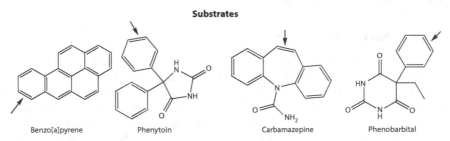

FIGURE 6.15   Catalytic mechanism of epoxide hydrolases.

Substrates and Inhibitors

mEH and sEH can hydrolyze a broad and complementary range of substrates. For example, mEH is the key hepatic enzyme that catalyzes the hydration of numerous xenobiotics such as the epoxides of 1,3-butadiene, styrene, naphthalene, benzo(a)pyrene, phenytoin, and carbamazepine. sEH on the other hand, appears to be selectively involved in the metabolism of arachidonic-acid derived epoxides and other endogenous epoxides [57]. Even though all these enzymes catalyze similar reactions, they are chemically and immunologically distinct. The microsomal and soluble forms of epoxide hydrolase show no evidence of sequence identity and, not surprisingly, are immunochemically distinct proteins [54].

Benzo[a]pyrene is one of most cited substrates eventually leading to cytotoxicity through activation by CYPs and epoxide hydrolases. Polycyclic aromatic hydrocarbons (PAHs), such as benzo[a]pyrene, benz[a] anthracene, chrysene, benzo[c]phenanthrene, 3-methylcholanthrene, and 1-hydroxy-3-methylcholanthrene as well as the aza-polycyclic dibenz[c, h]acridine, are oxidized by CYP enzymes to form epoxides, which are then converted to the corresponding trans dihydrodiol by epoxide hydrolase. The dihydrodiol is subsequently further oxidized to form a bay-region diolepoxide, which leads to toxicity (Figure 6.16). A feature common to all bay-region epoxides is their resistance to hydrolyation by epoxide hydrolase, resulting from steric hindrance from the nearby dihydrodiol group, thus leading to toxicity [61,62].

Substrates

Benzo[a]pyrene   Phenytoin   Carbamazepine   Phenobarbital

Arrows indicate the site of oxidation (epoxide) and subsequent hydrolysis by epoxide hydrolase.

Inhibitors

Benzoxazole derivative   1,1,1-trichloropropene-2,3-oxide

t-AUCB   cyclohexene oxide

FIGURE 6.16   Substrates and inhibitors of epoxide hydrolases.

Recently, Li et al. reported on a novel class of oxetane-containing molecule, AZD1979 [(3-(4-(2-oxa-6-azaspiro[3.3]heptan-6-ylmethyl)phenoxy)-azetidin-1-yl)(5-(4-ethoxyphenyl)-1,3,4-oxadiazol-2-yl) methanone], as a substrate of epoxide hydrolase. The interesting aspect of AZD1979 is that it does need not to be oxidized by CYP to form an epoxide before hydrolase activity can occur, as is the case with phenytoin and carbamazepine [63].

Several epoxide-containing compounds, such as 1,1,1-trichloropropene-2,3-oxide and cyclohexene oxide, are epoxide hydrolase inhibitors, as are some heavy metals such as divalent mercury and zinc (Figure 6.16). Benzoxazole-derived inhibitors with inhibition constants in the low nanomolar range have been identified through virtual and library screening. These agents represent useful *in vitro* tools for assessing the involvement of epoxide hydrolase activity in the characterization of xenobiotic biotransformations [60].

Reactions and Relevance to Human Drug Metabolism

Anticonvulsant drugs, such as phenobarbital, phenytoin, and carbamazepine, are some of the widely cited pharmaceuticals that are epoxide hydrolase substrates [54]. Biotransformation pathways for these drugs typically involve initial phase I metabolism by various CYPs that can then result in the generation of arene oxides, which are substrates for epoxide hydrolase [60]. The resulting epoxides can have teratogenic or tumorigenic properties or be involved in idiosyncratic drug reactions. Studies have shown a protective role for ethyl pyruvate in anticonvulsant hypersensitive syndrome, indicating that patients susceptible to anticonvulsant toxicity had decreased epoxide metabolism activity [64].

Carboxyl Esterases

Carboxyl esterases (CEs) (EC 3.1.1.1) are an important class of glycoprotein enzymes that typically catalyze the hydrolysis of carboxylic acid esters, thioesters, and amides. Ester hydrolysis results in the formation of the corresponding carboxylic acid and alcohol, thiol, or amine, respectively. CEs are involved in the hydrolysis of a wide variety of endogenous and exogenous substrates including various drugs, environmental toxicants, and carcinogens.

$$RCOOR' + H_2O \rightarrow RCOOH + R'\text{-}OH$$

Based on homology of the amino acid sequence, CE isozymes are classified into five families, CES 1, CES 2, CES 3, CES 4, and CES 5, and the majority of CEs that have been identified belong to the CES1 or CES2 family [65]. In humans, carboxylesterases, hCE1 and hCE2, are important mediators of drug metabolism.

Subcellular Location and Organ Distribution

CEs are present in virtually every tissue including liver, intestine, brain, heart, skin, lung, kidney, and also serum, with the highest hydrolase activity found in the liver and small intestine [61,66]. In the human liver, the expression of hCE1 greatly exceeds that of hCE2. In the intestine, only hCE2 is present and is highly expressed. Most of the carboxylesterase activity in liver is associated with the endoplasmic reticulum, although considerable carboxylesterase activity is present in lysosomes and cytosol [61].

Multiplicity and Species Differences

All mammalian species express multiple forms of CE, and the highest CE activity is present in the liver. There are notable differences between human CE and those from other mammalian species. The levels and isoforms of CE in rodents are high compared to humans. Rodents also have abundant serum CE compared to humans, which may contribute to inter species drug metabolism differences. For example, deltamethrin and esfenvalerate are pyrethroid insecticides, the rate of hydrolysis of deltamethrin in human liver microsomes is several fold faster than that in rat, whereas the hydrolysis of esfenvalerate in rat liver microsomes is twice as fast as it is human microsomes [67].

The rate of hydrolysis and the metabolites formed for an experimental oral radionuclide decorporation agent referred to as C2E5 (diethylene triamine pentaacetic acid pentaethyl ester) were remarkably different in S9 fractions and plasma incubations (human, dog, rat). Moderate to no C2E5 hydrolysis were observed in human and dog plasma, while in contrast, C2E5 was rapidly hydrolyzed in rat plasma and yielded a strikingly different metabolic profile [68].

Catalytic Mechanism

Like many hydrolases, CEs are serine hydrolases, which belong to the α,β-hydrolase family. All serine hydrolases possess a catalytic triad (Glu, His, Ser). The three major catalytic steps are substrate binding (reversible), acylation, and deacylation (Figure 6.17). The catalytic mechanism for CEs is the same as that for the serine hydrolase, chymotrypsin. Catalysis starts with a nucleophilic attack by the β-OH group on the Ser of the acyl carbonyl group. The oxyanion hole formed by the hydrogen bonds between the tetrahedral intermediate and the adjacent N-H groups stabilizes the negatively charged oxygen (O-). The ester bond breaks and the leaving alcohol group (R'-O⁻) picks up a proton from the imidazolium ion of His and diffuses away, completing the acylation stage of the hydrolytic reaction. The acyl portion of the original ester bond remains bound to the enzyme as an acyl-enzyme intermediate. A water molecule attacks the acyl-enzyme intermediate to give a second tetrahedral intermediate, which is stabilized by hydrogen bonds between His and Glu. His acts as a base and donates the proton to the oxygen atom of Ser, releasing the acid component of the substrate (R-COOH). The final deacylation step is essentially the reverse of the acylation step, with a water molecule substituting for the alcohol group of the original substrate [65,66].

Substrates and Inhibitors

CEs are phase I drug metabolizing enzymes that can hydrolyze a variety drugs, such as angiotensin-converting enzyme inhibitors (temocapril, enalapril, quinapril, and imidapril), anti-tumor drugs (irinotecan and capecitabin), narcotics (cocaine, heroin and meperidine), and antiplatelet agents (aspirin, clopidogrel and prasugrel) (Figure 6.18) [65].

Specific inhibitors that can inhibit hCE1 and hCE2 have been developed. Recent reports indicate that 27-hydroxycholesterol and digitonin can act as specific inhibitors of hCE1 activity in mammalian cells, whereas bisbenzene sulfonamides and loperamide, an anti-diarrheal, are specific inhibitors of hCE2 with inhibition constants in the low nanomolar to micromolar range [69,70].

Reactions and Relevance to Human Drug Metabolism

CEs are important determinants of the pharmacokinetic and pharmacodynamic behavior of drugs and prodrugs that contain an ester [65]. The most common drug substrates of these enzymes are ester prodrugs specifically designed to enhance oral bioavailability by hydrolysis to the active carboxylic acid after absorption from the gastrointestinal tract. The hydrolysis products of CEs can be active or inactive metabolites. For example, prasugrel, a prodrug, has no antiplatelet activity and must be hydrolyzed by CE to the thiolactone, an inactive intermediate metabolite that is subsequently oxidized to the active

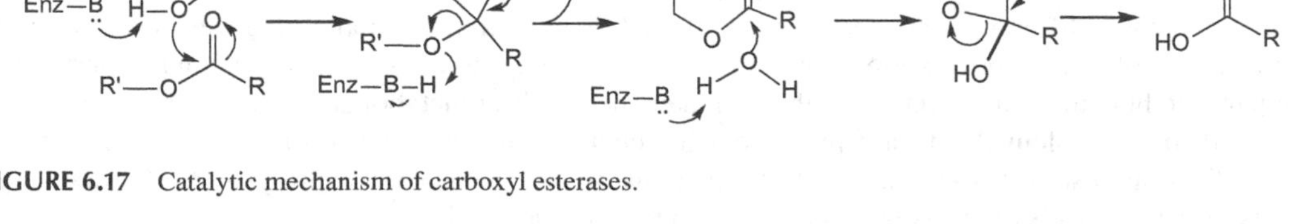

FIGURE 6.17   Catalytic mechanism of carboxyl esterases.

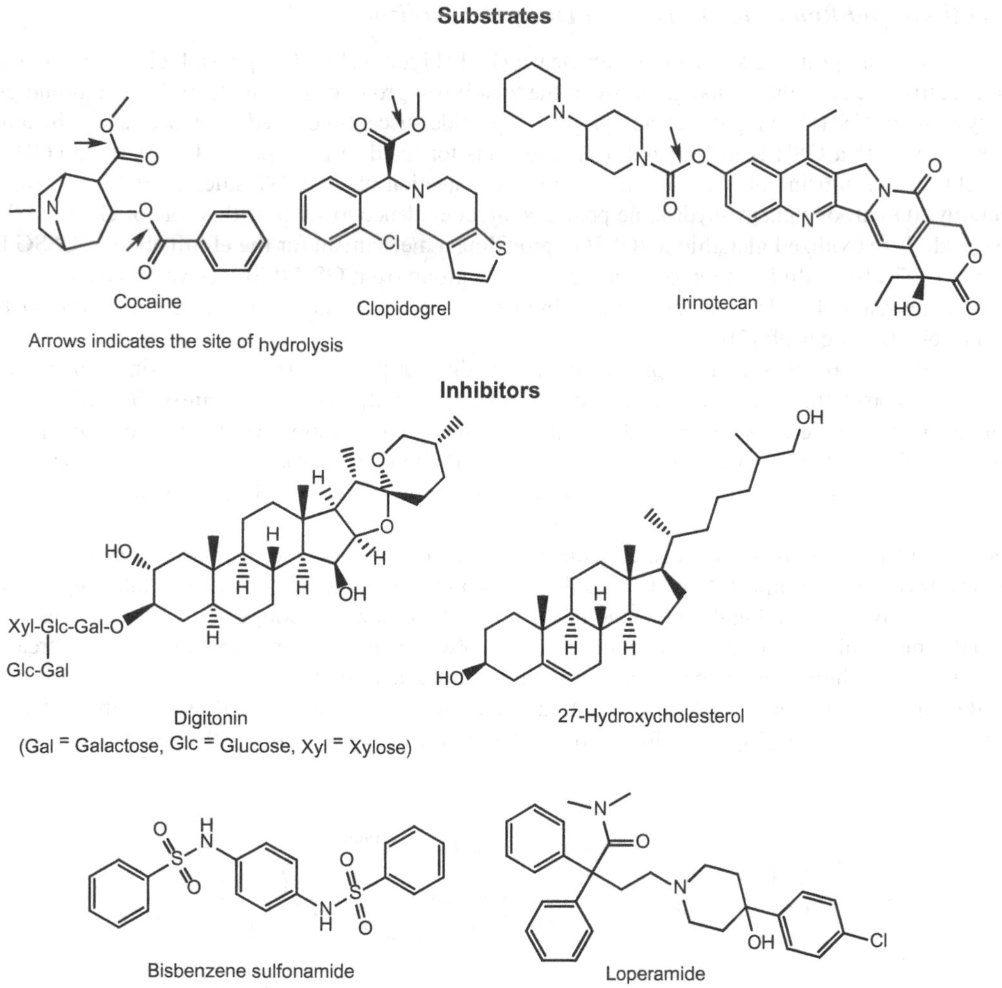

Substrates

Cocaine

Clopidogrel

Irinotecan

Arrows indicates the site of hydrolysis

Inhibitors

Digitonin
(Gal = Galactose, Glc = Glucose, Xyl = Xylose)

27-Hydroxycholesterol

Bisbenzene sulfonamide

Loperamide

FIGURE 6.18 Substrates and inhibitors of carboxyl esterases.

form [61]. Irinotecan, an anti-cancer pro drug, which is carbamate is also a substrate of CEs. Irinotecan hydrolysis results in the formation of the active metabolite, 7-ethyl-10-hydroxy camptothecin (SN-38) [61]. Cocaine, an opiate analgesic is also a substrate of CEs. It has two carboxylic ester bonds and both are hydrolyzed by CEs to inactive metabolites; hCE1 catalyzes the hydrolysis of the methyl ester to produce benzoylecgonine, whereas hCE2 catalyzes the hydrolysis of the benzoyl ester to produce ecgonine methyl ester [61].

γ-Glutamyl transpeptidase

γ-Glutamyl transpeptidase (GGT) (EC 2.3.2.2) is a membrane-bound glycoprotein consisting of two subunits of 51 and 22 kDa. This enzyme is present mainly on the luminal surface of the proximal tubules in the kidney as well as in bile ducts of the liver. Its main function is to hydrolyze glutathione (GSH). GGT-mediated hydrolysis of extracellular GSH (urine or serum) is essential for intracellular synthesis of GSH through re-absorption of its constituent amino acids (cysteine, aspartic, and glycine) especially in rapidly dividing cells.

Reactions and Relevance to Human Drug Metabolism

GGT is the only protease known that can cleave GSH (Figure 6.19). The physiological role of GGT is specifically to cleave the γ-linkage between the γ-carboxyl group of glutamate and the α-amino group of cysteine in GSH, leaving the cysteinyl-glycine peptide susceptible to additional cleavage by amino-peptidases so that GSH is hydrolyzed to amino acids for renal re-absorption. The elevated GSH level (by 3000-fold) in urine of mice within 1 hour after injection of the GGT suicide inhibitor L-gamma-glutamyl-(O-carboxy)phenyl-hydrazine provides direct evidence to support this role of GSH. GGT can also hydrolyze oxidized glutathione (GSSG), providing a mechanism for the elimination of GSSG from serum. GGT also hydrolyzes removal of the glutamyl group from GSH thiol-derivatives as the first step in the conversion of GSH conjugates of xenobiotics to mercapturic acids that are eliminated in urine as well as bile (Figure 6.19) [71].

Platinum compounds such as cisplatin (cis-diaminodichloroplatinum) and oxaliplatin are nephrotoxic. The dose of cisplatin is limited by its nephrotoxicity *in vivo* [72] and the mechanism by which cisplatin kills proximal tubule cells has been the subject of intense investigation for many years. One proposal involves GGT-mediated bioactivation of a cisplatin-GSH complex to produce more toxic species to damage the proximal tubule cells [73]. In this mechanism, highly expressed GGT at the luminal surface of proximal tubule cells hydrolyze the extracellular cisplatin-GSH complex in glomerular filtrate to produce a cisplatin-cysteinyl-glycine intermediate that is further hydrolyzed by another cell surface membrane enzyme amino-dipeptidase. The resulting cysteine-cisplatin conjugate is then taken up by tubule cells and converted to a highly toxic and reactive thiol by cysteine S-conjugate β-lyases. In agreement with this mechanism, no cisplatin nephrotoxicity was observed in GGT knockout mice and pre-treatment with the GGT inhibitor acivicin reduced cisplatin nephrotoxicity in mice.

GGT plays an important role in mediating nephrotoxicity of efavirenz (Sustiva), an HIV reverse transcriptase inhibitor [74]. The formation and subsequent processing of the GSH conjugate of a

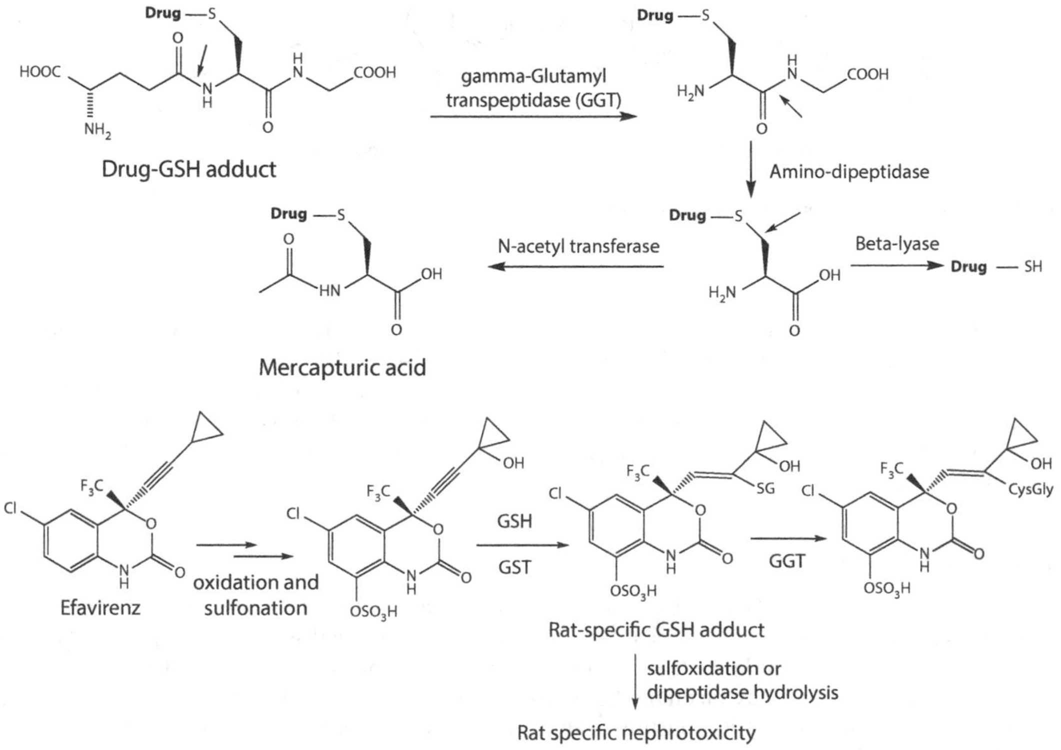

FIGURE 6.19 Metabolic reactions catalyzed by γ-glutamyl transpeptidase (GGT).

sulfate metabolite was postulated to be responsible for the species-specific renal toxicity in rats [75] (Figure 6.19). Elegant metabolism studies were conducted to show that a significant amount of the GSH conjugate was found in urine of rats and mice but not in that of monkey or humans, showing that rat-specific GSH S-transferase (GST) is responsible for formation of the metabolite. Interestingly, a cysteinylglycine conjugate that is also a GSH-related metabolite was found in rat urine and was formed by GGT in the kidneys of rats.

Cathepsins

Lysosomes are membrane-bound organelles that represent the main degradative compartment in animal cells and contain many types of cathepsin enzymes [76]. The human cathepsin family contains mainly cysteine proteases of cathepsins B, C, F, H, K, L, O, S, V, W, and X, the structure of which are similar to that of papain. For cysteine proteases, the conservative active site cleft of Cys25 and His163 are located at the interface opens of L-domain containing 3 alpha-helices and R-domain containing a beta-barrel that is enclosed by an alpha-helix. Cathepsins D and E are aspartic proteases and cathepsins A and G are serine proteases [77]. Cathepsins B and H are exopeptidases and endopeptidases. Cathepsins D, E, F, G, K, L, S, and V are endopeptidases, and Cathepsins A, C, and X are exopeptidases. All cathepsins are synthesized as inactive enzymes that are processed to active enzymes in lysosomes by protease enzymes [78]. The cathepsins activities are often tightly regulated by endogenous protein inhibitors, such as cystatins, stefins, thyropins, and serpins, which tightly bind to the target enzymes to prevent their activation. Cathepsins require a reducing and acidic environment such as lysosomes for optimal catalysis involved in a normal cellular protein degradation and turnover.

Cathepsin B (EC 3.4.22.1) is composed of a dimer of disulfide-linked heavy and light chains (~30 kDa) and belongs to the superfamily of papain-like cysteine proteases. Under certain pathological conditions, cathepsin B can be translocated to the peripheral cytoplasm and plasma membrane or excreted from cells. Access of the substrate to the active site of cathepsin B is controlled by an 18-residue-long insertion (Pro 107Asp 124, the occluding loop). In the lysosomes, cathepsin B is involved in the turnover of proteins and has various roles in maintaining the normal metabolism of cells. In addition, cathepsin B has a high expression in many human tumors and is involved in the immune response [79].

Cathepsin D (EC 3.4.23.5 is a soluble lysosomal aspartic endopeptidase. Aspartic proteases form of a group of enzymes that consist of two lobes separated by a cleft containing the active site of two aspartate residues. Similar to other aspartic proteases, such as pepsin, renin, cathepsin E, chymosin, and HIV protease, Cathepsin D can fit up to eight amino acid residues in the active site. Cathepsins also play important roles in the physiological processes of apoptosis. Cathepsin D is a key enzyme in neutrophil apoptosis by directly activating the initiator caspase-8.

Reactions and Relevance to Human Drug Metabolism

Figure 6.20 shows examples in which cathepsin B was used in prodrug designs. Satsangi et al. described an approach to conjugate paclitaxel to a hydrophilic macromolecular dendrimer through a cathepsin B cleavable tetrapeptide Gly-Phe-Leu-Gly [80]. The paclitaxel prodrug showed a higher cytotoxicity specific to cell lines with moderate to high expression than those with low expression of cathepsin B. The conjugate also showed a higher tumor reduction than paclitaxel in xenograft models. Shao et al. also used a novel prodrug, acetyl-Phe-lys-PABC-doxorubicin, to demonstrate the utility of cathepsin B cleavable linker [81]. This prodrug showed lower dose-dependent inhibitory effect on growth of gastric cancer cell line SGC-7901. Linking cytotoxic drugs to large molecule carriers is a strategy to deliver drugs to tumors [82]. The conjugation changed pharmacokinetic properties of cytotoxic drugs. Antibody drug conjugates (ADCs) consist of targeting moiety, a linker, and a cytotoxic drug. After internalization of the antigen-receptor complex, cytotoxic drugs such as calicheamycin, maytansine, duocarmycin, auristatin, or irinotecan are released intracellularly after linker cleavage. Brentuximab vedotin is an ADC that was approved to treat refractory Hodgkin's lymphoma and anaplastic large cell lymphoma. This ADC used an anti-CD30 IgG1 antibody linked to MMAE via a cathepsin B-cleavable val-cit-PAB linker [83].

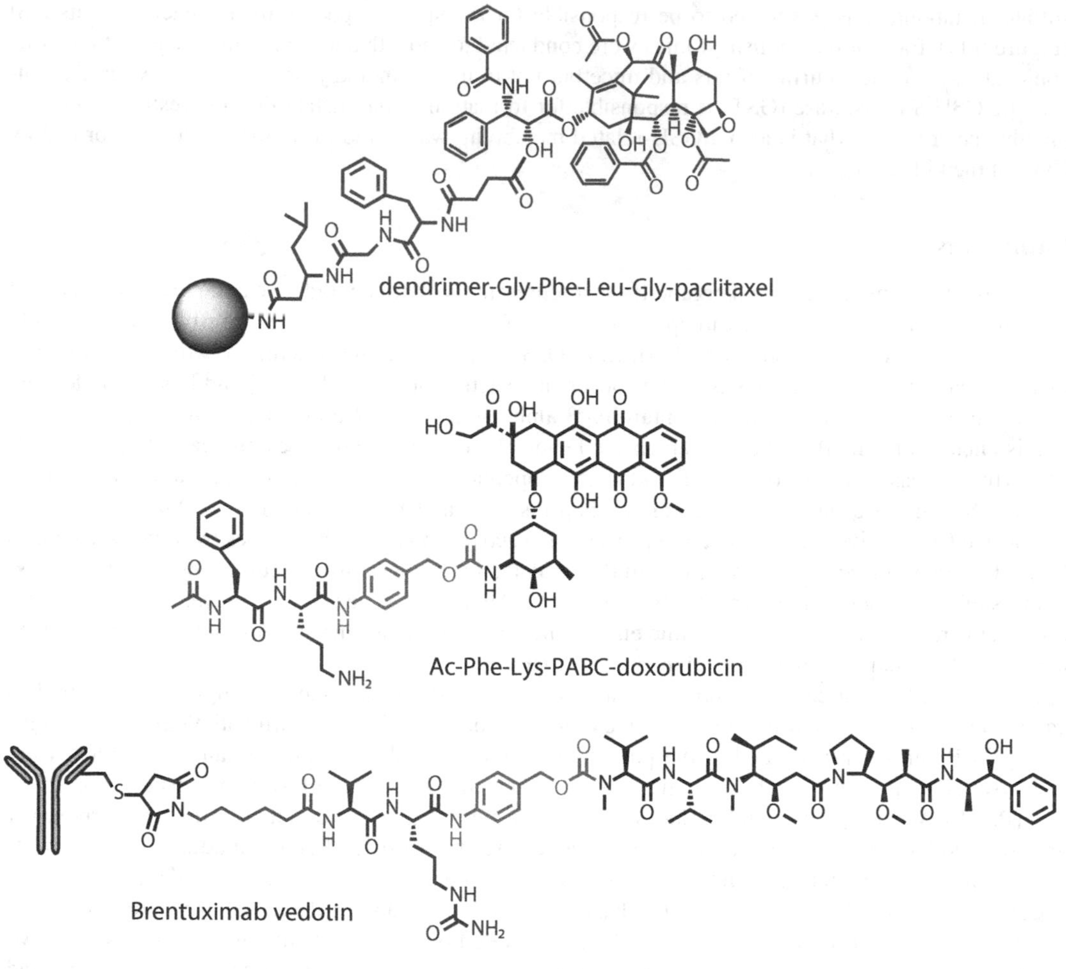

dendrimer-Gly-Phe-Leu-Gly-paclitaxel

Ac-Phe-Lys-PABC-doxorubicin

Brentuximab vedotin

FIGURE 6.20   Metabolic reactions catalyzed by cathepsin B.

Glutathione *S*-transferases

Glutathione *S*-transferases (GSTs) (EC 2.5.1.18) are a family of enzymes that are an integral part of defense mechanism protecting against electrophilic chemicals and oxidative stresses. The GST family consists of three subfamilies: cytosolic, mitochondrial, and microsomal (also known as MAPEG proteins), the former two are cytosolic proteins. Based on sequence similarity, cytosolic GSTs in mammals are grouped into subclasses: alpha, mu, pi, sigma, theta, omega, and zeta (Table 6.5). The cytosolic GST enzymes within a class typically have >40% sequence identity and those between classes share <25% identity [84].

Subcellular Location and Organ Distribution

In animals and humans, GSTs are extremely ubiquitous and constitute up to 10% of the total soluble protein. Hepatocytes contain high levels of alpha GST, and serum alpha GST has been used as an indicator of hepatocyte injury. Human renal proximal tubular cells contain high concentrations of alpha GST but distal tubular cells contain pi GST.

TABLE 6.5

Classification of Human Glutathione Transferases

	Class	Isoenzymes	Characteristic Reactions
Cytosolic GST	Alpha	GSTA1-1, A2-2, A3-3, A4-4, A5-5	A3-3: steroid isomerase, A4-4: HNE conjugation
	Mu	GSTM1-1, M2-2, M3-3, M4-4, M5-5	M1-1: aflatoxin B1-epoxide, CDNB conjugation
	Pi	GSTP1-1	Tetrahydro-benzo[a]pyrene, EA conjugation
	Theta	GSTT1-1, T2-2	T2-2: sulfatase
	Zeta	GSTZ1-1	Maleyacetoacetate isomerase
	Omega	GSTO1-1, O2-2	Dehydroascorbate reductase
	Sigma	GSTS1-1	Prostaglandin D synthase
Mitochondria GST	Kappa	GSTK1-1	Halide conjugation, perioxide reduction
Microosmal GST (MAPEG)		MGST1, MGST2, MGST3	CDNB, leukotriene C4 synthase

Catalytic Mechanism

The tertiary structures are highly conserved across all cytosolic GSTs. Mammalian cytosolic GSTs are dimeric with monomer of approximately 25 kDa in size. The dimer has a twofold axis with an extensive interface [85]. The N-terminal α/β-domains (G domain) contains GSH binding site. The GSH is bound in an extended confirmation by extensive hydrogen binding interactions that lower the thiol pKa from 9 to 7 by stabilizing the thiolate (GS$^-$) through hydrogen binding with an active amino acid: a tyrosine (alpha-, mu-, pi-, and sigma- classes), a serine (theta- and zeta-classes) and a cysteine (omega-class) for stronger nucleophilic activity. The α-helical domain (H domain) forms the binding pocket for hydrophobic substrates, which shows highly promiscuous substrate selectivity with catalytic activity for many structurally diverse chemicals. GSTs can also bind to non-substrate ligands such as bilirubin and steroids at the dimer interfaces, which could lead to inhibition of the enzymes.

Substrates and Inhibitors

GSTs catalyze conjugation of nonpolar xenobiotic and endogenous compounds containing electrophilic carbon, nitrogen, or sulfur atoms to glutathione (GSH) for detoxification. GSTs also involve many important biological processes such as prostaglandin and steroid biosynthesis, amino acid catabolism, and cell apoptosis [86].

GSTP1-1 is overexpressed in many cancers and appears to regulate JNK kinase pathways to block apoptosis and is a potential drug target. NBDHEX, a potent and specific GSTP1-1 inhibitor (IC50 ~ 0.8 μM), has demonstrated anti-proliferative activity in several cancer cell lines. Nocodazole is a novel GSTS1-1 inhibitor, which may be used as an anti-allergic or anti-inflammatory agent (Figure 6.21).

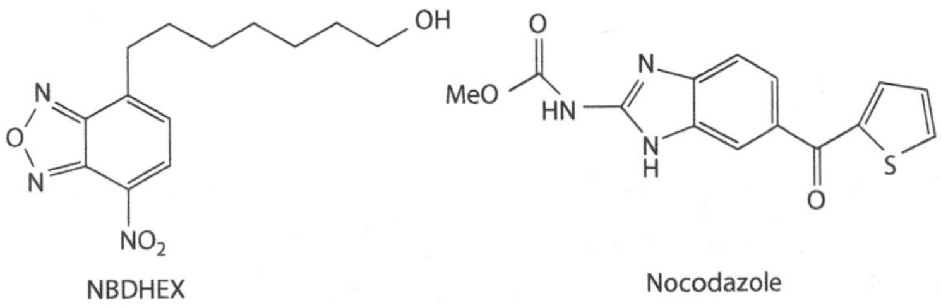

NBDHEX   Nocodazole

FIGURE 6.21 Inhibitors of glutathione *S*-transferases.

Reactions and Relevance to Human Drug Metabolism

GSTs catalyze diverse types of reactions (Figure 6.22) [86]. All GSTs catalyze the glutathione replacement reaction of 1-chloro-2,4-dinitrobenze (CDNB) (Figure 6.22a). GSTA4-4 catalyzes conjugation of 4-hydrononenal (HNE), a major lipid breakdown product that can modify proteins and DNA (Figure 6.22b). GSTZ1-1 is known as maleyacetoacetate isomerase, which is involved in the first step in the catabolism of phenylalanine and tyrosine metabolism (Figure 6.22c). In this catalysis, a Michael addition reaction turns a cis-double carbon-carbon bond to a single bond for rotation followed by a reversible Michael reaction to produce a trans-double bond isomer. GST3-3 is the most efficient enzyme to catalyze double-bound isomerization of Δ^5-androstene-3,17-dione to Δ^4-androstene-3,17-dione (Figure 6.22d). In this catalysis, a thiolate as an acid-base catalyst extracts a proton from C4 and inserts a proton to C6 in the steroid to form a double-bond positional isomer. GSTS1-1 catalyzes the conversation (prostaglandin D synthase) of prostaglandin H2 (PGH2) to prostaglandin D2 (PD2), a mediator of allergy and inflammation responses (Figure 6.22e). GSTs catalyze formation of ascorbic acid and detoxification of peroxide (Figure 6.22f and g). For reduction of dehydroascorbate acid, a proposed mechanism involves anionic

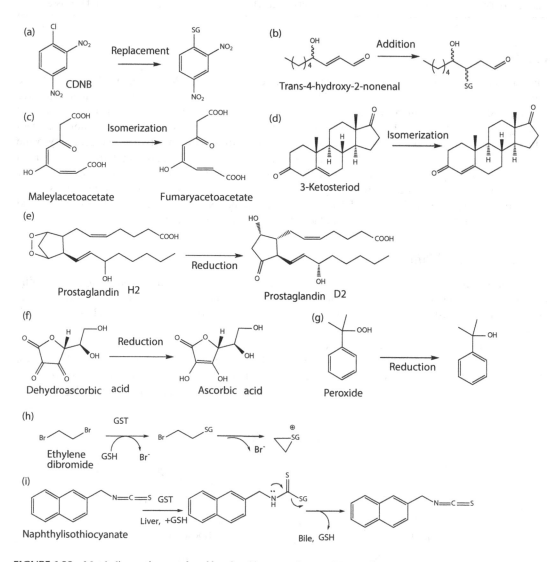

FIGURE 6.22 Metabolic reactions catalyzed by glutathione transferases (GSTs). This includes (a) replacement, (b) addition, (c) & (d) isomerization, and (e), (f), (g) reduction. (h) and (i) Examples of GSH addition facilitated by GST.

form of Cys 32 in the active site donates an electron to the C4 carbonyl, which abstracts a hydrogen from GSH to form ascorbic acid. GSTT2-2 also catalyzes sulfatase activity of benzylsulfate. GSTM1-1 detoxify aflatoxin B1-epoxide and benzo[a]pyrene diol epoxides.

GSH conjugation of xenobiotic compounds in general leads to formation of more water soluble products for detoxification and excretion. However, GSH conjugates can be more reactive or toxic than the parent compound (bioactivation) [87]. Ethylene dibromide is carcinogenic in animals. GST catalyzes the replacement of a bromide with glutathionyl to form a sulfur mustard analog that spontaneously cyclizes to form a highly reactive episulfonium ion (Figure 6.22h). Isocyanates, isothiocyanates, and α-β unsaturated ketones or aldehydes can form GSH conjugates; however, these GSH conjugates can release the substrates (the reactive species) that were originally detoxified. These GSH conjugates, therefore, serve as transporting agents [88–91]. α-Naphthylisothiocyanate (ANIT) is a classic example of isothiocyanate that induces intrahepatic cholestasis in rats by injury to biliary epithelial cells. This toxicity is believed to involve a thiocabamoyl-GSH conjugate of ANIT [92]. The reversible process of GSH adduct formation, Mrp-2-mediated transport to the bile duct, followed by degradation back to ANIT resulted in high concentrations of the toxic compound in the biliary ducts (Figure 6.22i). When ANIT was administered to Wistar and Mrp2-deficient TR(-) rats, the TR(-) rats were protected from ANIT induced cholestasis. These data show that Mrp2-mediated biliary secretion of GSH conjugate of ANIT is a prerequisite for development of cholestasis in rats [93].

Sulfotransferases

Sulfonation is the process of forming typically highly water-soluble sulfuric acid esters from phenols and aliphatic alcohols. In many cases, the hydroxyl group that is conjugated in this reaction has been revealed or introduced during a primary oxidative or hydrolytic reaction of a xenobiotic. Thus, sulfonation occurs as a second step, or phase II biotransformation, and is synonymous with the conjugation reaction of glucuronic acid with substrates by UDP-glucuronysyltransferases (UGT). Conjugation through an amine (*N*-sulfoconjugation) has been observed, but is infrequent compared to *O*-sulfoconjugation.

Sulfonation reaction is catalyzed by a large number of enzymes identified as sulfotransferases (SULT). Athough "SULT" is the internationally agreed upon abbreviation for the enzymes, the alternate abbreviation "ST" remains in use in some publications.

The nomenclature system of SULTs is based on amino acid homology.

Thirteen human genes code for the cytosolic SULT1, SULT2, SULT4, and SULT6 families. Each gene does not result in a single protein. For example, SULT1A3 and SULT1A4 encode for the identical protein SULT1A3/4, and the SULT2B1 gene encodes two functionally distinct proteins SULT2B1a and SULT2B1b.

Subcellular Location and Organ Distribution

Two types of SULTs exist and are differentiated based on their subcellular location: membrane bound and cytosolic. Membrane-bound SULTs at the Golgi apparatus of the cell are responsible for the sulfonation of peptides (e.g., CCK), proteins, lipids, and glycosaminoglycans. Due to their limited role in xenobiotic metabolism, membrane-bound SULTs will not be discussed in this chapter. Cytosolic SULTs are responsible for the sulfonation of xenobiotics and are of interest to the drug metabolism scientist. For example, the sulfonation of morphine may have important effects on its pharmacological efficacy. The cytosolic SULTs also use small endogenous substrates such as steroids, bile acids, and neurotransmitters, and, thereby, may act as important regulators of their actions at their respective transmitters.

The expression of the five major human SULTs involved in xenobiotic metabolism (SULT1A1, 1A3, 1B1, 1E1, and 2A1) were measured in various tissues from individual donors by immunoblotting [94]. SULT content was highest in small intestine (1.9–15.9 µg per mg cytosolic protein), then liver (2.3–7.9 µg/mg protein), and was much lower in kidney and lung (0.1–0.7 µg/mg protein). This indicates the potential role of presystemic sulfonation at both the gut and liver for orally administered drugs. In the small intestine, SULT1A3 and 1B1 were the most highly expressed isoforms; whereas, in the liver, SULT1A1 (approximately half of total SULT content of liver) and 2A1 were highly expressed. Interindividual variability in expression of SULTs exist, though no clear distinctions have been made based on sex or age of the donor.

Multiplicity and Species Differences

The expression pattern for SULTs in rats is unique in several ways. Rodents express multiple SULT2A transcripts [95]; whereas, humans have only SULT2A1. In contrast to the largely extrahepatic (i.e., small intestine) expression of SULTs in humans, expression is largely hepatic in rodents. Rats also show complex developmental and sex-related expression differences. SULT1 and 2 concentrations in juvenile rats are comparable, but adult male rats have significantly higher SULT1 activities, and adult females have higher SULT2 activities. Another example is SULT1E1, which is highly expressed in male rat liver; whereas, it is absent in female rat liver.

Catalytic Mechanism

SULTs mediate a sulfuryl transfer reaction that uses the co-substrate 3′-phosphoadenosine 5′-phosphsulfate (PAPS) (Figure 6.23). PAPS is generated through the reaction of inorganic sulfate and ATP by PAPS synthetases. The binding of PAPS by SULT may be a complex regulator for cofactor or substrate occupying the active site, and thereby may be a determinant of enzyme function [96].

Detailed kinetics studies by the Leyh group provide insight into the mechanistic function of SULTs [96–98]. Their work indicates that a rapid equilibrium random mechanism takes place; substrate binding is controlled by formation of a "gate" at the opening of the active site upon binding of the nucleotide, and substrate inhibition results from formation of an enzyme-PAP-substrate dead-end complex. The reader is directed to the references herein for detailed descriptions of the current understanding of the role of SULTs in sulfonation reactions.

Substrates and Inhibitors

The sulfonation of 17α-ethinylestradiol (EE2) in humans is readily catalyzed by cytosol in Sf9 cells that overexpress SULT1E1 at low nanomolar concentrations (K_m 6.7 nM). 2,6-Dichloro-p-nitrophenol (DCNP) and quercetin are effective *in vitro* inhibitors (IC_{50} 15.6 and 0.4 µM, respectively) of this reaction [99].

EE2 is also a potent inhibitor of SULT1A1. Tested in a single enzyme system with E. coli that express SULT1A1 in the presence of a relatively high PAPS concentration (10 µM), the sulfonation of 17β-estradiol, p-nitrophenol, and β-naphthol were inhibited, with measured K_i values of 15, 10, and 19 nM, respectively [100]. Interestingly, EE2 is not a good substrate for SULT1A1, requiring micromolar concentrations to observe its sulfonation.

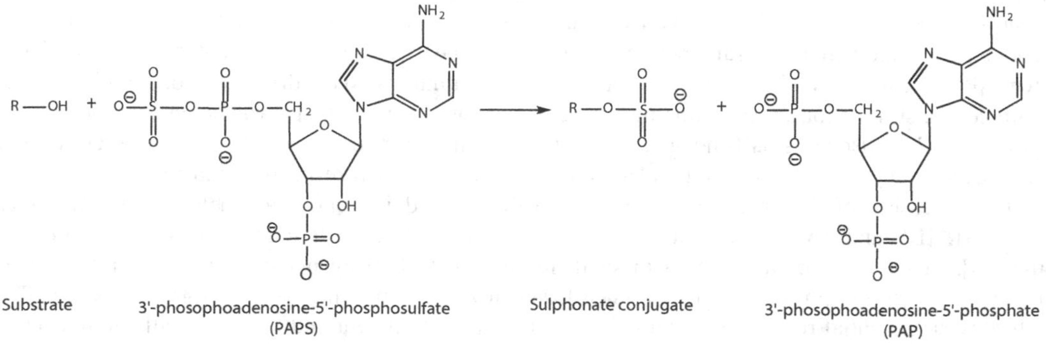

| Substrate | 3′-phosophoadenosine-5′-phosphosulfate (PAPS) | Sulphonate conjugate | 3′-phosophoadenosine-5′-phosphate (PAP) |

FIGURE 6.23 Catalytic mechanism of sulfonation mediated by sulfotransferases using PAPS as a cofactor.

Reactions and Relevance to Human Drug Metabolism

Crizotinib (PF-02341066, Figure 6.24) is a selective c-Met/Alk tyrosine kinase inhibitor that is marketed as an anticancer agent. *N*-Sulfonation is an important metabolic pathway that can impact crizotinib pharmacokinetics in rats [101]. Though total radioactivity recovered in excreta (urine and feces) was similar between male and female rats, a larger proportion of the radioactivity in females was accounted for by the sulfonate conjugate metabolite; the sulfonate conjugate in feces accounted for 44% of the administered dose in female rats and only 10% in male rats. This large sex difference was recapitulated *in vitro* with rat liver S9 incubations, which generated an abundant amount of the sulfonate conjugate (24% of total radioactivity) for females but only trace amounts for males. Sulfonation of crizotinib showed no gender differences in dogs and monkeys and was not an observed metabolic pathway in humans.

Apixaban (BMS-562247, Figure 6.24) is a reversible and selective direct Factor Xa inhibitor used as an anticoagulant for treating venous thromboembolic events. Its major circulating metabolite in humans is *O*-demethyl apixaban sulfate, which is formed by CYP-mediated *O*-demethylation followed by conjugation of the phenolic alcohol. The sulfonation step was studied in phenotyping experiments using commercially available, recombinantly expressed SULTs (SULT1A1, 1A2, 1A3, 1E1, and 2E1) and by selective chemical inhibition of SULTs in human liver S9 [102]. Sulfonation of *O*-demethyl apixaban was highest by SULT1A1 and 1A2 at 160 and 21 nmol/min/mg protein, respectively. Kinetic analysis with human liver S9, SULT1A1, and SULT1A2 showed comparable affinities (K_m 37–71 μM) but differed widely in maximal reaction velocities (V_{max} 7, 370, and 70 nmol/min/mg protein, respectively). In inhibition experiments, quercetin and 2,6-dichloro-4-nitrophenol inhibited the sulfonation reaction. These data show that SULT1A1 has a major role in the sulfonation of *O*-demethyl apixaban in humans.

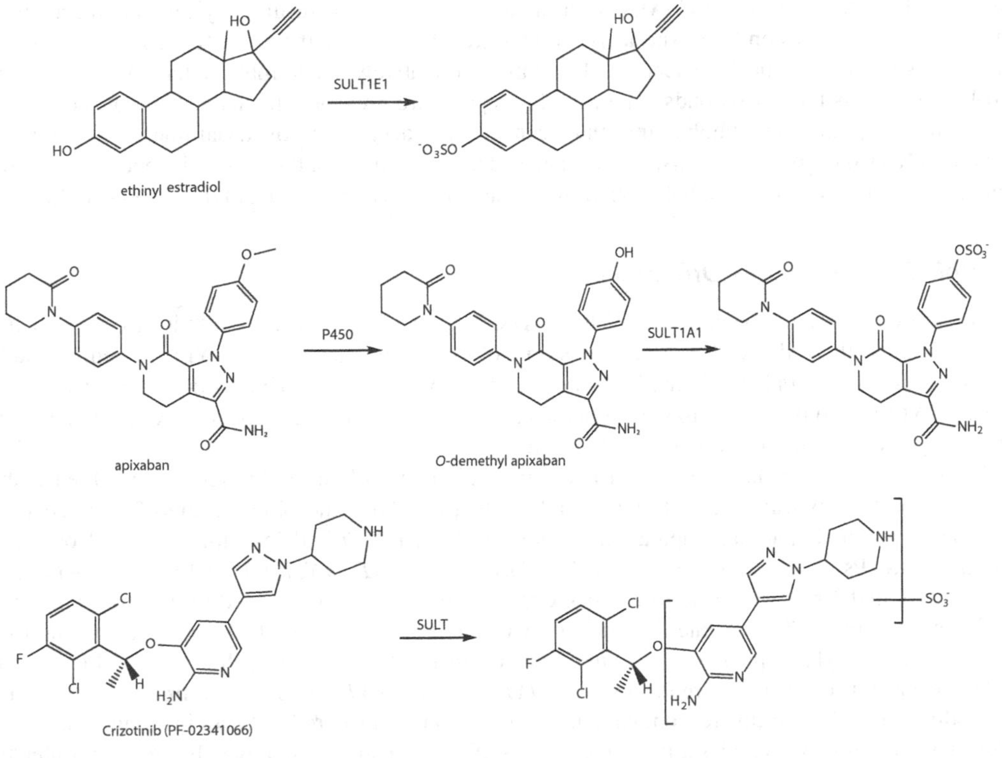

FIGURE 6.24 Metabolic reactions catalyzed by sulfotransferases (SULTs).

N-acetyltransferases

N-acetyltransferases (NATs) are enzymes that can transfer an acetyl group to an amine. Various *N*-acetyltransferases have been identified in human, and the substrates of *N*-acetylation include both small molecules and proteins. For example, aralkylamine *N*-acetyltransferase (AANAT) catalyzes the acetylation of serotonin, while GCN5-related *N*-acetyltransferases (GNATs) can transfer an acetyl group to protein substrates. In human, two NATs, NAT1, and NAT2, are significantly involved in the metabolism of drugs and other xenobiotics.

Subcellular Location and Organ Distribution

Human NAT1 and NAT2 are cytosolic enzymes. The molecular weights of mature human NAT1 and NAT2 proteins are approximately 34 and 31 kD, respectively. The two enzymes have different tissue distributions: NAT1 is distributed in almost all adult human tissues, while NAT2 is primarily expressed in human liver and gastrointestinal tract. Human NAT1 is also found in tissues such as red blood cells and lymphocytes, both of which are not normally associated with drug metabolism. Compared to NAT2, the much broader distribution of NAT1 in human tissues implies that NAT1 may be more involved in endogenous functions. For example, NAT1 potentially plays an endogenous role in human folate catabolism since the degradation products of folic acid, para-p aminobenzoyl glutamate (pABAglu) and 4-aminobenzoic acid (p-ABA) are acetylated by NAT1 [103].

Catalytic Mechanism

The reactions catalyzed by NATs have been shown to occur via a "Ping Pong Bi Bi" mechanism. This mechanism is comprised of two sequential steps. In the first step, the acetyl group is transferred from the acetyl donor (usually acetyl-CoA) to a certain amino acid residue (usually cysteine) in the active site cavity of NAT. In the second step, the acetyl group is transferred from the acetylated enzyme to an acetyl acceptor like an arylamine. The acetylated enzyme is a relatively stable intermediate with a hydrolysis half-life as long as tens of seconds if no acetyl acceptors are present. The active site pockets of NATs are usually deep and hydrophobic and, thus, can catalyze acetylation of arylamines. The stability of acetylated NAT intermediates is also at least partly due to the shape of the active site pocket because the acetylated residue is in a hydrophobic environment and deep inside away from the solvent [103].

Multiplicity and Species Differences

Species differences have been observed for NATs. NAT activity is totally absent in dogs and musk shrews. In cats, the only *NAT* gene encodes an isoform similar to human NAT1. Rodents including rats, mice, and hamsters have three *NAT* genes (*NAT1* to *NAT3*), but *NAT3* encodes an inactive protein. Rodent NAT1 is a homologous enzyme of human NAT2, while conversely, rodent NAT2 can metabolize certain typical substrates of human NAT1 [103,104].

The human *NAT1* gene is in human chromosome 8p22 and is polymorphic. According to the Database of Arylamine *N*-acetyltransferases (http://nat.mbg.duth.gr/), 28 polymorphic variants of *NAT1* gene have so far been identified in human populations. Among the human *NAT1* alleles with single nucleotide polymorphisms (SNPs) in the coding zones, *NAT1 * 14A*, *NAT1 * 14B*, *NAT1 * 15*, *NAT1 * 17*, *NAT1 * 19A*, *NAT1 * 19B*, and *NAT1 * 22* lead to inactive or less active proteins compared to the wild type human NAT1 encoded by *NAT1 * 4* (the reference of *NAT* alleles). Humans with these alleles belong to the "slow" NAT1 acetylator phenotype group. However, in most populations, the slow NAT1 acetylator alleles occur at a much lower frequency than *NAT1 * 4* and *NAT1 * 10* (containing two SNPs in the non-coding zone) do. For this reason, human *NAT1* was long considered to be an invariant gene, and its substrates, such as p-ABA and 4-aminosalicylate (4-AS), were usually thought to be "monomorphically" acetylated substrates.

The human *NAT2* gene is also in human chromosome 8p22 and is adjacent to the *NAT1* gene. The reference allele *NAT2 * 4* encodes the wild type human NAT2 and is a rapid acetylator. Besides *NAT2 * 4*, so far approximately 100 alleles of human *NAT2* have been identified and further categorized into 19 clusters according to the SNP(s) contained in each allele (http://nat.mbg.duth.gr). In each cluster, a common signature SNP can be found. A substantial proportion of the human *NAT2* alleles encode mutated NAT2 enzymes, which are less active than the wild type, resulting in the slow acetylator phenotype. Among different populations, the human *NAT2* gene shows considerable variation in allelic frequencies. For example, approximately 50% of people in Caucasian populations are slow acetylators, while the frequency in East Asian populations are 20%–30% [105]. The polymorphic drug metabolism by human NAT2 was recognized many years ago, and the related investigations greatly promoted our understanding of how pharmacogenetics impacts drug disposition in the human body.

Substrate, Inhibitors, and Inducers

Kawamura et al. established the substrate specificity for the NAT1 and NAT2 using various arylamines and aryl hydrazines as substrates. The two enzymes share over 80% similarity in their amino acid sequences, and overlapping but distinct substrate specificities were observed. Some substrates, like 5-aminosalicylate (5-AS), 4-ethoxyaniline, and 4-iodoaniline can be efficiently acetylated by both NATs. Meanwhile, each NAT binds to specific substrates that are not acetylated by the other NAT enzyme [106]. Human NAT1 shows high activity in the acetylation of p-ABA and 4-AS, but it does not catalyze the acetylation of aryl hydrazine compounds. In contrast, human NAT2 does not efficiently acetylate p-ABA and 4-AS, but hydrazine compounds can be excellent substrates of human NAT2.

Iodoacetate, *N*-ethylmaleimide, and p-chloromercuribenzoic acid are potent irreversible inhibitors of human NATs because these agents can covalently bind to the cysteine residue in the active site cavity [107]. Compounds that are structurally similar to the substrates of human NATs can act as reversible inhibitors, including salicylamide, 5-bromoslicylamide, 5-methylsalicylamide, and carboxyhydrazides [107,108]. In addition, phenolic compounds such as pentachlorophenol, 1-nitro-2-naphthol, phenolic acids, flavonoids, and coumarins may also inhibit the activity of human NATs [109]. The relevance of NAT1 in cancer, in particular breast cancer, has encouraged researchers to develop NAT1 inhibitors as promising therapeutic agents. Interestingly, a few existing drugs including tamoxifen, cisplatin, and disulfiram can inhibit NAT1 both *in vivo* and *in vitro*. For example, the inhibition of NAT1 by cisplatin is rapid and irreversible, and may contribute to the therapeutic effects of cisplatin [103].

In rabbits, the metabolism of sulfamethazine can be induced by glucocorticoids, such as hydrocortisone and immunostimulants (e.g., Freund's complete adjuvant) [110]. In rats, 3-methylcholanthrene and pregnenolone-16α-carbonitrile increase the acetylation of β-naphthylamine [111]. However, whether these NAT inducers in rodents can induce human NATs is largely unknown. Incubation of human peripheral blood mononuclear cells with NAT1 substrates such as p-ABA, 4-AS, benzocaine, or p-aminophenol decreased the cellular NAT1 expression without affecting NAT1 mRNA level, showing a post-transcriptional regulation [112].

Reactions and Relevance to Human Drug Metabolism

N-acetyltransferases use acetyl coenzyme A (acetyl-CoA) as the acetyl moiety donor to catalyze *N*-acetylation of arylamine/hydrazine, O-acetylation of aryl hydroxylamine, and also the intramolecular *N*-, *O*-acetyl transfer of *N*-acetylated aryl hydroxylamine (Figure 6.25) [104]. Among the acetylation products by NATs, *O*-acetylated aryl hydroxylamines are labile and carcinogenic because they easily degrade to nitrenium ions, which can covalently bind to DNA [7].

In humans, acetylation is an important pathway in the metabolism of arylamine or hydrazine drugs. Human NAT1, but not NAT2, is involved in the metabolism of 4-AS and p-ABA. In human urine, acetyl 4-AS was detected as a major metabolite of 4-AS, and acetyl p-ABA is detected as a minor metabolite of p-ABA [113,114]. Similarly, for 5-AS, the predominant metabolite in human serum and urine is acetyl 5-AS, and both human NAT1 and NAT2 may contribute to its metabolism [115].

Human NAT2 is involved in the metabolism of more drugs than human NAT1. Human *NAT2* genotypes together with non-genetic modulations result in phenotypes with various acetylating capabilities [104]. The anti-tuberculosis agent isoniazid is a hydrazine drug and is predominantly

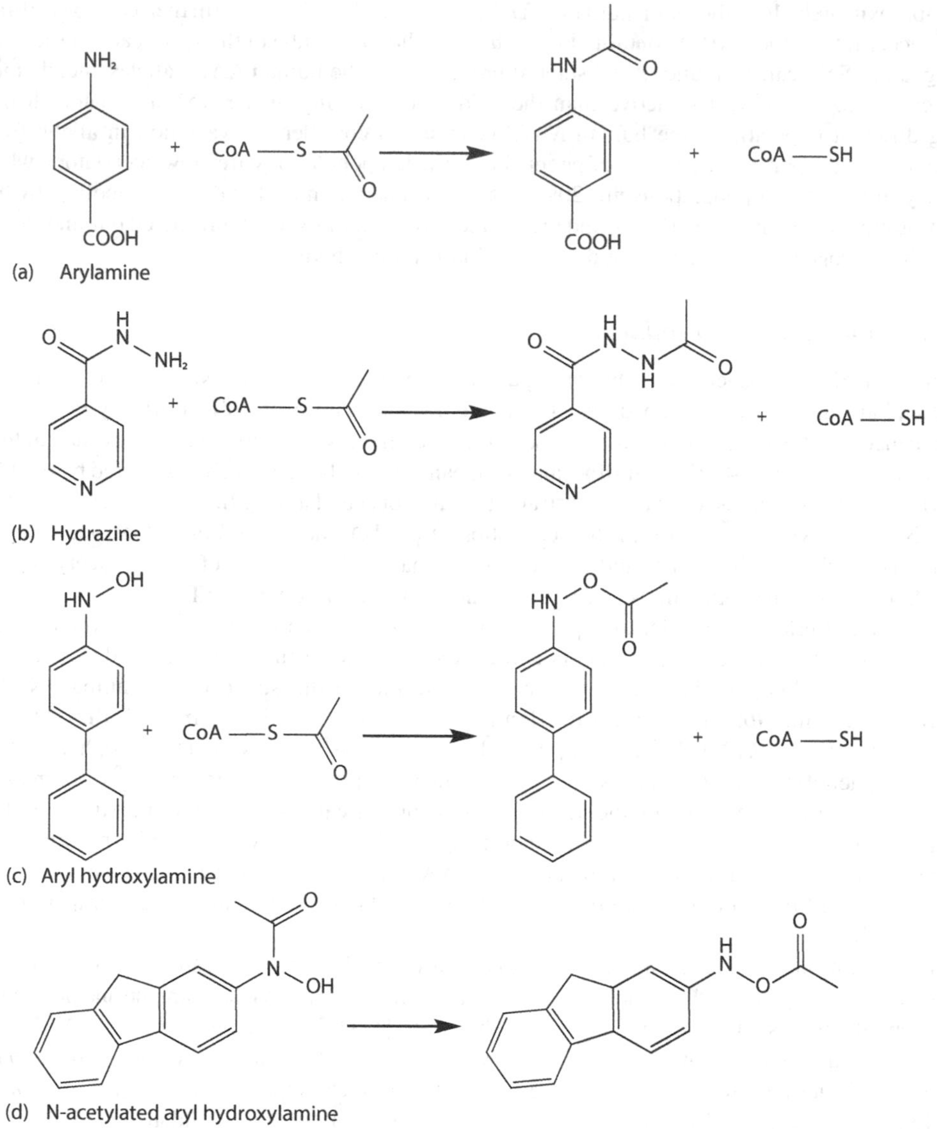

FIGURE 6.25 Metabolic reactions catalyzed by human *N*-acetyltransferases (NATs). (a), (b) Formation of *N*-acetylation and (c), (d) *O*-acetylation.

metabolized by human NAT2 to form inactive acetyl isoniazid *in vivo*. Inter-individual variability in the metabolism of isoniazid by patients has been ascribed to differences in NAT2 activities. In general, patients can be classified as "slow" or "rapid" isoniazid acetylators. In rapid acetylators, isoniazid is cleared rapidly from the circulation, and the majority of isoniazid is excreted in the urine as acetyl isoniazid. In the slow acetylators, only a much lower proportion of the isoniazid dose is acetylated and excreted in urine. Although a high plasma tuberculostatic activity is observed in slow acetylators, they are unfavorably more susceptible to dose-dependent toxicities of isoniazid than are the rapid acetylators. For example, the risk of isoniazid-induced hepatotoxicity is significantly higher in slow acetylators. Besides isoniazid, the other human NAT2 substrates including procainamide, sulphapyridine, dapsone, sulfamethazine, and hydralazine are also polymorphically acetylated.

Conclusions

While the majority of drugs and xenobiotics are metabolized and detoxified by CYP-mediated biotransformation pathways, non-CYP enzymes are becoming increasingly recognized to have important roles in the metabolism of drugs and drug candidates. This can be attributed to a rapid advancement in the research of metabolizing enzymes over the past four decades. The widespread use of metabolic stability screening in drug discovery has led to the identification of new chemical entities that rely on non-CYP enzymes for clearance; therefore, the number of drugs that undergo metabolism via these non-CYP enzymes has significantly increased. Like CYPs, non-CYP enzymes can also modulate drug efficacy, contribute to detoxification, or produce therapeutically active or reactive/toxic metabolites. The complementary roles of CYP and non-CYP enzymes are beneficial in drug development since they provide alternative clearance pathways that de-risk potential drug-drug interactions in the clinic.

ACKNOWLEDGMENT

The authors thank Ronitte Libedinsky for editorial support.

REFERENCES

1. Williams JA, Hyland R, Jones BC, Smith DA, Hurst S, Goosen TC, Peterkin V, Koup JR, Ball SE. Drug-Drug Interactions for Udp-Glucuronosyltransferase Substrates: A Pharmacokinetic Explanation for Typically Observed Low Exposure (Auci/Auc) Ratios. *Drug Metab Dispos* 2004; 32:1201–1208.
2. Beedham C. The Role of Non-P450 Enzymes in Drug Oxidation. *Pharm World Sci* 1997; 19:255–263.
3. Pryde DC, Dalvie D, Hu Q, Jones P, Obach RS, Tran TD. Aldehyde Oxidase: An Enzyme of Emerging Importance in Drug Discovery. *J Med Chem* 2010; 53:8441–8460.
4. Fan PW, Zhang D, Halladay JS, Driscoll JP, Khojasteh SC. Going Beyond Common Drug Metabolizing Enzymes: Case Studies of Biotransformation Involving Aldehyde Oxidase, Gamma-Glutamyl Transpeptidase, Cathepsin B, Flavin-Containing Monooxygenase, and Adp-Ribosyltransferase. *Drug Metab Dispos* 2016; 44:1253–1261.
5. Cerny MA. Prevalence of Non-Cytochrome P450-Mediated Metabolism in Food and Drug Administration-Approved Oral and Intravenous Drugs: 2006-2015. *Drug Metab Dispos* 2016; 44:1246–1252.
6. Strolin Benedetti M, Whomsley R, Baltes E. Involvement of Enzymes Other Than Cyps in the Oxidative Metabolism of Xenobiotics. *Expert Opin Drug Metab Toxicol* 2006; 2:895–921.
7. Gan J, Ma S, Zhang D. Non-Cytochrome P450-Mediated Bioactivation and Its Toxicological Relevance. *Drug Metab Rev* 2016; 48:473–501.
8. Cashman JR. Role of Flavin-Containing Monooxygenase in Drug Development. *Expert Opin Drug Metab Toxicol* 2008; 4:1507–1521.
9. Zhang J, Cashman JR. Quantitative Analysis of FMO Gene Mrna Levels in Human Tissues. *Drug Metab Dispos* 2006; 34:19–26.
10. Chen Y, Zane NR, Thakker DR, Wang MZ. Quantification of Flavin-Containing Monooxygenases 1, 3, and 5 in Human Liver Microsomes by Uplc-Mrm-Based Targeted Quantitative Proteomics and Its Application to the Study of Ontogeny. *Drug Metab Dispos* 2016; 44:975–983.
11. Fennema D, Phillips IR, Shephard EA. Trimethylamine and Trimethylamine N-Oxide, a Flavin-Containing Monooxygenase 3 (FMO3)-Mediated Host-Microbiome Metabolic Axis Implicated in Health and Disease. *Drug Metab Dispos* 2016; 44:1839–1850.
12. Cashman JR, Zhang J. Human Flavin-Containing Monooxygenases. *Annu Rev Pharmacol Toxicol* 2006; 46:65–100.
13. Janmohamed A, Hernandez D, Phillips IR, Shephard EA. Cell-, Tissue-, Sex- and Developmental Stage-Specific Expression of Mouse Flavin-Containing Monooxygenases (FMOs). *Biochem Pharmacol* 2004; 68:73–83.

14. Usmani KA, Chen WG, Sadeque AJ. Identification of Human Cytochrome P450 and Flavin-Containing Monooxygenase Enzymes Involved in the Metabolism of Lorcaserin, a Novel Selective Human 5-Hydroxytryptamine 2c Agonist. *Drug Metab Dispos* 2012; 40:761–771.
15. Lum CT, Stahl SM. Opportunities for Reversible Inhibitors of Monoamine Oxidase-a (Rimas) in the Treatment of Depression. *CNS Spectr* 2012; 17:107–120.
16. Robakis D, Fahn S. Defining the Role of the Monoamine Oxidase-B Inhibitors for Parkinson's Disease. *CNS Drugs* 2015; 29:433–441.
17. Chiba K, Trevor A, Castagnoli N, Jr. Metabolism of the Neurotoxic Tertiary Amine, Mptp, by Brain Monoamine Oxidase. *Biochem Biophys Res Commun* 1984; 120:574–578.
18. Duester G, Farres J, Felder MR, Holmes RS, Hoog JO, Pares X, Plapp BV, Yin SJ, Jornvall H. Recommended Nomenclature for the Vertebrate Alcohol Dehydrogenase Gene Family. *Biochem Pharmacol* 1999; 58:389–395.
19. Parkinson A, Ogilivie BW, Biotransformation of Xenobiotics. In *Casarett & Doull's Toxicology: The Basic Science of Poisons*, Klaassen CD, Ed. McGraw-Hill: New York, 2008; pp. 161–304.
20. Ceci JD, Lawther R, Duester G, Hatfield GW, Smith M, O'Malley MP, Felder MR. Androgen Induction of Alcohol Dehydrogenase in Mouse Kidney. Studies with a Cdna Probe Confirmed by Nucleotide Sequence Analysis. *Gene* 1986; 41:217–224.
21. Qulali M, Crabb DW. Estradiol Regulates Class I Alcohol Dehydrogenase Gene Expression in Renal Medulla of Male Rats by a Post-Transcriptional Mechanism. *Arch Biochem Biophys* 1992; 297:277–284.
22. Sandberg M, Yasar U, Stromberg P, Hoog JO, Eliasson E. Oxidation of Celecoxib by Polymorphic Cytochrome P450 2c9 and Alcohol Dehydrogenase. *Br J Clin Pharmacol* 2002; 54:423–429.
23. Walsh JS, Reese MJ, Thurmond LM. The Metabolic Activation of Abacavir by Human Liver Cytosol and Expressed Human Alcohol Dehydrogenase Isozymes. *Chem Biol Interact* 2002; 142:135–154.
24. Kapetanovic IM, Torchin CD, Thompson CD, Miller TA, McNeilly PJ, Macdonald TL, Kupferberg HJ, Perhach JL, Sofia RD, Strong JM. Potentially Reactive Cyclic Carbamate Metabolite of the Antiepileptic Drug Felbamate Produced by Human Liver Tissue *in Vitro*. *Drug Metab Dispos* 1998; 26:1089–1095.
25. Marchitti SA, Brocker C, Stagos D, Vasiliou V. Non-P450 Aldehyde Oxidizing Enzymes: The Aldehyde Dehydrogenase Superfamily. *Expert Opin Drug Metab Toxicol* 2008; 4:697–720.
26. Hempel J, Perozich J, Chapman T, Rose J, Boesch JS, Liu ZJ, Lindahl R, Wang BC. Aldehyde Dehydrogenase Catalytic Mechanism. A Proposal. *Adv Exp Med Biol* 1999; 463:53–59.
27. Wang MF, Han CL, Yin SJ. Substrate Specificity of Human and Yeast Aldehyde Dehydrogenases. *Chem Biol Interact* 2009; 178:36–39.
28. Koppaka V, Thompson DC, Chen Y, Ellermann M, Nicolaou KC, Juvonen RO, Petersen D, Deitrich RA, Hurley TD, Vasiliou V. Aldehyde Dehydrogenase Inhibitors: A Comprehensive Review of the Pharmacology, Mechanism of Action, Substrate Specificity, and Clinical Application. *Pharmacol Rev* 2012; 64:520–539.
29. Chen CH, Cruz LA, Mochly-Rosen D. Pharmacological Recruitment of Aldehyde Dehydrogenase 3a1 (Aldh3a1) to Assist Aldh2 in Acetaldehyde and Ethanol Metabolism *in Vivo*. *Proc Natl Acad Sci USA* 2015; 112:3074–3079.
30. Tafazoli S, O'Brien PJ. Peroxidases: A Role in the Metabolism and Side Effects of Drugs. *Drug Discovery Today* 2005; 10:617–625.
31. O'Brien PJ. Peroxidases. *Chem-Biol Interact* 2000; 129:113–139.
32. Tappel A. Selenium-Glutathione Peroxidase: Properties and Synthesis. *Curr Top Cell Regul* 2014; 24:87–96.
33. Fischer V, Haar JA, Greiner L, Lloyd RV, Mason RP. Possible Role of Free Radical Formation in Clozapine (Clozaril)-Induced Agranulocytosis. *Mol Pharmacol* 1991; 40:846.
34. Stiborová M, Poljaková J, Ryšlavá H, Dračínský M, Eckschlager T, Frei E. Mammalian Peroxidases Activate Anticancer Drug Ellipticine to Intermediates Forming Deoxyguanosine Adducts in DNA Identical to Those Found *In Vivo* and Generated from 12-Hydroxyellipticine and 13-Hydroxyellipticine. *Int J Cancer* 2007; 120:243–251.
35. Bäärnhielm C, Hansson G. Oxidation of 1,4-Dihydropyridines by Prostaglandin Synthase and the Peroxidic Function of Cytochrome P-450. *Biochem Pharmacol* 1986; 35:1419–1425.
36. Uetrecht JP. Myeloperoxidase as a Generator of Drug Free Radicals. *Biochem Soc Symp* 1995; 61:163.

37. O'Brien PJ, Khan S, Jatoe SD, Formation of Biological Reactive Intermediates by Peroxidases: Halide Mediated Acetaminophen Oxidation and Cytotoxicity. In *Biological Reactive Intermediates Iv: Molecular and Cellular Effects and Their Impact on Human Health*, Witmer CM, Snyder, RR, Jollow, DJ, Kalf, GF, Kocsis, JJ, Sipes, IG, Eds. Springer New York: Boston, MA, 1991; pp. 51–64.

38. Sharma S, Singh AK, Kaushik S, Sinha M, Singh RP, Sharma P, Sirohi H, Kaur P, Singh TP. Lactoperoxidase: Structural Insights into the Function, Ligand Binding and Inhibition. *Int J Biochem Mol Biol* 2013; 4:108–128.

39. Doerge DR, Divi RL. Porphyrin Π-Cation and Protein Radicals in Peroxidase Catalysis and Inhibition by Anti-Thyroid Chemicals. *Xenobiotica* 1995; 25:761–767.

40. Simmons DL, Botting RM, Hla T. Cyclooxygenase Isozymes: The Biology of Prostaglandin Synthesis and Inhibition. *Pharmacol Rev* 2004; 56:387–437.

41. Jin Y, Penning TM. Aldo-Keto Reductases and Bioactivation/Detoxication. *Annu Rev Pharmacol Toxicol* 2007; 47:263–292.

42. Penning TM, Bennett MJ, Smith-Hoog S, Schlegel BP, Jez JM, Lewis M. Structure and Function of 3 Alpha-Hydroxysteroid Dehydrogenase. *Steroids* 1997; 62:101–111.

43. Jez JM, Bennett MJ, Schlegel BP, Lewis M, Penning TM. Comparative Anatomy of the Aldo-Keto Reductase Superfamily. *Biochem J* 1997; 326(Pt 3):625–636.

44. O'connor T, Ireland LS, Harrison DJ, Hayes JD. Major Differences Exist in the Function and Tissue-Specific Expression of Human Aflatoxin B1 Aldehyde Reductase and the Principal Human Aldo-Keto Reductase Akr1 Family Members. *Biochem J* 1999; 343 Pt 2:487–504.

45. Penning TM, Burczynski ME, Jez JM, Hung CF, Lin HK, Ma H, Moore M, Palackal N, Ratnam K. Human 3alpha-Hydroxysteroid Dehydrogenase Isoforms (Akr1c1-Akr1c4) of the Aldo-Keto Reductase Superfamily: Functional Plasticity and Tissue Distribution Reveals Roles in the Inactivation and Formation of Male and Female Sex Hormones. *Biochem J* 2000; 351:67–77.

46. Charbonneau A, The VL. Genomic Organization of a Human 5beta-Reductase and Its Pseudogene and Substrate Selectivity of the Expressed Enzyme. *Biochim Biophys Acta* 2001; 1517:228–235.

47. Matsunaga T, Shintani S, Hara A. Multiplicity of Mammalian Reductases for Xenobiotic Carbonyl Compounds. *Drug Metab Pharmacokinet* 2006; 21:1–18.

48. Huang L, He R, Luo W, Zhu YS, Li J, Tan T, Zhang X, Hu Z, Luo D. Aldo-Keto Reductase Family 1 Member B10 Inhibitors: Potential Drugs for Cancer Treatment. *Recent Pat Anticancer Drug Discov* 2016; 11:184–196.

49. Verma K, Zang T, Gupta N, Penning TM, Trippier PC. Selective Akr1c3 Inhibitors Potentiate Chemotherapeutic Activity in Multiple Acute Myeloid Leukemia (Aml) Cell Lines. *ACS Med Chem Lett* 2016; 7:774–779.

50. Malátková P, Sokolová S, Chocholoušová Havlíková L, Wsól V. Carbonyl Reduction of Warfarin: Identification and Characterization of Human Warfarin Reductases. *Biochem Pharmacol* 2016; 109:83–90.

51. Dowty ME, Lin J, Ryder TF, Wang W, Walker GS, Vaz A, Chan GL, Krishnaswami S, Prakash C. The Pharmacokinetics, Metabolism, and Clearance Mechanisms of Tofacitinib, a Janus Kinase Inhibitor, in Humans. *Drug Metab Dispos* 2014; 42:759–773.

52. Le H, Fan PW, Wong S, Ma S, Driscoll JP, Hop CE, Cyrus Khojasteh S. Elucidating the Mechanism of Tofacitinib Oxidative Decyanation. *Drug Metab Lett* 2016; 10:136–143.

53. Ghosal A, Yuan Y, Tong W, Su AD, Gu C, Chowdhury SK, Kishnani NS, Alton KB. Characterization of Human Liver Enzymes Involved in the Biotransformation of Boceprevir, a Hepatitis C Virus Protease Inhibitor. *Drug Metab Dispos* 2011; 39:510–521.

54. Fretland AJ, Omiecinski CJ. Epoxide Hydrolases: Biochemistry and Molecular Biology. *Chem Biol Interact* 2000; 129:41–59.

55. Sims P, Grover PL, Swaisland A, Pal K, Hewer A. Metabolic Activation of Benzo(a)Pyrene Proceeds by a Diol-Epoxide. *Nature* 1974; 252:326–328.

56. Arand M, Cronin A, Adamska M, Oesch F. Epoxide Hydrolases: Structure, Function, Mechanism, and Assay. *Meth Enzymol* 2005; 400:569–588.

57. Morisseau C, Hammock BD. Epoxide Hydrolases: Mechanisms, Inhibitor Designs, and Biological Roles. *Annu Rev Pharmacol Toxicol* 2005; 45:311–333.

58. Meijer J, DePierre JW. Cytosolic Epoxide Hydrolase. *Chem Biol Interact* 1988; 64:207–249.

59. Meijer J, Lundqvist G, DePierre JW. Comparison of the Sex and Subcellular Distributions, Catalytic and Immunochemical Reactivities of Hepatic Epoxide Hydrolases in Seven Mammalian Species. *Eur J Biochem* 1987; 167:269–279.
60. Hammock BD, Grant DF, Storms DH, Epoxide Hydrolases. In *Comprehensive Toxicology*, Guengerich FP, Ed. Elsevier Science: Oxford, UK, 1997; pp. 283–305.
61. Laizure SC, Herring V, Hu Z, Witbrodt K, Parker RB. The Role of Human Carboxylesterases in Drug Metabolism: Have We Overlooked Their Importance? *Pharmacotherapy* 2013; 33:210–222.
62. Wislocki PG, Wood AW, Chang RL, Levin W, Yagi H, Hernandez O, Jerina DM, Conney AH. High Mutagenicity and Toxicity of a Diol Epoxide Derived from Benzo(a)Pyrene. *Biochem Biophys Res Commun* 1976; 68:1006–1012.
63. Li XQ, Hayes MA, Gronberg G, Berggren K, Castagnoli N, Jr., Weidolf L. Discovery of a Novel Microsomal Epoxide Hydrolase-Catalyzed Hydration of a Spiro Oxetane. *Drug Metab Dispos* 2016; 44:1341–1348.
64. Riley RJ, Kitteringham NR, Park BK. Structural Requirements for Bioactivation of Anticonvulsants to Cytotoxic Metabolites *in Vitro*. *Br J Clin Pharmacol* 1989; 28:482–487.
65. Hosokawa M. Structure and Catalytic Properties of Carboxylesterase Isozymes Involved in Metabolic Activation of Prodrugs. *Molecules* 2008; 13:412–431.
66. Satoh T, Hosokawa M. The Mammalian Carboxylesterases: From Molecules to Functions. *Annu Rev Pharmacol Toxicol* 1998; 38:257–288.
67. Godin SJ, Scollon EJ, Hughes MF, Potter PM, DeVito MJ, Ross MK. Species Differences in the *in Vitro* Metabolism of Deltamethrin and Esfenvalerate: Differential Oxidative and Hydrolytic Metabolism by Humans and Rats. *Drug Metab Dispos* 2006; 34:1764–1771.
68. Fu J, Pacyniak E, Leed MG, Sadgrove MP, Marson L, Jay M. Interspecies Differences in the Metabolism of a Multiester Prodrug by Carboxylesterases. *J Pharm Sci* 2016; 105:989–995.
69. Shimizu M, Fukami T, Nakajima M, Yokoi T. Screening of Specific Inhibitors for Human Carboxylesterases or Arylacetamide Deacetylase. *Drug Metab Dispos* 2014; 42:1103–1109.
70. Hatfield MJ, Potter PM. Carboxylesterase Inhibitors. *Expert Opin Ther Pat* 2011; 21:1159–1171.
71. Lohr JW, Willsky GR, Acara MA. Renal Drug Metabolism. *Pharmacol Rev* 1998; 50:107–141.
72. Corti A, Franzini M, Paolicchi A, Pompella A. Gamma-Glutamyltransferase of Cancer Cells at the Crossroads of Tumor Progression, Drug Resistance and Drug Targeting. *Anticancer Res* 2010; 30:1169–1181.
73. Hanigan MH, Lykissa ED, Townsend DM, Ou CN, Barrios R, Lieberman MW. Gamma-Glutamyl Transpeptidase-Deficient Mice Are Resistant to the Nephrotoxic Effects of Cisplatin. *Am J Pathol* 2001; 159:1889–1894.
74. Mutlib AE, Chen H, Nemeth G, Gan LS, Christ DD. Liquid Chromatography/Mass Spectrometry and High-Field Nuclear Magnetic Resonance Characterization of Novel Mixed Diconjugates of the Non-Nucleoside Human Immunodeficiency Virus-1 Reverse Transcriptase Inhibitor, Efavirenz. *Drug Metab Dispos* 1999; 27:1045–1056.
75. Mutlib AE, Gerson RJ, Meunier PC, Haley PJ, Chen H, Gan LS, Davies MH et al. The Species-Dependent Metabolism of Efavirenz Produces a Nephrotoxic Glutathione Conjugate in Rats. *Toxicol Appl Pharmacol* 2000; 169:102–113.
76. Quesada V, Ordonez GR, Sanchez LM, Puente XS, Lopez-Otin C. The Degradome Database: Mammalian Proteases and Diseases of Proteolysis. *Nucleic Acids Res* 2009; 37:D239–D243.
77. Conus S, Simon HU. Cathepsins and Their Involvement in Immune Responses. *Swiss Med Wkly* 2010; 140:w13042.
78. Turk V, Stoka V, Vasiljeva O, Renko M, Sun T, Turk B, Turk D. Cysteine Cathepsins: From Structure, Function and Regulation to New Frontiers. *Biochim Biophys Acta* 2012; 1824:68–88.
79. Mohamed MM, Sloane BF. Cysteine Cathepsins: Multifunctional Enzymes in Cancer. *Nat Rev Cancer* 2006; 6:764–775.
80. Satsangi A, Roy SS, Satsangi RK, Vadlamudi RK, Ong JL. Design of a Paclitaxel Prodrug Conjugate for Active Targeting of an Enzyme Upregulated in Breast Cancer Cells. *Mol Pharm* 2014; 11:1906–1918.
81. Shao LH, Liu SP, Hou JX, Zhang YH, Peng CW, Zhong YJ, Liu X, Liu XL, Hong YP, Firestone RA, Li Y. Cathepsin B Cleavable Novel Prodrug Ac-Phe-Lys-Pabc-Adm Enhances Efficacy at Reduced Toxicity in Treating Gastric Cancer Peritoneal Carcinomatosis: An Experimental Study. *Cancer* 2012; 118:2986–2996.

82. Weidle UH, Tiefenthaler G, Georges G. Proteases as Activators for Cytotoxic Prodrugs in Antitumor Therapy. *Cancer Genom Proteom* 2014; 11:67–79.

83. Chari RV, Miller ML, Widdison WC. Antibody-Drug Conjugates: An Emerging Concept in Cancer Therapy. *Angew Chem Int Ed Engl* 2014; 53:3796–3827.

84. Hayes JD, Flanagan JU, Jowsey IR. Glutathione Transferases. *Annu Rev Pharmacol Toxicol* 2005; 45:51–88.

85. Deponte M. Glutathione Catalysis and the Reaction Mechanisms of Glutathione-Dependent Enzymes. *Biochim Biophys Acta* 2013; 1830:3217–3266.

86. Wu B, Dong D. Human Cytosolic Glutathione Transferases: Structure, Function, and Drug Discovery. *Trends Pharmacol Sci* 2012; 33:656–668.

87. van Bladeren PJ. Glutathione Conjugation as a Bioactivation Reaction. *Chem Biol Interact* 2000; 129:61–76.

88. Zhang Y, Kolm RH, Mannervik B, Talalay P. Reversible Conjugation of Isothiocyanates with Glutathione Catalyzed by Human Glutathione Transferases. *Biochem Biophys Res Commun* 1995; 206:748–755.

89. Meyer DJ, Crease DJ, Ketterer B. Forward and Reverse Catalysis and Product Sequestration by Human Glutathione S-Transferases in the Reaction of Gsh with Dietary Aralkyl Isothiocyanates. *Biochem J* 1995; 306 (Pt 2):565–569.

90. Slatter JG, Rashed MS, Pearson PG, Han DH, Baillie TA. Biotransformation of Methyl Isocyanate in the Rat. Evidence for Glutathione Conjugation as a Major Pathway of Metabolism and Implications for Isocyanate-Mediated Toxicities. *Chem Res Toxicol* 1991; 4:157–161.

91. Baillie TA, Slatter JG. Glutathione: A Vehicle for the Transport of Chemically Reactive Metabolites In Vivo. *Acc Chem Res* 1991; 24:264–270.

92. Orsler DJ, Ahmed-Choudhury J, Chipman JK, Hammond T, Coleman R. Anit-Induced Disruption of Biliary Function in Rat Hepatocyte Couplets. *Toxicol Sci* 1999; 47:203–210.

93. Dietrich CG, Ottenhoff R, de Waart DR, Oude Elferink RP. Role of Mrp2 and Gsh in Intrahepatic Cycling of Toxins. *Toxicology* 2001; 167:73–81.

94. Riches Z, Stanley EL, Bloomer JC, Coughtrie MW. Quantitative Evaluation of the Expression and Activity of Five Major Sulfotransferases (Sults) in Human Tissues: The Sult "Pie". *Drug Metab Dispos* 2009; 37:2255–2261.

95. Blanchard RL, Freimuth RR, Buck J, Weinshilboum RM, Coughtrie MW. A Proposed Nomenclature System for the Cytosolic Sulfotransferase (Sult) Superfamily. *Pharmacogenetics* 2004; 14:199–211.

96. Wang T, Cook I, Leyh TS. 3′-Phosphoadenosine 5′-Phosphosulfate Allosterically Regulates Sulfotransferase Turnover. *Biochemistry* 2014; 53:6893–6900.

97. Wang T, Cook I, Falany CN, Leyh TS. Paradigms of Sulfotransferase Catalysis: The Mechanism of Sult2a1. *J Biol Chem* 2014; 289:26474–26480.

98. Cook I, Wang T, Leyh TS. Sulfotransferase 1a1 Substrate Selectivity: A Molecular Clamp Mechanism. *Biochemistry* 2015; 54:6114–6122.

99. Schrag ML, Cui D, Rushmore TH, Shou M, Ma B, Rodrigues AD. Sulfotransferase 1e1 Is a Low Km Isoform Mediating the 3-O-Sulfation of Ethinyl Estradiol. *Drug Metab Dispos* 2004; 32:1299–1303.

100. Rohn KJ, Cook IT, Leyh TS, Kadlubar SA, Falany CN. Potent Inhibition of Human Sulfotransferase 1a1 by 17α-Ethinylestradiol: Role of 3′-Phosphoadenosine 5′-Phosphosulfate Binding and Structural Rearrangements in Regulating Inhibition and Activity. *Drug Metab Dispos* 2012; 40:1588–1595.

101. Zhong WZ, Zhan J, Kang P, Yamazaki S. Gender Specific Drug Metabolism of Pf-02341066 in Rats--Role of Sulfoconjugation. *Curr Drug Metab* 2010; 11:296–306.

102. Wang L, Raghavan N, He K, Luettgen JM, Humphreys WG, Knabb RM, Pinto DJ, Zhang D. Sulfation of O-Demethyl Apixaban: Enzyme Identification and Species Comparison. *Drug Metab Dispos* 2009; 37:802–808.

103. Rodrigues-Lima F, Dairou J, Busi F, Dupret J-M. Human Arylamine N-Acetyltransferase 1: A Drug-Metabolizing Enzyme and a Drug Target? *Current Drug Targets* 2010; 11:759–766.

104. Sim E, Walters K, Boukouvala S. Arylamine N-Acetyltransferases: From Structure to Function. *Drug Metabol Rev* 2008; 40:479–510.

105. Elena G-M. Interethnic and Intraethnic Variability of Nat2 Single Nucleotide Polymorphisms. *Curr Drug Metabol* 2008; 9:487–497.

106. Kawamura A, Graham J, Mushtaq A, Tsiftsoglou SA, Vath GM, Hanna PE, Wagner CR, Sim E. Eukaryotic Arylamine N-Acetyltransferase: Investigation of Substrate Specificity by High-Throughput Screening. *Biochem Pharmacol* 2005; 69:347–359.

107. Weber WW, Levy GN, Hein DW, Acetylation. In *Conjugation Reactions in Drug Metabolism: An Integrated Approach*, Mulder GJ, Ed. CRC Press: 2003; pp 162–190.

108. Johnson W, Corte G. Inhibition of Isoniazid Acetylation *in vitro* and *in vivo*. *Proc Soc Exp Biol Med.* 1956; 92:446–448.

109. Kukongviriyapan V, Phromsopha N, Tassaneeyakul W, Kukongviriyapan U, Sripa B, Hahnvajanawong V, Bhudhisawasdi V. Inhibitory Effects of Polyphenolic Compounds on Human Arylamine N-Acetyltransferase 1 and 2. *Xenobiotica* 2006; 36:15–28.

110. du Souich P, Courteau H. Induction of Acetylating Capacity with Complete Freund's Adjuvant and Hydrocortisone in the Rabbit. *Drug Metabol Dispos* 1981; 9:279–283.

111. Thompson TN, Watkins JB, Gregus Z, Klaassen CD. Effect of Microsomal Enzyme Inducers on the Soluble Enzymes of Hepatic Phase Ii Biotransformation. *Toxicol Appl Pharmacol* 1982; 66:400–408.

112. Butcher NJ, Ilett KF, Minchin RF. Substrate-Dependent Regulation of Human Arylamine n-Acetyltransferase-1 in Cultured Cells. *Mol Pharmacol* 2000; 57:468–473.

113. Kitamura M, Nakao M, Yanagisawa I. Metabolism of Para-Aminobenzoic Acid. *J Biochem* 1960; 47:60–68.

114. Way EL, Peng C-T, Allawala N, Daniels TC. The Metabolism of P-Aminosalicylic Acid (Pas) in Man. *J Am Pharm Assoc* 1955; 44:65–69.

115. Myers B, Evans DN, Rhodes J, Evans BK, Hughes BR, Lee MG, Richens A, Richards D. Metabolism and Urinary Excretion of 5-Amino Salicylic Acid in Healthy Volunteers When Given Intravenously or Released for Absorption at Different Sites in the Gastrointestinal Tract. *Gut* 1987; 28:196–200.

7

The Genetic Basis of Variation in Drug Metabolism and Toxicity

Tore Bjerregaard Stage and Deanna L. Kroetz

CONTENTS

Background

It is well recognized that there is a large variability in drug response. It is estimated that around 50% of patients will not respond to treatment for a wide array of diseases such as migraine and diabetes; this proportion reaches nearly 75% for chemotherapy. This area of research has received much attention recently, culminating in President Barack Obama's State of the Union address in January 2015 announcing the Precision Medicine Initiative (https://www.nih.gov/precision-medicine-initiative-cohort-program). One of the goals is to "Help develop the right drug for the right person at the right dose," in stark contrast to the previous focus on developing drugs for a population. The key point in precision medicine is to target drugs to patients that have a high probability of responding well and to limit their use in those patients who will not respond or experience side effects.

There are many factors contributing to drug variability. Traditionally these are split into three categories; host factors (e.g., body weight, comorbidity), environmental factors (e.g., drug interactions, food intake), and genetic variation. This chapter will focus on pharmacogenetics, genetic variation causing variability in drug response, more specifically on genetic variants influencing drug pharmacokinetics, and risk of side effects.

A total of 52.5% of the small molecule drugs approved by the Food and Drug Administration (FDA) in the period from 2006–2015 ($n = 125$) were metabolized by P450, 30% were metabolized by non-P450 enzymes, and the remaining had no major metabolites [1]. The major enzymes involved in CYP-mediated drug metabolism are CYP3A4/5 > CYP2D6 > CYP2C9 > CYP1A2 > CYP2B6 > CYP2C19 > CYP2C8 > CYP2E1 $\approx$ CYP2J2 [2]. Genetic variation in these enzymes may lead to changes in efficacy and/or toxicity depending on whether the drug itself or a metabolite are active. For example, for a typical

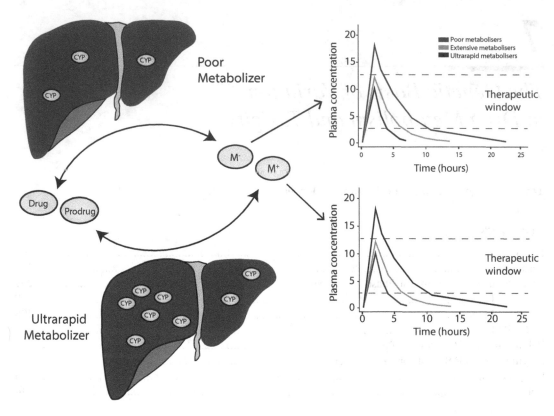

FIGURE 7.1 This figure highlights how drugs and prodrugs are metabolized to inactive (M-) and active (M+) metabolites. Additionally, hypothetical plasma concentration-time curves for different types of metabolizers are shown for pharmacologically active drugs (top panel) and prodrugs (bottom panel).

drug with activity associated with parent drug levels, poor metabolizers are expected to have higher plasma concentrations and increased risk of toxicity, while ultrarapid metabolizers will have reduced plasma levels that may lead to loss of efficacy (Figure 7.1). The opposite would be true for a prodrug, with ultrarapid metabolizers expected to have the highest levels of active drug and poor metabolizers the lowest levels.

All drugs provoke side effects (Paracelsus; "The dose makes the poison"). The most frequent and mild side effects are correlated directly to plasma concentrations (type A), while other side effects are more idiosyncratic, rarer, and more serious (type B). The latter presents an important clinical problem for many drug classes, such as antiepileptics that are known to provoke serious cutaneous reactions. Predicting and reducing the frequency of these types of hypersensitivity reactions would present a remarkable improvement in the clinical use of these drugs.

The frequency of genetic variants varies substantially between populations. Due to the large number of variants mentioned in this chapter, we do not find it feasible to discuss the frequency in this chapter. Minor allele frequencies can be easily found through public databases, such as ExAc (http://exac.broadinstitute.org), 1000 Genomes (http://1000genomes.org), the National Library of Medicine SNP Database (https://www.ncbi.nlm.nih.gov/snp), and the Pharmacogenomics Knowledge Base (PharmGKB, https://www.pharmgkb.org).

The field of pharmacogenetics contains a vast amount of literature and no single chapter can provide a comprehensive summary of all the data. This chapter will instead provide an introduction to the most well-established and clinically relevant variants in drug response genes. A summary of the gene-drug pairs for which currently published guidelines are available from the Clinical Pharmacogenetics Implementation Consortium (CPIC) for genotype-guided dosing is provided in Table 7.1. Many of these will be discussed in more detail below.

TABLE 7.1

Drugs with CPIC Guidelines Involving Drug Metabolism and HLA-B Alleles

Gene[a]	Drugs
CYP2D6	Tricyclic Antidepressants (Amitriptyline, Clomipramine, Desipramine, Doxepin, Imipramine, Nortriptyline, Trimipramine)
	Codeine
	Fluvoxamine
	Paroxetine
CYP2C9	Phenytoin
CYP2C9/VKORC1	Warfarin
CYP2C19	Tricyclic Antidepressants (Amitriptyline, Clomipramine, Desipramine, Doxepin, Imipramine, Nortriptyline, Trimipramine)
	Citalopram, Escitalopram
	Clopidogrel
	Sertraline
	Voriconazole
CYP3A5	Tacrolimus
TPMT	Azathioprine
	Mercaptopurine
	Thioguanine
UGT1A1	Atazanavir
DPYD	Capecitabine
	Fluorouracil
	Tegafur
HLA-B	Abacavir
	Allopurinol
	Carbamazepine
	Phenytoin

[a] Complete dosing guidelines for each of these gene-drug pairs can be found at https://cpicpgx.org/.

Terminology

Standard genetic nomenclature is used throughout this chapter. Genes are written in *italics* while proteins are written with normal text. A single nucleotide polymorphism (SNP) is the change of a single nucleotide to another in the genomic DNA. This may be described in several different ways, such as 163C>A, which means that in the indicated gene at position 163 a cytosine is replaced by an adenine. SNPs are also assigned a number with the prefix "rs," which maps the nucleotide change to a specific location on the genome. Nucleotide changes may result in changes in the encoded amino acids (non-synonymous), for example Lys262Arg, which means at the specific amino acid position a leucine is replaced by an arginine. Finally, one or multiple variants may be combined to make alleles. Alleles for *CYP* genes are indicated by an allelic number terminology, which can be found at http://www.cypalleles.ki.se.

Polymorphisms Relevant for Phase I Enzymes

Phase I metabolism is mainly characterized by modification of xenobiotics by introducing reactive and polar chemical groups via oxidation, reduction, or hydrolysis. In this section, we have highlighted the most important and relevant polymorphisms in genes encoding enzymes involved in Phase I metabolism of drugs. The discussion is focused on the three major enzyme families relevant for drug metabolism, the CYP1, CYP2, and CYP3 families.

CYP1 Family

CYP1A2 constitutes 13% of the total CYP liver content [3] and is involved in the metabolism of drugs such as clozapine, olanzapine, and theophylline. The probe substrate for CYP1A2 is caffeine as 80% of its total clearance is mediated via CYP1A2 demethylation [4]. Variation in caffeine metabolism is extensive, with a strong genetic heritability of the urinary metabolic ratio of 72.5% in a Danish twin study [5].

The most researched and relevant polymorphism for CYP1A2 is an intronic nucleotide substitution *CYP1A2*1F* (rs762551). In one study, smokers who carry the *CYP1A2*1F* allele had lower caffeine concentrations due to increased metabolism, while this effect was not detected in non-smokers [6]. A subsequent study failed to replicate these findings [7]. One possible explanation for these discordant findings may be that the variant is in linkage disequilibrium with other variants that are causal. Consistent with this hypothesis, another study showed no effect of *CYP1A2*1F* but did find an association with more complex *CYP1A2* haplotypes [8]. Clozapine is an atypical antipsychotic drug used in the treatment of schizophrenia and is metabolized by CYP1A2 and several other P450 enzymes. Treatment resistance due to low clozapine levels was observed among patients with the *CYP1A2*1F* allele [9,10]. Carriers of a haplotype containing the *CYP1A2*1F* and four other genetic variants (−3860 G>A, −2467del, −739 T>G, −729 C>T) have higher plasma concentrations of clozapine [11]. A similar trend was shown for olanzapine, as carriers of the *CYP1A2*1F* allele require lower body-weight adjusted dose [12]. Known side effects to antipsychotic treatment include QT prolongation and extrapyramidal side effects. Carriers of the *CYP1A2*1F* −163A variant have longer QTc prolongation than those with the reference allele during treatment with chlorpromazine, fluphenazine, trifluoperazine, and thioridazine [13] and experience more extrapyramidal side effects to antipsychotic treatment in a US [14] and a Chinese cohort [15]. These findings require further validation as this association was not replicated in a German cohort [16] or another Chinese cohort [17]. Finally, *CYP1A2*1F* has also been related to leflunomide-induced toxicity [18,19], which leads to an increased risk of discontinuing treatment due to side effects [20]. Taken together, these studies indicate that carriers of the *CYP1A2*1F* allele have increased CYP1A2 metabolic activity, leading to lower drug concentrations, fewer adverse events, and consequently a lower drug response.

Generally, the pharmacogenetic study of CYP1A2 variability is complicated by the influence of common environmental factors such as caffeine intake and smoking (a known CYP1A2 inducer). This has made interpretation of the literature difficult and likely contributed to the poor reproducibility of results. As a result, there are currently no established clinically relevant genetic variants in *CYP1A2*.

CYP2 Family

CYP2B6 comprises around 2%–5% of the hepatic P450 pool [2] with a large variability in both mRNA [21] and protein level [22]. CYP2B6 is involved in the metabolism of a wide array of drugs, including antiretroviral agents (e.g., efavirenz), antidepressants (e.g., bupropion), and anesthetics (e.g., propofol).

The most common and relevant genetic variation for *CYP2B6* is *CYP2B6*6* (rs3745274), which comprises two amino acid substitutions, Gln172His and Lys262Arg, and is common across all populations. *CYP2B6*6* is associated with lower CYP2B6 mRNA [21] and protein levels and activity [23]. The clinical significance of this genotype has been extensively studied for efavirenz, which is widely used in the treatment of human immunodeficiency virus (HIV). Carriers of the *CYP2B6*6* variant have higher plasma concentrations [24–27], efavirenz-induced side effects [28], and risk of discontinuation due to side effects [29,30]. This effect has successfully been countered in a prospective study, by prescribing lower doses to individuals carrying this variant [31]. A similar effect of this variant has been shown for another antiretroviral drug nevirapine [32–34] and the μ-opioid agonist methadone [35]. Interestingly, the opposite was shown for the anticancer drug cyclophosphamide, which is bioactivated via CYP2B6. In contrast to what was observed for other drugs, carriers of *CYP2B6*6* appear to have a higher rate of bioactivation of cyclophosphamide [36–38], which indicates an increased metabolic capacity among carriers of *CYP2B6*6*. This suggests substrate dependent effects of this variant.

CYP2C8 comprises approximately 7% of the hepatic P450 content [39] and plays a major role in the metabolism of many drugs, such as chemotherapeutics (e.g., paclitaxel) and antidiabetics (e.g., rosiglitazone).

For *CYP2C8*, the *2 and *3 alleles explain a large amount of the variability. In contrast to in vitro evidence, *CYP2C8*3* (two highly linked variants: rs10509681 and rs11572080) was linked to increased metabolism of repaglinide [40] but not at high doses [41,42]. Consistent with the repaglinide findings, carriers of *CYP2C8*3* have increased metabolism of the antidiabetic drugs rosiglitazone and pioglitazone [43–46]. A clinical study showed that carriers of this variant have lower rosiglitazone plasma concentrations and therapeutic efficacy and a higher risk of peripheral oedema in patients with type 2 diabetes [47]. This finding was recently reproduced in a large cohort of type 2 diabetes patients [48]. Interestingly, *CYP2C8*3* has been linked to slightly impaired clearance of the microtubule-stabilizing anticancer agent paclitaxel [49,50]. In line with this, some studies have indicated a higher risk of paclitaxel-induced peripheral neuropathy, but this was not consistently replicated [51–54]. Initially, no differences in efficacy or toxicity were observed among carriers of *CYP2C8*3* treated with the antimalarial drug amodiaquine [55], but recently a study showed higher resistance among *CYP2C8*3* carriers [56]. Thus *CYP2C8*3* is relevant for the metabolism of most drugs metabolized by CYP2C8, but the effect of the genetic variant is substrate-dependent.

*CYP2C8*2* (rs11572103) has not been investigated, most likely due to a low representation of this genotype outside of Africa. Carriers of this variant have lower area under the curve (AUC) of the M-III metabolite of pioglitazone in healthy individuals of African descent [57] and lower response to the antimalarial drug chloroquine [58]. These findings indicate that *CYP2C8*2* leads to a poor metabolizing phenotype, and this warrants further research, especially in African populations where the variant is frequently represented (a frequency of up to 20%).

CYP2C9 comprises approximately 15% of the hepatic P450 content [39] and is involved in the metabolism of ~15% of clinically used drugs [2]. The most widely used 2C9 substrates include non-steroidal anti-inflammatory drugs (NSAID, e.g., ibuprofen or diclofenac), anticoagulants (warfarin) and antidiabetics (tolbutamide). Due to the widespread use and the narrow therapeutic window for some CYP2C9 substrates, pharmacogenetics of *CYP2C9* has received significant attention.

Many variants have been described in *CYP2C9*, but the most common, widely researched and relevant are *2 (rs1799853) and *3 (rs1057910); the most widely studied drug regarding *CYP2C9* pharmacogenetics is warfarin. Carriers of *CYP2C9*2* or *CYP2C9*3* have decreased metabolism of warfarin, leading to higher plasma concentrations causing higher risk of bleeding [59–61]. This led to three large genotype-guided randomized clinical trials [62–64] that were all published in the same issue of the *New England Journal of Medicine*. To the disappointment of many pharmacogeneticists, the results were conflicting and not convincing. This complicated the clinical implementation of the use of clinical genotype-guided dosing of warfarin. Notably there were marked differences between the studies, especially in regard to the study populations, that could have led to some of the observed variability. It also highlights the difficulty in implementing clinical use of pharmacogenetics. The discussion of genotyping patients prior to treatment with warfarin to implement genotype-guided dosing continues.

Carriers of the *CYP2C9*2* and *CYP2C9*3* alleles also have decreased metabolism of NSAIDs, an effect seen for several NSAIDs [65]. Indeed, carriers of *CYP2C9*2* or *CYP2C9*3* alleles have decreased metabolic activity towards ibuprofen, which is further decreased in individuals also carrying the *CYP2C8*3* allele [66,67]. Individuals homozygous for *CYP2C9*3* have a nine-fold lower apparent oral clearance of meloxicam compared to those with the reference genotype [68]. A less dramatic, but similar trend was shown for celecoxib [69,70]. A serious adverse event to NSAID treatment is gastrointestinal bleeding. In line with pharmacokinetic studies, clinical observational studies showed increased risk of gastrointestinal bleeding among carriers of the *CYP2C9*2* and *CYP2C9*3* alleles [65,71], likely caused by increased plasma levels of NSAIDs.

CYP2C19 comprises only ~3% of the hepatic P450 content. Nonetheless, CYP2C19 is involved in the metabolism of important and widely used drug classes such as proton pump inhibitors (PPI, omeprazole), antiplatelet agents (clopidogrel), and selective serotonin reuptake inhibitors (SSRI, citalopram).

The most relevant and common genetic variants in *CYP2C19* are the poor metabolizing alleles *CYP2C19*2* (rs4244285) and *CYP2C19*3* (rs4986893) and the ultrarapid metabolizing allele *CYP2C19*17* (rs12248560). Clopidogrel is a prodrug transformed to active metabolites by CYP enzymes. Carriers of the poor metabolizing genotypes, *CYP2C19*2/*3*, have markedly reduced activation of clopidogrel, leading to a suppressed protective cardiovascular effect [72–76]. This led to studies trying to increase clopidogrel maintenance dose in poor metabolizers [77] and randomized controlled trials for genotype-guided clopidogrel treatment [78–81]. Strategies varied from dose-adjusting to switching from clopidogrel to prasugrel among poor metabolizers, and most studies were successful in reducing clopidogrel-associated bleeding or similar endpoints. The influence of *CYP2C19* variation on clopidogrel response seems to depend strongly on the indication, as the effect is largest for percutaneous coronary intervention (PCI) and almost absent for atrial fibrillation [82]. The FDA added a boxed warning to the clopidogrel label in 2010 alerting clinicians of the effect of poor metabolizing genetic variation on the response to clopidogrel. As for *CYP2C19*17*, some studies have shown an increase in clopidogrel response [75,83,84], while others did not replicate this association [85–87]. The poor metabolizing variants *CYP2C19*2/*3* have also been linked to reduced omeprazole metabolism [88–90], leading to a higher eradication of gastrointestinal bleeding among poor metabolizers [91,92]. The ultrarapid *CYP2C19*17* allele has also been linked with increased metabolism of omeprazole, although this effect seems to be variable [90,93].

CYP2D6 comprises around 3% of the hepatic CYP content [39], with a large variability in protein expression due to *CYP2D6* genetic variation [94]. Despite having a relatively low expression, CYP2D6 is involved in the metabolism of up to 20% of clinically used drugs and is known for being involved in the metabolism of many psychotropic drugs such as tricyclic antidepressants (TCA, e.g., nortriptyline/imipramine), SSRI (e.g., fluoxetine), and antipsychotics (risperidone). CYP2D6 is also involved in the metabolism of many other drugs, including opioids, stimulants (e.g., amphetamine), and beta-blockers (e.g., metoprolol). The first pharmacokinetic twin studies were performed with nortriptyline, a known CYP2D6 substrate [95,96], and showed that monozygotic twins had very similar plasma concentrations of nortriptyline, while plasma concentrations varied much more among dizygotic twin pairs. This led to the hypothesis that metabolism of drugs by CYP2D6 was strongly genetically linked. Forty years later, we know that genetic variation leads to four different phenotypes; poor metabolizers (PMs) are characterized by low or no expression of CYP2D6 due to null alleles in the *CYP2D6* gene, while ultrarapid metabolizers (UMs) carry multiple copies of the *CYP2D6* gene (up to 13 copies have been observed [97]). CYP2D6 intermediate metabolizers (IMs) carry one null allele and one reference allele, while extensive metabolizers (EMs) carry two copies of the reference allele. PMs and UMs are the most extreme phenotypic outliers, while IMs and EMs are more similar in terms of metabolic capacity. Multiple *CYP2D6* alleles can lead to each of these metabolizer phenotypes; the reader is referred to the PharmGKB website for listings of the various alleles associated with each phenotype.

As CYP2D6 is involved in the metabolism of many frequently used drugs, we have chosen to focus on one group in this chapter; psychotropic drugs. Psychiatric disorders have a high rate of therapeutic failure with up to 30%–50% of patients not responding sufficiently to initial treatment [98]. Twenty-six drugs psychotropic drugs have pharmacogenomic labeling (http://www.fda.gov/drugs/scienceresearch/researchareas/pharmacogenetics/ucm083378.htm), mostly involving *CYP2D6* polymorphisms. A clinical pharmacokinetic study showed a correlation between number of *CYP2D6* active alleles and the pharmacokinetics of the tricyclic antidepressant (TCA) nortriptyline [99]. Decreasing concentrations of nortriptyline were observed with increasing number of *CYP2D6* functional alleles; in contrast, levels of the 10-hydroxy metabolite of nortriptyline were inversely correlated with *CYP2D6* functional alleles. This has been consistently replicated and recently, the NIH-funded Clinical Pharmacogenetics Implementation Consortium (CPIC) published a guideline [100] suggesting that PMs receive a 50% lower initial dose of TCA, while IMs should receive a 25% lower initial dose. Increasing dose in UMs to accommodate the increased metabolic capacity may lead to accumulation of the 10-hydroxy metabolite, which may lead to toxicity, and thus increasing dose for UMs is not warranted if other options are available. Many similar examples have been reported for psychotropic drugs and extend to other types of drugs such as codeine. Codeine is metabolized by CYP2D6 to the active metabolite morphine. A pharmacogenetic study showed that CYP2D6 poor metabolizers had an abolished analgesic effect of codeine due to the prodrug not being converted to morphine by CYP2D6 [101], a finding further supported by the fact that no difference in analgesic effect was observed for morphine. This has since been replicated and CPIC guidelines recommend use of opioids not metabolized by CYP2D6 by individuals with UM and PM phenotypes [102].

CYP2E1 comprises ~15% of the hepatic CYP content and is involved in the metabolism of relatively few clinically used drugs. This enzyme is inducible by ethanol and even moderate exposure leads to rapidly increased expression which is reversible upon withdrawal [103]. The metabolism of the CYP2E1 probe substrate chlorzoxazone indicates relatively low interindividual variability with oral and fractional clearances varying four- to five-fold with slightly higher clearances among men compared to women [104]. The evidence for impact of genetic variants on enzyme function for CYP2E1 is generally underwhelming. Some studies have linked upstream genetic variants with CYP2E1 metabolic capacity or expression, but these have not been consistently replicated [105–108]. There is no current evidence for functionally important variants for drug metabolism, but some variants may be linked with disease susceptibility, such as lung cancer [109].

CYP3 Family

CYP3A4 is highly expressed in the liver (25% of hepatic CYP content) and intestines and is involved in the metabolism of up to 30% of clinically used drugs. Due to the involvement of CYP3A4 in the metabolism of many drugs, genetic variation was expected to have a substantial clinical impact. An early twin study of antipyrine hydroxylation indicated a substantial heritability of CYP3A4 metabolism [110]. However, many recent studies have not been able to readily replicate common variants impacting expression and metabolic capacity of CYP3A4 [111]. A recently described variant, *CYP3A4*22* (rs35599367), was linked to decreased hepatic CYP3A4 expression. Carriers of this variant required a lower dose of the cholesterol-lowering statins simvastatin, atorvastatin and lovastatin [112] indicating a reduced metabolic capacity consistent with the reported reduced expression. This variant has since been linked with decreased metabolism of tacrolicmus [113,114] and exemestane [115] among others.

CYP3A4 transcription is regulated by a number of nuclear receptors such as PXR, PPARα, and many others. Genetic variants in genes encoding nuclear receptors regulating *CYP3A4* transcription may play a role in hepatic expression and the metabolic capacity of the enzyme. Thus, a SNP in PPARα decreased mRNA and protein expression in human livers and reduced atorvastatin hydroxylation in volunteers carrying the variant [116].

CYP3A5 is distinguished from other CYP enzymes in that it is expressed in around 60% of Africans or African Americans, while only 5%–10% of Caucasians express CYP3A5 to an appreciable extent. CYP3A5 is structurally very similar to CYP3A4 as they share around 85% amino acid sequence identity and, thus, a large substrate overlap [117]. Lower concentrations of tacrolimus were observed among CYP3A5 expressors compared to non-expressors, indicating higher metabolic capacity for this drug when CYP3A5 contributes to metabolism [118,119]. A number of reduced function variants for CYP3A5 have been reported. A recent genome-wide association study (GWAS) identified *CYP3A5*3/*6/*7* as risk alleles for lower tacrolimus concentrations [120]. Associations with the *CYP3A5*3* (rs776746) variant have been frequently replicated, and this allele could be an important predictor for CYP3A metabolism among individuals expressing CYP3A5.

Polymorphisms Relevant for Phase II Enzymes

Following modification by Phase I metabolism, drugs are further modified via conjugation with larger molecules such as glutathione and glucuronic acid in Phase II metabolism. This leads to larger, less reactive, more polar and water-soluble drugs and enables elimination via bile/urine. There are a number of enzymes involved in Phase II metabolism, such as UDP-glucuronosyltransferase (UGT) and glutathione S-transferase (GSH).

The largest body of evidence for pharmacogenetic associations with Phase II enzymes regards the family of uridine diphosphate glucuronosyltransferases (UGTs), but recently other enzymes have received increasing attention. Of the UGTs, mainly UGT1 and UGT2 family members are involved in the glucuronidation of xenobiotics.

In the UGT1A family, the most highly expressed enzyme **UGT1A1** is found primarily in the liver and enterocytes. UGT1A1 plays a key role in the elimination of bile acids, a by-product of heme catabolism. The genetic variant *UGT1A1*28* (rs8175347) has been linked with Gilbert syndrome, characterized by mildly increased hyperbilirubinemia but otherwise mostly asymptomatic [121]. This variant has been linked with decreased UGT1A1 transcription causing reduced metabolism of bile acids leading to hyperbilirubinemia [121]. Atazanavir is an antiretroviral drug used to treat HIV and approved in 2008 by the FDA. The drug is generally well tolerated and efficacious but it interferes with bilirubin elimination, and around 40% of treated patients will have ALT/ALAT >2.5 times the upper normal limit [122]. Individuals homozygous for *UGT1A1*28* or *UGT1A1*37* (rs8175347) or rs887829 are at increased risk of bilirubin-associated discontinuation of the drug, which has been estimated at up to 60% [123]. Guidelines for dosing patients with reduced function variants of *UGT1A1* have been made for irinotecan [124,125] and atazanavir [123]. For atazanavir, it is recommended that poor metabolizers should be given another drug if possible, considering the very high likelihood that these patients will develop jaundice.

UGT2B7 has been studied to some extent, but most evidence regarding pharmacogenetic influence is conflicting at this point and there is no clear consensus as to relevant genetic determinants for drugs metabolized by this enzyme. The clinical relevance of any *UGT2B7* alleles will not be clear until further study.

Carboxylesterase (CES) 1 and 2 are involved in the hydrolysis of ester or amide bonds of xenobiotic compounds and endogenous substances. **CES1** is mainly expressed in the liver and reported to be 20% more highly expressed in females [126]. CES1 is implicated in the metabolism of widely used drugs such as dabigatran, methylphenidate, and clopidogrel [127]. A number of functional genetic variants in *CES1* have been linked to altered response of drugs [128], but the most consistently replicated variant is rs71647871, a non-synonymous SNP (428G>A, Gly143Glu) in the coding region of *CES1* found at low frequency in all populations (MAF <5%) [128]. This variant was initially shown to decrease the metabolism of methylphenidate in a carrier of the variant and to completely prevent metabolism in vitro [129], leading to a three-fold increase in area under the plasma-concentration curve and maximal concentration of methylphenidate. The variant has since been linked with decreased metabolism of oseltamivir [126,130], dabigatran [131], clopidogrel [132,133], and enalapril [134]. Due to the low frequency of this variant, the population effect may not be overwhelming, although this might explain variation on an individual basis.

Thiopurines are a group of drugs used as immunosuppressants or in the treatment of cancers. The group consists of mercaptopurine, azathioprine, and thioguanine that are all metabolized to some extent via thiopurine methyltransferase (TPMT). **TPMT** is polymorphic and three SNPs account for approximately 90% of the loss-of-function variation [135,136]. These loss-of-function variants lead to reduced metabolism of thiopurines, causing accumulation of the parent compound or toxic metabolites formed through secondary pathways. Carriers of two loss-of-function alleles have a 100% risk of developing severe dose-dependent myelosuppression at normal doses of mercaptopurine or azathioprine, while only ~50% of patients with one loss-of-function allele will tolerate normal doses [137–139]. A recent GWAS study showed that only variants in the *TPMT* gene were significant for activity and mercaptopurine tolerance, leading the authors to conclude that TPMT activity is a monogenic pharmacogenomic trait [140]. However, other genes may play a role in this toxicity, as variants in *NUDT15* have recently been associated with thiopurine toxicity, particularly in Asian populations [141–143]. A CPIC genotype-guided dosing algorithm [144] suggests that thiopurine dose should be reduced 10-fold and changed from daily dosing to three times weekly among individuals carrying two loss-of-function *TPMT* alleles. For carriers of one loss-of-function *TPMT* allele, the dose should be reduced by 30%–70% and titrated according to tolerance, while allowing time to reach steady-state before the next dose adjustment [144].

Polymorphisms Relevant for Drug Toxicity

Drugs may cause allergic reactions, which is a major clinical problem that may lead to an array of symptoms. Abacavir is an antiretroviral drug used in the treatment of HIV and is generally well tolerated. However, approximately 5%–8% of patients treated with abacavir experience hypersensitivity within six weeks of initiating treatment, which is characterized either clinically (presence of at least two of the following symptoms: fever, rash, gastrointestinal disturbance, fatigue, coughing, and/or dyspnea) or immunologically (skin-patch) and can be fatal [145]. In 2002, two studies reported that carriers of *HLA-B*57:01* [146,147] had markedly increased risk of abacavir hypersensitivity. These interesting results were replicated consistently in other ethnic groups in retrospective studies and led to a genotype-guided double-blind randomized prospective study (PREDICT-1, [148]). No immunologically confirmed cases of abacavir hypersensitivity reactions were observed among the patients who were screened for *HLA-B*57:01* vs. an incidence of 2.7% of the patients who were not screened [148]. This led to several guidelines suggesting that genetic testing for *HLA-B*57:01* should be performed prior to initiating abacavir treatment among naïve patients, and abacavir use should be avoided among carriers of the allele [149]. *HLA-B* encodes a class I human leukocyte antigen (HLA) molecule that is involved in presenting peptides to immune cells. The exact mechanism that increases the risk of abacavir hypersensitivity among carriers of *HLA-B*57:01* is not clear.

Skin hypersensitivity reactions are another example of allergic drug reactions. The symptoms range from mild eczema/rash to severe life-threatening disorders, such as Stevens-Johnson syndrome (SJS) or toxic epidermal necrolysis (TEN). The latter are characterized by skin cell death causing the epidermis to separate from the dermis, which results in dehydration and in serious cases death. If 2%–10% of the body surface is involved, it is characterized as SJS, and if more than 30% is involved, it is characterized as TEN.

Allopurinol is used in the treatment of gout as an inhibitor of xanthine oxidase, a crucial enzyme in the formation of uric acid. While generally well tolerated, allopurinol provokes skin-related hypersensitivity reactions like those described for abacavir. While rare (0.1%–0.4%), the mortality rate is up to 25%, and tools to predict this serious adverse event are warranted. Another *HLA-B* genotype, **58:01*, was reported to be significantly correlated with severe cutaneous adverse reactions (including SJS/TEN) in a Taiwan Han-Chinese population [150]. All individuals who experienced skin hypersensitivity symptoms carried the genotype, while the frequency was 15%–20% among tolerant controls and the background population. Despite the side effect only appearing among individuals with the variant, there was still a substantial number of patients with the variant tolerating treatment. This finding has since been replicated in various populations, leading to recommendations that patients with known *HLA-B*58:01* genotype be treated with other drugs due to an increased risk of allopurinol induced skin hypersensitivity reactions [151].

These are some examples of recent discoveries of pharmacogenetic prediction of side effects. This is not only relevant for patients being treated with these drugs, but also for drug development, as this knowledge may help predict these types of side effects among newly developed drugs. This may help reduce the rate of withdrawal of new drugs that may cause rare, but serious adverse events. Pharmacogenetic research regarding drug hypersensitivity is still in the early stages. It is complicated by the rarity and classification of side effects, but recent findings have given important insight into mechanisms that were previously largely unknown. This type of pharmacogenetic research into type II adverse events holds much promise for the future.

Perspectives

In this chapter, we have focused on pharmacogenetic variants relevant for drug metabolism and toxicity. It is important to note that the frequency of genetic variants differs significantly between populations. For example, the frequency of CYP2D6 UMs is very low in East Asian populations, while up to 10% of Oceanic populations are UMs. This also means that genetic variants relevant in an African population may not extend to Asian or Caucasian populations. For this reason, replication in different ethnic cohorts is very important in pharmacogenetics.

Due to the exploratory nature and relatively small sample size in many pharmacogenetic studies, treating physicians require a higher grade of evidence before implementing the obtained knowledge into clinical practice. This includes randomized controlled trials and pharmacoeconomic evaluation to take both efficacy as well as economic factors into account before routine implementation of genotyping in clinical practice. Many investigators are currently working on projects to improve evidence of patient benefits and to evaluate economic perspectives of pharmacogenetic application in the clinic.

Another recurring problem in pharmacogenetic research is the lack of reproducibility, likely caused by many factors. First, pharmacokinetic and pharmacodynamic variability is very complex. A full understanding of this variability is required in order to interpret study results. Performing pharmacogenetic studies in populations with multiple comorbidities and concomitant use of drugs will add to variability and mask pharmacogenetic signals. Furthermore, clinical studies have historically focused on the effect of single variants. While this is easier, many variants often need to be considered in relation to the full genotype of the patient as some variants have opposing or synergistic effects leading to misinterpretation when only looking at a single variant. New evidence is constantly emerging regarding factors important in drug variability, such as epigenetics and the microbiome, which may also play a crucial role in inter-individual variability in drug response and toxicity. This highlights the need for tools that are able to convert the noise into relevant signals, considering all relevant factors to account for differences in drug metabolism and toxicity. It appears likely that the future for pharmacogenomics will consist of more complex treatment algorithms as our knowledge expands, and that these will integrate other types of information besides just the genetics of an individual. While a substantial amount of pharmacogenetic research has already been undertaken, it appears that the most widely used sentence in research, "More research in this area is warranted," still applies.

REFERENCES

1. Cerny MA. Prevalence of non–cytochrome P450–mediated metabolism in food and drug administration–approved oral and intravenous drugs: 2006–2015. *Drug Metab Dispos*. 2016;44(8):1246–1252.
2. Zanger UM, Schwab M. Cytochrome P450 enzymes in drug metabolism: Regulation of gene expression, enzyme activities, and impact of genetic variation. *Pharmacol Ther*. 2013;138(1):103–141.
3. Shimada T, Yamazaki H, Mimura M, Inui Y, Guengerich FP. Interindividual variations in human liver cytochrome P-450 enzymes involved in the oxidation of drugs, carcinogens and toxic chemicals: studies with liver microsomes of 30 Japanese and 30 Caucasians. *J Pharmacol Exp Ther*. 1994;270(1):414–423.
4. Butler MA, Iwasaki M, Guengerich FP, Kadlubar FF. Human cytochrome P-450PA (P-450IA2), the phenacetin O-deethylase, is primarily responsible for the hepatic 3-demethylation of caffeine and N-oxidation of carcinogenic arylamines. *Proc Natl Acad Sci USA*. 1989;86(20):7696–700.
5. Rasmussen BB, Brix TH, Kyvik KO, Brøsen K. The interindividual differences in the 3-demthylation of caffeine alias CYP1A2 is determined by both genetic and environmental factors. *Pharmacogenetics*. 2002;12(6):473–478.
6. Sachse C, Brockmöller J, Bauer S, Roots I. Functional significance of a C-->A polymorphism in intron 1 of the cytochrome P450 CYP1A2 gene tested with caffeine. *Br J Clin Pharmacol*. 1999;47(4):445–449.
7. Nordmark A, Lundgren S, Ask B, Granath F, Rane A. The effect of the CYP1A2*1F mutation on CYP1A2 inducibility in pregnant women. *Br J Clin Pharmacol*. 2002;54(5):504–510.
8. Aklillu E, Carrillo JA, Makonnen E, Hellman K, Pitarque M, Bertilsson L, Ingelman-Sundberg M. Genetic polymorphism of CYP1A2 in ethiopians affecting induction and expression: Characterization of novel haplotypes with single-nucleotide polymorphisms in intron 1. *Mol Pharmacol*. 2003;64(3):659–669.
9. Ozdemir V, Kalow W, Okey AB, Lam MS, Albers LJ, Reist C, Fourie J, Posner P, Collins EJ, Roy R. Treatment-resistance to clozapine in association with ultrarapid CYP1A2 activity and the C-->A polymorphism in intron 1 of the CYP1A2 gene: Effect of grapefruit juice and low-dose fluvoxamine. *J Clin Psychopharmacol*. 2001;21(6):603–607.
10. Eap CB, Bender S, Jaquenoud Sirot E, Cucchia G, Jonzier-Perey M, Baumann P, Allorge D, Broly F. Nonresponse to clozapine and ultrarapid CYP1A2 activity: Clinical data and analysis of CYP1A2 gene. *J Clin Psychopharmacol*. 2004;24(2):214–219.
11. Melkersson KI, Scordo MG, Gunes A, Dahl M-L. Impact of CYP1A2 and CYP2D6 polymorphisms on drug metabolism and on insulin and lipid elevations and insulin resistance in clozapine-treated patients. *J Clin Psychiatry*. 2007;68(5):697–704.
12. Laika B, Leucht S, Heres S, Schneider H, Steimer W. Pharmacogenetics and olanzapine treatment: CYP1A2*1F and serotonergic polymorphisms influence therapeutic outcome. *Pharmacogenomics J*. 2010;10(1):20–29.

13. Tay JKX, Tan CH, Chong S-A, Tan E-C. Functional polymorphisms of the cytochrome P450 1A2 (CYP1A2) gene and prolonged QTc interval in schizophrenia. *Prog Neuropsychopharmacol Biol Psychiatry*. 2007;31(6):1297–1302.

14. Basile VS, Ozdemir V, Masellis M, Walker ML, Meltzer HY, Lieberman JA, Potkin SG, Alva G, Kalow W, Macciardi FM, Kennedy JL. A functional polymorphism of the cytochrome P450 1A2 (CYP1A2) gene: Association with tardive dyskinesia in schizophrenia. *Mol Psychiatry*. 2000;5(4):410–417.

15. Fu Y, Fan C, Deng H, Hu S, Lv D, Li L, Wang J, Lu X. Association of CYP2D6 and CYP1A2 gene polymorphism with tardive dyskinesia in Chinese schizophrenic patients. *Acta Pharmacol Sin*. 2006;27(3):328–332.

16. Schulze TG, Schumacher J, Müller DJ, Krauss H, Alfter D, Maroldt A, Ahle G et al. Lack of association between a functional polymorphism of the cytochrome P450 1A2 (CYP1A2) gene and tardive dyskinesia in schizophrenia. *Am J Med Genet*. 2001;105(6):498–501.

17. Chong S-A, Tan E-C, Tan CH. Smoking and tardive dyskinesia: Lack of involvement of the CYP1A2 gene. *J Psychiatry Neurosci*. 2003;28(3):185–189.

18. Bohanec Grabar P, Rozman B, Tomsic M, Suput D, Logar D, Dolzan V. Genetic polymorphism of CYP1A2 and the toxicity of leflunomide treatment in rheumatoid arthritis patients. *Eur J Clin Pharmacol*. 2008;64(9):871–876.

19. Soukup T, Dosedel M, Nekvindova J, Toms J, Vlcek J, Pavek P. Genetic polymorphisms in metabolic pathways of leflunomide in the treatment of rheumatoid arthritis. *Clin Exp Rheumatol*. 2015;33(3):426–432.

20. Hopkins AM, Wiese MD, Proudman SM, O'Doherty CE, Upton RN, Foster DJR. Genetic polymorphism of CYP1A2 but not total or free teriflunomide concentrations is associated with leflunomide cessation in rheumatoid arthritis. *Br J Clin Pharmacol*. 2016;81(1):113–123.

21. Hofmann MH, Blievernicht JK, Klein K, Saussele T, Schaeffeler E, Schwab M, Zanger UM. Aberrant splicing caused by single nucleotide polymorphism c.516G>T [Q172H], a marker of CYP2B6*6, is responsible for decreased expression and activity of CYP2B6 in liver. *J Pharmacol Exp Ther*. 2008;325(1):284–292.

22. Gervot L, Rochat B, Gautier JC, Bohnenstengel F, Kroemer H, de Berardinis V, Martin H, Beaune P, de Waziers I. Human CYP2B6: Expression, inducibility and catalytic activities. *Pharmacogenetics*. 1999;9(3):295–306.

23. Desta Z, Saussele T, Ward B, Blievernicht J, Li L, Klein K, Flockhart DA, Zanger UM. Impact of CYP2B6 polymorphism on hepatic efavirenz metabolism in vitro. *Pharmacogenomics*. 2007;8(6):547–558.

24. Tsuchiya K, Gatanaga H, Tachikawa N, Teruya K, Kikuchi Y, Yoshino M, Kuwahara T, Shirasaka T, Kimura S, Oka S. Homozygous CYP2B6*6 (Q172H and K262R) correlates with high plasma efavirenz concentrations in HIV-1 patients treated with standard efavirenz-containing regimens. *Biochem Biophys Res Commun*. 2004;319(4):1322–1326.

25. Bienczak A, Cook A, Wiesner L, Olagunju A, Mulenga V, Kityo C, Kekitiinwa A et al. The impact of genetic polymorphisms on the pharmacokinetics of efavirenz in African children. *Br J Clin Pharmacol*. 2016;82(1):185–198.

26. Oluka MN, Okalebo FA, Guantai AN, McClelland RS, Graham SM. Cytochrome P450 2B6 genetic variants are associated with plasma nevirapine levels and clinical response in HIV-1 infected Kenyan women: A prospective cohort study. *AIDS Res Ther*. 2015;12:10.

27. Sinxadi PZ, Leger PD, McIlleron HM, Smith PJ, Dave JA, Levitt NS, Maartens G, Haas DW. Pharmacogenetics of plasma efavirenz exposure in HIV-infected adults and children in South Africa. *Br J Clin Pharmacol*. 2015;80(1):146–156.

28. Haas DW, Ribaudo HJ, Kim RB, Tierney C, Wilkinson GR, Gulick RM, Clifford DB, Hulgan T, Marzolini C, Acosta EP. Pharmacogenetics of efavirenz and central nervous system side effects: An Adult AIDS Clinical Trials Group study. *AIDS Lond Engl*. 2004;18(18):2391–2400.

29. Lubomirov R, Colombo S, di Iulio J, Ledergerber B, Martinez R, Cavassini M, Hirschel B et al. Association of pharmacogenetic markers with premature discontinuation of first-line anti-HIV therapy: An observational cohort study. *J Infect Dis*. 2011;203(2):246–257.

30. Wyen C, Hendra H, Siccardi M, Platten M, Jaeger H, Harrer T, Esser S et al. German Competence Network for HIV/AIDS Coordinators. Cytochrome P450 2B6 (CYP2B6) and constitutive androstane receptor (CAR) polymorphisms are associated with early discontinuation of efavirenz-containing regimens. *J Antimicrob Chemother*. 2011;66(9):2092–2098.

31. Gatanaga H, Hayashida T, Tsuchiya K, Yoshino M, Kuwahara T, Tsukada H, Fujimoto K et al. Successful efavirenz dose reduction in HIV type 1-infected individuals with cytochrome P450 2B6*6 and *26. *Clin Infect Dis Off Publ Infect Dis Soc Am*. 2007;45(9):1230–1237.

32. Penzak SR, Kabuye G, Mugyenyi P, Mbamanya F, Natarajan V, Alfaro RM, Kityo C, Formentini E, Masur H. Cytochrome P450 2B6 (CYP2B6) G516T influences nevirapine plasma concentrations in HIV-infected patients in Uganda. *HIV Med*. 2007;8(2):86–91.

33. Mahungu T, Smith C, Turner F, Egan D, Youle M, Johnson M, Khoo S, Back D, Owen A. Cytochrome P450 2B6 516G-->T is associated with plasma concentrations of nevirapine at both 200 mg twice daily and 400 mg once daily in an ethnically diverse population. *HIV Med*. 2009;10(5):310–317.

34. Ciccacci C, Di Fusco D, Marazzi MC, Zimba I, Erba F, Novelli G, Palombi L, Borgiani P, Liotta G. Association between CYP2B6 polymorphisms and Nevirapine-induced SJS/TEN: A pharmacogenetics study. *Eur J Clin Pharmacol*. 2013;69(11):1909–1916.

35. Kharasch ED, Regina KJ, Blood J, Friedel C. Methadone pharmacogenetics: CYP2B6 polymorphisms determine plasma concentrations, clearance, and metabolism. *Anesthesiology*. 2015;123(5):1142–1153.

36. Xie H, Griskevicius L, Ståhle L, Hassan Z, Yasar U, Rane A, Broberg U, Kimby E, Hassan M. Pharmacogenetics of cyclophosphamide in patients with hematological malignancies. *Eur J Pharm Sci Off J Eur Fed Pharm Sci*. 2006;27(1):54–61.

37. Nakajima M, Komagata S, Fujiki Y, Kanada Y, Ebi H, Itoh K, Mukai H, Yokoi T, Minami H. Genetic polymorphisms of CYP2B6 affect the pharmacokinetics/pharmacodynamics of cyclophosphamide in Japanese cancer patients. *Pharmacogenet Genomics*. 2007;17(6):431–445.

38. Helsby NA, Hui C-Y, Goldthorpe MA, Coller JK, Soh MC, Gow PJ, De Zoysa JZ, Tingle MD. The combined impact of CYP2C19 and CYP2B6 pharmacogenetics on cyclophosphamide bioactivation. *Br J Clin Pharmacol*. 2010;70(6):844–853.

39. Achour B, Barber J, Rostami-Hodjegan A. Expression of hepatic drug-metabolizing cytochrome P450 enzymes and their intercorrelations: A meta-analysis. *Drug Metab Dispos*. 2014;42(8):1349–1356.

40. Niemi M, Leathart JB, Neuvonen M, Backman JT, Daly AK, Neuvonen PJ. Polymorphism in CYP2C8 is associated with reduced plasma concentrations of repaglinide. *Clin Pharmacol Ther*. 2003;74(4):380–387.

41. Bidstrup TB, Damkier P, Olsen AK, Ekblom M, Karlsson A, Brøsen K. The impact of CYP2C8 polymorphism and grapefruit juice on the pharmacokinetics of repaglinide. *Br J Clin Pharmacol*. 2006;61(1):49–57.

42. Tomalik-Scharte D, Fuhr U, Hellmich M, Frank D, Doroshyenko O, Jetter A, Stingl JC. Effect of the CYP2C8 genotype on the pharmacokinetics and pharmacodynamics of repaglinide. *Drug Metab Dispos Biol Fate Chem*. 2011;39(5):927–932.

43. Kirchheiner J, Thomas S, Bauer S, Tomalik-Scharte D, Hering U, Doroshyenko O, Jetter A et al. Pharmacokinetics and pharmacodynamics of rosiglitazone in relation to CYP2C8 genotype. *Clin Pharmacol Ther*. 2006;80(6):657–667.

44. Tornio A, Niemi M, Neuvonen PJ, Backman JT. Trimethoprim and the CYP2C8*3 allele have opposite effects on the pharmacokinetics of pioglitazone. *Drug Metab Dispos Biol Fate Chem*. 2008;36(1):73–80.

45. Aquilante CL, Bushman LR, Knutsen SD, Burt LE, Rome LC, Kosmiski LA. Influence of SLCO1B1 and CYP2C8 gene polymorphisms on rosiglitazone pharmacokinetics in healthy volunteers. *Hum Genomics*. 2008;3(1):7–16.

46. Aquilante CL, Kosmiski LA, Bourne DWA, Bushman LR, Daily EB, Hammond KP, Hopley CW et al. Impact of the CYP2C8*3 polymorphism on the drug-drug interaction between gemfibrozil and pioglitazone. *Br J Clin Pharmacol*. 2013;75(1):217–226.

47. Stage TB, Christensen MMH, Feddersen S, Beck-Nielsen H, Brøsen K. The role of genetic variants in CYP2C8, LPIN1, PPARGC1A and PPARγ on the trough steady-state plasma concentrations of rosiglitazone and on glycosylated haemoglobin A1c in type 2 diabetes. *Pharmacogenet Genomics*. 2013;23(4):219–227.

48. Dawed AY, Donnelly L, Tavendale R, Carr F, Leese G, Palmer CNA, Pearson ER, Zhou K. CYP2C8 and SLCO1B1 variants and therapeutic response to thiazolidinediones in patients with Type 2 diabetes. *Diabetes Care*. 2016:dc152464.

49. Henningsson A, Marsh S, Loos WJ, Karlsson MO, Garsa A, Mross K, Mielke S et al. Association of CYP2C8, CYP3A4, CYP3A5, and ABCB1 polymorphisms with the pharmacokinetics of paclitaxel. *Clin Cancer Res Off J Am Assoc Cancer Res*. 2005;11(22):8097–8104.

50. Bergmann TK, Brasch-Andersen C, Gréen H, Mirza M, Pedersen RS, Nielsen F, Skougaard K et al. Impact of CYP2C8*3 on paclitaxel clearance: A population pharmacokinetic and pharmacogenomic study in 93 patients with ovarian cancer. *Pharmacogenomics J.* 2011;11(2):113–120.

51. Leskelä S, Jara C, Leandro-García LJ, Martínez A, García-Donas J, Hernando S, Hurtado A et al. Polymorphisms in cytochromes P450 2C8 and 3A5 are associated with paclitaxel neurotoxicity. *Pharmacogenomics J.* 2011;11(2):121–129.

52. Hertz DL, Motsinger-Reif AA, Drobish A, Winham SJ, McLeod HL, Carey LA, Dees EC. CYP2C8*3 predicts benefit/risk profile in breast cancer patients receiving neoadjuvant paclitaxel. *Breast Cancer Res Treat.* 2012;134(1):401–410.

53. Hertz DL, Roy S, Jack J, Motsinger-Reif AA, Drobish A, Clark LS, Carey LA, Dees EC, McLeod HL. Genetic heterogeneity beyond CYP2C8*3 does not explain differential sensitivity to paclitaxel-induced neuropathy. *Breast Cancer Res Treat.* 2014;145(1):245–254.

54. Lee M-Y, Apellániz Ruiz M, Johansson I, Vikingsson S, Bergmann TK, Brøsen K, Green H, Rodríguez-Antona C, Ingelman-Sundberg M. Role of cytochrome P450 2C8*3 (CYP2C8*3) in paclitaxel metabolism and paclitaxel-induced neurotoxicity. *Pharmacogenomics.* 2015;16(9):929–937.

55. Adjei GO, Kristensen K, Goka BQ, Hoegberg LCG, Alifrangis M, Rodrigues OP, Kurtzhals JAL. Effect of concomitant artesunate administration and cytochrome P4502C8 polymorphisms on the pharmacokinetics of amodiaquine in ghanaian children with uncomplicated malaria. *Antimicrob Agents Chemother.* 2008;52(12):4400–4406.

56. Cavaco I, Mårtensson A, Fröberg G, Msellem M, Björkman A, Gil JP. CYP2C8 status of patients with malaria influences selection of Plasmodium falciparum pfmdr1 alleles after amodiaquine-artesunate treatment. *J Infect Dis.* 2013;207(4):687–688.

57. Aquilante CL, Wempe MF, Spencer SH, Kosmiski LA, Predhomme JA, Sidhom MS. Influence of CYP2C8*2 on the pharmacokinetics of pioglitazone in healthy African-American volunteers. *Pharmacotherapy.* 2013;33(9):1000–1007.

58. Paganotti GM, Gallo BC, Verra F, Sirima BS, Nebié I, Diarra A, Coluzzi M, Modiano D. Human genetic variation is associated with Plasmodium falciparum drug resistance. *J Infect Dis.* 2011;204(11):1772–1778.

59. Rettie AE, Wienkers LC, Gonzalez FJ, Trager WF, Korzekwa KR. Impaired (S)-warfarin metabolism catalysed by the R144C allelic variant of CYP2C9. *Pharmacogenetics.* 1994;4(1):39–42.

60. Aithal GP, Day CP, Kesteven PJ, Daly AK. Association of polymorphisms in the cytochrome P450 CYP2C9 with warfarin dose requirement and risk of bleeding complications. *Lancet Lond Engl.* 1999;353(9154):717–719.

61. Higashi MK, Veenstra DL, Kondo LM, Wittkowsky AK, Srinouanprachanh SL, Farin FM, Rettie AE. Association between CYP2C9 genetic variants and anticoagulation-related outcomes during warfarin therapy. *JAMA.* 2002;287(13):1690–1698.

62. Pirmohamed M, Burnside G, Eriksson N, Jorgensen AL, Toh CH, Nicholson T, Kesteven P et al. A randomized trial of genotype-guided dosing of warfarin. *N Engl J Med.* 2013;369(24):2294–2303.

63. Verhoef TI, Ragia G, de Boer A, Barallon R, Kolovou G, Kolovou V, Konstantinides S et al. A randomized trial of genotype-guided dosing of acenocoumarol and phenprocoumon. *N Engl J Med.* 2013;369(24):2304–2312.

64. Kimmel SE, French B, Kasner SE, Johnson JA, Anderson JL, Gage BF, Rosenberg YD et al. A Pharmacogenetic versus a clinical algorithm for warfarin dosing. *N Engl J Med.* 2013;369(24):2283–2293.

65. Agúndez JAG, García-Martín E, Martínez C. Genetically based impairment in CYP2C8- and CYP2C9-dependent NSAID metabolism as a risk factor for gastrointestinal bleeding: Is a combination of pharmacogenomics and metabolomics required to improve personalized medicine? *Expert Opin Drug Metab Toxicol.* 2009;5(6):607–620.

66. García-Martín E, Martínez C, Tabarés B, Frías J, Agúndez JAG. Interindividual variability in ibuprofen pharmacokinetics is related to interaction of cytochrome P450 2C8 and 2C9 amino acid polymorphisms. *Clin Pharmacol Ther.* 2004;76(2):119–127.

67. Karaźniewicz-łada M, łuczak M, Gł´owka F. Pharmacokinetic studies of enantiomers of ibuprofen and its chiral metabolites in humans with different variants of genes coding CYP2C8 and CYP2C9 isoenzymes. *Xenobiotica.* 2009;39(6):476–485.

68. Lee H-I, Bae J-W, Choi C-I, Lee Y-J, Byeon J-Y, Jang C-G, Lee S-Y. Strongly increased exposure of meloxicam in CYP2C9*3/*3 individuals. *Pharmacogenet Genomics.* 2014;24(2):113–117.

69. Kirchheiner J, Störmer E, Meisel C, Steinbach N, Roots I, Brockmöller J. Influence of CYP2C9 genetic polymorphisms on pharmacokinetics of celecoxib and its metabolites. *Pharmacogenetics.* 2003;13(8):473–480.

70. Liu R, Gong C, Tao L, Yang W, Zheng X, Ma P, Ding L. Influence of genetic polymorphisms on the pharmacokinetics of celecoxib and its two main metabolites in healthy chinese subjects. *Eur J Pharm Sci Off J Eur Fed Pharm Sci.* 2015;79:13–19.

71. Blanco G, Martínez C, Ladero JM, Garcia-Martin E, Taxonera C, Gamito FG, Diaz-Rubio M, Agundez JAG. Interaction of CYP2C8 and CYP2C9 genotypes modifies the risk for nonsteroidal anti-inflammatory drugs-related acute gastrointestinal bleeding. *Pharmacogenet Genomics.* 2008;18(1):37–43.

72. Brandt JT, Close SL, Iturria SJ, Payne CD, Farid NA, Ernest CS, Lachno DR, Salazar D, Winters KJ. Common polymorphisms of CYP2C19 and CYP2C9 affect the pharmacokinetic and pharmacodynamic response to clopidogrel but not prasugrel. *J Thromb Haemost JTH.* 2007;5(12):2429–2436.

73. Kim KA, Park PW, Hong SJ, Park J-Y. The effect of CYP2C19 polymorphism on the pharmacokinetics and pharmacodynamics of clopidogrel: A possible mechanism for clopidogrel resistance. *Clin Pharmacol Ther.* 2008;84(2):236–242.

74. Umemura K, Furuta T, Kondo K. The common gene variants of CYP2C19 affect pharmacokinetics and pharmacodynamics in an active metabolite of clopidogrel in healthy subjects. *J Thromb Haemost JTH.* 2008;6(8):1439–1441.

75. Mega JL, Close SL, Wiviott SD, Shen L, Hockett RD, Brandt JT, Walker JR, Antman EM, Macias W, Braunwald E, Sabatine MS. Cytochrome p-450 polymorphisms and response to clopidogrel. *N Engl J Med.* 2009;360(4):354–362.

76. Collet J-P, Hulot J-S, Pena A, Villard E, Esteve J-B, Silvain J, Payot L, Brugier D, Cayla G, Beygui F, Bensimon G, Funck-Brentano C, Montalescot G. Cytochrome P450 2C19 polymorphism in young patients treated with clopidogrel after myocardial infarction: a cohort study. *Lancet Lond Engl.* 2009 24;373(9660):309–317.

77. Collet J-P, Hulot J-S, Anzaha G, Pena A, Chastre T, Caron C, Silvain J et al. High doses of clopidogrel to overcome genetic resistance: The randomized crossover CLOVIS-2 (Clopidogrel and Response Variability Investigation Study 2). *JACC Cardiovasc Interv.* 2011;4(4):392–402.

78. Roberts JD, Wells GA, Le May MR, Labinaz M, Glover C, Froeschl M, Dick A et al. Point-of-care genetic testing for personalisation of antiplatelet treatment (RAPID GENE): A prospective, randomised, proof-of-concept trial. *Lancet Lond Engl.* 2012;379(9827):1705–1711.

79. Ahn SG, Yoon J, Kim J, Uh Y, Kim KM, Lee JH, Lee J-W et al. Genotype- and phenotype-directed personalization of antiplatelet treatment in patients with non-ST elevation acute coronary syndromes undergoing coronary stenting. *Korean Circ J.* 2013;43(8):541–549.

80. Xie X, Ma Y-T, Yang Y-N, Li X-M, Zheng Y-Y, Ma X, Fu Z-Y et al. Personalized antiplatelet therapy according to CYP2C19 genotype after percutaneous coronary intervention: A randomized control trial. *Int J Cardiol.* 2013;168(4):3736–3740.

81. So DYF, Wells GA, McPherson R, Labinaz M, Le May MR, Glover C, Dick AJ et al. A prospective randomized evaluation of a pharmacogenomic approach to antiplatelet therapy among patients with ST-elevation myocardial infarction: The RAPID STEMI study. *Pharmacogenomics J.* 2016;16(1):71–78.

82. Paré G, Mehta SR, Yusuf S, Anand SS, Connolly SJ, Hirsh J, Simonsen K, Bhatt DL, Fox KAA, Eikelboom JW. Effects of CYP2C19 genotype on outcomes of clopidogrel treatment. *N Engl J Med.* 2010;363(18):1704–1714.

83. Frere C, Cuisset T, Morange P-E, Quilici J, Camoin-Jau L, Saut N, Faille D, Lambert M, Juhan-Vague I, Bonnet J-L, Alessi M-C. Effect of cytochrome p450 polymorphisms on platelet reactivity after treatment with clopidogrel in acute coronary syndrome. *Am J Cardiol.* 2008;101(8):1088–1093.

84. Sibbing D, Gebhard D, Koch W, Braun S, Stegherr J, Morath T, Von Beckerath N, Mehilli J, Schömig A, Schuster T, Kastrati A. Isolated and interactive impact of common CYP2C19 genetic variants on the antiplatelet effect of chronic clopidogrel therapy. *J Thromb Haemost JTH.* 2010;8(8):1685–1693.

85. Simon T, Verstuyft C, Mary-Krause M, Quteineh L, Drouet E, Méneveau N, Steg PG et al. Genetic determinants of response to clopidogrel and cardiovascular events. *N Engl J Med.* 2009;360(4):363–375.

86. Sorich MJ, Polasek TM, Wiese MD. Systematic review and meta-analysis of the association between cytochrome P450 2C19 genotype and bleeding. *Thromb Haemost.* 2012;108(1):199–200.

87. Lewis JP, Stephens SH, Horenstein RB, O'Connell JR, Ryan K, Peer CJ, Figg WD et al. The CYP2C19*17 variant is not independently associated with clopidogrel response. *J Thromb Haemost JTH.* 2013;11(9):1640–1646.
88. Ieiri I, Kubota T, Urae A, Kimura M, Wada Y, Mamiya K, Yoshioka S et al. Pharmacokinetics of omeprazole (a substrate of CYP2C19) and comparison with two mutant alleles, C gamma P2C19m1 in exon 5 and C gamma P2C19m2 in exon 4, in Japanese subjects. *Clin Pharmacol Ther.* 1996;59(6):647–653.
89. Qiao H-L, Hu Y-R, Tian X, Jia L-J, Gao N, Zhang L-R, Guo Y-Z. Pharmacokinetics of three proton pump inhibitors in Chinese subjects in relation to the CYP2C19 genotype. *Eur J Clin Pharmacol.* 2006;62(2):107–112.
90. Román M, Ochoa D, Sánchez-Rojas SD, Talegón M, Prieto-Pérez R, Rivas Â, Abad-Santos F, Cabaleiro T. Evaluation of the relationship between polymorphisms in CYP2C19 and the pharmacokinetics of omeprazole, pantoprazole and rabeprazole. *Pharmacogenomics.* 2014;15(15):1893–1901.
91. Tanigawara Y, Aoyama N, Kita T, Shirakawa K, Komada F, Kasuga M, Okumura K. CYP2C19 genotype-related efficacy of omeprazole for the treatment of infection caused by Helicobacter pylori. *Clin Pharmacol Ther.* 1999;66(5):528–534.
92. Kurzawski M, Gawrońska-Szklarz B, Wrześniewska J, Siuda A, Starzyńska T, Droździk M. Effect of CYP2C19*17 gene variant on helicobacter pylori eradication in peptic ulcer patients. *Eur J Clin Pharmacol.* 2006;62(10):877–880.
93. Sim SC, Risinger C, Dahl M-L, Aklillu E, Christensen M, Bertilsson L, Ingelman-Sundberg M. A common novel CYP2C19 gene variant causes ultrarapid drug metabolism relevant for the drug response to proton pump inhibitors and antidepressants. *Clin Pharmacol Ther.* 2006;79(1):103–113.
94. Zanger UM, Fischer J, Raimundo S, Stüven T, Evert BO, Schwab M, Eichelbaum M. Comprehensive analysis of the genetic factors determining expression and function of hepatic CYP2D6. *Pharmacogenetics.* 2001;11(7):573–585.
95. Alexanderson B, Evans DA, Sjöqvist F. Steady-state plasma levels of nortriptyline in twins: Influence of genetic factors and drug therapy. *Br Med J.* 1969;4(5686):764–768.
96. Alexanderson B. Prediction of steady-state plasma levels of nortriptyline from single oral dose kinetics: A study in twins. *Eur J Clin Pharmacol.* 1973;6(1):44–53.
97. Johansson I, Lundqvist E, Bertilsson L, Dahl ML, Sjöqvist F, Ingelman-Sundberg M. Inherited amplification of an active gene in the cytochrome P450 CYP2D locus as a cause of ultrarapid metabolism of debrisoquine. *Proc Natl Acad Sci USA.* 1993;90(24):11825–11829.
98. Thase ME. Achieving remission and managing relapse in depression. *J Clin Psychiatry.* 2003;64 (Suppl 18):3–7.
99. Dalén P, Dahl ML, Bernal Ruiz ML, Nordin J, Bertilsson L. 10-Hydroxylation of nortriptyline in white persons with 0, 1, 2, 3, and 13 functional CYP2D6 genes. *Clin Pharmacol Ther.* 1998;63(4):444–452.
100. Hicks JK, Swen JJ, Thorn CF, Sangkuhl K, Kharasch ED, Ellingrod VL, Skaar TC et al. Clinical pharmacogenetics implementation consortium guideline for CYP2D6 and CYP2C19 genotypes and dosing of tricyclic antidepressants. *Clin Pharmacol Ther.* 2013;93(5):402–408.
101. Poulsen L, Brøsen K, Arendt-Nielsen L, Gram LF, Elbæk K, Sindrup SH. Codeine and morphine in extensive and poor metabolizers of sparteine: Pharmacokinetics, analgesic effect and side effects. *Eur J Clin Pharmacol.* 1996;51(3–4):289–295.
102. Crews KR, Gaedigk A, Dunnenberger HM, Leeder JS, Klein TE, Caudle KE, Haidar CE et al. Clinical pharmacogenetics implementation consortium guidelines for cytochrome P450 2D6 genotype and codeine therapy: 2014 update. *Clin Pharmacol Ther.* 2014;95(4):376–382.
103. Oneta CM, Lieber CS, Li J, Rüttimann S, Schmid B, Lattmann J, Rosman AS, Seitz HK. Dynamics of cytochrome P4502E1 activity in man: Induction by ethanol and disappearance during withdrawal phase. *J Hepatol.* 2002;36(1):47–52.
104. Kim RB, O'Shea D. Interindividual variability of chlorzoxazone 6-hydroxylation in men and women and its relationship to CYP2E1 genetic polymorphisms. *Clin Pharmacol Ther.* 1995;57(6):645–655.
105. McCarver DG, Byun R, Hines RN, Hichme M, Wegenek W. A genetic polymorphism in the regulatory sequences of human CYP2E1: Association with increased chlorzoxazone hydroxylation in the presence of obesity and ethanol intake. *Toxicol Appl Pharmacol.* 1998;152(1):276–281.
106. Plee-Gautier E, Foresto F, Ferrara R, Bodénez P, Simon B, Manno M, Berthou F, Lucas D. Genetic repeat polymorphism in the regulating region of CYP2E1: Frequency and relationship with enzymatic activity in alcoholics. *Alcohol Clin Exp Res.* 2001;25(6):800–884.

107. Hu Y, Oscarson M, Johansson I, Yue QY, Dahl ML, Tabone M, Arincò S, Albano E, Ingelman-Sundberg M. Genetic polymorphism of human CYP2E1: Characterization of two variant alleles. *Mol Pharmacol.* 1997;51(3):370–376.

108. Vuilleumier N, Rossier MF, Chiappe A, Degoumois F, Dayer P, Mermillod B, Nicod L, Desmeules J, Hochstrasser D. CYP2E1 genotype and isoniazid-induced hepatotoxicity in patients treated for latent tuberculosis. *Eur J Clin Pharmacol.* 2006;62(6):423–429.

109. Wang Y, Yang H, Li L, Wang H, Zhang C, Yin G, Zhu B. Association between CYP2E1 genetic polymorphisms and lung cancer risk: A meta-analysis. *Eur J Cancer Oxf Engl 1990.* 2010;46(4):758–764.

110. Penno MB, Dvorchik BH, Vesell ES. Genetic variation in rates of antipyrine metabolite formation: A study in uninduced twins. *Proc Natl Acad Sci USA.* 1981;78(8):5193–5196.

111. Sadée W. The relevance of "missing heritability" in pharmacogenomics. *Clin Pharmacol Ther* 2012;92(4):428–430.

112. Wang D, Guo Y, Wrighton SA, Cooke GE, Sadee W. Intronic polymorphism in CYP3A4 affects hepatic expression and response to statin drugs. *Pharmacogenomics J.* 2011;11(4):274–286.

113. Bruckmueller H, Werk AN, Renders L, Feldkamp T, Tepel M, Borst C, Caliebe A, Kunzendorf U, Cascorbi I. Which genetic determinants should be considered for tacrolimus dose optimization in kidney transplantation? A combined analysis of genes affecting the CYP3A locus. *Ther Drug Monit.* 2015;37(3):288–295.

114. Vanhove T, Annaert P, Lambrechts D, Kuypers DRJ. Effect of ABCB1 diplotype on tacrolimus disposition in renal recipients depends on CYP3A5 and CYP3A4 genotype. *Pharmacogenomics J.* 2016;17(6):556.

115. Hertz DL, Kidwell KM, Seewald NJ, Gersch CL, Desta Z, Flockhart DA, Storniolo A-M, Stearns V, Skaar TC, Hayes DF, Henry NL, Rae JM. Polymorphisms in drug-metabolizing enzymes and steady-state exemestane concentration in postmenopausal patients with breast cancer. *Pharmacogenomics J.* 2016;17(6):521.

116. Klein K, Thomas M, Winter S, Nussler AK, Niemi M, Schwab M, Zanger UM. PPARA: A novel genetic determinant of CYP3A4 in vitro and in vivo. *Clin Pharmacol Ther.* 2012;91(6):1044–1052.

117. Williams JA, Ring BJ, Cantrell VE, Jones DR, Eckstein J, Ruterbories K, Hamman MA, Hall SD, Wrighton SA. Comparative metabolic capabilities of CYP3A4, CYP3A5, and CYP3A7. *Drug Metab Dispos Biol Fate Chem.* 2002;30(8):883–891.

118. Prytuła AA, Cransberg K, Bouts AHM, van Schaik RHN, de Jong H, de Wildt SN, Mathôt RAA. The effect of weight and CYP3A5 genotype on the population pharmacokinetics of tacrolimus in stable paediatric renal transplant recipients. *Clin Pharmacokinet.* 2016;55(9):1129–1143.

119. Deininger KM, Vu A, Page RL, Ambardekar AV, Lindenfeld J, Aquilante CL. CYP3A pharmacogenetics and tacrolimus disposition in adult heart transplant recipients. *Clin Transplant.* 2016;30(9):1074–1081.

120. Oetting WS, Schladt DP, Guan W, Miller MB, Remmel RP, Dorr C, Sanghavi K, et al. Genomewide association study of tacrolimus concentrations in african american kidney transplant recipients identifies multiple CYP3A5 alleles. *Am J Transplant Off J Am Soc Transplant Am Soc Transpl Surg.* 2016;16(2):574–582.

121. Strassburg CP. Pharmacogenetics of Gilbert's syndrome. *Pharmacogenomics.* 2008;9(6):703–715.

122. Torti C, Lapadula G, Antinori A, Quirino T, Maserati R, Castelnuovo F, Maggiolo F et al. Hyperbilirubinemia during atazanavir treatment in 2,404 patients in the Italian atazanavir expanded access program and MASTER Cohorts. *Infection.* 2009;37(3):244–249.

123. Gammal RS, Court MH, Haidar CE, Iwuchukwu OF, Gaur AH, Alvarellos M, Guillemette C et al. Clinical Pharmacogenetics Implementation Consortium (CPIC) Guideline for UGT1A1 and Atazanavir Prescribing. *Clin Pharmacol Ther.* 2016;99(4):363–369.

124. Etienne-Grimaldi M-C, Boyer J-C, Thomas F, Quaranta S, Picard N, Loriot M-A, Narjoz C et al. Collective work by Groupe de Pharmacologie Clinique Oncologique (GPCO-Unicancer), French Réseau National de Pharmacogénétique Hospitalière (RNPGx). UGT1A1 genotype and irinotecan therapy: General review and implementation in routine practice. *Fundam Clin Pharmacol.* 2015;29(3):219–237.

125. Swen JJ, Nijenhuis M, de Boer A, Grandia L, Maitland-van der Zee AH, Mulder H, Rongen G a. PJM, van Schaik RHN, Schalekamp T, Touw DJ, van der Weide J, Wilffert B, Deneer VHM, Guchelaar H-J. Pharmacogenetics: from bench to byte–an update of guidelines. *Clin Pharmacol Ther.* 2011;89(5):662–673.

126. Shi J, Wang X, Eyler RF, Liang Y, Liu L, Mueller BA, Zhu H-J. Association of oseltamivir activation with gender and carboxylesterase 1 genetic polymorphisms. *Basic Clin Pharmacol Toxicol.* 2016;119(6):555–561.

127. Redinbo MR, Bencharit S, Potter PM. Human carboxylesterase 1: From drug metabolism to drug discovery. *Biochem Soc Trans.* 2003;31(Pt 3):620–624.

128. Rasmussen HB, Bjerre D, Linnet K, Jürgens G, Dalhoff K, Stefansson H, Hankemeier T et al. Individualization of treatments with drugs metabolized by CES1: Combining genetics and metabolomics. *Pharmacogenomics.* 2015;16(6):649–665.

129. Zhu H-J, Patrick KS, Yuan H-J, Wang J-S, Donovan JL, DeVane CL, Malcolm R et al. Two CES1 gene mutations lead to dysfunctional carboxylesterase 1 activity in man: Clinical significance and molecular basis. *Am J Hum Genet.* 2008;82(6):1241–1248.

130. Zhu H-J, Markowitz JS. Activation of the antiviral prodrug oseltamivir is impaired by two newly identified carboxylesterase 1 variants. *Drug Metab Dispos.* 2009;37(2):264–267.

131. Shi J, Wang X, Nguyen J, Bleske BE, Liang Y, Liu L, Zhu H-J. Dabigatran etexilate activation is affected by the CES1 genetic polymorphism G143E (rs71647871) and gender. *Biochem Pharmacol.* 2016;119:76–84.

132. Lewis JP, Horenstein RB, Ryan K, O'Connell JR, Gibson Q, Mitchell BD, Tanner K et al. The functional G143E variant of carboxylesterase 1 is associated with increased clopidogrel active metabolite levels and greater clopidogrel response. *Pharmacogenet Genomics.* 2013;23(1):1–8.

133. Tarkiainen EK, Holmberg MT, Tornio A, Neuvonen M, Neuvonen PJ, Backman JT, Niemi M. Carboxylesterase 1 c.428G>A single nucleotide variation increases the antiplatelet effects of clopidogrel by reducing its hydrolysis in humans. *Clin Pharmacol Ther.* 2015;97(6):650–658.

134. Tarkiainen EK, Tornio A, Holmberg MT, Launiainen T, Neuvonen PJ, Backman JT, Niemi M. Effect of carboxylesterase 1 c.428G>A single nucleotide variation on the pharmacokinetics of quinapril and enalapril. *Br J Clin Pharmacol.* 2015;80(5):1131–1138.

135. Schaeffeler E, Fischer C, Brockmeier D, Wernet D, Moerike K, Eichelbaum M, Zanger UM, Schwab M. Comprehensive analysis of thiopurine S-methyltransferase phenotype-genotype correlation in a large population of German-Caucasians and identification of novel TPMT variants. *Pharmacogenetics.* 2004;14(7):407–417.

136. Yates CR, Krynetski EY, Loennechen T, Fessing MY, Tai HL, Pui CH, Relling MV, Evans WE. Molecular diagnosis of thiopurine S-methyltransferase deficiency: Genetic basis for azathioprine and mercaptopurine intolerance. *Ann Intern Med.* 1997;126(8):608–614.

137. Relling MV, Hancock ML, Rivera GK, Sandlund JT, Ribeiro RC, Krynetski EY, Pui CH, Evans WE. Mercaptopurine therapy intolerance and heterozygosity at the thiopurine S-methyltransferase gene locus. *J Natl Cancer Inst.* 1999;91(23):2001–2008.

138. Evans WE, Hon YY, Bomgaars L, Coutre S, Holdsworth M, Janco R, Kalwinsky D et al. Preponderance of thiopurine S-methyltransferase deficiency and heterozygosity among patients intolerant to mercaptopurine or azathioprine. *J Clin Oncol Off J Am Soc Clin Oncol.* 2001;19(8):2293–2301.

139. Stocco G, Cheok MH, Crews KR, Dervieux T, French D, Pei D, Yang W, Cheng C, Pui C-H, Relling MV, Evans WE. Genetic polymorphism of inosine triphosphate pyrophosphatase is a determinant of mercaptopurine metabolism and toxicity during treatment for acute lymphoblastic leukemia. *Clin Pharmacol Ther.* 2009;85(2):164–172.

140. Liu C, Yang W, Pei D, Cheng C, Smith C, Landier W, Hageman L et al. A genome-wide approach validates that thiopurine methyltransferase activity is a monogenic pharmacogenomic trait. *Clin Pharmacol Ther.* 2016;101:373–381.

141. Yang S-K, Hong M, Baek J, Choi H, Zhao W, Jung Y, Haritunians T et al. A common missense variant in NUDT15 confers susceptibility to thiopurine-induced leukopenia. *Nat Genet.* 2014;46(9):1017–1020.

142. Yang JJ, Landier W, Yang W, Liu C, Hageman L, Cheng C, Pei D et al. Inherited NUDT15 variant is a genetic determinant of mercaptopurine intolerance in children with acute lymphoblastic leukemia. *J Clin Oncol Off J Am Soc Clin Oncol.* 2015;33(11):1235–1242.

143. Moriyama T, Nishii R, Perez-Andreu V, Yang W, Klussmann FA, Zhao X, Lin T-N et al. NUDT15 polymorphisms alter thiopurine metabolism and hematopoietic toxicity. *Nat Genet.* 2016;48(4):367–373.

144. Relling MV, Gardner EE, Sandborn WJ, Schmiegelow K, Pui C-H, Yee SW, Stein CM, Carrillo M, Evans WE, Klein TE. Clinical pharmacogenetics implementation consortium guidelines for thiopurine methyltransferase genotype and thiopurine dosing. *Clin Pharmacol Ther.* 2011;89(3):387–391.

145. Hetherington S, McGuirk S, Powell G, Cutrell A, Naderer O, Spreen B, Lafon S, Pearce G, Steel H. Hypersensitivity reactions during therapy with the nucleoside reverse transcriptase inhibitor abacavir. *Clin Ther.* 2001;23(10):1603–1614.
146. Mallal S, Nolan D, Witt C, Masel G, Martin AM, Moore C, Sayer D, Castley A, Mamotte C, Maxwell D, James I, Christiansen FT. Association between presence of HLA-B*5701, HLA-DR7, and HLA-DQ3 and hypersensitivity to HIV-1 reverse-transcriptase inhibitor abacavir. *Lancet Lond Engl.* 2002;359(9308):727–732.
147. Hetherington S, Hughes AR, Mosteller M, Shortino D, Baker KL, Spreen W, Lai E et al. Genetic variations in HLA-B region and hypersensitivity reactions to abacavir. *Lancet Lond Engl.* 2002;359(9312):1121–1122.
148. Mallal S, Phillips E, Carosi G, Molina J-M, Workman C, Tomazic J, Jägel-Guedes E et al. HLA-B*5701 screening for hypersensitivity to abacavir. *N Engl J Med.* 2008;358(6):568–579.
149. Martin MA, Klein TE, Dong BJ, Pirmohamed M, Haas DW, Kroetz DL. Clinical pharmacogenetics implementation consortium guidelines for HLA-B genotype and abacavir dosing. *Clin Pharmacol Ther.* 2012;91(4):734–738.
150. Hung S-I, Chung W-H, Liou L-B, Chu C-C, Lin M, Huang H-P, Lin Y-L et al. HLA-B*5801 allele as a genetic marker for severe cutaneous adverse reactions caused by allopurinol. *Proc Natl Acad Sci USA.* 2005;102(11):4134–4139.
151. Hershfield MS, Callaghan JT, Tassaneeyakul W, Mushiroda T, Thorn CF, Klein TE, Lee MTM. Clinical pharmacogenetics implementation consortium guidelines for human leukocyte antigen-B genotype and allopurinol dosing. *Clin Pharmacol Ther.* 2013;93(2):153–158.

8

Inhibition of Drug Metabolizing Enzymes

F. Peter Guengerich

CONTENTS

Introduction

The topic of the inhibition of the enzymes of drug metabolism is of great interest to enzymologists, chemists, pharmacologists, and clinicians. Two major practical applications of this knowledge of inhibition are important in the pharmaceutical industry. One is drug-drug interactions, i.e., one drug may inhibit the biotransformation of another when two are taken concurrently (Correia and Hollenberg 2015,

Guengerich 1997). Such interactions can be fatal, and the possibilities are scrutinized by regulatory agencies. The other major interest in enzyme inhibition is based on the selection of enzymes as targets for drug action (Yu et al. 2014). For instance, monoamine oxidase and some of the cytochrome P450 (P450) enzymes are targets because the products of their normal reactions can be deleterious under certain conditions (Guengerich 2017). However, the focus of this chapter will be on inhibition of drug metabolism as opposed to drug targets.

Basic Mechanisms of Enzyme Inhibition

The general treatments presented here in this update of the first and second editions (Guengerich 1999b, 2009) are rather introductory, and the reader is referred to more comprehensive, classical treatments of the subject (Cornish-Bowden 1979, Dixon and Webb 1964, Kuby 1991, Segel 1975b, Silverman 1988). Classifications used here are oriented toward major mechanisms known for the enzymes of drug metabolism. Inhibition has its basis in the enzymology itself, including the field of enzyme kinetics. Overviews of major mechanisms and their principles will be presented, followed by a few prominent examples involving various enzymes, particularly the P450s.

Competitive Inhibition

The classic view of competitive inhibition is that the inhibitor shares structural similarity with the normal substrate (although defining a "normal" substrate for many of the enzymes under consideration is not always easy). The inhibitor may or may not be a substrate itself; i.e., be transformed to a product by the enzyme:

$$ E+S \xrightleftharpoons[k_{-1}]{k^1} ES \xrightleftharpoons[k_{-2}]{k_2} ES^* \xrightleftharpoons[k_{-3}]{k_3} EP \xrightleftharpoons[k_{-4}]{k_4} E+P $$

$$ E+I \xrightleftharpoons[k_{-1}']{k_1'} EI $$

where an intermediate ES* may or may not be present. Sometimes k_1, k_1, and k_4 are termed "k_{on}" and k_{-1}, k_{-1}, and k_4 are "k_{off}" rates. In classic competitive inhibition, the steady-state $k_{m,apparent}$ value (for the reaction with the "typical" substrate) increases when the inhibitor is present, and examination of steady-state kinetics with increasing concentrations of inhibitor and concommitant increasing $k_{m,apparent}$ values allow estimation of an inhibition constant K_i because they are related by the expression

$$ v = \frac{V_{max}}{K_m(1+[I]/K_i)+[S]} $$

where $k_{m,apparent} = K_m (1 + [I]/K_i)$. (Recall that $V_{max} = k_{cat} \times$ enzyme concentration/mg protein; k_{cat} will be used in this chapter.) This behavior is readily identified by a common intersection point (ordinate) in a Lineweaver-Burk (1/v vs. 1/S) plot or various characteristics of other linear transformations of the Michaelis-Menten equation.

   The classic approach to characterization of competitive inhibition and the associated parameters is to do enzyme assays with varying concentrations of both the substrate S and inhibitor I, fitting to the above equations or their derivatives. An alternative method is the Dixon plot, in which 1/v is plotted vs. S (Kuby 1991). Historically, linearized transforms were used in order to do fitting "by eye" or linear regression. All of the linear plots have weighting deficiencies (Cornish-Bowden 1979), and many convenient and useful non-linear regression software programs are now commercially available. However, screening for inhibition is very common in the pharmaceutical industry today and new approaches have been introduced to handle the increased load of drug candidates. One statistical experimental approach is usually termed "virtual kinetics" (Bronson et al. 1995).

In principle, K_i is an actual binding constant, as opposed to K_m, which is usually not. When the inhibitor is a substrate itself, the two substrates show competitive inhibition of each other. In some idealized and simple cases, if the $K_m \sim K_d$ then $K_m \sim K_i$. However, there are many reasons why such a relationship may not be seen with a complex enzyme system.

Competitive inhibition is a relatively commonly encountered phenomenon in drug metabolism work, and there are means of characterizing *in vivo* situations through pharmacokinetic parameters (Black et al. 1996, Renwick 1994, von Moltke et al. 1994). Many of the enzymes under consideration have multiple drug substrates (e.g., P450s 2C9, 2D6, 3A4) that can compete with each other (Guengerich 2015). Drug-drug interactions of this sort can be expected in individuals who are administered several drugs simultaneously.

Non-competitive Inhibition

In classic non-competitive inhibition, the inhibitor binds to the enzyme at a site distinct from that of the substrate. The expected result is that a decrease in k_{cat} or (V_{max}) is observed without a change in K_m. For instance, one might expect an electrophilic inhibitor (binding outside of the active site) to poison the enzyme in such a manner. Although this example is often presented in introductory biochemistry courses, clear examples of such inhibition are not so common and are not often encountered in studies with enzymes of drug metabolism. *In vitro*, one might expect such results by adding heavy metals to or heating an enzyme. What is often encountered is "mixed inhibition," where it is usually the case that K_{cat} decreases and K_m increases. The physical meaning of such changes may vary, and simply describing a phenomenon as mixed inhibition is not very meaningful. For example, such behavior might be observed if one were dealing with two different enzymes in a population (e.g., microsomes) that both catalyzed the same reaction and one was inhibited competitively while the other was being inactivated by mechanistic inactivation. Interpretation of such results must be done carefully with a single enzyme system.

A comprehensive discussion of all of the features of competitive and non-competitive inhibition is beyond the scope of this chapter. Competitive inhibition is commonly considered to reflect a single site but the potential for compounds binding to different parts of a larger active site is also possible. For more on the complex possibilities for competitive (and non-competitive and uncompetitive) inhibition, see Segel (1975c).

In a case from the author's own laboratory (Shinkyo and Guengerich 2011), cholesterol, quinidine, and nifedipine are all substrates for P450 3A4 but cholesterol behaved as a non-competitive inhibitor of the oxidations of nifedipine and quinidine. The results can be rationalized in a model (Figure 8.1) based on a system originally proposed by Segel (1975a).

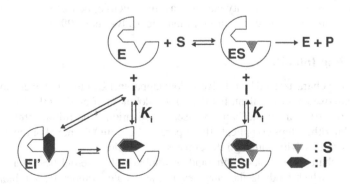

FIGURE 8.1 Model used to explain the apparently non-competitive inhibition of drug (quinidine) oxidation by cholesterol with P450 3A4 (Shinkyo and Guengerich 2011). A 2-site model is used, with overlap of the sites (Segel 1975a). The substrate(s) is quinidine and the inhibitor (I) is cholesterol. However, cholesterol can also occupy the substrate site and undergo 4β-hydroxylation.

Uncompetitive Inhibition

As in the case of non-competitive inhibition, classic uncompetitive inhibition is defined but seldom seen in practice. The principle is that the inhibitor binds *only* to the enzyme-substrate complex. Both k_{cat} and K_m are decreased proportionately, and the ratio k_{cat}/K_m remains constant. For instance, in a Lineweaver-Burk plot parallel lines should be seen in the absence and presence of the inhibitor. The enzyme efficiency (and, by extension, the intrinsic clearance of the drug substrate) would not really change. However, there are few clear examples of this phenomenon in the field.

Product Inhibition

In some cases, a product of a reaction of a drug-metabolizing enzyme may inhibit the reaction. For instance, $NADP^+$ is a competitive inhibitor of NADPH-P450 reductase (Vermilion and Coon 1978). (For this reason, an NADPH-generating system (Guengerich 2014a) is preferred to adding a bolus of NADPH as a cofactor in *in vitro* incubations.) In a cellular system, this case would not exist because there are reduction systems that work well on the oxidized cofactor. However, in other cases, the product may not have physical characteristics very different from the substrate and competitively inhibits, sometimes being further transformed. For instance, benzene is oxidized by P450 2E1 to phenol and then on to hydroquinone (Guengerich et al. 1991), and P450 17A1 oxidizes pregnenolone to 17α-hydroxypregnenolone and then to dehydroepiandrosterone. Thus, benzene and phenol compete, as do pregnenolone, 17α-hydroxypregnenolone, and dehydroepiandrosterone (Pallan et al. 2015). Polycyclic aromatic hydrocarbons and their dihydrodiols compete for Family 1 P450 enzymes (Shimada and Guengerich 2006, Shimada et al. 2007).

Transition-State Analogs

Transition-state analogs are tight-binding, non-covalently bound inactivators that resemble the transition state for the enzymatic reaction; that is, the transient complex formed in a single step within the catalytic cycle with the maximum free energy. The axiom that the enzyme has the highest affinity for this putative entity (which cannot be directly observed) was developed by Haldane (Haldane 1930) and Pauling (Pauling 1948) and was the basis for the development of catalytic antibodies (Lerner and Benkovic 1988).

$$E + I \underset{k_{off}}{\overset{k_{on}}{\rightleftharpoons}} E - I$$

The k_{on} rate is rapid and k_{off} is slow. Inactivation is rapid and no time dependence is observed under typical assay conditions. Enzyme activity can, at least in principle, be restored by removal of inhibitor using dialysis, gel filtration, centrifugal concentration, etc. (Silverman 1995).

Slow, Tight-Binding Inhibitors

These compounds are characterized by relatively slow (apparent) k_{on} rates and even slower k_{off} rates. The binding can be non-covalent or covalent, but due to the slowness of binding the loss of activity may be time-dependent and mistaken for mechanism-based inactivation. The initial interaction is, of course, diffusion-limited, but other steps complicate the apparent "k_{on}" rate.) Removal of the inhibitor by dialysis etc. will restore enzyme activity, although the process may be slow.

An example of a characterized slow, tight-binding inhibitor of a steroid (testosterone) 5α-reductase is finasteride (Proscar®), which binds to the enzymes at a slow rate, competitively inhibits, and effectively irreversibly inactivates the enzyme (Tian et al. 1995). Another example involves "coxib" prostaglandin synthase ("COX-2") inhibitors (Marnett 2000). Possible causes for the slow, tight binding include a conformational change of the enzyme imposed by binding, a change in the protonation state of the enzyme, displacement of a water molecule at the active site, or reversible formation of a covalent bond (Silverman 1995).

Mechanism-Based Enzyme Inactivators

Silverman (2004) has stated that a broad definition of this term includes any inactivators that utilize the enzyme mechanism but invokes a stricter definition, one that will be adhered to in this chapter. A definition is "an unreactive compound whose structure resembles that of either the substrate or the product of the target enzyme, and which undergoes a catalytic transformation by the enzyme to a species that, prior to release from the active site, inactivates the enzyme" (Silverman 1995). A key point here is the need to inactivate the enzyme before leaving the active site. The definition, taken as a whole, restricts the grouping from the transition state analogs, affinity labels, and slow, tight-binding inhibitors.

Mechanism-based inactivation is sometimes encountered inadvertently with existing drugs. There are several major intentional uses of these compounds, and this group will be covered in some detail (for more extensive discussion see Abeles and Alston 1990, Abeles and Maycock 1976, Rando 1984, Silverman 1988, 2004, Waley 1980, 1985, Walsh 1984). Mechanism-based inactivators have been of considerable interest because of their usefulness in the delineation of enzyme mechanisms. They are also of interest in the design of new drugs because, in principle, only the activity of the target enzyme will be attenuated (Silverman 2004, Singh et al. 2011). Many of the better diagnostic inhibitors of the drug-metabolizing enzymes are mechanism-based inactivators. For instance, these can be used to gain valuable *in vitro* information about which of the P450s are involved in a particular reaction (Correia and Hollenberg 2015, Guengerich 2015, Halpert and Guengerich 1997).

The relevant scheme for mechanism-based inactivation is

$$\text{E} + \text{I} \underset{k_{1}}{\overset{k_{1}}{\rightleftharpoons}} \text{E} - \text{I} \underset{k_{-2}}{\overset{k_{2}}{\rightleftharpoons}} \text{E} - \text{I}' \xrightarrow{k_{4}} \begin{array}{c} \text{EI}' \\ \downarrow k_{3} \\ \text{E} - \text{I} \end{array},$$

where I is the mechanism-based inactivator, E–I* is an intermediate derived by transformation of the initial complex, EI is inactivated enzyme, and P is a stable product that leaves the enzyme. Sometimes these inhibitors are called "suicide inactivators" although the term is not generally accepted by purists. It is the enzyme, not the inhibitor, that is dying.

Several parameters are experimentally determined and used to describe these inhibitors. The ratio k_4/k_3 is the "partition ratio," which can be thought of as the number of times that the enzyme must cycle, on the average, for one inactivation to occur. However, the ratio can range from several thousand to less than one, even approaching zero.

The inactivation process shows first-order kinetics; that is, a plot of the logarithm of the remaining enzyme activity *vs* time gives a straight line (first order, or single exponential kinetics) (Figure 8.2). The half-life, $t_{1/2}$, can be determined at each inhibitor concentration used and used to calculate k, using the relationship $t_{1/2} = 0.693/k_{\text{inact}} + 0.693\,2K_{\text{I}}/k_{\text{inact}} \cdot \text{I}$ (Silverman 1995). The plot of k *vs* [I] is hyperbolic, and a linear transformation (e.g., plot of $1/k$ *vs* $1/[\text{I}]$) yields k_{inact}, the maximum rate of inactivation, and K_{I}, the concentration of inhibitor required for half-maximal inhibition. In the above scheme, $k_{\text{inact}} = k_2$ if k_2 is rate-limiting in the overall reaction. K_{I} is a complex expression of microscopic rate constants but is useful in estimating the potential usefulness of an inhibitor.

A number of criteria can be used to determine if mechanism-based inactivation is actually occurring. Although not all of these tests are applicable to every situation, the case for mechanism-based inactivation is stronger when several can be demonstrated.

One of the simplest tests is whether or not the typical cofactors are required. (Note: In the strict sense, "cofactors" are co-substrates, which appear in the overall stoichiometry of a reaction, e.g., NADH/NAD⁺, as opposed to "prosthetic groups," which bind tightly to the enzyme but do not figure in the stoichiometry.) For instance, in a P450-dependent reaction, is pre-incubation with NADPH necessary in order to see inhibition by the compound under consideration? In most cases, a mechanism-based inactivator also has a strictly competitive component and results can be misleading. The generally accepted way of discerning

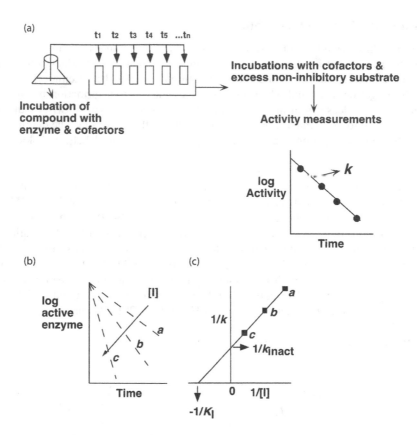

FIGURE 8.2 Determination of k_{inact} for a mechanism-based inactivator. (a) The compound under investigation is incubated with the enzyme (plus all relevant cofactors); at various time points the solution is diluted into an excess of (non-inhibitory) substrate to determine the amount of remaining "active enzyme." (b) Plots of log10 [active enzyme] *vs* time give the plots designated *a*, *b*, and *c* at various concentrations of the inhibitory substrate I. *a*, *b*, and *c* have constants, k, defined by the slopes ($k = 0.693/t_{1/2}$). (c) The values of k from lines *a*, *b*, and *c* are related to [I] in the double reciprocal "Kitz-Wilson" plot. The intercept on the ordinate in this plot gives k_{inact}, the extrapolated rate of inactivation at infinite inhibitor concentration, and the intercept on the x axis gives K_I, the inhibitor concentration at which a half-maximal rate of inactivation is seen.

the two aspects is to preincubate the concentrated enzyme with cofactors and a certain concentration of the inhibitor and then, at a certain time, to dilute this enzyme (e.g., 50-fold) into a solution containing a non-inhibitory substrate (and cofactors) and assay product formation, either continuously, if possible, or after a set time (Figure 8.2).

One characteristic of mechanism-based inactivation is the first-order kinetic pattern mentioned above. In practice, aliquots are withdrawn at indicated times from an incubation of enzyme, the inhibitor, and any necessary cofactors are diluted into excess substrate as mentioned above. The rate of inactivation (k) should increase when the experiment is repeated with a higher concentration of inhibitor, as mentioned above (Figure 8.2). In a plot of the logarithm of residual enzyme activity *versus* time, the intercept ($t = 0$) indicates the extent of inhibition that is of a competitive nature.

The enzyme should be protected from inactivation by a "normal" (non-inhibitory) substrate. Of course, this criterion may not distinguish a mechanism-based inhibitor from a competitive one, unless the time-dependence of inhibition is examined.

Another criterion is irreversibility. However, in some cases, a slow reactivation is seen, usually occurring over a period of days. Exactly what time period of reactivation does or does not constitute mechanism-based inactivation is not specifically defined. In practice, one usually removes excess inhibitor from the enzyme (e.g., dialysis, gel filtration, centrifugal filtration) and assays the activity of the enzyme to determine if it has been restored.

The inhibitor is usually covalently bound to the enzyme in mechanism-based inactivation, either to the protein or a prosthetic group. The stoichiometry of binding should be unimolecular; that is, only one molecule should be bound per enzyme (subunit). The extent of labeling should be correlated with the degree of inactivation; e.g., a ratio of 0.7 labeled inhibitor bound per enzyme subunit should correspond to a 70% loss of activity (corrected for any competitive inhibition). Further, labeling should be specific in the sense that "scavenger" nucleophiles (e.g., glutathione) and other proteins (that do have access to the enzyme active site) are not labeled. A general rule of thumb is that a specific radioactivity of 0.5 μCi (^{14}C)/μmol is needed for labeling studies of this type, in order to obtain sufficient counts for analysis (using liquid scintillation counting or similar drug methods). Other isotopes can be used; tritium is acceptable if the hydrogen is stable in all involved processes. In some cases, it is possible to use other labels such as fluorescent chromophores or mass spectrometry, although quantitation is more difficult.

True mechanism-based inactivators use the same catalytic step in partitioning between product formation and inactivation. Thus, both should show the same cofactor requirements and any kinetic isotope effects (e.g., deuterium) should be common to both.

More extensive treatments of the theory and practice of mechanism-based inactivation have appeared elsewhere (Abeles and Maycock 1976, Rando 1984, Silverman 1988, 1995, 2004, Waley 1980, 1985), as well as examples of applications to various enzymes (Abeles and Alston 1990, Abeles and Maycock 1976, Correia and Hollenberg 2015, Rando 1984, Schechter and Sjoerdsma 1990, Silverman 1995, 2004, Walsh 1984, Xiao and Prestwich 1991).

Inhibitors that Generate Reactive Products that Become Covalently Attached to the Enzyme

This group of compounds is often grouped with the mechanism-based inactivators discussed above. Many of the same criteria apply, such as the need for cofactors and the irreversible nature of the inactivation. However, labeling may be more extensive and less specific. Also, careful analysis of the kinetics may show critical differences from linearity in plots of log (enzyme activity) *vs* time (Silverman 1995, 2004). For instance, there might be a lag in the inhibition and then an apparent first-order plot, as the concentration of reactive product increases. If fresh enzyme is added to the mixture at this point, then no lag will be observed due to the build-up of electrophilic product in the medium. However, it should be emphasized that discerning deviations from pseudo-first-order kinetics may not be easy, especially if the assays are subject to error or if relatively few data points are collected.

Experiments in which mechanism-based inactivation and inhibition of the type discussed here need not be restricted to purified enzymes. They can be done with relatively crude preparations, e.g., microsomes or cytosolic fractions, if appropriate caveats are used. Labeling studies can be done with such preparations to examine the specificity of the process.

Inhibitors of Various Enzymes

This section is intended not to be comprehensive but to provide some examples of the previously discussed types of enzyme inhibition as they relate to several of the enzymes involved in the biotransformation of drugs and xenobiotics. The reader is referred to other articles for more comprehensive lists of inhibitors (Correia and Hollenberg 2015, Guengerich 2010, 2015).

Monoamine Oxidases

There are two forms of monoamine oxidase, termed A and B (Bach et al. 1988, Cashman and Motika 2010). These have long been recognized to show differences in inhibition by various drugs and are recognized to be the products of different genes. Mechanism-based inactivation is common among many of the inhibitors of these enzymes, and drugs have been developed in order to treat problems related to the nervous system (Dostert et al. 1989, Silverman 1995).

Monoamine oxidase A oxidizes biogenic amines and is selectively inhibited by the mechanism-based inactivator clorgyline. The B form of the enzyme is involved in the oxidation of non-catecholamines and is inhibited by pargyline and deprenyl, also mechanism-based inactivators. These compounds all contain an *N*-propynyl (propanyol) group (-N-C≡C-CH$_3$), which leads to a covalent adduct (Silverman 1995).

Another inhibitor of monoamine oxidase is the anticonvulsant milacemide, CH$_3$(CH$_2$) 4NHCH$_2$CONH$_2$, which is also a substrate (Silverman 1995). The compound is thought to be oxidized to an aminium radical (1-electron oxidation) with attack on an α-carbon to generate a protein adduct (Silverman 1995).

Another popular group of inhibitors has been ring-strained cycloalkylamines, which rearrange to reactive products following 1-electron oxidation (Silverman 1983, Silverman and Ding 1993). The anti-depressant tranylcypromine was one of the first compounds in this class. Postulated mechanisms for some of these are shown in Figure 8.3. There are two paths (a, b). One (a) leads to modification of a protein Cys group. The other pathway (b) leads to modification of the flavin prosthetic group, either at the C-4a or N-5 atom (Mitchell et al. 2001). The former (a) appears to be a reversible process, with the enzyme losing the group after 24 h (see the section Mechanism-based Inactivation for discussion of the issue of reversibility). A series of cyclopropyl derivatives of *N*-methyl-4-phenyl-1,2,5,6-tetrahydropyridine have been studied (Rimoldi et al. 1995, Tipton et al. 1986).

The development of monoamine oxidase inhibitors continues to be an area of active interest. For more recent developments in this field see Boppana et al. (2009), Carradori and Silvestri (2015), Valente et al. (2011).

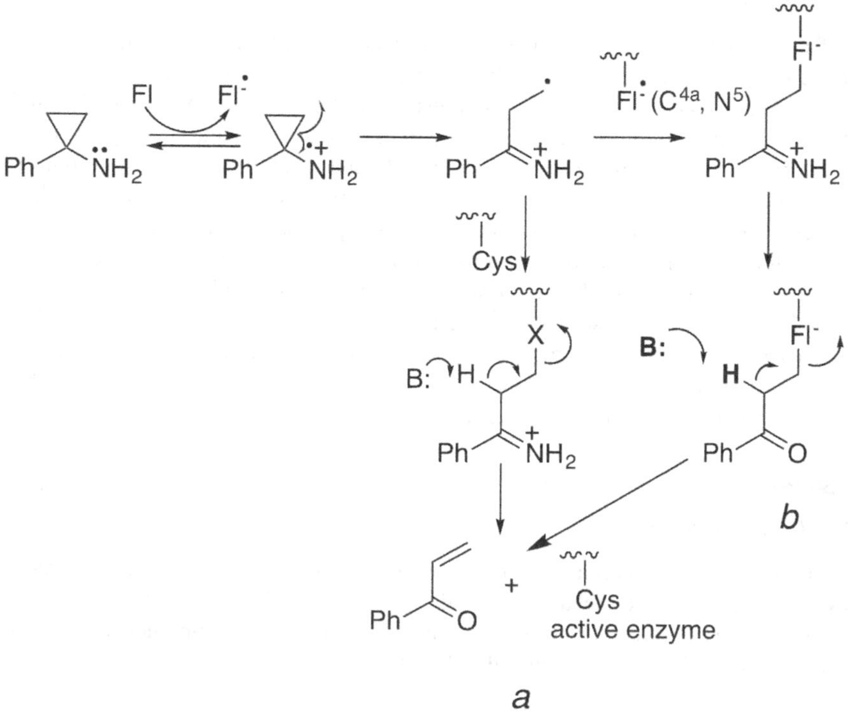

FIGURE 8.3 Proposed scheme for oxidation of 1-phenylcyclopropylamine by monoamine oxidase, with both pathways leading to inactivation by binding to a cysteine (a) and flavin (b) (Silverman 1995). In the case of the flavin, both the C-4a and N-5 adducts. (From Mitchell, D.J. et al., *Biochemistry*, 40, 5447–5456, 2001; Mitchell, D.J. et al., *Bioorg. Med. Chem. Lett.*, 11, 1757–1760, 2001a.)

Cytochromes P450

Inhibitors of P450s have been studied with regard to several aspects. Some aspects are quite basic. First, many different P450 enzymes are found in humans and experimental animals and diagnostic inhibitors have been used to ascertain the roles of individual P450s in catalysis of reactions (Correia and Hollenberg 2015). Due to the overlapping catalytic specificity of many of the P450s, inhibitors are usually not totally selective, although these have improved with time. Nevertheless, the selectivity can be examined and the use of diagnostic inhibition of individual P450s is possible, with appropriate caveats (Bourrié et al. 1996, Newton et al. 1994). A list of generally accepted "probe" inhibitors is presented in Table 8.1 (Correia and Hollenberg 2015). Further, inhibitors have provided considerable insight into function, both in terms of chemical aspects of catalysis and structural details of the proteins that contribute to selectivity (Correia and Hollenberg 2015, Halpert 1995).

Other aspects of P450 inhibition are more practical (Vanden Bossche et al. 1995). For instance, one prominent strategy in therapy of estrogen-dependent tumors is the inhibition of P450 19A1, the "aromatase" that catalyzes the 3-step conversion of androgens to estrogens (Guengerich 2015, Ortiz de Montellano 2015). Aminoglutethimide is a classic but not ideal inhibitor, and better drugs are on the market today, e.g., exemestane, letrazole, anastrozole (Correia and Hollenberg 2015, Santen et al. 2009). Another target in yeast and fungal infections is P450 51, the lanosterol 14α-demethylase (Aoyama et al. 1987, Pikuleva and Waterman 2013). Many azoles (e.g., ketoconazole) are used as drugs in this regard (Vanden Bossche 1992). Selectivity for the fungal enzyme is observed, but these drugs can also inhibit mammalian P450 51 and other P450s at higher concentrations (Baldwin et al. 1995, Hargrove et al. 2016, Sonino 1987). Another example of a P450 inhibitor is piperonyl butoxide, which has long been used as an insecticide "synergist" to block the detoxication of chemicals by insect P450s (Figure 8.4) (Casida 1970). As more information becomes available about the P450s present in noxious insects, the design and development of pesticides (and synergists) with more selectivity for the insect enzymes should be possible.

Another practical area in which the development of better inhibitors of P450s may be useful is in cancer prevention. Some inhibitors (e.g., ethynyls) can block rodent and human P450s that activate carcinogens (Hammons et al. 1989) and can be shown to block carcinogen-induced cancers in rodents (Viaje et al. 1990). The drug oltipraz and the natural compound sulforophane have been studied in cancer prevention studies because of their abilities to induce conjugation enzymes (e.g., GSH transferase, NADPH-quinone reductase) (Davidson et al. 1990, Zhang et al. 1992). More importantly, perhaps, they have both been shown to block P450s involved in the activation of carcinogens, e.g., aflatoxin B_1 (Langouet et al. 1995).

Several types of inhibition are seen for the P450s. A relatively common mechanism is competitive inhibition. For instance, quinidine and most other P450 2D6 inhibitors seem to act in this way (Koymans et al. 1992); a basic nitrogen in the inhibitor seems to bind in the same site as the substrates in most, but not all cases (Guengerich et al. 2002, Strobl et al. 1993, Wolff et al. 1985). Azoles have already been mentioned and are one example of nitrogen heterocycles that ligand to the heme iron (Murray and Wilkinson 1984, Vanden Bossche 1992). Sulfaphenazole is a competitive inhibitor of P450 2C9 and has selectivity (compared to other P450 2C enzymes) (Brian et al. 1989, Miners et al. 1988). Many organic solvents inhibit P450 2E1 by competing as substrates (Chauret et al. 1998, Yoo et al. 1987), so care must be taken in *in vitro* experimental designs.

Another group of inhibitors are not particularly effective themselves but are oxidized to "metabolic intermediates" that bind tightly to the heme and prevent further involvement of the iron atom in catalysis. For instance, some amines are oxidized to *C*-nitroso derivatives (e.g., troleandomycin) (Danan et al. 1981, Jönsson and Lindeke 1992) and piperonyl butoxide (*vide supra*) yields a carbene (Figure 8.4) (Murray et al. 1983). This process might be termed mechanism-based inactivation but perhaps a better description would be transformation by the enzyme(s) to very tight-binding inhibitors. The linkages are not covalent in the usual sense, since addition of a strong oxidant [e.g., $Fe(CN)_6^{3-}$] oxidizes such a ferrous complex to ferric and releases the ligand.

Mechanism-based inactivators have been studied extensively, primarily from a basic standpoint (Halpert and Guengerich 1997, Ortiz de Montellano and Correia 1983). Many vinyl and acetylenic

TABLE 8.1

Some Diagnostic Inhibitors of Human P450 Enzymes

P450	Inhibitor	Apparent Mechanism
1A1	7,8-Benzoflavone	Competitive[a]
	Ellipticine	Competitive
1A2	Furafylline	Mechanism-based
	7,8-Benzoflavone	Competitive[a]
	Fluvoxamine	Competitive
	Methoxsalen	
	Tranylcypromine	
2A6	Diethyldithiocarbamate	Mechanism-based
	Pilocarpine	
	Tryptamine	
	Pyridine analogs of nicotine	Competitive[b]
2B6	3-Isopropenyl-3-methyldiamantane	
	2-Isopropenyl-2-methyldiamantane	
	Phenacyclidene	
	Thio-TEPA	
	Clopidogrel	
	Ticlopidine	
2C8	Montelukast	Competitive
	Quercitin	Competitive
	Pioglitazone	Competitive
2C9	Sulfaphenazole	Competitive[c]
	Tienilic acid	Mechanism-based
	Fluconazole	
2C19	Ticlopidine	
	Nootkatone	
2D6	Quinidine, several others[d]	Competitive[e]
2E1	4-Methylpyrazole	Competitive
	Diethyldithiocarbamate	Mechanism-based[a]
	Clomethiozole	
	Diallysulfide	
	Many organic solvents	Competitive[a]
3A4, 3A5	Ketoconazole[a]	
	Itraconazole	
	Troleandomycin	Conversion to heme ligand
	Azamulin	
	Erythromycin	Conversion to heme ligand
	Verapamil	
	Gestodene	Mechanism-based

Note: U.S. Food and Drug Administration 2006, Correia 2005, Correia and Hollenberg 2015.

[a] Known to be oxidized by the enzyme. Also, some of the results with these compounds reported in (Chang et al. 1994) are not supported in subsequent work (Bourrié et al. 1996, Newton et al. 1994).

[b] Denton et al. 2005.

[c] Apparently not a heme ligand (Mancy et al. 1996).

[d] Strobl et al. 1993.

[e] Apparently not oxidized (Guengerich et al. 1986).

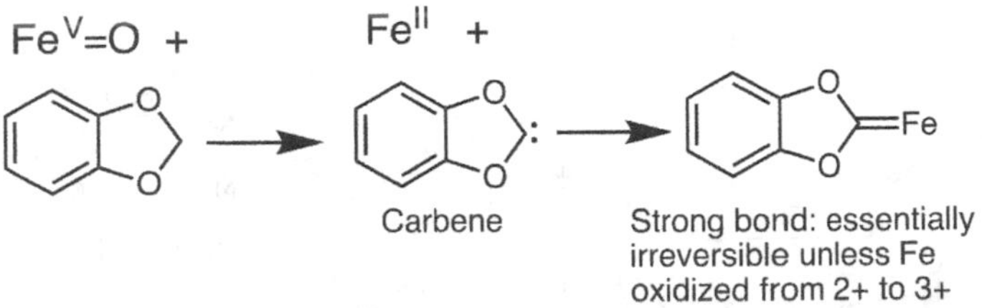

FIGURE 8.4 Oxidation of piperonyl butoxide by P450 to a carbene that yields a stable ferrous ligand. (From Casida, J.E., *J Agr Food Chem.*, 18, 753–772, 1970.)

inhibitors have been characterized as yielding heme and/or protein adducts (Figure 8.4). Some of these have practical consequences with drugs (e.g., secobarbital (Ortiz de Montellano and Correia 1983)). A dihalomethylene group (Halpert et al. 1986) can also be involved in mechanism-based inactivation, although it is not clear whether chloramphenicol should be classified in this group or among the inhibitors that is converted to a reactive product (Miller and Halpert 1986). Inhibition by cyclopropylamines is considered to involve oxidation to an aminium radical that rearranges to a reactive methylene radical, as in the case of the postulated mechanism for monoamine oxidase (Figure 8.3), although adducts remain to be characterized (Bondon et al. 1989, Hanzlik and Tullman 1982, Macdonald et al. 1982).

4-Alkyl-1,4-dihydropyridines are readily oxidized by P450s by 1-electron oxidation (Augusto et al. 1982). Rearrangement of the putative aminium radical to the pyridine generates an alkyl radical, which modifies a pyrrole nitrogen of the prosthetic heme (Ortiz de Montellano et al. 1981). If an aromatic group is at the 4-position it is retained, and such compounds are used as drugs (Böcker and Guengerich 1986). This is, strictly speaking, not an example of mechanism-based inactivation, since (i) alkyl radicals can react with spin traps outside of the protein (Augusto et al. 1982) and (ii) other P450s that cannot oxidize the 4-alkyl-1,4-dihydropyridines can also be inactivated when an enzyme capable of oxidation (e.g., P450 3A4) is also present. Ortiz de Montellano and his associates have also characterized other compounds (e.g., 1-aminobenzotriazole) that are oxidized by P450s to yield covalent heme adducts (Lukton et al. 1988, Ortiz de Montellano 2005, Stearns and Ortiz de Montellano 1985). It is possible to use 1-aminobenzotriazole to lower total hepatic P450 levels in rats to <30% that of the normal for 13 weeks without significant physiological effects (Meschter et al. 1994), and 1-aminobenztinazole is still used as a general inhibitor of P450 in laboratory animals (Dostalek et al. 2007, 2008).

Mechanism-based inhibition is of considerable inhibition of P450s, in the context of leading to drug-drug interactions, particularly with P450 3A4. For more details see ref. (Correia and Hollenberg 2015). Collectively these inhibitors may be grouped into several families of effects: (i) oxidation to compounds that bind heme reversibly but very tightly (i.e., methylene dioxyphenyl compounds (*vide supra*), amines that are oxidized to C-nitroso derivatives (Jönsson and Lindeke 1992); (ii) oxidation to intermediates that react with P450 heme and generate porphyrin derivatives (Correia and Hollenberg 2015, Ortiz de Montellano and Correia 1983); (iii) oxidation to products that react with the (apo) protein (as opposed to heme), and (iv) oxidation to products that crosslink the heme to the protein (Correia and Hollenberg 2015). A list of some of the chemical moieties that have demonstrated mechanism-based inactivation includes olefins, acetylenes (and proparyls), thiophenes, furans, strained cycloalkylamines, some thiols and thionosulfurs, and dihalomethylenes (Correia and Hollenberg 2015).

Most of the compounds that have been studied fall into classes ii and iii. Some mechanisms are shown in Figure 8.5. At this time prediction of whether an olefin or acetylene will act as a mechanism-based inactivator is not possible nor is the prediction as to whether heme modification, protein modification, or a mixture of both may occur. Few examples of group iv, with heme-protein crosslinking, have been characterized in any detail.

During the time elapsed since the last edition of this monograph was published (Guengerich 2009), more examples of P450-based inactivation have been characterized in some detail (Table 8.2).

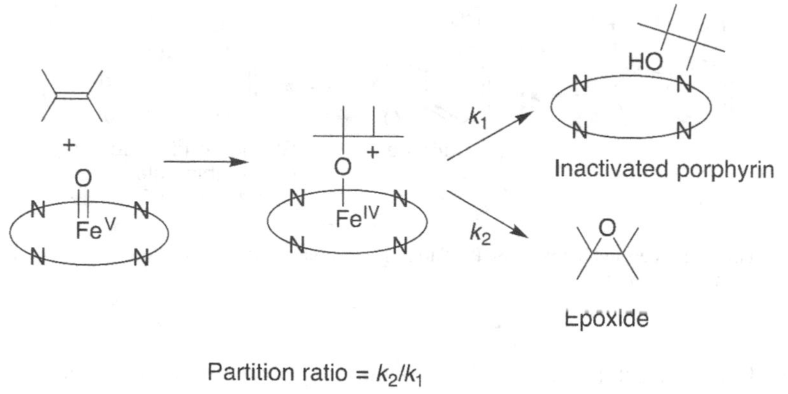

Partition ratio = k_2/k_1

FIGURE 8.5 Mechanism-based inactivation of P450 by heme destruction during the epoxidation of an olefin (Ortiz de Montellano and Reich 1986). The partition ratio is given by k_2/k_1. Several of the N-alkyl porphyrin adducts arising from the heme have been rigorously characterized by NMR and mass spectrometry.

TABLE 8.2

P450 Mechanism-Based Inhibitors

Compound	Putative Activated Moiety	P450	Mode of Binding	References
Ritonavir		3A4, 2B6	Heme	Lin et al. (2013)
OSI-930	Thiophene	3A4		Lin et al. (2011b)
Raloxifene				VandenBrink et al. (2012)
Phenylisothiocyanate	Isothiocyanate	2E1		Yoshigae et al. (2013)
Diethyldithiocarbamate		2E1		Pratt-Hyatt et al. (2010)
Clopidogrel	Thiophene	2B6	Heme, Cys-475	Zhang et al. (2011)
tert-Butylphenylacetylene	Acetylene	2B6	Thr-302	Lin et al. (2011)
Selegiline	Acetylene	2B6	Protein	Sridar et al. (2012)
Bergamottin	Benzofuran	3A4	Protein	Lin et al. (2012)

Note: Concentrated on human P450 results published since 2009. This list is not intended to be comprehensive. For more, see (Correia and Hollenberg 2015, Guengerich 2009, Guengerich 2015, Ortiz de Montellano and Correia 1983).

In several cases, the specific P450 residues involved in covalent binding have been identified. Although we have a reasonably good understanding of the chemistry involved in some of these processes (*vide supra*), there are several chemicals for which the chemistry involved in inhibition/binding is still not well understood (e.g., imines, piperazines).

The discussion above is focused on the matter of dealing with inhibition of P450s by drugs and drug candidates during development, which is usually an undesirable phenomenon, in that drug-drug interactions are often unfavorable. However, there are situations in which P450 inhibition can be favorable, e.g., when an expensive drug is used, and the goal is to decrease cleavance and increase exposure. This is often the case with drugs used for HIV-1 treatment. The protease inhibitor of P450 3A4, the major drug-metabolizing P450 in liver and small intestine (Guengerich 1999a). Cobicistat (Figure 8.6) is also a strong inhibitor but without its own pharmacological activity. Poulos's laboratory (Kaur et al. 2016) developed other, more inhibitory molecules based on structural data. The interactions of two P450 3A4 phenylalanine residues with drug phenyl rings is important, and this knowledge led

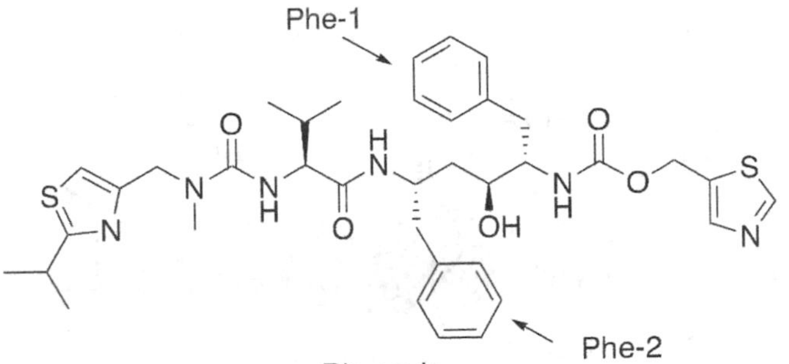

Ritonavir

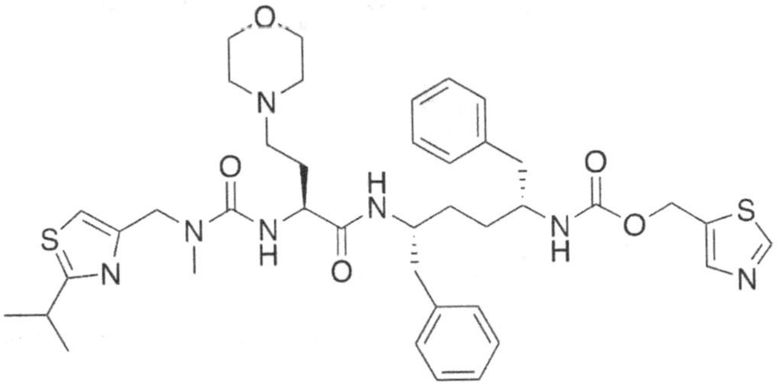

Cobicistat

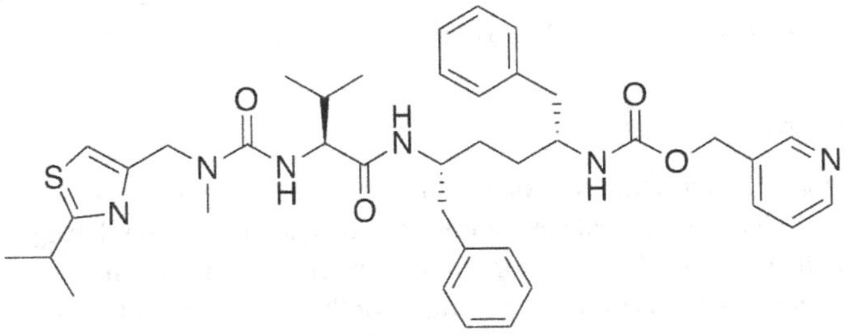

GS3

FIGURE 8.6 Potent inhibitors of P450 3A4. The phenyl side-chains proximal to and distal from the heme-liganding moiety are designated Phe-1 and Phe-2, respectively. (From Kaur, P. et al., *J. Med. Chem.*, 59, 4210–4220, 2016.)

to the design of GS3 (Figure 8.6). A pharmacophore for P450 3A4 inhibition is shown in Figure 8.7, which can be of use not only in developing strong inhibitors but also avoiding binding with other drugs in which inhibition should be avoided.

NADPH-P450 Reductase

This flavoprotein is involved in the transfer of electrons from NADPH to P450s (Masters 1980). The enzyme also functions in electron transfer to some other hemoproteins, e.g., heme oxygenase (Yoshida et al. 1974).

Inhibition has not been studied extensively. The oxidation product $NADP^+$ is a competitive inhibitor (Vermilion and Coon 1978). The 2′-phosphate group is important in binding; 2′-AMP is also a competitive inhibitor and the enzyme is the basis for the use of 2′,5′-ADP affinity chromatography in purification (Yasukochi and Masters 1976).

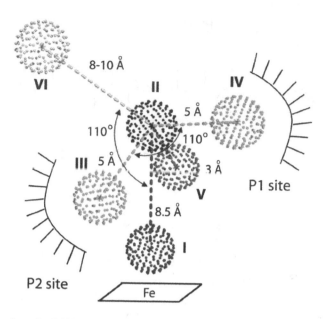

FIGURE 8.7 Pharmacophore for P450 3A4 inhibition (Kaur et al. 2016). The pharmacophore was developed from ritonavir and analogues (Figure 8.6).

Diphenyliodonium has been reported to be a mechanism-based inactivator of the enzyme (Tew 1993). The mechanism is postulated to involve 1-electron reduction of the iodonium to give an iodide/flavin radical pair that combines to give an N_5-phenylflavin adduct, along with a labeled amino acid (Trp-419).

Flavin-Containing Monooxygenases

In contrast to the flavoprotein monoamine oxidase, little is known about inhibitors of this enzyme (Cashman 2018), and a recent search did not reveal new inhibitors. Some are known but have poor affinities (Clement et al. 1996). No mechanism-based inactivators have been characterized. The various substrates seem to inhibit each other, at least insofar as they are substrates for the same form of the enzyme (at least five forms can exist in a single animal species) (Cashman and Motika 2010, Hines et al. 1994).

Aldehyde Oxidase and Xanthine Oxidoreductase

Aldehyde oxidase, and the related molybdenum-flavin-iron sulfur protein xanthine oxidoreductase, is involved in the oxidation of a number of drugs, particularly heterocycles (Panoutsopoulos et al. 2004). The mechanism differs clearly from P450 and other mixed function oxidases in that electrons are removed from a substrate and transferred to an electron donor, generally NAD^+ or O_2 (Beedham 2010, Rajagopalan 1997). The oxygen atom incorporated into the substrate is derived from H_2O, not O_2.

Allopurinol is a reversible inhibitor that can be used to distinguish between the involvement of aldehyde oxidase and xanthine oxidoreductase *in vitro* or *in vivo*, preferentially inhibiting the latter enzyme (Beedham 2010). Aldehyde oxidase is preferentially inhibited by isovanillin (Beedham 2010) and hydralazine (Strelevitz et al. 2012).

There is considerable interest in the development of xanthine oxidoreductase inhibitors that can be used clinically (Chen et al. 2015, Rodrigues et al. 2016, Song et al. 2016). The major indication is gout, which results from an excess of the product, uric acid. In addition, inhibition of xanthine oxidoreductase has been considered in the treatment of inflammation as it relates to atherosclerosis (Oyama et al. 2016) and hypertension (Kohagura et al. 2016). Some plant polyphenols have inhibitory activity (Stepanic et al. 2015).

In contrast to xanthine oxidoreductase, aldehyde oxidase has no defined physiological function yet, and there seems to be no reason to develop inhibitors. This enzyme, however, is of interest because some drugs are oxidized, generally heterocycles. In most reactions, the nature of the products is not immediately discerned from P450 reactions. X-ray structures of human aldehyde oxidase (AOX1) have been reported (2.6–2.7 Å) with a substrate, phthalazine, and an inhibitor, thioridazine (Coelho et al. 2015). Strategies have been reported to change drug candidate structures to avoid oxidation by aldehyde oxidase (Linton et al. 2011). Finally, dietary constituents have been identified as inhibitors of aldehyde oxidase (Barr et al. 2015, Hamzeh-Mivehroud et al. 2013).

The neonicotinoid insecticide imidacloprid has been shown to be reduced from a nitro to a nitroso substitution. The nitroso compound, in turn, is an irreversible, mechanism-based inactivator of rabbit aldehyde oxidase, as judged by several kinetic and other criteria, including covalent binding (Dick et al. 2007).

Carbonyl Dehydrogenases and Reductases

Pyrazole is an inhibitor of alcohol dehydrogenase. Disulfiram is a well-known inhibitor of aldehyde dehydrogenase. This drug, Antabuse®, has been given to recovering alcoholics to produce unpleasant physiological effects when the individuals consume ethanol. Disulfiram is reduced to diethyldithiocarbamate, which seems to be bound to Cys-302 of the enzyme in disulfide linkage (Vasilou and Petersen 2010). Diethyldithiocarbamate is also an inhibitor of some P450s (esp. 2E1, 2A6) (Yamazaki et al. 1992). It may have a mechanism-based action, at least as judged by the kinetics seen in limited investigations (Guengerich et al. 1991). *In vivo*, diethyldithiocarbamate is methylated and then oxygenated to yield a more effective inhibitor (Hart and Faiman 1993, Madan et al. 1995).

The sedative chloral (2,2,2-trichloroacetaldehyde) is a competitive inhibitor of aldehyde dehydrogenase, with a K_i value of 1–10 µM. A stable thiohemiacetal is formed with Cys-302. Because of the electronegativity of the chlorine atoms, transfer of a hydride ion is effectively blocked.

Other drugs that inhibit aldehyde dehydrogenase include cyanamide and pargyline (Vasilou and Petersen 2010). Cyanamide is activated in the presence of H_2O_2 and catalase to generate N-hydroxycyanamide (HO-NH-CN), which decomposes to cyanide and nitroxyl (NH=O), which inhibits aldehyde dehydrogenase. Pargyline is activated by P450 2E1 to propioaldehyde, which attacks aldehyde dehydrogenase. Aldehyde dehydrogenase is also inhibited in its action on nitroglycerin, in a mechanism that is not completely understood (Vasilou and Petersen 2010).

The systemic fungicide benomyl has been found to be a selective inhibitor of ADH2 (Staub et al. 1999, Vasilou and Petersen 2010).

The drug sulindac is selective for AKR1B10 (Cousido-Siah et al. 2015), salicylates inhibit AKR1C1 (Dhagat et al. 2007), ursodeoxycholate and bile acids inhibit AKR1C2 (Jin 2011), indomethacin inhibits AKR1C3 (Byrns et al. 2008), and phenolphthalein inhibits AKR1C4 (Ohta et al. 2000, Penning 2018). Flufemic acid and 6-medroxypregesterone acetate are general Subfamily 1C AKR inhibitors (Byrns et al. 2008, Khanim et al. 2014, Penning 2018).

Aldose reductase (AKR1B1) is a target for inhibition in the treatment of certain types of diabetes. The drugs sorbinil (Bohren et al. 2000), alrestatin (Ehrig et al. 1994), and tolrestat (Rastelli and Costantino 1998) are effective in diabetic rats but have not been as useful in humans (Flynn and Kubiseski 1997). Ponalrestat (Sato and Kador 1990) may have more specificity for AKR1B1 > AKR1A1 (Penning 2018).

Esterases and Amidases

The mechanisms of inhibition of acetylcholinesterase have long been of interest because chemical warfare agents (nerve gases) and organophosphate insecticides can interfere with cholinergic transmission and lead to respiratory failure. The basic principles have been known for some time and involve nucleophilic attack by a Ser in the active site (Lockridge and Quinn 2010, Lockridge et al. 2018) (Figure 8.8). In contrast to most of the examples of drug inhibition, this is a "non-competitive" mechanism where reaction with an active site Ser occurs. The reaction is somewhat reversible in that hydrolysis can occur to reactivate the enzyme. However, a rearrangement usually referred to as "aging" can occur to fix the damage by generation of a non-hydrolyzable linkage (Lockridge and Quinn 2010, Lockridge et al. 2018). Transition-state analog inhibitors of acetylcholinesterase have been developed by replacing the ester moiety with ketones (Ordentlich et al. 1998).

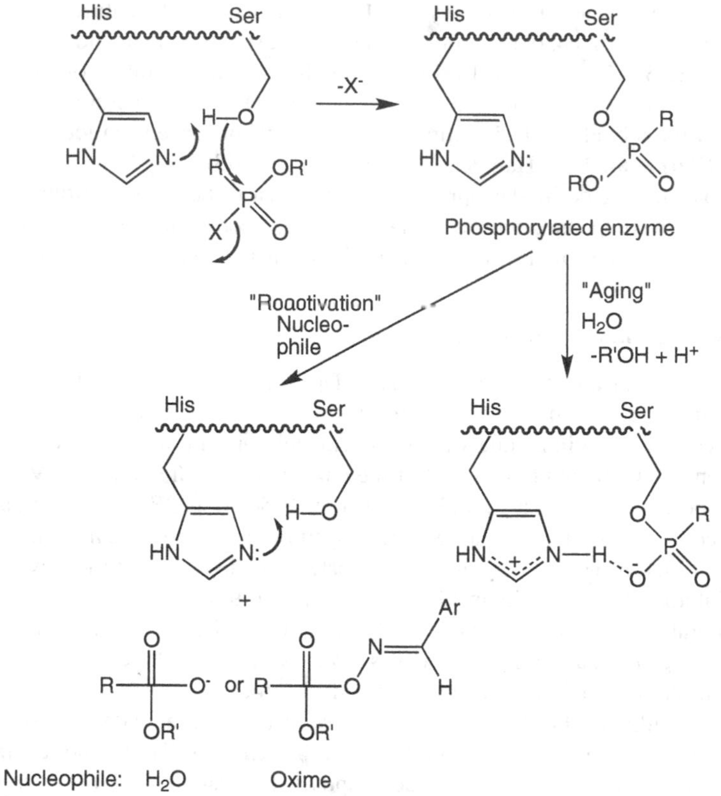

FIGURE 8.8 Inactivation of acetylcholinesterase by organophosphates and enzyme reactivation and "aging". (From Quinn, D.M., Esterases of the *a/b* hydrolase fold family, in *Biotransformation, Vol. 3, Comprehensive Toxicology*, edited by F.P. Guengerich, 243–264, Elsevier Science Ltd, Oxford, UK, 1997.)

Other esterases (e.g., butyrylcholinesterase, paraoxonase, carboxylesterase, esterase D) have no unique physiological function but are involved in the metabolism of drugs and pesticides. Esterases follow only P450s and UDP-glycosyl transferases in their contribution to drug metabolism (Williams et al. 2004). Covalent binding of the nerve agent sarin occurs to Ser-198 of butylcholinesterase (Lockridge et al. 2018).

Serine esterases are inhibited by a number of organophosphates and related compounds, including diisopropyl fluorophosphate, paraoxon, malaoxon, dichlorvos, chlorpyrifos oxon, phenylmethyl sulfonyl fluoride, and other nerve agents, as well as NaF itself (Lockridge et al. 2018). Paraoxonase is not very sensitive to these agents, however, but is sensitive to calcium chelators, e.g., EDTA. Ethopropazine inhibits paraoxonase but not acetylcholineesterase, but the opposite holds for compound BW294C51 (Lockridge et al. 2018). Eserine inhibits both (Lockridge et al. 2018).

Epoxide Hydrolase

The epoxide hydrolases are now recognized to be a subfamily of the α,β-lyase family that have certain features that make epoxides good substrates (Lacourciere and Armstrong 1994). The discovery that a covalent ester intermediate is formed has had considerable implication for mechanistic studies (Lacourciere and Armstrong 1993). Early reports of modes of inhibition should be re-examined in this context.

A number of supposedly competitive inhibitors of microsomal epoxide hydrolase have been reported (Oesch 1974). Of these, 3,3,3-trichloropropylene oxide was historically considered the most diagnostic, although it seems to have disappeared from the commercial market because of unknown regulatory issues. If an ester intermediate is formed, the rate of hydrolysis of this may be the issue, and this may be better classified as a slow, tight-binding inhibitor. Other non-epoxide "stable" inhibitors have been developed, beginning with valpromide (Pacifici et al. 1986). A potent one is 2-nonylsulfonyl propionamide (K_i 72 nM) (Morisseau et al. 2008).

Soluble epoxide hydrolase, a cytosolic enzyme, has an important physiological role in the hydrolysis of epoxides of fatty acids (Marowsky and Arand 2018, Marowsky et al. 2010). The soluble epoxide hydrolase has inhibitors with lower K_i values, particularly among the chalcone oxides (Hammock et al. 1997). Hammock's group has developed inhibitors that are being considered for treatment of a number of disease states (Goswami et al. 2016, Guedes et al. 2016, Hye Khan et al. 2016, Nording et al. 2015, Ren et al. 2016).

Glutathione (GSH) Transferases

These enzymes are very abundant (Jakoby and Habig 1980), and the crystal structures of many are now known (Armstrong 1991, 2010). Some hydrophobic compounds are good ligands (hence one of the original names, "ligandin" (Litwack et al. 1971)), which probably act as competitive inhibitors (Jakoby and Habig 1980). GSH has a K_d for several of the GSH transferases of ~20 μM, facilitating the use of affinity chromatography for purification (Simons and Vander Jagt 1977). Replacement of the R_2CH-CH_2-SH moiety of GSH with $R_2CH_2CO_2^-$ provides an analog of a key intermediate (thiolate anion), which has a K_i of 0.9 μM (Graminski et al. 1989b). A somewhat similar approach was used by Mulder, who replaced the entire L-Cys-Gly moiety with D-aminoadipate (Adang et al. 1991) (K_i 8 μM). Also, a Meisenheimer complex of GSH with 1,3,5-trinitrobenzene appears to behave as a transition state analog (Graminski et al. 1989). Product complexes can also be used as inhibitors (Armstrong 2010). For instance, S-(3′-iodobenzyl)GSH had a K_i of 0.2 μM and was used to solve the structure of GST 3-3, as a source of a heavy atom in diffraction studies. Some GSH conjugates have been used as affinity labels (Katusz et al. 1992). The GSH conjugate 2-(S-glutathionyl)-3,5,6-trichloro-1,4-benzoquinone is an effective irreversible inhibitor (K_i < 1 μM, k_{inact} 0.3 min^{-1}) and modifies active site Tyr groups (Ploemen et al. 1994). Since GSH transferases are generally beneficial, the question can be raised as to why they should be targets for inhibition. The antischistosomal drug praziquantel is used to inhibit the parasite *Schistosoma japonica* (McTigre et al. 1995). It appears to compete by binding to a hydrophobic substrate site near the subunit interface of the dimer. Also, GSH transferase overexpression may contribute to multiple drug resistance in cancer cells and is a potential therapeutic target (McTigre et al. 1995, Tew 2016).

Sulfotransferase

The phenols 2,6-dichloro-4-nitrophenol and pentachlorophenol have been described as competitive, "dead-end" inhibitors of Family 1 sulfotransferase (Duffel 2010, 2017). Hydroxylated metabolites of polychlorinated biphenyls (PCBs) are inhibitors of hSULT1E1 and other Family 1 sulfotransferases (Duffel 2017). Triclosan, a polycyclic aromatic hydrocarbon phenol, inhibits thyroid hormone sulfation (Duffel 2017). A variety of drugs, food components, food additives, and endogenous chemicals have been shown to inhibit sulfotransferases (Duffel 2017).

UDP-Glycosyl Transferase (UGT)

Many drugs have been characterized as competitive inhibitors of the steroid-, bilirubin-, and drug-conjugation activities of UDP-glycosyltransferases (formerly called UDP-glucuronosyltransferases, UGTs) (see Table 7 of Mackenzie et al. 2010). The roles of these interactions in practical drug metabolism issues are largely unexplored. Both transition-state analog inhibitors (Noort et al. 1990) and photoaffinity labels (Radominska et al. 1994, Thomassin and Tephly 1990, Xiong et al. 2006) have been designed and used to characterize these enzymes (Mackenzie et al. 2010).

One of the deficiencies in the UGT field is the limited number of inhibitors specific for individual UGT enzymes (Meech et al. 2017). The UGTs are second only to P450s in terms of the fraction of drugs metabolized (Williams et al. 2004). Some selectivity has been noted with drugs (Meech et al. 2017): UGT1A4 is selectively inhibited by hecogenin (Uchaipichat et al. 2006a), UGT2B7 by fluconazole (Uchaipichat et al. 2006), and UGT1A1 by nilotinib (Ai et al. 2014). Relatively limited information is available about *in vivo* drug-drug interactions involving UGTs (Meech et al. 2017).

Examples of Relevance of Inhibition to Drug-Drug Interactions

Clinical aspects of drug-drug interactions are covered elsewhere in this book and, therefore, only a few classical examples of *in vivo* problems will be mentioned here. The reader is also referred to other treatments of the subject (Guengerich 2015, Ito et al. 2005).

As mentioned already, in some cases, the enzymes are targets and inhibition is intended. In other cases, some inhibition may be expected based on preliminary *in vitro* assays. Nevertheless, most pharmaceutical companies would rather not put a drug with the potential for interaction problems on the market, if another that did not have such potential were available. What one would like to avoid is the development of a potential inhibition/interaction problem with a drug already on the market (or heavily invested in the developmental process). A few examples will be mentioned.

The H_2 receptor antagonist cimetidine has been widely prescribed for ulcers. This compound can inhibit P450-catalyzed reactions, although it is a relatively weak inhibitor (Knodell et al. 1991). Nevertheless, a considerable market share was lost to the non-inhibitory alternative ranitidine through advertising, on the basis of the prospect of drug-drug interactions.

Terfenadine was the first non-sedating antihistamine on the market and was highly successful (Guengerich 2014b). Nevertheless, some adverse incidents have been reported, and the basis of some seems to be related to metabolism. Terfenadine is usually extensively oxidized, and in most individuals none of the parent drug is found circulating in plasma. One of the two main oxidation routes yields the inactive N-dealkylation products. The product of the other oxidation route, a carboxylic acid, retains its ability to block the histamine receptor. The acid is actually a zwitterion and does not readily cross the blood brain barrier, so it is non-sedating. If P450 3A4 is inhibited, then terfenadine can accumulate and may cause arrythmias (Kivistö et al. 1994, Yun et al. 1993). Adverse effects had been reported (Woosley et al. 1993), and the FDA withdrew registration, mainly based on experiences with the concurrent use of known P450 3A4 inhibitors, e.g., erythromycin and ketoconazole (Guengerich 2014b, Stinson 1997).

Another example of P450 3A4 inhibition involves the progestin gestodene, which had been used with the estrogen 17α-ethynylestradiol in some oral contraceptive formulations. All 17α-acetylenic steroids seem to have some inherent capability of acting as P450 mechanism-based inactivators (Guengerich 1988, Ortiz de Montellano et al. 1979), but gestodene was more effective than many others (Guengerich 1990). The inhibition of P450 3A4 has been offered as an explanation for some of the thrombolytic problems attributed to gestodene (Jung-Hoffmann and Kuhl 1990), because inhibition of 17β-estradiol and 17β-ethynylestradiol oxidation (catalyzed by P450 3A4) could raise estrogen levels, a known factor in thrombolytic problems. The levels of gestodene ingested daily are not high enough to account for destruction of a substantial fraction of the hepatic P450 3A4 pool (Guengerich 1990) but could account for loss of the intestinal pool, as in the case of grapefruit juice and bergomottin and related compounds (Ainslie et al. 2014, Schmiedlin-Ren et al. 1997, Seden et al. 2010).

Considerations of Enzyme Inhibition in Medicinal Chemistry and Drug Development

Today many pharmaceutical companies routinely screen libraries of new chemical entities for inhibition early in the drug development process. The major concern is inhibition of P450 enzymes and the potential for drug-drug interactions. Five P450 enzymes—1A2, 2C9, 2C19, 2D6, and 3A4—account for ~90% of all P450 metabolism of drugs, and these are used in initial screens (Guengerich 2015, Rendic and Guengerich 2015). One strategy is to use individual recombinant P450s; the other is to use human liver microsomes. With either, one can use either model fluorescent or luminescent substrates for individual P450s (Crespi et al. 1998), although these have largely been supplanted by diagnostic marker reactions (Correia and Hollenberg 2015), usually with LC-MS methods. Most pharmaceutical companies have moved in favor of the LC-MS approaches because of better predictability of interactions with company compounds.

Reversible inhibition can be analyzed rapidly. In general, IC_{50} values of >10 μM are considered unimportant, IC_{50} values $<1\mu$M are considered problematic, and IC_{50} values of 1–10 μM are considered possible issues, depending upon the predicted plasmal tissue C_{max}, although plasma concentrations of drugs are usually $<1\mu$M. However, today it is appreciated that tissue levels can be much higher than plasma levels due to the action of uptake transporters (Ho and Kim 2010). For more extensive discussion of *in vitro/in vivo* extrapolation of inhibition parameters, see (Houston and Galetin 2003, Ito et al. 1998a, Shiran et al. 2006).

Compounds that are still of interest are further examined for the contribution of preincubation with NADPH on metabolism of P450 diagnostic substrates. The consideration of mechanism-based inactivation is more complex. For a list of some of the typical chemical moieties associated with P450 mechanism-based inactivation, see Table 8.2. One approach is to experimentally obtain *in vitro* parameters for inhibition in human liver microsomes, purified human P450 systems, or human hepatocytes. The parameters of most interest are the partition coefficient, $k_{inactivation}$, and K_i (Figure 8.2). The ratio $k_{inactivation}/K_i$ is perhaps the most useful parameter, being rather analogous to k_{cat}/K_m for catalysis, which is prediction of Cl_{int} *in vivo*.

The ratio $k_{inactivation}/K_i$ does not give a definite answer regarding whether a drug candidate will be a problem *in vivo*. The dose will be one issue, as will the partition ratio. However, a very useful strategy is to compare $k_{inactivation}/K_i$ (and other parameters) to drugs already used in practice and experience with those. For instance, $k_{inactivation}/K_i$ varies from 2 (17α-ethynylestradiol) to 126,000 (ritonavir) (Zhou et al. 2005) or possibly even more (Kaur et al. 2016). The former compound is generally not considered to be a problem, due to low doses but the latter is recognized as producing major *in vivo* drug interactions. Further development of databases such as this should help guide decisions about prediction of drug-drug interactions Ito et al. (1998b).

Conclusions

Inhibition of the enzymes usually associated with drug metabolism is a subject of both basic and practical interest. Basic studies involve studies of mechanisms of catalysis and the utilization of selective inhibitors of individual forms of enzymes in multigene families. Practical aspects of inhibition include drug-drug interactions and enzymes as therapeutic targets. Among the more common modes of enzyme inhibition seen are competitive inhibition, product inhibition, slow, tight-binding inhibition, mechanism-based inactivation, and products that become covalently attached. Discrimination among these is necessary for a proper understanding of action. However, in some cases, the classification into a particular mode may not be obvious. A better understanding of inhibition mechanisms and selectivity has led to more efficient screening for drug-drug interactions in the pharmaceutical industry and appreciation of the phenomenon in the regulatory agencies.

ACKNOWLEDGMENT

Research in the author's laboratory has been supported in the past by USPHS grant R37 CA090426 and currently by R01 GM118122. Thanks are extended to K. Trisler for assistance in preparation of the manuscript.

REFERENCES

Abeles, R.H. and T.A. Alston. "Enzyme inhibition by fluoro compounds." *Journal of Biological Chemistry* 265 (1990):16705–16708.

Abeles, R.H. and A.L. Maycock. "Suicide enzyme inactivators." *Accounts of Chemical Research* 9 (1976):313–319.

Adang, A.E.P., J. Brussee, A. van der Gen, and G.J. Mulder. "Inhibition of rat liver glutahione S-transferase isoenzymes by peptides stabilized against degradation by γ-glutamyl transpeptidases." *Journal of Biological Chemistry* 266 (1991):830–836.

Ai, L., L. Zhu, L. Yang, G. Ge, Y. Cao, Y. Liu, Z. Fang, and Y. Zhang. "Selectivity for inhibition of nilotinib on the catalytic activity of human UDP-glucuronosyltransferases." *Xenobiotica* 44 (4) (2014):320–325.

Ainslie, G.R., K.K. Wolf, Y. Li, E. A. Connolly, Y.V. Scarlett, J.H. Hull, and M.F. Paine. "Assessment of a candidate marker constituent predictive of a dietary substance-drug interaction: Case study with grapefruit juice and CYP3A4 drug substrates." *Journal of Pharmacology and Experimental Therapeutics* 351 (3) (2014):576–584.

Aoyama, Y., Y. Yoshida, T. Nishino, H. Katsuki, U.S. Maitra, V.P. Mohan, and D.B. Sprinson. "Isolation and characterization of an altered cytochrome P-450 from a yeast mutant defective in lanosterol 14α-demethylation." *Journal of Biological Chemistry* 262 (1987):14260–14264.

Armstrong, R.N. "Glutathione S-transferases: Reaction mechanism, structure, and function." *Chemical Research in Toxicology* 4 (1991):131–140.

Armstrong, R.N. 2010. "Glutathione transferases." In *Bioransformation*, edited by F.P. Guengerich, 295–321. Oxford, UK: Elsevier.

Augusto, O., H.S. Beilan, and P.R. Ortiz de Montellano. "The catalytic mechanism of cytochrome P-450: Spin-trapping evidence for one-electron substrate oxidation." *Journal of Biological Chemistry* 257 (1982):11288–11295.

Bach, A.W.J., N.C. Lan, D.L. Johnson, C.W. Abell, M.E. Bembenek, S.W. Kwan, P.H. Seeburg, and J.C. Shih. "cDNA cloning of human liver monoamine oxidase A and B: Molecular basis of differences in enzymatic properties." *Proceedings of the National Academy of Sciences, USA* 85 (1988):4934–4938.

Baldwin, S.J., J.C. Bloomer, G.J. Smith, A.D. Ayrton, S.E. Clarke, and R.J. Chenery. "Ketoconazole and sulphaphenazole as the respective selective inhibitors of P450 3A and 2C9." *Xenobiotica* 25 (1995):261–270.

Barr, J.T., J.P. Jones, N.H. Oberlies, and M.F. Paine. "Inhibition of human aldehyde oxidase activity by diet-derived constituents: Structural influence, enzyme-ligand interactions, and clinical relevance." *Drug Metabolism and Disposition* 43 (1) (2015):34–41.

Beedham, C. 2010. "Xanthine oxidoreductase and aldehyde oxidase." In *Biotransformation*, edited by F.P. Guengerich, 185–205. New York: Elsevier.

Black, D.J., K.L. Kunze, L.C. Wienkers, B.E. Gidal, T.L. Seaton, N.D. Mcdonnell, J.S. Evans, J.E. Bauwens, and W.F. Trager. "Warfarin-fluconazole II. A metabolically based drug interaction: *In vivo* studies." *Drug Metabolism and Disposition* 24 (1996):422–428.

Böcker, R.H. and F.P. Guengerich. "Oxidation of 4-aryl- and 4-alkyl-substituted 2,6-dimethyl-3,5-bis(alkoxycarbonyl)-1,4-dihydropyridines by human liver microsomes and immunochemical evidence for the involvement of a form of cytochrome P-450." *Journal of Medicinal Chemistry* 29 (1986):1596–1603.

Bohren, K.M. and C.E. Grimshaw. "The Sorbinil Trap: A Predicted Dead-End Complex Confirms the Mechanism of Aldose Reductase Inhibition." *Biochemistry* 39 (32) (2000):9967–9974.

Bondon, A., T.L. Macdonald, T.M. Harris, and F.P. Guengerich. "Oxidation of cycloalkylamines by cytochrome P-450. Mechanism-based inactivation, adduct formation, ring expansion, and nitrone formation." *Journal of Biological Chemistry* 264 (4) (1989):1988–1997.

Boppana, K., P.K. Dubey, S.A. Jagarlapudi, S. Vadivelan, and G. Rambabu. "Knowledge based identification of MAO-B selective inhibitors using pharmacophore and structure based virtual screening models." *European Journal of Medicinal Chemistry* 44 (9) (2009):3584–3590.

Bourrié, M., V. Meunier, Y. Berger, and G. Fabre. "Cytochrome P450 isoform inhibitors as a tool for the investigation of metabolic reactions catalyzed by human liver microsomes." *Journal of Pharmacology and Experimental Therapeutics* 277 (1996):321–332.

Brian, W.R., P.K. Srivastava, D.R. Umbenhauer, R.S. Lloyd, and F.P. Guengerich. "Expression of a human liver cytochrome P-450 protein with tolbutamide hydroxylase activity in *Saccharomyces cerevisiae*." *Biochemistry* 28 (12) (1989):4993–4999.

Bronson, D.D., D.M. Daniels, J.T. Dixon, C.C. Redick, and P.D. Haaland. "Virtual kinetics: Using statistical experimental design for rapid analysis of enzyme inhibitor mechanisms." *Biochemical Pharmacology* 50 (1995):823–831.

Byrns, M.C., S. Steckelbroeck, and T.M. Penning. "An indomethacin analogue, N-(4-chlorobenzoyl)-melatonin, is a selective inhibitor of aldo-keto reductase 1C3 (type 2 3α-HSD, type 5 17β-HSD, and prostaglandin F synthase), a potential target for the treatment of hormone dependent and hormone independent malignancies." *Biochemical Pharmacology* 75 (2) (2008):484–493.

Carradori, S. and R. Silvestri. "New frontiers in selective human MAO-B inhibitors." *Journal of Medicinal Chemistry* 58 (17) (2015):6717–6732.

Cashman, J.R. 2018. "Monoamine oxidases and flavin-containing monooxygenases." In *Biotransformation*, edited by F.P. Guengerich, 87–124. Oxford, UK: Elsevier.

Cashman, J.R. and M.S. Motika. 2010. "Monamine oxidases and flavin-containing monooxygenases." In *Biotransformation*, edited by F.P. Guengerich, 77–109. Oxford, UK: Elsevier.

Casida, J.E. "Mixed function oxidase involvement in the biochemistry of insecticide synergists." *Journal of Agricultural and Food Chemistry* 18 (1970):753–772.

Chang, T.K.H., F.J. Gonzalez, and D.J. Waxman. "Evaluation of triacetyloleandomycin, α-naphthoflavone and diethyldithiocarbamate as selective chemical probes for inhibition of human cytochrome P450." *Archives of Biochemistry and Biophysics* 311 (1994):437–442.

Chauret, N., A. Gauthier, and D.A. Nicoll-Griffith. "Effect of common organic solvents on in vitro cytochrome P450-mediated metabolic activities in human liver microsomes." *Drug Metabolism and Disposition* 26 (1998):1–4.

Chen, S., T. Zhang, J. Wang, F. Wang, H. Niu, C. Wu, and S. Wang. "Synthesis and evaluation of 1-hydroxy/methoxy-4-methyl-2-phenyl-1*H*-imidazole-5-carboxylic acid derivatives as non-purine xanthine oxidase inhibitors." *European Journal of Medicinal Chemistry* 103 (2015):343–353.

Clement, B., M. Weide, and D.M. Ziegler. "Inhibition of purified and membrane-bound flavin-containing monooxygenase 1 by (*N,N*-dimethylamino)stilbene carboxylates." *Chemical Research in Toxicology* 9 (1996):599–604.

Coelho, C., A. Foti, T. Hartmann, T. Santos-Silva, S. Leimkuhler, and M.J. Romao. "Structural insights into xenobiotic and inhibitor binding to human aldehyde oxidase." *Nature Chemical Biology* 11 (10) (2015):779–783.

Cornish-Bowden, A. 1979. *Fundamentals of Enzyme Kinetics*. London, UK: Butterworths.

Correia, M.A. 2005. "Inhibition of cytochrome P450 enzymes." In *Cytochrome P450: Structure, Mechanism, and Biochemistry*, edited by P.R. Ortiz de Montellano, 247–322. New York: Kluwer Academic.

Correia, M.A. and P.F. Hollenberg. 2015. "Inhibition of cytochrome P450 enzymes." In *Cytochrome P450: Structure, Mechanism, and Biochemistry*, edited by P.R. Ortiz de Montellano, 177–259. New York: Springer.

Cousido-Siah, A., F.X. Ruiz, I. Crespo, S. Porte, A. Mitschler, X. Pares, A. Podjarny, and J. Farres. "Structural analysis of sulindac as an inhibitor of aldose reductase and AKR1B10." *Chemico-Biological Interactions* 234 (2015):290–296.

Crespi, C.L., V.P. Miller, and B.W. Penman. "High throughput screening for inhibition of cytochrome P450 metabolism." *Medicinal Chemistry Research* 8 (1998):457–471.

Danan, G., V. Descatoire, and D. Pessayre. "Self-induction by erythromycin of its own transformation into a metabolite forming an inactive complex with reduced cytochrome P-450." *Journal of Pharmacology and Experimental Therapeutics* 218 (1981):509–514.

Davidson, N.E., P.A. Egner, and T.W. Kensler. "Transcriptional control of glutathione S-transferase gene expression by the chemoprotective agent 5-(2-pyrazinyl)-4-methyl-1,2-dithiole-3-thione (oltipraz) in rat liver." *Cancer Research* 50 (1990):2251–2255.

Denton, T.T., X. Zhang, and J.R. Cashman. "5-Substituted, 6-substituted, and unsubstituted 3-heteroaromatic pyridine analogues of nicotine as selective inhibitors of cytochrome P-450 2A6." *Journal of Medicinal Chemistry* 48 (1) (2005):224–239.

Dhagat, U., V. Carbone, R.P. Chung, T. Matsunaga, S. Endo, A. Hara, and O. El-Kabbani. "A salicylic acid-based analogue discovered from virtual screening as a potent inhibitor of human 20*a*-hydroxysteroid dehydrogenase." *Medicinal Chemistry* 3 (6) (2007):546–550.

Dick, R.A., D.B. Kanne, and J.E. Casida. "Nitroso-imidacloprid irreversibly inhibits rabbit aldehyde oxidase." *Chemical Research in Toxicology* 20 (12) (2007):1942–1946.

Dixon, M. and E.C. Webb. 1964. *Enzymes*. 2nd ed. London, UK: Longman's, Green and Co Ltd.

Dostalek, M., J.D. Brooks, K.D. Hardy, G.L. Milne, M.M. Moore, S. Sharma, J.D. Morrow, and F.P. Guengerich. "In vivo oxidative damage in rats is associated with barbiturate response but not other cytochrome P450 inducers." *Molecular Pharmcaology* 72 (6) (2007):1419–1424.

Dostalek, M., K.D. Hardy, G.L. Milne, J.D. Morrow, C. Chen, F.J. Gonzalez, J. Gu, X. Ding, D.A. Johnson, J.A. Johnson, M.V. Martin, and F.P. Guengerich. "Development of oxidative stress by cytochrome P450 induction in rodents is selective for barbiturates and related to loss of pyridine nucleotide-dependent protective systems." *Journal of Biological Chemistry* 283 (25) (2008):17147–17157.

Dostert, P.L., M.S. Benedetti, and K.F. Tipton. "Interactions of monoamine oxidase with substrates and inhibitors." *Medicinal Research Reviews* 9 (1989):45–89.

Duffel, M.W. 2010. "Sulfotransferases." In *Biotransformation*, edited by F.P. Guengerich, 367–384. Oxford, UK: Elsevier.

Duffel, M.W. 2017. "Sulfotransferases." In *Biotransformation*, edited by F.P. Guengerich, in press. Oxford, UK: Elsevier.

Ehrig, T., K.M. Bohren, F.G. Prendergast, and K.H. Gabbay. "Mechanism of aldose reductase inhibition: Binding of NADP+/NADPH and alrestatin-like inhibitors." *Biochemistry* 33 (23) (1994):7157–7165.

Flynn, T.G. and T.J. Kubiseski. 1997. "Aldo-ketoreductases: Structure, mechanism, and function." In *Comprehensive Toxicology*, edited by I.G. Sipes, C.A. McQueen, and A.J. Gandolfi, 133–147. New York: Elsevier Sciences.

Goswami, S.K., D. Wan, J. Yang, C.A. Trindade da Silva, C. Morisseau, S.D. Kodani, G.Y. Yang, B. Inceoglu, and B.D. Hammock. "Anti-ulcer efficacy of soluble epoxide hydrolase inhibitor TPPU on diclofenac-induced intestinal ulcers." *Journal of Pharmacology and Experimental Therapeutics* 357 (3) (2016):529–536.

Graminski, G.F., Y. Kubo, and R.N. Armstrong. "Spectroscopic and kinetic evidence for the thiolate anion of glutathione at the active site of glutathione S-transferase." *Biochemistry* 28 (1989a):3562–3568.

Graminski, G.F., P. Zhang, M.A. Sesay, H.L. Ammon, and R.N. Armstrong. "Formation of the 1-(S-glutathionyl)-2,4,6-trinitrocyclohexadienate anion at the active site of glutathione S-transferase: Evidence for enzymic stabilization of S-complex intermediates in nucleophilic aromatic substitution reactions." *Biochemistry* 28 (1989b):6252–6258.

Guedes, A., L. Galuppo, D. Hood, S.H. Hwang, C. Morisseau, and B.D. Hammock. "Soluble epoxide hydrolase activity and pharmacologic inhibition in horses with chronic severe laminitis." *Equine Veterinary Journal* 49 (3) (2016):345–351.

Guengerich, F.P. "Oxidation of 17α-ethynylestradiol by human liver cytochrome P-450." *Molecular Pharmacology* 33 (5) (1988):500–508.

Guengerich, F.P. "Mechanism-based inactivation of human liver microsomal cytochrome P-450 IIIA4 by gestodene." *Chemical Research in Toxicology* 3 (4) (1990):363–371.

Guengerich, F.P. "Role of cytochrome P450 enzymes in drug-drug interactions." *Advances in Pharmacology* 43 (1997):7–35.

Guengerich, F.P. "Cytochrome P-450 3A4: Regulation and role in drug metabolism." *Annual Review of Pharmacology and Toxicology* 39 (1999a):1–17.

Guengerich, F.P. 2014a. "Analysis and characterization of enzymes and nucleic acids relevant to toxicology." In *Hayes' Principles and Methods of Toxicology*, edited by A.W. Hayes and C.L. Kruger, 1905–1964. Boca Raton, FL: CRC Press-Taylor & Francis.

Guengerich, F.P. 2014b. "Cytochrome P450-mediated drug interactions and cardiovascular toxicity: The Seldane to Allegra transformation." In *Predictive ADMET: Integrated Approaches in Drug Discovery and Development*, edited by J. Wang and L. Urban, 523–534. New York: Wiley.

Guengerich, F.P. 2015. "Human cytochrome P450 enzymes." In *Cytochrome P450: Structure, Mechanism, and Biochemistry*, edited by P.R. Ortiz de Montellano, 523–785. New York: Springer.

Guengerich, F.P. "Intersection of roles of cytochrome P450 enzymes with xenobiotic and endogenous substrates. Relevance to toxicity and drug interactions." *Chemical Research in Toxicology* 30 (1) (2017):2–12.

Guengerich, F.P., D.H. Kim, and M. Iwasaki. "Role of human cytochrome P-450 IIE1 in the oxidation of many low molecular weight cancer suspects." *Chemical Research in Toxicology* 4 (2) (1991):168–179.

Guengerich, F.P., G.P. Miller, I.H. Hanna, M.V. Martin, S. Leger, C. Black, N. Chauret, J.M. Silva, L.A. Trimble, J.A. Yergey, and D.A. Nicoll-Griffith. "Diversity in the oxidation of substrates by cytochrome P450 2D6: Lack of an obligatory role of aspartate 301-substrate electrostatic bonding." *Biochemistry* 41 (36) (2002):11025–11034.

Guengerich, F.P., D. Muller-Enoch, and I.A. Blair. "Oxidation of quinidine by human liver cytochrome P-450." *Molecular Pharmcaology* 30 (3) (1986):287–295.

Guengerich, F.P. 1999b. "Inhibition of drug metabolizing enzymes: Molecular and biochemical aspects." In *Handbook of Drug Metabolism*, edited by T.F. Woolf, 203–227. New York: Marcel Dekker.

Guengerich, F.P. 2009. "Inhibition of drug metabolizing enzymes: Molecular and biochemical aspects." In *Handbook of Drug Metabolism*, 2nd ed, edited by L. Wienkers and P. Pearson, 203–226, New York: Marcel Dekker.

Guengerich, F.P. 2010. "Mechanisms of enzyme catalysis and inhibition." In *Biotransformation, Vol. 4, Comprehensive Toxicology*, 2nd ed, Vol. 4, 31–39, edited by F.P. Guengerich, McQueen, C.A. Science Ed.

Haldane, J.B.S. 1930. *Enzymes*. London, UK: Longmans, Green.

Halpert, J.R. "Structural basis of selective cytochrome P450 inhibition." *Annual Review of Pharmacology and Toxicology* 35 (1995):29–53.

Halpert, J.R., C. Balfour, N.E. Miller, and L.S. Kaminsky. "Dichloromethyl compounds as mechanism-based inactivators of rat liver cytochromes P-450 in vitro." *Molecular Pharmcaology* 30 (1986):19–24.

Halpert, J.R. and F.P. Guengerich. 1997. "Enzyme inhibition and stimulation." In *Biotransformation, Vol. 3, Comprehensive Toxicology*, edited by F.P. Guengerich, 21–35. Oxford, UK: Elsevier Science Ltd.

Hammock, B.D., D.F. Grant, and D.H. Storms. 1997. "Epoxide hydrolases." In *Biotransformation, Vol. 3, Comprehensive Toxicology*, edited by F.P. Guengerich, 283–305. Oxford, UK: Elsevier Science Ltd.

Hammons, G.J., W.L. Alworth, N.E. Hopkins, F.P. Guengerich, and F.F. Kadlubar. "2-Ethynylnaphthalene as a mechanism-based inactivator of the cytochrome P-450 catalyzed N-oxidation of 2-naphthylamine." *Chemical Research in Toxicology* 2 (6) (1989):367–374.

Hamzeh-Mivehroud, M., S. Rahmani, M.R. Rashidi, M.A. Hosseinpour Feizi, and S. Dastmalchi. "Structure-based investigation of rat aldehyde oxidase inhibition by flavonoids." *Xenobiotica* 43 (8) (2013):661–670.

Hanzlik, R.P. and R.H. Tullman. "Suicidal inactivation of cytochrome P-450 by cyclopropylamines. Evidence for cation-radical intermediates." *Journal of the American Chemical Society* 104 (1982):2048–2050.

Hargrove, T.Y., L. Friggeri, Z. Wawrzak, S. Sivakumaran, Yazlovitskaya, S.W. Heibert, F.P. Guengerich, M.R. Waterman, and G.I. Lepesheva. "Probing human cytochrome P450 sterol 14α-demethylase (CYP51) as a target for anticancer chemotherapy: Towards structure-aided drug design." *Journal of Lipid Research* 57 (2016):1552–1563.

Hart, B.W. and M.D. Faiman. "Bioactivation of *S*-methyl *N,N*-diethylthiolcarbamate to *S*-methyl *N, N*-diethylthiolcarbamate sulfoxide." *Biochemical Pharmacology* 46 (1993):2285–2290.

Hines, R.N., J.R. Cashman, R.M. Philpot, D.E. Williams, and D.M. Ziegler. "The mammalian flavin-containing monooxygenases: Molecular charcterization and regulation of expression." *Toxicology and Applied Pharmacology* 125 (1994):1–6.

Ho, R.H. and R.B. Kim. 2010. "Uptake transporters." In *Biotransfomration*, edited by F.P. Guengerich, 519–555. Oxford, UK: Elsevier.

Houston, J.B. and A. Galetin. "Progress towards prediction of human pharmacokinetic parameters from in vitro technologies." *Drug Metabolism Reviews* 35 (4) (2003):393–415.

Hye Khan, M.A., S.H. Hwang, A. Sharma, J.A. Corbett, B.D. Hammock, and J.D. Imig. "A dual COX-2/sEH inhibitor improves the metabolic profile and reduces kidney injury in Zucker diabetic fatty rat." *Prostaglandins and Other Lipid Mediators* 125 (2016):40–47.

Ito, K., D. Hallifax, R.S. Obach, and J.B. Houston. "Impact of Parallel Pathways of Drug Elimination and Multiple Cytochrome P450 Involvement on Drug-Drug Interactions: Cyp2d6 Paradigm." *Drug Metabolism and Disposition* 33 (6) (2005):837–844.

Ito, K., T. Iwatsubo, S. Kanamitsu, Y. Nakajima, and Y. Sugiyama. "Quantitative prediction of in vivo drug clearance and drug interactions from in vitro data on metabolism, together with binding and transport." *Annual Review of Pharmacology and Toxicology* 38 (1998a):461–499.

Ito, K., T. Iwatsubo, S. Kanamitsu, K. Ueda, H. Suzuki, and Y. Sugiyama. "Prediction of pharmacokinetic alterations caused by drug-drug interactions: Metabolic interaction in the liver." *Pharmacological Reviews* 50 (1998b):387–411.

Jakoby, W.B. and W.H. Habig. 1980. "Glutathione transferases." In *Enzymatic Basis of Detoxication, Vol. 2*, edited by W.B. Jakoby, 63–94. New York: Academic Press.

Jin, Y. "Activities of aldo-keto reductase 1 enzymes on two inhaled corticosteroids: Implications for the pharmacological effects of inhaled corticosteroids." *Chemico-Biological Interactions* 191 (1–3) (2011):234–238.

Jönsson, K.H. and B. Lindeke. "Cytochrome P-455 nm complex formation in the metabolism of phenylalkylamines. XII. Enantioselectivity and temperature dependence in microsomes and reconstituted cytochrome P-450 systems from rat liver." *Chirality* 4 (1992):469–477.

Jung-Hoffmann, C., and H. Kuhl. "Pharmacokinetics and pharmacodynamics of oral contraceptive steroids: Factors influencing steroid metabolism." *American Journal of Obstetrics and Gynecology* 163 (1990):2183–2197.

Katusz, R.M., B. Bono, and R.F. Colman. "Affinity labeling of Cys[111] of glutathione *S*-transferase, isoenzyme 1-1, by *S*-(4-bromo-2,3-dioxobutyl)glutathione." *Biochemistry* 31 (1992):8984–8990.

Kaur, P., A.R. Chamberlin, T.L. Poulos, and I.F. Sevrioukova. "Structure-based inhibitor design for evaluation of a CYP3A4 pharmacophore model." *Journal of Medicinal Chemistry* 59 (9) (2016):4210–4220.

Khanim, F., N. Davies, P. Velica, R. Hayden, J. Ride, C. Pararasa, M.G. Chong, U. Gunther, N. Veerapen, P. Winn, R. Farmer, E. Trivier, L. Rigoreau, M. Drayson, and C. Bunce. "Selective AKR1C3 inhibitors do not recapitulate the anti-leukaemic activities of the pan-AKR1C inhibitor medroxyprogesterone acetate." *British Journal of Cancer* 110 (6) (2014):1506–1516.

Kivistö, K.T., P.J. Neuvonen, and U. Klotz. "Inhibition of terfenadine metabolism: Pharmacokinetic and pharmacodynamic consequences." *Clinical Pharmacokinetics* 27 (1994):1–5.

Knodell, R.G., D.G. Browne, G.P. Gwozdz, W.R. Brian, and F.P. Guengerich. "Differential inhibition of individual human liver cytochromes P-450 by cimetidine." *Gastroenterology* 101 (6) (1991):1680–1691.

Kohagura, K., T. Tana, A. Higa, M. Yamazato, A. Ishida, K. Nagahama, A. Sakima, K. Iseki, and Y. Ohya. "Effects of xanthine oxidase inhibitors on renal function and blood pressure in hypertensive patients with hyperuricemia." *Hypertension Research* 39 (8) (2016):593–597.

Koymans, L., N.P.E. Vermeulen, S.A.B.E. van Acker, J.M. te Koppele, J.J.P. Heykants, K. Lavrijsen, W. Meuldermans, and G.M. Donné-Op den Kelder. "A predictive model for substrates of cytochrome P450-debrisoquine (2D6)." *Chemical Research in Toxicology* 5 (1992):211–219.

Kuby, S.A. 1991. *A Study of Enzymes, Vol. I, Enzyme Catalysis, Kinetics, and Substrate Binding*. Boca Raton, FL: CRC Press.

Lacourciere, G.M. and R.N. Armstrong. "The catalytic mechanism of microsomal epoxide hydrolase involves an ester intermediate." *Journal of the American Chemical Society* 115 (1993):10466–10467.

Lacourciere, G.M. and R.N. Armstrong. "Microsomal and soluble epoxide hydrolases are members of the same family of C-X bond hydrolase enzymes." *Chemical Research in Toxicology* 7 (1994):121–124.

Langouët, S., B. Coles, F. Morel, L. Becquemont, P. Beaune, F.P. Guengerich, B. Ketterer, and A. Guillouzo. "Inhibition of CYP1A2 and CYP3A4 by oltipraz results in reduction of aflatoxin B_1 metabolism in human hepatocytes in primary culture." *Cancer Research* 55 (23) (1995):5574–5579.

Lerner, R.A. and S.J. Benkovic. "Principles of antibody catalysis." *Bioessays* 9 (1988):107–112.

Lin, H.L., J.D'Agostino, C. Kenaan, D. Calinski, and P.F. Hollenberg. "The effect of ritonavir on human CYP2B6 catalytic activity: Heme modification contributes to the mechanism-based inactivation of CYP2B6 and CYP3A4 by ritonavir." *Drug Metabolism and Disposition* 41 (10) (2013):1813–1824.

Lin, H.L., C. Kenaan, and P.F. Hollenberg. "Identification of the residue in human CYP3A4 that is covalently modified by bergamottin and the reactive intermediate that contributes to the grapefruit juice effect." *Drug Metabolism and Disposition* 40 (5) (2012):998–1006.

Lin, H.L., H.M. Zhang, M.J. Pratt-Hyatt, and P.F. Hollenberg. "Thr302 is the site for the covalent modification of human cytochrome P450 2B6 leading to mechanism-based inactivation by *tert*-butylphenylacetylene." *Drug Metabolism and Disposition* 39 (12) (2011a):2431–2439.

Lin, H.L., H. Zhang, C. Medower, P.F. Hollenberg, and W.W. Johnson. "Inactivation of cytochrome P450 (P450) 3A4 but not P450 3A5 by OSI-930, a thiophene-containing anticancer drug." *Drug Metabolism and Disposition* 39 (2) (2011b):345–350.

Linton, A., P. Kang, M. Ornelas, S. Kephart, Q. Hu, M. Pairish, Y. Jiang, and C. Guo. "Systematic structure modifications of imidazo[1,2-*a*]pyrimidine to reduce metabolism mediated by aldehyde oxidase (AO)." *Journal of Medicinal Chemistry* 54 (21) (2011):7705–7712.

Litwack, G., B. Ketterer, and I.M. Arias. "Ligandin: A hepatic protein which binds steroids, bilirubin, carcinogens, and a number of exogenous anions." *Nature* 234 (1971):466–467.

Lockridge, O. and D.M. Quinn. 2010. "Esterases." In *Biotransformation*, edited by F.P. Guengerich, 243–273. Oxford, UK: Elsevier.

Lockridge, O., D.M. Quinn, and Z. Radić. 2018. "Esterases." In *Biotransformation*, edited by F.P. Guengerich, 277–307. Oxford, UK: Elsevier.

Lukton, D., J.E. Mackie, J.S. Lee, G.S. Marks, and P.R. Ortiz de Montellano. "2,2-Dialkyl-1,2-dihydroquinolines: Cytochrome P-450 catalyzed N-alkylporphyrin formation, ferrochelatase inhibition, and induction of 5-aminolevulinic acid synthase activity." *Chemical Research in Toxicology* 1 (1988):208–215.

Macdonald, T.L., K. Zirvi, L.T. Burka, P. Peyman, and F.P. Guengerich. "Mechanism of cytochrome P-450 inhibition by cyclopropylamines." *Journal of the American Chemical Society* 104 (1982):2050–2052.

Mackenzie, P.I., D.A. Gardner-Stephen, and J.O. Miners. 2010. "UDP-glucuronosyltransferases." In *Biotransformation*, edited by F.P. Guengerich, 413–433. Oxford, UK: Elsevier.

Madan, A., A. Parkinson, and M.D. Faiman. "Identification of the human and rat P450 enzymes responsible for the sulfoxidation of *S*-methyl *N, N*-diethylthiolcarbamate (DETC-Me): The terminal step in the bioactivation of disulfiram." *Drug Metabolism and Disposition* 23 (1995):1153–1162.

Mancy, A., S. Dijols, S. Poli, P. Guengerich, and D. Mansuy. "Interaction of sulfaphenazole derivatives with human liver cytochromes P450 2C: Molecular origin of the specific inhibitory effects of sulfaphenazole on CYP 2C9 and consequences for the substrate binding site topology of CYP 2C9." *Biochemistry* 35 (50) (1996):16205–16212.

Marnett, L.J. "Cyclooxygenase mechanisms." *Current Opinion in Chemical Biology* 4 (5) (2000): 545–552.

Marowsky, A. and M. Arand. 2018. "Mammalian epoxide hydrolases." In *Biotransformation*, edited by F.P. Guengerich, 275–294. Oxford, UK: Elsevier.

Marowsky, A., A. Cronin, F. Frere, M. Adamska, and M. Arand. 2010. "Mammalian epoxide hydrolases." In *Biotransformation*, edited by F.P. Guengerich, 275–294. Oxford, UK: Elsevier.

Masters, B.S.S. 1980. "The role of NADPH-cytochrome *c* (P-450) reductase in detoxication." In *Enzymatic Basis of Detoxication, Vol. I*, edited by W.B. Jakoby, 183–200. New York: Academic Press.

McTigre, M.A., D.R. Williams, and J.A. Tainer. "Crystal structures of a Schistomal drug vaccine target: Glutathione S-transferase from *Schistoma japonica* and its complex with the leading antischistosomal drug praziquantel." *Journal of Molecular Biology* 246 (1995):21.

Meech, R., D.-G. Hu, J.O. Miners, and P.I. Mackenzie. 2018. "UDP-glycosyltransferases." In *Biotransformation*, edited by F.P. Guengerich, 469–496. Oxford, UK: Elsevier.

Meschter, C.L., B.A. Mico, M. Mortillo, D. Feldman, W.A. Garland, J.A. Riley, and L.S. Kaufman. "A 13-week toxicologic and pathologic evaluation of prolonged cytochromes P450 inhibition by 1-aminobenzotriazole in male rats." *Fundamental and Applied Toxicology* 22 (1994):369–381.

Miller, N.E. and J. Halpert. "Analogues of chloramphenicol as mechanism-based inactivators of rat liver cytochrome P-450: Modifications of the propanediol side chain, the *p*-nitro group, and the dichloromethyl moiety." *Molecular Pharmcaology* 29 (1986):391–398.

Miners, J.O., K.J. Smith, R.A. Robson, M.E. McManus, M.E. Veronese, and D.J. Birkett. "Tolbutamide hydroxylation by human liver microsomes: Kinetic characterisation and relationship to other cytochrome P-450 dependent xenobiotic oxidations." *Biochemical Pharmacology* 37 (1988):1137–1144.

Mitchell, D.J., D. Nikolic, E. Rivera, S.O. Sablin, S. Choi, R.B. van Breemen, T.P. Singer, and R.B. Silverman. "Spectrometric evidence for the flavin-1-phenylcyclopropylamine inactivator adduct with monoamine oxidase N." *Biochemistry* 40 (18) (2001a):5447–5456.

Mitchell, D.J., D. Nikolic, R.B. van Breemen, and R.B. Silverman. "Inactivation of monoamine oxidase B by 1-phenylcyclopropylamine: Mass spectral evidence for the flavin adduct." *Bioorganic & Medicinal Chemistry Letters* 11 (13) (2001b):1757–1760.

Morisseau, C., J.W. Newman, C.E. Wheelock, T. Hill Iii, D. Morin, A.R. Buckpitt, and B.D. Hammock. "Development of metabolically stable inhibitors of mammalian microsomal epoxide hydrolase." *Chemical Research in Toxicology* 21 (4) (2008):951–957.

Murray, M. and C.F. Wilkinson. "Interactions of nitrogen heterocycles with cytochrome P-450 and monooxygenase activity." *Chemico-Biological Interactions* 50 (1984):267–275.

Murray, M., C.F. Wilkinson, C. Marcus, and C.E. Dubé. "Structure-activity relationships in the interactions of alkoxymethylenedioxybenzene derivatives with rat hepatic microsomal mixed-function oxidases in vivo." *Molecular Pharmcaology* 24 (1983):129–136.

Newton, D.J., R.W. Wang, and A.Y.H. Lu. "Cytochrome P450 inhibitors: Evaluation of specificities in the *in vitro* metabolism of therapeutic agents by human liver microsomes." *Drug Metabolism and Disposition* 23 (1994):154–158.

Noort, D., M.W.H. Coughtrie, B. Burchell, G.A. van der Morel, J.H. van Boom, A. van der Gen, and G.J. Mulder. "Inhibition of UDP-glucuronosyltransferase activity by possible transition state analogues in rat liver microsomes." *European Journal of Biochemistry* 281 (1990):170.

Nording, M.L., J. Yang, L. Hoang, V. Zamora, D. Uyeminami, I. Espiritu, K.E. Pinkerton, B.D. Hammock, and A. Luria. "Bioactive lipid profiling reveals drug target engagement of a soluble epoxide hydrolase inhibitor in a murine model of tobacco smoke exposure." *Journal of Metabolomics* 1 (2015):1–14.

Oesch, F. "Purification and specificity of a human microsomal epoxide hydratase." *Biochemical Journal* 139 (1974):77–88.

Ohta, T., S. Ishikura, S. Shintani, N. Usami, and A. Hara. "Kinetic alteration of a human dihydrodiol/3alpha-hydroxysteroid dehydrogenase isoenzyme, AKR1C4, by replacement of histidine-216 with tyrosine or phenylalanine." *Biochemical Journal* 352 Pt 3 (2000):685–691.

Ordentlich, A., D. Barak, C. Kronman, N. Ariel, Y. Segall, B. Velan, and A. Shafferman. "Functional characteristics of the oxyanion hole in human acetylcholinesterase." *Journal of Biological Chemistry* 273 (31) (1998):19509–19517.

Ortiz de Montellano, P.R., ed. 2005. 3rd ed, *Cytochrome P450: Structure, Mechanism, and Biochemistry*. New York: KluwerAcademic/Plenum Publishers.

Ortiz de Montellano, P.R. 2015. "Substrate oxidation." In *Cytochrome P450: Structure, Mechanism, and Biochemistry*, edited by P.R. Ortiz de Montellano, 111–176. New York: Springer.

Ortiz de Montellano, P.R., H.S. Beilan, and K.L. Kunze. "N-Alkylprotoporphyrin IX formation in 3,5-dicarbethoxy-1,4-dihydrocollidine-treated rats: Transfer of the alkyl group from the substrate to the porphyrin." *Journal of Biological Chemistry* 256 (1981):6708–6713.

Ortiz de Montellano, P.R. and M.A. Correia. "Suicidal destruction of cytochrome P-450 during oxidative drug metabolism." *Annual Review of Pharmacology and Toxicology* 23 (1983):481–503.

Ortiz de Montellano, P.R., K.L. Kunze, G.S. Yost, and B.A. Mico. "Self-catalyzed destruction of cytochrome P-450: Covalent binding of ethynyl sterols to prosthetic heme." *Proceedings of the National Academy Sciences USA* 76 (1979):746–749.

Ortiz de Montellano, P.R. and N.O. Reich. 1986. "Inhibition of cytochrome P-450 enzymes." In *Cytochrome P-450*, edited by P.R. Ortiz de Montellano, 273–314. New York: Plenum Press.

Oyama, J., A. Tanaka, Y. Sato, H. Tomiyama, M. Sata, T. Ishizu, I. Taguchi, T. Kuroyanagi, H. Teragawa, N. Ishizaka et al. "Rationale and design of a multicenter randomized study for evaluating vascular function under uric acid control using the xanthine oxidase inhibitor, febuxostat: The PRIZE study." *Cardiovascular Diabetology* 15 (2016):87.

Pacifici, G.M., M. Franchi, C. Bencini, and A. Rane. "Valpromide inhibits human epoxide hydrolase." *British Journal of Clinical Pharmacology* 22 (3) (1986):269–274.

Pallan, P.S., L.D. Nagy, L. Lei, E. Gonzalez, V.M. Kramlinger, C.M. Azumaya, Z. Wawrzak, M.R. Waterman, F.P. Guengerich, and M. Egli. "Structural and kinetic basis of steroid 17α,20-lyase activity in teleost fish cytochrome P450 17A1 and its absence in cytochrome P450 17A2." *Journal of Biological Chemistry* 290 (6) (2015):3248–3268.

Panoutsopoulos, G.I., D. Kouretas, and C. Beedham. "Contribution of aldehyde oxidase, xanthine oxidase, and aldehyde dehydrogenase on the oxidation of aromatic aldehydes." *Chemical Research in Toxicology* 17 (10) (2004):1368–1376.

Pauling, L. "Chemical achievement and hope for the future." *American Scientist* 36 (1948):51–58.

Penning, T.M. 2018. "The aldo-keto reductase superfamily." In *Biotransformation*, edited by F.P. Guengerich, 149–167. Oxford, UK: Elsevier.

Pikuleva, I.A. and M.R. Waterman. "Cytochromes P450: Roles in diseases." *Journal of Biological Chemistry* 288 (24) (2013):17091–17098.

Ploemen, J.H.T.M., W.W. Johnson, S. Jespersen, D. Vanderwall, B. van Ommen, J. van der Greef, P.J. van Bladeren, and R.N. Armstrong. "Active-site tyrosyl residues are targets in the irreversible inhibition of a class mu glutathione transferase by 2-(*S*-glutathionyl)-3,5,6-trichloro-1,4-benzoquinone." *Journal of Biological Chemistry* 269 (1994):26890–26897.

Pratt-Hyatt, M., H.L. Lin, and P.F. Hollenberg. "Mechanism-based inactivation of human CYP2E1 by diethyldithiocarbamate." *Drug Metabolism and Disposition* 38 (12) (2010):2286–2292.

Quinn, D.M. 1997. "Esterases of the α/β hydrolase fold family." In *Biotransformation, Vol. 3, Comprehensive Toxicology*, edited by F.P. Guengerich, 243–264. Oxford, UK: Elsevier Science Ltd.

Radominska, A., P. Paul, S. Treat, H. Towbin, C. Pratt, J. Little, J. Magdalou, R. Lester, and R. Drake. "Photoaffinity labeling for evaluation of uridinyl analogs as specific inhibitors of rat liver UDP-glucuronosyltransferase." *Biochimica Biophysica Acta* 1205 (1994):336.

Rajagopalan, K.V. 1997. "Xanthine dehydrogenase and aldehyde oxidase." In *Biotransformation, Vol. 3, Comprehensive Toxicology*, edited by F.P. Guengerich, 165–178. New York: Elsevier Science.

Rando, R.R. "Mechanism-based enzyme inactivators." *Pharmacological Reviews* 36 (1984):111–142.

Rastelli, G. and L. Costantino. "Molecular dynamics simulations of the structure of aldose reductase complexed with the inhibitor tolrestat." *Bioorganic & Medicinal Chemistry Letters* 8 (6) (1998):641–646.

Ren, Q., M. Ma, T. Ishima, C. Morisseau, J. Yang, K.M. Wagner, J.C. Zhang, C. Yang, W. Yao, C. Dong, M. Han, B.D. Hammock, and K. Hashimoto. "Gene deficiency and pharmacological inhibition of soluble epoxide hydrolase confers resilience to repeated social defeat stress." *Proceeding of the National Academy of Sciences USA* 113 (13) (2016):E1944–E1952.

Rendic, S. and F.P. Guengerich. "Survey of human oxidoreductases and cytochrome P450 enzymes involved in the metabolism of xenobiotic and natural chemicals." *Chemical Research in Toxicology* 28 (1) (2015):38–42.

Renwick, A.G. 1994. "Toxicokinetics and pharmacokinetics in toxicology." In *Principles and Methods of Toxicology*, edited by A.W. Hayes, 101–147. New York: Raven Press.

Rimoldi, J.M., Y.X. Wang, S.K. Nimkar, S.H. Kuttab, A.H. Anderson, H. Burch, and N. Castagnoli, Jr. "Probing the mechanism of bioactivation of MPTP type analogs by monoamine oxidase B: Structure-activity studies on substituted 4-phenoxy-, 4-phenyl-, and 4-thiophenoxy-1-cyclopropyl-1,2,3,6-tetrahydropyridines." *Chemical Research in Toxicology* 8 (1995):703–710.

Rodrigues, M.V., A.F. Barbosa, J.F. da Silva, D.A. dos Santos, K.L. Vanzolini, M.C. de Moraes, A.G. Correa, and Q.B. Cass. "9-Benzoyl 9-deazaguanines as potent xanthine oxidase inhibitors." *Bioorganic & Medicinal Chemistry* 24 (2) (2016):226–231.

Santen, R.J., H. Brodie, E.R. Simpson, P.K. Siiteri, and A. Brodie. "History of aromatase: Saga of an important biological mediator and therapeutic target." *Endocrine Reviews* 30 (4) (2009):343–375.

Sato, S. and P.F. Kador. "Inhibition of aldehyde reductase by aldose reductase inhibitors." *Biochemical Pharmacology* 40 (5) (1990):1033–1042.

Schechter, P.J. and A. Sjoerdsma. 1990. "Therapeutic utility of selected enzyme-activated irreversible inhibitors." In *Enzymes as Targets for Drug Design*, 201–210. New York: Academic Press.

Schmiedlin-Ren, P., D.J. Edwards, M.E. Fitzsimmons, K. He, K.S. Lown, P.M. Woster, A. Rahman, K.E. Thummel, J.M. Fisher, P.F. Hollenberg, and P.B. Watkins. "Mechanisms of enhanced oral availability of CYP3A4 substrates by grapefruit constituents." *Drug Metabolism and Disposition* 25 (1997):1228–1233.

Seden, K., L. Dickinson, S. Khoo, and D. Back. "Grapefruit-drug interactions." *Drugs* 70 (18) (2010):2373–2407.

Segel, I.H. 1975a. "Multisite and allosteric enzymes." In *Enzyme Kinetics: Behavior and Analysis of Rapid Equilibrium and Steady-state Enzyme Systems*, 355–356. New York: John Wiley & Sons, Inc.

Segel, I.H. 1975b. *Enzyme Kinetics*. New York: Wiley.

Segel, I.H. 1975c. "Behavior and analysis of rapid equilibrium and steady-state enzyme systems." *Enzyme Kinetics*. New York: John Wiley & Sons, Inc.

Shimada, T. and F.P. Guengerich. "Inhibition of human cytochrome P450 1A1-, 1A2-, and 1B1-mediated activation of procarcinogens to genotoxic metabolites by polycyclic aromatic hydrocarbons." *Chemical Research in Toxicology* 19 (2) (2006):288–294.

Shimada, T., N. Murayama, K. Okada, Y. Funae, H. Yamazaki, and F. P. Guengerich. "Different mechanisms for inhibition of human cytochromes P450 1A1, 1A2, and 1B1 by polycyclic aromatic inhibitors." *Chemical Research in Toxicology* 20 (3) (2007):489–496.

Shinkyo, R. and F.P. Guengerich. "Inhibition of human cytochrome P450 3A4 by cholesterol." *Journal of Biological Chemistry* 286 (21) (2011):18426–18433.

Shiran, M.R., N.J. Proctor, E.M. Howgate, K. Rowland-Yeo, G.T. Tucker, and A. Rostami-Hodjegan. "Prediction of metabolic drug clearance in humans: In vitro-in vivo extrapolation vs allometric scaling." *Xenobiotica* 36 (7) (2006):567–580.

Silverman, R.B. "Mechanism of inactivation of monoamine oxidase by *trans*-2-phenylcyclopropylamine and the structure of the enzyme-inactivator adduct." *Journal of Biological Chemistry* 258 (1983):14766–14769.

Silverman, R.B. 1988. *Mechanism-based Enzyme Inactivation: Chemistry & Enzymology*. Boca Raton, FL: CRC Press.

Silverman, R.B. "Mechanism-based enzyme inactivators." *Methods in Enzymology* 249 (1995):240–283.

Silverman, R.B. 2004. *The Organic Chemistry of Drug Design and Drug Action*. 2nd ed. Boston, Massachusetts: Elsevier.

Silverman, R.B. and C.Z. Ding. "Chemical model for a mechanism of inactivation of monoamine oxidase by heterocyclic compounds. Electronic effects on acetal hydrolysis." *Journal of the American Chemical Society* 115 (1993):4571–4576.

Simons, P.C. and D.L. Vander Jagt. "Purification of glutathione S-transferases from human liver by glutathione-affinity chromatography." *Analitical Biochemistry* 82 (1977):334–341.

Singh, J., R.C. Petter, T.A. Baillie, and A. Whitty. "The resurgence of covalent drugs." *Nature Reviews in Drug Discovery* 10 (4) (2011):307–317.

Song, J.U., J.W. Jang, T.H. Kim, H. Park, W.S. Park, S.H. Jung, and G.T. Kim. "Structure-based design and biological evaluation of novel 2-(indol-2-yl) thiazole derivatives as xanthine oxidase inhibitors." *Bioorganic & Medicinal Chemistry Letters* 26 (3) (2016):950–954.

Sonino, N. "The use of ketoconazole as an inhibitor of steroid production." *New England Journal of Medicine* 317 (1987):812–818.

Sridar, C., C. Kenaan, and P.F. Hollenberg. "Inhibition of bupropion metabolism by selegiline: Mechanism-based inactivation of human CYP2B6 and characterization of glutathione and peptide adducts." *Drug Metabolism and Disposition* 40 (12) (2012):2256–2266.

Staub, R.E., G.B. Quistad, and J.E. Casida. "S-Methyl N-butylthiocarbamate sulfoxide: Selective carbamoylating agent for mouse mitochondrial aldehyde dehydrogenase." *Biochemical Pharmacology* 58 (9) (1999):1467–1473.

Stearns, R.A. and P.R. Ortiz de Montellano. "Inactivation of cytochrome P-450 by a catalytically generated cyclobutadiene species." *Journal of the American Chemical Society* 107 (1985):234–240.

Stepanić, V., A.C. Gasparovic, K.G. Troselj, D. Amic, and N. Zarkovic. "Selected attributes of polyphenols in targeting oxidative stress in cancer." *Current Topics in Medicinal Chemistry* 15 (5) (2015):496–509

Stinson, S.C. "Uncertain climate for antihistamines." *Chemical & Engineering News* 75 (1997):43–45.

Strelevitz, T.J., C.C. Orozco, and R.S. Obach. "Hydralazine as a selective probe inactivator of aldehyde oxidase in human hepatocytes: Estimation of the contribution of aldehyde oxidase to metabolic clearance." *Drug Metabolism and Disposition* 40 (7) (2012):1441–1448.

Strobl, G.R., S. von Kruedener, J. Stockigt, F.P. Guengerich, and T. Wolff. "Development of a pharmacophore for inhibition of human liver cytochrome P-450 2D6: Molecular modeling and inhibition studies." *Journal of Medicinal Chemistry* 36 (9) (1993):1136–1145.

Tew, D.G. "Inhibition of cytochrome P450 reductase by the diphenyliodonium cation. Kinetic analysis and covalent modifications." *Biochemistry* 32 (1993):10209–10215.

Tew, K.D. "Glutathione-associated enzymes in anticancer drug resistance." *Cancer Research* 76 (1) (2016):7–9.

Thomassin, J. and T.R. Tephly. "Photoafinity labeling of rat liver microsomal morphine UDP-glucuronosyltransferase by [³H]flunitrazepam." *Molecular Pharmacology* 38 (1990):294–298.

Tian, G.C., R.A. Mook, M.L. Moss, and S.V. Frye. "Mechanism of time-dependent inhibition of 5a-reductases by Δ¹-4-azasteroids: Toward perfection of rates of time-dependent inhibition by using ligand-binding energies." *Biochemistry* 34 (1995):13453–13459.

Tipton, K.F., J.M. McCrodden, and M.B.H. Youdim. "Oxidation and enzyme-activated irreversible inhibition of rat liver monoamine oxidase-B by 1-methyl-4-phenyl-1,2,3,6-tetrahydropyridine (MPTP)." *Biochemical Journal* 240 (1986):379–383.

Uchaipichat, V., P.I. Mackenzie, D.J. Elliot, and J.O. Miners. "Selectivity of substrate (trifluoperazine) and inhibitor (amitriptyline, androsterone, canrenoic acid, hecogenin, phenylbutazone, quinidine, quinine, and sulfinpyrazone) "probes" for human UDP-glucuronosyltransferases." *Drug Metabolism and Disposition* 34 (3) (2006a):449–456.

Uchaipichat, V., L.K. Winner, P.I. Mackenzie, D.J. Elliot, J.A. Williams, and J.O. Miners. "Quantitative prediction of in vivo inhibitory interactions involving glucuronidated drugs from in vitro data: The effect of fluconazole on zidovudine glucuronidation." *British Journal of Clinical Pharmacology* 61 (4) (2006b):427–439.

U. S. Food and Drug Administration, 2006. "Drug development and drug innteractions: Table of substrates, inhibitors and inducers." http://www.fda.gov/Drugs/DevelopmentApprovalProcess/DevelopmentResources/DrugInteractionsLabeling/ucm093664.htm (accessed 16 September 2016).

Valente, S., S. Tomassi, G. Tempera, S. Saccoccio, E. Agostinelli, and A. Mai. "Novel reversible monoamine oxidase A inhibitors: Highly potent and selective 3-(1H-pyrrol-3-yl)-2-oxazolidinones." *Journal of Medicinal Chemistry* 54 (23) (2011):8228–8232.

Vanden Bossche, H. "Inhibitors of P450-dependent steroid biosynthesis: From research to medical treatment." *Journal of Steroid Biochemistry and Molecular Biology* 43 (1992):1003–1021.

Vanden Bossche, H., L. Koymans, and H. Moereels. "P450 inhibitors of use in medical treatment: Focus on mechanisms of action." *Pharmacology and Therapeutics* 67 (1995):79–100.

VandenBrink, B.M., J.A. Davis, J.T. Pearson, R.S. Foti, L.C. Wienkers, and D.A. Rock. "Cytochrome P450 architecture and cysteine nucleophile placement impact raloxifene-mediated mechanism-based inactivation." *Molecular Pharmcaology* 82 (5) (2012):835–842.

Vasilou, V. and D.R. Petersen. 2010. "Aldehyde dehydrogenases." In *Biotransformation*, edited by F.P. Guengerich, 131–147. Oxford, UK: Elsevier.

Vermilion, J.L. and M.J. Coon. "Purified liver microsomal NADPH-cytochrome P-450 reductase: Spectral characterization of oxidation-reduction states." *Journal of Biological Chemistry* 253 (1978):2694–2704.

Viaje, A., J.Y.L. Lu, N.E. Hopkins, A.N. Nettikumara, J. DiGiovanni, W.L. Alworth, and T.J. Slaga. "Inhibition of the binding of 7,12-dimethylbenz[*a*]anthracene and benzo[*a*]pyrene to DNA in mouse skin epidermis by 1-ethynylpyrene." *Carcinogenesis* 11 (1990):1139–1143.

von Moltke, L.L., D.J. Greenblatt, S.X. Duan, J.S. Harmatz, and R.I. Shader. "*In vitro* prediction of the terfenadine-ketoconazole pharmacokinetic interaction." *Journal of Clinical Pharmacology* 34 (1994):1222–1227.

Waley, S.G. "Kinetics of suicide substrates." *Biochemical Journal* 185 (1980):771–773.

Waley, S.G. "Kinetics of suicide substrates: Practical procedures for determining parameters." *Biochemical Journal* 227 (1985):843–849.

Walsh, C.T. "Suicide substrates, mechanism-based enzyme inactivators: Recent developments." *Annual Review of Biochemistry* 53 (1984):493–535.

Williams, J.A., R. Hyland, B.C. Jones, D.A. Smith, S. Hurst, T.C. Goosen, V. Peterkin, J.R. Koup, and S.E. Ball. "Drug-drug interactions for UDP-glucuronosyltransferase substrates: A pharmacokinetic explanation for typically observed low exposure (AUC_i/AUC) ratios." *Drug Metabolism and Disposition* 32 (11) (2004):1201–1208.

Wolff, T., L.M. Distlerath, M.T. Worthington, J.D. Groopman, G.J. Hammons, F.F. Kadlubar, R.A. Prough, M.V. Martin, and F.P. Guengerich. "Substrate specificity of human liver cytochrome P-450 debrisoquine 4-hydroxylase probed using immunochemical inhibition and chemical modeling." *Cancer Research* 45 (5) (1985):2116–2122.

Woosley, R.L., Y. Chen, J.P. Freiman, and R.A. Gillis. "Mechanism of the cardiotoxic actions of terfenadine." *Journal of the American Medical Association* 269 (1993):1532–1536.

Xiao, X. and G.D. Prestwich. "29-Methylidene-2,3-oxidosqualene: A potent mechanism-based inactivator of oxidosqualene cyclase." *Journal of the American Chemical Society* 113 (1991):9673–9674.

Xiong, Y., D. Bernardi, S. Bratton, M.D. Ward, E. Battaglia, M. Finel, R.R. Drake, and A. Radominska-Pandya. "Phenylalanine 90 and 93 are localized within the phenol binding site of human UDP-glucuronosyltransferase 1A10 as determined by photoaffinity labeling, mass spectrometry, and site-directed mutagenesis." *Biochemistry* 45 (7) (2006):2322–2332.

Yamazaki, H., Y. Inui, C.H. Yun, F.P. Guengerich, and T. Shimada. "Cytochrome P450 2E1 and 2A6 enzymes as major catalysts for metabolic activation of N-nitrosodialkylamines and tobacco-related nitrosamines in human liver microsomes." *Carcinogenesis* 13 (10) (1992):1789–1794.

Yasukochi, Y. and B.S.S. Masters. "Some properties of a detergent-solubilized NADPH-cytochrome *c* (cytochrome P-450) reductase purified by biospecific affinity chromatography." *Journal of Biological Chemistry* 251 (1976):5337–5344.

Yoo, J.S.H., R.J. Cheung, C.J. Patten, D. Wade, and C.S. Yang. "Nature of *N*-nitrosodimethylamine demethylase and its inhibitors." *Cancer Research* 47 (1987):3378–3383.

Yoshida, T., S. Takahashi, and G. Kikuchi. "Partial Purification and Reconstitution of the Heme Oxygenase System from Pig Spleen Microsomes." *Journal of Biochemistry (Tokyo)* 75 (1974):1187–1191.

Yoshigae, Y., C. Sridar, U.M. Kent, and P.F. Hollenberg. "The inactivation of human CYP2E1 by phenethyl isothiocyanate, a naturally occurring chemopreventive agent, and its oxidative bioactivation." *Drug Metabolism and Disposition* 41 (4) (2013):858–869.

Yu, J., T.K. Ritchie, A. Mulgaonkar, and I. Ragueneau-Majlessi. "Drug disposition and drug-drug interaction data in 2013 FDA new drug applications: A systematic review." *Drug Metabolism and Disposition* 42 (12) (2014):1991–2001.

Yun, C.H., R.A. Okerholm, and F.P. Guengerich. "Oxidation of the antihistaminic drug terfenadine in human liver microsomes. Role of cytochrome P-450 3A(4) in N-dealkylation and C-hydroxylation." *Drug Metabolism and Disposition* 21 (3) (1993):403–409.

Zhang, H., H. Amunugama, S. Ney, N. Cooper, and P.F. Hollenberg. "Mechanism-based inactivation of human cytochrome P450 2B6 by clopidogrel: Involvement of both covalent modification of cysteinyl residue 475 and loss of heme." *Molecular Pharmacology* 80 (5) (2011):839–847.

Zhang, Y., P. Talalay, C.G. Cho, and G.H. Posner. "A major inducer of anticarcinogenic protective enzyme from broccoli: Isolation and elucidation of structure." *Proceedings of the National Academy of Sciences USA* 89 (1992):2399–2403.

Zhou, S., S. Yung Chan, B. Cher Goh, E. Chan, W. Duan, M. Huang, and H.L. McLeod. "Mechanism-based inhibition of cytochrome P450 3A4 by therapeutic drugs." *Clinical Pharmacokinetics* 44 (3) (2005):279–304.

9

Quantitative Approaches to Human Clearance Projection in Drug Research and Development

Nigel J. Waters

CONTENTS

Introduction

In the discovery and development of new medicines, the ability to accurately predict human pharmacokinetic (PK) properties is a critical part of the translational R&D process, enabling (i) differentiation of clinical candidates, (ii) facilitating first-in-human studies, (iii) projection of efficacious dose regimens (dose size and frequency), and (iv) insight into safety margins. A wide range of approaches have been developed, proposed, and qualified over many years to predict the fundamental PK parameters, clearance, volume of distribution, oral absorption, and bioavailability. The focus of this chapter is on one of the more challenging PK properties to predict in human, drug clearance (CL), which is integral to understanding whether a compound will have an adequate half-life and oral bioavailability to support safe and efficacious therapy. Drug clearance is a proportionality constant between the rate of elimination from the body (systemic clearance) or an organ (organ clearance) and its concentration at the site of measurement, i.e. blood or plasma. A physiologically more meaningful definition is the apparent volume of blood (or plasma or plasma water) cleared of drug per unit time and can be expressed as blood CL, plasma CL, or unbound CL, respectively, as well as in terms of systemic (total body) CL or specific organ CL. The major pathways of elimination for most drugs are hepatic metabolism, biliary excretion, and renal excretion.

Predicting human CL represents a significant challenge because it is dependent on both physiological processes (e.g. organ blood flows, glomerular filtration rate, hepatic, and renal function) and biochemical/molecular determinants (e.g. affinity for the broad array of enzymes and transporters involved in drug disposition). Furthermore, there can be significant species differences in each of these processes that complicates prospective efforts to predict CL in human. The first insight into the possible CL in man usually takes place early in drug discovery with the routine screening of compounds in human liver microsome stability assays. This initial readout is then further informed with PK data in one or two preclinical species during lead optimization before more detailed analyses using multiple, integrated data sources during late lead optimization and development candidate nomination phases. Further refinement of the predictions may also occur through preclinical development as more is learned about the compound in question during investigational new drug application (IND)-enabling studies.

Methods used in prediction of human CL have included scaling using *in vitro* data from human tissue preparations, interspecies scaling and allometry using animal PK data, physiologically-based pharmacokinetic (PBPK) modelling, and species-invariant time approaches such as Dedrick analysis. There are fundamental differences between the various methods. For example, the latter two methodologies utilize concentration-time data, while others involve the primary parameter, CL, or a derivation, e.g. intrinsic clearance (CLint). Computational methods, such as quantitative structure-activity relationships (QSAR), which rely solely on chemical structure and calculated molecular properties as model inputs, have also received attention recently and shown early promise in predicting human CL in the drug discovery setting.

Microdosing has also been a strategy employed to yield CL estimates in human, in which a dose much lower than that which would lead to pharmacologically-relevant concentrations is administered in order to derive PK parameters (Lappin et al., 2006, 2008). Such an approach requires only a minimal investment in animal toxicology studies and less bulk API synthesis. However, it has fallen out of favor in recent years due to concerns over non-linearity between dose and exposure. Global retrospective analyses have highlighted that the predictive performance is not markedly improved over methods using animal PK or human *in vitro* data, although there are specific case studies where it has proved valuable when preclinical CL estimates have been disparate (Beaumont and Smith, 2009), particularly when allied with PBPK modeling (Jones et al., 2016).

In recent years, the prediction of CL in human has become a more quantitative exercise, integrating data from a multitude of *in silico*, *in vitro*, and *in vivo* experiments. In addition, as with much of the work in a modern DMPK laboratory, it has also become more mechanistic in nature with the availability of tools and approaches enabling the prediction of specific organ clearances, or metabolism by a specific enzyme pathway. As a result, the industry has evolved from a time when PK in animal species was directional of the likely PK in man in a descriptive, empirical fashion. Presently data from a variety of sources; computational, biochemical, cellular, and whole organism, are integrated into a holistic and quantitative framework. As such, the predictive science has developed to a point where statistical rigor is becoming an area of increasing focus; e.g. moving towards confidence intervals and variance on any point estimate, and further appreciation of the potential for error propagation in methods using multiple data inputs (Sundqvist et al., 2015).

A mechanistic basis to understanding CL in human also lends itself to predicting specific organ or pathway CL and, therefore, enables estimation of fraction metabolized (fm) by a specific pathway or fraction excreted (fe) by a particular transporter. This approach can be hugely informative in understanding the risk of drug interactions (as a victim) as well as the potential for inter-subject variability in a human population, e.g. CL by a polymorphic enzyme. In drug discovery, it is preferable to select compounds for further development with clearance by multiple routes to mitigate these issues associated with variable CL in man. This also extends to hepatic and/or renal impairment as a source of interpatient variability in drug exposure.

A number of recent industry initiatives, including several by the PhRMA CPCDC group, have explored the predictive accuracy of the various methods that are used to predict human PK and, in particular, human CL using large datasets of both publicly available and proprietary compounds with intravenous PK data in man (Poulin et al., 2011; Ring et al., 2011; Vuppugalla et al., 2011; Lombardo et al., 2013a). The PhRMA CPCDC initiative looked at 29 different methods (interspecies scaling with rat and/or dog and IVIVE with liver microsomes and hepatocytes) using a dataset of 19 compounds with i.v. clinical PK data. Another large analysis of this type was reported recently, in which 37 different methods (interspecies scaling with rat, dog and/or monkey) were applied to a dataset of approximately 400 compounds with i.v. clinical PK data (Lombardo et al., 2013a). These independent analyses led to similar conclusions on the most accurate methods based on global concordance, with FCIM allometry standing out amongst the interspecies scaling approaches. Further details on how these methods performed in a global context will be described in the relevant sections below, as well as individual case reports for specific compounds. It should be noted that although a method may show superior predictive accuracy in a comprehensive analysis, like those described above, the prospective prediction of human CL requires

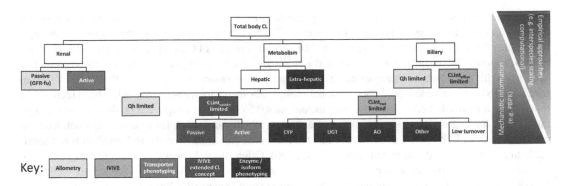

FIGURE 9.1   Schematic illustrating potential mechanisms of clearance for drugs, annotated with the methods generally considered most effective in prediction of human clearance.

the DMPK scientist to carefully consider the most appropriate methods based on what is known about the properties of the particular compound in question (Figure 9.1).

Interspecies Scaling and Allometry

Allometry is the study of the relationship of body size to anatomy and physiology and is well documented for pharmacokinetic prediction applications, which attempts to account for interspecies differences in PK. The basis for allometry is a power law that relates body weight to the PK parameter of interest (Equation 9.1);

$$y = a \cdot W^b \qquad (9.1)$$

where y is the PK parameter of interest (typically CL, VD, or $t_{1/2}$), a is the coefficient, W is body weight, and b is the exponent. This is often graphically represented as a log-log plot of clearance (volume per unit time) in each species against body weight. Compelling allometric relationships between body weight and drug clearance can be achieved since fundamentally there is a strong allometric relationship between body weight and physiological factors imperative in drug clearance, e.g. cardiac output, eliminating organ blood flows, basal metabolic rate, and glomerular filtration rate (Boxenbaum, 1982). The exponent for these rate- and flow-based physiological parameters is around 0.67–0.75 and provides a frame of reference for prospective predictions of drug clearance using simple allometry. Recently, it has been shown that the relationship between body weight and basal metabolic rate has a convex curvature on a logarithmic scale and is, therefore, not a pure power law, which could explain the variability reported in the allometric exponent (Kolokotrones et al., 2010). Well-documented examples where simple allometry has worked well include fluconazole (Jezequel, 1994) and methotrexate (Boxenbaum, 1982), both of which are predominantly renally excreted in preclinical species and man.

Simple allometry does not always produce a convincing cross-species correlation or an exponent falling in the physiologically-relevant range, and in addition, supporting data of a species difference in CL for a particular compound may indicate that simple allometry is not appropriate. As a result, various groups have proposed alternative allometric methods utilizing a wide range of correction factors to improve the cross-species correlation of CL. These have included using additional physiological parameters (e.g. rule of exponents), plasma protein binding (e.g. unbound clearance allometry, fu-corrected intercept method), and *in vitro* metabolism data (e.g. Lave approach) as correction factors to the simple allometric relationship, as well as modifying the underlying power law (e.g. multi-exponential allometry).

The rule of exponents (RoE) approach seeks to improve the allometric prediction of human CL by systematically utilizing brain weight and maximum life potential (MLP) as correction factors, the former being largely empirical and the latter being an attempt to normalize for species differences in metabolic capacity (Boxenbaum, 1982; Mahmood and Balian, 1996). If the exponent from simple allometry lies between 0.55

and 0.7, then simple allometry is considered appropriate. However, if the simple allometry exponent lies between 0.71 and 1.0, then the product of CL and MLP is recommended as the ordinate term. Likewise, if the simple allometry exponent is even higher (>1.0), then the product of CL and brain weight as the ordinate term is proposed. This approach has been tested with a wide variety of drugs and shown improved predictive accuracy. Although there are many examples where predictions obtained from this method were not accurate, it tended to produce less prediction error than simple allometry for a given drug. It has been recognized that although prediction error for drugs with exponents <0.55 is not very high, the prediction error can be large when the exponents of simple allometry are >1.3, which can be helpful in assessing confidence in prediction. It should be noted, as highlighted by the authors of this work, that the RoE method is not applicable to renally excreted compounds (Mahmood, 2006). Other physiological correction factors have been proposed for compounds cleared predominantly in urine (kidney blood flow, GFR, and kidney weight) or bile (RoE with bile flow rate) (Mahmood, 1998; Mahmood and Sahajwalla, 2002; Mahmood, 2012).

The fu-corrected intercept method (FCIM) is a version of fixed exponent allometry developed by Tang and Mayersohn (Tang and Mayersohn, 2005), as shown below (Equation 9.2).

$$\text{Predicted human CL (mL/min)} = 33.35 \times (a/Rfu)^{0.77} \tag{9.2}$$

where a is the coefficient from simple allometry, i.e. intercept from the log-log plot of CL versus body weight using at least three animal species, and Rfu is the ratio of unbound fraction in plasma between rats and humans. In this method, rat plasma free fraction represents a surrogate of the average free fraction in preclinical species and, therefore, provides the basis for a correction factor in cases of large species differences in plasma protein binding between animal species and human. That said, this approach has been shown to have a comparatively high predictive accuracy in many of the global analyses of human CL prediction with average fold errors of ca. 2 (Poulin et al., 2011; Ring et al., 2011; Vuppugalla et al., 2011; Lombardo et al., 2013a), making it a good first option in prospective CL prediction. Unlike other allometric methods, FCIM has also shown excellent predictive accuracy for compounds that exhibit vertical allometry, which is discussed further below (Tang and Mayersohn, 2005).

The use of *in vitro* metabolism data as a correction factor in allometry has been proposed by Lave and coworkers (Lave et al., 1997), wherein the CL in each species is normalized by the ratio of *in vitro* intrinsic clearance (CLint) between human and the animal species. This product term CL·(*in vitro* CLint-human/*in vitro* CLint-animal) is plotted against body weight to derive the allometric relationship and extrapolate human CL. Using either liver microsomal or hepatocyte CLint data, this method showed superior predictive accuracy for ten extensively metabolized compounds including the endothelin receptor antagonist, bosentan (Lave et al., 1996, 1997).

Modification to the underlying power law has been proposed by Goteti et al. (Goteti et al., 2008, 2010) using a multiple exponential equation of the general form below (Equation 9.3).

$$\text{Predicted human CL (mL/min)} = a \cdot W^b + c \cdot W^d \tag{9.3}$$

where a and c are the coefficients, and b and d are the exponents from the log-log plot of CL versus body weight (W). This approach has been advocated when the exponent from simple allometry is >1.3 and performed reasonably well in a larger global analysis of CL prediction methods with a GMFE of 2.4 on a 97 compound dataset with rat, dog, and monkey PK data (Lombardo et al., 2013a).

Prospective application of interspecies scaling methods relies on using diagnostic parameters, such as the allometric exponent to ascertain some degree of confidence in the resulting projection. It should be noted that concerns have been raised among investigators of using the coefficient of determination (r^2) as a statistical metric for judging the predictability of human CL (Tang and Mayersohn, 2007). Analysis of literature data indicated that the prediction accuracy of human CL was not correlated with values of r^2. Therefore, it is concluded that r^2 is a limited statistical measure when assessing allometric scaling for the purpose of predicting human CL.

A phenomenon commonly observed in interspecies scaling is that of vertical allometry, which refers to instances where the predicted human clearance is substantially higher than the observed human clearance (Mahmood and Boxenbaum, 2014). Vertical allometry was initially reported for diazepam based on

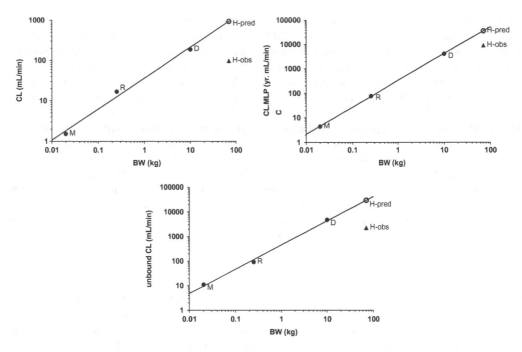

FIGURE 9.2 Scaling of pinometostat clearance demonstrates vertical allometry by simple allometry (a); RoE-MLP correction (b) and simple allometry of unbound clearance (c). Key: body weight (BW), mouse (M), rat (R), dog (D), predicted human clearance (H-pred), observed human clearance (H-obs). (With kind permission from Taylor & Francis: *Xenobiotica.*, Mechanistic investigations into the species differences in pinometostat clearance: Impact of binding to alpha-1-acid glycoprotein and permeability-limited hepatic uptake 10, 2016, 1–9, Smith, S.A. et al.)

a 33-fold higher predicted human clearance than the observed value. More recently, it has been observed for a number of drugs including UCN-01 (Fuse et al., 1998), tamsulosin (Hoogdalem et al., 1997), susalimod (Pahlman et al., 1998), and pinometostat (Smith et al., 2016; Figure 9.2). Tang and Mayersohn illustrated that all examples of vertical allometry (defined as a prediction error > 10-fold) occurred only for compounds with very low observed CL in man (Tang and Mayersohn, 2006a). This increased incidence in drug development has led to questions of how to define and identify vertical allometry in a prospective manner, and if so, when accurate clearance predictions can be obtained. As mentioned above, it has been established that FCIM shows improved predictive accuracy for compounds exhibiting vertical allometry exemplified with UCN-01 (Tang and Mayersohn, 2006b) and pinometostat (Smith et al., 2016). This is not the case with the RoE method. Furthermore, diagnostic parameters for vertical allometry have been proposed including the ratio of unbound fraction in plasma between rat and human of >5 (consistent with the key term in FCIM) and clogP (calculated octanol:water partition coefficient of neutral form) >2. In addition, drugs displaying vertical allometry tend to be extensively bound to plasma proteins. And more specifically, there is a tendency for these compounds to bind preferentially to alpha1-acid glycoprotein (AAG). Notably, there is a disproportionately higher expression of AAG in human plasma (0.55–1.8 mg/mL) relative to preclinical species (e.g. mouse, 0.1 mg/mL; rat, 0.1–0.3 mg/mL; dog, 0.3–1 mg/mL), which is likely a major contributing factor alone, in addition to potential species-specific differences in AAG binding affinity. There is evidence in the literature that tamsulosin (Koiso et al., 1996) and UCN-01 (Fuse et al., 1998) extensively bind to AAG and, as such, is responsible for the low human clearance of these two drugs. The plasma clearance of pinometostat was also shown to be markedly lower in human compared to the preclinical species, mouse, rat, and dog, with *in vitro* kinetic analysis demonstrating a high affinity interaction with human AAG (Smith et al., 2016).

In recent years, there has been much debate in the literature on the appropriate number and type of animal species needed in an allometric relationship to achieve a satisfactory prediction accuracy. It is typical in drug development that PK data would be available in rat, dog, and monkey (and perhaps one other species if used in pharmacology studies). Other animal species have been proposed for interspecies scaling including mini-pig (Yoshimatsu et al., 2016) and African green monkey (Ward et al., 2008), and species selection, in general, has garnered much debate (Wong et al., 2012). In late lead optimization and early development, the availability of PK data in both dog and monkey is not uncommon to support selection of the non-rodent species for preclinical toxicology assessment. Several groups have demonstrated that allometry with three species provides superior predictions, with the two species approach being highly variable and dependent on the two species chosen (Goteti et al., 2010: Nagilla and Ward, 2004). Other groups have supported that data in three species may not be necessary (Tang et al., 2007) or that data in monkey is not a prerequisite for good predictions (Hosea, 2011). Additionally, it has been reported that the availability of data from both common non-rodent species (dog and monkey) does not ensure enhanced predictive quality compared with having only monkey data (Ward and Smith, 2004). Scaling using data from two species offers advantages in terms of cost, time, and animal use and this has led to further exploration of single species scaling approaches to further these goals and enable human CL prediction earlier in drug discovery. One such evaluation has been single species fixed-exponent allometry of the general form below (Equation 9.4).

$$\text{Predicted CL in human (mL/min)} = CL_{animal} \left(W_{human}/W_{animal}\right)^{0.66}, \quad (9.4)$$

which when CL is expressed in a body weight normalized form simplifies to coefficients of 0.16, 0.41, and 0.40 for rat, dog, and monkey CL (body weight normalized), respectively. Caldwell and colleagues demonstrated the value of this approach early in drug discovery using rat data alone and the fixed exponent allometric approach; on a dataset of 176 compounds the average fold error (AFE) for human CL was 2.25 with 79% of compounds within 3-fold (Caldwell et al. 2004). Other groups have corroborated this finding (Hosea et al. 2009), including Tang et al. (2007), using a different proprietary compound dataset, which also showed that fixed exponent allometry using monkey CL gave an AFE of 1.9 with 80% falling within 3-fold. The other key finding from this work was that liver blood flow (LBF) correction (Equation 9.5) using data in monkey performed equally well, and unlike rat and dog, the fixed exponent and LBF correction approaches converged in monkey with similar coefficients (0.41 vs. 0.47).

$$CL_{human}/LBF_{human} = CL_{animal}/LBF_{animal} \quad (9.5)$$

The LBF-correction approach using monkey CL data was also advocated by other groups, showing superior performance to simple allometry and RoE (Nagilla and Ward 2004; Ward and Smith, 2004). In a recent global analysis of CL prediction methods, fixed exponent allometry and LBF correction, both using monkey data, performed better than many of the other interspecies scaling methods, including all single species approaches with or without incorporation of plasma free fraction terms (Lombardo et al., 2013a).

With such a wide diversity of interspecies scaling methods and permutations with conflicting reports on the predictive accuracy of some of these approaches, identifying determinants of extrapolative success has been an active area of research. The identification of calculated molecular properties that may help inform a particular approach to interspecies scaling has been one area of focus (Jolivette and Ward, 2005). Wajima and coworkers took this a step further and developed a hybrid approach; a multiple linear regression equation that included terms for rat CL, dog CL, molecular weight, and hydrogen bond acceptors, which showed some improvements over simple allometry (Wajima et al., 2002). The other major contributing factor that can help improve prospective selection of the most appropriate scaling method is understanding the primary mechanism of CL in preclinical species. In addition to the modified forms of allometry to scale excretory CL mentioned earlier, investigations into other interspecies scaling methods have been proposed. For example, Paine and colleagues demonstrated that renal CL in dog together with correction for species differences in renal blood flow and plasma free fraction performed well in predicting human renal CL for a set of 36 drugs (Paine et al., 2011). Conversely, monkey has been shown to be a good model for predicting human CL of UGT substrates, with a similar fm_{UGT} demonstrated between monkey and human using a dataset of 12 drugs (Deguchi et al., 2011). Adding further complexity to animal scale-up methods is the case of compounds such as antipyrine, which despite species differences in the relative contribution of metabolic pathways, unbound CLint is well described by an allometric relationship (Boxenbaum, 1986).

In summary, the collective experience of many researchers in the field has been that allometric scaling works well for CL primarily driven by physiological parameters; e.g. hepatic blood flow-limited CL or passive renal filtration. Early in drug discovery, in the absence of understanding around CL mechanisms in preclinical species, single species scaling methods can be a useful initial guidepost. Further work is needed to aid in the *a priori* selection of interspecies scaling methods with the best chance of predictive accuracy for a given compound of interest. Analyses in that direction are starting to emerge (Liu et al., 2016).

Species-Invariant Time Methods

In chronological time, smaller short-lived animals generally clear drugs from their bodies more rapidly per unit of body weight than larger long-lived animals. When expressed according to each species' internal biological clock, drug clearance tends to be similar (Mordenti, 1986). This is the basis for species-invariant time approaches derived from concentration-time data in preclinical species and human, in which the time scale is transformed from chronological time to biological time (Boxenbaum, 1986; Dedrick, 1973). Normalization of the time scale from a time that is physically determined (i.e. the rotation of the Earth) to one that is biologically relevant renders the PK data invariant to space-time. As described in the earlier section, biologically relevant processes can occur on different species-specific chronological time scales, and so the mathematical transformation of the concentration-time axes, accounts for the allometrically-scalable species differences described earlier (e.g. heartbeat time, respiratory cycle time, etc.). For example, the terminal $t_{1/2}$ of hexobarbital is 24, 210, and 328 minutes in mouse, dog, and human, respectively. The allometric relationship for this parameter has an exponent of 0.348. Gut beat duration in mammals has an allometric exponent of 0.31. Given the similarity in allometric exponent between the physiological parameter and the PK parameter, it can be ascertained by allometric cancellation that the terminal $t_{1/2}$ for hexobarbital equates to ~1684 gut beats, i.e. time invariant across species.

The first application of the concept of biological time to PK processes was reported in 1970 by Dedrick et al. using interspecies variation in methotrexate PK as the basis for analysis (Dedrick et al., 1970). The elementary Dedrick plot, as it was later termed by Boxenbaum, is illustrated below. Assuming simple allometric relationships for CL ($= aW^x$) and volume of distribution ($V = bW^y$) and first-order kinetics, the elimination rate constant (k) would be as defined in Equation 9.6, and the plasma concentration (C) after iv bolus administration in Equation 9.7.

$$k = CL/V = (a/b)W^{x-y} \tag{9.6}$$

$$C = (D/V)e^{-kt} = (D/bW^y)e^{-(a/b)(W^{x-y})t} \tag{9.7}$$

where D is the dose. Assuming y = 1 (V exponent of unity), then Equation 9.7 can be rearranged so that the PK profiles for each species would be expected to become superimposable when concentration is plotted normalized for dose per unit bodyweight (i.e. C/(D/W)) as a function of time normalized by W^{1-x} (Equation 9.8). This unit of time is referred to as a kallynochron (*kallyno* from the Greek "to make clean;" *chron*, the Greek root for time).

$$C/(D/W) = (1/b)e^{-(a/b)(t/W^{1-x})} \tag{9.8}$$

The complex Dedrick plot accounts for the situation in which V is not directly proportional to body weight, i.e. where y ≠ 1. In this case, C is normalized as C/(D/W^y) and plotted as a function of time normalized by W^{y-x} (Equation 9.9). This unit of time is referred to as an apolysichron (*apolysi* from the Greek "to release").

$$C/(D/W^y) = (1/b)e^{-(a/b)(t/W^{y-x})} \tag{9.9}$$

In one apolysichron, each species eliminates the same fraction of drug from the body whereas in one kallynochron each species clears the same volume of blood (or plasma) per unit bodyweight. Therefore, the kallynochron derives its significance from clearance whereas the apolysichron is a species-independent measure of half-life or mean residence time.

It should be noted that the elementary and complex Dedrick plots have been illustrated here using monoexponential kinetics for simplicity, but superimposable data can be obtained with multiexponential decay (e.g. chlordiazepoxide, Boxenbaum and Ronfeld, 1983). Two additional unit of time parameters have been proposed by Boxenbaum; the dienetichron and the syndesichron, which are similar to the apolysichron with incorporation of MLP and brain weight, respectively (Boxenbaum, 1983, 1984). The application of Dedrick analysis was recently demonstrated with the anticancer compound, SJ-8029, an amide-containing molecule that is hydrolyzed to an aminoacridine derivative with topoisomerase activity (SJ-8026) and a piperazine derivative with microtubule activity (SJ-8031) (Shin et al., 2003). The i.v. PK were generated in mouse, rat, rabbit, and dog where the compound had a CL of 200, 105, 92, and 43 mL/min/kg, respectively. The Dedrick plots based on kallynochron, apolysichron, and dienetichron transformations are illustrated in Figure 9.3, showing the superposition of the profiles in preclinical species for this high extraction compound. No information was available

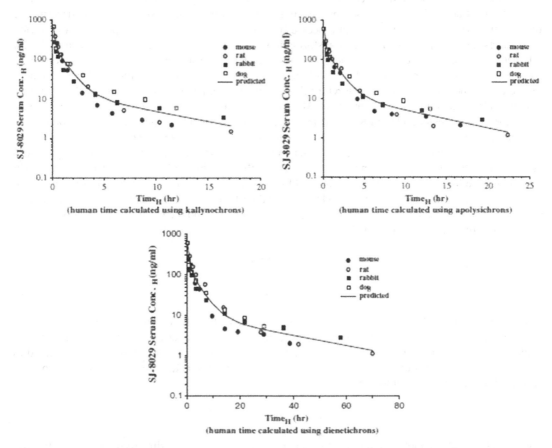

FIGURE 9.3 Serum concentration-time curves predicted following i.v. injection of the anti-cancer agent, SJ-8029 (1 mg/kg dose) to a 70 kg human based on kallynochron, apolysichron and dienetichron time transformations. The concentration-time profiles for the preclinical species show good superposition and goodness-of-fit parameters. (From Shin, B.S. et al.: Pharmacokinetic Scaling of SJ-8029, A Novel Anticancer Agent Possessing Microtubule and Topoisomerase Inhibiting Activities, By Species-Invariant Time Methods. *Biopharmaceutics & Drug Disposition*. 2003. 24. 191–197. Copyright John Wiley & Sons Publications. Reproduced with permission.)

on the PK disposition of SJ-8029 in humans to further support the validity of the methods that has been achieved with compounds such as methotrexate and chlordiazepoxide. Analogous reports have been presented for epirubicin (Shin et al., 2015), oltipraz (Bae, et al., 2005), ethosuximide, cyclosporine, and ciprofloxacin (Mahmood and Yuan, 1999).

Dedrick methods rely on the accuracy of the underlying allometric relationship, and so attempts have been made to find alternative ways to transform to biological time. In the method developed by Wajima and colleagues (Wajima et al., 2004), the i.v. concentration-time data is normalized by Css and MRT, respectively, in each species (where Css = Dose/Vss and MRT = Vss/CL). The superposition of the C/Css versus t/MRT data is then assessed, and if this is compelling (e.g. based on coefficient of variation or AIC), a reverse-transformation of the average profile is achieved using estimates of Vss, CL, and dose in human. Consequently, Vss and CL estimates determined by any method can be used to derive i.v. concentration-time profiles in human. Wajima et al. demonstrated the utility of this approach on four antibiotics (ceftizoxime, cefodizime, cefotetan, and cefmenoxime) with data in preclinical species and human and showed improved superposition for these compounds over the elementary Dedrick plot. Human CL and Vss estimates were based on the earlier described MLR approach (Wajima et al., 2002). As the authors of this work eluded to, the drugs used in the study have low Vss and are predominantly excreted unchanged in urine, implicating the need for further validation of the method with compounds displaying a broader range of drug disposition properties. The PhRMA CPCDC initiative explored the Wajima species-invariant time method using 18 compounds for which human i.v. PK data was available (Vuppugalla et al., 2011). In this analysis, human CL and Vss estimates were either allometry-based (e.g. FCIM) or QSAR-based. Focusing on the outcome of the model fit to the i.v. data (n = 18), the overall degree of accuracy (based on a composite of several statistical measures) was 34% high to high/medium and 37% medium to medium/low and 30% low, suggesting the overall ability of the Wajima approach to predict the shape of the PK profile was in general poor. An additional independent analysis of the Wajima approach using a larger set of cross-species i.v. PK data on 54 marketed drugs with diverse physicochemical properties was reported recently (Lombardo et al., 2016). Using the average of the best methods for human CL and Vss prediction demonstrated in earlier reports (Lombardo et al., 2013a, 2013b), yielded 88% and 70% of the predictions within 2-fold error for Vss and CL, respectively. The prediction of the human i.v. PK profile using Wajima superpositioning of rat, dog, and monkey concentration-time profiles showed that 63% of the compounds yielded a geometric mean fold error below 2-fold, and an additional 19% yielded a geometric mean fold error between 2- and 3-fold, leaving only 18% of the compounds with a relatively poor prediction. Interestingly, good superposition was observed in all cases signifying the cause for poor prediction of the human i.v. PK profile was attributable to the human CL estimates used in the reverse transformation of the data.

In Vitro Scaling of Metabolic Clearance

The increased availability of human tissue for *in vitro* drug metabolism studies has greatly enhanced our understanding of drug disposition in human. Liver microsomes and cryopreserved hepatocytes are now "off the shelf" reagents that are widely utilized in high-throughput screens in early drug discovery through to late stage definitive nonclinical ADME studies supporting compound characterization. From a CL prediction perspective, the typical approach involves pooled (multiple donor) liver microsome preparations supplemented with excess NADPH (or a NADPH regenerating system), or alternatively pooled hepatocyte suspensions, are co-incubated with test compound at a concentration initially assumed to be sub-Km (e.g. low single digit micromolar). Over a relatively short timeframe (ca. 45 mins for microsomes, ca. 2–4 hours for hepatocytes), aliquots of the reaction mixture are taken and quenched in organic solvent. This study design allows for measurement of parent analyte, typically by LC-MS/MS, and calculation of the elimination rate constant (kel) from the resulting parent depletion timecourse. The kel measured *in vitro* must then be transformed to an intrinsic clearance (CLint) (Equation 9.10), and then a scaled CLint using factors such as microsomal protein per gram liver, hepatocellularity and gram liver per kilogram bodyweight (Equation 9.11). This scaled CLint is then incorporated into a physiological model of CL, such as the well-stirred model (Pang and Rowland, 1977), which includes terms for liver blood flow (Qh), free fraction in blood (fub), and incubational binding (fuinc) (Equation 9.12);

$$\text{Apparent } \textit{in vitro } \text{CLint} = \text{kel/mg microsomal protein per mL} \qquad (9.10)$$

$$= \text{kel/million hepatocytes per mL}$$

$$\text{Scaled CLint} = \textit{in vitro } \text{CL}_{int} \cdot \text{MMPGL} \cdot \text{LWPBW} \qquad (9.11)$$

$$= \textit{in vitro } \text{CL}_{int} \cdot \text{HPGL} \cdot \text{LWPBW}$$

where MMPGL is mg microsomal protein per gram liver, HPGL is million hepatocytes per gram liver, and LWPBW is grams liver per kilogram bodyweight. The appropriate scaling factors to use for human has been reviewed recently (Barter et al., 2007).

$$CL_H = \frac{Q_H \cdot \dfrac{f_{ub}}{f_{uinc}} \cdot CL_{int}}{Q_H + \dfrac{f_{ub}}{f_{uinc}} \cdot CL_{int}} \qquad (9.12)$$

Therefore, a CL prediction can be achieved with data from metabolic stability, plasma protein binding, and blood-plasma partitioning assays. Incubational binding can be measured directly using similar methods to plasma protein binding or calculated computationally based on physicochemical descriptors (Waters et al., 2014).

As a compound progresses through development, the assay approach may be modified to better characterize CLint via Vmax and Km determination (Clint = Vmax/Km) or define a pathway-specific CLint, both accomplished by measurement of metabolite formation kinetics where quantitation with analytical standards or via radiolabeled compound is desirable.

The CL value from *in vitro* scaling provides an estimate of the hepatic metabolic clearance. Since a large proportion of marketed drugs are primarily cleared via CYP metabolism, many studies have explored the experimental and scaling aspects of *in vitro-in vivo* extrapolation of clearance for CYP substrates, such that this is a well-established approach for predicting hepatic metabolic CL in drug research (Houston, 1994; Iwatsubo et al., 1997; Obach, 1999; Riley et al., 2005). As well as microsomes and hepatocytes, recombinant human CYP enzymes have also shown utility in the prediction of CL (Stringer et al., 2009).

Much like that of interspecies scaling, the current state-of-the-art specifies robust predictions are generally considered to fall with the twofold to threefold window of the observed value. The potential for disparity between *in vitro* and *in vivo* CL, and the possible contributing sources of experimental variability or factors that may not reflect the *in vivo* situation is well appreciated including enzyme source, experimental conditions, and inter-individual variation such as genetic polymorphism (Wang and Gibson, 2014). The culmination of much work in this area suggests there is a general tendency for underprediction with hepatocytes and this has been attributed to impaired uptake or cofactor exhaustion (Hallifax et al., 2010).

Notwithstanding, it is prudent to assess confidence in human CL prediction by *in vitro* methods and this is typically addressed prospectively through the development of a cross-species *in vitro-in vivo* correlation (IVIVC). A comparison of the fold difference between the CL observed in each preclinical species and that from *in vitro* scaling in the corresponding species matrix can lend confidence in the prediction of human CL by *in vitro* scaling. This has been demonstrated with the Substance P receptor antagonist, ezlopitant, where the IVIVC fold error in rat, guinea pig, dog, and monkey were 0.98, 0.45, 0.56, and 1.05, with a human predicted CL of 6.3 mL/min/kg and an observed human oral CL of 8 mL/min/kg (Obach, 2000). In some cases, there may be a systematic fold error in the IVIVC for preclinical species, and some investigators have used this as an empirical correction factor in the *in vitro* scaling for human CL. Alternatively, an empirical scaling offset based on linear regression analyses of observed versus predicted CL for a dataset of compounds has also been proposed (Naritomi et al., 2001, 2003; Riley et al., 2005). In the optimization of the IVIVC approach, there has been much debate on the application of the factors influencing free concentration in the well-stirred model. Depending on the physicochemical properties of the compound in question, the plasma free fraction and/or incubational binding can be important determinants of a successful CL prediction. Inclusion of these factors is typically performed *a priori* and can be validated through a cross-species IVIVC, as described above. This topic has recently been reviewed in detail (Waters et al., 2014). Using the parent depletion approach to measure CLint is dependent on the substrate concentration. Typically, a low micromolar concentration is used and assumed to be below Km and sub-saturating, as mentioned above. However, for drugs with high systemic exposure, marked hepatic uptake or during first pass following oral administration, the intrahepatic concentrations *in vivo* could be saturating and *in vitro* CLint could be overestimated.

While the experimental protocols for determining CLint of CYP substrates using liver microsome and hepatocyte preparations is well established, consideration of the appropriate *in vitro* matrix and experimental conditions for other drug metabolizing enzymes is critical. For example, the flavin monooxygenase enzyme family is present in liver microsomal preparations and utilizes NADPH as a cofactor but is sensitive to heat when NADPH is not present. Uridine glucuronosyltransferase (UGT) enzymes are expressed on the luminal side of the microsomal preparation and so require addition of reagents that allow compound access to the active site of these enzymes, and the pore-forming peptidic antibiotic, alamethicin, is often used. In microsomal assays, this enzyme family obviously also requires availability of an activated glucuronic acid cofactor in the form of uridine diphospho glucuronic acid (UDPGA). Cytosolic enzymes such as aldehyde oxidase are also emerging as increasingly relevant in drug metabolism, and so hepatocytes and cytosolic fractions become key reagents in determining CLint for compounds metabolized by these enzymes.

In recent years, the increased availability of metabolic stability screens in drug discovery, enhanced application of this data by medicinal chemists towards drug design, and the progression to increasingly novel, druggable targets has led to a general trend of compounds with less propensity to CYP metabolism. The natural consequence of this has been an increase in the involvement of other, lesser studied drug metabolizing enzymes, presenting new challenges to the DMPK scientist and the robust prediction of human CL. Quantitative prediction of CL by human UGTs is now emerging and was recently illustrated using liver microsomes activated for both CYP and UGT metabolism (Kilford et al., 2009; Figure 9.4). Furthermore, a promising cross-species IVIVC was reported for AMG232, a novel inhibitor of the p53-MDM2 protein-protein interaction, where the major metabolic route was to an acyl glucuronide (Ye et al., 2015). Some progress has been made in quantifying human CL by the cytosolic molybdenum oxidases such as aldehyde oxidase, implicated in the oxidation of electron-deficient carbons of azaheterocycles prevalent in newer drug classes such as kinase inhibitors (Zientek and Youdim, 2015). It is usually the case that liver is the major organ of drug extraction by metabolism, but drug metabolizing enzymes (DMEs) are expressed extrahepatically and, therefore, can be an underlying assumption in many IVIVC analyses. Recently, Cubitt et al. showed a successful IVIVC case study with liver and intestinal microsomes using a set of compounds in which multiple routes of metabolic conjugation in different tissues (liver and intestine) were the major routes of elimination (Cubitt et al., 2011).

There has been a resurgence in the development of targeted covalent inhibitors with the recent approvals of ibrutinib, afatinib, and neratinib. These types of compounds represent a special case since the CL mechanism can be predominantly extrahepatic metabolism driven by glutathione conjugation of the Michael acceptor (e.g. acrylamide group) typically present in targeted covalent inhibitors. The extrahepatic CL in rat, dog, and monkey, calculated as the difference between observed total body clearance and predicted hepatic clearance in cryopreserved hepatocytes suspended in 100% serum, showed a strong allometric relationship for afatinib and neratinib and compared favorably with clinical PK data. Comparisons of extrahepatic and hepatic CLs predicted that extrahepatic CL largely determined the PK of afatinib (>90% as a proportion of total body clearance) and neratinib (~34%) in humans (Shibata and Chiba, 2015).

As highlighted above, there has been a significant advancement in our understanding of CYP mediated metabolism of drugs and approaches to block metabolic soft-spots or reduce active site affinity. Consequently, this has led to a marked increase in the number of compounds demonstrating clearance by alternative lesser-studied metabolic pathways or exhibiting low metabolic CL that approaches the limit of the current assay designs outlined earlier. The rapid loss of drug metabolizing enzyme activity in these

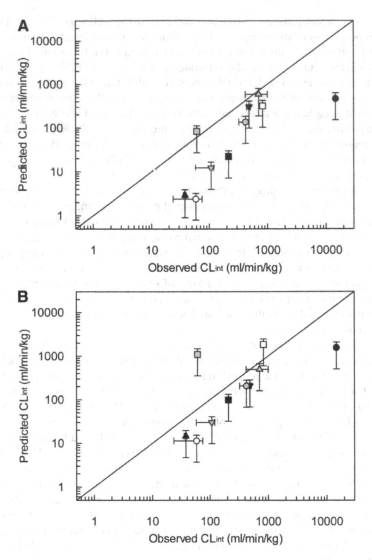

FIGURE 9.4 Prediction of clearance from *in vitro* data obtained in the presence of combined CYP and UGT cofactors and in the absence (A) and presence (B) of 2% bovine serum albumin. Compounds included buprenorphine, carvedilol, codeine, diclofenac, gemfibrozil, ketoprofen, midazolam, naloxone, raloxifene and zidovudine. Error bars indicate range of scaling factors on the *y*-axis from 13 to 54 mg/g liver (Barter et al., 2007) and a range of Qh on the *x*-axis from 17 to 25.5 mL/min/kg. (Reproduced from Kilford, P.J. et al., *Drug Metab. Dispos.*, 37, 82–89, 2009, ASPET Publications.)

conventional assay formats has led research groups to address this problem with the development and validation of *in vitro* assays enabling quantitative estimates of metabolic CL for compounds with low turnover. One approach that has been proposed, and is readily accessible, is the relay method in which successive suspended hepatocyte assays are performed in a series of up to five, 4-hour incubations. The incubation mixture at the end of each 4-hour period is centrifuged to pellet the hepatocytes, and the supernatant is isolated and introduced into a freshly prepared hepatocyte suspension (or alternatively frozen until the next incubation can be performed). In this way, turnover can be assessed over a 20-hour window with metabolic competency assured over the entire time-course (Di et al., 2012, 2013).

Plated hepatocytes as monolayer or sandwich cultures also offer the opportunity to extend incubation time (e.g. days to weeks), as the plating allows the liver-like function of these cells to recover from the isolation procedure (Griffin and Houston, 2005). However, studies using this model to estimate metabolic clearance for compounds with low turnover is lacking. Nevertheless, more innovative approaches such as hepatocyte-fibroblast co-culture systems have been developed (Khetani and Bhatia, 2008) and shown encouraging results for quantitative prediction of low metabolic CL compounds (Chan et al., 2013). A micropatterned co-culture of human hepatocytes is enabled by seeding cells on collagen-patterned matrices, unattached cells are washed off after a 2–3 hour period, followed by seeding of supportive mouse 3T3-J2 fibroblasts. This HepatoPac™ system shows good morphology, viability, and functionality including hepatic-specific CYP and Phase II enzyme expression for up to 6 weeks. The HuREL™ co-culture system is an analogous approach using stromal cells as the supportive milieu and has also shown similar promising results (Bonn et al., 2016; Hultman et al., 2016). A recent cross-study comparative analysis further supports these newer approaches for low CL compounds indicating 100%, 71%, and 86% of predicted values within 3-fold of observed for HepatoPac™, suspension and relay methods, respectively (Hutzler et al., 2015). It should also be emphasized that the relay method, HepatoPac™ and HuREL™ systems are also showing promise in recapitulating the qualitative metabolite profile observed in human *in vivo* relative to liver microsomes and hepatocyte suspensions.

Understanding the fractional clearance by metabolic pathways (fm) is also an important endeavor in drug development to assess the impact of genetic polymorphism, DDI potential as a victim, and intrinsic covariates such as hepatic impairment. Prior to a definitive human A(D)ME study, which is usually performed later in clinical development, the use of *in vitro* tools to estimate fm represents the best option in early development. From the regulatory perspective, evaluating the metabolic profile and understanding the enzymology of the major clearance mechanisms is considered paramount, with the consensus threshold of $\geq 25\%$ of systemic clearance based on results from *in vitro* enzyme phenotyping experiments, human pharmacokinetic studies following intravenous administration, a mass-balance study, and pharmacokinetic studies in which renal/biliary clearances are determined (*FDA Guidance for Industry: Drug Interaction Studies – Study Design, Data Analysis, Implications for Dosing, and Labeling Recommendations*, 2012; *EMA Guideline on the Investigation of Drug Interactions*, 2012). The relationship between fm and the theoretical maximum change in AUC or CL is shown in Figure 9.5, demonstrating that increasingly high precision is required in a quantitative fm estimate as it approaches unity.

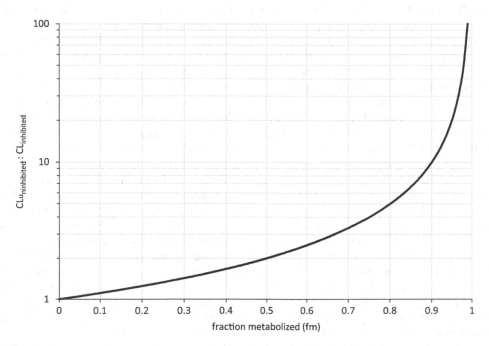

FIGURE 9.5 Relationship between fraction metabolized and the theoretical maximum fold-change in CL between the presence and absence of the specific metabolic pathway. Shown as a semi-log plot to illustrate the steepness in the curve as fm approaches unity.

The prevalence of CYP metabolism has led to three well-established *in vitro* approaches to the estimation of fm. Some prior understanding of the qualitative metabolite profile can be informative and, typically, at least two of the three methods are performed to aid in interpretation and assess consistency. The three assay approaches can be summarized as: (i) human liver microsomes in the presence and absence of CYP isoform-specific chemical inhibitors and/or inhibitory antibodies, (ii) rate of metabolism determined in heterologously expressed recombinant human CYP isoforms, and (iii) correlation analysis comparing the reaction rate of interest with a specific CYP isoform marker activity across a liver microsome panel from individual donors. The approach using recombinant enzymes requires scaling to translate the rate of reaction observed to that measured in human liver microsomes. The first scalar proposed was RAF (relative activity factor), which defines the amount of recombinant CYP to elicit the equivalent reaction rate in HLM (Crespi, 1995). A more recent scalar is the ISEF (intersystem extrapolation factor) that integrates the variables of intrinsic activity and accessory protein expression between two systems (Chen et al., 2011; Proctor et al., 2004). When the ratio of metabolic rates in rhP450 and HLM are calculated for ISEF, the turnover numbers in HLM are expressed as per picomole of P450 by including the hepatic P450 abundance. This approach allows the prediction of metabolism due to the variability of P450 abundance in HLM and rhP450 systems. Both approaches have demonstrated utility and so there is currently no general consensus for either approach, although predictive success of each method appears to be largely dependent on the experimental conditions used (Zientek and Youdim, 2015).

Amongst the CYP superfamily, the isoforms of most interest to the DMPK scientist include CYP1A2, 2C9, 2C19, 2D6, and 3A4 because of their prevalence in drug biotransformation in the liver and the potential to be major contributors to fm_{CYP}. Other isoforms may be of interest depending on the chemical class and if there is evidence for extrahepatic metabolism. In addition, CYP3A5 has received more attention recently and is of emerging importance, as its involvement in the metabolism of CYP3A substrates *in vivo* is more than previously recognized. CYP3A5 is polymorphic with a *CYP3A5*1* wild-type frequency of 5%–15% in Caucasians, 24%–40% in various Asian ethnicities, and 40%–60% in African ethnicities. The CYP3A5 genotype has been shown to be a major covariate in the oral clearance of a number of CYP3A substrates including tacrolimus where the magnitude is such that dose increases of 2-fold would be needed in patients carrying CYP3A5 variants to achieve the required trough concentration (Barry and Levine, 2010). This has led to recent efforts to better understand the contribution of CYP3A5 *in vitro* during drug development. If initial data support a major CYP3A contribution to clearance, recombinant CYP3A5 enzyme and individual donor liver microsomes for the CYP3A5 variants can be utilized. Furthermore, recent efforts to identify specific CYP3A4 inhibitors have resulted in the discovery of CYP3cide, a potent and specific time-dependent inactivator of CYP3A4 (kinact/KI 3300–3800 mL/min/μmol, partition ratio approaching unity). Use of this inhibitor together with the potent CYP3A4/5 inhibitor, ketoconazole, can be used to differentiate between CYP3A4 and CYP3A5 activities, enabling an estimate of fm_{CYP3A5} (Walsky et al., 2012). Similar reports have been described using the specific CYP3A4 MBI inhibitor azamulin (Parmentier et al., 2016) and SR-9186 (Li et al., 2012).

As for CYPs, UGT phenotyping has been conducted using specific chemical inhibitors, recombinant human UGTs, and correlation analysis. However, the identification of specific inhibitors has only advanced slowly, with the most specific being reported for UGT1A1 (atazanavir), 1A4 (hecogenin), 1A9 (niflumic acid), and 2B7 (fluconazole). In the area of recombinant UGTs, the tissue abundance data has been lacking or disparate, precluding rigorous scaling application in drug development. Although that is starting to change with the recent application of proteomics to quantify UGT expression in various tissues (Margaillan et al., 2015a, 2015b). A recent case study of laropiprant demonstrated the successful use of RAFs to scale recombinant UGT1A1, 1A9, and 2B7 to hepatic clearance as well as scaling UGT1A9 and 2B7 to renal clearance (Gibson et al., 2013). As mentioned earlier, aldehyde oxidase is also an enzyme of increasing importance in drug metabolism. Scaling the contribution of AO has been attempted but has been hampered by the extrahepatic component to AO-mediated clearance, human AO polymorphisms driving population variability, and the *in vitro* enzyme stability. If an AO-mediated reaction is implicated from metabolite structural information or stability assays in liver cytosol or S9, an estimate of fm_{AO} can be attained using chemical inhibitors such as hydralazine in incubations of pooled human liver S9 or hepatocytes. Cytosol or S9 assays with chemical inhibitors are also useful in differentiating AO (e.g. hydralazine as inhibitor) and the related enzyme xanthine oxidase (e.g. allopurinol as inhibitor) contributions (Zientek and Youdim, 2015). Estimating fm for drug metabolizing enzymes other than CYP is clearly evolving and an active area of research as illustrated for UGT and AO.

Approaches for Transporter-Mediated Clearance

The role of active transport processes in the disposition of drugs has been recognized for many years through demonstration of the clinical relevance of transporter genetic polymorphism and drug interactions. Not until the recent revolution in molecular biology techniques have the proteins responsible been able to be identified, characterized, sequenced, and cloned. This has provided a number of *in vitro* tools that when integrated with evolving modeling approaches have improved the extrapolative success for transporter-mediated drug clearance in human. A contemporary view of the proteins shown to have a major role in the hepatobiliary and renal disposition of drugs are illustrated in Figure 9.6. In both hepatocytes and renal proximal tubular cells, there is a localized expression of transporter isoforms that can drive the concerted movement of drugs from the blood to the intracellular milieu and from there into

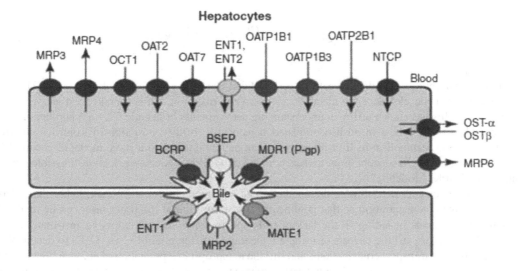

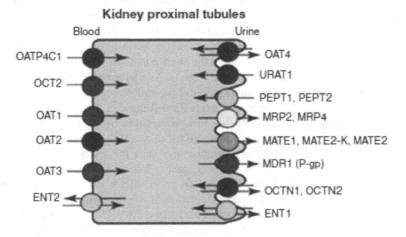

FIGURE 9.6 Transporter isoforms implicated in the hepatobiliary and renal disposition of drugs. (Reproduced from Hillgren et al. (2013), courtesy of John Wiley & Sons Publications.)

the bile caniculus or urine, respectively. The important members of the solute carrier family are OATP (SLCO), OCT (SLC22), OAT (SLC22), and MATE (SLC47), and the ATP-binding cassette transporters, such as P-glycoprotein (ABCB1), MRP (ABCC), and BCRP (ABCG2). Cumulative studies have highlighted the cooperative roles of uptake transporters, metabolic enzymes, and efflux transporters and, as such, developed the concept of a rate-limiting process in hepatic and renal elimination (Kusuhara and Sugiyama, 2009; Giacomini and Huang, 2013).

The *in vitro* systems typically used to study uptake and efflux kinetics fall into two categories: (i) expression systems such as immortalized cell lines (e.g. CHO, LLC-PK1, or MDCK) or vesicles, and (ii) primary or cultured cells (e.g. plated or sandwich-cultured hepatocytes) or derived cell lines (e.g. Caco-2, HepG2). Expression systems allow the determination of kinetic parameters for the overexpressed transporter of interest, while cellular matrices enable transport kinetics to be measured in the context of the interplay of uptake, efflux, and metabolism. For compounds with low passive membrane permeability, the scaled CL_{int} from hepatocytes can be significantly lower than that from liver microsomes. In addition, active transport processes active at the cell membrane level *in vivo* are obviously not present in subcellular preparations, can be of suboptimal activity in hepatocyte suspensions and are better reflected in plated hepatocytes. This has led to the development of the extended CL concept, a modification to the well-stirred model as shown below (Equation 9.13).

$$CL_{int,app} = CL_{int,met} * \frac{CL_{int,uptake} + CL_{int,pass}}{CL_{int,met} + CL_{int,pass} + CL_{int,efflux}} \qquad (9.13)$$

where the apparent intrinsic clearance, $CL_{int,app}$, is defined by $CL_{int,met}$, $CL_{int,pass}$, $CL_{int,uptake}$, and $CL_{int,efflux}$ referring to intrinsic clearance by metabolism, passive permeation, active uptake, and active efflux, respectively. This has shown utility in understanding determinants of hepatic CL for a number of compounds. Measuring uptake in suspended/plated hepatocytes, biliary excretion in sandwich-cultured hepatocytes, and metabolism in liver microsomes can be integrated into a static model of hepatic CL, such as the extended CL concept, prior to incorporation into PBPK models (see Section "Physiologically-Based PK (PBPK) Modeling").

It is vital to consider determining the uptake kinetic parameters, Km and Vmax, rather than CLint based on a single concentration so that nonlinearity and saturation of the transporter can be modeled. A number of reasons including (i) the lack of truly specific chemical inhibitors against many of the transporter isoforms, (ii) the caveats of using a temperature differential (4°C vs. 37°C) to deconvolute active and passive transport contributions, and (iii) the inappropriate application of enzyme kinetic principles to the bidirectional nature of monolayer membrane transport has led investigators to recommend compartmental modeling approaches. These models include media and cellular compartments for fitting the dynamic changes in drug concentration due to passive permeation, active uptake and efflux, as well as metabolism and binding processes (Zamek-Gliszczynski et al., 2013). Scaling these data effectively requires not only both appropriate study and design, but also the necessary scaling factors to bridge the functional and protein expression differences between the *in vitro* test system and the *in vivo* situation, as well as understanding the uncertainty around these parameters. As for the non-P450 enzymes, abundance data for drug transporters is now emerging from quantitative proteomic analyses to characterize *in vitro*-to-*in vivo* scaling factors and species differences in expression (Prasad et al., 2016; Fallon et al., 2016). Sandwich-cultured human hepatocytes (SCHH) have proven useful in modeling the multiple transport and metabolism processes that are involved in hepatobiliary disposition. Using a SCHH *in vitro* system together with available clinical plasma concentration-time data for seven compounds, Jones et al. established a prediction approach for active liver uptake and efflux (Jones et al., 2012). These SCHH *in vitro* data were dynamically modeled including estimation of biliary efflux and active and passive uptake from the same *in vitro* experiment through modulation of calcium ions. The *in vitro* parameters were then scaled to *in vivo* and were subsequently integrated into a whole-body PBPK model, together with other absorption, distribution, metabolism, and excretion properties to simulate the human plasma concentrations. In this analysis, active uptake and biliary excretion were underpredicted (~60-fold) and overpredicted (~20-fold), respectively; so, the investigators proposed empirical scaling factors for prospective applications in the future with these correction factors being laboratory-specific to the experimental SCHH system. The basis for the scaling factors is unclear and warrants further investigation but may be related to expression and/or activity differences between *in vitro* and *in vivo* settings.

The ability to model multiple dispositional processes at the level of the hepatocyte using *in vitro* data has improved greatly in recent years. Recapitulating the structural and functional features of the nephron *in vitro* has proven more challenging, but conceptually would follow Equation 9.14 such that glomerular filtration, active tubular secretion, and active reabsorption could be quantified. This topic has been the subject of two recent reviews (Scotcher et al., 2016a, 2016b).

$$CL_R = Q_R \times \left[\frac{f_{u,b} \times GFR}{Q_R} + \left(1 - \frac{f_{u,b} \times GFR}{Q_R} \right) \left(\frac{f_{u,b} \times CL_{sec,u}}{Q_R + f_{u,b} \times CL_{sec,u}} \right) \right] \times \left(1 - f_{Re\text{-}abs} \right) \qquad (9.14)$$

Preclinical knock-out models for all transporters shown in Figure 9.6 have been characterized and are commercially available (Zamek-Gliszczynski et al., 2013). These can provide useful information if there is confidence that the excretory clearance in preclinical species translates to man, since the contribution of secretion to the total body clearance (i.e. fractional excretory clearance, fe, a concept analogous to that of fm and follows an identical relationship to that shown in Figure 9.5) is prone to species differences. For example, metformin is cleared entirely by urinary excretion of parent, in both mouse and human, of which 20% is glomerular filtration and 80% is active tubular secretion via the concerted action of OCT and MATE isoforms. As such, comparative PK in Oct1/2- and Mate1- knock-out and wild-type mice is reflective of the contribution of OCT and MATE to the human CL of metformin. By contrast, pemetrexed is cleared by urinary excretion in human (OAT3/4 mediated active secretion), but predominantly by metabolism in mouse; therefore, the human excretory CL is not well described by preclinical transporter knock-out models. The interspecies extrapolation of biliary CL is similarly challenging and further confounded by the loss of intestinal reabsorption in bile-duct cannulated studies in preclinical species. Biliary clearance in rat often overestimates clearance in human largely due to higher expression levels of hepatobiliary transporters and higher bile flow in rat (Lai, 2009).

Physiologically-Based PK (PBPK) Modeling

PBPK modeling provides a quantitative and systems-based framework with each compartment representing a physiological volume interconnected by flow rates that are anatomically representative of the circulatory system (Figure 9.7). Mass balance equations describe the transfer of drug from the arterial blood into tissues and from tissues into venous blood. As such, simulations are dynamic in nature with model fitting and prediction focused on concentration-time data. Essentially, PBPK models are more comprehensive than empirical PK models, incorporating both system-specific parameters as well as drug-specific parameters. Although not a new approach, PBPK modeling applied in pharmaceutical research and development has gained increasing attention in recent years with the availability of robust *in vitro* and *in silico* data, advancements in *in vitro-in vivo* extrapolation, and the substantial investment that has been made in the curated databases of system-dependent and probe drug-dependent parameters that are the foundation of the commercially available software packages. This technological progress has enhanced the number and breadth of robust applications in the area of clinical pharmacology including first-in-man, special populations, drug interactions, and biopharmaceutics/formulations (Jones et al., 2015; Huang et al., 2013). Considerable experience has now accumulated with the development of PBPK models to describe drug concentration-time profiles. The construction of PBPK models has typically utilized the various *in vitro* and physicochemical data available in early preclinical drug development in what is often termed a "bottom-up" approach to recapitulate the concentration-time data. Alternatively, there may be reasons to consider a "top-down" approach where the underlying drug-specific parameterization of the PBPK model is accomplished by optimizing the fit of the concentration-time data in question. In practice, there is usually an approach that lands somewhere between the two, termed

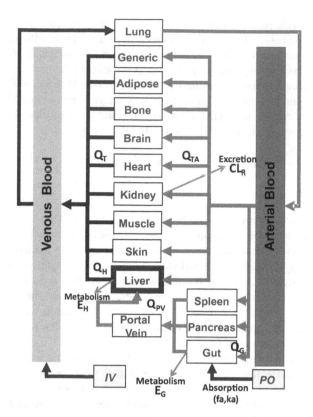

FIGURE 9.7 Generalized PBPK model scheme illustrating the connectivity (blood flows) between compartments (tissues and organs), as well as the typical routes of entry and elimination.

"middle-out," where some of the drug-specific parameters based on *in vitro* or *in silico* data may not scale appropriately or there are missing data and incomplete information regarding some aspects of drug disposition, and an element of "top-down" model optimization is necessary. Furthermore, mechanistic understanding can be gained through parameter sensitivity analysis and asking "what if" questions of the optimized model. The prospective application to human CL prediction prior to first-in-human studies, precludes the use of a "top-down" approach and relies on parameters derived from *in vitro* and *in vivo* characterization described earlier. And because PBPK modeling is focused on fitting concentration-time profiles, multiple data inputs are required beyond CL properties, integrating data on compound absorption and distribution as well. Model validation in the *a priori* prediction of CL for a particular compound has typically been achieved through modeling the corresponding data in preclinical species, confirming the underlying model recapitulates the concentration-time profiles in rodent and non-rodent species prior to transforming the model to physiology and drug-specific parameters relevant to human, and performing simulations. This approach was recommended by Jones et al. (Jones et al., 2006). In their study, PBPK modeling was compared with the Dedrick approach using 19 F. Hoffmann-La Roche compounds, in order to determine the best approaches and strategies for the prediction of human pharmacokinetics. Total body clearance was predicted as the sum of scaled rat renal clearance (GFR-normalized unbound renal CL) or alternatively simple allometry of CLr when data from ≥ four species were available, and hepatic clearance projected from *in vitro* metabolism data. In the majority of cases, PBPK gave more accurate predictions of pharmacokinetic parameters and plasma concentration-time profiles than the Dedrick approach. By following the proposed strategy of PBPK model validation using animal data, a prediction would have been made prospectively for approximately 70% of the compounds. The prediction accuracy for these compounds, i.e. percentage of compounds with an average-fold error of <2-fold was 83% for apparent oral clearance (CL/F), 75% for terminal elimination half-life, and 92% for AUC. For the other 30% of compounds, unacceptable prediction accuracy was obtained in animals, and therefore, a prospective prediction of human pharmacokinetics would not have been made using PBPK. For these compounds, prediction accuracy was also poor using the Dedrick approach.

The PhRMA CPCDC initiative reported on the effectiveness of PBPK models for simulating human plasma concentration-time profiles on a blinded dataset of 108 compounds (Poulin et al., 2011). The shape of the plasma concentration-time courses as a measure of model quality indicated up to 69% of the simulations demonstrated a medium to high degree of accuracy for intravenous pharmacokinetics, whereas this number decreased to 23% after oral administration. A general underestimation of drug exposure (Cmax and AUC0-t) was attributed to an underprediction of absorption parameters and/or overprediction of distribution or oral first-pass. The CL prediction, in general, had less of an impact on the simulations, with *in vitro* CLint or FCIM methods showing equivalent performance. An analogous study by De Buck and colleagues (De Buck et al., 2007) used a dataset of 26 clinically tested drugs to assess the utility of generic PBPK modeling in predictions of human PK. Total body clearance was predicted as the sum of scaled rat renal clearance (GFR-normalized unbound renal CL) and hepatic clearance projected from *in vitro* metabolism data. The best CL predictions were obtained by disregarding both blood and microsomal or hepatocyte binding, whereas strong bias was seen using both blood and microsomal or hepatocyte binding. The PBPK model, which combined the best performing Vd and CL methods yielded the most accurate predictions of *in vivo* terminal half-life (69% within 2-fold).

The predictive accuracy of PBPK modeling towards first-in-human PK projections is very much determined by the properties of the compound in question. For compounds cleared predominant by CYP metabolism and exhibiting high passive membrane permeation, the level of confidence in PBPK simulations is relatively high (Jones et al., 2015). The level of confidence for compound disposition mediated by non-CYP enzymes or transporters is comparatively lower and can be attributed to current limitations around the scaling of activity and abundance for these pathways, as described earlier. Conceptually at least, PBPK modeling lends itself well to understanding more complex drug disposition by providing an integrative framework to predict CL by multiple pathways, or where multiple moieties need to be characterized, e.g. prodrugs, drugs with active metabolites, etc. A recent example includes that of ganciclovir and its prodrug valganciclovir (Lukacova et al., 2016). The initial "bottom-up" modeling based on physicochemical properties and measured *in vitro* inputs was verified in animal species, before a clinical model was corroborated in a stepwise fashion with pharmacokinetic data in adult, children, and neonatal patients. The final model incorporated conversion of valganciclovir to ganciclovir through esterases and permeability-limited tissue distribution of both drugs with active transport processes added in gut, liver, and kidney.

Once CL data are obtained from initial clinical studies in healthy volunteers or early phase trials in patients these same model/s can be refined using a "top-down" component and/or with additional data generated during development to support CL prediction in special populations e.g. pediatrics, hepatic and renal impairment, pharmacogenetics, and the effect of disease (Rioux and Waters, 2016; Jones et al., 2015). This is an area of active research as PBPK modeling and simulation has evolved into a regulatory science and has been extensively reviewed elsewhere (Zhao et al., 2012).

Computational Approaches

The availability of high-quality datasets for computational modeling of human CL (Obach et al., 2008) together with the recent momentum in computational ADME modeling, more specifically with quantitative structure-activity relationships (QSAR), has led to some encouraging findings in this area. QSAR attempts to find relationships between the molecular properties of molecules and the biological responses they elicit when applied to a biological system. The advancements in computer hardware and software now allow the molecular properties of molecules to be easily estimated without the need to synthesize the molecules in question. Thus, the use of predictive computational (*in silico*) QSAR models allows the biological properties of virtual structures to be predicted and a more informed choice of target to be selected for synthesis. Considerable progress has been made in computational QSAR models for predicting ADME properties in recent years (Gleeson et al., 2011). However, the accurate prediction of human CL remains a challenge due to the complexity of the underlying physiological and biochemical mechanisms. QSAR studies are usually carried out using supervised methods—those in which the model is trained using the measured values of the property to be modeled. Supervised methods used in QSAR modeling range from simple statistical regression methods such as multiple linear regression (MLR), principal components regression (PCR), or partial least squares (PLS), through to more flexible non-linear methods such as artificial and Bayesian neural networks (ANN and BNN), as well as recursive partitioning methods such as classification and regression trees (CART). In the absence of measured data, QSAR model predictions can be extremely useful and provide a means of identifying molecules that may be problematic. QSAR models are more than a literature curiosity, and successful ones offer the potential to be used as a virtual screen to filter design targets before synthesis; thus, improving the efficiency of pharmaceutical R&D.

A number of studies have been reported in this area (Yap et al., 2006; Yu, 2010) with the most recent study leading to the development of a completely *in silico* linear PLS model to predict the human plasma clearance, built from a dataset of 754 compounds using physicochemical descriptors and structural fragments (Berellini et al., 2012). Model validation included using a leave-class-out approach (structural, therapeutic or ionization based) and yielded a geometric mean fold error (GMFE) of 2.1 with 59% and 80% of compounds predicted within 2- and 3-fold error (Figure 9.8). The *in silico* model performance also compared favorably with interspecies scaling methods; on an identical external test set of 69 compounds the GMFE was 1.8, 1.9, and 1.9 for the *in silico*, monkey LBF, and FCIM methods, respectively, while % < 2-fold was 70, 62, and 62, respectively. This work was extended to include an additional modeling tier, which classified compounds by their primary route of elimination; metabolism or renal, with similar encouraging results (Lombardo et al., 2014).

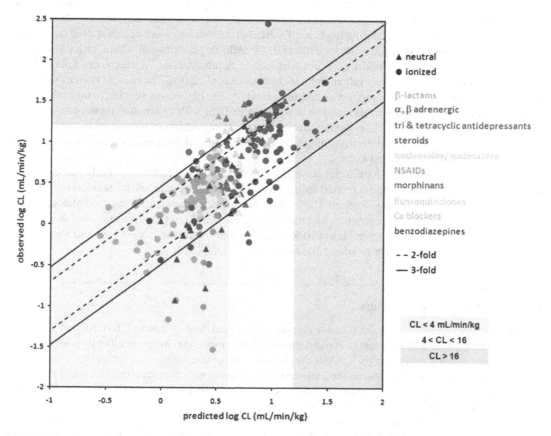

FIGURE 9.8   Observed versus predicted plot for total human plasma clearance using a QSAR computational model based on a leave-class-out validation approach. Data-points are colored according to therapeutic class, shape denotes charge type; neutral (triangle-up) and ionized at pH 7.5 (circle). (Reprinted with permission Berellini, G. et al., *J. Chem. Inf. Model.*, 52, 2069–2078, 2012. Copyright 2012 American Chemical Society.)

Somewhat analogous was the computational approach explored by Kusama and coworkers who developed an *in silico* classification system for the likely major clearance pathway based on four calculated properties, molecular weight, charge, lipophilicity (expressed as logD), and fraction unbound in plasma (predicted) (Kusama et al., 2010). The major clearance pathways were assigned for a training set of 141 approved drugs using five categories; metabolism by CYP3A4, metabolism by CYP2C9, metabolism by CYP2D6, hepatic uptake by OATPs, or renal excretion as unchanged parent drug. The dataset was initially grouped by charge type before subsequently plotting in a 3D space with axes of molecular weight, logD, and fraction unbound in plasma. The data were plotted so that each clearance pathway could be clustered into groups, with statistical significance confirmed using leave-one-out and external test set validations.

These contemporary computational models are showing predictive performance comparable with more experimentally intensive methods and should be useful in drug design for the optimization of candidate compounds as well as providing an orthogonal means to assess confidence in prediction, prior to first-in-human clinical studies.

Conclusions & Future Directions

The current state-of-the-art in prospective human CL prediction commonly involves using multiple methodologies carefully guided based on what is known about the disposition properties of the compound in question. With those CL estimates available, an assessment of consistency in prediction looking for convergence or divergence in the predictions across multiple methods is typically required. A consensus CL prediction with a sense of the potential range (i.e. mean, SD, %CV) is warranted as this data is then used as a subsequent input, together with estimates of VD, oral absorption, and target exposure, into a projection of the clinically efficacious dose and regimen. Presently, the exercise of human CL prediction is founded on three orthogonal but complementary bases: *in vitro* approaches deriving kinetic data for human enzymes and transporters, PK data in preclinical species as models for the impact of the whole organism, and computational methods that leverage learnings from the known disposition of chemically-related drugs in man. Congruence in CL estimates from diverse methods that span these three systems lends confidence in any prospective prediction. As discussed earlier, information on the mechanisms of clearance in preclinical species can help inform appropriate selection of prediction methodologies. Furthermore, potentially human-specific determinants of CL have been reported in retrospective analyses and are now being investigated prospectively, e.g. the extent of drug binding to human AAG. Obviously, the accuracy of CL predictions becomes evident once PK data are available from early clinical studies. With some understanding of the PK properties in healthy volunteers or the initial patient population, the focus moves to predicting CL in special populations, such as pediatrics, renal and hepatic impairment, and subjects with genetic polymorphisms, to further support clinical development. This area has benefited greatly from the advancements in PBPK modeling described earlier.

Contemporary drug discovery has created several areas of emerging importance to the accurate prediction of human CL. Firstly, medicinal chemistry strategies have become increasingly successful at reducing CYP-mediated metabolism of drug candidates to a point that renders some of these compounds susceptible to lesser studied or poorly understood elimination pathways. That scenario presents a greater challenge to the drug metabolism scientist in terms of the availability of validated *in vitro* tools or understanding around interspecies differences. Furthermore, high metabolic stability of newer drug candidates has presented analytical challenges in the accurate determination of CLint by substrate depletion. Alternatively, transporter-mediated CL may be invoked as the primary or rate-limiting elimination pathway with the associated issues of scaling CL by this pathway, either from *in vitro* data or from data generated in preclinical species. All of these aspects are active areas of research as highlighted in this chapter. There is also a renewed emphasis in bringing a more robust statistical framework to the prediction of human PK and dose given some of the challenges in deriving and communicating point estimates as well as defining the error and confidence intervals on a prediction (Sundqvist et al., 2015). There are a number of emerging technologies in development that have the potential to impact the quantitative prediction of human CL in the future, including 3D and microfluidic cell culture (e.g. organ-on-a-chip) systems. The further application of ómic technologies will also aid in understanding species differences in the molecular determinants of CL and provide scaling factors for the future mechanistic prediction of human CL.

REFERENCES

Bae SK, Lee SJ, Kim YG, et al. Interspecies pharmacokinetic scaling of oltipraz in mice, rats, rabbits and dogs, and prediction of human pharmacokinetics. *Biopharm. Drug Dispos.* 2005;26:99–115.

Barry A, Levine M. A systematic review of the effect of CYP3A5 genotype on the apparent oral clearance of tacrolimus in renal transplant recipients, *Ther. Drug Monit.* 2010;32:708–714.

Barter ZE, Bayliss MK, Beaune PH, et al. Scaling factors for the extrapolation of in vivo metabolic drug clearance from in vitro data: Reaching a consensus on values of human microsomal protein and hepatocellularity per gram of liver. *Curr. Drug Metab.* 2007;8(1):33–45.

Beaumont K, Smith DA. Does human pharmacokinetic prediction add significant value to compound selection in drug discovery research? *Curr. Opin. Drug Discov. Dev.* 2009;12(1):61–71.

Berellini G, Waters NJ, Lombardo F. *In silico* prediction of total human plasma clearance. *J. Chem. Inf. Model.* 2012;52(8):2069–2078.

Bonn B, Svanberg P, Janefeldt A, et al. Determination of human hepatocyte intrinsic clearance for slowly metabolized compounds: Comparison of a primary hepatocyte/stromal cell co-culture with plated primary hepatocytes and HepaRG. *Drug Metab. Dispos.* 2016;44:527–533.

Boxenbaum H. Time concepts in physics, biology, and pharmacokinetics. *J. Pharm. Sci.* 1986;75(11):1053–1062.

Boxenbaum H. Interspecies pharmacokinetic scaling and the evolutionary-comparative paradigm. *Drug Metab. Rev.* 1984;15(5–6):1071–1121.

Boxenbaum H. Evolutionary biology, animal behavior, fourth-dimensional space, and the raison d'etre of drug metabolism and pharmacokinetics. *Drug Metab. Rev.* 1983;14(5):1057–1097.

Boxenbaum H, Ronfeld R. Interspecies pharmacokinetic scaling and the Dedrick plots. *Am. J. Physiol.* 1983;245(6):R768–R775.

Boxenbaum H. Interspecies scaling, allometry, physiological time, and the ground plan of pharmacokinetics. *J. Pharmacokinet. Biopharm.* 1982; 10(2):201–227.

Caldwell GW, Masucci JA, Yan Z, et al. Allometric scaling of pharmacokinetic parameters in drug discovery: Can human CL, Vss and t1/2 be predicted from in-vivo rat data? *Eur. J. Drug Metab. Pharmacokinet.* 2004;29(2):133–143.

Chan TS, Yu H, Moore A, et al. Meeting the challenge of predicting hepatic clearance of compounds slowly metabolized by cytochrome P450 using a novel hepatocyte model, HepatoPac. *Drug Metab. Dispos.* 2013;41:2024–2032.

Chen Y, Liu L, Nguyen K, et al. Utility of intersystem extrapolation factors in early reaction phenotyping and the quantitative extrapolation of human liver microsomal intrinsic clearance using recombinant cytochromes P450. *Drug Metab. Dispos.* 2011;39:373–382.

Crespi CL. Xenobiotic-metabolizing human cells as tools for pharmacological and toxicological research. In *Advances in Drug Research*, 179–235. Academic Press, 1995.

Cubitt HE, Houston JB, Galetin A. Prediction of human drug clearance by multiple metabolic pathways: Integration of hepatic and intestinal microsomal and cytosolic data. *Drug Metab. Dispos.* 2011;39:864–873.

De Buck SS, Sinha VK, Fenu LA, et al. Prediction of human pharmacokinetics using physiologically based modeling: A retrospective analysis of 26 clinically tested drugs. *Drug Metab. Dispos.* 2007;35(10):1766–1780.

Dedrick RL. Animal scale-up. *J. Pharmacokinet. Biopharm.* 1973;1(5):435–461.

Dedrick R, Bischoff KB, Zaharko DS. Interspecies correlation of plasma concentration history of methotrexate (NSC-740). *Cancer Chemother. Rep.* 1970;54(2):95–101.

Deguchi T, Watanabe N, Kurihara A, et al. Human pharmacokinetic prediction of UDP-glucuronosyltransferase substrates with an animal scale-up approach. *Drug Metab. Dispos.* 2011;39(5):820–829.

Di L, Atkinson K, Orozco CC, et al. In vitro–in vivo correlation for low-clearance compounds using hepatocyte relay method. *Drug Metab. Dispos.* 2013;41:2018–2023.

Di L, Trapa P, Obach RS, et al. A novel relay method for determining low-clearance values. *Drug Metab. Dispos.* 2012;40:1860–1865.

Fallon JK, Smith PC, Xia CQ, et al. Quantification of four efflux drug transporters in liver and kidney across species using targeted quantitative proteomics by isotope dilution nanoLC-MS/MS. *Pharm Res.* 2016;33(9):2280–2288.

Fuse E, Tanii H, Kurata N, et al. Unpredicted clinical pharmacology of UCN-01 caused by specific binding to human alpha1-acid glycoprotein. *Cancer Res.* 1998;58(15):3248–3253.

Giacomini KM, Huang S-M. Transporters in drug development and clinical pharmacology. *Clin. Pharmacol. Ther.* 2013;94(1):3–9.

Gibson CR, Lu P, Maciolek C, et al. Using human recombinant UDP-glucuronosyltransferase isoforms and a relative activity factor approach to model total body clearance of laropiprant (MK-0524) in humans. *Xenobiotica.* 2013;43:1027–1036.

Gleeson MP, Hersey A, Hannongbua S. In-silico ADME models: A general assessment of their utility in drug discovery applications. *Curr. Top. Med. Chem.* 2011;11(4):358–381.

Goteti K, Brassil PJ, Good SS, et al. Estimation of human drug clearance using multiexponential techniques. *J. Clin. Pharmacol.* 2008;48(10):1226–1236.

Goteti K, Garner CE, Mahmood I. Prediction of human drug clearance from two species: A comparison of several allometric methods. *J. Pharm. Sci.* 2010;99(3):1601–1613.

Griffin SJ, Houston JB. Prediction of *in vitro* intrinsic clearance from hepatocytes: Comparison of suspensions and monolayer cultures. *Drug Metab. Dispos.* 2005;33(1):115–120.

Hallifax D, Foster JA, Houston JB. Prediction of human metabolic clearance from *in vitro* systems: Retrospective analysis and prospective view. *Pharm Res.* 2010;27(10):2150–2161.

Hillgren KM, Keppler D, Zur AA, et al. Emerging transporters of clinical importance: An update from the international transporter consortium. *Clin. Pharmacol. Ther.* 2013;94(1):52–63.

Hoogdalem EJ, Soeish Y, Matsushima H, et al. Disposition of the selective alpha-1A adrenoceptor antagonist tamsulosin in humans: Comparison with data from interspecies scaling. *J. Pharm. Sci.* 1997;86:1156–1161.

Hosea NA, Collard WT, Cole S, et al. Prediction of human pharmacokinetics from preclinical information: Comparative accuracy of quantitative prediction approaches. *J. Clin. Pharmacol.* 2009;49(5):513–533.

Hosea NA. Drug design tools – in silico, *in vitro* and *in vivo* ADME/PK prediction and interpretation: Is PK in monkey an essential part of a good human PK prediction? *Curr. Top. Med. Chem.* 2011;11:351–357.

Houston JB. Utility of *in vitro* drug metabolism data in predicting *in vivo* metabolic clearance. *Biochem. Pharmacol.* 1994;47(9):1469–1479.

Huang SM, Abernethy DR, Wang Y, et al. The utility of modeling and simulation in drug development and regulatory review. *J. Pharm. Sci.* 2013;102:2912–2923.

Hultman I, Vedin C, Abrahamsson A, et al. Use of HμREL human coculture system for prediction of intrinsic clearance and metabolite formation for slowly metabolized compounds. *Mol. Pharm.* 2016;13(8):2796–2807.

Hutzler JM, Ring BJ, Anderson SR. Low-turnover drug molecules: A current challenge for drug metabolism scientists. *Drug Metab. Dispos.* 2015;43:1917–1928.

Iwatsubo T, Hirota N, Ooie T, et al. Prediction of *in vivo* drug metabolism in the human liver from *in vitro* metabolism data. *Pharmacol. Ther.* 1997;73(2):5147–5171.

Jezequel SG. Fluconazole: Interspecies scaling and allometric relationships of pharmacokinetic properties. *J. Pharm. Pharmacol.* 1994;46(3):196–199.

Jolivette LJ, Ward KW. Extrapolation of human pharmacokinetic parameters from rat, dog, and monkey data: Molecular properties associated with extrapolative success or failure. *J. Pharm. Sci.* 2005;94(7):1467–1483.

Jones HM, Barton HA, Lai Y, et al. Mechanistic pharmacokinetic modeling for the prediction of transporter-mediated disposition in humans from sandwich culture human hepatocyte data. *Drug Metab. Dispos.* 2012;40(5):1007–1017.

Jones HM, Butt RP, Webster RW, et al. Clinical micro-dose studies to explore the human pharmacokinetics of four selective inhibitors of human Nav1.7 voltage-dependent sodium channels. *Clin. Pharmacokinet.* 2016;55(7):875–887.

Jones HM, Chen Y, Gibson C, et al. Physiologically based pharmacokinetic modeling in drug discovery and development: A pharmaceutical industry perspective. *Clin. Pharmacol. Ther.* 2015;97:247–262.

Jones HM, Parrott N, Jorga K, et al. A novel strategy for physiologically based predictions of human pharmacokinetics. *Clin. Pharmacokinet.* 2006;45(5):511–542.

Khetani SR, Bhatia SN. Microscale culture of human liver cells for drug development. *Nat. Biotechnol.* 2008;26:120–126.

Kilford PJ, Stringer R, Sohal B, et al. Prediction of drug clearance by glucuronidation from *in vitro* data: Use of combined cytochrome P450 and UDP-glucuronosyltransferase cofactors in alamethicin-activated human liver microsomes. *Drug Metab. Dispos.* 2009;37(1):82–89.

Koiso K, Akaza H, Kikuchi K, et al. Pharmacokinetics of tamsulosin hydrochloride in patients with renal impairment: Effects of alpha 1-acid glycoprotein. *J. Clin. Pharmacol.* 1996;36(11):1029–1038.

Kolokotrones T, Savage V, Deeds EJ, et al. Curvature in metabolic scaling. *Nature.* 2010;464:753–756.

Kusama M, Toshimoto K, Maeda K, et al. *In silico* classification of major clearance pathways of drugs with their physiochemical parameters. *Drug Metab. Dispos.* 2010;38:1362–1370.

Kusuhara H, Sugiyama Y. *In vitro-in vivo* extrapolation of transporter mediated clearance in the liver and kidney. *Drug Metab. Pharmacokinet.* 2009;24(1):37–52.

Lai Y. Identification of interspecies difference in hepatobiliary transporters to improve extrapolation of human biliary secretion. *Expert Opin. Drug Metab. Toxicol.* 2009;5:1175–1187.

Lappin G, Garner RC. The utility of microdosing over the past 5 years. *Expert Opin. Drug Metab. Toxicol.* 2008;4(12):1499–1506.

Lappin G, Kuhnz W, Jochemsen R, et al. Use of microdosing to predict pharmacokinetics at the therapeutic dose: Experience with 5 drugs. *Clin. Pharmacol. Ther.* 2006;80(3):203–215.

Lave T, Dupin S, Schmitt C, et al. Integration of *in vitro* data into allometric scaling to predict hepatic metabolic clearance in man: Application to 10 extensively metabolized drugs. *J. Pharm. Sci.* 1997;86:584–590.

Lave T, Coassolo P, Ubeaud G, et al. Interspecies scaling of bosentan, a new endothelin receptor antagonist and integration of *in vitro* data into allometric scaling. *Pharm. Res.* 1996;13(1):97–101.

Li X, Song X, Kamenecka TM, et al. Discovery of a highly selective CYP3A4 inhibitor suitable for reaction phenotyping studies and differentiation of CYP3A4 and CYP3A5. *Drug Metab. Dispos.* 2012;40:1803–1809.

Liu D, Song H, Song L, et al. A unified strategy in selection of the best allometric scaling methods to predict human clearance based on drug disposition pathway. *Xenobiotica.* 2016;46(12):1105–1111.

Lombardo F, Berellini G, Labonte LR, et al. Systematic evaluation of Wajima superposition (steady-state concentration to mean residence time) in the estimation of human intravenous pharmacokinetic profile. *J. Pharm. Sci.* 2016;105(3):1277–1287.

Lombardo F, Obach RS, Varma MV, et al. Clearance mechanism assignment and total clearance prediction in human based upon *in silico* models. *J. Med. Chem.* 2014;57(10):4397–4405.

Lombardo F, Waters NJ, Argikar UA, et al. Comprehensive assessment of human pharmacokinetic prediction based on *in vivo* animal pharmacokinetic data, part 2: Clearance. *J. Clin. Pharmacol.* 2013a;53(2):178–191.

Lombardo F, Waters NJ, Argikar UA, et al. Comprehensive assessment of human pharmacokinetic prediction based on *in vivo* animal pharmacokinetic data, part 1: Volume of distribution at steady state. *J. Clin. Pharmacol.* 2013b;53(2):167–177.

Lukacova V, Goelzer P, Reddy M, et al. A physiologically based pharmacokinetic model for ganciclovir and its prodrug valganciclovir in adults and children. *AAPS J.* 2016;18(6):1453–1463.

Mahmood I. Interspecies scaling of renally secreted drugs. *Life Sci.* 1998;63:2365–2371.

Mahmood I. Prediction of human drug clearance from animal data: Application of the rule of exponents and "fu Corrected Intercept Method" (FCIM). *J. Pharm. Sci.* 2006;95(8):1810–1821.

Mahmood I. Interspecies scaling of biliary excreted drugs: Prediction of human clearance and volume of distribution. *Drug Metabol. Drug Interact.* 2012;27(3):157–164.

Mahmood I, Balian JD. Interspecies scaling: Predicting clearance of drugs in humans. Three different approaches. *Xenobiotica.* 1996;26:887–895.

Mahmood I, Boxenbaum H. Vertical allometry: Fact or fiction? *Reg. Toxicol. Pharmacol.* 2014;68:468–474.

Mahmood I, Sahajwalla C. Interspecies scaling of biliary excreted drugs. *J. Pharm. Sci.* 2002;91:1908–1914.

Mahmood I, Yuan R. A comparative study of allometric scaling with plasma concentrations predicted by species-invariant time methods. *Biopharm. Drug Dispos.* 1999;20(3):137–144.

Margaillan G, Rouleau M, Fallon JK, et al. Quantitative profiling of human renal UDP-glucuronosyltransferases and glucuronidation activity: A comparison of normal and tumoral kidney tissues. *Drug Metab. Dispos.* 2015b;43(4):611–619.

Margaillan G, Rouleau M, Klein K, et al. Multiplexed targeted quantitative proteomics predicts hepatic glucuronidation potential. *Drug Metab. Dispos.* 2015a;43(9):1331–1335.

Mordenti J. Man versus beast: Pharmacokinetic scaling in mammals. *J. Pharm. Sci.* 1986;75(11):1028–1040.

Nagilla R, Ward KW. A comprehensive analysis of the role of correction factors in the allometric predictivity of clearance from rat, dog, and monkey to humans. *J. Pharm. Sci.* 2004;93(10):2522–2534.

Naritomi Y, Terashita S, Kagayama A, et al. Utility of hepatocytes in predicting drug metabolism: Comparison of hepatic intrinsic clearance in rats and humans *in vivo* and in vitro. *Drug Metab. Dispos.* 2003;31:580–588.

Naritomi Y, Terashita S, Kimura S, et al. Prediction of human hepatic clearance from *in vivo* animal experiments and *in vitro* metabolic studies with liver microsomes from animals and humans. *Drug Metab. Dispos.* 2001;29:1316–1324.

Obach RS. Metabolism of ezlopitant, a nonpeptidic substance P receptor antagonist, in liver microsomes: Enzyme kinetics, cytochrome P450 isoform identity, and *in vitro-in vivo* correlation. *Drug Metab. Dispos.* 2000;28(9):1069–1076.

Obach RS. Prediction of human clearance of twenty-nine drugs from hepatic microsomal intrinsic clearance data: An examination of *in vitro* half-life approach and nonspecific binding to microsomes. *Drug Metab. Dispos.* 1999;27(11):1350–1359.

Obach RS, Lombardo F, Waters NJ. Trend analysis of a database of intravenous pharmacokinetic parameters in humans for 670 drug compounds. *Drug Metab. Dispos.* 2008;36(7):1385–1405.

Pahlman I, Edholm M, Kankaanranta S, et al. Pharmacokinetics of susalimod, a highly biliary-excreted sulphasalazine analogue, in various species: Non-predictable human clearance by allometric scaling. *J. Pharm. Pharmacol.* 1998;49:494–498.

Paine SW, Ménochet K, Denton R, et al. Prediction of human renal clearance from preclinical species for a diverse set of drugs that exhibit both active secretion and net reabsorption. *Drug Metab. Dispos.* 2011;39(6):1008–1013.

Pang KS, Rowland M. Hepatic clearance of drugs. I. Theoretical considerations of a "well-stirred" model and a "parallel tube" model. Influence of hepatic blood flow, plasma and blood cell binding, and the hepatocellular enzymatic activity on hepatic drug clearance. *J. Pharmacokinet. Biopharm.* 1977;5(6):625–653.

Parmentier Y, Pothier C, Delmas A, et al. Direct and quantitative evaluation of the human CYP3A4 contribution (fm) to drug clearance using the *in vitro* SILENSOMES model. *Xenobiotica.* 2016;47(7):562–575.

Poulin P, Jones RD, Jones HM, et al. PhRMA CPCDC initiative on predictive models of human pharmacokinetics, part 5: Prediction of plasma concentration-time profiles in human by using the physiologically-based pharmacokinetic modeling approach. *J. Pharm. Sci.* 2011;100(10):4127–4157.

Prasad B, Johnson K, Billington S, et al. Abundance of drug transporters in the human kidney cortex as quantified by quantitative targeted proteomics. *Drug Metab. Dispos.* 2016;dmd-116.

Proctor NJ, Tucker GT, Rostami-Hodjegan A. Predicting drug clearance from recombinantly expressed CYPs: Intersystem extrapolation factors. *Xenobiotica.* 2004;34:151–178.

Riley RJ, McGinnity DF, Austin RP. A unified model for predicting human hepatic, metabolic clearance from *in vitro* intrinsic clearance data in hepatocytes and microsomes. *Drug Metab. Dispos.* 2005;33:1304–1311.

Ring BJ, Chien JY, Adkison KK, et al. PhRMA CPCDC initiative on predictive models of human pharmacokinetics, part 3: Comparative assessment of prediction methods of human clearance. *J. Pharm. Sci.* 2011;100(10):4090–4110.

Rioux N, Waters NJ. Physiologically based pharmacokinetic modeling in pediatric oncology drug development. *Drug Metab. Dispos.* 2016;44(7):934–943.

Scotcher D, Jones C, Posada M, et al. Key to opening kidney for *in vitro-in vivo* extrapolation entrance in health and disease: Part I: *In vitro* systems and physiological data. *AAPS J.* 2016a;18(5):1067–1081.

Scotcher D, Jones C, Posada M, et al. Key to opening kidney for *in vitro-in vivo* extrapolation entrance in health and disease: Part II: Mechanistic models and *in vitro-in vivo* extrapolation. *AAPS J.* 2016b;18(5):1082–1094.

Shibata Y, Chiba M. The role of extrahepatic metabolism in the pharmacokinetics of the targeted covalent inhibitors afatinib, ibrutinib, and neratinib. *Drug Metab. Dispos.* 2015;43:375–384.

Shin BS, Kima DH, Choa CY, et al. Pharmacokinetic scaling of SJ-8029, a novel anticancer agent possessing microtubule and topoisomerase inhibiting activities, by species-invariant time methods. *Biopharm. Drug Dispos.* 2003;24:191–197.

Shin DH, Park SH, Jeong SW, et al. Pharmacokinetic scaling of epirubicin using allometric and species-invariant time methods. *J. Pharm. Investig.* 2015;45(5):441–448.

Smith SA, Gagnon S, Waters NJ. Mechanistic investigations into the species differences in pinometostat clearance: Impact of binding to alpha-1-acid glycoprotein and permeability-limited hepatic uptake. *Xenobiotica.* 2016;10:1–9.

Stringer RA, Strain-Damerell C, Nicklin P, et al. Evaluation of recombinant cytochrome P450 enzymes as an *in vitro* system for metabolic clearance predictions. *Drug Metab. Dispos.* 2009;37(5):1025–1034.

Sundqvist M, Lundahl A, Någård MB, et al. Quantifying and communicating uncertainty in preclinical human dose-prediction. *CPT Pharmacometrics Syst. Pharmacol.* 2015;4:243–254.

Tang H, Hussain A, Leal M, et al. Interspecies prediction of human drug clearance based on scaling data from one or two animal species. *Drug Metab. Dispos.* 2007;35:1886–1893.

Tang H, Mayersohn M. A novel model for prediction of human drug clearance by allometric scaling. *Drug Metab. Dispos.* 2005;33.1297–1303.

Tang H, Mayersohn M. A global examination of allometric scaling for predicting human drug clearance and the prediction of large vertical allometry. *J. Pharm. Sci.* 2006a;95:1783–1799.

Tang H, Mayersohn M. On the observed large interspecies overprediction of human clearance ("vertical allometry") of UCN-01: Further support for a proposed model based on plasma protein binding. *J. Clin. Pharmacol.* 2006b;46:398–400.

Tang H, Mayersohn M. Utility of the coefficient of determination (r^2) in assessing the accuracy of interspecies allometric predictions: Illumination or illusion? *Drug Metab. Dispos.* 2007;35:2139–2142.

Vuppugalla R, Marathe P, He H, et al. PhRMA CPCDC initiative on predictive models of human pharmacokinetics, part 4: Prediction of plasma concentration-time profiles in human from *in vivo* preclinical data by using the Wajima approach. *J. Pharm. Sci.* 2011;100(10):4111–4126.

Wajima T, Fukumura K, Yano Y, et al. Prediction of human clearance from animal data and molecular structural parameters using multivariate regression analysis. *J. Pharm. Sci.* 2002;91(12):2489–2499.

Wajima T, Yano Y, Fukumura K, et al. Prediction of human pharmacokinetic profile in animal scale up based on normalizing time course profiles. *J. Pharm. Sci.* 2004; 93(7):1890–1900.

Walsky RL, Obach RS, Hyland R, et al. Selective mechanism-based inactivation of CYP3A4 by CYP3cide (PF-04981517) and its utility as an *in vitro* tool for delineating the relative roles of CYP3A4 versus CYP3A5 in the metabolism of drugs. *Drug Metab. Dispos.* 2012;40:1686–1697.

Wang YH, Gibson CR. Variability in human *in vitro* enzyme kinetics. In *Enzyme Kinetics in Drug Metabolism*, 337–362. Humana Press, 2014.

Ward KW, Coon DJ, Magiera D, et al. Exploration of the African green monkey as a preclinical pharmacokinetic model: Intravenous pharmacokinetic parameters. *Drug Metab. Dispos.* 2008;36:715–720.

Ward KW, Smith BR. A comprehensive quantitative and qualitative evaluation of extrapolation of intravenous pharmacokinetic parameters from rat, dog, and monkey to humans. I. Clearance. *Drug Metab. Dispos.* 2004;32(6):603–611.

Waters NJ, Obach RS, Di L. Consideration of the unbound drug concentration in enzyme kinetics. In *Enzyme Kinetics in Drug Metabolism*, 119–145. Humana Press, 2014.

Wong H, Lewin-Koh S, Theil F, et al. Influence of the compound selection process on the performance of human clearance prediction methods. *J. Pharm. Sci.* 2012;101(2):509–515.

Yap CW, Li ZR, Chen YZ. Quantitative structure-pharmacokinetic relationships for drug clearance by using statistical learning methods. *J. Mol. Graphics Modell.* 2006;24:383–395.

Ye Q, Jiang M, Huang WT, et al. Pharmacokinetics and metabolism of AMG 232, a novel orally bioavailable inhibitor of the MDM2-p53 interaction, in rats, dogs and monkeys: *In vitro-in vivo* correlation. *Xenobiotica.* 2015;45(8):681–692.

Yoshimatsu H, Konno Y, Ishii K, et al. Usefulness of minipigs for predicting human pharmacokinetics: Prediction of distribution volume and plasma clearance. *Drug Metab. Pharmacokinet.* 2016;31(1):73–81.

Yu MJ. Predicting total clearance in humans from chemical structure. *J. Chem. Inf. Model.* 2010;50:1284–1295.

Zamek-Gliszczynski M, Lee C, Poirier A, et al. ITC Recommendations for transporter kinetic parameter estimation and translational modeling of transport-mediated PK and DDIs in humans. *Clin. Pharmacol. Ther.* 2013;94(1):64–79.

Zhao P, Rowland M, Huang SM. Best practice in the use of physiologically based pharmacokinetic modeling and simulation to address clinical pharmacology regulatory questions. *Clin. Pharmacol. Ther.* 2012;92:17–20.

Zientek MA, Youdim K. Reaction phenotyping: Advances in the experimental strategies used to characterize the contribution of drug-metabolizing enzymes. *Drug Metab. Dispos.* 2015;43:163–181.

10

Sites of Extra Hepatic Metabolism, Part I: The Airways and Lung

John G. Lamb and Christopher A. Reilly

CONTENTS

Introduction

As in every tissue, the metabolism of xenobiotic compounds in pulmonary tissues is both complex and often cell specific and selective. Despite years of research the precise mechanisms and factors that determine pulmonary-specific metabolism and associated consequences for xenobiotic disposition in humans remain relatively undefined. Several excellent reviews dedicated to this topic were highlighted in the previous version of this chapter [1–9]. While dated, these authoritative reviews remain highly relevant to the field. A more up to date review has recently been published [10]. When possible, additional sub-topic specific reviews are referenced throughout the sections of this updated chapter.

The complexity associated with pulmonary metabolism of xenobiotics arises, in part because of the many different cell types (estimates of ~40), diverse cellular functions and differences in gene expression patterns that exist for each cell type at any given time, as a function of cell age and an ever-changing microenvironment [8]. Lung cells include immune cells responsible for recognizing and destroying foreign chemical and biological agents, secretory cells that maintain airway surface hydration, ciliated cells, which move foreign particles up and out the tracheobronchial tract, and epithelial and endothelial cells that line the airways, alveoli, and pulmonary vasculature and comprise the junction between vascular fluids and the external environment. The drug-metabolizing functions of many of these cells have not been fully revealed, but continually expanding scientific literature indicates that significant differences exist among different cell types [1–9].

Metabolic processes in the lung are still often studied using whole-lung homogenates. These studies are plentiful in the scientific literature and have been reasonably helpful to evaluate the overall metabolic capacity of the lung. However, these studies usually conclude that lung tissues are far less active in the metabolism of xenobiotics compared to the liver; exhibiting both a decrease in the overall ability to clear xenobiotics and a loss of metabolic diversity due to limited expression of many xenobiotic metabolizing enzymes. However, studies using lung homogenates are overly simplistic because they fail to accurately illustrate the gamut of unique interactions that occur between xenobiotics and lung cells. In many instances erroneous conclusions about the susceptibility of the lung and selected lung cell types to toxic insult, or the capability of certain cells or regions of the respiratory tract to metabolize xenobiotics, have been drawn from such studies. The use of precision cut lung slices has been proposed as an improved tool to study lung toxicity [11,12] and studies using primary cells as models have been informative with respect to the specific metabolic capacity and diversity of different lung cells [13,14]; albeit the expression of many drug metabolizing enzymes, and even the ability to induce certain enzymes, is lost in cultured cells compared to native tissues [13,15].

Generally, pulmonary metabolism of xenobiotics plays a relatively minor role in determining the overall systemic bioavailability and distribution of xenobiotics. The majority of xenobiotic metabolism occurs in other organs such as the liver, although significant first-pass metabolism by the lung can be observed for selected agents that are delivered via inhalation (e.g., ester hydrolysis of beclomethasone and remifentanil) [14,16], those actively sequestered by lung cells (e.g., amiodarone and paraquat), or those selectively acted upon by drug metabolizing enzymes expressed solely in the lung (e.g., 3-methylindole and CYP2F enzymes). Examples of physiological compounds that are subject to accumulation or metabolic clearance by the lung include eicosanoids [17,18] and endogenous oligoamines such as spermine [6]. Examples of therapeutic xenobiotics where pulmonary metabolism is important include glucocorticoids [13,14,19–21], which can accumulate in lung cells as fatty-acid esters [22–28], and toxic xenobiotics such as components of cigarette smoke and inhaled environmental pollutants. The accumulation of nitrogen-containing drugs, such as paraquat [6,29,30], propranolol [6,31,32], fentanyl, and related agents [33–35], ipomeanol [6,36], amioderone [37], and imipramine [38–40] by first-pass retention has also been observed. A prototypical example of selective metabolism of a xenobiotic by lung tissues is the metabolism of inhaled butadiene for which both the monoxide and di-epoxide metabolites were found at higher concentrations in lung tissues than in liver tissues of mice, presumably due to metabolism in the lung and not by selective accumulation of the metabolites by lung cells [41,42]. Additional lung toxicants that involve metabolic bioactivation within specific cell types in the respiratory tract include coumarin, 1,1-dichloroethylene, ethyl carbamate, 3-methylindole, naphthalene, styrene, and trichloroethylene [43].

Xenobiotic metabolism in respiratory tissues can be examined by comparing the chemical classes that are metabolized or by focusing on the enzymes responsible for the biotransformations. This chapter will primarily focus on the expression of pulmonary drug metabolizing enzymes and associated consequences. Frequently genes coding for xenobiotic metabolizing enzymes that are associated with pulmonary pharmacotherapy and/or pneumotoxicity, including cytochrome P450s, flavin-containing monooxygenases, and UDP-glucuronosyltransferases are solely expressed in the respiratory tract, where they play definitive roles in determining the ultimate actions of xenobiotics in respiratory cells and the respiratory tract as a whole.

Redox Enzymes

NADPH Cytochrome P450 Reductase

NADPH cytochrome P450 reductase (POR) is a flavoprotein enzyme that catalyzes the sequential transfer of electrons from nicotinamide adenine dinucleotide phosphate (NADPH) to the heme of cytochrome P450 enzymes. NADPH cytochrome P450 reductase is required for P450 enzyme function and ultimately substrate oxidation, dehydrogenation, dealkylation, etc. Only one gene product has been identified for NADPH cytochrome P450 reductase, and its expression is generally considered ubiquitous. The essential role of POR in driving the pneumotoxicity of chemicals is illustrated by two examples: (1) a reduction in styrene toxicity in mice lacking hepatic expression of POR, causing a decrease in circulating pneumotoxic styrene oxide [44] and (2) in mice lacking POR in Club cells of the airways, where substantially reduced pulmonary specific bioactivation of nicotine-derived nitrosamine ketone (4-(methylnitrosamino)-1-(3-pyridyl)-1-butanone; NNK) and associated tumor formation was observed [45].

Mutations in NADPH cytochrome P450 reductase contribute to numerous human diseases often involving disruption to endogenous steroid metabolism [46–57]. In fact, POR deficiency (PORD) was recognized as a new form of congenital adrenal hyperplasia in 2004. As one might expect, changes in

POR activity also impact the metabolism of xenobiotics and toxicants, albeit at times in a seemingly substrate-dependent manner [58–71]. POR*28 (A503V) has been shown to alter the pharmacokinetics and action of numerous CYP3A substrates including midazolam, erythromycin, tacrolimus, cyclosporine A, sirolimus, and atorvastatin, particularly in cases where CYP3A inactivating polymorphisms such as CYP3A4*22 and CYP3A5*3 also occurred. Numerous other POR variants (e.g., *5/A287P, *2/R457H) have also been shown to alter drug metabolism by CYPs [67–69,72]. Additional information on this topic is available through the CYP alleles database (http://www.cypalleles.ki.se/). Although the reductase enzyme is assumed to be ubiquitously expressed and tightly coupled to P450 enzymes on the endoplasmic reticulum membrane, reductase has not been immunochemically detected in all cells within the lung, including type I alveolar cells and vascular endothelial cells that possess demonstrable P450 protein [73–76]. Therefore, it is doubtful that the P450 enzymes in these cells (if truly expressed) are catalytically active. Localization of reductase to bronchiolar and bronchial epithelial cells, Club cells and alveolar type II cells has also been demonstrated in human lung tissues [77].

Because NADPH cytochrome P450 reductase is essentially (but not always) required for P450 enzyme function, its individual contributions to xenobiotic metabolism are often overlooked. A classic example of pulmonary xenobiotic metabolism directly catalyzed by NADPH cytochrome P450 reductase is the NADPH-dependent bioactivation and toxicity of paraquat in pneumocytes [29,30]. Paraquat is actively accumulated in alveolar type II cells via polyamine transporters. NADPH cytochrome P450 reductase catalyzes the one-electron reduction of paraquat to form the highly reducing paraquat cation radical, a potent cytotoxicant by virtue of its ability to readily reduce molecular oxygen (O_2) to form the superoxide anion radical (O_2^-) as well as to liberate iron from ferritin [78,79]. Superoxide ultimately dismutates (enzymatically via superoxide dismutase or spontaneously) to form hydrogen peroxide (H_2O_2) and through the Fenton reaction with ferrous iron (Fe^{2+}) produces the hydroxyl radical ($\cdot$OH), a potent oxidant that reacts with cellular nucleophiles at diffusion limited rates. Metabolism of paraquat by NADPH cytochrome P450 reductase has been shown to promote cell death through the depletion of reducing agents, lipid peroxidation and DNA and protein oxidation. Paraquat is one example of how NADPH cytochrome P450 reductase-dependent metabolism directly influences the biological effects of a selected agent in the lung, and other examples of this same mechanism exist for different drug/tissue combinations (e.g., doxorubicin in the heart). Of significance many POR variants with reduced enzyme activity (*8/Y181D, *5/A287P, *2/R457H, *4/V492E and *7/V608F) have been found to attenuate paraquat toxicity in a model of cellular injury, while *6/C569Y had no effect [80]. Interestingly and contradictory to what has been suggested by multiple studies, a recent study demonstrated that cardiomyocyte-specific knock-out of POR had no effect on doxorubicin toxicity [81].

Cytochrome P450

Cytochrome P450 enzymes are a family of heme-containing proteins that catalyze a variety of oxidative metabolic processes. There are 57 unique P450 genes in humans and each gene product exhibits unique distribution and function, including selective expression in tissues and the ability or inability to metabolize a given endogenous or xenobiotic agent [82]. There are also at least 59 pseudogenes among the 18 CYP families and 43 subfamilies. Certain mutations in most cytochrome P450 enzymes have been implicated in human disease states and variations in drug disposition [83]. Various aspects of P450 enzyme catalysis/biochemistry have been reviewed throughout the years. The classic example of a P450-catalyzed reaction is the addition of oxygen to a carbon-carbon bond to render the molecule more water soluble and amenable to conjugation reactions that further hasten the excretion of the xenobiotic from the body via specific excretion mechanisms. Cytochrome P450 reactions are also used for steroid and bile acid synthesis, as well as in the production and degradation of many other critical endogenous substances. The oxidation of a hydrocarbon substrate by P450 is represented by the following equation: $RH + O_2 + NADPH + H^+ \rightarrow ROH + H_2O + NADP^+$. P450-catalyzed reactions are not limited to hydrocarbon hydroxylation/oxygenation; heteroatom (O-, N-, and S-) dealkylation, dehydrogenation/desaturation, aliphatic and aromatic epoxidation, heteroatom (O-, N-, and S-) oxidation, hydrolysis (amide and ester), decarboxylation, and dehalogenation reactions are all possible for P450 enzymes, depending upon the chemical properties of the substrate and the specific P450 enzyme.

P450 enzymes are expressed to varying degrees throughout the human body with the greatest concentration in the liver. The P450 content in whole-lung microsomal fractions range from 0.01 nmol/mg microsomal protein for humans [84,85] to 1.04 nmol/mg protein for goats [86]. These values are 1/10th the P450 content of hepatic microsomes from the same species [2]. Therefore, key factors governing significant contributions of P450 enzymes in the pharmacology and toxicology of xenobiotics in the respiratory tract include the concentration of specific enzymes in certain cells or regions of the respiratory tract and the concentration of the agent in metabolically competent lung cells.

The number of P450 enzymes that are known to be expressed as functional proteins in respiratory tissues has increased in recent years as more studies using advanced methodologies, technologies and improved chemical probes have investigated xenobiotic metabolism in lung tissue. P450s that have been found in human respiratory tissue using either mRNA analysis, immunohistology, or functional assays include CYP1A1, 1A2, 1B1, 2A6, 2A7, 2A13, 2B6, 2C8, 2C18, 2C19, 2D6, 2E1, 2F1, 2S1, 2J2, 3A5, 3A7, 4B1, and many others (Table 10.1) [3,5,9,87–91]. Several more recent comprehensive mRNA profiling studies of CYP and other xenobiotic metabolizing enzymes in normal lung and cancer tissue, liver and lung cells commonly used in *in vitro* toxicology assays are recommended reading for anyone interested in the expression profiles of a specific drug metabolizing enzyme [92–94]. A similar CYP mRNA profiling study was performed using a comprehensive panel of mouse tissues [95]. Most CYP and other drug-metabolizing enzyme genes are expressed in the lung in addition to other organs. However, some P450 genes are selectively expressed in the lung and more specifically in specific regions of the

TABLE 10.1

Summary of Xenobiotic Metabolizing Enzymes in the Respiratory Tract

Enzyme	Species	Substrates/Toxicants	Localization
Cytochrome P450 1A1	All	Ethoxyresorufin, multiple PAHs, aromatic amines, arachidonic and docosahexaenoic acids, theophylline	Olfactory epithelium, bronchial epithelium, Club cells, type II cells, induced macrophages. Inducible by AhR ligands
Cytochrome P450 1A2	All	PAHs, aflatoxin B1, APAP, heterocyclic amines, nitro aromatics, arachidonic and docosahexaenoic acids, caffeine, zileuton, others	Induced by AhR ligands in bronchial epithelium, Club cells, pulmonary parenchyma by smoking, air pollutants, etc.
Cytochrome P450 1B1	Rat, mouse, human	PAHs, 17β-estradiol, sterols, nitroarenes, arylenes, aromatic and aryl amines, some lipids	Expressed by human cells from airways and parenchyma. Inducible by cigarette smoke.
Cytochrome P450 2A5/6/13	Mouse, human	Coumarin, diethylnitrosmine, aflatoxin B1, NNK, nicotine, naphthalene, 3MI, styrene, 1,3-butadiene, 2,6-dichlorobenzonitrile hexamethylphosphoramide, others	Trachea, bronchial epithelium, olfactory mucosa, pulmonary parenchyma
Cytochrome P450 2B1/4/6/7	Rabbit, rat, human	Arachidonic acid, BHT, NNK, bupropion, nicotine, alfentanil, propofol, tamoxifen, others	Bronchial epithelium Club cells, parenchyma
Cytochrome P450 2C8	Human	Arachidonic acid and other long chain PUFAs (linoleic, docosohexaenoic, eicosapentaenoic acids), montelukast, others	Bronchial epithelium-low
Cytochrome P450 2C9	Human	Warfarin, phenytoin, motelukast, limonene, 5-HT, multiple arachidonic acid and PUFAs, benzo[a]pyrene and other PAHs, others	Bronchial epithelium, parenchyma
Cytochrome P450 2C18	Human	Arachidonic acid and other long chain PUFAs (linoleic, docosohexaenoic, eicosapentaenoic acids), sterols, others	Bronchial epithelium

(Continued)

TABLE 10.1 *(Continued)*

Summary of Xenobiotic Metabolizing Enzymes in the Respiratory Tract

Enzyme	Species	Substrates/Toxicants	Localization
Cytochrome P450 2C19	Human	Arachidonic acid and other long chain PUFAs (linoleic, docosohexaenoic, eicosapentaenoic acids), clopidogrel, diazepam, others	Bronchial epithelium, pulmonary parenchyma
Cytochrome P450 2D6	Human	Hydroxytryptamines, neurosteroids, and both m- and p-tyramine, nicotine, opioids, others	Bronchial epithelium—low
Cytochrome P450 2E1	All	4-Nitrophenol, dimethyl-nitrosamine, DDD, dichloroethylene, and other small halogenated organics, benzene, arachidonic acid, 3MI, others	Nasal tissues, bronchial epithelium Club cells, pulmonary parenchyma
Cytochrome P450 2F1/2/3/4	All	Ethoxycoumarin, naphthalene, styrene, 3MI, dichloroethylene	Club cells, trachea, bronchial epithelium Club cells, pulmonary parenchyma
Cytochrome P450 2G1	Rabbit, mouse	Testosterone, progesterone, aflatoxin B1	Olfactory mucosa [96]
Cytochrome P450 2J2	All	Arachidonic, linoleic, docosohexaenoic, eicosapentaenoic acids	Ciliated epithelial
Cytochrome P450 2S1	All	Retinoic acid, Arachidonic, linoleic, docosohexaenoic, eicosapentaenoic acids, Prostaglandins G2 and H2 benzo[a]pyrene, ellipticine	Epithelial cells
Cytochrome P450 3A4	Human	Benzo[a]pyrene, arachidonic acid, testosterone, glucocorticoids, many others	N.D.
Cytochrome P450 3A5	Human	Benzo[a]pyrene, arachidonic acid, testosterone, glucocorticoids, many others	Bronchial and alveolar epithelium. Induced by glucocorticoids
Cytochrome P450 3A7	Human	Benzo[a]pyrene, arachidonic acid, testosterone, glucocorticoids, many others	Parenchyma
Cytochrome P450 4B1/2	All	2-Aminoflourene, 4-ipomeanol, valproic acid	Club cells, bronchial epithelium, and pulmonary parenchyma
Prostaglandin H synthase (COX2)	All	Benzo[a]pyrene-7,8-diol, arachidonic acid	Endothelial and epithelial cells
Flavin-containing monooxygenases 1-5	All	Soft nucleophiles, such as basic amines, phosphines, sulfides, thioureas, ethionamide, indoles, others	Entire respiratory system, mainly FMO4 and 5 in cultured cells
Epoxide hydrolases 1/2	All	PAH and other epoxides (e.g., styrene oxide)	Widely distributed in cultured cells and tissue
UDP-Glucuronosyltransferases (all UGT members)	All	1-Naphthol, 4-methyl-umbelliferone, eugenol, and many other xenobiotics with oxygen, nitrogen, sulfur, or carboxyl functional groups	Clara cells, variable in bronchial epithelium and perencyma
Glutathione S-transferases (All members)	All	1-Chloro-2,4-dinitrobenzene, benzo[a]pyrene epoxide, other aromatic epoxides, styrene oxide, other electrophilic centers on xenoibiotics	Club cells and ciliated cells, bronchial epithelium, Parenchyma
NAD(P)H quinone dehydrogenase 1/2 (Diaphorase)	Human	Two-electron reduction of many quinones to hydroquinones, benzoquinone, others	Widely distributed in cultured cells and tissue
Sulfotransferases (all members)	Human	Alcohol or amine groups on xenobiotics (many substrates)	1A1, 1A2, 1A3/41B1, 1C4, 1E1, 2B1 in bronchial epithelium and parenchyma

lung including the nose, trachea, bronchi, and distal tissue. Some enzymes exhibiting selective expression in the human lung include CYP2A13, 2F1, 4B1, and 2S1.

Recent work described in greater detail below shows the significance of site-specific expression of these enzymes in chemical injury. In general, similar properties and expression profiles are observed for P450 orthologues, thus allowing many studies of pulmonary xenobiotic metabolism to be performed in rodents and other animal models. However, it should be noted that in common models (e.g., mice) there is less distinction between locations of cells that populate the airway epithelium than in humans. In the case of mice there is abundant expression of Club cells, which generally contain some of the highest levels of P450 enzymes in the major airways, whereas in humans these cells are primarily found in the more distal airways. Further, enzyme specific metabolism, such as the intrinsic efficiency of specific CYPs, and the presence and/or absence of functionally coupled metabolic processes that promote or prevent toxicities can vary across species often greatly affecting how chemicals act in different models. For example, *Cyp2f2* is associated with the acute pneumotoxic properties of styrene and tumor formation in mouse lungs [44,97–101], but CYP2F1 humanized mice did not initiate lung tumors when treated with styrene [99] due, presumably, in part to inherent issues with CYP2F1 stability [102]. Thus, despite the general similarities in expression profiles researchers are cautioned when extrapolating results across species since differences exist in overall metabolic potential, P450 enzyme selectivity, catalytic efficiency, and interactions between multiple enzymes and cell targets.

The selective expression and catalytic participation of certain P450 enzymes in human lung cells is a major factor for the pneumotoxicity and/or carcinogenicity of several prototypical xenobiotic pneumotoxins [7,103] including naphthalene [104], 4-ipomeanol [105–108], 3-methylindole [109–114], butylated hydroxytoluene [115,116], 1,1-dichloroethylene [117,118], and 4-(methylnitrosamino)-l-(3-pyridyl)-l-butanone (NNK) [119–121]. Examples of several of these toxicants, their putative reactive intermediates, and the P450 enzymes that catalyze the bioactivation processes are shown in Figures 10.1 through 10.4.

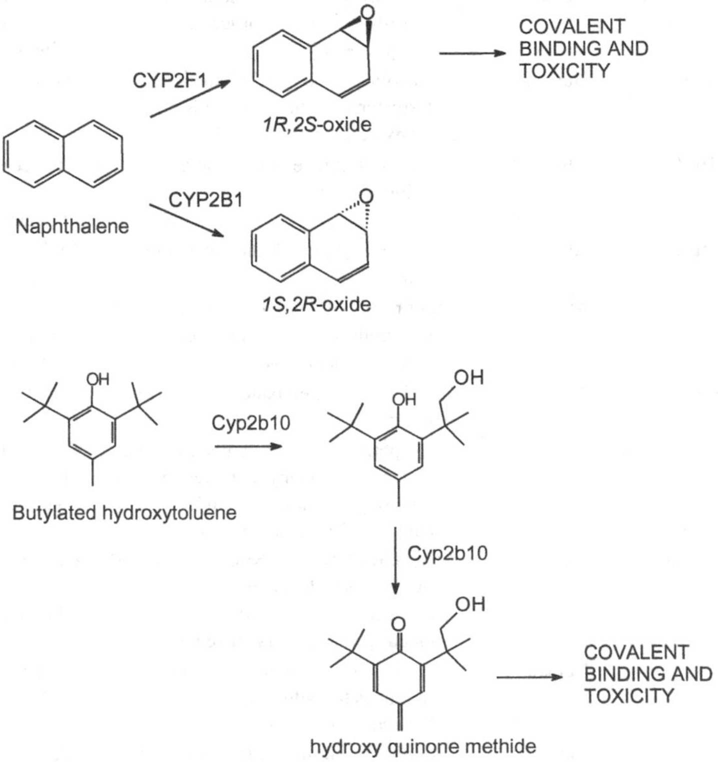

FIGURE 10.1 Bioactivation of naphthalene and butylated hydroxytoluene by CYP enzymes from the CYP2B and CYP2F sub-families. The postulated ultimate reactive intermediates of each toxicant are shown. Abbreviation: CYP, cytochrome P450.

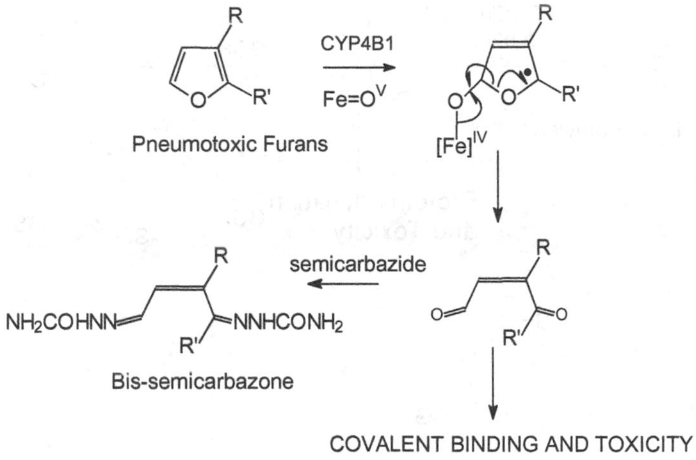

Furan	R	R'
4-Ipomeanol	$CO(CH_2)_2CHOHCH_3$	H
3-Methylfuran	CH_3	H
2-Methylfuran	H	CH_3
Perilla Ketone	$CO(CH_2)_2CH(CH_3)_2$	H
Menthofuran	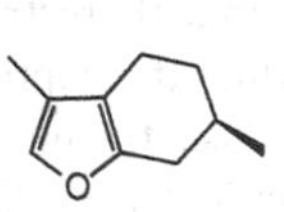	

FIGURE 10.2 Pneumotoxic furans are bioactivated through formation of highly reactive unsaturated *bis*-carbonyl intermediates. The furans are usually toxic to hepatic cells in addition to lung cells. The glutathione adducts of these intermediates are highly unstable, so they were trapped and identified as their semicarbazone adducts.

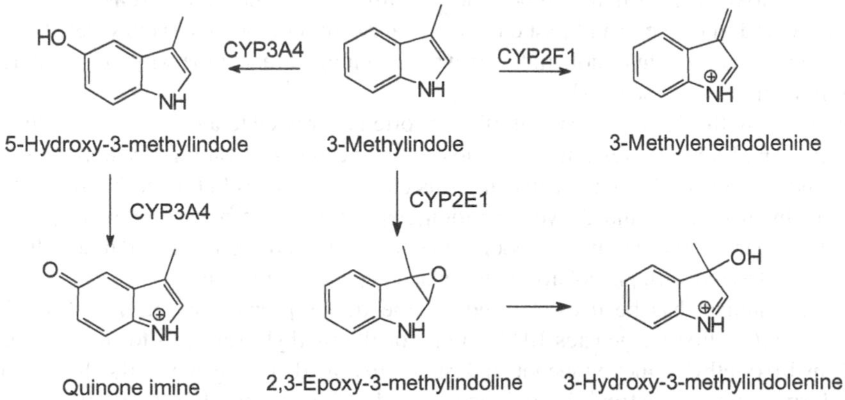

FIGURE 10.3 The prototypical pneumotoxin 3MI is bioactivated by CYP2F enzymes. Four reactive intermediates that may participate in the pneumotoxicity of 3MI are 3-methyleneindolenine, 2,3-epoxy-3-methylindoline, 3-hydroxy-3-methylindolenine, and the quinone imine of 5-hydroxy-3-methylindole. The quinone imine of 5-hydroxy-3-methylindole was identified from incubations of 3MI with human liver microsomes, and CYP3A4 is implicated as the most likely mediator of this bioactivation pathway. Oxidation of 3MI in the respiratory tract can proceed through two distinct pathways, dehydrogenation and ring oxygenation that appear to be predominantly mediated by different CYP enzymes. 3-methyindolenine is a product of CYP2F enzymes and results from many experiments suggest that this intermediate is primarily responsible for the pneumotoxic effects of 3MI. Abbreviations: CYP, cytochrome P450; 3MI, 3-methylindole.

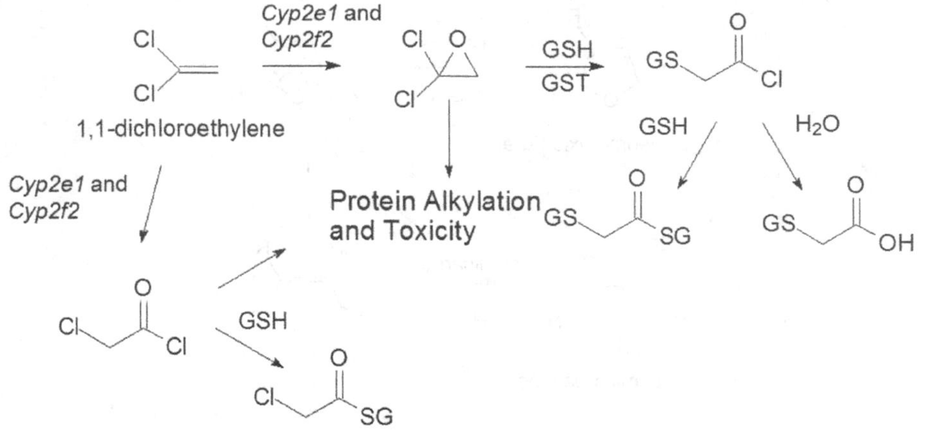

FIGURE 10.4　1,1-Dichloroethylene is a pneumotoxicant in mice and its bioactivation by the mouse *Cyp2f2* and *Cyp2e1* enzymes is remarkably complex for such a small and simple molecule. The epoxide and two putative acyl halide reactive intermediates are shown, along with the glutathione adducts of the electrophiles. The glutathione adducts and the mercapturates that are the excreted forms of these adducts have been used *in vitro* and *in vivo* as biomarkers of alkylation events. Abbreviations: CYP, cytochrome P450; GSH, glutathione; GST, glutathione S-transferase.

Many examples of regional and/or cell type specific expression of P450s exist. For example, in humans the expression of CYP1A1 gene is primarily restricted to the bronchial and alveolar epithelial and capillary endothelial cells of the lung, while the expression of 2A6, 2A13, 2B6, 2C, 2J2, 2S1, and 3A genes is observed throughout the nasal mucosa, trachea, and lung tissues [5,9,88,122,123]. In rabbits, CYP2A10, 2A11, and 2G1 enzymes are specifically expressed in nasal tissues, particularly the olfactory epithelium, where CYP2A10 and CYP2A11 constitute over 90% of total P450 in this anatomical region. In addition, the 2B4 and 4B1 enzymes constitute over 90% of the total P450 content of rabbit lung [124], and the orthologues of these enzymes in other species often appear to be major contributors to the P450 contents and catalytic activities of lung tissues. Similarly, the 2F subfamily genes are selectively expressed in human and some animal lung tissues and human placenta [88,122,125]. Several polymorphic variants of CYP2F1 also have been identified indicating the possibility of inter-individual responses to lung toxicants [126]. It is important to highlight that for each P450 enzyme selective toxicities can be observed in the cells and tissue regions that express unique P450 enzymes. For example, in mice *Cyp2f2* activates 3-methylindole in the airways and lung parenchyma while *Cyp2a5* activates this compound in the nasal mucosa [127].

The enzymes from the 2B and 4B subfamilies are often expressed to a much higher extent in the lung than in the liver and higher expression often leads to enhanced bioactivation of xenobiotics. Mouse lung *Cyp2b10* is highly expressed in Club cells, and this enzyme oxidizes butylated hydroxytoluene (BHT) by subsequent hydroxylation and dehydrogenation steps to produce a pneumotoxic quinone methide (Figure 10.1) [115,116]. This enzyme was not found to be expressed extensively in mouse liver unless the animals were pre-treated with phenobarbital to induce hepatic expression.

A unique mechanism has been established for the tumor promoting activity of BHT [128,129]. Presumably, *Cyp2b10* first oxygenates BHT on one of the methyl groups to form 6-*tert*-butyl-2-(1′,1′-dimethyl-2′-hydroxy)ethyl-4-methylphenol and subsequently dehydrogenates the hydroxylated intermediate to form a potent electrophilic quinone methide. This electrophile then alkylates cysteine or histidine residues on crucial protective enzymes, including peroxiredoxin 6 and superoxide dismutase 1 and possibly other antioxidant enzymes in mouse lung. Inactivation of these vital enzymes leads to high levels of reactive oxygen species and inflammation, conditions that facilitate tumor promotion in the mouse lung.

CYP4B1 is selectively expressed in rat lung not liver. This enzyme is known for metabolism of chemicals that include 2-aminofluorene, 2-naphthylamine, and benzidine. It has been shown that CYP4B1*1/*2 or *2/*2 genotypes carry a 1.75-fold increased risk of bladder cancer [130], but a similar association for

4B1 has not yet been found for lung cancer [131]. CYP4B1 efficiently catalyzes the bioactivation of 4-ipomeanol [6,104–107] to a pneumotoxic unsaturated *bis*-carbonyl electrophile. Several other substituted furans are bioactivated in a similar manner (Figure 10.2) and most are pneumotoxic and usually hepatotoxic as well. In contrast with rabbit CYP4B1, human CYP4B1 does not bioactivate 4-ipomeanol or promote cytotoxicity in HepG2 cells and primary human T-cells that overexpress this enzyme [132]. The basis for this appears to be the due to specific amino acid residues on the B-C loop to F-helix regions that destabilize the human enzyme and limit its catalytic capabilities. Specifically, it was shown that an 18 amino acid segment of the wild-type rabbit CYP4B1 protein conferred high 4-ipomeanol metabolism, and introduction of 12 of the 18 amino acids into human CYP4B1 increased its stability and conferred the ability to active 4-ipomeanol at levels comparable to the rabbit enzyme. Like CYP4B1, CYP4B2 is selectively transcribed in lung tissues of goats [110] and bioactivation of 3-methylindole (3MI) to the electrophilic 3-methyleneindolenine intermediate is partially catalyzed by this enzyme [109,112,133,134]. The goat 4B2 enzyme uniquely oxidized the pneumotoxin 3MI at the methyl group to form the methylene imine and indole-3-carbinol without detectable production of 3-methyloxindole or any other oxygenated products [135]. Other enzymes tested in this study either produced the methylene imine (CYP2F1 and CYP2F3), ring-oxygenated products only (CYP2E1) or oxygenated products and the methylene imine (CYP1A1 and CYP1A2) [134]. The mechanism by which 3-methyindole causes pneumotoxicity is shown in Figure 10.3.

The human CYP1 family contains three genes, CYP1A1, 1A2, and 1B1. These P450s are expressed to varying degrees in the human respiratory tract. CYP1A1 is the major extrahepatic gene and it is ubiquitously expressed at trace levels in many cell types populating the major and peripheral airways (<1 mm in diameter) and the alveoli in human lungs [9,88,136–139]. CYP1A1 is highly induced by several compounds in tobacco smoke (polycyclic aromatic hydrocarbons and aromatic amines) [136,140,141], TCDD [142,143] and 3-methylindole metabolites via activation of the aryl hydrocarbon receptor (AhR) [144]. Both AhR and CYP1A1 may play important roles in environmentally-induced and/or exacerbated asthma [145,146] as well as PAH-induced lung carcinogenesis [147], but direct correlations between gene/protein expression do not always follow a logical association. For example, CYP1A1 mRNA is increased, and enzyme level decreased in the toluene diisocyanate-induced asthma model [148], but the significance of these changes has yet to be determined. CYP1A1 metabolizes polycyclic aromatic hydrocarbons (PAHs) including benzo[a]pyrene [149], 5- and 6-methylchrysene [150], and aromatic amines [151]. The sequential two-step metabolism of benzo[a]pyrene to the benzo[a]pyrene-7,8-diol-9,10-epoxide is a prototypical example of how a P450 enzyme can determine the toxicity, in this case carcinogenicity, of an otherwise inactive agent in the lung. CYP1A1-mediated metabolism of 3-methyindole has also been associated with DNA damage by this potent acute pneumotoxin and potential carcinogen [144,152,153]. CYP1A1 expression levels are directly correlated with aryl hydrocarbon hydroxylase activity in human tissues [154–156], CYP1A1 expression levels are correlated with increased risk for lung cancer in humans and higher levels of expression or the expression of the *2A/T3801C (Msp1), and *2A/*2C/I462V allelic variants are believed to increase risks for developing lung cancer [157–160].

Like CYP1A1, CYP1A2 is expressed in human lung tissue primarily in smokers [5,9,161,162]. Evaluations of human lung samples routinely list CYP1A1 and CYP1B1 as the most highly transcribed P450 enzymes [9,122] albeit this may not be true at the single cell level. CYP1A2 metabolizes caffeine, aflatoxin B1, acetaminophen, and some pro-carcinogenic PAHs. CYP1A2 likely plays a broad role in the pulmonary metabolism of other aromatic and heterocyclic amines, nitroaromatic compounds, mycotoxins, and estrogens particularly in lungs of smokers [5,9]. CYP1A2 is readily induced in lung cells by components of cigarette smoke and other environmental combustion-by products containing PAHs such as diesel exhaust particles. Like CYP1A1, 1A2 may also play roles in asthma with some evidence that variations in CYP1A2 (CYP1A2*IC) can impact the pharmacokinetics of theophylline [163]. However, the significance of this finding remains to be validated as similar results were not found in a related study [164]. In terms of lung cancer risks the CYP1A2*IC allele was not associated with elevated risk (slow caffeine metabolism) [165], while the CYP1A2*IF (fast caffeine metabolism) allele was associated with increased risk [166].

CYP1B1 is expressed in bronchial and alveolar epithelial cells as well as in alveolar macrophages [9]. Like CYP1A1 and 1A2, 1B1 is induced by tobacco smoke [167] and TCDD [88,168].

CYP1B1 catalyzes the 2- and 4-hydroxylation of 17β-estradiol as well as the bioactivation of numerous PAHs, including benzo[a]pyrene, nitroarenes, arylarenes, and aromatic and aryl amines [9,169,170]. There is some evidence that differences in CYP1B1 variant expression influence susceptibility to lung cancer [171] since the CYP1B1 polymorphism (CYP1B1*3/L432V) has been associated with increased risk for lung cancer [172].

A number of CYP2A gene products are expressed in animal and human respiratory tract [173–175]. CYP2A6, 2A7, and CYP2A13 genes are expressed in the human respiratory tract particularly in the nasal epithelium [176]. CYP2A6 is expressed in nasal, tracheal and bronchial epithelial cells [9,174] while CYP2A13 is also expressed at low levels in the airways and alveolar epithelial cells [177]. CYP2A6 is capable of bioactivating the cigarette smoke component 3-methyindole to electrophiles [178] and CYP2A13 bioactivates 3MI to 3-methyleneindolenine the putative toxic electrophile of 3MI. 3-methyleneindolenine may be responsible for CYP2A13 inactivation and DNA damage [152,179]. Mouse *Cyp2a5* appears to have similar tissue and cellular distribution as human CYP2A6 [180] and *Cyp2a5* has been shown to be important in the metabolism of nicotine [181,182], naphthalene [183], NNK [184] and 3-methyindole [185], primarily in the olfactory mucosa of mice. Interestingly, comparison of 3-methyindole metabolism in *Cyp2a5* and *Cyp2f2* mice demonstrated the production of primarily stable hydroxylated/oxygenated metabolites in olfactory mucosal microsomes, while in lung microsomes containing more *Cyp2f2* produced primarily unstable reactive epoxide and dehydrogenated metabolites.

There is strong evidence that CYP2A enzymes, particularly CYP2A13 [186], play critical roles in the metabolic bioactivation of tobacco specific nitrosamines the major pro-carcinogenic substances in cigarette smoke. CYP2A6 efficiently catalyzes the 7-hydroxylation of coumarin [187] the metabolism of nicotine to cotinine [188,189] and is responsible, in part, for the bioactivation of 4-methynitrosamino-1,3-pyridyl-1-butanone (NNK) [190–192], the tobacco-specific pro-carcinogenic nitrosamine. CYP2As also metabolize the nasal carcinogen hexamethylphosphoramide [175]. The genetic polymorphism CYP2A6*4C (2A6-deleted/null allele) has been shown to correlate with a decreased odds ratio for lung cancer suggesting a key role for catalytically active CYP2A6 in the development of lung cancer by environmental pneumotoxicants [193,194]. Furthermore, CYP2A6 expression may influence smoking behavior [194,195] and this idea has been supported by studies using a *Cyp2a5*-null mouse [182].

CYP2A13 is active towards a number of chemical agents and lung carcinogens including aflatoxin B1 [196], hexamethylphosphoramide [175], 2'-methoxyacetophenone, N,N'-dimethylanaline, N-nitrosodiethylamine, N-nitrosomethylphenylamine, 2,6-dichlorobenzonitrile [197], NNK [198,199], naphthalene [200], styrene [200], and toluene [200]. Recent studies have led to the conclusion that CYP2A13 is the most efficient catalyst of NNK bioactivation [201] and expression of the R257C variant form of CYP2A13 (found in CYP2A13*2A and *2B), which exhibits reduced turnover efficiency for NNK, was associated with a decreased risk for lung adenocarcinoma in heavy smokers due presumably to a change in nicotine clearance and desire [201].

CYP2B6 is expressed in Club and other bronchial epithelial cells of the human lung and as an inactive splice variant called CYP2B7 [137,202,203]. CYP2B6 has also been implicated in the bioactivation of NNK in the lung [190,204] and in 2B6 humanized mice hepatic expression and induction was associated with bupropion and nicotine metabolism [205]. A pilot study has also associated CYP2B6 polymorphisms with changes in risk for lung cancer [206].

CYP2C8 and CYP2C18 may also be expressed in human lungs [162], possibly localized to the serous cells of bronchial glands [207]. CYP2C8 may participate in the regulation of vascular and bronchial tone via the synthesis of endothelium-derived hyperpolarizing factor [208–210], possibly epoxyeicosatrienoic acids (EETs). Variants of CYP2C19 have been associated with micro vascular angina through the metabolism of EETs [211]. Studies of the CYP2C9*2/R144C and *3/I359L variants and relative risk for lung cancer have not shown strong associations [212,213]. However, a recent study suggests a possible association between CYP2C19*3/containing W212X, I331V (*1A) and/or D360N (*3B/*20), and M136K (*3C), smoking and lung cancer [214].

The expression of CYP2D6 in lung is debated [9], although there is support for low-level expression in bronchial mucosal cells [92–94]. CYP2D6 is a highly polymorphic enzyme and the expression of the "extensive metabolizer" phenotype arising from gene duplication is associated with increased risk for lung cancer in heavy smokers [157]. Recently the T188C variant has also been associated with increased risk of lung cancer in Chinese [215]. CYP2D6 metabolizes a number of pharmaceutical agents [216] including basic amine-containing drugs, nicotine, opiates, and structurally related substances. CYP2D6 may also bioactivate NNK and other carcinogens [217,218].

CYP2E1 is ubiquitously expressed in lung tissue particularly in Club, bronchial, bronchiolar, alveolar epithelial and endothelial cells. Some studies have suggested that this enzyme can be induced by ethanol [219] or pyridine [98] in lung tissues and in nasal tissues. In rats it has been shown that chronic alcohol exposure induced CYP2E1 and blocking CYP2E1 attenuated pulmonary immune dysfunction and lipid accumulation [220]. The CYP2E1 enzyme is primarily active towards small halogenated hydrocarbons [221–225], and several of these chemicals cause Club cell damage in animals via the formation of electrophilic intermediates. CYP2E1 bioactivates ethyl carbamate, urethane [226,227] and nitrosamines [228] to produce carcinogenic electrophiles. CYP2E1 catalyzes the epoxidation of 1,1-dichloroethylene (DCE) to its ultimate electrophilic intermediates (Figure 10.4) [117,118]. Pulmonary damage elicited by CYP2E1-induced processes are typically not as selective for lung tissue damage because 2E1 is usually expressed more extensively in the liver, but the selective necrosis of Club cells caused by some agents (e.g., dichloroethylene/DCE) indicates that expression of 2E1 in Club cells is the primary mechanism of toxicity for several pneumotoxicants. Indeed, the toxicity of DCE to Club cells has been linked specifically to the expression of *Cyp2e1* in mice [225], although evidence suggests that *Cyp2f2* also contributes to the observed metabolism-dependent toxicity for DCE [117,118]. Metabolism of DCE by *2e1* and *2f2* produces both chloral and the epoxide of DCE, 1,1-dichlorooxirane. Studies have quantified the formation of the glutathione adduct of DCE epoxide *in vitro* and *in vivo* and have demonstrated that the primary ultimate electrophile in the cytotoxic process is the epoxide [117,118]. CYP2E1 is also most likely the catalyst for the oxidation of 1,1-dichloro-2,2-bis(*p*-chlorophenyl) ethane (DDD) to a reactive acyl halide intermediate that causes necrosis in isolated Club cells and human bronchial epithelial cells [229,230].

A prominent example of P450 enzymes that are selectively expressed in pulmonary tissues is provided by the CYP2F subfamily. Four members of this subfamily have been identified from human (CYP2F1) [125], mouse (*Cyp2f2*) [231], goat (CYP2F3) [112] and rat (CYP2F4) [232]. Mice, rats, goats and humans show high selectivity for CYP2F transcription in pulmonary tissues [110,125]. CYP2F1, and other orthologues, catalyzes the metabolism of ethoxycoumarin, propoxycoumarin, and pentoxyresorufin [125] and the bioactivation of benzene [233,234], 3-methylindole [111–113,133,134,144,152,153,178,185,235], naphthalene [112,183,232,236], styrene [44,97,100,101], 1,1-dichloroethylene [117], and NNK [112,133,134,152,237]. CYP2F1 is expressed in alveolar macrophages, epithelial (Club), and endothelial cells in the lung [9,238]. The production of 3-methyleneindolenine, the putative pneumotoxic electrophilic intermediate of 3MI (Figure 10.3), has been shown to be highest for CYP2F1 (and other 2F orthologues) compared to many other human P450 enzymes, including CYP4B1, 1A2, 3A4, and 2E1 [235]. Production of the methylene imine intermediate of 3MI by CYP2F1 has been shown to induce DNA damage and apoptosis in human bronchial epithelial cells expressing CYP2F1 [109,153] and covalent binding of the methylene imine intermediate to cellular nucleophiles in lung tissues is directly correlated with the expression and activity of CYP2F enzymes [125]. 3-Methyleneindolenine alkylates, both DNA [239] and proteins [86,111], and the electrophile is potent enough to cause mechanism-based inactivation of both CYP2F1 and CYP2F3 [114]. Assessment of the pulmonary metabolism of 3-methylindole in mice has revealed a key role for *Cyp2f2* in the bioactivation of 3MI to 3-methyleneindolenine in the airways. Further, the goat 2F3 enzyme has been cloned and characterized [112] and similar to CYP2F1 and *2f2*, 2F3 demonstrated catalytic specificity for the dehydrogenation of 3MI, without formation of the primary oxygenated products observed with other CYPs such as 2E1. Thus, the organ-selective pneumotoxicity of 3MI can be explained in part by the selective expression of the CYP2F enzymes and its efficient production of the toxic methylene imine intermediate, coupled with a relatively lower capacity of lung cells to effectively detoxify the 3-metheneindolenine reactive intermediate. Interestingly, 3MI is also metabolized to an extensive array of reactive quinoid intermediates in the liver [113]. However, the hepatotoxicity of 3MI is minimal even when GSH is depleted, where renal toxicity has been reported develop, due presumably to circulating metabolites [240].

Similar to CYP2F1 and CYP2F3, the mouse *Cyp2f2* enzyme is an efficient catalyst of 3MI dehydrogenation and DCE epoxidation [117,118]. *Cyp2f2* is also the primary stereo-selective catalyst of the *1R,2S*-naphthalene oxide (Figure 10.1), the putative reactive epoxide that produces Club cell necrosis in mice.

This enzyme is highly localized to the Club cells in distal bronchioles of mouse lung [241] and the production of the reactive epoxide was much higher in the micro-dissected distal airways from mice than from hamsters or rats, two species with less susceptibility to naphthalene toxicity. *Cyp2f2* knock-out mice were resistant to naphthalene induced pulmonary toxicity. However, toxicity was still observed in the olfactory mucosa due to other *Cyp* enzymes [236].

Mechanistic studies of CYP2F1-mediated bioactivation of 3-methyindole and the ability to study CYP2F1-related processes in humans have been hindered do to the inability to efficiently express this enzyme *in vitro* and even in humanized mice, where fairly low levels of expression of CYP2F1 are achieved [102,133,232,242]. Recently, Behrendorff and colleagues [102] utilized a directed evolution approach to identify sites on 3MI that limited its expression in *E. coli* by creating chimera with the caprine CYP2F3 orthologue, which expresses at reasonable levels in *E. coli*. A library of P450 2F1/2F3 mutants was created by DNA family shuffling and screened for expression in *E. coli*. Three generations of DNA shuffling revealed a mutant that expressed at high levels, with 96.5% nucleotide sequence identity to 2F1. Two regions of CYP2F1 were identified as problematic for expression and insertion of 2F3-derived sequences at nucleotides 191–278 (amino acids 65–92) and 794–924 (amino acids 265–305) increased levels of expression of an active enzyme; other residues outside these regions also had effects on expression. The chimeric enzyme containing changes in these two key regions was catalytically active producing the prototypical dehydrogenated and pneumotoxic product of 3MI bioactivation by CYP2F enzymes, 3-methyleneindolenine, as determined by analysis of glutathione adducts. A study reporting the activity of CYP2F1 as a mediator of naphthalene pneumotoxicity in CYP2F1-humanized mice should also be forthcoming.

With respect to the mechanism for metabolic bioactivation of 3MI to its pneumotoxic metabolite 3-methyeneindolenine, there exists a very specific but not fully understood structure-function relationship that promotes both initial and secondary hydrogen/proton abstraction from 3MI during catalysis. This is opposed to the more common P450-catalyzed hydroxyl rebound mechanism that in the case of 3MI leads to the formation of non-reactive indole-3-carbinol from the same initial radical intermediate. Deuterium isotope studies show that the formation of 3-methyindolenine occurs via metabolism at the 3-methyl position [113,243–245]. Also, modifications to specific residues in CYP2F3 drastically affect partitioning between dehydrogenation and oxygenation of 3MI at the 3-methyl position. Specifically, enzymes harboring single amino acid mutations in substrate recognition sites (SRS) 5, SRS 6, and near SRS 2 (S474H and D361T) were capable of oxygenating 3MI with a concomitant increase in dehydrogenation rates. Conversely, G214L, E215Q and S475I only catalyzed 3MI oxygenation, highlighting their roles in directing dehydrogenation of 3MI. Double mutations in these same regions also introduced oxygenase activity to CYP2F3 and the D361T mutant retained the high intramolecular kinetic deuterium isotope effect (K_H/K_D) of 6.8 observed for wild-type CYP2F3.

CYP2J2 is another extrahepatic P450 expressed in the lung, particularly in ciliated epithelial cells of the human airway [246]. CYP2J2 catalyzes the epoxidation of arachidonic acid to bioactive EETs and conversion of other polyunsaturated fatty acids (PUFAs) to biologically active substances. Therefore, CYP2J2 is believed to play a key role in modulating airway smooth muscle tone, inflammatory signaling and cellular ion homeostasis [247–251]. CYP2J2 also metabolize anti-inflammatory and antihypertensive drugs [88] and metabolism of antihistamine drugs has been implicated in the pathogenesis of cardiac conditions. 2J2 is also highly expressed in tumor cells [252].

CYP2S1 mRNA is highly expressed in epithelial cells of the nasal passages, trachea, bronchi, and bronchioles with limited expression in alveolar cells [253,254]. CYP2S1 expression can be induced by TCDD binding to the AhR receptor [255], as well as by all-*trans*-retinoic acid [256], UV light [256], carcinogenic PAHs present in coal tar [255] and negatively regulated by glucocorticoids [257]. CYP2S1 also appears to be up-regulated in tumor cells [258] leading some to believe that it is integral in the metabolism of endogenous substrates involved in cell cycle control. CYP2S1 has been shown to metabolize benzo[a]pyrene, ellipticine [259], and other environmental carcinogens including naphthalene [260]. Endogenous substrates include retinoic acid [261] fatty acid endoperoxides, hydroperoxides [262] and prostaglandin G_2 [263]. Metabolism of prostaglandin G_2 by CYP2S1 has been shown to have effects on the proliferation and migration of bronchial epithelial cells [263] and to promote cell proliferation in colon cancer cells [264].

CYP3A4 and 3A5 have also been reported to be expressed in human lungs. However, the dominant (perhaps only) CYP3A isoform expressed in most human lungs is CYP3A5. CYP3A gene/enzyme expression is highest in bronchial and alveolar epithelial cells, alveolar macrophages and bronchial glands [9,265,266]. Many report a lack of expression of CYP3A4 in human lung [13,14,122,267–269], but one report has indicated that CYP3A4 was expressed in about 20% of individuals [265]. Conversely, 3A5 is almost always found in human lung samples. CYP3A5 expression in the lung is dramatically induced by glucocorticoids through binding to the glucocorticoid receptor in human adenocarcinoma cells [13] and is repressed by cigarette smoke [13,14,270]. However, CYP3A4 expression appears to be selectively repressed in lung cells by differential binding of transcription factors including pregnane X receptor (PXR), the constitutive androstane receptor (CAR) [269], as well as a yet unidentified lung-selective factor that binds to a specific 57-base pair region in the promoter region of CYP3A4, but not 3A5 because CYP3A5 lacks this motif [267]. CYP3A enzymes are abundant and have the broadest substrate selectivity of all P450 enzymes metabolizing approximately 60% of all therapeutics, often showing little limitation in their ability to metabolize a chemical [88]. However, differences in intrinsic metabolic capacity for a given CYP3A substrate occur, with the general trend that CYP3A4 is more active than CYP3A5 and both are more active than CYP3A7 [19,271,272]. Bioactivation of aflatoxin B1 to its carcinogenic epoxide [273,274] has been attributed to CYP3A4/5 expression in the lung and CYP3A5 may bioactivate NNK [190]. In general, however, few differences in substrate selectivity have been documented for these enzymes and differential effects of xenobiotics in lung cells as a function of CYP3A enzymes is most likely due to variations in CYP3A activity and expression.

Inhaled and oral glucocorticoids (GCs) are CYP3A enzyme substrates for which variations in metabolism in the lung may be important. GCs are also potent inducers of CYP3A5 gene expression in lung epithelial cells [13,14]. The importance of CYP3A enzymes in the disposition of chemicals in the lungs has recently been illustrated by studies showing a relationship between altered CYP3A enzyme expression and asthma symptom control among children being treated with GCs. Patients with >1 copy of the inactive CYP3A4*22 variant reported improved symptom control when using fluticasone propionate [20], which is metabolized to a large extent by CYP3A4 [19]. Interestingly, metabolism of fluticasone propionate by CYP3A5 resulted in potent mechanism-based inactivation of the enzyme [275] suggesting that the beneficial effects of the CYP3A4*22 allele may be related to both a decrease in local clearance by CYP3A5 in lung cells as well as reduced systemic clearance by both CYP3A4 and CYP3A5 in other organs, mainly the liver (Figure 10.5). Similarly, patients expressing the non-functional CYP3A5*3 variant reported better asthma symptom control compared to those expressing the active 3A5*1 when using beclomethasone dipropionate [276]. Beclomethasone dipropionate was found to be metabolized mainly by esterase-dependent pathways leading to the therapeutic metabolite beclomethasone 17-monopropionate

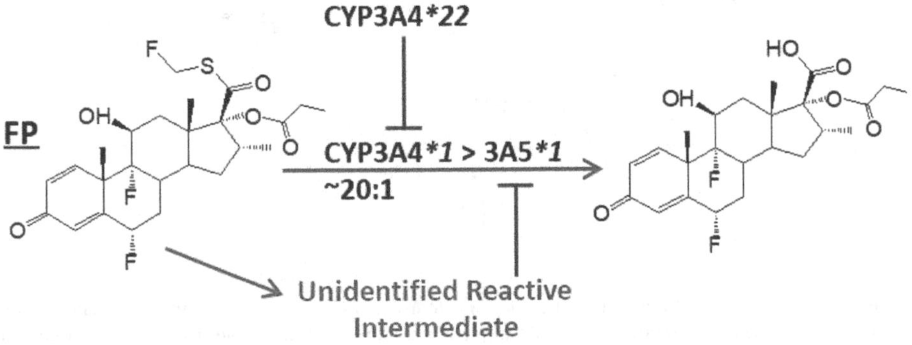

FIGURE 10.5 Metabolic scheme for CYP3A mediated metabolism and clearance of fluticasone propionate. An unidentified metabolic intermediate of fluticasone propionate, presumably arising by metabolism at or near the C6-C7 position of the B-ring, has been shown to be a potent mechanism-based inhibitor of CYP3A5*1 and to a lesser extent CYP3A4*1. Concurrent expression of the inactive CYP3A4*22 variant in conjunction with CYP3A5 inhibition and/or CYP3A5*3 expression has been suggested to reduce the clearance of fluticasone propionate in the lungs and systemically, resulting in improved asthma symptom control in children. Abbreviations: FP, fluticasone propionate.

in lung epithelial cells as well as to inactive C6-OH and Δ6-dehydrogenated metabolites by CYP3A5 [14,19]. It was concluded that CYP3A5 may effectively decrease the level of parent prodrug available for production of the active therapeutic molecule in lung cells; thus, attenuation of beclomethasone dipropionate clearance in lung cells and elsewhere throughout the body due to CYP3A5*3 expression was likely the basis for the observed clinical benefit (Figure 10.6). It is currently hypothesized that both the CYP3A4*22 and 3A5*3 scenarios likely involve higher intra-pulmonary and blood levels of steroid as a basis for improved asthma control. Paradoxically, this could also influence hypothalamic-pituitary-adrenal axis suppression that can occur with these drugs. However, the actual effects of the CYP3A4*22 and CYP3A5*3 polymorphisms on GC pharmacokinetics have not yet been established.

CYP4B1 mRNA is routinely detected in human lung samples, although the expression of a functional enzyme in human lung tissue has been debated [9,277]. CYP4B1 expression has been detected in differentiated human bronchial epithelial cells in an air liquid interface culture [278]. The prototypical substrate for the CYP4B1 enzyme from rabbit lung is 2-aminofluorene [279] and 4-ipomeanol, a classic pneumotoxicant, is metabolized effectively by this enzyme in rabbit and rat lung tissues. Recombinant human 4B1 did not bioactivate 4-ipomeanol, although the rabbit enzyme expressed in the same system was an efficient catalyst of 4-ipomeanol bioactivation [280]. This likely the effect of issues related to expression of CYP4B1 as described above [105]. The rabbit cDNA has been expressed in mouse C3H/10T1/2 cells, and in these cells the enzyme bioactivated 4-ipomeanol to a cytotoxic intermediate [281]. CYP4B1 also metabolized 2-aminoanthracene in these cells to produce cytotoxicity. Recombinant

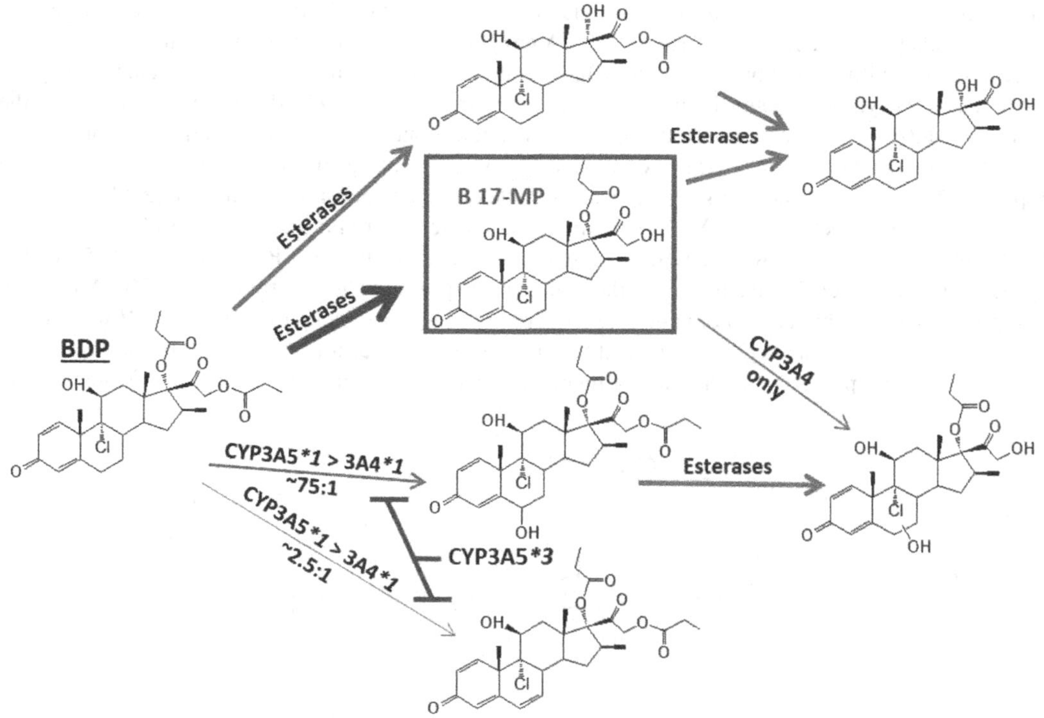

FIGURE 10.6 Metabolic scheme highlighting the roles of esterase and CYP3A enzymes in the metabolism of the glucocorticoid beclomethasone dipropionate, with CYP3A5 playing a more prominent role than CYP3A4. Beclomethasone is bioactivated to the pharmacologically active metabolite beclomethasone 17-monopropionate by esterase enzymes (bold arrows) and inactivated in a competitive manner by de-esterification at C-21 or CYP3A-mediated oxygenation and dehydrogenation at the C6-C7 position (lower structure). Beclomethasone 17-monopropionate is also degraded by esterases and CYP3A4. Attenuation of CYP3A5 metabolism by expression of the CYP3A5*3 variant has been suggested to attenuate the clearance of both beclomethasone dipropionate and beclomethasone 17-monopropionate in lung cells and systemically resulting in improved asthma symptom control in children. Abbreviations: BDP, beclomethasone dipropionate; B 17-MP, beclomethasone 17-monopropionate.

goat CYP4B2 was expressed primarily in the lung and catalyzed the oxygenation of 2-aminofluorene, the prototype substrate for CYP4B1 enzymes, as well as preferential dehydrogenation of 3MI to the pneumotoxic methylene imine metabolite [135]. It is possible that CYP4B2 is a major contributor to the pneumotoxicity of 3MI in goats. In animal models, ocular expression of CYP4B1 is important in the synthesis of eicosanoids, which mediate oxidative stress [282].

Prostaglandin Synthases/Cyclooxygenases

Prostaglandin endoperoxide synthases or cyclooxygenases PTGS1/COX1 and PTGS2/COX2 are another important group of xenobiotic metabolizing enzymes present in the lung. These enzymes are responsible for the biosynthesis of prostaglandins and thromboxanes [283–286]. COX3 is a splice variant of COX1 originally found in the CNS of dogs but is not functional in humans, and partial COX1 (PCOX1A and 1B), for which roles in physiology and drug metabolism have not yet been described, also exist [287]. *bis*-Dioxygenation of arachidonic acid by the cyclooxygenase function of PGH synthases yields the hydroperoxide-endoperoxide PGG_2. Subsequent 2-electron reduction of the hydroperoxide by the peroxidase function of PGH synthases produces PGH_2. PGH_2 is the precursor of other prostaglandins (D_2, E_2, $F_{2\alpha}$, and I_2) and thromboxane A_2. Arachidonic acid metabolites have been shown to be produced by human alveolar type II cells [288] and essentially many other cells to varying degrees.

The peroxidase function of PGH synthases is similar in nature to that of other heme peroxidases that metabolize xenobiotics. PGH synthases form activated iron-oxo intermediates analogous to compounds I and II of horseradish peroxidase and exhibit relatively broad substrate specificity, reducing alkyl and lipid hydroperoxides as well as H_2O_2 [289,290]. The relatively high oxidation potentials of the intermediate iron-oxo heme compounds that form during PGH synthase turnover can often facilitate the co-oxidation of xenobiotics, including the 1-electron oxidation of potentially pneumotoxic phenols and aromatic amines like 2-aminofluorene and benzidine, a potent bladder carcinogen [291,292]. Products of PGH synthase-mediated co-oxidation reactions are frequently shown to be identical to those produced by P450- and peroxidase-catalyzed reactions [293]. Classic examples of PGH synthase-mediated co-oxidation of human lung toxicants and carcinogens are aflatoxin B1 metabolism [294–296] and the conversion of benzo[a]pyrene 7,8-dihydrodiol to the genotoxic benzo[a]pyrene-7,8-diol-9,10-epoxide metabolite via hydroperoxide-dependent mechanisms [297,298]. Epoxidation of the benzo[a]pyrene 7,8-dihydrodiol appears to be predominantly catalyzed by PGH synthase, not P450s, in type II alveolar cells from rats [299]. PGH synthase has also been shown to catalyze the epoxidation of the diol to tetrols (after hydrolysis of the epoxide) at approximately half the rate of P450-mediated turnover in hamster trachea and human lung explants [297]. PGH synthase is also being explored as a potential therapeutic target for the treatment of asthma [300] and lung cancer [301].

Flavin-Containing Monooxygenases

The flavin-containing monooxygenases (FMO) are another class of xenobiotic metabolizing enzymes. The participation of the FMO enzymes in the metabolism of xenobiotics has been well documented but the contribution of FMOs to oxidative metabolism is limited relative to P450 enzymes. However, in some instances, metabolism by FMOs is dominant especially for the oxidation of N-, P-, and S-containing chemicals. In humans, the FMO family consists of six genes whose protein products catalyze N-, P- and S-oxidation of nucleophilic small molecule xenobiotics to the corresponding N-, P-, and S-oxides [302,303]. The active site of FMOs is an activated C(4a)-hydroperoxide flavin generated by addition of oxygen to reduced flavin adenine dinucleotide ($FADH_2$) [304]. This intermediate is relatively stable and FMOs typically reside in the activated form until a suitable substrate enters the enzyme active site [305,306]. Primary and secondary amines are good substrates for FMOs, but several other unusual substrates, such as secondary and tertiary amines, hydrazines, phosphines, iodides, and sulfides, are oxidized by these enzymes [302,303]. FMO3 has been shown to catalyze the N-oxidation of indoline to form N-hydroxyindole, N-hydroxyindoline, and an interesting novel dimer of indoline, [1,4,2,5] dioxadiazino[2,3-*a*:5,6-*a'*]diindole [307]. Similar to P450 enzymes, FMOs generally convert lipophilic xenobiotics to more polar, oxygenated metabolites that are more readily excreted.

The expression of FMO1, FMO2, FMO2.1, and FMO3 and FMO5 are generally considered to be organ-selective [302,303,308]. In the human lung FMO2 is the primary FMO enzyme. Quantitative PCR analysis has shown that FMO2 mRNA is present at 50-fold higher concentrations than FMO3 and FMO5 and 150-fold higher than FMO1 and FMO4 [308]. In mice FMO2 is also the dominant lung enzyme. However, FMO1 is also expressed at moderate levels representing ~34% of the total FMO transcripts compared to the expression of approximately 59% for FMO2 [309]. FMO6 is also expressed at low levels in the human lung but FMO6 is a non-functional pseudogene [302,303]. Similarly, the FMO2 gene (the FMO2*2 allele) in Caucasians and Asians codes for a prematurely truncated protein that is readily degraded. FMO2.1, the full-length and functional form of FMO2 arising from the FMO2*1 genotype is expressed in ~13%–26% of African Americans [303,310,311] and ~5% in Hispanics [171,303,311]. The significance of FMO2.1 expression in human lungs remains incompletely defined, but African Americans or Hispanics are likely to be significantly more susceptible to thiourea-mediated pneumotoxicity.

FMO-dependent metabolism is generally considered protective and it typically reduces both the toxicological and pharmacological potency of substrates [9,303]. However, examples of bioactivation of xenobiotics to electrophiles have been demonstrated. Examples include the conversion of thioureas like phenylthiourea (Figure 10.7) to its sulfenic acid and in a subsequent oxidation step to the sulfinic acid [312,313]. The toxicity of the thiourea was postulated to occur by redox cycling of the sulfenic acid with the parent thiourea, coupled to the oxidation of glutathione to its dimer. The pulmonary selective FMO2.1 protein is functional and catalytically unique compared to the other FMOs, in that it exhibits significant thermal stability and more stringent substrate selectivity, due presumably to a restricted substrate access channel. FMO2.1 readily catalyzes the N-oxidation of primary alkyl amines, including *n*-dodecylamine, to produce N-hydroxy primary amines that can be oxidized to oximes [302,303,308]. Human FMO2.1 also catalyzes the oxidation of lipoic acid [302,303,308] and organophosphate insecticides, including the efficient oxidation of phorate, disulfoton [311], and the lung toxicant, ethylenethiourea [312].

Finally, the physiological role of FMO enzymes has also been explored, particularly the role of FMOs in the metabolism of endogenous cysteamine to regulate cellular thiol status and H_2O_2 levels, as well as their metabolism of farnesylated proteins, and trimethylamine [302,303]. As such, it is possible that FMO2.1 may contribute significantly to pulmonary homoeostasis during oxidative stress induced by selected pneumotoxic xenobiotics in addition to the direct role in the metabolic modification of selected substrates. Whether differential expression of FMO2 and FMO2.1 play a major role in determining individual differences in susceptibility to selected pneumotoxicants is not fully understood. However, FMO2.1 is highly expressed in populations in sub-Saharan Africa (European and Asian populations do

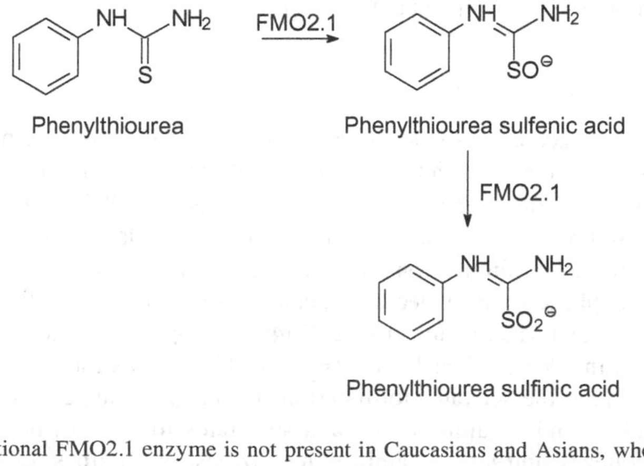

Phenylthiourea   Phenylthiourea sulfenic acid

Phenylthiourea sulfinic acid

FIGURE 10.7 The functional FMO2.1 enzyme is not present in Caucasians and Asians, who have the FMO*2 allele, which codes for a prematurely truncated protein. The functional enzyme is only present in respiratory cells of approximately 13%–26% of African Americans and 5% of Hispanics. Oxidation of phenylthiourea to its sulfenic acid metabolite and reduction back to the thiourea by glutathione oxidation to its disulfide leads to potent acute lung injury by reactive oxygen species and NADPH depletion. FMO2.1 also catalyzes the subsequent oxidation to the sulfinic acid metabolite. Abbreviation: FMO, Flavin-containing monooxygenases.

not express FMO2.1) and metabolizes the antitubercular drugs thiacetazone and ethionamide, possibly contributing to therapy resistant tuberculosis [314].

Hydrolysis and Conjugation Enzymes

Epoxide Hydrolases

Epoxide hydrolases (EPHX1 and EPHX2), also known as epoxide hyratases, are well known for catalyzing the hydration of arene, alkene, and aliphatic epoxides of PAHs and aromatic amines to form *trans*-dihydrodiols. The epoxide hydrolases and roles in human diseases have been reviewed [315–317]. EPHX1 is the endoplasmic reticulum-localized form while EPHX2 (also called soluble epoxide hydrolase or sEH) is cytosolic [318]. EPHXs contribute to both bioactivation and detoxification processes depending upon the substrate and cellular context. For example, while epoxide hydrolysis is key in the detoxification of many toxins and pneumotoxins (e.g., styrene oxide, PAH-epoxides, etc.), sEH/EPHX2 has been found to play a potentially important role in promoting LPS-induced acute lung injury, based on findings that inhibition of this enzyme was associated with a reduction in multiple pro-inflammatory and injury-associated markers [152]. The basis for the protective effect of the inhibitor was attributed to an increase in pulmonary EETs from inhibiting the decomposition of these molecules to the corresponding dihydroxyeicosatrienoic acids (DHETs) and potentially favoring the biosynthesis of, for example, anti-inflammatory 15-epi-lipoxin A4 from 14,15-EET. In general, the levels of these enzymes are lower in lung homogenates relative to liver preparations; however, EPHX expression and function is detectable in most lung cells and tissue fractions. Recently, it has been shown that 3-methylcholanthrene induces microsomal EPHX1 activity in both rat lung and liver, albeit induction in the lung was ~50% that of the liver [319]. Furthermore, analysis of EPHX1 and EPHX2 gene expression in primary lung parenchymal cells confirmed the expression of both EPHX1 and EPHX2, and a number of CYP genes [268]. EPHX1 was expressed at a level similar to that for cryopreserved hepatocytes, while EPHX2 was ~50% [268].

A recurring theme of this chapter is that the cellular distribution of most drug metabolizing enzymes is variable in the lung. EPHX-mediated hydrolysis of styrene oxide was highest in the distal airways of beagle dog lungs and the observed levels were twice that of liver preparations [320]. High EPHX activities in the distal airways corresponded to increases in Club cell abundance and EPHX activity was significantly higher in isolated Club cells versus alveolar type II cells [321] and presumably other epithelial cell types. As such, it seems that EPHXs are expressed more abundantly in more metabolically competent cells that generate higher amounts of reactive cytotoxic or genotoxic epoxides. Here EPHXs likely play critical roles in the detoxification of potentially deleterious electrophilic epoxide intermediates generated by the P450 enzymes. This concept is supported by findings that EPHX1 expression was markedly induced in broncho-alveolar lavage samples of smokers but repressed in bronchial biopsy samples taken from anterior portions of the lung; BAL samples consisted primarily of macrophages, but bronchial biopsy samples were comprised of epithelial cells [167]. The authors speculated that repression of EPHX1 in smokers was potentially beneficial in the context of bioactivation of benzo[a]pyrene. However, it is likely that reduced EPHX1 expression may have other adverse consequences in smokers as discussed below.

The balance between bioactivation and detoxification is the principal determinant of metabolism-dependent toxicities and ultimately in the frequency of formation of neoplastic lesions. In this context, EPHXs are a double-edged sword. A direct role for epoxide hydrolase in pulmonary drug toxicities is demonstrated by the hydration of benzo[a]pyrene-7,8-epoxide following oxidation of benzo[a]pyrene by selected P450 enzymes. The product of epoxide hydrolysis is the benzo[a]pyrene-7,8-diol that can be readily conjugated and detoxified by conjugation enzymes. However, subsequent oxidation of the benzo[a]pyrene-7,8-diol to the benzo[a]pyrene-7,8-diol-9,10-epoxide by P450s represents the principal mechanism leading to DNA mutations and lung cancer. Despite the role of pulmonary EPHXs in the detoxification of selected epoxide intermediates elevated EPHX1 activity has been associated with an increased risk for lung cancer [322], particularly when CYP1A1 expression is high [323]. Decreased EPHX1 activity, either through low levels of expression or through the expression of poor functioning polymorphic variants (i.e., Y113H and H139R), has been associated with slightly decreased risks for lung cancer [324]. It has been demonstrated that smokers with EPHX1-H139R (which is associated with a higher enzyme activity) had significantly higher DNA adduct levels [325], while expression of >1 copy of the H139R variant was associated with increased risks of lifetime asthma [326].

Roles for EPHX in pneumotoxicity have also been further evaluated using styrene and styrene oxide [97,98]. Styrene is metabolized in mouse lungs to the toxin styrene oxide (an epoxide), to a large extent by *Cyp2f2* [97,101]. Epoxide hydrolysis by mEH/EPHX1 is recognized as a critical detoxification pathway. In mEH/*Ephx1*-defifcient mice it was found that metabolism of styrene oxide to glycol was suppressed, indices of both hepato- and pneumotoxicity were higher and mice were more susceptible to lethality. Interestingly, EPHX1 seemed to have less of an effect on exogenously delivered styrene oxide versus that which was metabolically generated from styrene *in vivo*. Finally, it should be noted that the *Cyp2f2/Ephx1*/styrene oxide pathway may not be involved in the carcinogenic effects of styrene in mouse lungs [327] that could explain the somewhat contradictory relationships between EPHX1, acute pneumotoxicity, and cancer risks.

UDP-Glucuronosyltransferases

Uridine diphosphate glucuronosyltransferases (UGT) are a super-family of microsomal xenobiotic metabolizing enzymes that catalyze the addition of UDP-glucuronic acid to small hydrophobic molecules with highly diverse structures. Some endogenous compounds such as bilirubin and bile acids can be conjugated with UDP-glucose and UDP-xylose [328]. However, the clinical significance of these conjugates is unclear. UGTs provide a primary mechanism of protection against the accumulation of unfolded proteins in the endoplasmic reticulum [329] and toxic xenobiotics and/or their oxidative products to render potentially toxic substances inactive and amenable for excretion [330]. UGT enzymes are found in bacteria, yeast, and plants, which catalyze the transfer of a glycosyl chemical group from a nucleotide sugar. The UGT family of genes is divided into four sub-families, UGT1, UGT2, UGT3, and UGT8 [328,331–333]. The human UGT1 sub-family is distinctively derived from a single gene locus and consists of UGT1A1, 1A3, 1A4, 1A5, 1A6, 1A7, 1A8, 1A9, and 1A10. The UGT2 sub-family is comprised of multiple, similar genes that have evolved from gene duplication. The UGT2 family is comprised of UGT2A1, 2A2, 2A3, 2B4, 2B7, 2B10, 2B11, 2B15, 2B17, and 2B28. Members of the UGT3 (UGT3A1, and 3A2) and UGT8 (UGT8A1) are thought to play a minimal role in the metabolism of drugs [328]. The different UGT enzymes often exhibit overlapping substrate profiles [334], but UGT2B proteins exhibit reduced capacity to metabolize phenolic and heterocyclic compounds, such as the known carcinogens and pro-carcinogens found in cigarette smoke [331]. Conversely, UGT1 enzymes are highly active towards these substances.

UGT1A1, 1A3, 1A4, 1A6, 1A9, 2B4, 2B7, and 2B11 transcripts are considerably more abundant in human liver, while UGT1A6, 1A7, 1A8, 1A10, and 2A1 are primarily extrahepatic UGTs that are expressed at moderate levels in human pulmonary tissues [268,335–337]. Transcripts for UGT1A1, 1A3, 1A5, 1A7, 1A8, and 2B12 were amplified from rat lung [336], while UGT1A1, 1A4, 1A6, 2A1, 2B4, 2B7, and 2B11 were detected in human lung samples and in most upper aero-digestive tract tissues including the mouth and tongue [268,337]. In general, the overall extent of glucuronidation of xenobiotics by pulmonary tissues is considered to be minimal but not insignificant with respect to xenobiotic toxicology. For example, 4-nitrophenol glucuronidation in rat lung microsomes is only 30% of the rat liver microsomal rate of glucuronidation [338]. However, cell-type selective differences in metabolic capacity were observed, because rat Club cells glucuronidated 4-methylumbelliferone to a greater extent than did isolated alveolar type II cells [339]. Again, the overall metabolic capacity of Club cells is generally higher than other cells in the lung. Recently it has been shown that a mixture of PAHs was able to induce the expression of rat lung UGT1A6 and 1A9. However, the glucuronidation activities of UGT1A6 and 1A9 were considerably lower and were highly variable in human lungs [340]. Unfortunately, other UGT activities were not evaluated in this study, but the authors [268] showed similar results using multiple probe substrates. In 2002, no member of the UGT1A genes had been found to be expressed in human lung tissue [337], but more recent studies [94], and those described above, confirm the expression of a number of UGT1 enzymes. In contrast, UGT2A1, 2B4, 2B7, 2B10, 2B11, 2B15, and 2B17 are expressed in human and animal nasal epithelium and lung at levels equal to or even greater than in liver [268,337,341,342].

In fact, UGT2A1 may be selectively expressed at high levels in the nasal epithelium [336,341] and to a lesser extent in the whole lung, albeit still higher than in hepatocytes [268]. Recombinant UGT2A1 gene expressed in mammalian cells has broad substrate selectivity and it shows activity towards a number of phenolic, aliphatic, and monoterpenoid alcohols, selected steroids and androgens, and carcinogens [341]. Therefore, it is possible that this enzyme plays a direct role in the inactivation of odorants such as eugenol [343].

Examples of bioactivation of xenobiotics to toxins by UGTs are limited and contributions to toxicity are typically due to a lack of efficient detoxification of xenobiotics by UGT enzymes rather than a gain of toxicity. A mechanism (Figure 10.6) for the pneumotoxicity and pulmonary carcinogenicity of trichloroethylene has been proposed to be mediated by deficient UGT activities in lung Club cells [344]. The authors showed that isolated Club cells from mice did not possess sufficient UGT activity to glucuronidate trichloroethanol, while isolated hepatocytes efficiently formed this inactive metabolite (Figure 10.8). The lack of glucuronidation of trichloroethanol was proposed to lead to the build-up of the cytotoxic P450-generated intermediate, chloral, in the Club cells. Thus, the lack of detoxification by glucuronidation in susceptible cells was proposed as an operative mechanism for the toxicity of trichloroethylene and likely applies to many other pneumotoxins. It is also possible that bioactivation by glucuronidation may produce toxicities to respiratory tissues, by mechanisms analogous to acyl linked glucuronide toxicities to hepatic tissues [345] and renal tissues [346]. UGT polymorphisms have been implicated as risk factors for cancers of the lung (as well as other tissues) [347].

Glutathione S-Transferases

A recent and informative review of Glutathione S-Transferases (GSTs) is provided by Hayes et al. [348]. GSTs catalyze the nucleophilic addition of reduced glutathione to hydrophobic compounds that contain electrophilic carbon, nitrogen, and sulfur atoms. Prototypical substrates include halogen or nitrobenzenes (e.g., 1-chloro-2,4-dinitrobenzene/CDNB), arene oxides, quinones, and α,β-unsaturated carbonyls. Furthermore, GSTs catalyze the isomerization of unsaturated compounds and participate in

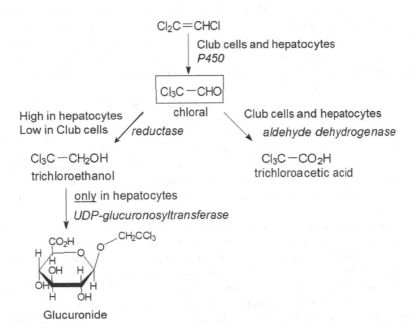

FIGURE 10.8 Mechanism of selective Club cell damage by trichloroethylene, caused by the lack of detoxification. Although chloral, the putative toxic intermediate from trichloroethylene can be formed in both mouse lung Club cells and hepatocytes; efficient detoxification of this aldehyde by reductase and by UGT is lacking in the lung epithelial cells. Abbreviation: UGT, uridine diphosphate glucuronosyltransferases.

the synthesis of various prostaglandins and leukotrienes [349–351]. Cytosolic, microsomal, and mitochondrial forms of GST exist. Cytosolic GSTs are the largest family of enzymes and are comprised of two subunits of 199–244 amino acids each. Cytosolic GSTs are divided into the following seven major sub-classes: alpha (GSTA1 through A5), mu (GSTM1 through M5), kappa (GSTK1), theta (GSTT1 and T2), omega (GSTO1 and O2), pi (GSTP1), sigma (GSTS1), and zeta (GSTZ1), based on amino acid similarities and antibody cross-reactivity. At least 16 different cytosolic GSTs are expressed by humans, due in part to the fact that alpha and mu class GST subunits form heterodimers [349]. Microsomal GSTs are dimeric enzymes comprised of 226 amino acid kappa class subunits and belong a family of proteins collectively referred to as membrane associated proteins involved in eicosanoid and glutathione metabolism (MAPEGs) [349,350,352]. There are six MAPEG proteins, microsomal GSTs (MGST1-3, leukotriene C4 synthase, 5-lipoxygenase activating protein/FLAP, and prostaglandin E synthase/PTGS). It is the MGSTs 1-3 that have glutathione S-transferase and peroxidase activities and are involved in cellular defense against toxic, carcinogenic, and pharmacologically active electrophilic compounds. Chloride Ion Channel (CLIC) proteins (CLIC 1-5) and ganglioside-induced differentiation-associated proteins (GAPD1 and GAPD1-like 1) are also members of the cytosolic GST family, based on structural similarities. However, these proteins do not catalyze GSH-dependent reactions with common GST substrates [348].

The expression of GSTs in respiratory tissues has been evaluated in animals and in humans. The precise elucidation of which GSH transferase exists in which cells of the respiratory system have not been accurately determined, because most studies simply determine the aggregate CDNB activities of gene expression in lung homogenates or mixed populations of cells. CDNB activity distribution in the lung was slightly higher in proximal airways than in distal airways of the mouse and monkey [353]. It appears that at least the alpha, mu, and pi classes are expressed in rat [354] and human [355] lung samples. It has been shown that the pi, mu, and alpha classes of GSTs represent approximately 94%, 3%, and 3%, respectively, of the total human lung activity toward CDNB [356], although differences in the ability to catalyze CDNB conjugation likely confounded determination of the true ratios of enzyme expression. Regardless, immunochemical staining of GST enzymes in human lungs demonstrated expression of the alpha and pi forms in large and small airway epithelial tissues [355] and recent studies of BAL and bronchial biopsy samples from smokers and non-smokers confirmed the expression of GSTP1, GSTA2, and GSTM1. Cytosolic GST alpha was mildly induced by 3-methylcholanthere in rat lungs [319]. As with many other drug-metabolizing enzymes, Club cells tend have considerably higher GST activity than alveolar type II cells, using CDNB as a probe [339,357], consistent with the expected elevated production of reactive electrophiles by resident P450 (and other) enzymes in Club cells.

Conjugation of xenobiotics by GST enzymes is typically considered protective. GSTs, particularly GSTP1, are over-expressed during lung cancer, rendering the cancer cells less susceptible to some anti-cancer drugs. Several studies have attempted to link polymorphisms of the mu class of GSTs in human lung tissues with susceptibility to lung cancer induced by cigarette smoking [358] as well as possibly ambient pollutant toxicities [359–366]. A particularly strong association has been shown between genetic polymorphisms in the CYP1A1 gene and a deficient genotype of a mu GSTs, relative to lung cancer induced by cigarette smoking [367]. Individuals with both genetic alterations had elevated risks for lung cancer from smoking.

Similarly, GSTA4 null mice have been shown to be more sensitive to the pneumotoxicant paraquat and to exhibit a reduced capacity to conjugate the toxic α,β-unsaturated aldehyde 4-hydroxynonenal [368]. Conjugation with GSH has been shown to be protective in the lung against toxicities elected by DCE [117,222], naphthalene [369–371], 3MI [111], and isocyanates [372,373]. However, there are some instances where conjugation promotes toxicity, such as that observed with formation of the unstable electrophilic DNA modifying agent S-chloromethylglutathione from dichloromethane [374,375] or the depletion of intracellular GSH stores via recycling of selected isothiocyanate conjugates (i.e., thiocarbamates).

Variations in GSTs have also been investigated as risk factors for respiratory diseases including asthma, particularly asthma associated with environmental exposure to high levels of pollutants [359–366]. Many studies have suggested relationships between GST variations and asthma. However, recent meta-analyses do not necessarily support such associations [376,377]. It is unclear whether the lack of associations in the meta analyses versus many independent studies was due to a true lack of association or simply a product of inadequately controlling for variable such as specific asthma sub-types/endotypes, which should be considered in future studies.

Conclusions

This chapter is intended to provide an overview of the metabolic enzymes that exist in respiratory tissues and to distinguish metabolism of drugs in this organ system from other anatomical regions that also participate to a greater or lesser extent in the metabolism of xenobiotics. The lung should not be viewed as a metabolic organ with lower activities than liver but rather as an active, dynamic, and often highly selective metabolic tissue with important contributions to xenobiotic disposition and toxicity. The complexity of cellular distribution and function and gene expression in respiratory tissues provides a unique paradigm for scientists involved in drug metabolism, toxicology, risk assessment, and pharmaceutical development. As we continue to learn more about the mechanisms of selective gene expression in certain lung cells, and the functional consequences of the enzymology of the gene products, predictions of metabolic processes and toxicological consequences will become possible.

REFERENCES

1. Bond, J.A., Metabolism of xenobiotics by the respiratory tract, in *Toxicology of the Lung* J.D.C.D.E. Gardner, and R.O. McClellan, Editor 1993, Raven Press: New York. pp. 187–215.
2. Buckpitt, A.R.a. C., M.K., Biochemical function of the respiratory tract: Metabolism of xenobiotics, in *Comprehensive Toxicology*, C.A.M. I. G. Sipes, and A. J. Gandolfi, Editor 1997, Elsevier Science: New York. p. 159–186.
3. Castell, J.V., M.T. Donato, and M.J. Gomez-Lechon, Metabolism and bioactivation of toxicants in the lung. The *in vitro* cellular approach. *Exp Toxicol Pathol*, 2005. **57**(Suppl 1): 189–204.
4. Dahl, A.R. and J.L. Lewis, Respiratory tract uptake of inhalants and metabolism of xenobiotics. *Annu Rev Pharmacol Toxicol*, 1993. **33**: 383–407.
5. Ding, X. and L.S. Kaminsky, Human extrahepatic cytochromes P450: Function in xenobiotic metabolism and tissue-selective chemical toxicity in the respiratory and gastrointestinal tracts. *Annu Rev Pharmacol Toxicol*, 2003. **43**: 149–173.
6. Foth, H., Role of the lung in accumulation and metabolism of xenobiotic compounds–implications for chemically induced toxicity. *Crit Rev Toxicol*, 1995. **25**(2): 165–205.
7. Yost, G.S., Bioactivation and selectivity of pneumotoxic chemicals, in *Tissue Specific Toxicity: Biochemical Mechanisms*, W.D.a. H.-G. Neumann, Editor 1992, Academic Press: London, UK. pp. 195–220.
8. Yost, G.S., Sites of metabolism: Lung, in *Handbook of Drug metabolism*, T.F. Wolf, Editor 1999, Marcel Dekker, Inc: New York. pp. 263–278.
9. Zhang, J.Y., Y. Wang, and C. Prakash, Xenobiotic-metabolizing enzymes in human lung. *Curr Drug Metab*, 2006. **7**(8): 939–948.
10. Gundert-Remy, U., et al., *Extrahepatic metabolism at the body's internal–external interfaces*. *Drug Metab Rev*, 2014. **46**(3): 291–324.
11. Morin, J.-P., et al., Precision cut lung slices as an efficient tool for *in vitro* lung physio-pharmacotoxicology studies. *Xenobiotica*, 2013. **43**(1): 63–72.
12. Nave, R., R. Fisher, and N. McCracken, *In vitro* metabolism of beclomethasone dipropionate, budesonide, ciclesonide, and fluticasone propionate in human lung precision-cut tissue slices. *Respir Res*, 2007. **8**: 65.
13. Roberts, J.K., et al., Regulation of CYP3A genes by glucocorticoids in human lung cells. *F1000Res*, 2013. **2**: 173.
14. Roberts, J.K., et al., Metabolism of beclomethasone dipropionate by cytochrome P450 3A enzymes. *J Pharmacol Exp Ther*, 2013. **345**(2): 308–316.
15. Courcot, E., et al., Xenobiotic metabolism and disposition in human lung cell models: Comparison with *in vivo* expression profiles. *Drug Metab Dispos*, 2012. **40**(10): 1953.

16. Bevans, T., et al., Inhaled remifentanil in rodents. *Anesth Analg*, 2016. **122**(6): 1831–1838.

17. Weissmann, N., et al., Effects of arachidonic acid metabolism on hypoxic vasoconstriction in rabbit lungs. *Eur J Pharmacol*, 1998. **356**(2–3): 231–237.

18. Yaghi, A., et al., Cytochrome P450 metabolites of arachidonic acid but not cyclooxygenase-2 metabolites contribute to the pulmonary vascular hyporeactivity in rats with acute Pseudomonas pneumonia. *J Pharmacol Exp Ther*, 2001. **297**(2): 479–488.

19. Moore, C.D., et al., Metabolic pathways of inhaled glucocorticoids by the CYP3A enzymes. *Drug Metab Dispos*, 2013. **41**(2): 379–389.

20. Stockmann, C., et al., Fluticasone propionate pharmacogenetics: CYP3A4*22 polymorphism and pediatric asthma control. *J pediatr*, 2013. **162**(6): 1222–1227.e2.

21. Stockmann, C., et al., Effect of CYP3A5*3 on asthma control among children treated with inhaled beclomethasone. *J Allergy Clin Immunol*, 2015. **136**(2): 505–507.

22. Tunek, A., K. Sjodin, and G. Hallstrom, Reversible formation of fatty acid esters of budesonide, an antiasthma glucocorticoid, in human lung and liver microsomes. *Drug Metab Dispos*, 1997. **25**(11): 1311–1317.

23. Nonaka, T., et al., Ciclesonide uptake and metabolism in human alveolar type II epithelial cells (A549). *BMC Pharmacol*, 2007. **7**: 12.

24. Nave, R., et al., Formation of fatty acid conjugates of ciclesonide active metabolite in the rat lung after 4-week inhalation of ciclesonide. *Pulm Pharmacol Ther*, 2005. **18**(6): 390–396.

25. Miller-Larsson, A., et al., Reversible fatty acid conjugation of budesonide. Novel mechanism for prolonged retention of topically applied steroid in airway tissue. *Drug Metab Dispos*, 1998. **26**(7): 623–630.

26. Hubbard, W.C., et al., Detection and quantitation of fatty acid acyl conjugates of triamcinolone acetonide via gas chromatography-electron-capture negative-ion mass spectrometry. *Anal Biochem*, 2003. **322**(2): 243–250.

27. Edsbacker, S. and R. Brattsand, Budesonide fatty-acid esterification: A novel mechanism prolonging binding to airway tissue. Review of available data. *Ann Allergy Asthma Immunol*, 2002. **88**(6): 609–616.

28. Brattsand, R. and A. Miller-Larsson, The role of intracellular esterification in budesonide once-daily dosing and airway selectivity. *Clin Ther*, 2003. **25**(Suppl C): C28–C41.

29. Dinis-Oliveira, R.J., et al., Paraquat poisonings: Mechanisms of lung toxicity, clinical features, and treatment. *Crit Rev Toxicol*, 2008. **38**(1): 13–71.

30. Gram, T.E., Chemically reactive intermediates and pulmonary xenobiotic toxicity. *Pharmacol Rev*, 1997. **49**(4): 297–341.

31. Howell, R.E. and P.N. Lanken, Pulmonary accumulation of propranolol *in vivo*: Sites and physiochemical mechanism. *J Pharmacol Exp Ther*, 1992. **263**(1): 130–135.

32. Vestal, R.E., D.M. Kornhauser, and D.G. Shand, Active uptake of propranolol by isolated rabbit alveolar macrophages and its inhibition by other basic amines. *J Pharmacol Exp Ther*, 1980. **214**(1): 106–111.

33. Waters, C.M., T.C. Krejcie, and M.J. Avram, Facilitated uptake of fentanyl, but not alfentanil, by human pulmonary endothelial cells. *Anesthesiology*, 2000. **93**(3): 825–831.

34. Waters, C.M., et al., Uptake of fentanyl in pulmonary endothelium. *J Pharmacol Exp Ther*, 1999. **288**(1): 157–163.

35. Boer, F., et al., Pulmonary uptake of sufentanil during and after constant rate infusion. *Br J Anaesth*, 1996. **76**(2): 203–208.

36. Larsson, P. and H. Tjalve, Tracing tissues with 4-ipomeanol-metabolizing capacity in rats. *Chem Biol Interact*, 1988. **67**(1–2): 1–24.

37. Antonini, J.M. and M.J. Reasor, Accumulation of amiodarone and desethylamiodarone by rat alveolar macrophages in cell culture. *Biochem Pharmacol*, 1991. **42**(Suppl): S151–S156.

38. Suhara, T., et al., Lung as reservoir for antidepressants in pharmacokinetic drug interactions. *Lancet*, 1998. **351**(9099): 332–335.

39. Yoshida, H., K. Okumura, and R. Hori, Subcellular distribution of basic drugs accumulated in the isolated perfused lung. *Pharm Res*, 1987. **4**(1): 50–53.

40. Junod, A.F., Accumulation of 14 C-imipramine in isolated perfused rat lungs. *J Pharmacol Exp Ther*, 1972. **183**(1): 182–187.

41. Himmelstein, M.W., et al., Toxicology and epidemiology of 1,3-butadiene. *Crit Rev Toxicol*, 1997. **27**(1): 1–108.

42. Himmelstein, M.W., B. Asgharian, and J.A. Bond, High concentrations of butadiene epoxides in livers and lungs of mice compared to rats exposed to 1,3-butadiene. *Toxicol Appl Pharmacol*, 1995. **132**(2): 281–288.

43. Pelkonen, O., et al., Local kinetics and dynamics of xenobiotics. *Cr Rev Toxicol*, 2008. **38**(8): 697–720.

44. Carlson, G.P., Modification of the metabolism and toxicity of styrene and styrene oxide in hepatic cytochrome P450 reductase deficient mice and CYP2F2 deficient mice. *Toxicology*, 2012. **294**(2–3): 104–108.

45. Weng, Y., et al., Determination of the role of target tissue metabolism in lung carcinogenesis using conditional cytochrome P450 reductase-null mice. *Cancer Res*, 2007. **67**(16): 7825–7832.

46. Pandey, A.V. and C.E. Flück, NADPH P450 oxidoreductase: Structure, function, and pathology of diseases. *Pharmacol Therapeut*, 2013. **138**(2): 229–254.

47. Parween, S., et al., P450 oxidoreductase deficiency: Loss of activity caused by protein instability from a novel L374H mutation. *J Clin Endocrinol Metab*, 2016: jc20161928.

48. Krone, N., et al., Genotype-phenotype analysis in congenital adrenal hyperplasia due to P450 oxidoreductase deficiency. *J Clin Endocrinol Metab*, 2012. **97**(2): E257–E267.

49. Iijima, S., A. Ohishi, and T. Ohzeki, Cytochrome P450 oxidoreductase deficiency with Antley-Bixler syndrome: Steroidogenic capacities. *J Pediatr Endocrinol Metab*, 2009. **22**(5): 469–475.

50. Fukami, M. and T. Ogata, Cytochrome P450 oxidoreductase deficiency: Rare congenital disorder leading to skeletal malformations and steroidogenic defects. *Pediatr Int*, 2014. **56**(6): 805–808.

51. Fukami, M., et al., Anorectal and urinary anomalies and aberrant retinoic acid metabolism in cytochrome P450 oxidoreductase deficiency. *Mol Genet Metab*, 2010. **100**(3): 269–273.

52. Burkhard, F.Z., et al., P450 Oxidoreductase deficiency: Analysis of mutations and polymorphisms. *J Steroid Biochem Mol Biol*, 2016. **165**: 38–50.

53. Pandey, A.V. and P. Sproll, Pharmacogenomics of human P450 oxidoreductase. *Front Pharmacol*, 2014. **5**: 103.

54. Herkert, J.C., et al., A rare cause of congenital adrenal hyperplasia: Antley-Bixler syndrome due to POR deficiency. *Neth J Med*, 2011. **69**(6): 281–283.

55. Fluck, C.E., et al., Mutant P450 oxidoreductase causes disordered steroidogenesis with and without Antley-Bixler syndrome. *Nat Genet*, 2004. **36**(3): 228–230.

56. Adachi, M., et al., POR R457H is a global founder mutation causing Antley-Bixler syndrome with autosomal recessive trait. *Am J Med Genet A*, 2006. **140**(6): 633–635.

57. Tomalik-Scharte, D., et al., Impaired hepatic drug and steroid metabolism in congenital adrenal hyperplasia due to P450 oxidoreductase deficiency. *Eur J Endocrinol*, 2010. **163**(6): 919–924.

58. Zhang, X., et al., Identification of cytochrome P450 oxidoreductase gene variants that are significantly associated with the interindividual variations in warfarin maintenance dose. *Drug Metab Dispos*, 2011. **39**(8): 1433–1439.

59. Zhang, J.J., et al., Effect of the P450 oxidoreductase 28 polymorphism on the pharmacokinetics of tacrolimus in Chinese healthy male volunteers. *Eur J Clin Pharmacol*, 2013. **69**(4): 807–812.

60. Zhang, J.J., et al., The genetic polymorphisms of POR*28 and CYP3A5*3 significantly influence the pharmacokinetics of tacrolimus in Chinese renal transplant recipients. *Int J Clin Pharmacol Ther*, 2015. **53**(9): 728–736.

61. Woillard, J.B., et al., Effect of CYP3A4*22, POR*28, and PPARA rs4253728 on sirolimus *in vitro* metabolism and trough concentrations in kidney transplant recipients. *Clin Chem*, 2013. **59**(12): 1761–1769.

62. Lesche, D., et al., CYP3A5*3 and POR*28 genetic variants influence the required dose of tacrolimus in heart transplant recipients. *Ther Drug Monit*, 2014. **36**(6): 710–715.

63. Elens, L., et al., Single-nucleotide polymorphisms in P450 oxidoreductase and peroxisome proliferator-activated receptor-alpha are associated with the development of new-onset diabetes after transplantation in kidney transplant recipients treated with tacrolimus. *Pharmacogenet Genom*, 2013. **23**(12): 649–657.

64. Elens, L., et al., Impact of POR*28 on the clinical pharmacokinetics of CYP3A phenotyping probes midazolam and erythromycin. *Pharmacogenet Genom*, 2013. **23**(3): 148–155.

65. Elens, L., et al., Impact of POR*28 on the pharmacokinetics of tacrolimus and cyclosporine A in renal transplant patients. *Ther Drug Monit*, 2014. **36**(1): 71–79.

66. Drogari, E., et al., POR*28 SNP is associated with lipid response to atorvastatin in children and adolescents with familial hypercholesterolemia. *Pharmacogenomics*, 2014. **15**(16): 1963–1972.

67. Subramanian, M., et al., Effect of P450 oxidoreductase variants on the metabolism of model substrates mediated by CYP2C9.1, CYP2C9.2, and CYP2C9.3. *Pharmacogenet Genom*, 2012. **22**(8): 590–597.

68. Sandee, D., et al., Effects of genetic variants of human P450 oxidoreductase on catalysis by CYP2D6 *in vitro.Pharmacogenet Genom*, 2010. **20**(11): 677–686.

69. Miller, W.L., et al., Consequences of POR mutations and polymorphisms. *Mol Cell Endocrinol*, 2011. **336**(1–2): 174–179.

70. Kuypers, D.R., et al., Combined effects of CYP3A5*1, POR*28, and CYP3A4*22 single nucleotide polymorphisms on early concentration-controlled tacrolimus exposure in de-novo renal recipients. *Pharmacogenet Genom*, 2014. **24**(12): 597–606.

71. de Jonge, H., et al., The P450 oxidoreductase *28 SNP is associated with low initial tacrolimus exposure and increased dose requirements in CYP3A5-expressing renal recipients. *Pharmacogenomics*, 2011. **12**(9): 1281–1291.

72. Chen, X., et al., Influence of various polymorphic variants of cytochrome P450 oxidoreductase (POR) on drug metabolic activity of CYP3A4 and CYP2B6. *PLoS One*, 2012. **7**(6): e38495.

73. Lee, M.J. and D. Dinsdale, The subcellular distribution of NADPH-cytochrome P450 reductase and isoenzymes of cytochrome P450 in the lungs of rats and mice. *Biochem Pharmacol*, 1995. **49**(10): 1387–1394.

74. Overby, L., et al., Cellular localization of flavin-containing monooxygenase in rabbit lung. *Exp Lung Res*, 1992. **18**(1): 131–144.

75. Overby, L.H., et al., Distribution of cytochrome P450 1A1 and NADPH-cytochrome P450 reductase in lungs of rabbits treated with 2,3,7,8-tetrachlorodibenzo-p-dioxin: Ultrastructural immunolocalization and in situ hybridization. *Mol Pharmacol*, 1992. **41**(6): 1039–1046.

76. Serabjit-Singh, C.J., et al., Cytochrome p-450: Localization in rabbit lung. *Science*, 1980. **207**(4438): 1469–1470.

77. Hall, P.M., et al., Immunohistochemical localization of NADPH-cytochrome P450 reductase in human tissues. *Carcinogenesis*, 1989. **10**(3): 521–530.

78. Thomas, C.E. and S.D. Aust, Rat liver microsomal NADPH-dependent release of iron from ferritin and lipid peroxidation. *J Free Radic Biol Med*, 1985. **1**(4): 293–300.

79. Thomas, C.E. and S.D. Aust, Reductive release of iron from ferritin by cation free radicals of paraquat and other bipyridyls. *J Biol Chem*, 1986. **261**(28): 13064–13070.

80. Han, J.F., et al., Effect of genetic variation on human cytochrome p450 reductase-mediated paraquat cytotoxicity. *Toxicol Sci*, 2006. **91**(1): 42–48.

81. Fang, C., et al., Deletion of the NADPH-cytochrome P450 reductase gene in cardiomyocytes does not protect mice against doxorubicin-mediated acute cardiac toxicity. *Drug Metab Dispos*, 2008. **36**(8): 1722–1728.

82. Nelson, D.R., et al., Comparison of cytochrome P450 (CYP) genes from the mouse and human genomes, including nomenclature recommendations for genes, pseudogenes and alternative-splice variants. *Pharmacogenetics*, 2004. **14**(1): 1–18.

83. Nebert, D.W., K. Wikvall, and W.L. Miller, Human cytochromes P450 in health and disease. *Philo Trans R Soc B Biol Sci*, 2013. **368**(1612): 20120431.

84. Wheeler, C.W. and T.M. Guenthner, Spectroscopic quantitation of cytochrome P-450 in human lung microsomes. *J Biochem Toxicol*, 1990. **5**(4): 269–272.

85. Wheeler, C.W. and T.M. Guenthner, Cytochrome P-450-dependent metabolism of xenobiotics in human lung. *J Biochem Toxicol*, 1991. **6**(3): 163–169.

86. Ruangyuttikarn, W., G.L. Skiles, and G.S. Yost, Identification of a cysteinyl adduct of oxidized 3-methylindole from goat lung and human liver microsomal proteins. *Chem Res Toxicol*, 1992. **5**(5): 713–719.

87. Hukkanen, J., et al., Detection of mRNA encoding xenobiotic-metabolizing cytochrome P450s in human bronchoalveolar macrophages and peripheral blood lymphocytes. *Mol Carcinog*, 1997. **20**(2): 224–230.

88. Hukkanen, J., et al., Expression and regulation of xenobiotic-metabolizing cytochrome P450 (CYP) enzymes in human lung. *Crit Rev Toxicol*, 2002. **32**(5): 391–411.

89. Hukkanen, J., O. Pelkonen, and H. Raunio, Expression of xenobiotic-metabolizing enzymes in human pulmonary tissue: Possible role in susceptibility for ILD. *Eur Respir J Suppl*, 2001. **32**: 122s–126s.

90. Piipari, R., et al., Expression of CYP1A1, CYP1B1 and CYP3A, and polycyclic aromatic hydrocarbon-DNA adduct formation in bronchoalveolar macrophages of smokers and non-smokers. *Int J Cancer*, 2000. **86**(5): 610–616.

91. Raunio, H., et al., Expression of xenobiotic-metabolizing CYPs in human pulmonary tissue. *Exp Toxicol Pathol*, 1999. **51**(4–5): 412–417.

92. Leclerc, J., et al., Profiling gene expression of whole cytochrome P450 superfamily in human bronchial and peripheral lung tissues: Differential expression in non-small cell lung cancers. *Biochimie*, 2010. **92**(3): 292–306.

93. Leclerc, J., et al., Xenobiotic metabolism and disposition in human lung: Transcript profiling in non-tumoral and tumoral tissues. *Biochimie*, 2011. **93**(6): 1012–1027.

94. Courcot, E., et al., Xenobiotic metabolism and disposition in human lung cell models: Comparison with *in vivo* expression profiles. *Drug Metab Dispos*, 2012. **40**(10): 1953–1965.

95. Renaud, H.J., et al., Tissue distribution and gender-divergent expression of 78 cytochrome P450 mRNAs in mice. *Toxicol Sci*, 2011. **124**(2): 261–277.

96. Zhuo, X., et al., Targeted disruption of the olfactory mucosa-specific Cyp2g1 gene: Impact on acetaminophen toxicity in the lateral nasal gland, and tissue-selective effects on Cyp2a5 expression. *J Pharmacol Exp Ther*, 2004. **308**(2): 719–728.

97. Carlson, G.P., Metabolism and toxicity of styrene in microsomal epoxide hydrolase-deficient mice. *J Toxicol Environ Health A*, 2010. **73**(24): 1689–1699.

98. Carlson, G.P., Comparison of styrene oxide enantiomers for hepatotoxic and pneumotoxic effects in microsomal epoxide hydrolase-deficient mice. *J Toxicol Environ Health A*, 2011. **74**(6): 347–350.

99. Carlson, G.P. and B.J. Day, Induction by pyridine of cytochrome P450IIE1 and xenobiotic metabolism in rat lung and liver. *Pharmacology*, 1992. **44**(3): 117–123.

100. Cruzan, G., et al., Studies of styrene, styrene oxide and 4-hydroxystyrene toxicity in CYP2F2 knockout and CYP2F1 humanized mice support lack of human relevance for mouse lung tumors. *Regul Toxicol Pharm*, 2013. **66**(1): 24–29.

101. Cruzan, G., et al., Styrene respiratory tract toxicity and mouse lung tumors are mediated by CYP2F-generated metabolites. *Regul Toxicol Pharmacol*, 2002. **35**(3): 308–319.

102. Behrendorff, J.B., et al., Directed evolution reveals requisite sequence elements in the functional expression of P450 2F1 in Escherichia coli. *Chem Res Toxicol*, 2012. **25**(9): 1964–1974.

103. Yost, G.S., Mechanisms of cytochrome P450-mediated formation of pneumotoxic electrophiles, in *Biological Reactive Intermediates V*, R. Snyder, Editor 1996, Plenum Press: New York. pp. 221–229.

104. Buckpitt, A., et al., Naphthalene-induced respiratory tract toxicity: Metabolic mechanisms of toxicity. *Drug Metab Rev*, 2002. **34**(4): 791–820.

105. Baer, B.R., A.E. Rettie, and K.R. Henne, Bioactivation of 4-ipomeanol by CYP4B1: Adduct characterization and evidence for an enedial intermediate. *Chem Res Toxicol*, 2005. **18**(5): 855–864.

106. Plopper, C.G., et al., Elevated susceptibility to 4-ipomeanol cytotoxicity in immature Clara cells of neonatal rabbits. *J Pharmacol Exp Ther*, 1994. **269**(2): 867–880.

107. Verschoyle, R.D., et al., CYP4B1 activates 4-ipomeanol in rat lung. *Toxicol Appl Pharmacol*, 1993. **123**(2): 193–198.

108. Chen, L.J., E.F. DeRose, and L.T. Burka, Metabolism of furans *in vitro*: Ipomeanine and 4-ipomeanol. *Chem Res Toxicol*, 2006. **19**(10): 1320–1329.

109. Nichols, W.K., et al., 3-methylindole-induced toxicity to human bronchial epithelial cell lines. *Toxicol Sci*, 2003. **71**(2): 229–236.

110. Ramakanth, S., et al., Correlation between pulmonary cytochrome P450 transcripts and the organ-selective pneumotoxicity of 3-methylindole. *Toxicol Lett*, 1994. **71**(1): 77–85.

111. Thornton-Manning, J.R., et al., Metabolism and bioactivation of 3-methylindole by Clara cells, alveolar macrophages, and subcellular fractions from rabbit lungs. *Toxicol Appl Pharmacol*, 1993. **122**(2): 182–190.

112. Wang, H., D.L. Lanza, and G.S. Yost, Cloning and expression of CYP2F3, a cytochrome P450 that bioactivates the selective pneumotoxins 3-methylindole and naphthalene. *Arch Biochem Biophys*, 1998. **349**(2): 329–340.

113. Yan, Z., et al., Metabolism and bioactivation of 3-methylindole by human liver microsomes. *Chem Res Toxicol*, 2007. **20**(1): 140–148.

114. Kartha, J.S. and G.S. Yost, Mechanism-based inactivation of lung-selective cytochrome P450 CYP2F enzymes. *Drug Metab Dispos*, 2008. **36**(1): 155–162.
115. Bolton, J.L., et al., Metabolic activation of butylated hydroxytoluene by mouse bronchiolar Clara cells. *Toxicol Appl Pharmacol*, 1993. **123**(1): 43–49.
116. Witschi, H., A.M. Malkinson, and J.A. Thompson, Metabolism and pulmonary toxicity of butylated hydroxytoluene (BHT). *Pharmacol Ther*, 1989. **42**(1): 89–113.
117. Simmonds, A.C., et al., Bioactivation of 1,1-dichloroethylene by CYP2E1 and CYP2F2 in murine lung. *J Pharmacol Exp Ther*, 2004. **310**(3): 855–864.
118. Simmonds, A.C., et al., Bioactivation of 1,1-dichloroethylene to its epoxide by CYP2E1 and CYP2F enzymes. *Drug Metab Dispos*, 2004. **32**(9): 1032–1039.
119. Akopyan, G. and D. Bonavida, Understanding tobacco smoke carcinogen NNK and lung tumorigenesis. *Int J Oncol*, 2006. **29**(4): 745–752.
120. Hecht, S.S., Recent studies on mechanisms of bioactivation and detoxification of 4-(methylnitrosamino)-1-(3-pyridyl)-1-butanone (NNK), a tobacco-specific lung carcinogen. *Crit Rev Toxicol*, 1996. **26**(2): 163–181.
121. Nishikawa, A., et al., Cigarette smoking, metabolic activation and carcinogenesis. *Curr Drug Metab*, 2004. **5**(5): 363–373.
122. Bieche, I., et al., Reverse transcriptase-PCR quantification of mRNA levels from cytochrome (CYP)1, CYP2 and CYP3 families in 22 different human tissues. *Pharmacogenet Genom*, 2007. **17**(9): 731–742.
123. Nishimura, M., et al., Tissue distribution of mRNA expression of human cytochrome P450 isoforms assessed by high-sensitivity real-time reverse transcription PCR. *Yakugaku Zasshi*, 2003. **123**(5): 369–375.
124. Domin, B.A., T.R. Devereux, and R.M. Philpot, The cytochrome P-450 monooxygenase system of rabbit lung enzyme components, activities, and induction in the nonciliated bronchiolar epithelial (Clara) cell, alveolar type II cell, and alveolar macrophage. *Mol Pharmacol*, 1986. **30**(3): 296–P303.
125. Nhamburo, P.T., et al., The human CYP2F gene subfamily: Identification of a cDNA encoding a new cytochrome P450, cDNA-directed expression, and chromosome mapping. *Biochemistry*, 1990. **29**(23): 5491–5499.
126. Tournel, G., et al., Molecular analysis of the CYP2F1 gene: Identification of a frequent non-functional allelic variant. *Mutat Res/Fund Mol M*, 2007. **617**(1–2): 79–89.
127. Zhou, X., et al., Respective roles of CYP2A5 and CYP2F2 in the bioactivation of 3-methylindole in mouse olfactory mucosa and lung: Studies using Cyp2a5-null and Cyp2f2-null mouse models. *Drug Metab Dispos*, 2012. **40**(4): 642.
128. Kupfer, R., et al., Lung toxicity and tumor promotion by hydroxylated derivatives of 2,6-di-tert-butyl-4-methylphenol (BHT) and 2-tert-butyl-4-methyl-6-iso-propylphenol: Correlation with quinone methide reactivity. *Chem Res Toxicol*, 2002. **15**(8): 1106–1112.
129. Meier, B.W., et al., Mechanistic basis for inflammation and tumor promotion in lungs of 2,6-di-tert-butyl-4-methylphenol-treated mice: Electrophilic metabolites alkylate and inactivate antioxidant enzymes. *Chem Res Toxicol*, 2007. **20**(2): 199–207.
130. Sasaki, T., et al., Possible relationship between the risk of Japanese bladder cancer cases and the CYP4B1 genotype. *Jpn J Clin Oncol*, 2008. **38**(9): 634–640.
131. Tamaki, Y., et al., Association between cancer risk and drug-metabolizing enzyme gene (CYP2A6, CYP2A13, CYP4B1, SULT1A1, GSTM1, and GSTT1) polymorphisms in cases of lung cancer in Japan. *Drug Metab Pharmacokinet*, 2011. **26**(5): 516–522.
132. Wiek, C., et al., Identification of amino acid determinants in CYP4B1 for optimal catalytic processing of 4-ipomeanol. *Biochem J*, 2015. **465**(1): 103–114.
133. Lanza, D.L., et al., Specific dehydrogenation of 3-methylindole and epoxidation of naphthalene by recombinant human CYP2F1 expressed in lymphoblastoid cells. *Drug Metab Dispos*, 1999. **27**(7): 798–803.
134. Lanza, D.L. and G.S. Yost, Selective dehydrogenation/oxygenation of 3-methylindole by cytochrome p450 enzymes. *Drug Metab Dispos*, 2001. **29**(7): 950–953.
135. Carr, B.A., et al., Characterization of pulmonary CYP4B2, specific catalyst of methyl oxidation of 3-methylindole. *Mol Pharmacol*, 2003. **63**(5): 1137–1147.
136. Wheeler, C.W., S.S. Park, and T.M. Guenthner, Immunochemical analysis of a cytochrome P-450IA1 homologue in human lung microsomes. *Mol Pharmacol*, 1990. **38**(5): 634–643.

137. Willey, J.C., et al., Xenobiotic metabolism enzyme gene expression in human bronchial epithelial and alveolar macrophage cells. *Am J Respir Cell Mol Biol*, 1996. **14**(3): 262–271.

138. Willey, J.C., et al., Quantitative RT-PCR measurement of cytochromes p450 1A1, 1B1, and 2B7, microsomal epoxide hydrolase, and NADPH oxidoreductase expression in lung cells of smokers and nonsmokers. *Am J Respir Cell Mol Biol*, 1997. **17**(1): 114–124.

139. Saarikoski, S.T., et al., Localization of CYP1A1 mRNA in human lung by in situ hybridization: Comparison with immunohistochemical findings. *Int J Cancer*, 1998. **77**(1): 33–39.

140. McLemore, T.L., et al., Expression of CYP1A1 gene in patients with lung cancer: Evidence for cigarette smoke-induced gene expression in normal lung tissue and for altered gene regulation in primary pulmonary carcinomas. *J Natl Cancer Inst*, 1990. **82**(16): 1333–1339.

141. Anttila, S., et al., Smoking and peripheral type of cancer are related to high levels of pulmonary cytochrome P450IA in lung cancer patients. *Int J Cancer*, 1991. **47**(5): 681–685.

142. Wei, C., et al., Induction of CYP1A1 and CYP1A2 expressions by prototypic and atypical inducers in the human lung. *Cancer Lett*, 2002. **178**(1): 25–36.

143. Hukkanen, J., et al., Induction and regulation of xenobiotic-metabolizing cytochrome P450s in the human A549 lung adenocarcinoma cell line. *Am J Respir Cell Mol Biol*, 2000. **22**(3): 360–366.

144. Weems, J.M. and G.S. Yost, 3-Methylindole metabolites induce lung CYP1A1 and CYP2F1 enzymes by AhR and non-AhR mechanisms, respectively. *Chem Res Toxicol*, 2010. **23**(3): 696–704.

145. Beamer, C.A. and D.M. Shepherd, Role of the aryl hydrocarbon receptor (AhR) in lung inflammation. *Semin Immunopathol*, 2013. **35**(6): 693–704.

146. Chiba, T., J. Chihara, and M. Furue, Role of the Arylhydrocarbon Receptor (AhR) in the Pathology of Asthma and COPD. *J Allergy (Cairo)*, 2012. **2012**: 372384.

147. Moorthy, B., C. Chu, and D.J. Carlin, Polycyclic aromatic hydrocarbons: From metabolism to lung cancer. *Toxicol Sci*, 2015. **145**(1): 5–15.

148. Haag, M., et al., Increased expression and decreased activity of cytochrome P450 1A1 in a murine model of toluene diisocyanate-induced asthma. *Arch Toxicol*, 2002. **76**(11): 621–627.

149. Shou, M., et al., The role of 12 cDNA-expressed human, rodent, and rabbit cytochromes P450 in the metabolism of benzo[a]pyrene and benzo[a]pyrene trans-7,8-dihydrodiol. *Mol Carcinog*, 1994. **10**(3): 159–168.

150. Koehl, W., et al., Metabolism of 5-methylchrysene and 6-methylchrysene by human hepatic and pulmonary cytochrome P450 enzymes. *Cancer Res*, 1996. **56**(2): 316–324.

151. Hammons, G.J., et al., Metabolism of carcinogenic heterocyclic and aromatic amines by recombinant human cytochrome P450 enzymes. *Carcinogenesis*, 1997. **18**(4): 851–854.

152. Weems, J.M., et al., Potent mutagenicity of 3-methylindole requires pulmonary cytochrome P450-mediated bioactivation: A comparison to the prototype cigarette smoke mutagens B(a)P and NNK. *Chem Res Toxicol*, 2010. **23**(11): 1682–1690.

153. Weems, J.M., et al., 3-Methylindole is mutagenic and a possible pulmonary carcinogen. *Toxicol Sci*, 2009. **112**(1): 59–67.

154. Anttila, S., et al., Immunohistochemical detection of pulmonary cytochrome P450IA and metabolic activities associated with P450IA1 and P450IA2 isozymes in lung cancer patients. *Environ Health Perspect*, 1992. **98**: 179–182.

155. Bartsch, H., et al., Expression of pulmonary cytochrome P4501A1 and carcinogen DNA adduct formation in high risk subjects for tobacco-related lung cancer. *Toxicol Lett*, 1992. **64–65**: 477–483.

156. Chang, K.W., et al., Differential response to benzo[A]pyrene in human lung adenocarcinoma cell lines: The absence of aryl hydrocarbon receptor activation. *Life Sci*, 1999. **65**(13): 1339–1349.

157. Vineis, P., The relationship between polymorphisms of xenobiotic metabolizing enzymes and susceptibility to cancer. *Toxicology*, 2002. **181–182**: 457–462.

158. Mollerup, S., et al., Sex differences in risk of lung cancer: Expression of genes in the PAH bioactivation pathway in relation to smoking and bulky DNA adducts. *Int J Cancer*, 2006. **119**(4): 741–744.

159. Kawajiri, K., et al., The CYP1A1 gene and cancer susceptibility. *Crit Rev Oncol Hematol*, 1993. **14**(1): 77–87.

160. Nakachi, K., et al., Association of cigarette smoking and CYP1A1 polymorphisms with adenocarcinoma of the lung by grades of differentiation. *Carcinogenesis*, 1995. **16**(9): 2209–2213.

161. Wei, C., et al., CYP1A2 is expressed along with CYP1A1 in the human lung. *Cancer Lett*, 2001. **171**(1): 113–120.

162. Bernauer, U., et al., Characterisation of the xenobiotic-metabolizing Cytochrome P450 expression pattern in human lung tissue by immunochemical and activity determination. *Toxicol Lett*, 2006. **164**(3): 278–288.

163. Yim, E.Y., et al., CYP1A2 polymorphism and theophylline clearance in Korean non-smoking asthmatics. *Asia Pac Allergy*, 2013. **3**(4): 231–240.

164. Wang, L., et al., Association between common CYP1A2 polymorphisms and theophylline metabolism in non-smoking healthy volunteers. *Basic Clin Pharmacol Toxicol*, 2013. **112**(4): 257–263.

165. Ren, J., et al., Meta-analysis of correlation between the CYP1A2 -3860 G > A polymorphism and lung cancer risk. *Genet Mol Res*, 2016. **15**(2).

166. Ma, Z., et al., CYP1A2 rs762551 polymorphism contributes to risk of lung cancer: A meta-analysis. *Tumour Biol*, 2014. **35**(3): 2253–2257.

167. Thum, T., et al., Expression of xenobiotic metabolizing enzymes in different lung compartments of smokers and nonsmokers. *Environ Health Perspect*, 2006. **114**(11): 1655–1661.

168. Jiang, H., et al., Competing roles of cytochrome P450 1A1/1B1 and aldo-keto reductase 1A1 in the metabolic activation of (+/−)-7,8-dihydroxy-7,8-dihydro-benzo[a]pyrene in human bronchoalveolar cell extracts. *Chem Res Toxicol*, 2005. **18**(2): 365–374.

169. McFadyen, M.C. and G.I. Murray, Cytochrome P450 1B1: A novel anticancer therapeutic target. *Future Oncol*, 2005. **1**(2): 259–263.

170. Tsuchiya, Y., M. Nakajima, and T. Yokoi, Cytochrome P450-mediated metabolism of estrogens and its regulation in human. *Cancer Lett*, 2005. **227**(2): 115–124.

171. Aklillu, E., et al., Characterization of common CYP1B1 variants with different capacity for benzo[a]pyrene-7,8-dihydrodiol epoxide formation from benzo[a]pyrene. *Cancer Res*, 2005. **65**(12): 5105–5111.

172. Chen, P.-F., et al., Association between the CYP1B1 polymorphisms and lung cancer risk: A meta-analysis. *Technol Cancer Res T*, 2016. **15**(5): NP73–NP82.

173. Peng, H.M., X. Ding, and M.J. Coon, Isolation and heterologous expression of cloned cDNAs for two rabbit nasal microsomal proteins, CYP2A10 and CYP2A11, that are related to nasal microsomal cytochrome P450 form a. *J Biol Chem*, 1993. **268**(23): 17253–17260.

174. Su, T., et al., Expression of CYP2A genes in rodent and human nasal mucosa. *Drug Metab Dispos*, 1996. **24**(8): 884–890.

175. Thornton-Manning, J.R., et al., Nasal cytochrome P450 2A: Identification, regional localization, and metabolic activity toward hexamethylphosphoramide, a known nasal carcinogen. *Toxicol Appl Pharmacol*, 1997. **142**(1): 22–30.

176. Chen, Y., et al., Immunoblot analysis and immunohistochemical characterization of CYP2A expression in human olfactory mucosa. *Biochem Pharmacol*, 2003. **66**(7): 1245–1251.

177. Zhu, L.R., et al., CYP2A13 in human respiratory tissues and lung cancers: An immunohistochemical study with a new peptide-specific antibody. *Drug Metab Dispos*, 2006. **34**(10): 1672–1676.

178. Thornton-Manning, J., et al., Metabolism of 3-methylindole by vaccinia-expressed P450 enzymes: Correlation of 3-methyleneindolenine formation and protein-binding. *J Pharmacol Exp Ther*, 1996. **276**(1): 21–29.

179. D'Agostino, J., et al., The pneumotoxin 3-methylindole is a substrate and a mechanism-based inactivator of CYP2A13, a human cytochrome P450 enzyme preferentially expressed in the respiratory tract. *Drug Metab Dispos*, 2009. **37**(10): 2018–2027.

180. Piras, E., et al., Cell-specific expression of CYP2A5 in the mouse respiratory tract: Effects of olfactory toxicants. *J Histochem Cytochem*, 2003. **51**(11): 1545–1555.

181. Zhou, X., et al., Role of CYP2A5 in the clearance of nicotine and cotinine: Insights from studies on a Cyp2a5-null mouse model. *J Pharmacol Exp Ther*, 2010. **332**(2): 578–587.

182. Li, L., et al., Impact of nicotine metabolism on nicotine's pharmacological effects and behavioral responses: Insights from a Cyp2a(4/5)bgs-null mouse. *J Pharmacol Exp Ther*, 2013. **347**(3): 746–754.

183. Hu, J., et al., Essential role of the cytochrome P450 enzyme CYP2A5 in olfactory mucosal toxicity of naphthalene. *Drug Metab Dispos*, 2014. **42**(1): 23–27.

184. Zhou, X., et al., Role of CYP2A5 in the bioactivation of the lung carcinogen 4-(methylnitrosamino)-1-(3-pyridyl)-1-butanone in mice. *J Pharmacol Exp Ther*, 2012. **341**(1): 233–241.

185. Zhou, X., et al., Respective roles of CYP2A5 and CYP2F2 in the bioactivation of 3-methylindole in mouse olfactory mucosa and lung: Studies using Cyp2a5-null and Cyp2f2-null mouse models. *Drug Metab Dispos*, 2012. **40**(4): 642–647.

186. Megaraj, V., et al., Role of CYP2A13 in the bioactivation and lung tumorigenicity of the tobacco-specific lung procarcinogen 4-(methylnitrosamino)-1-(3-pyridyl)-1-butanone: *In vivo* studies using a CYP2A13-humanized mouse model. *Carcinogenesis*, 2014. **35**(1): 131–137.

187. Pelkonen, O., et al., CYP2A6: A human coumarin 7-hydroxylase. *Toxicology*, 2000. **144**(1–3): 139–147.

188. Messina, E.S., R.F. Tyndale, and E.M. Sellers, A major role for CYP2A6 in nicotine C-oxidation by human liver microsomes. *J Pharmacol Exp Ther*, 1997. **282**(3): 1608–1614.

189. Murphy, S.E., L.M. Johnson, and D.A. Pullo, Characterization of multiple products of cytochrome P450 2A6-catalyzed cotinine metabolism. *Chem Res Toxicol*, 1999. **12**(7): 639–645.

190. Smith, G.B., et al., Biotransformation of 4-(methylnitrosamino)-1-(3-pyridyl)-1-butanone (NNK) in peripheral human lung microsomes. *Drug Metab Dispos*, 2003. **31**(9): 1134–1141.

191. Tiano, H.F., et al., Human CYP2A6 activation of 4-(methylnitrosamino)-1-(3-pyridyl)-1-butanone (NNK): Mutational specificity in the gpt gene of AS52 cells. *Carcinogenesis*, 1994. **15**(12): 2859–2866.

192. Hecht, S.S., Biochemistry, biology, and carcinogenicity of tobacco-specific N-nitrosamines. *Chem Res Toxicol*, 1998. **11**(6): 559–603.

193. Kamataki, T., et al., Genetic polymorphism of CYP2A6 as one of the potential determinants of tobacco-related cancer risk. *Biochem Biophys Res Commun*, 2005. **338**(1): 306–310.

194. Fujieda, M., et al., Evaluation of CYP2A6 genetic polymorphisms as determinants of smoking behavior and tobacco-related lung cancer risk in male Japanese smokers. *Carcinogenesis*, 2004. **25**(12): 2451–2458.

195. Malaiyandi, V., E.M. Sellers, and R.F. Tyndale, Implications of CYP2A6 genetic variation for smoking behaviors and nicotine dependence. *Clin Pharmacol Ther*, 2005. **77**(3): 145–158.

196. He, X.Y., et al., Efficient activation of aflatoxin B1 by cytochrome P450 2A13, an enzyme predominantly expressed in human respiratory tract. *Int J Cancer*, 2006. **118**(11): 2665–2671.

197. Su, T., et al., Human cytochrome P450 CYP2A13: Predominant expression in the respiratory tract and its high efficiency metabolic activation of a tobacco-specific carcinogen, 4-(methylnitrosamino)-1-(3-pyridyl)-1-butanone. *Cancer Res*, 2000. **60**(18): 5074–5079.

198. Wong, H.L., et al., Metabolic activation of the tobacco carcinogen 4-(methylnitrosamino)-(3-pyridyl)-1-butanone by cytochrome P450 2A13 in human fetal nasal microsomes. *Chem Res Toxicol*, 2005. **18**(6): 913–918.

199. Jalas, J.R., X. Ding, and S.E. Murphy, Comparative metabolism of the tobacco-specific nitrosamines 4-(methylnitrosamino)-1-(3-pyridyl)-1-butanone and 4-(methylnitrosamino)-1-(3-pyridyl)-1-butanol by rat cytochrome P450 2A3 and human cytochrome P450 2A13. *Drug Metab Dispos*, 2003. **31**(10): 1199–1202.

200. Fukami, T., et al., Human cytochrome P450 2A13 efficiently metabolizes chemicals in air pollutants: Naphthalene, styrene, and toluene. *Chem Res Toxicol*, 2008. **21**(3): 720–725.

201. Wang, H., et al., Substantial reduction in risk of lung adenocarcinoma associated with genetic polymorphism in CYP2A13, the most active cytochrome P450 for the metabolic activation of tobacco-specific carcinogen NNK. *Cancer Res*, 2003. **63**(22): 8057–8061.

202. Gervot, L., et al., Human CYP2B6: Expression, inducibility and catalytic activities. *Pharmacogenetics*, 1999. **9**(3): 295–306.

203. Mace, K., et al., Characterisation of xenobiotic-metabolising enzyme expression in human bronchial mucosa and peripheral lung tissues. *Eur J Cancer*, 1998. **34**(6): 914–920.

204. Dicke, K.E., S.M. Skrlin, and S.E. Murphy, Nicotine and 4-(methylnitrosamino)-1-(3-pyridyl)-butanone metabolism by cytochrome P450 2B6. *Drug Metab Dispos*, 2005. **33**(12): 1760–1764.

205. Liu, Z., et al., Characterization of CYP2B6 in a CYP2B6-humanized mouse model: Inducibility in the liver by phenobarbital and dexamethasone and role in nicotine metabolism *in vivo.Drug Metab Dispos*, 2015. **43**(2): 208–216.

206. Wassenaar, C.A., et al., Pilot study of CYP2B6 genetic variation to explore the contribution of nitrosamine activation to lung carcinogenesis. *Int J Mol Sci*, 2013. **14**(4): 8381–8392.

207. Yokose, T., et al., Immunohistochemical study of cytochrome P450 2C and 3A in human non-neoplastic and neoplastic tissues. *Virchows Arch*, 1999. **434**(5): 401–411.

208. Fisslthaler, B., I. Fleming, and R. Busse, EDHF: A cytochrome P450 metabolite in coronary arteries. *Semin Perinatol*, 2000. **24**(1): 15–19.

209. Fisslthaler, B., et al., Nifedipine increases cytochrome P4502C expression and endothelium-derived hyperpolarizing factor-mediated responses in coronary arteries. *Hypertension*, 2000. **36**(2): 270–275.

210. Vriens, J., et al., Modulation of the Ca2 permeable cation channel TRPV4 by cytochrome P450 epoxygenases in vascular endothelium. *Circ Res*, 2005. **97**(9): 908–915.

211. Akasaka, T., et al., Association of CYP2C19 variants and epoxyeicosatrienoic acids on patients with microvascular angina. *Am J Physiol Heart Circ Physiol*, 2016. **311**(6): H1409-H1415.

212. Garcia-Martin, E., et al., Influence of cytochrome P450 CYP2C9 genotypes in lung cancer risk. *Cancer Lett*, 2002. **180**(1): 41–46.

213. London, S.J., et al., Lung cancer risk in relation to the CYP2C9*1/CYP2C9*2 genetic polymorphism among African-Americans and Caucasians in Los Angeles County, California. *Pharmacogenetics*, 1996. **6**(6): 527–533.

214. Yan, F., et al., Interaction between smoking and CYP2C19*3 polymorphism increased risk of lung cancer in a Chinese population. *Tumour Biol*, 2014. **35**(6): 5295–5298.

215. Huang, Y., et al., CYP2D6 T188C variant is associated with lung cancer risk in the Chinese population. *Tumour Biol*, 2013. **34**(4): 2189–2193.

216. Samer, C.F., et al., Applications of CYP450 testing in the clinical setting. *Mol Diagn Ther*, 2013. **17**(3): 165–184.

217. Bouchardy, C., S. Benhamou, and P. Dayer, The effect of tobacco on lung cancer risk depends on CYP2D6 activity. *Cancer Res*, 1996. **56**(2): 251–253.

218. Laforest, L., et al., CYP2D6 gene polymorphism in caucasian smokers: Lung cancer susceptibility and phenotype-genotype relationships. *Eur J Cancer*, 2000. **36**(14): 1825–1832.

219. Ding, X.X. and M.J. Coon, Induction of cytochrome P-450 isozyme 3a (P-450IIE1) in rabbit olfactory mucosa by ethanol and acetone. *Drug Metab Dispos*, 1990. **18**(5): 742–745.

220. Romero, F., et al., Chronic alcohol ingestion in rats alters lung metabolism, promotes lipid accumulation, and impairs alveolar macrophage functions. *Am J Resp Cell Mol*, 2014. **51**(6): 840–849.

221. Raucy, J.L., J.C. Kraner, and J.M. Lasker, Bioactivation of halogenated hydrocarbons by cytochrome P4502E1. *Crit Rev Toxicol*, 1993. **23**(1): 1–20.

222. Forkert, P.G., Mechanisms of 1,1-dichloroethylene-induced cytotoxicity in lung and liver. *Drug Metab Rev*, 2001. **33**(1): 49–80.

223. Forkert, P.G., S.M. Boyd, and J.B. Ulreich, Pulmonary bioactivation of 1,1-dichloroethylene is associated with CYP2E1 levels in A/J, CD-1, and C57BL/6 mice. *J Pharmacol Exp Ther*, 2001. **297**(3): 1193–1200.

224. Lee, R.P. and P.G. Forkert, *In vitro* biotransformation of 1,1-dichloroethylene by hepatic cytochrome P-450 2E1 in mice. *J Pharmacol Exp Ther*, 1994. **270**(1): 371–376.

225. Lee, R.P. and P.G. Forkert, Pulmonary CYP2E1 bioactivates 1,1-dichloroethylene in male and female mice. *J Pharmacol Exp Ther*, 1995. **273**(1): 561–567.

226. Forkert, P.G., et al., Oxidation of vinyl carbamate and formation of 1,N6-ethenodeoxyadenosine in murine lung. *Drug Metab Dispos*, 2007. **35**(5): 713–720.

227. Hoffler, U., H.A. El-Masri, and B.I. Ghanayem, Cytochrome P450 2E1 (CYP2E1) is the principal enzyme responsible for urethane metabolism: Comparative studies using CYP2E1-null and wild-type mice. *J Pharmacol Exp Ther*, 2003. **305**(2): 557–564.

228. Yang, C.S., et al., Cytochrome P450IIE1: Roles in nitrosamine metabolism and mechanisms of regulation. *Drug Metab Rev*, 1990. **22**(2–3): 147–159.

229. Nichols, W.K., et al., Bioactivation of halogenated hydrocarbons by rabbit pulmonary cells. *Pharmacol Toxicol*, 1992. **71**(5): 335–339.

230. Nichols, W.K., et al., Oxidation at C-1 controls the cytotoxicity of 1,1-dichloro-2,2- bis(p-chlorophenyl) ethane by rabbit and human lung cells. *Drug Metab Dispos*, 1995. **23**(5): 595–599.

231. Ritter, J.K., et al., Mouse pulmonary cytochrome P-450 naphthalene hydroxylase: cDNA cloning, sequence, and expression in Saccharomyces cerevisiae. *Biochemistry*, 1991. **30**(48): 11430–11437.

232. Baldwin, R.M., M.A. Shultz, and A.R. Buckpitt, Bioactivation of the pulmonary toxicants naphthalene and 1-nitronaphthalene by rat CYP2F4. *J Pharmacol Exp Ther*, 2005. **312**(2): 857–865.

233. Powley, M.W. and G.P. Carlson, Cytochromes P450 involved with benzene metabolism in hepatic and pulmonary microsomes. *J Biochem Mol Toxicol*, 2000. **14**(6): 303–309.

234. Sheets, P.L., G.S. Yost, and G.P. Carlson, Benzene metabolism in human lung cell lines BEAS-2B and A549 and cells overexpressing CYP2F1. *J Biochem Mol Toxicol*, 2004. **18**(2): 92–99.

235. Thornton-Manning, J.R., et al., Metabolic activation of the pneumotoxin, 3-methylindole, by vaccinia-expressed cytochrome P450s. *Biochem Biophys Res Commun*, 1991. **181**(1): 100–107.

236. Li, L., et al., Generation and characterization of a Cyp2f2-null mouse and studies on the role of CYP2F2 in naphthalene-induced toxicity in the lung and nasal olfactory mucosa. *J Pharmacol Exp Ther*, 2011. **339**(1): 62–71.

237. Smith, T.J., et al., Metabolism of 4-(methylnitrosamino)-1-(3-pyridyl)-1-butanone in human lung and liver microsomes and cytochromes P-450 expressed in hepatoma cells. *Cancer Res*, 1992. **52**(7): 1757–1763.

238. Baldwin, R.M., et al., Comparison of pulmonary/nasal CYP2F expression levels in rodents and rhesus macaque. *J Pharmacol Exp Ther*, 2004. **309**(1): 127–136.

239. Regal, K.A., et al., Detection and characterization of DNA adducts of 3-methylindole. *Chem Res Toxicol*, 2001. **14**(8): 1014–1024.

240. Yost, G.S., D.J. Kuntz, and L.D. McGill, Organ-selective switching of 3-methylindole toxicity by glutathione depletion. *Toxicol Appl Pharmacol*, 1990. **103**(1): 40–51.

241. Buckpitt, A., et al., Relationship of cytochrome P450 activity to Clara cell cytotoxicity. IV. Metabolism of naphthalene and naphthalene oxide in microdissected airways from mice, rats, and hamsters. *Mol Pharmacol*, 1995. **47**(1): 74–81.

242. Wei, Y., et al., Generation and characterization of a CYP2A13/2B6/2F1-transgenic mouse model. *Drug Metab Dispos*, 2012. **40**(6): 1144–1150.

243. Kartha, J.S., et al., Single mutations change CYP2F3 from a dehydrogenase of 3-methylindole to an oxygenase. *Biochemistry*, 2008. **47**(37): 9756–9770.

244. Skiles, G.L. and G.S. Yost, Mechanistic studies on the cytochrome P450-catalyzed dehydrogenation of 3-methylindole. *Chem Res Toxicol*, 1996. **9**(1): 291–297.

245. Skordos, K.W., J.D. Laycock, and G.S. Yost, Thioether adducts of a new imine reactive intermediate of the pneumotoxin 3-methylindole. *Chem Res Toxicol*, 1998. **11**(11): 1326–1331.

246. Zeldin, D.C., et al., CYP2J subfamily P450s in the lung: Expression, localization, and potential functional significance. *Mol Pharmacol*, 1996. **50**(5): 1111–1117.

247. Capdevila, J.H., J.R. Falck, and R.C. Harris, Cytochrome P450 and arachidonic acid bioactivation. Molecular and functional properties of the arachidonate monooxygenase. *J Lipid Res*, 2000. **41**(2): 163–181.

248. Scarborough, P.E., et al., P450 subfamily CYP2J and their role in the bioactivation of arachidonic acid in extrahepatic tissues. *Drug Metab Rev*, 1999. **31**(1): 205–234.

249. Spiecker, M. and J.K. Liao, Vascular protective effects of cytochrome p450 epoxygenase-derived eicosanoids. *Arch Biochem Biophys*, 2005. **433**(2): 413–420.

250. Xiao, Y.F., Cyclic AMP-dependent modulation of cardiac L-type Ca2+ and transient outward K+ channel activities by epoxyeicosatrienoic acids. *Prostaglandins Other Lipid Mediat*, 2007. **82**(1–4): 11–18.

251. Zeldin, D.C., Epoxygenase pathways of arachidonic acid metabolism. *J Biol Chem*, 2001. **276**(39): 36059–36062.

252. Xu, M., et al., Cytochrome P450 2J2: Distribution, function, regulation, genetic polymorphisms and clinical significance. *Drug Metab Rev*, 2013. **45**(3): 311–352.

253. Rylander, T., et al., Identification and tissue distribution of the novel human cytochrome P450 2S1 (CYP2S1). *Biochem Biophys Res Commun*, 2001. **281**(2): 529–535.

254. Saarikoski, S.T., et al., Localization of cytochrome P450 CYP2S1 expression in human tissues by in situ hybridization and immunohistochemistry. *J Histochem Cytochem*, 2005. **53**(5): 549–556.

255. Rivera, S.P., S.T. Saarikoski, and O. Hankinson, Identification of a novel dioxin-inducible cytochrome P450. *Mol Pharmacol*, 2002. **61**(2): 255–259.

256. Smith, G., et al., Cutaneous expression of cytochrome P450 CYP2S1: Individuality in regulation by therapeutic agents for psoriasis and other skin diseases. *Lancet*, 2003. **361**(9366): 1336–1343.

257. Bebenek, I.G., et al., CYP2S1 is negatively regulated by corticosteroids in human cell lines. *Toxicol Lett*, 2012. **209**(1): 30–34.

258. Downie, D., et al., Profiling cytochrome P450 expression in ovarian cancer: Identification of prognostic markers. *Clin Cancer Res*, 2005. **11**(20): 7369–7375.

259. Mrízová, I., et al., Heterologous expression of human cytochrome P450 2S1 in Escherichia coli and investigation of its role in metabolism of benzo[a]pyrene and ellipticine. *Monatshefte Fur Chemie*, 2016. **147**: 881–888.

260. Bui, P.H. and O. Hankinson, Functional characterization of human cytochrome P450 2S1 using a synthetic gene-expressed protein in Escherichia coli. *Mol Pharmacol*, 2009. **76**(5): 1031–1043.

261. Saarikoski, S.T., et al., CYP2S1: A short review. *Toxicol Appl Pharm*, 2005. **207**(2, Supplement): 62–69.
262. Bui, P., et al., Human CYP2S1 metabolizes cyclooxygenase- and lipoxygenase-derived Eicosanoids. *Drug Metab Dispos*, 2011. **39**(2): 180–190.
263. Madanayake, T.W., et al., *Cytochrome P450 2S1 depletion enhances cell proliferation and migration in bronchial Epithelial cells, in part, through modulation of prostaglandin E2 synthesis.Drug Metab Dispos*, 2012. **40**(11): 2119.
264. Yang, C., et al., CYP2S1 depletion enhances colorectal cell proliferation is associated with PGE2-mediated activation of β-catenin signaling. *Exp Cell Res*, 2015. **331**(2): 377–386.
265. Anttila, S., et al., Expression and localization of CYP3A4 and CYP3A5 in human lung. *Am J Respir Cell Mol Biol*, 1997. **16**(3): 242–249.
266. Raunio, H., et al., Expression of xenobiotic-metabolizing cytochrome P450s in human pulmonary tissues. *Arch Toxicol Suppl*, 1998. **20**: 465–469.
267. Biggs, J.S., et al., Transcription factor binding to a putative double E-box motif represses CYP3A4 expression in human lung cells. *Mol Pharmacol*, 2007. **72**(3): 514–525.
268. Somers, G.I., et al., A comparison of the expression and metabolizing activities of phase I and II enzymes in freshly isolated human lung parenchymal cells and cryopreserved human hepatocytes. *Drug Metab Dispos*, 2007. **35**(10): 1797–1805.
269. Raunio, H., J. Hakkola, and O. Pelkonen, Regulation of CYP3A genes in the human respiratory tract. *Chem Biol Interact*, 2005. **151**(2): 53–62.
270. Hukkanen, J., et al., Regulation of CYP3A5 by glucocorticoids and cigarette smoke in human lung-derived cells. *J Pharmacol Exp Ther*, 2003. **304**(2): 745–752.
271. Reilly, C.A., et al., Reactive intermediates produced from the metabolism of the vanilloid ring of capsaicinoids by p450 enzymes. *Chem Res Toxicol*, 2013. **26**(1): 55–66.
272. Williams, J.A., et al., Comparative metabolic capabilities of CYP3A4, CYP3A5, and CYP3A7. *Drug Metab Dispos*, 2002. **30**(8): 883–891.
273. Aoyama, T., et al., Five of 12 forms of vaccinia virus-expressed human hepatic cytochrome P450 metabolically activate aflatoxin B1. *Proc Natl Acad Sci USA*, 1990. **87**(12): 4790–4793.
274. Kelly, J.D., et al., Aflatoxin B1 activation in human lung. *Toxicol Appl Pharmacol*, 1997. **144**(1): 88–95.
275. Murai, T., et al., The inhaled glucocorticoid fluticasone propionate efficiently inactivates cytochrome P450 3A5, a predominant lung P450 enzyme. *Chem Res Toxicol*, 2010. **23**(8): 1356–1364.
276. Stockmann, C., et al., Effect of CYP3A5*3 on asthma control among children treated with inhaled beclomethasone. *J Allergy Clin Immun*, 2015. **136**(2): 505–507.
277. Nhamburo, P.T., et al., Identification of a new P450 expressed in human lung: Complete cDNA sequence, cDNA-directed expression, and chromosome mapping. *Biochemistry*, 1989. **28**(20): 8060–8066.
278. Boei, J.J.W.A., et al., Xenobiotic metabolism in differentiated human bronchial epithelial cells. *Arch Toxicol*, 2016: 1–13.
279. Wolf, C.R., et al., The rabbit pulmonary monooxygenase system: Characteristics and activities of two forms of pulmonary cytochrome P-450. *Chem Biol Interact*, 1978. **21**(1): 29–43.
280. Czerwinski, M., et al., Metabolic activation of 4-ipomeanol by complementary DNA-expressed human cytochromes P-450: Evidence for species-specific metabolism. *Cancer Res*, 1991. **51**(17): 4636–4638.
281. Smith, P.B., et al., 4-Ipomeanol and 2-aminoanthracene cytotoxicity in C3H/10T1/2 cells expressing rabbit cytochrome P450 4B1. *Biochem Pharmacol*, 1995. **50**(10): 1567–1575.
282. Nakano, M., et al., Ocular cytochrome P450s and transporters: Roles in disease and endobiotic and xenobiotic disposition. *Drug Metab Rev*, 2014. **46**(3): 247–260.
283. Lipsky, P.E., Role of cyclooxygenase-1 and -2 in health and disease. *Am J Orthop*, 1999. **28**(3 Suppl): 8–12.
284. Marnett, L.J., Cyclooxygenase mechanisms. *Curr Opin Chem Biol*, 2000. **4**(5): 545–552.
285. Marnett, L.J., Structure, function and inhibition of cyclo-oxygenases. *Ernst Schering Res Found Workshop*, 2000(31): 65–83.
286. Simmons, D.L., R.M. Botting, and T. Hla, Cyclooxygenase isozymes: The biology of prostaglandin synthesis and inhibition. *Pharmacol Rev*, 2004. **56**(3): 387–437.
287. Chandrasekharan, N.V., et al., COX-3, a cyclooxygenase-1 variant inhibited by acetaminophen and other analgesic/antipyretic drugs: Cloning, structure, and expression. *Proc Natl Acad Sci USA*, 2002. **99**(21): p. 13926–13931.

288. van Overveld, F.J., et al., Release of arachidonic acid metabolites from isolated human alveolar type II cells. *Prostaglandins*, 1992. **44**(2): 101–110.

289. Samokyszyn, V.M. and L.J. Marnett, Hydroperoxide-dependent cooxidation of 13-cis-retinoic acid by prostaglandin H synthase. *J Biol Chem*, 1987. **262**(29): 14119–14133.

290. Samokyszyn, V.M., et al., Cooxidation of 13-cis-retinoic acid by prostaglandin H synthase. *Biochem Biophys Res Commun*, 1984. **124**(2): 430–436.

291. Wise, R.W., T.V. Zenser, and B.B. Davis, Prostaglandin H synthase metabolism of the urinary bladder carcinogens benzidine and ANFT. *Carcinogenesis*, 1983. 4(3): 285–289.

292. Yamazoe, Y., et al., DNA adducts formed by ring-oxidation of the carcinogen 2-naphthylamine with prostaglandin H synthase *in vitro* and in the dog urothelium *in vivo*.*Carcinogenesis*, 1985. **6**(9): 1379–1387.

293. Zenser, T.V., et al., Metabolism of N-acetylbenzidine and initiation of bladder cancer. *Mutat Res*, 2002. **506–507**: 29–40.

294. Donnelly, P.J., et al., Biotransformation of aflatoxin B1 in human lung. *Carcinogenesis*, 1996. **17**(11): 2487–2494.

295. Liu, L. and T.E. Massey, Bioactivation of aflatoxin B1 by lipoxygenases, prostaglandin H synthase and cytochrome P450 monooxygenase in guinea-pig tissues. *Carcinogenesis*, 1992. **13**(4): 533–539.

296. Massey, T.E., G.B. Smith, and A.S. Tam, Mechanisms of aflatoxin B1 lung tumorigenesis. *Exp Lung Res*, 2000. **26**(8): 673–683.

297. Reed, G.A., et al., Prostaglandin H synthase-dependent co-oxygenation of (+/−)-7,8-dihydroxy-7,8-dihydrobenzo[a]pyrene in hamster trachea and human bronchus explants. *Carcinogenesis*, 1984. **5**(7): 955–960.

298. Reed, G.A. and L.J. Marnett, Metabolism and activation of 7,8-dihydrobenzo[a]pyrene during prostaglandin biosynthesis. Intermediacy of a bay-region epoxide. *J Biol Chem*, 1982. **257**(19): 11368–11376.

299. Sivarajah, K., et al., Prostaglandin synthetase and cytochrome P-450-dependent metabolism of (+/−) benzo(a)pyrene 7,8-dihydrodiol by enriched populations of rat Clara cells and alveolar type II cells. *Cancer Res*, 1983. **43**(6): 2632–2636.

300. Claar, D., T.V. Hartert, and R.S. Peebles, The role of prostaglandins in allergic lung inflammation and asthma. *Expert Rev Resp Med*, 2015. **9**(1): 55–72.

301. Liu, R., K.-P. Xu, and G.-S. Tan, Cyclooxygenase-2 inhibitors in lung cancer treatment: Bench to bed. *Eur J Pharmacol*, 2015. **769**: 127–133.

302. Cashman, J.R. and J. Zhang, Human flavin-containing monooxygenases. *Annu Rev Pharmacol Toxicol*, 2006. **46**: 65–100.

303. Krueger, S.K. and D.E. Williams, Mammalian flavin-containing monooxygenases: Structure/function, genetic polymorphisms and role in drug metabolism. *Pharmacol Ther*, 2005. **106**(3): 357–387.

304. Massey, V., Activation of molecular oxygen by flavins and flavoproteins. *J Biol Chem*, 1994. **269**(36): 22459–22462.

305. Beaty, N.B. and D.P. Ballou, Transient kinetic study of liver microsomal FAD-containing monooxygenase. *J Biol Chem*, 1980. **255**(9): 3817–3819.

306. Williams, D.E., et al., Rabbit lung flavin-containing monooxygenase is immunochemically and catalytically distinct from the liver enzyme. *Biochem Biophys Res Commun*, 1984. **125**(1): 116–122.

307. Sun, H., et al., Dehydrogenation of indoline by cytochrome P450 enzymes: A novel "aromatase" process. *J Pharmacol Exp Ther*, 2007. **322**(2): 843–851.

308. Zhang, J. and J.R. Cashman, Quantitative analysis of FMO gene mRNA levels in human tissues. *Drug Metab Dispos*, 2006. **34**(1): 19–26.

309. Siddens, L.K., et al., Characterization of mouse flavin-containing monooxygenase transcript levels in lung and liver, and activity of expressed isoforms. *Biochem Pharmacol*, 2008. **75**(2): 570–579.

310. Whetstine, J.R., et al., Ethnic differences in human flavin-containing monooxygenase 2 (FMO2) polymorphisms: Detection of expressed protein in African-Americans. *Toxicol Appl Pharmacol*, 2000. **168**(3): 216–224.

311. Henderson, M.C., et al., S-oxygenation of the thioether organophosphate insecticides phorate and disulfoton by human lung flavin-containing monooxygenase 2. *Biochem Pharmacol*, 2004. **68**(5): 959–967.

312. Henderson, M.C., et al., Human flavin-containing monooxygenase form 2 S-oxygenation: Sulfenic acid formation from thioureas and oxidation of glutathione. *Chem Res Toxicol*, 2004. **17**(5): 633–640.

313. Smith, P.B. and C. Crespi, Thiourea toxicity in mouse C3H/10T1/2 cells expressing human flavin-dependent monooxygenase 3. *Biochem Pharmacol*, 2002. **63**(11): 1941–1948.

314. Francois, A.A., et al., Human flavin-containing monooxygenase 2.1 catalyzes oxygenation of the antitubercular drugs thiacetazone and ethionamide. *Drug Metab Dispos*, 2009. **37**(1): 178–186.

315. El-Sherbeni, A.A. and A.O. El-Kadi, The role of epoxide hydrolases in health and disease. *Arch Toxicol*, 2014. **88**(11): 2013–2032.

316. He, J., et al., Soluble epoxide hydrolase: A potential target for metabolic diseases. *J Diabetes*, 2016. **8**(3): 305–313.

317. Vaclavikova, R., D.J. Hughes, and P. Soucek, Microsomal epoxide hydrolase 1 (EPHX1): Gene, structure, function, and role in human disease. *Gene*, 2015. **571**(1): 1–8.

318. El-Sherbeni, A.A. and A.O.S. El-Kadi, The role of epoxide hydrolases in health and disease. *Arch Toxicol*, 2014. **88**(11): 2013–2032.

319. Kondraganti, S.R., et al., Persistent induction of hepatic and pulmonary phase II enzymes by 3-methylcholanthrene in rats. *Toxicol Sci*, 2008. **102**(2): 337–344.

320. Bond, J.A., J.R. Harkema, and V.I. Russell, Regional distribution of xenobiotic metabolizing enzymes in respiratory airways of dogs. *Drug Metab Dispos*, 1988. **16**(1): 116–124.

321. Devereux, T.R., J.J. Diliberto, and J.R. Fouts, Cytochrome P-450 monooxygenase, epoxide hydrolase and flavin monooxygenase activities in Clara cells and alveolar type II cells isolated from rabbit. *Cell Biol Toxicol*, 1985. **1**(2): 57–65.

322. Park, J.Y., et al., Genetic analysis of microsomal epoxide hydrolase gene and its association with lung cancer risk. *Eur J Cancer Prev*, 2005. **14**(3): 223–230.

323. Lin, P., et al., Association of CYP1A1 and microsomal epoxide hydrolase polymorphisms with lung squamous cell carcinoma. *Br J Cancer*, 2000. **82**(4): 852–857.

324. Kiyohara, C., et al., EPHX1 polymorphisms and the risk of lung cancer: A HuGE review. *Epidemiology*, 2006. **17**(1): 89–99.

325. Peluso, M.E.M., et al., DNA adducts and combinations of multiple lung cancer at-risk alleles in environmentally exposed and smoking subjects. *Environ Mol Mutagen*, 2013. **54**(6): 375–383.

326. Tung, K.Y., C.H. Tsai, and Y.L. Lee, Microsomal epoxide hydroxylase genotypes/diplotypes, traffic air pollution, and childhood asthma. *Chest*, 2011. **139**(4): 839–848.

327. Cruzan, G., et al., CYP2F2-generated metabolites, not styrene oxide, are a key event mediating the mode of action of styrene-induced mouse lung tumors. *Regul Toxicol Pharmacol*, 2012. **62**(1): 214–220.

328. Rowland, A., J.O. Miners, and P.I. Mackenzie, The UDP-glucuronosyltransferases: Their role in drug metabolism and detoxification. *Int J Biochem Cell B*, 2013. **45**(6): 1121–1132.

329. Arnold, S.M., et al., Two homologues encoding human UDP-glucose: Glycoprotein glucosyltransferase differ in mRNA expression and enzymatic activity. *Biochemistry*, 2000. **39**(9): 2149–2163.

330. Burchell, B., et al., Drug-mediated toxicity caused by genetic deficiency of UDP-glucuronosyltransferases. *Toxicol Lett*, 2000. **112–113**: 333–340.

331. Tukey, R.H. and C.P. Strassburg, Human UDP-glucuronosyltransferases: metabolism, expression, and disease. *Annu Rev Pharmacol Toxicol*, 2000. **40**: 581–616.

332. Mackenzie, P.I., et al., Nomenclature update for the mammalian UDP glycosyltransferase (UGT) gene superfamily. *Pharmacogenet Genom*, 2005. **15**(10): 677–685.

333. Mackenzie, P.I., et al., The UDP glycosyltransferase gene superfamily: recommended nomenclature update based on evolutionary divergence. *Pharmacogenetics*, 1997. **7**(4): 255–269.

334. Batt, A.M., et al., Drug metabolizing enzymes related to laboratory medicine: Cytochromes P-450 and UDP-glucuronosyltransferases. *Clin Chim Acta*, 1994. **226**(2): 171–190.

335. Strassburg, C.P., et al., Differential expression of the UGT1A locus in human liver, biliary, and gastric tissue: Identification of UGT1A7 and UGT1A10 transcripts in extrahepatic tissue. *Mol Pharmacol*, 1997. **52**(2): 212–220.

336. Shelby, M.K., et al., Tissue mRNA expression of the rat UDP-glucuronosyltransferase gene family. *Drug Metab Dispos*, 2003. **31**(3): 326–333.

337. Zheng, Z., J.L. Fang, and P. Lazarus, Glucuronidation: An important mechanism for detoxification of benzo[a]pyrene metabolites in aerodigestive tract tissues. *Drug Metab Dispos*, 2002. **30**(4): 397–403.

338. Yoshimura, T., S. Tanaka, and T. Horie, Species difference and tissue distribution of uridine diphosphate-glucuronyltransferase activities toward E6080, 1-naphthol and 4-hydroxybiphenyl. *J Pharmacobiodyn*, 1992. **15**(8): 387–393.

339. Jones, K.G., et al., Xenobiotic metabolism in Clara cells and alveolar type II cells isolated from lungs of rats treated with beta-naphthoflavone. *J Pharmacol Exp Ther*, 1983. **225**(2): 316–319.

340. Elovaara, E., et al., Polycyclic aromatic hydrocarbon (PAH) metabolizing enzyme activities in human lung, and their inducibility by exposure to naphthalene, phenanthrene, pyrene, chrysene, and benzo(a)pyrene as shown in the rat lung and liver. *Arch Toxicol*, 2007. **81**(3): 169–182.

341. Jedlitschky, G., et al., Cloning and characterization of a novel human olfactory UDP-glucuronosyltransferase. *Biochem J*, 1999. **340**(Pt 3): 837–843.

342. Turgeon, D., et al., Relative enzymatic activity, protein stability, and tissue distribution of human steroid-metabolizing UGT2B subfamily members. *Endocrinology*, 2001. **142**(2): 778–787.

343. Lazard, D., et al., Odorant signal termination by olfactory UDP glucuronosyl transferase. *Nature*, 1991. **349**(6312): 790–793.

344. Odum, J., J.R. Foster, and T. Green, A mechanism for the development of Clara cell lesions in the mouse lung after exposure to trichloroethylene. *Chem Biol Interact*, 1992. **83**(2): 135–153.

345. Hargus, S.J., et al., Covalent modification of rat liver dipeptidyl peptidase IV (CD26) by the nonsteroidal anti-inflammatory drug diclofenac. *Chem Res Toxicol*, 1995. **8**(8): 993–996.

346. McGurk, K.A., et al., Reactivity of mefenamic acid 1-o-acyl glucuronide with proteins *in vitro* and *ex vivo.Drug Metab Dispos*, 1996. **24**(8): 842–849.

347. Hu, D.G., et al., Genetic polymorphisms of human UDP-glucuronosyltransferase (UGT) genes and cancer risk. *Drug Metab Rev*, 2016. **48**(1): 47–69.

348. Board, P.G. and D. Menon, Glutathione transferases, regulators of cellular metabolism and physiology. *Biochim Biophys Acta (BBA) – Gen Subj*, 2013. **1830**(5): 3267–3288.

349. Hayes, J.D., J.U. Flanagan, and I.R. Jowsey, Glutathione transferases. *Annu Rev Pharmacol Toxicol*, 2005. **45**: 51–88.

350. Jakobsson, P.J., et al., Common structural features of MAPEG – a widespread superfamily of membrane associated proteins with highly divergent functions in eicosanoid and glutathione metabolism. *Protein Sci*, 1999. **8**(3): 689–692.

351. Khojasteh-Bakht, S.C., S.D. Nelson, and W.M. Atkins, Glutathione S-transferase catalyzes the isomerization of (R)-2-hydroxymenthofuran to mintlactones. *Arch Biochem Biophys*, 1999. **370**(1): 59–65.

352. Bresell, A., et al., Bioinformatic and enzymatic characterization of the MAPEG superfamily. *FEBS J*, 2005. **272**(7): 1688–1703.

353. Duan, X., A.R. Buckpitt, and C.G. Plopper, Variation in antioxidant enzyme activities in anatomic sub-compartments within rat and rhesus monkey lung. *Toxicol Appl Pharmacol*, 1993. **123**(1): 73–82.

354. Lee, M.J. and D. Dinsdale, Immunolocalization of glutathione S-transferase isoenzymes in bronchiolar epithelium of rats and mice. *Am J Physiol*, 1994. **267**(6 Pt 1): L766–L774.

355. Anttila, S., et al., Immunohistochemical localization of glutathione S-transferases in human lung. *Cancer Res*, 1993. **53**(23): 5643–5648.

356. Singhal, S.S., et al., Glutathione S-transferases of human lung: Characterization and evaluation of the protective role of the alpha-class isozymes against lipid peroxidation. *Arch Biochem Biophys*, 1992. **299**(2): 232–241.

357. Forkert, P.G., et al., Morphologic changes and covalent binding of 1,1-dichloroethylene in Clara and alveolar type II cells isolated from lungs of mice following *in vivo* administration. *Drug Metab Dispos*, 1990. **18**(4): 534–539.

358. Nakajima, T., et al., Expression and polymorphism of glutathione S-transferase in human lungs: Risk factors in smoking-related lung cancer. *Carcinogenesis*, 1995. **16**(4): 707–711.

359. Wang, I.J., et al., Glutathione S-transferase, incense burning and asthma in children. *Eur Respir J*, 2011. **37**(6): 1371–1377.

360. Piacentini, S., et al., Glutathione S-transferase gene polymorphisms and air pollution as interactive risk factors for asthma in a multicentre Italian field study: A preliminary study. *Ann Hum Biol*, 2010. **37**(3): 427–439.

361. McCunney, R.J., Asthma, genes, and air pollution. *J Occup Environ Med*, 2005. **47**(12): 1285–1291.

362. Lee, Y.L., et al., Glutathione S-transferase P1 gene polymorphism and air pollution as interactive risk factors for childhood asthma. *Clin Exp Allergy*, 2004. **34**(11): 1707–1713.

363. Islam, T., et al., Glutathione-S-transferase (GST) P1, GSTM1, exercise, ozone and asthma incidence in school children. *Thorax*, 2009. **64**(3): 197–202.

364. Hwang, B.F., et al., Fine particle, ozone exposure, and asthma/wheezing: Effect modification by gluta-thione S-transferase P1 polymorphisms. *PLoS One*, 2013. **8**(1): e52715.

365. Hersoug, L.G., et al., The relationship of glutathione-S-transferases copy number variation and indoor air pollution to symptoms and markers of respiratory disease. *Clin Respir J*, 2012. **6**(3): 175–185.

366. Bowatte, G., et al., Do variants in GSTs modify the association between traffic air pollution and asthma in adolescence? *Int J Mol Sci*, 2016. **17**(4): 485.

367. Nakachi, K., et al., Polymorphisms of the CYP1A1 and glutathione S-transferase genes associated with susceptibility to lung cancer in relation to cigarette dose in a Japanese population. *Cancer Res*, 1993. **53**(13): 2994–2999.

368. Engle, M.R., et al., Physiological role of mGSTA4-4, a glutathione S-transferase metabolizing 4-hydroxynonenal: Generation and analysis of mGsta4 null mouse. *Toxicol Appl Pharmacol*, 2004. **194**(3): 296–308.

369. Phimister, A.J., et al., Glutathione depletion is a major determinant of inhaled naphthalene respiratory toxicity and naphthalene metabolism in mice. *Toxicol Sci*, 2004. **82**(1): 268–278.

370. Phimister, A.J., et al., Prevention of naphthalene-induced pulmonary toxicity by glutathione prodrugs: Roles for glutathione depletion in adduct formation and cell injury. *J Biochem Mol Toxicol*, 2005. **19**(1): 42–51.

371. Phimister, A.J., et al., Consequences of abrupt glutathione depletion in murine Clara cells: Ultrastructural and biochemical investigations into the role of glutathione loss in naphthalene cytotoxicity. *J Pharmacol Exp Ther*, 2005. **314**(2): 506–513.

372. Wisnewski, A.V., et al., Isocyanate-conjugated human lung epithelial cell proteins: A link between exposure and asthma? *J Allergy Clin Immunol*, 1999. **104**(2 Pt 1): 341–347.

373. Wisnewski, A.V., et al., Glutathione protects human airway proteins and epithelial cells from iso-cyanates. *Clin Exp Allergy*, 2005. **35**(3): 352–357.

374. Guengerich, F.P., W.A. McCormick, and J.B. Wheeler, Analysis of the kinetic mechanism of halo-alkane conjugation by mammalian theta-class glutathione transferases. *Chem Res Toxicol*, 2003. **16**(11): 1493–1499.

375. Wheeler, J.B., et al., Conjugation of haloalkanes by bacterial and mammalian glutathione transferases: Mono- and dihalomethanes. *Chem Res Toxicol*, 2001. **14**(8): 1118–1127.

376. Piacentini, S., et al., Glutathione S-transferase polymorphisms, asthma susceptibility and confounding variables: a meta-analysis. *Mol Biol Rep*, 2013. **40**(4): 3299–3313.

377. Minelli, C., et al., Glutathione-S-transferase genes and asthma phenotypes: A Human Genome Epidemiology (HuGE) systematic review and meta-analysis including unpublished data. *Int J Epidemiol*, 2010. **39**(2): 539–562.

11

Sites of Extra Hepatic Metabolism, Part II: Gut

Dan-Dan Tian, Emily J. Cox, and Mary F. Paine

CONTENTS

Introduction

The oral route remains the most common, convenient, economical, and generally safest means for drug administration. However, for drugs intended to act systemically, this route is not always the most efficient due to the numerous anatomic and physiologic barriers that drugs can encounter from the time of ingestion until the time of entry into the general circulation. Consequently, before an orally administered drug enters the systemic circulation and elicits pharmacologic effects in the target tissue(s), significant loss of the original dose can occur during sequential passage through the gastrointestinal (GI) tract, the liver, and the cardiopulmonary system. These barriers can preclude the use of some drugs as oral agents. Isoproterenol, dihydroergotamine, lidocaine, nitroglycerin, fentanyl, and naloxone are examples of drugs that are susceptible to a high *first-pass effect*, which refers to the loss of drug as the dose passes, for the first time, through organs of elimination during transit from the site of administration to the systemic circulation [1]. Processes known to cause significant loss of active drug during first-pass include incomplete release from the dosage form, degradation in the GI lumen, poor permeation through the GI wall, active export into the GI lumen, biliary excretion, and metabolism. Of these processes, only metabolism can take place in all of the aforementioned organs.

Metabolism represents the major means by which the body eliminates drugs [2,3]. Enzymatic modification of the drug generally produces inactive metabolites with increased polarity and water-solubility to enhance excretion. The extent of conversion of several drugs to inactive metabolites can be large enough such that circulating concentrations of active drug are reduced significantly, which in turn can cause a significant decrease in pharmacologic activity and, ultimately, a reduced clinical response.

Drugs with a narrow therapeutic window that undergo extensive first-pass metabolism are particularly vulnerable to a reduced clinical response. In addition, the extent of first-pass metabolism can vary substantially between individuals, further hampering the optimization of oral drug therapy.

Of the first-pass organs of drug elimination, the liver is the most often implicated, in large part because it expresses the highest specific contents of drug metabolizing enzymes. Next to the liver, the small intestinal mucosa is undoubtedly the most important extrahepatic site of drug metabolism [3]. Although the role of the relevant enzymes in the liver has been established for some time, relatively less is known about the complement of enzymes in the small intestine. Nevertheless, considerable progress has been made within the last three decades regarding the identification and characterization of different subfamilies and individual isoforms. In parallel, the potential impact of intestinal first-pass metabolism on oral drug disposition has become increasingly recognized. Before discussing the various enzymes and the clinical implications, an understanding of drug movement through the GI wall is warranted.

Drug Movement through the Gastrointestinal Wall

The GI tract is the first in the sequence of organs that drugs encounter when taken orally. Most drugs are administered as solid dosage forms. As such, dissolution of the dosage form must occur in the GI lumen before the molecules are absorbed through the GI wall. Several physicochemical properties of both the drug and the GI environment govern the rate of dissolution. Drug properties include solubility, particle size, salt form, complexation, and crystal form; environmental properties include pH and lumenal stirring [4]. Following dissolution of the dosage form, the drug molecules must then traverse the contents of the lumen (e.g., water, food, bacteria) and a mucous layer before they are absorbed through the epithelial layer into the lamina propria, which contains the capillaries that eventually lead to the portal vein.

Most drugs are weak acids or weak bases and are absorbed by passive diffusion. Based on the pH partition hypothesis, which assumes that only unionized drug can traverse biological membranes, weak acids should be absorbed more rapidly from the stomach (pH 1–3) than from the small intestine (pH 6–8) or large intestine (pH 6–7) [5]. The converse is predicted for weak bases. Contrary to this hypothesis, the majority of drugs are absorbed predominately in the small intestine, regardless of whether they are weak acids or weak bases, and whether in the unionized or ionized form. This discrepancy between actual sites of drug absorption and those predicted by the pH partition hypothesis can be explained by two key factors that render the small intestine more receptive to drug absorption than the stomach or the large intestine: surface area and permeability.

The adult small intestine, which has an anatomical length (i.e., length at autopsy or after surgical removal) of approximately 500 cm, is divided into three segments: duodenum, jejunum, and ileum [6]. The duodenum measures 25–30 cm in length, begins just distal to the pyloric sphincter of the stomach, and ends at the ligament of Treitz [6]. Whereas the ligament of Treitz distinguishes the duodenum from the jejunum, no such anatomical landmark distinguishes the jejunum from the ileum; however, the jejunum is generally assumed to represent the proximal two-fifths, and the ileum the distal three-fifths, of the remainder of the small intestine (approximately 200 and 300 cm, respectively). The length of the entire large intestine is approximately 160 cm [6,7].

The major function of the small intestine is to absorb nutrients. The unique morphology of the mucosal surface facilitates this task. A cross-section of the small intestine shows extensive folding (Figure 11.1). These folds of Kerkering, or plicae circulares, are circular folds created by mucosal/submucosal invaginations into the lumen. These structures, which are predominant in the duodenum and jejunum and are essentially absent by the middle ileum, are lined with finger-like projections, or villi. At the base of the villi are the crypts of Lieberkuhn, which consist of undifferentiated (crypt) cells. Over the course of two to three days, crypt cells migrate to the villous tips while maturing into various cell types, including mucus-secreting goblet cells, enteroendocrine cells, and absorptive cells (enterocytes); after three more days, the mature cells of the villous tips are shed into the lumen [6,8]. Enterocytes, which are the predominant cell types that compose the single layer of epithelial cells lining the villi, are further lined with microvilli. Taken together, this combination of circular folds, villi, and microvilli creates a tremendous absorptive surface area. In adults, this area has historically been estimated at 200 m^2,

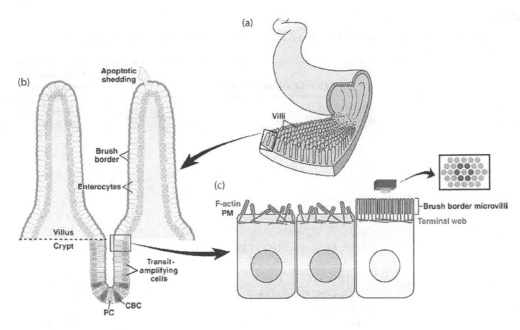

FIGURE 11.1 *Functional architecture of the intestinal epithelium.* (a) The lumen is lined with villi. (b) Enterocytes are generated in a stem cell niche composed of crypt base columnar (CBC) cells and flanking Paneth cells (PC). (c) The enterocytes are lined with microvilli. (Reproduced with permission from Crawley, S.W. et al., *J. Cell Biol.*, 207, 441–451, 2014.)

roughly the size of a tennis court, but more recent estimates suggest an area closer to one-half of a badminton court (30 m²) [9]. In comparison, the surface area of the stomach is approximately 0.053 m², and that of the large intestine is approximately 0.35 m² [7].

In addition to having a much greater surface area than the stomach and large intestine, the small intestine is more permeable, due in part to having both a relatively thin epithelial layer and a lower electrical resistance [1]. Thus, as with nutrients, the small intestine is the prime site for the absorption of drugs. Additionally, because surface area and permeability decline from proximal to distal regions, it can be argued that, at least for immediate-release formulations, drug absorption occurs predominately in the duodenum and jejunum.

Absorption of drug molecules through the small intestinal epithelial layer occurs *via* paracellular or transcellular mechanisms. That is, the molecule can either passively diffuse between enterocytes (paracellular), or it can passively diffuse or be actively transported through the apical (lumenal) and basolateral membranes of enterocytes (transcellular). Most hydrophilic, polar drugs are absorbed by the paracellular route (exceptions are polar drugs that are actively transported across the epithelial cell), whereas most lipophilic, nonpolar drugs are absorbed by the transcellular route [10]. For drugs absorbed by the latter route, the opportunity exists for first-pass metabolism, as the relevant enzymes are located intracellularly, predominantly in the endoplasmic reticulum or cytosol of enterocytes. As such, evidence has amassed that the small intestine can contribute significantly to the overall first-pass metabolism of drugs, potentially with clinical ramifications.

Clinical Implications of Intestinal First-Pass Metabolism

Many commonly prescribed drugs undergo extensive first-pass metabolism upon oral administration (Table 11.1). Regarding those listed in Table 11.1, at least 45% of the original dose is lost, on average, before entering the systemic circulation. That is, all have a low average *oral bioavailability* (F_{oral}), which refers to the fraction of the oral dose that reaches the systemic circulation in the unchanged form. Because metabolism is frequently the major driver of first-pass drug elimination, F_{oral} is often used to assess the

TABLE 11.1

Selected Drugs with Low and Variable Oral Bioavailability Believed to Be due in Part to Intestinal First-Pass Metabolism

Drug	Intestinal Enzyme(s)	Oral Bioavailability (%) (Average ± SD)
Alfentanil	CYP3A [71,77]	43 ± 19
Amiodarone	CYP3A	46 ± 22
Atorvastatin	CYP3A	12
Buspirone	CYP3A	3.9 ± 4.3
Cyclosporine	CYP3A	28 ± 18
Diclofenac	CYP2C9	54 ± 2
Dihydroergotamine	CYP3A [178,179]	0.5 ± 0.1
Diltiazem	CYP3A	38 ± 11
Erythromycin	CYP3A	35 ± 25
Ethinyl estradiol	CYP3A, SULT1E1, UGT1A1 [142,152,163]	42
Felodipine	CYP3A	15 ± 8
Fluvastatin	CYP2C9	29 ± 18
Irinotecan	CYP3A, CES2 [137,138,180]	8
Isoproterenol	SULT1A3 [142,148]	28
Lidocaine	CYP3A	35 ± 11
Losartan	CYP2C9, CYP3A	36 ± 16
Lovastatin	CYP3A	≤5
Midazolam	CYP3A	44 ± 17
Nicardipine	CYP3A	18 ± 11
Nifedipine	CYP3A	50 ± 13
Omeprazole	CYP2C19, CYP3A	53 ± 29
Oxybutinin	CYP3A	1.6–10.9
Raloxifene	UGT1A1, UGT1A8, UGT1A10 [164,165]	2
Saquinavir	CYP3A	4–13
Sirolimus	CYP3A	15
Tacrolimus	CYP3A	25 ± 10
Terbutaline	SULT1A3 [150]	14 ± 2
Triazolam	CYP3A	44
Verapamil	CYP3A, CYP2C9	22 ± 8

Enzyme(s) and bioavailability values are from reference [181] unless indicated otherwise.

extent of first-pass metabolism. F_{oral} can be calculated from the ratio of the area under the blood or plasma concentration-time curve following oral administration (AUC_{oral}) to that following intravenous administration (AUC_{iv}) after correcting for dose (Equation 11.1):

$$F_{oral} = \frac{AUC_{oral}}{AUC_{iv}} \times \frac{Dose_{iv}}{Dose_{oral}} \tag{11.1}$$

When drug metabolizing organs are arranged sequentially (e.g., the small intestine and liver), F_{oral} may be viewed as the product of the fractions of the oral dose that escape first-pass metabolism by each organ (Eq. 11.2):

$$F_{oral} = F_{abs} \times F_I \times F_L \tag{11.2}$$

where F_{abs} is the fraction of an oral dose absorbed intact through the apical membrane of the enterocyte, and F_I and F_L are the fractions of the absorbed dose that escape metabolism by the intestine (enterocytes) and liver, respectively. In terms of extraction ratios (fractions of the absorbed dose that do not escape first-pass metabolism), Eq. 11.2 can be rewritten as follows (Eq. 11.3):

$$F_{oral} = F_{abs} \times (1-E_I) \times (1-E_L) \tag{11.3}$$

where E_I and E_L are the extraction ratios associated with the intestine and liver, respectively. Equation 11.2 illustrates the impact of a second presystemic site of metabolism on F_{oral}. For example, if the entire dose of a drug is absorbed into the enterocytes intact ($F_{abs} = 1$), the F_I is 60%, and the F_L is 40%, then an F_{oral} of 24% is predicted. If only first-pass metabolism by the liver is considered ($1 \times 1 \times 40\%$), then an F_{oral} of 40% is predicted. Thus, omission of the intestinal component would result in an overestimation of F_{oral}, which could potentially lead to suboptimal dosing and potential therapeutic failure due to ineffective concentrations at the site(s) of action. For drugs that have a wide therapeutic window, simply increasing the dose can rectify this situation. However, for drugs that have a narrow therapeutic window, optimization of oral dosing regimens becomes more challenging. Factors that significantly alter metabolism, including other xenobiotics that induce or inhibit drug metabolizing enzymes, thus altering F_I and/or F_L, present additional challenges to optimal oral drug therapy.

The above equation also illustrates the potential impact of a second presystemic site of metabolism on the interindividual variation in F_{oral}. For example, if a drug has an F_I that varies from 30% to 60% (2-fold range), an F_L that varies from 20% to 80% (4-fold range), and the extraction efficiencies of the gut and liver vary independently, then F_{oral} will vary from 6% to 48% (8-fold range), resulting in a 100% increase in the variation in F_{oral} (if only F_L were considered initially). Data collected from 143 pharmacokinetic studies showed a significant inverse correlation between F_{oral} and the interindividual variation in F_{oral}, as measured by the coefficient of variation in F_{oral} [11]. This relationship indicated that the greater the extent of first-pass elimination, the greater the variation in F_{oral}. Accordingly, knowledge of the degree of variation in the expression of major drug metabolizing enzymes in the human intestine is essential, as these enzymes can represent a key determinant of not only the extent of first-pass metabolism, but also the interindividual variation in F_{oral} and the probability and magnitude of drug-xenobiotic interactions [12,13].

Drug Metabolizing Enzymes in the Gut Wall

The human GI tract shares several of the same drug metabolizing enzymes as the liver and includes both phase I and phase II enzymes (Table 11.2). As with enzymes in the hepatocyte, enzymes in the enterocyte generally reside in either the microsomal or cytosolic fraction (Table 11.2). Compared to enzymes in the liver, research on the expression and catalytic properties of the complement of enzymes in the

TABLE 11.2

Drug Metabolizing Enzymes in the Human Small Intestine that Are Known to Be Expressed at the Protein Level and to have Catalytic Activity

Enzyme	Location in Subcellular Fraction
Phase I	
Cytochromes P450 (CYPs)	Microsomes
Carboxylesterases (CESs)	Microsomes, Cytosol
Epoxide Hydrolases (EHs)	Microsomes, Cytosol
Flavin Monooxygenases (FMOs)	Microsomes
Phase II	
Sulfotransferases (SULTs)	Cytosol
UDP-Glucuronosyltransferases (UGTs)	Microsomes
Catechol-*O*-methyltransferases (COMTs)	Microsomes, Cytosol
N-Acetyltransferases (NATs)	Cytosol
Glutathione *S*-Transferases (GSTs)	Microsomes, Cytosol

intestine has lagged, largely due to a limited supply of high quality tissue, as well as a lack of sensitive methods for detecting the relatively lower expression and catalytic activity of gut enzymes compared to liver enzymes. However, over the past two decades, a variety of human intestine-derived tissue preparations have become available, including subcellular fractions (microsomes, cytosol), precision-cut tissue slices, shed enterocytes, Ussing chamber preparations, and intestinal cell lines [14–16]. In parallel, ongoing identification of selective catalytic probe substrates and inhibitors and improved methods of detection have permitted rigorous characterization of specific intestinal enzymes.

Phase I Enzymes

Cytochromes P450

The cytochromes P450 (CYPs) are the most prominent of the enteric phase I enzymes. The existence of CYP protein and associated monooxygenase activity (7-ethoxycoumarin O-deethylation) in the human small intestine was first reported in 1979 by Hoensch and coworkers [17], who determined total CYP content in a small number of surgical specimens. Average ($\pm$ SD) content, as measured by carbon monoxide difference spectra, declined from proximal to distal regions and ranged from 93 ± 19 to 35 ± 4 pmol/mg microsomal protein; 7-ethoxycoumarin O-deethylase activity paralleled this pattern. Similar values were reported later by other investigators [18,19]. Thus, per mg microsomal protein, total CYP content in the average adult small intestine ranges from approximately 10%–30% of that in the average human liver. Almost a decade following the report by Hoensch et al., a series of pivotal *in vitro* and *in vivo* studies by Watkins and coworkers identified CYP3A as the major CYP subfamily expressed in human enterocytes.

CYP3A

In Vitro Studies   Using mucosae isolated from jejunal sections from four surgical patients, Watkins et al. identified a CYP enzyme and associated mRNA that were recognized selectively by an anti-CYP3A1 murine monoclonal antibody (which detected all human CYP3A forms) and HLp (CYP3A4) cDNA, respectively [20]. Using purified HLp as the reference standard, average ($\pm$ SD) CYP3A protein content in microsomes prepared from the specimens was comparable to that for liver microsomes prepared from four separate organ donors/surgical patients (70 ± 20 vs 65 ± 20 pmol/mg). The average CYP3A-catalyzed rate of erythromycin N-demethylation in jejunal microsomes was comparable to that for liver microsomes and was inhibited by anti-CYP3A1. Three years later, de Waziers and coworkers [21] quantified, by immunoblot analysis, the expression of various CYP isoforms/subfamilies in microsomes prepared from the following human extrahepatic tissues: esophagus, stomach, duodenum, jejunum, ileum, colon, and kidney. These investigators reported that, next to the liver, the duodenum was the highest with respect to immunoreactive CYP3A protein, followed by the jejunum, followed by the ileum. Average duodenal, jejunal, and ileal CYP3A content represented approximately 50%, 30%, and 10%, respectively, of average hepatic CYP3A content. Corresponding values for the remaining extrahepatic organs were less than 5%. Consistent with the report by Watkins et al., CYP3A was the dominant CYP expressed in all three regions of the small intestine. More recently, a comprehensive analysis of microsomes prepared from the duodenal/proximal jejunal portion of 31 unrelated human donor small intestines demonstrated CYP3A as the major "piece" of the intestinal CYP "pie", representing ~80% of total immunoquantified CYP protein [22] (Figure 11.2). Subsequent to the earlier *in vitro* studies, the significance of intestinal CYP3A to first-pass drug metabolism *in vivo* was demonstrated.

In Vivo Studies   The widely used immunosuppressive agent, cyclosporine, is plagued with having a large interindividual variation in F_{oral}, which has been reported to range from 5% to 89% for the conventional formulation (Sandimunne®) [23] and from 21% to 73% for the microemulsion formulation (Neoral®) [24–27]. This property, coupled with a narrow therapeutic window, can lead to an under- or overdosing of the patient, which in turn can lead to graft rejection or toxicity. The low and unpredictable F_{oral} of cyclosporine was believed initially to result from erratic absorption through the intestinal lumen

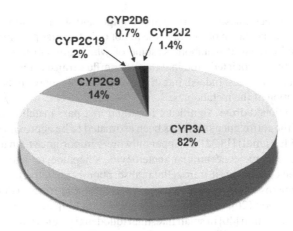

FIGURE 11.2 *The average human proximal small intestinal cytochrome P450 "pie".* The percent contributions of individual enzymes are based on average total immunoquantified CYP content (61 pmol/mg). (Adapted with permission from Paine, M.F. et al., *Drug Metab. Dispos.*, 34, 880–886, 2006.)

coupled with variable hepatic first-pass metabolism (i.e., a low and variable F_{abs} and F_L). However, Watkins and coworkers [28], after instilling cyclosporine into the duodenum of two patients during the anhepatic phase of their liver transplant operations, measured appreciable concentrations of two CYP3A-mediated primary metabolites in hepatic portal and systemic blood. The investigators concluded that the extrahepatic site of metabolism was the gut because organs other than the gut (i.e. kidney and lung) express low levels of CYP3A, and portal metabolite concentrations exceeded systemic concentrations at the end of the anhepatic phase of the operation. These observations provided direct evidence that the small intestine contributes significantly to the first-pass metabolism of a CYP3A substrate. A subsequent pharmacokinetic analysis of cyclosporine AUC after oral and intravenous administration suggested that the intestine, rather than the liver, was largely responsible for the first-pass elimination of cyclosporine [29]. However, cyclosporine is now known to be a substrate for the efflux transporter P-glycoprotein (P-gp), which is expressed on the apical membranes of enterocytes and other cell types. As such, this indirect approach would not distinguish between intestinal CYP3A-mediated metabolism and P-gp-mediated efflux.

Unlike cyclosporine, the sedative-hypnotic agent and CYP3A substrate midazolam is not a substrate for P-gp [30] and thus should serve as a "clean" *in vivo* CYP3A probe. Using a study design similar to that for the cyclosporine study, the disposition of midazolam and primary metabolite, 1′-hydroxymidazolam, was examined in a larger group of anhepatic transplant recipients following either intravenous (n = 5) or intraduodenal (n = 5) administration [31]. Blood was collected simultaneously from the hepatic portal vein and a peripheral artery during the approximately one-hour anhepatic phase. Using the difference between the arterial and hepatic portal venous midazolam AUCs (intravenous) or between the hepatic portal venous and arterial midazolam and 1′-hydroxymidazolam AUCs (intraduodenal), an average (± SD) extraction fraction of 8% ± 12% and 43% ± 18% was calculated for subjects who received midazolam by the intravenous and intraduodenal route, respectively. The low and variable extraction fraction following intravenous administration indicated that the intestine contributed somewhat to the systemic metabolism of midazolam. Importantly, the fivefold greater value following oral administration was consistent with the average intestinal extraction ratio estimated in healthy volunteers (43%–47%) [32,33]. These values also were consistent with the average hepatic extraction ratio estimated in healthy volunteers (44% ± 14%) [32]. These data strongly indicated that the small intestine is a major determinant of the overall extent of the first-pass metabolism of midazolam and can rival the liver.

Using the indirect approach, enteric CYP3A also has been shown to contribute significantly to the first-pass metabolism of alfentanil, atorvastatin, buspirone, cisapride, felodipine, nifedipine, and verapamil [34–36]. The comparable contributions of the intestine and liver (mean extraction ratio of 49% and 48%, respectively) to the overall first-pass elimination of verapamil was confirmed subsequently using a method involving a multilumen intestinal perfusion technique and stable isotope-labeled drug [37]. This method demonstrated the importance of the intestine to not only the first-pass metabolism of verapamil, but also the secretion of verapamil metabolites, some of which are substrates for P-gp and possibly MRP2 (multidrug resistance associated protein 2), another efflux transporter known to be expressed on the apical membranes of enterocytes. Indeed, intestinal secretion was shown to be as important as biliary excretion for the elimination of the metabolites.

For all of the aforementioned drugs, significant intestinal first-pass metabolism occurred despite that total CYP3A content of the entire gut mucosa has been estimated to be approximately 1% of total hepatic CYP3A content (70 vs 5490 nmol) [18,38]. Of apparently more importance than total enzyme mass is the comparable intracellular enzyme concentration (enterocyte vs hepatocyte) and the obligatory nature of drug passage through the enterocyte (if transcellular absorption is operative). Thus, a more appropriate comparison might be microsomal intrinsic activities. For example, mean CYP3A-mediated rates of erythromycin N-demethylation [20], tacrolimus O-demethylation [39], midazolam 1'-hydroxylation [18], and testosterone 6β-hydroxylation [40] in small intestinal (duodenal/jejunal) microsomes were 45%–120% of corresponding metabolic rates in hepatic microsomes. Based on these data, mean intestinal mucosal intrinsic clearances may be comparable to corresponding hepatic intrinsic clearances. Whether or not such a similarity will occur *in vivo* is more difficult to predict, as total oral dose, enzyme saturability, and absorption rate become relevant. Should the dose be large enough, and the K_m of the drug for the enzyme active site be low enough, it is possible that the majority of absorbed drug could escape intestinal first-pass metabolism. Some of the HIV protease inhibitors (e.g., indinavir, saquinavir, and the active metabolite of fosamprenavir, amprenavir) may represent such drugs.

CYP3A4 versus CYP3A5   As in the liver, CYP3A4 protein appears to be expressed constitutively in the small intestine of all individuals, whereas CYP3A5 expression is polymorphic. Immunoreactive CYP3A5 protein was detected readily at a frequency of 20%–30% in intestinal tissue obtained from adult Caucasians [18,41,42]. Moreover, if detected, the enzyme was expressed along the length of the small intestinal tract [18]. As has been shown for the liver [43], the frequency of CYP3A5 expression in the small intestine varies among different racial/ethnic groups [42]. With the advent of specific, commercially available antibodies and suitable reference standards for immunoblot analysis, CYP3A5 was reported to constitute 3%–80% of total intestinal CYP3A (CYP3A4+CYP3A5) protein content [22,44]. Accordingly, like hepatic CYP3A5 [43,45], enteric CYP3A5 may contribute significantly to the first-pass metabolism of drugs in some individuals. Identification of a selective *in vivo* CYP3A5 probe substrate is needed to test this hypothesis.

Significant expression of CYP3A4 in the GI tract appears to be restricted to the small intestine. Both CYP3A5 mRNA and protein expression in the mucosa of the stomach and colon were more prominent than corresponding CYP3A4 measures [46,47]. Consistent with these observations, in two full-length human donor small intestines that were CYP3A5-positive, the ratio of CYP3A5–CYP3A4 immunoreactive protein decreased from duodenum to jejunum, then increased in distal ileum to values comparable to or greater than those observed for the duodenum [48]. Finally, Gervot et al. [49] detected CYP3A5 protein, but not CYP3A4 protein, in colonic mucosa from 40 unrelated and uninduced tissue donors. The authors suggested that any CYP3A4 in colonic tissue is likely to be a consequence of prior treatment of the donor with an enzyme inducer.

Localization   CYP3A4 protein expression along the length of the small intestine is not uniform. Enzyme content is generally highest from duodenum to middle jejunum, then declines progressively to distal ileum [18,19,21]. Median CYP3A4 content in microsomes prepared from mucosal scrapings obtained from 20 donor small intestines decreased from 31 to 23 to 17 pmol/mg protein in duodenum, jejunum, and ileum, respectively [18]. CYP3A-catalyzed midazolam 1'-hydroxlation activity paralleled this pattern [18]. Likewise, erythromycin N-demethylase activity decreased from proximal to distal regions [19]. These data suggested that the extent of CYP3A-mediated first-pass metabolism may depend in part on the site of absorption.

CYP3A4 expression from the crypt to the tip of the small intestinal villus also is not uniform. By immunohistochemical analysis, CYP3A4 protein was not detected in the crypt cells or goblet cells but was readily detected in enterocytes, with the most intense staining evident in the mature enterocytes lining the villous tips [46,50]. By *in situ* hybridization, a similar pattern was reported for CYP3A4 mRNA [47]. Within the enterocyte, CYP3A4 protein was located predominately at the apex of the cell, adjacent to the microvillous border [47]. The strategic location of CYP3A4 in mature enterocytes further highlights the small intestine as uniquely suited for the task of first-pass drug metabolism.

Modifying Agents and Conditions　Localization of CYP3A within only the mature enterocytes of the small intestinal mucosa is consistent with a wider pattern of differentiation of cell function as cells formed within the crypts migrate towards the villus tip and are eventually shed. Total CYP3A content even within a defined region of the small intestine varies considerably. CYP3A protein content measured in duodenal pinch biopsies obtained from CYP3A inducer/inhibitor-free healthy volunteers has been reported to vary approximately 10-fold [41,42]. Even greater variability (>30-fold) was reported for CYP3A protein content and catalytic activity in duodenal, jejunal, and ileal mucosal scrapings obtained from 20 organ donors [18]. Although some of the extreme variability in the latter study could have been due to events preceding organ procurement (e.g., reduced nutritional intake, antibiotic administration, brain death, and ischemia), these observations suggest that CYP3A is remarkably sensitive to a variety of modifying factors or conditions that can alter enzyme expression.

Dietary Factors. One of the most extensively studied dietary substances in terms of CYP3A-mediated drug metabolism is grapefruit juice, which, when consumed in usual volumes, has been shown to elevate systemic concentrations of a variety of drugs by inhibiting intestinal, but not hepatic, CYP3A-mediated first-pass metabolism [51–54]. The lack of an effect on hepatic CYP3A has been attributed to dilution of the causative ingredients in portal blood to concentrations below the effective inhibitory concentrations (K_i or IC_{50}) and/or to avid binding of the causative ingredients to plasma and/or cellular proteins in portal blood [55,56]. The magnitude of the grapefruit juice effect can be large enough to cause untoward effects, such as severe muscle pain with some HMG-CoA reductase inhibitors ("statins") [57–59] and hypotension/dizziness with some calcium channel antagonists [60]. Accordingly, the labeling of several drug products contains precautionary statements about the concomitant intake of grapefruit juice. Using a "furanocoumarin-free" grapefruit juice suitable for human consumption and the CYP3A probe substrate felodipine, furanocoumarins were demonstrated unequivocally as major causative ingredients, several of which are potent reversible and mechanism-based inhibitors of enteric CYP3A catalytic activity [54,61]. In addition, the pioneering study by Lown and colleagues [62] showed that grapefruit juice significantly reduced average enteric CYP3A4 immunoreactive protein (measured in duodenal pinch biopsies) by 60% in 10 healthy volunteers; the lack of a decrease in corresponding mRNA suggested a post-transcriptional mechanism. *In vitro* studies involving CYP3A4-expressing Caco-2 cells confirmed that two candidate furanocoumarins (bergamottin and 6′,7′-dihydroxybergamottin) reduced CYP3A4 protein by accelerating enzyme degradation without affecting enzyme synthesis [63]. The list of drugs shown to interact with grapefruit and related citrus juices is expansive and is described in several comprehensive reviews [51–54, 64–67].

Therapeutic Agents. Therapeutic agents that have been shown to inhibit intestinal CYP3A in vivo include the azole antifungals ketoconazole [68] and fluconazole [69]; the macrolide antibiotics erythromycin [70], troleandomycin [71], and clarithromycin [72–74]; the calcium channel antagonist diltiazem [75]; and the HIV protease inhibitors ritonavir and indinavir [76,77]. Exposure of human subjects to the enzyme inducer rifampin (7–10 days) and to the popular herbal product St. John's wort (14 days) increased average duodenal CYP3A protein content by ≥4- and 1.5-fold, respectively, relative to baseline [50,78,79]. Moreover, a comparison of the effect of rifampin on the systemic and apparent oral clearance of the CYP3A substrates midazolam [33,71,80], triazolam [81], verapamil [78], nifedipine [34], and alfentanil [35,71] suggested that the inducer increased enteric enzyme levels to an extent comparable to or greater than hepatic levels. This effect of enzyme inhibitors and inducers on enteric CYP3A activity compared to hepatic CYP3A activity may be due to higher intracellular concentrations and greater receptor occupancy in the enterocyte that occurs during absorption of the modifying agent.

Pathophysiologic Conditions. Although less is known about the effect of disease on enteric CYP3A relative to hepatic CYP3A, some human studies have shown that pathophysiologic conditions can markedly alter enteric CYP3A protein expression/catalytic activity. For example, Lang et al. [82] reported that adult patients with celiac disease had reduced levels of jejunal mucosal CYP3A protein as a consequence of widespread epithelial cell destruction. Treatment with a gluten-free diet reversed this aberration. Similar observations were reported for pediatric patients with celiac disease [83]. In the pediatric patients, after gluten re-challenge, a further decrease in enteric CYP3A expression was observed. More recently, Morón et al. [84] reported a decrease in intestinal CYP3A activity using simvastatin as the CYP3A probe. The average C_{max} of orally administered simvastatin for untreated celiac patients was significantly higher (46 ± 24 nM) than that for patients on a gluten-free diet (21 ± 16 nM) or healthy subjects (19 ± 11 nM). Chalasani et al. [85] compared the disposition of midazolam between cirrhotic patients, cirrhotic patients with transjugular intrahepatic portosystemic shunts (TIPS), and healthy volunteers. The significantly higher mean F_{oral} in the cirrhotic patients with TIPS compared with the cirrhotic patients and healthy volunteers (0.76 vs 0.27 and 0.30) was largely due to the significantly higher F_I in the TIPS patients compared with the cirrhotic and healthy subjects (0.83 vs 0.32 and 0.42). The markedly lower extent of midazolam first-pass metabolism in the TIPS patients was concluded to result from diminished enteric CYP3A activity.

Intestinal versus Hepatic CYP3A   In view of the many differing responses between enteric and hepatic CYP3A to various regulatory factors, it follows that intestinal and hepatic CYP3A appear to be regulated independently. Such noncoordinate regulation was first demonstrated by Lown and coworkers [41], who reported that neither duodenal CYP3A protein content nor catalytic activity correlated with hepatic CYP3A activity in 20 healthy subjects. Likewise, no rank order correlation was observed between intestinal and hepatic CYP3A protein content or midazolam 1'-hydroxylation activity in microsomes prepared from eight matched intestine-liver donor pairs [18]. Finally, independent groups of investigators found no correlation between the F_I and F_L of midazolam in healthy volunteers [32,33,73]. This noncoordinate regulation between intestinal and hepatic CYP3A indicates that a measure of one should not be used to predict the other. However, the possibility of overlapping mechanisms of constitutive and inducible CYP3A expression cannot be excluded.

CYP1A1

CYP1A1 is expressed predominantly in extrahepatic tissues, including the lungs [86–88], placenta [89,90], stomach, and small intestine [22,91–93]. In two independent investigations in which duodenal biopsies were obtained from healthy volunteers, CYP1A1 mRNA was expressed constitutively in all specimens; as with other CYP isoforms, large interindividual variation was evident among the specimens, at least 6-fold [92,94]. CYP1A1 protein and catalytic (ethoxyresorufin O-deethylase, or EROD) activity were undetectable or low. Following treatment with the CYP1A inducers omeprazole [92] or chargrilled meat [94], enteric CYP1A1 protein and catalytic activity became readily detectable. Similarly, median duodenal EROD activity was higher in smokers and omeprazole-treated patients compared to non-smoking control subjects (2.1 and 1.1 vs 0.5 pmol/min/mg homogenate protein) [93]. More recently, the CYP1A inducer, β-naphthoflavone, was shown to increase CYP1A1 mRNA expression in precision-cut slices of proximal jejunum (362-fold; n = 3) and colon (132-fold; n = 3) [95]. EROD activity in proximal jejunum slices (n = 5) increased from 33 to 67 pmol/min/mg, whereas activity in colon slices was below the limit of detection.

Characterization of a bank of microsomes prepared from the proximal region of 18 human donor small intestines showed measurable rates of EROD activity in one-third of the donors, with a median and range (23.7 and 1.4–124 pmol/min/mg, respectively) [48] comparable to those reported for CYP1A2-catalyzed EROD activity in human liver microsomes (39.4 and 10.1–224 pmol/min/mg, respectively) [96]. Median CYP1A1 protein content for the three preparations in which immunoreactive CYP1A1 was detected readily (5.6 pmol/mg) [22] was 14% of the average CYP1A2 protein content reported for a large panel of human liver microsomes (41 pmol/mg) [97]. The differing protein contents between enteric CYP1A1 and hepatic CYP1A2 despite comparable EROD activities was attributed to CYP1A1 having a greater catalytic efficiency than CYP1A2 towards the *O*-deethylation of ethoxyresorufin, as evidenced by recombinant CYP1A1 having both a lower K_m and a higher V_{max} compared to recombinant CYP1A2 (87 nM and 7.6 min^{-1} vs 240 nM and 1.9 min^{-1}) [98]. A greater catalytic efficiency for CYP1A1 compared to CYP1A2 also has been demonstrated for ethoxycoumarin *O*-deethylation and benzo(a)pyrene hydroxylation [99]. In contrast, the catalytic efficiency of CYP1A1 towards the CYP1A drug substrates caffeine [100], theophylline [101], phenacetin [102], and *R*-warfarin [103] was reported to be much lower than that compared to CYP1A2. Consistent with these observations, there are no examples reported in the literature describing enteric CYP1A1 as having a significant role in the first-pass metabolism of drugs.

CYP2C9

Although CYP2C mRNAs have been detected in a number of human extrahepatic tissues (e.g., kidney, testes, adrenal gland, prostate, brain, duodenum), significant protein expression appears to be limited to the small intestine [21,104]. de Waziers et al. [21] first detected what was described as "CYP2C8-10" in small intestinal microsomes, which, like CYP3A, was expressed predominantly in the proximal region. Other investigators later confirmed the descending pattern of expression of a CYP2C enzyme along the length of the small intestine [19]. However, in both studies, it was unclear which enzyme (CYP2C8, CYP2C9, or CYP2C19) was detected. Based on the relative amount of each CYP2C enzyme in human liver, the intestinal form identified was most likely CYP2C9. From an analysis of 31 duodenal/jejunal microsomal preparations, two proteins were detected that reacted with a CYP2C-selective anti-CYP2C19 antibody and that comigrated with recombinant CYP2C9 and CYP2C19 protein reference standards [22]. CYP2C9 protein content varied 9-fold among the different preparations, with a mean specific content (8.4 pmol/mg) that was nearly one-tenth of reported average hepatic microsomal specific content (73 pmol/mg protein) [105].

With respect to intestinal CYP2C9 catalytic activity, Prueksaritanont et al. [106] reported a >20-fold variation in tolbutamide methylhydroxylase activity (<0.5–9.8 pmol/min/mg) for five duodenal/jejunal microsomal preparations; average (± SD) activity (5.1 ± 3.8 pmol/min/mg) was at least one-tenth of the hepatic counterpart. Other investigators subsequently reported a similarly large interindividual variation in CYP2C9-catalyzed diclofenac 4'-hydroxylase activity (7.3–129 pmol/min/mg) for 10 human jejunal microsomal preparations; median activity was 55 pmol/min/mg [40], which was roughly one-sixth of that reported for a panel of 16 human liver microsomal preparations (~320 pmol/min/mg) [107]. Collectively, these *in vitro* data suggest that the small intestine would have minimal contribution to the first-pass metabolism of drugs. However, due to the wide range in both specific content and activity, enteric CYP2C9 could be important in some individuals for substrates with a low oral bioavailability, e.g., fluvastatin [108]. In addition, the low expression/catalytic activity of CYP2C9 in the intestine relative to the liver does not preclude the potential importance of enteric CYP2C9 to the first-pass metabolism of substrates ingested in trace amounts, e.g., pesticides [109,110].

CYP2C19

CYP2C19 immunoreactive protein content for the aforementioned 31 human duodenal/jejunal microsomal preparations ranged from <0.6 to 3.9 and averaged 1.0 pmol/mg [22], which was one-fifteenth of average hepatic microsomal content (14 pmol/mg) [105]. Large interindividual variation in enteric CYP2C19 catalytic activity also has been reported. CYP2C19-catalyzed *S*-mephenytoin 4'-hydroxylase activity varied from 0.8 to 13.1 pmol/min/mg in the same panel of human small intestinal microsomal preparations that were analyzed previously for CYP2C9 activity [40]. Average enteric catalytic activity (5.2 pmol/min/mg) was approximately one-tenth of the average activity reported for a panel of 10 human liver microsomal preparations (~45 pmol/min/mg) [111]. As with enteric CYP2C9, these data suggest a minimal role for enteric CYP2C19 in the first-pass metabolism of drugs. The scarcity of CYP2C19 drug substrates with a low oral bioavailability supports this contention. One report involving liver transplant recipients in which CYP2C19 genotype differed between the native intestine and graft liver suggested that the intestine may contribute appreciably to the metabolism of omeprazole [112], but controlled clinical studies are needed to confirm this result. In addition, although enteric CYP2C19 expression/activity is low relative to hepatic CYP2C19, the potential importance of enteric CYP2C19 to the first-pass metabolism of xenobiotics ingested in trace amounts, e.g., pesticides and insect repellents, cannot be dismissed [113].

CYP2D6

CYP2D6 expression in the human intestine was first reported in 1990 by de Waziers and coworkers [21]. Like CYP3A4, CYP2D6 protein was most concentrated in the proximal region and was localized in the enterocytes. The enzyme was not detected in ileum or colon. Prueksaritanont and coworkers later confirmed the expression of CYP2D6 protein in microsomes prepared from the proximal portion of two [114] and five [106] human donor small intestines. Moreover, CYP2D6-catalyzed (+)-bufuralol 1'-hydroxylation activity was measurable in all preparations. From a comprehensive comparison involving 19 human jejunal and 31 human liver microsomal preparations, CYP2D6 immunoreactive protein was detected readily in 18 of the intestinal preparations, with a median specific content (0.9 pmol/mg) that was one-fifteenth of the median content measured in the liver preparations (12.8 pmol/mg) [115]. Median catalytic activity, as assessed by the intrinsic clearance of metoprolol oxidation, was also much lower in jejunal compared to hepatic microsomes (0.7 vs 19.7 µL/min/mg). Likewise, the predicted average *in vivo* intestinal extraction ratio for metoprolol was negligible compared to the predicted average hepatic extraction ratio (0.01 vs 0.48). The authors concluded that, unless a CYP2D6 substrate has a long residence time in the intestinal mucosa or undergoes futile cycling *via* an efflux transporter, enteric CYP2D6 would be expected to contribute minimally to the first-pass metabolism of drugs. The negligible catalytic activity of enteric CYP2D6 was confirmed by the *O*-demethylation of oxycodone [116]. However, enteric CYP2D6 may become clinically relevant if it mediates the formation of a cytotoxic metabolite that could cause mucosal damage [115].

CYP2J2

CYP2J2 is a relatively recently identified human CYP that is expressed predominately in extrahepatic tissues [117,118]. Although most abundant in the heart, CYP2J2 is also expressed at appreciable levels (both mRNA and immunoreactive protein) in the GI tract [119]. Immunoreactive CYP2J2 protein has been detected in microsomes prepared from the human esophagus, stomach, small intestine, and colon. Unlike other small intestinal CYPs, CYP2J2 expression was qualitatively highest in the esophagus. Expression was slightly lower, but relatively uniform throughout the remainder of the GI tract from stomach to colon [119]. In addition, interindividual variation in CYP2J2 expression in jejunal microsomes is negligible [119]. Although the role of CYP2J2 in drug metabolism remains largely unknown, *in vitro* studies have suggested that intestinal CYP2J2 contributes to the first-pass metabolism of the non-sedating antihistamines astemizole and ebastine.

Using human intestinal and liver microsomes, Matsumoto et al. [120] showed *O*-demethylation as the primary metabolic pathway for astemizole, with the average (± SD) rate in enteric microsomes comparable with that in liver microsomes (171 ± 57 vs 207 ± 82 pmol/min/mg). With recombinant CYP2J2 as the reference standard, immunoreactive CYP2J2 protein in microsomes prepared from five human small intestines averaged 2.1 (±0.6) pmol/mg, consistent with that measured in a larger number of small intestinal microsomal preparations (1.0 ± 0.1 pmol/mg; n = 31) [22,121]. These observations are comparable with average CYP2J2 content measured in liver microsomes from 20 Japanese and 29 Caucasian donors (2.0 ± 1.5 and 1.2 ± 2.1 pmol/mg, respectively) [122]. A role for intestinal CYP2J2 in the *O*-demethylation of astemizole was supported further by the excellent correlation between CYP2J2 protein content and *O*-demethylastemizole formation rate in intestinal microsomes (r = 0.90, p <0.05), as well as the strong inhibition of *O*-demethylastemizole formation by the CYP2J2 substrates ebastine and arachidonic acid. Using similar strategies, along with an inhibitory anti-CYP2J2 antibody, Hashizume et al. [123] demonstrated that CYP2J2 is the major ebastine hydroxylase in human intestinal microsomes. A screening of 139 prescription drugs showed that six (albendazole, amiodarone, cyclosporine, danazol, mesoridazine, tamoxifen, and thioridazine) were metabolized by CYP2J2 [124]. However, CYP2J2 had a relatively minor contribution to the clearance of these drugs, which are also CYP3A4 substrates. For example, the intrinsic clearance ratio for *N*-desethyl amiodarone formation was 4.6 for human liver microsomes/human intestinal microsomes and was 17 for recombinant CYP3A4/recombinant CYP2J2. Thus, although CYP2J2 appears to have a relatively minor contribution to hepatic drug metabolism, its abundance in the intestine suggests that this enzyme influences first-pass metabolism of select substrates, especially astemizole and ebastine.

CYP4F

CYP4F enzymes catalyze the biotransformation of several endogenous compounds, including arachidonic acid and its leukotriene, prostaglandin, lipoxin, and hydroxyeicosatetraenoic acid derivatives [125,126]. Accordingly, the CYP4Fs are important regulators of vascular tone and inflammation, as well as other physiologic functions. The CYP4Fs also metabolize some drug substrates. For example, CYP4F12 mRNA was detected in human liver and small intestine [127], and the enzyme catalyzed ebastine hydroxylation. However, a subsequent report by the same investigators showed that intestinal CYP2J2 was the predominate enzyme contributing to ebastine hydroxylation [123]. More recently, Wang and coworkers identified CYP4Fs as the major enzymes in human proximal small intestinal microsomes that catalyze the initial *O*-demethylation of the antiparasitic agent pafuramidine [128]. However, the much lower average intrinsic clearance of this reaction (0.3 mL/min/mg) relative to that for pooled human liver microsomes (7.6 mL/min/mg) suggested that enteric CYP4Fs do not contribute significantly to the initial *O*-demethylation of pafuramidine during first-pass. A role for enteric CYP4F in subsequent *O*-demethylation reactions remains to be determined. Interestingly, quantitative Western blot analysis of these intestinal preparations indicated appreciable CYP4F protein expression in the small intestine, with a mean (range) of 7 (3–18) pmol/mg, which was comparable to that for CYP2C9. This observation suggested that CYP4F could represent an appreciable portion of the human intestinal CYP "pie" [128].

Other CYPs

Other CYP mRNAs expressed in the human small intestine include CYP1B1 [19], CYP2C8, CYP2C18 [104], and CYP1A2, the latter of which is expressed only after treatment with omeprazole [92]. The importance of these enzymes *in vivo* remains to be determined. Immunoblot analysis showed that CYP2A6, CYP2B6, CYP2C8, CYP2E1, and CYP4A11 were undetectable or were expressed in only trace amounts in the human small intestine [21,22,128,129]. The roles of these enzymes in enteric first-pass drug metabolism are likely to be negligible.

Other Phase I Enzymes

Other phase I enzymes reported to be expressed in the human intestine include carboxylesterases (CESs) [130], epoxide hydrolases [21,131], and flavin monooxygenases (FMOs) [132]. Of these enzymes, the CESs have been implicated in the first-pass metabolism of some drugs. Whereas the CES1 family predominates in the liver, the CES2 family predominates in the small intestine and preferentially hydrolyzes substrates with a relatively small acyl group, e.g., prasugrel and irinotecan [130,133]. CES2 is uniformly distributed throughout the intestine and exhibits developmental regulation such that mRNA and protein levels increase with age [134,135]. Human intestinal microsomes have been shown to catalyze the hydrolysis of the CES substrates betamethasone valerate and aspirin at comparable (aspirin) or greater (betamethasone valerate) rates than human liver microsomes [133]. Using fluorescein diacetate as a CES2 substrate, the K_m and V_{max} values for human intestinal microsomes were 4.04 ± 0.96 μM and 39.5 ± 2.5 μmol/mg/min, respectively, whereas the values for human liver microsomes were 4.87 ± 0.51 μM and 18.5 ± 0.5 μmol/mg/min, respectively [136]. Similarly, intestinal biopsy tissues were as proficient as liver biopsy tissues in converting the prodrug and CES substrate irinotecan to the active chemotherapeutic metabolite, SN-38 [137,138]. Approximately one-third of an intravenous radiolabeled dose of irinotecan is excreted in human bile as unchanged drug [139]. Therefore, because the bile duct empties into the duodenum, direct conversion of the prodrug to SN-38 could occur in the intestine, followed by bacterial β-glucuronidase-mediated deconjugation of SN-38 glucuronide, leading to accumulation of SN-38 in the intestine and potential toxicity (i.e., severe diarrhea). Large interindividual variability in systemic exposure of irinotecan and SN-38 following oral administration of irinotecan has been attributed in part to interindividual variation in the extent of intestinal CES-mediated first-pass metabolism [140].

Epoxide hydrolases have been detected in the human small intestine, but protein levels and catalytic activity were much lower (≥6%) relative to the liver [21,131,141]. Although a significant role for intestinal epoxide hydrolases in the first-pass metabolism of drugs has not been identified, these enzymes could play a protective role in the detoxification of procarcinogenic epoxides generated from environmental xenobiotics [142]. Like epoxide hydrolases, flavin monooxygenases (to date only FMO1) have been detected in the human small intestine, but the much lower catalytic activity (*p*-tolyl methyl sulfoxidation) relative to the liver (0.11 ± 0.04 vs 2.8 ± 1.4 nmol/min/mg microsomal protein, respectively) indicates a minimal role for these enzymes in the first-pass metabolism of drugs [132,143].

Phase II Enzymes

Sulfotransferases

Five SULTs are known to be expressed and to have functional activity in the human GI tract: SULT1A1, SULT1A3, SULT1B1, SULT1E1, and SULT2A1. Using cytosolic fractions prepared from the stomach, small intestine, and colon of 23 unrelated organ donors, Chen et al. [144] showed the stomach and colon to have low sulfation activity toward 2-naphthol (SULT1A1) and dopamine (SULT1A3) and to have very low to no activity toward estradiol (SULT1E1) and dehydroepiandrosterone (DHEA) (SULT2A1). Comparatively, sulfation activity toward all probe substrates was higher in the small intestine. These results were confirmed by Teubner et al. [145]. Given the much greater surface area of the small intestine, sulfation activity in this section of the GI tract is undoubtedly the most important with respect to drug metabolism.

Average (± SD) small intestinal SULT1A1 and SULT2A1 activities were less than one-half and approximately one-fifth, respectively, of the corresponding activities measured in four human liver cytosolic preparations (2.1 ± 1.4 vs 5.3 ± 1.0 nmol/min/mg and 32 ± 33 vs 140 ± 28 pmol/min/mg, respectively) [144]. In contrast, small intestinal SULT1A3 and SULT1E1 activities were approximately three-fold higher than and comparable to, respectively, the corresponding hepatic activities (0.45 ± 0.25 vs 0.17 ± 0.05 nmol/min/mg and 3.3 ± 0.9 vs 2.6 ± 1.6 pmol/min/mg, respectively) [144]. These results were confirmed by Riches et al., who reported expression levels of SULT1A1, SULT1B1, SULT1E1, and SULT2A1 in the small intestine of 0.41-, 2.9-, 1.4-, and 0.24-fold that of liver SULT2A1 [146], respectively, calculated as a percentage of the total amount of immunoquantified SULT (n = 6 donors). SULT1A3 protein was not detected in the liver but was highly expressed in the small intestine (770–3300 ng/mg cytosolic protein). Expression levels of intestinal SULT isozymes are shown in Figure 11.3 [146]. Intestinal sulfation activity toward all probes substrates showed large interindividual variation, as exemplified by coefficients of variation of at least 60%, consistent with an earlier report involving 62 human jejunal preparations analyzed for SULT1E1 and SULT2A1 immunoreactive protein [147]. SULT activity along the length of the small intestine varied among different donors; some donors showed higher activity in the proximal portion, whereas others showed higher activity in the distal portion [144]. Age, sex, underlying pathology, and time of tissue storage appeared not to influence SULT activity and/or protein expression [144,147]. No significant correlation was evident between any

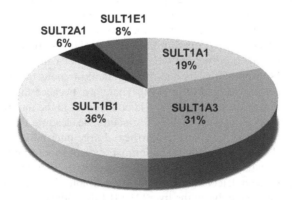

FIGURE 11.3 *The average human small intestinal SULT "pie".* The percent contributions of individual enzymes are based on average total immunoquantified SULT content (7800 ± 4600 ng/mg cytosol protein; n = 6 donors). (Reproduced with permission from Riches, Z. et al., *Drug Metab. Dispos.*, 37, 2255–2261, 2009.)

of these enzymes with respect to catalytic activity or protein expression, suggesting the enzymes are regulated independently [144,147].

Of the aforementioned intestinal SULTs, SULT1A3 and SULT1E1 have been implicated to contribute significantly to the first-pass metabolism of some drugs. Intestinal SULT1A3-mediated metabolism likely contributes to the low oral bioavailability of the β-adrenergic agents isoproterenol and terbutaline [148–150] (Table 11.1). SULT1E1 is likely the major intestinal SULT involved in the first-pass metabolism of ethinyl estradiol [147,151,152] (Table 11.1).

UDP-Glucuronosyltransferases

The UDP-Glucuronosyltransferases (UGTs) are ubiquitous in a number of extrahepatic tissues, including the GI tract [153,154]. As with sulfation activity, relative to the small intestine, glucuronidation activity in general appears to be much lower in the stomach and colon (and esophagus) [153]. The expression of UGT mRNAs has been confirmed in the small intestine by multiple laboratories using the same or different approaches: UGT1A1, UGT1A3, UGT1A5, UGT1A6, UGT1A7, UGT1A8, UGT1A9, UGT1A10, UGT2B7, UGT2B15, and UGT2B17 [155,156]. In addition, selective expression of UGT1A8 and UGT1A10 mRNAs in the small intestine and/or colon versus the liver has been reported by multiple investigators [155–157]. Specific antibodies are not yet available except for UGT1A1 and UGT1A6. Recently, Oda et al. generated a specific monoclonal antibody against UGT1A9 and observed that UGT1A9 protein is not expressed in the jejunum and ileum [158]. Of all of these enzymes, UGT1A1, UGT1A3, UGT1A4, UGT1A6, UGT1A7, UGT1A8, UGT1A9, UGT1A10, UGT2B7, UGT2B15, and UGT2B17 have been detected at the protein level in small intestinal microsomes, albeit in varied extents between different studies [154,159,160]. Using microsomes prepared from the three regions of three unrelated donor intestines, Fisher and coworkers showed UGT1A1 activity, as measured by estradiol 3-glucuronidation, was generally much higher than that in pooled human liver microsomes (0.2–3.9 vs 0.4 nmol/min/mg) [154], suggesting an important role for intestinal UGT1A1 in the first-pass metabolism of relevant drug substrates. In contrast, intestinal UGT2B7 activity, as measured by morphine 3-glucuronidation, was at most one-fifth of that measured in the pooled liver microsomes (0–0.5 vs 2.3 nmol/min/mg), suggesting a minor role for intestinal UGT2B7 in the first-pass metabolism of morphine and other UGT2B7 substrates. Multiple investigators have shown many enteric UGTs to be polymorphic and/or have large interindividual variation in expression level and catalytic activity [155,159–161]. Moreover, UGT activity along the length of the small intestine appears to vary with different substrates and UGT isoforms [155,162]. For example, UGT activity toward testosterone (a UGT2B substrate) increased gradually from proximal jejunum to colon, whereas that toward bilirubin (a UGT1A1 substrate) decreased sharply from proximal to distal intestine [155].

Of the aforementioned intestinal UGTs, several of the UGT1As have been implicated to contribute significantly to the extensive first-pass metabolism, and hence low oral bioavailability, of some drugs. For example, evidence suggests that enteric UGT1A1, in addition to enteric CYP3A and SULT1E1, may contribute to the first-pass metabolism of ethinyl estradiol [151,163] (Table 11.1). The intestine-specific forms, UGT1A8 and UGT1A10, likely are the major contributors to the low oral bioavailability of raloxifene [164,165] (Table 11.1). Enteric UGT1As (e.g., UGT1A1, UGT1A3) may influence the efficiency of the enterohepatic cycling of SN-38 [166] and ezetimibe [167,168].

Other Phase II Enzymes

Other phase II enzymes that have been identified in the human GI tract include members of the catechol-*O*-methyltransferase (COMT), *N*-acetyltransferase (NAT), and glutathione *S*-transferase (GST) families [21,161,169–172]. Catechol-*O*-methyltransferase (COMT), which has specificity toward catechol type substrates and transfer a methyl group to one of the hydroxyl groups, acts as a barrier to detoxifying xenobiotics [169,173]. COMT protein in vertebrates consists of a soluble form (S-COMT) and a minor fraction of membrane-bound form (MB-COMT) in various tissues except brain. S-COMT activity in the intestine was higher than MB-COMT activity by a factor of 8–20. Using 3,4-dihydroxybenzoic acid as a substrate, S-COMT activity along the small intestine appears comparable in the mucous layer of the duodenum, ileum, and colon, with turnover rates of 435, 382, and 360 pmol/min/mg protein, respectively [174]. COMT activity in the kidney and duodenum was approximately 30% and 10%, respectively, of that in the liver [175], suggesting a minor role for the intestine in COMT-mediated metabolism.

Mesalazine (5-aminosalicylic acid), indicated for the treatment of inflammatory bowel disease, undergoes extensive first-pass acetylation. Intestinal NAT, most likely NAT1 [171], is believed to contribute to this process [176]. Although expression and activity of both NAT1 and NAT2 have been detected in the small intestine, NAT1 activity, as measured by *p*-aminobenzoic acid acetylation, was always higher than NAT2 activity, as measured by sulfamethazine acetylation [171]. NAT1 and NAT2 activity levels also show considerable variation, such that the ratio of NAT1:NAT2 activity varied from two- to 70-fold. Among four human donor small intestines, NAT1 activity was relatively uniform or increased slightly along the length of the GI tract, whereas NAT2 activity tended to decrease from the duodenum to the rectum.

The GSTs are commonly implicated in the detoxification or bioactivation of environmental toxins, carcinogens, and some chemotherapeutic agents. Microsomal GST1, GST2, and GST3, content in human intestinal microsomes were approximately 4%, 28%, and 125% of that in liver, respectively [141]. Using cytosolic fractions prepared from the GI tracts (stomach to colon) of 16 organ donors, Coles et al. showed GSTP1, GSTA1, and GSTA2 to be the major GST proteins expressed in the small intestine [172]. All three of these enzymes showed large interindividual variation in all regions of the GI tract; however, the GST enzymes exhibited consistent patterns of expression along the length of the GI tract. Specifically, GSTP1 was expressed throughout the GI tract and decreased progressively from stomach to colon. In contrast, GSTA1 and GSTA2 were expressed at very low levels in the stomach and colon relative to the small intestinal regions, where levels were high in the duodenum and decreased to distal ileum. Similar differences in expression between stomach and duodenum for GSTA and GSTP were reported by other investigators who examined antral and duodenal biopsy specimens obtained from 202 patients [177]. It has been speculated that the low levels of GSTA in the stomach and colon contribute to the greater susceptibility of these GI tissues to some cancers compared to the small intestine [161,172]. With respect to chemotherapeutic agents, Gibbs and coworkers, using cytosolic fractions prepared from 12 small intestines and 23 livers, reported comparable busulfan conjugation intrinsic clearances (GSTA activity) between the two organs (0.17 ± 0.07 vs 0.18 ± 0.09 μL/min/mg), suggesting a role for intestinal GSTA in the first-pass metabolism of busulfan [170].

Summary and Perspectives

Most drugs are taken orally. For those intended to act systemically, a significant fraction of the dose can be eliminated during its first passage through a sequence of organs prior to entering the systemic circulation. For some drugs, the extent of first-pass elimination can be large enough to significantly compromise oral bioavailability, with the consequent potential for a reduced clinical response. Next to the liver, the small intestine can represent a major organ of first-pass drug elimination, the means of which occurs primarily *via* metabolism.

Like the liver, the small intestinal mucosa is replete with myriad drug biotransformation enzymes, including both phase I and phase II enzymes. Of all of these enzymes, the CYPs are the most extensively studied. Of the CYP enzymes, CYP3A is the most extensively studied and represents, on average, approximately 80% of total immunoquantified CYP content in the proximal human small intestine. In addition, microsomal CYP3A catalytic activity and immunoreactive protein content in the proximal region (duodenum to mid-jejunum) are within the ranges reported for human liver microsomes. These *in vitro* observations are consistent with clinical studies demonstrating that the intestinal contribution to the low and variable F_{oral} of some CYP3A substrates can rival the hepatic contribution. However, because intestinal and hepatic CYP3A appear to be regulated independently, and thus do not correlate, CYP3A activity measured in one organ will not necessarily predict CYP3A activity in the other. Taken together, the development and refinement of *in vivo* methods capable of delineating intestinal from hepatic first-pass metabolism, as well as capable of delineating CYP3A-mediated metabolism from transporter-mediated efflux, is of clinical importance. Such methods constitute an ongoing and active area of research, as the successful prediction of intestinal first-pass metabolism could aid in the therapeutic management of drugs with a low and variable F_{oral}, particularly those with a narrow therapeutic window.

Other human enteric CYP enzymes have been identified and characterized *in vitro* (CYP1A1, CYP2C9, CYP2C19, CYP2D6, CYP2J2, and CYP4F), but their role in drug disposition *in vivo* remains to be determined. Regarding other enteric phase I enzymes, CESs have been implicated in the first-pass metabolism of some drugs, whereas roles for the epoxide hydrolases and FMOs remain to be determined. Regarding phase II enzymes, whereas a number of such families have been known to be expressed in the human intestine for some time (e.g., SULTs, UGTs, COMT, NATs, GSTs), progress on the identification and quantification of individual isoforms has lagged behind that of the CYPs. With the increasing availability of quality human intestinal tissue, along with the ongoing identification of selective probe substrates, inhibitors, and antibodies, it is anticipated that a comprehensive characterization of these enzymes will soon become achievable. Meanwhile, further refinement of human intestinal cell culture models and/or the identification of an appropriate animal model should improve our understanding of the unique nature of intestinal drug metabolizing enzymes. These advances will allow not only improved prediction of the impact of the intestine on overall first-pass elimination of existing drugs, but also to improvement of the drug selection process during pre-clinical development.

REFERENCES

1. Rowland, M. and T.N. Tozer, *Clinical Pharmacokinetics and Pharmacodynamics: Concepts and Applications*. Fourth ed. 2011, Philadelphia, PA: Lippincott Williams & Wilkins.
2. Wienkers, L.C. and T.G. Heath, Predicting *in vivo* drug interactions from *in vitro* drug discovery data. *Nat Rev Drug Discov*, 2005. **4**(10): 825–833.
3. Bohnert, T. et al., Evaluation of a new molecular entity as a victim of metabolic drug-drug interactions-an industry perspective. *Drug Metab Dispos*, 2016. **44**(8): 1399–1423.
4. Thelen, K. and J.B. Dressman, Cytochrome P450-mediated metabolism in the human gut wall. *J Pharm Pharmacol*, 2009. **61**(5): 541–558.
5. Nugent, S.G. et al., Intestinal luminal pH in inflammatory bowel disease: Possible determinants and implications for therapy with aminosalicylates and other drugs. *Gut*, 2001. **48**(4): 571–577.
6. Rubin, D. and A. Shaker, Small intestine: Anatomy and structural anomalies, in *Yamada's Textbook of Gastroenterology*, D. Podolsky, Camilleri, M, Fitz, JG, Kalloo, AN, Shanahan, F, Wang, TC, Editor. 2016, Wiley Blackwell: Oxford, UK. pp. 73–92.
7. DeSesso, J.M. and C.F. Jacobson, Anatomical and physiological parameters affecting gastrointestinal absorption in humans and rats. *Food Chem Toxicol*, 2001. **39**(3): 209–228.
8. Crawley, S.W., M.S. Mooseker, and M.J. Tyska, Shaping the intestinal brush border. *J Cell Biol*, 2014. **207**(4): 441–451.
9. Helander, H.F. and L. Fandriks, Surface area of the digestive tract—Revisited. *Scand J Gastroenterol*, 2014. **49**(6): 681–689.
10. Griffin, B. and C. O'Driscoll, Models of the small intestine, in *Volume VII: Drug Absorption Studies: In Situ, In Vitro and In Silico Models*, C. Ehrhardt, Kim, KJ, Editor. 2008, American Association of Pharmaceutical Scientists: New York. pp. 34–76.
11. Hellriegel, E.T., T.D. Bjornsson, and W.W. Hauck, Interpatient variability in bioavailability is related to the extent of absorption: Implications for bioavailability and bioequivalence studies. *Clin Pharmacol Ther*, 1996. **60**(6): 601–607.
12. Varma, M.V. et al., Dealing with the complex drug-drug interactions: Towards mechanistic models. *Biopharm Drug Dispos*, 2015. **36**(2): 71–92.
13. Chow, E.C. and K.S. Pang, Why we need proper PBPK models to examine intestine and liver oral drug absorption. *Curr Drug Metab*, 2013. **14**(1): 57–79.
14. de Graaf, I.A. et al., Preparation and incubation of precision-cut liver and intestinal slices for application in drug metabolism and toxicity studies. *Nat Protoc*, 2010. **5**(9): 1540–1551.
15. Peters, S.A. et al., Predicting drug extraction in the human gut wall: Assessing contributions from drug metabolizing enzymes and transporter proteins using preclinical models. *Clin Pharmacokinet*, 2016. **55**(6): 673–696.

16. Jones, C.R. et al., Gut wall metabolism. Application of pre-clinical models for the prediction of human drug absorption and first-pass elimination. *AAPS J*, 2016. **18**(3): 589–604.
17. Hoensch, H.P., R. Hutt, and F. Hartmann, Biotransformation of xenobiotics in human intestinal mucosa. *Environ Health Perspect*, 1979. **33**: 71–78.
18. Paine, M.F. et al., Characterization of interintestinal and intraintestinal variations in human CYP3A-dependent metabolism. *J Pharmacol Exp Ther*, 1997. **283**(3): 1552–1562.
19. Zhang, Q.Y. et al., Characterization of human small intestinal cytochromes P-450. *Drug Metab Dispos*, 1999. **27**(7): 804–809.
20. Watkins, P.B. et al., Identification of glucocorticoid-inducible cytochromes P-450 in the intestinal mucosa of rats and man. *J Clin Invest*, 1987. **80**(4): 1029–1036.
21. de Waziers, I. et al., Cytochrome P 450 isoenzymes, epoxide hydrolase and glutathione transferases in rat and human hepatic and extrahepatic tissues. *J Pharmacol Exp Ther*, 1990. **253**(1): 387–394.
22. Paine, M.F. et al., The human intestinal cytochrome P450 "pie". *Drug Metab Dispos*, 2006. **34**(5): 880–886.
23. Ptachcinski, R.J., R. Venkataramanan, and G.J. Burckart, Clinical pharmacokinetics of cyclosporin. *Clin Pharmacokinet*, 1986. **11**(2): 107–132.
24. Wallemacq, P.E. et al., Clinical pharmacokinetics of Neoral in pediatric recipients of primary liver transplants. *Transpl Int*, 1997. **10**(6): 466–470.
25. Chueh, S.C. and B.D. Kahan, Pretransplant test-dose pharmacokinetic profiles: Cyclosporine microemulsion versus corn oil-based soft gel capsule formulation. *J Am Soc Nephrol*, 1998. **9**(2): 297–304.
26. Ku, Y.M., D.I. Min, and M. Flanigan, Effect of grapefruit juice on the pharmacokinetics of microemulsion cyclosporine and its metabolite in healthy volunteers: Does the formulation difference matter? *J Clin Pharmacol*, 1998. **38**(10): 959–965.
27. Lee, M. et al., Effect of grapefruit juice on pharmacokinetics of microemulsion cyclosporine in African American subjects compared with Caucasian subjects: Does ethnic difference matter? *J Clin Pharmacol*, 2001. **41**(3): 317–323.
28. Kolars, J.C. et al., First-pass metabolism of cyclosporin by the gut. *Lancet*, 1991. **338**(8781): 1488–1490.
29. Hebert, M.F. et al., Bioavailability of cyclosporine with concomitant rifampin administration is markedly less than predicted by hepatic enzyme induction. *Clin Pharmacol Ther*, 1992. **52**(5): 453–457.
30. Kim, R.B. et al., Interrelationship between substrates and inhibitors of human CYP3A and P-glycoprotein. *Pharm Res*, 1999. **16**(3): 408–414.
31. Paine, M.F. et al., First-pass metabolism of midazolam by the human intestine. *Clin Pharmacol Ther*, 1996. **60**(1): 14–24.
32. Thummel, K.E. et al., Oral first-pass elimination of midazolam involves both gastrointestinal and hepatic CYP3A-mediated metabolism. *Clin Pharmacol Ther*, 1996. **59**(5): 491–502.
33. Quinney, S.K. et al., Interaction between midazolam and clarithromycin in the elderly. *Br J Clin Pharmacol*, 2008. **65**(1): 98–109.
34. Holtbecker, N. et al., The nifedipine-rifampin interaction. Evidence for induction of gut wall metabolism. *Drug Metab Dispos*, 1996. **24**(10): 1121–1123.
35. Kharasch, E.D. et al., Concurrent assessment of hepatic and intestinal cytochrome P450 3A activities using deuterated alfentanil. *Clin Pharmacol Ther*, 2011. **89**(4): 562–570.
36. Gertz, M. et al., Prediction of human intestinal first-pass metabolism of 25 CYP3A substrates from *in vitro* clearance and permeability data. *Drug Metab Dispos*, 2010. **38**(7): 1147–1158.
37. von Richter, O. et al., Determination of *in vivo* absorption, metabolism, and transport of drugs by the human intestinal wall and liver with a novel perfusion technique. *Clin Pharmacol Ther*, 2001. **70**(3): 217–227.
38. Yang, J., G.T. Tucker, and A. Rostami-Hodjegan, Cytochrome P450 3A expression and activity in the human small intestine. *Clin Pharmacol Ther*, 2004. **76**(4): 391.
39. Lampen, A. et al., Metabolism of the immunosuppressant tacrolimus in the small intestine: Cytochrome P450, drug interactions, and interindividual variability. *Drug Metab Dispos*, 1995. **23**(12): 1315–1324.
40. Obach, R.S. et al., Metabolic characterization of the major human small intestinal cytochrome p450s. *Drug Metab Dispos*, 2001. **29**(3): 347–352.
41. Lown, K.S. et al., Interpatient heterogeneity in expression of CYP3A4 and CYP3A5 in small bowel. Lack of prediction by the erythromycin breath test. *Drug Metab Dispos*, 1994. **22**(6): 947–955.
42. Paine, M.F. et al., Do men and women differ in proximal small intestinal CYP3A or P-glycoprotein expression? *Drug Metab Dispos*, 2005. **33**(3): 426–433.

43. Kuehl, P. et al., Sequence diversity in CYP3A promoters and characterization of the genetic basis of polymorphic CYP3A5 expression. *Nat Genet*, 2001. **27**(4): 383–391.
44. Lin, Y.S. et al., Co-regulation of CYP3A4 and CYP3A5 and contribution to hepatic and intestinal midazolam metabolism. *Mol Pharmacol*, 2002. **62**(1): 162–172.
45. Isoherranen, N. et al., The influence of CYP3A5 expression on the extent of hepatic CYP3A inhibition is substrate-dependent: An *in vitro-in vivo* evaluation. *Drug Metab Dispos*, 2008. **36**(1): 146–154.
46. Kolars, J.C. et al., CYP3A gene expression in human gut epithelium. *Pharmacogenetics*, 1994. **4**(5): 247–259.
47. McKinnon, R.A. et al., Characterisation of CYP3A gene subfamily expression in human gastrointestinal tissues. *Gut*, 1995. **36**(2): 259–267.
48. Paine, M.F., P. Schmiedlin-Ren, and P.B. Watkins, Cytochrome P-450 1A1 expression in human small bowel: Interindividual variation and inhibition by ketoconazole. *Drug Metab Dispos*, 1999. **27**(3): 360–364.
49. Gervot, L. et al., CYP3A5 is the major cytochrome P450 3A expressed in human colon and colonic cell lines. *Environ Toxicol Pharmacol*, 1996. **2**(4): 381–388.
50. Kolars, J.C. et al., Identification of rifampin-inducible P450IIIA4 (CYP3A4) in human small bowel enterocytes. *J Clin Invest*, 1992. **90**(5): 1871–1878.
51. Holmberg, M.T. et al., Grapefruit juice markedly increases the plasma concentrations and antiplatelet effects of ticagrelor in healthy subjects. *Br J Clin Pharmacol*, 2013. **75**(6): 1488–1496.
52. Won, C.S., N.H. Oberlies, and M.F. Paine, Influence of dietary substances on intestinal drug metabolism and transport. *Curr Drug Metab*, 2010. **11**(9): 778–792.
53. Bailey, D.G. et al., Grapefruit juice-drug interactions. *Br J Clin Pharmacol*, 1998. **46**(2): 101–110.
54. Paine, M.F. and N.H. Oberlies, Clinical relevance of the small intestine as an organ of drug elimination: Drug-fruit juice interactions. *Expert Opin Drug Metab Toxicol*, 2007. **3**(1): 67–80.
55. Paine, M.F., A.B. Criss, and P.B. Watkins, Two major grapefruit juice components differ in intestinal CYP3A4 inhibition kinetic and binding properties. *Drug Metab Dispos*, 2004. **32**(10): 1146–1153.
56. Paine, M.F., A.B. Criss, and P.B. Watkins, Two major grapefruit juice components differ in time to onset of intestinal CYP3A4 inhibition. *J Pharmacol Exp Ther*, 2005. **312**(3): 1151–1160.
57. Lee, J.W., J.K. Morris, and N.J. Wald, Grapefruit juice and statins. *Am J Med*, 2016. **129**(1): 26–9.
58. Karch, A.M., The grapefruit challenge: the juice inhibits a crucial enzyme, with possibly fatal consequences. *Am J Nurs*, 2004. **104**(12): 33–35.
59. Dreier, J.P. and M. Endres, Statin-associated rhabdomyolysis triggered by grapefruit consumption. *Neurology*, 2004. **62**(4): 670.
60. Bailey, D.G. and G.K. Dresser, Interactions between grapefruit juice and cardiovascular drugs. *Am J Cardiovasc Drugs*, 2004. **4**(5): 281–297.
61. Paine, M.F. et al., A furanocoumarin-free grapefruit juice establishes furanocoumarins as the mediators of the grapefruit juice-felodipine interaction. *Am J Clin Nutr*, 2006. **83**(5): 1097–1105.
62. Lown, K.S. et al., Grapefruit juice increases felodipine oral availability in humans by decreasing intestinal CYP3A protein expression. *J Clin Invest*, 1997. **99**(10): 2545–2453.
63. Malhotra, S., Schmiedlin-Ren, P, Paine, MF, Criss, AB, Watkins, PB, The furocoumarin 6',7'-dihydroxybergamottin (DHB) accelerates CYP3A4 degradation via the proteasomal pathway. *Drug Metab Rev*, 2001. **33**: 97.
64. Satoh, H. et al., Citrus juices inhibit the function of human organic anion-transporting polypeptide OATP-B. *Drug Metab Dispos*, 2005. **33**(4): 518–523.
65. Mertens-Talcott, S.U. et al., Polymethoxylated flavones and other phenolic derivates from citrus in their inhibitory effects on P-glycoprotein-mediated transport of talinolol in Caco-2 cells. *J Agric Food Chem*, 2007. **55**(7): 2563–2568.
66. Hanley, M.J. et al., The effect of grapefruit juice on drug disposition. *Expert Opin Drug Metab Toxicol*, 2011. **7**(3): 267–286.
67. Seden, K. et al., Grapefruit-drug interactions. *Drugs*, 2010. **70**(18): 2373–2407.
68. Seidegard, J., L. Nyberg, and O. Borga, Differentiating mucosal and hepatic metabolism of budesonide by local pretreatment with increasing doses of ketoconazole in the proximal jejunum. *Eur J Pharm Sci*, 2012. **46**(5): 530–536.
69. Ahonen, J., K.T. Olkkola, and P.J. Neuvonen, Effect of route of administration of fluconazole on the interaction between fluconazole and midazolam. *Eur J Clin Pharmacol*, 1997. **51**(5): 415–419.
70. Olkkola, K.T. et al., A potentially hazardous interaction between erythromycin and midazolam. *Clin Pharmacol Ther*, 1993. **53**(3): 298–305.

71. Kharasch, E.D. et al., Intravenous and oral alfentanil as *in vivo* probes for hepatic and first-pass cytochrome P450 3A activity: Noninvasive assessment by use of pupillary miosis. *Clin Pharmacol Ther*, 2004. **76**(5): 452–466.

72. Quinney, S.K. et al., Rate of onset of inhibition of gut-wall and hepatic CYP3A by clarithromycin. *Eur J Clin Pharmacol*, 2013. **69**(3): 439–448.

73. Gorski, J.C. et al., The contribution of intestinal and hepatic CYP3A to the interaction between midazolam and clarithromycin. *Clin Pharmacol Ther*, 1998. **64**(2): 133–143.

74. Pinto, A.G. et al., Inhibition of human intestinal wall metabolism by macrolide antibiotics: Effect of clarithromycin on cytochrome P450 3A4/5 activity and expression. *Clin Pharmacol Ther*, 2005. **77**(3): 178–188.

75. Pinto, A.G. et al., Diltiazem inhibits human intestinal cytochrome P450 3A (CYP3A) activity *in vivo* without altering the expression of intestinal mRNA or protein. *Br J Clin Pharmacol*, 2005. **59**(4): 440–446.

76. Kharasch, E.D. et al., Methadone pharmacokinetics are independent of cytochrome P4503A (CYP3A) activity and gastrointestinal drug transport: Insights from methadone interactions with ritonavir/indinavir. *Anesthesiology*, 2009. **110**(3): 660–672.

77. Kharasch, E.D. et al., Lack of indinavir effects on methadone disposition despite inhibition of hepatic and intestinal cytochrome P4503A (CYP3A). *Anesthesiology*, 2012. **116**(2): 432–447.

78. Fromm, M.F. et al., Differential induction of prehepatic and hepatic metabolism of verapamil by rifampin. *Hepatology*, 1996. **24**(4): 796–801.

79. Durr, D. et al., St John's Wort induces intestinal P-glycoprotein/MDR1 and intestinal and hepatic CYP3A4. *Clin Pharmacol Ther*, 2000. **68**(6): 598–604.

80. Backman, J.T., K.T. Olkkola, and P.J. Neuvonen, Rifampin drastically reduces plasma concentrations and effects of oral midazolam. *Clin Pharmacol Ther*, 1996. **59**(1): 7–13.

81. Villikka, K. et al., Triazolam is ineffective in patients taking rifampin. *Clin Pharmacol Ther*, 1997. **61**(1): 8–14.

82. Lang, C.C. et al., Decreased intestinal CYP3A in celiac disease: Reversal after successful gluten-free diet: A potential source of interindividual variability in first-pass drug metabolism. *Clin Pharmacol Ther*, 1996. **59**(1): 41–46.

83. Johnson, T.N. et al., Enterocytic CYP3A4 in a paediatric population: Developmental changes and the effect of coeliac disease and cystic fibrosis. *Br J Clin Pharmacol*, 2001. **51**(5): 451–460.

84. Moron, B. et al., CYP3A4-catalyzed simvastatin metabolism as a non-invasive marker of small intestinal health in celiac disease. *Am J Gastroenterol*, 2013. **108**(8): 1344–1351.

85. Chalasani, N. et al., Hepatic and intestinal cytochrome P450 3A activity in cirrhosis: Effects of transjugular intrahepatic portosystemic shunts. *Hepatology*, 2001. **34**(6): 1103–1108.

86. Wheeler, C.W., S.S. Park, and T.M. Guenthner, Immunochemical analysis of a cytochrome P-450IA1 homologue in human lung microsomes. *Mol Pharmacol*, 1990. **38**(5): 634–643.

87. Shimada, T. et al., Characterization of human lung microsomal cytochrome P-450 1A1 and its role in the oxidation of chemical carcinogens. *Mol Pharmacol*, 1992. **41**(5): 856–864.

88. Ding, X. and L.S. Kaminsky, Human extrahepatic cytochromes P450: Function in xenobiotic metabolism and tissue-selective chemical toxicity in the respiratory and gastrointestinal tracts. *Annu Rev Pharmacol Toxicol*, 2003. **43**: 149–173.

89. Hakkola, J. et al., Xenobiotic-metabolizing cytochrome P450 enzymes in the human feto-placental unit: Role in intrauterine toxicity. *Crit Rev Toxicol*, 1998. **28**(1): 35–72.

90. Syme, M.R., J.W. Paxton, and J.A. Keelan, Drug transfer and metabolism by the human placenta. *Clin Pharmacokinet*, 2004. **43**(8): 487–514.

91. Peters, W.H. and P.G. Kremers, Cytochromes P-450 in the intestinal mucosa of man. *Biochem Pharmacol*, 1989. **38**(9): 1535–1538.

92. McDonnell, W.M., J.M. Scheiman, and P.G. Traber, Induction of cytochrome P450IA genes (CYP1A) by omeprazole in the human alimentary tract. *Gastroenterology*, 1992. **103**(5): 1509–1516.

93. Buchthal, J. et al., Induction of cytochrome P4501A by smoking or omeprazole in comparison with UDP-glucuronosyltransferase in biopsies of human duodenal mucosa. *Eur J Clin Pharmacol*, 1995. **47**(5): 431–435.

94. Fontana, R.J. et al., Effects of a chargrilled meat diet on expression of CYP3A, CYP1A, and P-glycoprotein levels in healthy volunteers. *Gastroenterology*, 1999. **117**(1): 89–98.

95. van de Kerkhof, E.G. et al., Induction of metabolism and transport in human intestine: Validation of precision-cut slices as a tool to study induction of drug metabolism in human intestine *in vitro*. *Drug Metab Dispos*, 2008. **36**(3): 604–613.

96. Pelkonen, O. et al., The effect of cigarette smoking on 7-ethoxyresorufin *O*-deethylase and other monooxygenase activities in human liver: Analyses with monoclonal antibodies. *Br J Clin Pharmacol*, 1986. **22**(2): 125–134.

97. Shimada, T. et al., Interindividual variations in human liver cytochrome P-450 enzymes involved in the oxidation of drugs, carcinogens and toxic chemicals: Studies with liver microsomes of 30 Japanese and 30 Caucasians. *J Pharmacol Exp Ther*, 1994. **270**(1): 414–423.

98. Penman, B.W. et al., Development of a human lymphoblastoid cell line constitutively expressing human CYP1A1 cDNA: Substrate specificity with model substrates and promutagens. *Carcinogenesis*, 1994. **15**(9): 1931–1937.

99. Miners, J., McKinnon, RA, CYP1A, in *Metabolic Drug Interactions*, R. Levy, Thummel, KE, Trager, WF, Hansten, PD, Eichelbaum, M, Editor. 2000, Lippincott Williams & Wilkins: Philadelphia, PA. pp. 61–73.

100. Tassaneeyakul, W. et al., Caffeine as a probe for human cytochromes P450: validation using cDNA-expression, immunoinhibition and microsomal kinetic and inhibitor techniques. *Pharmacogenetics*, 1992. **2**(4): 173–183.

101. Ha, H.R. et al., Metabolism of theophylline by cDNA-expressed human cytochromes P-450. *Br J Clin Pharmacol*, 1995. **39**(3): 321–326.

102. Tassaneeyakul, W. et al., Specificity of substrate and inhibitor probes for human cytochromes P450 1A1 and 1A2. *J Pharmacol Exp Ther*, 1993. **265**(1): 401–407.

103. Kaminsky, L.S. and Z.Y. Zhang, Human P450 metabolism of warfarin. *Pharmacol Ther*, 1997. **73**(1): 67–74.

104. Klose, T.S., J.A. Blaisdell, and J.A. Goldstein, Gene structure of CYP2C8 and extrahepatic distribution of the human CYP2Cs. *J Biochem Mol Toxicol*, 1999. **13**(6): 289–295.

105. Galetin, A. and J.B. Houston, Intestinal and hepatic metabolic activity of five cytochrome P450 enzymes: Impact on prediction of first-pass metabolism. *J Pharmacol Exp Ther*, 2006. **318**(3): 1220–1229.

106. Prueksaritanont, T. et al., Comparative studies of drug-metabolizing enzymes in dog, monkey, and human small intestines, and in Caco-2 cells. *Drug Metab Dispos*, 1996. **24**(6): 634–642.

107. Bort, R. et al., Hepatic metabolism of diclofenac: Role of human CYP in the minor oxidative pathways. *Biochem Pharmacol*, 1999. **58**(5): 787–796.

108. Scripture, C.D. and J.A. Pieper, Clinical pharmacokinetics of fluvastatin. *Clin Pharmacokinet*, 2001. **40**(4): 263–281.

109. Hu, Y. et al., CYP2C subfamily, primarily CYP2C9, catalyses the enantioselective demethylation of the endocrine disruptor pesticide methoxychlor in human liver microsomes: Use of inhibitory monoclonal antibodies in P450 identification. *Xenobiotica*, 2004. **34**(2): 117–132.

110. Usmani, K.A. et al., *In vitro* sulfoxidation of thioether compounds by human cytochrome P450 and flavin-containing monooxygenase isoforms with particular reference to the CYP2C subfamily. *Drug Metab Dispos*, 2004. **32**(3): 333–339.

111. Pearce, R.E. et al., Effects of freezing, thawing, and storing human liver microsomes on cytochrome P450 activity. *Arch Biochem Biophys*, 1996. **331**(2): 145–169.

112. Hosohata, K. et al., Impact of intestinal CYP2C19 genotypes on the interaction between tacrolimus and omeprazole, but not lansoprazole, in adult living-donor liver transplant patients. *Drug Metab Dispos*, 2009. **37**(4): 821–826.

113. Tang, J. et al., Metabolism of chlorpyrifos by human cytochrome P450 isoforms and human, mouse, and rat liver microsomes. *Drug Metab Dispos*, 2001. **29**(9): 1201–1204.

114. Prueksaritanont, T., L.M. Dwyer, and A.E. Cribb, (+)-bufuralol 1′-hydroxylation activity in human and rhesus monkey intestine and liver. *Biochem Pharmacol*, 1995. **50**(9): 1521–1525.

115. Madani, S. et al., Comparison of CYP2D6 content and metoprolol oxidation between microsomes isolated from human livers and small intestines. *Pharm Res*, 1999. **16**(8): 1199–1205.

116. Lalovic, B. et al., Quantitative contribution of CYP2D6 and CYP3A to oxycodone metabolism in human liver and intestinal microsomes. *Drug Metab Dispos*, 2004. **32**(4): 447–454.

117. Xu, M. et al., Cytochrome P450 2J2: Distribution, function, regulation, genetic polymorphisms and clinical significance. *Drug Metab Rev*, 2013. **45**(3): 311–352.

118. El-Serafi, I. et al., Cytochrome P450 2J2, a new key enzyme in cyclophosphamide bioactivation and a potential biomarker for hematological malignancies. *Pharmacogenomics J*, 2015. **15**(5): 405–413.

119. Zeldin, D.C. et al., CYP2J subfamily cytochrome P450s in the gastrointestinal tract: Expression, localization, and potential functional significance. *Mol Pharmacol*, 1997. **51**(6): 931–943.

120. Matsumoto, S. et al., *In vitro* inhibition of human small intestinal and liver microsomal astemizole O-demethylation: Different contribution of CYP2J2 in the small intestine and liver. *Xenobiotica*, 2003. **33**(6): 615–623.

121. Matsumoto, S. et al., Involvement of CYP2J2 on the intestinal first-pass metabolism of antihistamine drug, astemizole. *Drug Metab Dispos*, 2002. **30**(11): 1240–1245.

122. Yamazaki, H. et al., Inter-individual variation of cytochrome P4502J2 expression and catalytic activities in liver microsomes from Japanese and Caucasian populations. *Xenobiotica*, 2006. **36**(12): 1201–1209.

123. Hashizume, T. et al., Involvement of CYP2J2 and CYP4F12 in the metabolism of ebastine in human intestinal microsomes. *J Pharmacol Exp Ther*, 2002. **300**(1): 298–304.

124. Lee, C.A. et al., Identification of novel substrates for human cytochrome P450 2J2. *Drug Metab Dispos*, 2010. **38**(2): 347–356.

125. Michaels, S. and M.Z. Wang, The revised human liver cytochrome P450 "Pie": Absolute protein quantification of CYP4F and CYP3A enzymes using targeted quantitative proteomics. *Drug Metab Dispos*, 2014. **42**(8): 1241–1251.

126. Kalsotra, A. and H.W. Strobel, Cytochrome P450 4F subfamily: At the crossroads of eicosanoid and drug metabolism. *Pharmacol Ther*, 2006. **112**(3): 589–611.

127. Hashizume, T. et al., cDNA cloning and expression of a novel cytochrome p450 (cyp4f12) from human small intestine. *Biochem Biophys Res Commun*, 2001. **280**(4): 1135–1141.

128. Wang, M.Z. et al., Human enteric microsomal CYP4F enzymes O-demethylate the antiparasitic prodrug pafuramidine. *Drug Metab Dispos*, 2007. **35**(11): 2067–2075.

129. Mouly, S. et al., Hepatic but not intestinal CYP3A4 displays dose-dependent induction by efavirenz in humans. *Clin Pharmacol Ther*, 2002. **72**(1): 1–9.

130. Laizure, S.C. et al., The role of human carboxylesterases in drug metabolism: Have we overlooked their importance? *Pharmacotherapy*, 2013. **33**(2): 210–222.

131. Krishna, D.R. and U. Klotz, Extrahepatic metabolism of drugs in humans. *Clin Pharmacokinet*, 1994. **26**(2): 144–160.

132. Yeung, C.K. et al., Immunoquantitation of FMO1 in human liver, kidney, and intestine. *Drug Metab Dispos*, 2000. **28**(9): 1107–1111.

133. Imai, T. et al., Substrate specificity of carboxylesterase isozymes and their contribution to hydrolase activity in human liver and small intestine. *Drug Metab Dispos*, 2006. **34**(10): 1734–1741.

134. Taketani, M. et al., Carboxylesterase in the liver and small intestine of experimental animals and human. *Life Sci*, 2007. **81**(11): 924–932.

135. Chen, Y.T. et al., Ontogenic expression of human carboxylesterase-2 and cytochrome P450 3A4 in liver and duodenum: Postnatal surge and organ-dependent regulation. *Toxicology*, 2015. **330**: 55–61.

136. Wang, J. et al., Characterization of recombinant human carboxylesterases: Fluorescein diacetate as a probe substrate for human carboxylesterase 2. *Drug Metab Dispos*, 2011. **39**(8): 1329–1333.

137. Khanna, R. et al., Proficient metabolism of irinotecan by a human intestinal carboxylesterase. *Cancer Res*, 2000. **60**(17): 4725–4728.

138. Gupta, E. et al., Pharmacokinetics of orally administered camptothecins. *Ann N Y Acad Sci*, 2000. **922**: 195–204.

139. Slatter, J.G. et al., Pharmacokinetics, metabolism, and excretion of irinotecan (CPT-11) following I.V. infusion of [(14)C]CPT-11 in cancer patients. *Drug Metab Dispos*, 2000. **28**(4): 423–433.

140. Soepenberg, O. et al., Phase I and pharmacokinetic study of oral irinotecan given once daily for 5 days every 3 weeks in combination with capecitabine in patients with solid tumors. *J Clin Oncol*, 2005. **23**(4): 889–898.

141. Song, W., L. Yu, and Z. Peng, Targeted label-free approach for quantification of epoxide hydrolase and glutathione transferases in microsomes. *Anal Biochem*, 2015. **478**: 8–13.

142. Shen, D.D., K.L. Kunze, and K.E. Thummel, Enzyme-catalyzed processes of first-pass hepatic and intestinal drug extraction. *Adv Drug Deliv Rev*, 1997. **27**(2–3): 99–127.

143. Haining, R.L. et al., Baculovirus-mediated expression and purification of human FMO3: Catalytic, immunochemical, and structural characterization. *Drug Metab Dispos*, 1997. **25**(7): 790–797.

144. Chen, G. et al., Human gastrointestinal sulfotransferases: identification and distribution. *Toxicol Appl Pharmacol*, 2003. **187**(3): 186–197.

145. Teubner, W. et al., Identification and localization of soluble sulfotransferases in the human gastrointestinal tract. *Biochem J*, 2007. **404**(2): 207–215.

146. Riches, Z. et al., Quantitative evaluation of the expression and activity of five major sulfotransferases (SULTs) in human tissues: The SULT "pie". *Drug Metab Dispos*, 2009. **37**(11): 2255–2261.
147. Her, C. et al., Human jejunal estrogen sulfotransferase and dehydroepiandrosterone sulfotransferase: Immunochemical characterization of individual variation. *Drug Metab Dispos*, 1996. **24**(12): 1328–1335.
148. Kurogi, K. et al., Concerted actions of the catechol O-methyltransferase and the cytosolic sulfotransferase SULT1A3 in the metabolism of catecholic drugs. *Biochem Pharmacol*, 2012. **84**(9): 1186–1195.
149. Mizuma, T. et al., Differentiation of organ availability by sequential and simultaneous analyses: Intestinal conjugative metabolism impacts on intestinal availability in humans. *J Pharm Sci*, 2005. **94**(3): 571–575.
150. Hartman, A.P. et al., Enantioselective sulfation of beta 2-receptor agonists by the human intestine and the recombinant M-form phenolsulfotransferase. *Chirality*, 1998. **10**(9): 800–803.
151. Back, D.J. et al., The gut wall metabolism of ethinyloestradiol and its contribution to the pre-systemic metabolism of ethinyloestradiol in humans. *Br J Clin Pharmacol*, 1982. **13**(3): 325–330.
152. Schrag, M.L. et al., Sulfotransferase 1E1 is a low km isoform mediating the 3-O-sulfation of ethinyl estradiol. *Drug Metab Dispos*, 2004. **32**(11): 1299–1303.
153. Tukey, R.H. and C.P. Strassburg, Genetic multiplicity of the human UDP-glucuronosyltransferases and regulation in the gastrointestinal tract. *Mol Pharmacol*, 2001. **59**(3): 405–414.
154. Fisher, M.B. et al., The role of hepatic and extrahepatic UDP-glucuronosyltransferases in human drug metabolism. *Drug Metab Rev*, 2001. **33**(3–4): 273–297.
155. Ritter, J.K., Intestinal UGTs as potential modifiers of pharmacokinetics and biological responses to drugs and xenobiotics. *Expert Opin Drug Metab Toxicol*, 2007. **3**(1): 93–107.
156. Ohno, S. and S. Nakajin, Determination of mRNA expression of human UDP-glucuronosyltransferases and application for localization in various human tissues by real-time reverse transcriptase-polymerase chain reaction. *Drug Metab Dispos*, 2009. **37**(1): 32–40.
157. Nakamura, A. et al., Expression of UGT1A and UGT2Bs mRNA in human normal tissues and various cell lines. *Drug Metab Dispos*, 2008. **36**(8): 1461–1464.
158. Oda, S. et al., Preparation of a specific monoclonal antibody against human UDP-glucuronosyltransferase (UGT) 1A9 and evaluation of UGT1A9 protein levels in human tissues. *Drug Metab Dispos*, 2012. **40**(8): 1620–1627.
159. Harbourt, D.E. et al., Quantification of human uridine-diphosphate glucuronosyl transferase 1A isoforms in liver, intestine, and kidney using nanobore liquid chromatography-tandem mass spectrometry. *Anal Chem*, 2012. **84**(1): 98–105.
160. Miyauchi, E. et al., Quantitative atlas of cytochrome P450, UDP-glucuronosyltransferase, and transporter proteins in jejunum of morbidly obese subjects. *Mol Pharm*, 2016. **13**(8): 2631–2640.
161. Kaminsky, L.S. and Q.Y. Zhang, The small intestine as a xenobiotic-metabolizing organ. *Drug Metab Dispos*, 2003. **31**(12): 1520–1525.
162. Strassburg, C.P. et al., Identification of cyclosporine A and tacrolimus glucuronidation in human liver and the gastrointestinal tract by a differentially expressed UDP-glucuronosyltransferase: UGT2B7. *J Hepatol*, 2001. **34**(6): 865–872.
163. Ebner, T., R.P. Remmel, and B. Burchell, Human bilirubin UDP-glucuronosyltransferase catalyzes the glucuronidation of ethinylestradiol. *Mol Pharmacol*, 1993. **43**(4): 649–654.
164. Mizuma, T., Intestinal glucuronidation metabolism may have a greater impact on oral bioavailability than hepatic glucuronidation metabolism in humans: A study with raloxifene, substrate for UGT1A1, 1A8, 1A9, and 1A10. *Int J Pharm*, 2009. **378**(1–2): 140–141.
165. Gufford, B.T. et al., Milk thistle constituents inhibit raloxifene intestinal glucuronidation: A potential clinically relevant natural product-drug interaction. *Drug Metab Dispos*, 2015. **43**(9): 1353–1359.
166. Stingl, J.C. et al., Relevance of UDP-glucuronosyltransferase polymorphisms for drug dosing: A quantitative systematic review. *Pharmacol Ther*, 2014. **141**(1): 92–116.
167. Ghosal, A. et al., Identification of human UDP-glucuronosyltransferase enzyme(s) responsible for the glucuronidation of ezetimibe (Zetia). *Drug Metab Dispos*, 2004. **32**(3): 314–320.
168. Kosoglou, T. et al., Ezetimibe: A review of its metabolism, pharmacokinetics and drug interactions. *Clin Pharmacokinet*, 2005. **44**(5): 467–494.
169. Kiss, L.E. and P. Soares-da-Silva, Medicinal chemistry of catechol O-methyltransferase (COMT) inhibitors and their therapeutic utility. *J Med Chem*, 2014. **57**(21): 8692–8717.
170. Gibbs, J.P., J.S. Yang, and J.T. Slattery, Comparison of human liver and small intestinal glutathione S-transferase-catalyzed busulfan conjugation *in vitro*. *Drug Metab Dispos*, 1998. **26**(1): 52–55.

171. Hickman, D. et al., Expression of arylamine N-acetyltransferase in human intestine. *Gut*, 1998. **42**(3): 402–409.
172. Coles, B.F. et al., Interindividual variation and organ-specific patterns of glutathione S-transferase alpha, mu, and pi expression in gastrointestinal tract mucosa of normal individuals. *Arch Biochem Biophys*, 2002. **403**(2): 270–276.
173. Tian, D.D. et al., Methylation and its role in the disposition of tanshinol, a cardiovascular carboxylic catechol from Salvia miltiorrhiza roots (Danshen). *Acta Pharmacol Sin*, 2015. **36**(5): 627–643.
174. Nissinen, E. et al., Catechol-O-methyltransferase activity in human and rat small intestine. *Life Sci*, 1988. **42**(25): 2609–2614.
175. Mannisto, P.T. and S. Kaakkola, Catechol-O-methyltransferase (COMT): Biochemistry, molecular biology, pharmacology, and clinical efficacy of the new selective COMT inhibitors. *Pharmacol Rev*, 1999. **51**(4): 593–628.
176. Vree, T.B. et al., Liver and gut mucosa acetylation of mesalazine in healthy volunteers. *Int J Clin Pharmacol Ther*, 2000. **38**(11): 514–522.
177. Hoensch, H. et al., Influence of clinical factors, diet, and drugs on the human upper gastrointestinal glutathione system. *Gut*, 2002. **50**(2): 235–240.
178. Delaforge, M. et al., Metabolism of dihydroergotamine by a cytochrome P-450 similar to that involved in the metabolism of macrolide antibiotics. *Xenobiotica*, 1989. **19**(11): 1285–1295.
179. Little, P.J. et al., Bioavailability of dihydroergotamine in man. *Br J Clin Pharmacol*, 1982. **13**(6): 785–790.
180. Garcia-Carbonero, R. and J.G. Supko, Current perspectives on the clinical experience, pharmacology, and continued development of the camptothecins. *Clin Cancer Res*, 2002. **8**(3): 641–661.
181. Thummel, K., D.D. Shen, and N. Isoherranen, Design and optimization of dosage regimens: Pharmacokinetic data, in *Goodman & Gilman's The Pharmacological Basis of Therapeutics*, L. Brunton, Chabner, BA, Knollman, BC, Editor. 2011, McGraw-Hill: New York. pp. 1891–1990.

12

Sites of Extra Hepatic Metabolism, Part III: Kidney

Lawrence H. Lash

CONTENTS

Introduction

Although the kidneys only comprise 1%–2% of total body weight, they can play an important, if not critical, role in overall drug metabolism in the body. There are several factors that are responsible for the ability of the kidneys to play such a disproportionately important role. First, despite their weight, the kidneys receive approximately 25% of the cardiac output, thereby delivering a large proportion of blood-borne chemicals to the renal circulation. A second major factor is that by multiple mechanisms that are a central, underlying part of the basic physiology of the kidneys, drugs and chemicals may become concentrated within renal epithelial cells to levels that are often markedly higher than those to which the tissue is exposed. These concentrating mechanisms include glomerular filtration, the counter-current circulatory system that operates in the distal nephron and has the physiological function of concentrating the tubular fluid several-fold over that in the plasma, and the existence of a large array of transporters for organic anions and cations on the basolateral and luminal membranes of renal epithelial cells.

A third reason for the importance of the kidneys in drug metabolism is that once inside the renal cell, many of the same enzymes that have been classically studied in liver are also present, enabling metabolism to occur. A review of many of these enzymes, as well as some that are unique to the kidneys or that have unique characteristics compared to those in other organs because of renal morphology or physiology, are the primary areas of focus for this chapter.

In studying renal drug metabolism, it is critical to consider the impact of nephron heterogeneity [1,2]. The mammalian kidney is complex and can be structurally and functionally subdivided into multiple, distinct parts. At the simplest level, kidneys are subdivided into cortex, outer medulla (further subdivided into inner stripe and outer stripe), and inner medulla (or papilla). The nephron, which is the basic building block of the kidney, can exist as either short-looped or long-looped types, the frequency of which varies among species. To understand the importance of this sub-organellar organization, one can compare nephron segment-specific differences in metabolism, cellular energetics, and other parameters of physiological function (Table 12.1). The different segments of the nephron, three of which are highlighted here, provide a perfect example of form corresponding with function. In terms of morphology, the proximal tubule is ideally suited for extensive reabsorption and secretion of anions, cations, and metabolites because of the large surface area provided by the microvilli on the luminal or brush-border plasma membrane and the extensive infoldings on the serosal or basolateral plasma membrane. Mitochondrial density is high in nephron segments that exhibit particularly high activities of energy-dependent processes, such as active transport and biosynthetic reactions.

Of particular interest for the primary focus of this chapter, significant segment-specific differences exist in pathways of drug metabolism. For the majority of reactions that are of interest for drugs and other xenobiotics, the highest amounts of the key reaction pathways are present in the proximal tubules. It should be noted, however, that certain enzymatic pathways in other nephron segments also play a critical role for the bioactivation of certain drugs and chemicals. For the majority of drugs and chemicals of interest, it is the proximal tubules that are the primary sites of metabolism. As listed in Table 12.1, the various Phase I

TABLE 12.1

Selected Biochemical, Morphological and Functional Properties of Some Key Nephron Segments of Mammalian Kidney

Nephron Cell Type	Morphology	Physiology	Metabolism
Proximal tubule	Tall, prominent microvilli on luminal membrane; cuboidal shape; extensive basolateral infoldings; high density of mitochondria	Active Na^+ reabsorption; organic anion and cation secretion; most glucose and amino acid reabsorption; passive water and Cl^- reabsorption	Oxidative phosphorylation, citric acid cycle, gluconeogenesis; substrates = fatty acids, ketone bodies, lactate, glutamine, pyruvate, citrate, acetate; Drug metabolism: High CYP, FMO, UGT, SULT, GSH-dependent
Thick ascending limb	Extensive interdigitations; large number of elongated, rod-shaped mitochondria	Water-impermeable; Na^+-K^+-$2Cl^-$ cotransport; active Ca^{2+} and Mg^{2+} transport; dilution of hyperosmotic tubular urine	Oxidative phosphorylation and glycolysis; substrates = lactate, glucose, ketone bodies, fatty acids, acetate; Drug metabolism: Low CYP, FMO, UGT, SULT; high PGS (mTAL)
Distal tubule (distal convoluted tubule and cortical collecting duct)	DCT: appears bright under microscope; numerous, long mitochondria. CCT: appears granular under microscope; wider than DCT.	High rates of Na^+ reabsorption; thiazide-inhibitable Na^+-Cl^- cotransport; K^+-Cl^- cotransport; Ca^{2+} reabsorption; DCT: water impermeable; CCT: vasopressin-dependent water channel	Glycolysis; substrates = glucose, lactate, β-hydroxybutyrate, fatty acids (CCT only); Drug metabolism: Generally all low

Abbreviations: CCT, cortical collecting duct; CYP, cytochrome P450; DCT, distal convoluted tubule; FMO, flavin-containing monooxygenase; mTAL, medullary thick ascending limb; PGS, prostaglandin synthetase; SULT, sulfotransferase; UGT, UDP-glucuronosyltransferase.

and Phase II pathways, as well as enzymes such as the cysteine conjugate β-lyase (CCBL), are predominantly localized in the proximal tubules.

Experimental Models to Study Kidney Drug Metabolism

The segment-specific distribution of many drug metabolism enzymes sometimes makes it difficult to properly study or even detect certain reaction pathways. This is particularly true for pathways that are present at relatively low activities. For clinical studies, one is of course limited to non-invasive methods to determine metabolism. Metabolites of certain chemicals in either blood or urine can be considered as biomarkers for the presence of a particular enzyme. It is often difficult, however, to distinguish renal metabolism from the more prominent hepatic metabolism. Moreover, the subsequent action of additional enzymes that generate reactive and unstable metabolites may make detection of metabolism difficult.

A suitable alternative to *in vivo* study of metabolism can be the use of a variety of *in vitro* models. A key advantage of using such models is that renal metabolism can be measured separately from hepatic metabolism. When *in vitro* models are used to measure renal metabolism, however, care is needed in choosing the model because of the selective distribution of drug metabolism enzymes and transporters along the nephron. Thus, a model that contains multiple nephron cell types may result in either measurement of low metabolic rates or failure to detect metabolism because of dilution of the pathway enzymes due to the presence of cell types that do not express them.

A detailed discussion of the various *in vitro* models that are available to study renal drug metabolism is beyond the scope of this chapter. The reader is referred to two reviews [3,4] that describe various model systems and consider their advantages, disadvantages, primary uses, and limitations. A few comments will be made here, with the focus being on their applicability for the study and quantitation of drug metabolism reactions.

The simplest *in vitro* model in terms of its preparation is that of the isolated perfused kidney. It has the advantage that extrarenal metabolism is eliminated. As with many of the freshly isolated *in vitro* models, its use is limited to relatively short time periods because of gradual and progressive functional impairment. Another limitation for study of drug metabolism is that one cannot always distinguish processes that occur in specific nephron segments (the dilution effect mentioned above). The isolated perfused kidney is also relatively expensive in that a single animal (typically the rat) is used for all measurements.

Renal slices are a convenient and relatively simple model that enables better assessment of metabolism occurring in specific nephron segments. Substrate transport is conveniently measured as the slice-to-medium ratio, and is often used as an assessment of tubular viability when actively transported substrates are used. While slices are easy to prepare and have relatively low cost, they are limited by a relatively short lifetime, the potential for collapsed lumens and poor oxygenation, and the presence of multiple cell populations despite the ability to prepare slices from discrete regions of the kidney (i.e., cortex, outer stripe and inner stripe of the outer medulla, inner medulla).

The most convenient *in vitro* models to enable measurement of drug metabolism pathways in specific nephron cell types, thereby minimizing the "dilution effect," are freshly isolated tubular fragments and isolated cells. Both can be prepared from specific nephron segments using various physical separation methods, such as microdissection, density-gradient centrifugation, or electrophoresis. Enzymatic digestion with collagenase and/or hyaluronidase is often used as a first step prior to separation of cell types. Although both methods can provide similar data, it is usually easiest to prepare tubular fragments from rabbits and isolated cells from rats. As with the isolated perfused kidney and renal slices, isolated tubular fragments and isolated cells can only be maintained in a viable state for a limited time period, which is typically up to 4 hr.

While the relatively short lifetime of isolated tubular fragments or isolated cells is not a limitation if one wants to simply quantify metabolism, other types of assays such as enzyme induction or study of gene regulation require models that retain viability for longer periods of time. To accomplish this, many investigators have established primary cultures of renal epithelial cells from the proximal tubule [3,5–18] and distal tubule and thick ascending limb [14,19,20] of rat, mouse or rabbit. The advantage of primary cultures is that they can be maintained in a viable state for at least 4–5 days and are derived directly from the *in vivo* tissue. Unfortunately, primary cell cultures, particularly those from epithelial cells, tend to lose some of their differentiated functions during the course of culture. Expression of drug metabolism enzymes are particularly prone to being lost during culture. To combat this problem, investigators have used serum-free, hormonally-defined media with limited success.

Another important issue about the experimental model used concerns the known species-dependent differences in drug metabolism enzymes, which will be discussed in the sections below. Inasmuch as we are primarily interested in drug metabolism in the human kidney, the availability of human kidneys or human kidney slices (e.g., surgical waste) has enabled investigators to use freshly isolated renal cells or primary cultures of proximal tubular cells from the primary species of interest [21–28]. Primary cultures of human proximal tubular cells also suffer from the same potential problem of de-differentiation as do those from rats, mice, or rabbits. The primary advantage in the use of human proximal tubular cells for primary culture is, of course, the absence of the need for consideration of species differences in responses.

Another type of *in vitro* renal cellular model is that of continuous or immortalized cell lines. Distinct advantages with use of these cell lines are that they are easy to use and are reproducible. Renal cell lines that are commonly used in study of metabolism, transport, and toxicity derive from various species and multiple nephron segments, including the glomerulus, proximal tubule, medullary thick ascending limb, and distal tubule. As discussed elsewhere [29], these cell lines, by being immortalized, have undergone genotypic and phenotypic changes that may make them questionable as models of *in vivo* renal metabolism. As compared with primary cell cultures, immortalized cell lines possess even more uncertainties as to their value for *in vivo* drug metabolism.

An alternative experimental model that is currently being developed and becoming more popular involves human stem cell-based approaches to generate proximal tubule-like cells [30–34]. Renal progenitor cells appear to play important roles in renal repair under various pathological conditions, such as repair of ischemia-reperfusion injury in mice [35–37]. Human induced pluripotent stem cells have been developed and used to demonstrate protection from ischemia-reperfusion and some forms of drug-induced injury [30,38]. Such cells have gained in popularity because of the safety and ethical concerns with the use of human embryonic stem cells. Further development of these models and validation of end points used to predict renal damage are still needed but may lead to their more extensive application in the study of chemically induced nephrotoxicity and drug metabolism [37,38].

Membrane Transport

Although membrane transport processes are not, strictly speaking, a part of drug metabolism, no discussion of the renal handling of drugs can be complete without some consideration of how drugs gain access to enzymes in renal epithelial cells. Figure 12.1 schematically summarizes some of the major carrier proteins on the basolateral (BLM) and brush-border (BBM) plasma membranes of renal proximal tubular cells that are important in the renal tubular uptake or efflux of organic anions and organic cations. Most drugs of interest for therapeutics or toxicology studies are charged, so that the carrier proteins shown are responsible for the majority of their transport in the renal proximal tubule.

The various carriers are either primary, secondary, or tertiary active or facilitated transporters. Primary active transporters are those that directly couple ATP hydrolysis to the movement of substrate; relevant examples include the multidrug-resistance-associated proteins (MRPs), the multiple drug resistance protein (MDR1; also known as P-glycoprotein), the $(Na^+ + K^+)$-stimulated ATPase, and the Na^+/H^+ exchanger (NHE). Secondary active transporters are those that couple or exchange substrate with an ion (generally either Na^+ or H^+ ion) whose gradient is generated by a primary active transporter. These include the sodium-dicarboxylate 3 (*SLC13A3*; NaC3) carrier and the organic cation transporters (OCTs) N1 and N2. Tertiary active transporters include the organic anion transporters (OATs) 1 and 3, which couple uptake of organic anions, bile salts, and some organic cations with efflux of 2-oxoglutarate (2-OG⁻), which is generated by NaC3. The remaining carriers are either facilitated exchangers or uniporters. Similar to many of the drug metabolism enzymes that are discussed below (particularly the cytochrome P450s), the various OATs, OCTs, MRPs, and MDR1 have broad and often overlapping substrate specificities,

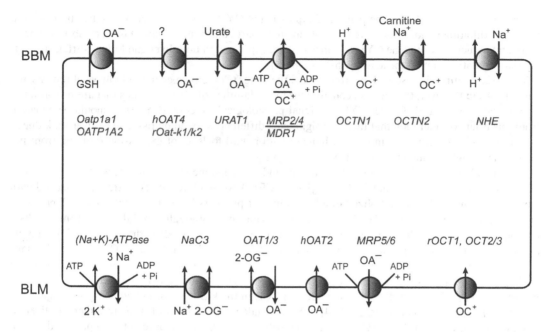

FIGURE 12.1 Organic anion and cation transport in renal proximal tubule. This scheme illustrates the major transporters found on the basolateral (BLM) and brush-border (BBM) plasma membranes that mediate the uptake or efflux of organic anions (OA⁻) and organic cations (OC⁺). Also shown are the (Na⁺ + K⁺)-stimulated ATPase, the sodium-dicarboxylate 3 (NaC3) carrier, and the sodium-hydrogen exchanger (NHE), which provide the driving force for many of the carriers involved in the transport of drugs. Other abbreviations: GSH, glutathione; MDR, multiple drug resistance protein; MRP, multidrug resistance-associated protein; OAT, organic anion transporter; OCT, organic cation transporter; Oat-k1/2, kidney-specific organic anion transporter; OATP, organic anion transporting polypeptide; 2-OG⁻, 2-oxoglutarate; URAT, urate transporter. Note that when the carrier name is preceded by "h" or "r," this indicates that it is only found in human or rat, respectively.

resulting in some degree of functional redundancy. However, there are some discrete substrate specificities for the various carriers. Readers are referred to several recent reviews on the identity, function, and regulation of mammalian renal organic anion and cation transporters [39–47].

Phase I Metabolism in the Kidneys

The major Phase I or oxidative metabolism enzymes in the kidneys exhibit similar biochemistry as those in the liver, although there are significant differences based on patterns of expression and nephron heterogeneity [48,49]. This section will review three major enzyme systems, cytochrome P450s (CYPs), flavin-containing monooxygenases (FMO), and prostaglandin synthetase (PGS). The focus will be to describe the patterns of expression of the different enzymes among cell types of the nephron and sex- and species-dependent differences that are known to exist. The species-dependent differences have important implications for the use of metabolism data from laboratory animals for making predictions for metabolism in humans. In some cases, particularly for some drugs and chemicals that are bioactivated to reactive intermediates that elicit nephrotoxicity, metabolic pathways in rats or mice cannot be used to make predictions for humans.

Cytochrome P450

The most obvious difference between the better studied CYP enzymes in liver and those in kidney is that overall expression of CYP enzymes in kidney are generally only 5%–20% of those in the liver. Another difference is that CYP enzymes are not uniformly distributed throughout the nephron but exhibit discrete localizations (cf. Table 12.1). The pattern of expression of CYP enzymes differs in the two tissues, with the liver exhibiting a more extensive array of enzymes, particularly in humans. Further, substrate specificity and inducibility of some CYP enzymes that are expressed in both liver and kidney differ, suggesting that regulation of enzyme activity differs [48–51].

Table 12.2 summarizes some key properties of the major CYP enzymes in the kidneys of rodents and humans. As in the liver, the kidneys contain four major families of CYP enzymes that are important in drug metabolism (CYP1, CYP2, CYP3) or renal physiological function (CYP4). It should be apparent from this brief consideration that there are significant differences based on tissue (e.g., liver vs. kidney), sex, and species (e.g., rat vs. mouse vs. human) with regard to level of expression (ranging from not detectable to high), inducibility, and nephron cell type localization.

An example that highlights some of the tissue- and species-dependent differences in CYP is that of the environmental contaminant trichloroethylene (TCE). Adverse effects of TCE are all associated with metabolism, and TCE is metabolized to a large range of products by both CYP ("oxidative" pathway) or glutathione S-transferase (GST; "conjugation" pathway), although CYP-dependent metabolism predominates at all but the highest substrate concentrations [52]. CYP2E1 is the primary CYP enzyme that metabolizes small halogenated solvents such as TCE. CYP2C11 in the rat or CYP2C19 in humans is also reasonably active towards TCE. TCE has several potential target organs, which varies according to sex, species, and dose, and is considered a "known human carcinogen" by the National Toxicology Program (NTP) [53]. All of the adverse effects of TCE in the kidneys are linked solely to its glutathione (GSH)-dependent metabolism [52,54]. CYP-dependent metabolism of TCE in either the liver or kidneys may, however, influence GSH-dependent metabolism, which can have both a hepatic and a renal component even though the terminal products are formed in the kidneys. Thus, we find that rat kidney readily metabolizes TCE to its oxidative metabolites as both CYP2E1 and CYP2C11 are expressed at fairly high levels in the proximal tubules [55]. In contrast to this situation, little or no detectable oxidative metabolism of TCE occurs in the human kidney [22], which is consistent with the inability to detect either CYP2E1 or CYP2C19 in human proximal tubular cells [23,56]. Hence, we can modulate GSH-dependent metabolism and toxicity of TCE in rat proximal tubular cells by altering CYP status [57]. This is an example of a case where metabolism data cannot be extrapolated from rodents to humans at all because of species-dependent differences.

As suggested by its broad substrate specificities, enzymes of the CYP2 family are a diverse set of enzymes. Differences exist between species and tissues in a given species. As summarized in Table 12.2, CYP2A enzymes are expressed in mouse kidney but not in rat or human kidney [48]. CYP2B1/2 illustrates both species and tissue differences. Whereas CYP2B1/2 is inducible by phenobarbital in rat liver, it is not induced by it in rat kidney and is undetectable in human kidney. As mentioned above,

TABLE 12.2

Selected Cytochrome P450 (Cyp) Enzymes Expressed in Rodent and Human Kidney

CYP Enzyme	Rats and/or Mice	Humans
CYP1A1/2	Low constitutive; CYP1A1 inducible	Not detected or poorly inducible
CYP1B1/2	Present at modest levels	Present at modest levels
CYP2A	Present in mice; not detected in rats	Not detected
CYP2B1/2	Inducible by clofibrate in rats	Not detected
CYP2C11 (CYP2C19)	Constitutive; sex and developmental differences	Not detected
CYP2D6	Low levels	Low levels
CYP2E1	Present; inducible	Not detected or barely detectable
CYP3A1/2 (CYP3A4/5)	Primarily in glomerulus	Glomerulus, proximal tubule; genetic polymorphisms
CYP4A2/3 (CYP4A11)	Proximal tubule; inducible by fibrates	Proximal tubule; inducible by ethanol, dexamethasone

The major CYP enzymes that are important in drug metabolism or in renal physiology are listed for rats, mice, and, where applicable, the human orthologue is listed in parentheses.

CYP2C enzymes and CYP2E1 also demonstrate significant species differences. Whereas CYP2E1 is readily detected in rat and mouse kidney [51,58], its expression has not been detected in human kidney [22,23,56,59]. In rat and mouse kidney, CYP2E1 expression is under androgenic control and males have significantly more enzyme than females. A consequence of this gender-dependent difference is that male mice are markedly more susceptible than female mice to nephrotoxicity caused by certain CYP2E1 substrates [60].

The CYP3 gene family is highly expressed in kidneys of both rodents and humans, although there may be some difference in nephron localization across species, with a higher proportion being expressed in the glomerulus vs. the proximal tubules in rodent kidney and the reverse in human kidney [58,61,62]. The human orthologue of rodent CYP3A1/2 is CYP3A4/5; it is readily detected in microsomes from human kidney cortex homogenates [56,62] but appears to exhibit a high degree of variability among human kidney samples [56], consistent with the known genetic polymorphisms for CYP3A4 and other CYP enzymes [63,64].

Enzymes of the CYP4A family are primarily involved in metabolism of fatty acids, such as arachidonic acid, and are prominently expressed in the kidneys [65–67]. Although they do not metabolize drugs and other xenobiotics, this CYP family is mentioned here because their expression is strongly influenced by hypolipidemic drugs, such as the fibrates, and other drugs that are known to cause peroxisome proliferation. One should note, however, that the effectiveness of such peroxisome proliferators is much greater in liver than in kidney and in rats than in humans.

Flavin-Containing Monooxygenase

Like the CYPs, flavin-containing monooxygenases (FMOs) are a multigene family of enzymes found in the endoplasmic reticulum that are highly expressed in the liver, but also in extrahepatic tissues, including the kidneys [68,69]. While there are five active isoforms (FMO1–5) that have been identified in mammals, they are not ubiquitously expressed, with significant species-, sex-, tissue-, and developmental-dependent differences [70–73]. Although the FMOs have a fairly broad substrate specificity, they are most active in catalyzing the oxidation of sulfur-, selenium-, and nitrogen-containing drugs and xenobiotics. While many FMO substrates are also metabolized by various CYPs, there are several types of substrates that are restricted to FMO.

In contrast to human liver, which expresses primarily FMO3 as well as several other FMO enzymes, human kidney (in particular, the proximal tubules) expresses primarily FMO1, somewhat lower levels of FMO5, and very low levels of FMO3 [74]. Similarly, Nishimura and Naito [75] assessed profiles of FMO mRNA expression in human kidney, and found that FMO1 mRNA was the most abundantly expressed form whereas FMO2, FMO3, FMO4, and FMO5 mRNAs were expressed at 4%, 0.09%, 25%, and 13%, respectively, of the levels found for FMO1. Another interesting finding was that FMO1 protein levels varied considerably in a limited number of samples of human kidney, consistent with the existence of genetic polymorphisms [74]. Moreover, single nucleotide polymorphisms and splicing variants have been identified for all of the FMOs in several human tissues, including the kidneys [68].

It has been known for many years that sulfoxides are stable, urinary metabolites of many cysteine S-conjugates. It was only with the studies of Elfarra and colleagues [76–78] that it became apparent that these sulfoxide metabolites may play a different role than just being a stable end-product. In the kidneys, in particular, many of the studies over the past nearly two decades have focused on the role of FMOs in the bioactivation of nephrotoxic cysteine S-conjugates, which are converted to reactive sulfoxides [22,76–81]. The function of FMOs in bioactivation of cysteine S-conjugates and the role of this in nephrotoxicity are discussed further, in the sections on the GSH conjugation pathway and in the example of how TCE and perchloroethylene (Perc) cause nephrotoxicity.

Prostaglandin Synthase

Prostaglandins play a number of critical roles in renal physiology and pathophysiology, involving volume and sodium homeostasis, with the various lipid-derived products functioning as important signaling molecules [82,83]. The biosynthesis of prostaglandins involves a two-step process, catalyzed by the

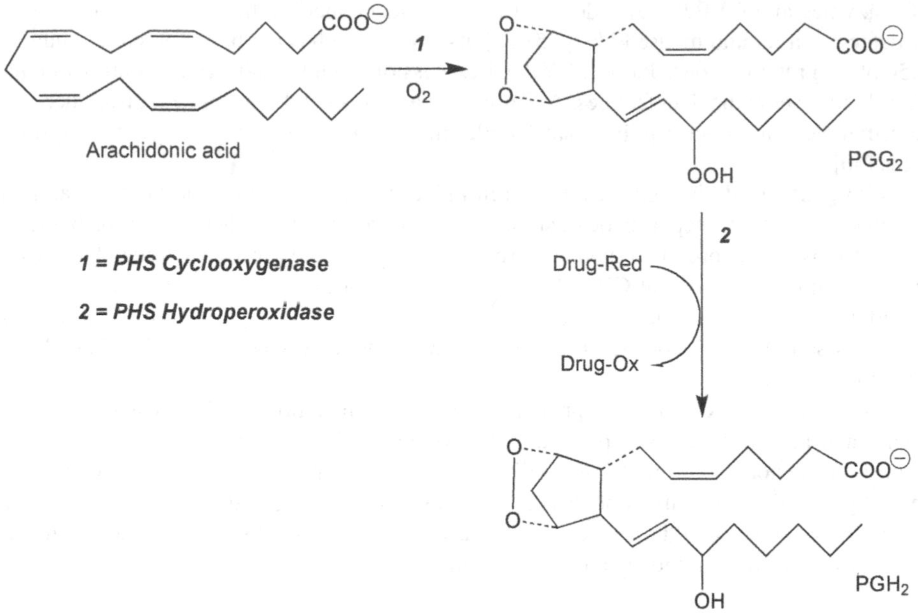

FIGURE 12.2 Prostaglandin synthase reaction pathway for drug co-oxidation. Scheme showing how certain drugs are oxidized during the hydroperoxidase step of the prostaglandin synthase (PHS) reaction.

bifunctional prostaglandin H synthase (PHS): the cyclooxygenase-dependent oxidation of a polyunsaturated fatty acid, such as arachidonic acid, to a hydroperoxy endoperoxide, prostaglandin G_2 (PGG$_2$), and the subsequent reduction to a hydroxy endoperoxide prostaglandin H_2 (PGH$_2$) (Figure 12.2). In the kidneys, PHS is localized in the microsomal fraction of cells of the inner and outer medulla [84,85].

Although the primary focus of studies on this pathway has been that of subsequent products (e.g., various eicosanoids) that influence renal function, it was realized in the late-1970s that a number of drugs can undergo co-oxidation in the hydroperoxidase step of the PHS reaction [86,87]. The diverse group of drugs that can oxidized in this manner include analgesics such as acetaminophen (APAP) and aminopyrene, and carcinogens such as benzidine and benzo(a)pyrene. PHS-catalyzed oxidation of benzidine has been associated with increased risk of bladder cancer [87–90].

Phase II Metabolism in the Kidneys

Phase II metabolism reactions include the various conjugation reactions, such as glucuronidation, sulfation, and GSH conjugation. A drug or xenobiotic is linked by a covalent bond to an endogenous group through a functional group (e.g., hydroxyl or amino group) that is either present in the parent molecule or is introduced by a Phase I reaction (e.g., CYP- or FMO-catalyzed oxidation, reduction, or hydrolysis). While these pathways occur in the liver, they are also present in select regions of the kidney, although isozyme patterns differ. Although it is generally true that the conjugates formed by Phase II reactions are highly water soluble and are readily excreted in either bile or urine, there are some notable exceptions, particularly for renal metabolism; some of these exceptions will be discussed below in the section on specific examples.

Glucuronidation

This Phase II reaction is catalyzed by a family of enzymes called the UDP-glucuronosyltransferases (UGTs), which are localized in the endoplasmic reticulum and are expressed in most tissues, but in varying amounts. Glucuronidation is an Sn2 reaction in which an acceptor group on the substrate (nucleophile) attacks an electrophilic carbon on the glucuronic acid moiety. Glucuronides may form on N-, S-, and C-groups of both endogenous and xenobiotic substrates. The glucuronidation pathway occurs in three steps, the first two for formation of UDP-glucuronic acid (UDPGA) from glucose-1-phosphate and UTP with NAD^+-dependent oxidation, and the third for formation of the conjugate. UDPGA is considered to be limiting in extrahepatic tissues, whereas ample substrate levels are usually present in the liver [49].

UGTs were originally divided into two gene families, UGT1 and UGT2, based on sequence homology. Recently, the nomenclature used for the UDP-glycosyltransferases, which include the UGTs, was updated [91]. Thus, the mammalian UGT gene superfamily, as of October, 2005, has 117 members that are divided into four gene families, UGT1, UGT2, UGT3, and UGT8. UGTs from the UGT1 and UGT2 family are the most efficient at using UDPGA as donor substrate so are the ones that are of most interest in drug metabolism. The sugar specificity of the UGT3 members is unclear as this group has only recently been identified. The UGT8 family is a single gene that encodes UDP-galactose ceramide galactosyltransferase and is not likely to be involved in drug metabolism.

Substrates for the UGTs include a broad range of both endogenous (e.g., steroid hormones, bile acids, biogenic amines) and xenobiotic chemicals (e.g., fat-soluble vitamins, carcinogens, acetaminophen, salicylic acid). Klaassen and colleagues [92] studied the mRNA expression of several members of the UGT1 and UGT2 gene families in several rat tissues. As summarized by Shelby et al. [92], UGT1 family members are encoded from a single gene that has multiple first exons followed by four common exons. Individual UGT1A gene products are formed by the splicing of one of the first exons with the four common exons. Identification of distinct gene promoter regions for the multiple first exon is consistent with tissue-specific patterns of expression and inducibility of specific UGT1A isoforms. In the rat, nine different first exons have been identified, generating UGT1A1 through UGT1A9, although UGT1A4 and UGT1A9 are pseudogenes (i.e., they do not encode for functional proteins). Members of the UGT2 gene family, in contrast to those of the UGT1 gene family, are encoded from individual genes, with each gene containing six exons. The UGT2 gene family is further subdivided into two subfamilies, UGT2A and UGT2B. In humans, a total of 17 UGTs have been characterized as of a 2004 review [93]. The potential importance of UGTs in human health and disease was also emphasized in that review. A check of the UGT homepage (https://www.flinders.edu.au/medicine/sites/clinical-pharmacology/ugt-homepage.cfm) in December 2016 shows 21 human UGTs.

Renal UGTs are microsomal enzymes of 54–56 kDa molecular weight and are found predominantly in the proximal tubules. Comparison of UGT activities in liver and kidney microsomes from several species shows that rates of metabolism are invariably higher in the liver than the kidney, sometimes by >10-fold, and those in rodents were generally higher than those in humans [49]. Similar to the situation with several CYPs, renal and hepatic UGTs exhibit different patterns of inducibility; in some cases, certain inducers are just more effective in liver whereas in other cases, chemicals may induce in one tissue and not at all in the other.

The studies of Shelby et al. [92] showed that individual genes of both the UGT1 and UGT2 families exhibit distinct patterns of expression that vary with both tissue and gender. mRNA expression was determined in liver, kidney, lung, stomach, small intestine (duodenum, jejunum, ileum), colon, and brain (cerebellum, cerebral cortex). Of the seven functional UGT1A gene products, UGT1A1 mRNA was detected in all tissues studied and was found at similar levels for both males and females, with the exception of lung tissue, which was relatively low. UGT1A2, UGT1A3, and UGT1A7 were detected primarily in the gastrointestinal tract with no significant gender differences for the former and possibly some for the latter. UGT1A5 mRNA was primarily limited to the liver with higher levels in females. UGT1A6 mRNA was found in most tissues, but was highest in the kidneys and large intestine; expression in rat kidney from females was significantly higher than that in males. UGT1A8 mRNA was detected almost exclusively in liver and kidney and was about 2-fold higher in females in both tissues. Thus, from the UGT1 gene family, rat kidney expresses primarily UGT1A1, UGT1A6, and UGT1A8. In human kidneys, Nishimura and Naito [75] found UGT1A6 and UGT1A9 (a pseudogene) to be the major mRNA species detected. Lash et al. [56] detected UGT1A1 and UGT1A6 proteins in primary cultures of human proximal tubular cells.

Shelby et al. [92] found more prominent tissue-specific differences in mRNA expression for members of the UGT2 gene family. UGT2A1 was detected almost exclusively in the nasal epithelium whereas

UGT2B1 and UGT2B2 were detected almost exclusively in liver with >2-fold higher levels found in female rats as compared to male rats. UGT2B3 mRNA was found predominantly in liver with 10%–20% as much found in the small intestine. UGT2B6 mRNA was also predominantly expressed in liver with low levels (<10% of liver) detected in small intestine and brain. The only isoform mRNAs detected in kidney were those for UGT2B8 (very low levels) and UGT2B12. The latter was found ubiquitously but was most prominent in kidney and liver. In human kidney, relatively low levels of mRNA for UGT2B10, UGT2B15, and UGT2B17 were detected [75]. In primary cultures of human proximal tubular cells, UGT2B7 protein was readily detected as well [46]. UGT8 mRNA was also detected in human kidney [75], but its function has not yet been characterized.

Sulfation

The sulfation pathway results in the sulfonation of a broad range of drugs, hormones, and neurotransmitters. As with the glucuronidation pathway, the sulfation pathway occurs in three steps, the first two being those that activate the donor substrate, forming 3′-phosphoadenosine-5′-phosphosulfate (PAPS), and the third being the sulfonation or sulfation reaction, which is catalyzed by a family of cytoplasmic enzymes called the sulfotransferases (SULTs). The known gene products are spread across six gene families (SULT1–6), although Sult3 is only found in mice and rabbits and Sult5a1 is only found in mice (see 94, 95 for recent reviews). Thus, there are 13 human cytosolic SULTs currently known that include members of the SULT1, SULT2, SULT4, and SULT6 gene families. Only those SULT enzymes that are found in the kidneys will be briefly discussed below. Much like other major drug metabolism enzyme systems, genetic polymorphisms and single nucleotide polymorphisms (SNPs) have been found for the SULTs [96], suggesting that individual variations in SULT activity may both contribute to disease or sensitivity to toxic chemicals or may be used to individualize new therapeutic approaches.

Products of the SULT1 family have a broad substrate specificity and can sulfonate simple, small planar phenols, such as estradiol, thyroid hormones, and a broad variety of drugs and environmental chemicals. SULT1A1 is the major adult liver SULT1A subfamily member and is also found in the kidneys. Both SULT1A1 and SULT1A3 are reported to be abundant in fetal liver and kidney, but the latter one is said to disappear in the adult, although expression of SULT1A3 protein was recently reported in primary cultures of human proximal tubular cells [56] and both SULT1A1 and SULT1A3 mRNA were reported in adult kidney [75], with SULT1A1 being by far the most highly expressed. Although SULT1A2 mRNA is found in several tissues, including the liver and kidneys, the consensus is that it is not translated into a functional protein in humans and, thus, is likely a pseudogene. SULT1E1 is also expressed in the kidneys [56,75,94], but is primarily active with phenols such as estradiol.

SULT2 family members are most active in the sulfonation of hydroxyl groups of steroids such as androsterone. SULT2A1 has been localized to the kidney by immunostaining and was found not only in the proximal tubules but in several more distal nephron segments. SULT2A1 protein was readily detected in primary cultures of human proximal tubular cells [56]. SULT2B1 exists as two variants and has been found in human kidney [75,94]. Thus, enzymes of the SULT2 family do not seem to have a major role in drug metabolism.

Glutathione Conjugation

Mercapturate Pathway

Along with glucuronidation and sulfation, GSH conjugation functions as a major detoxification pathway for many drugs and other xenobiotics. In the classical view, GSH S-transferases (GSTs) catalyze the conjugation of reactive electrophiles with GSH in the initial step of a detoxication pathway that ultimately results in formation of N-acetylcysteine conjugates (mercapturates), which are ultimately excreted in urine (Figure 12.3). Although GSTs are expressed in most cell types, including renal tubular epithelial cells, hepatocytes express the highest levels of any organ.

In mammals, multiple families of GSTs are found in cytoplasm, mitochondria, and endoplasmic reticulum (microsomes). Isoforms of importance for renal drug metabolism are those found in the cytoplasm

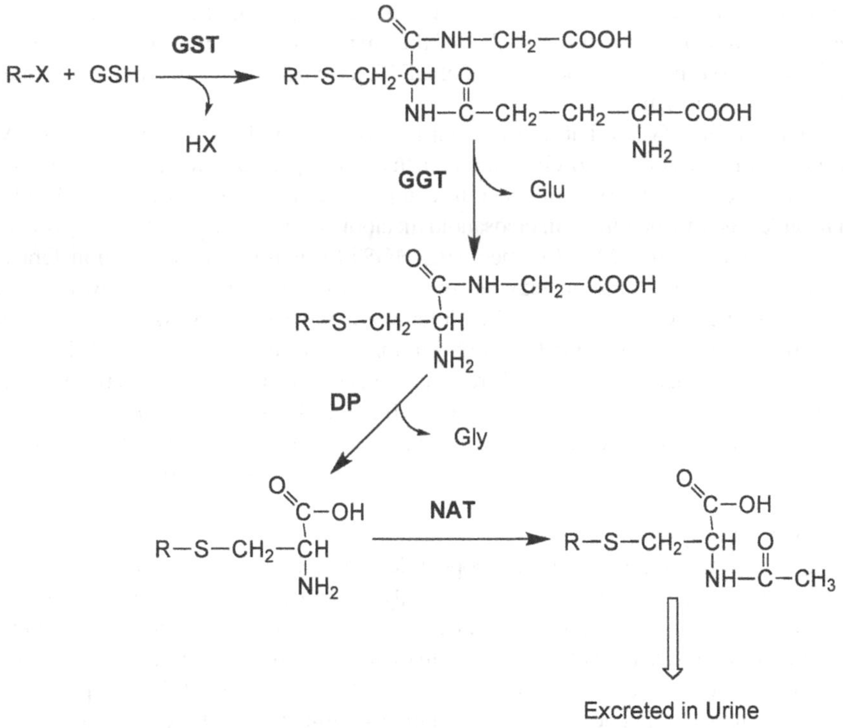

$$R–X + GSH \xrightarrow[HX]{GST} R–S–CH_2–CH$$

(GSH conjugate)

$$\downarrow \text{GGT} \searrow \text{Glu}$$

(cysteinylglycine conjugate)

$$\downarrow \text{DP} \searrow \text{Gly}$$

(cysteine conjugate)

$$R–S–CH_2–CH(NH_2)–C(=O)OH \xrightarrow{NAT} R–S–CH_2–CH(NH–C(=O)–CH_3)–C(=O)OH$$

$$\Downarrow$$

Excreted in Urine

FIGURE 12.3 Classical mercapturic acid pathway for drug detoxication. Drug (R-X; X is a good leaving group) are conjugated with GSH to form the GSH conjugate, either in the liver or kidney. Subsequent reactions occur in the kidneys, and include hydrolysis of the γ-glutamyl isopeptide bond by γ-glutamyltransferase (GGT) and the cysteinylglycine peptide bond by dipeptidase (DP) activity to yield the cysteine conjugate. The cysteine conjugate undergoes *N*-acetylation by the cysteine conjugate *N*-acetyltransferase (NAT) to form the *N*-acetylcysteine conjugate, or mercapturate. The mercapturate, because of its polarity, is readily excreted into the urine.

and microsomes. Cytoplasmic GSTs are dimers with subunits of 199–244 amino acids in length and are divided into seven families based on amino acid sequence (i.e., >40% homology). These families are designated as Alpha, Mu, Pi, Sigma, Theta, Omega, and Zeta. The convention is to refer to rodent GSTs by Greek letters (i.e., GSTα, μ, π, σ, τ, and ζ) and human GSTs by capital Arabic letters (i.e., GSTA, M, P, S, T, O, and Z). At present, 16 cytoplasmic GST subunits are known in humans. The mature protein can exist as a variety of homo- and heterodimers, indicating that a large variety of isoenzymes are ultimately generated.

Three families of cytoplasmic GSTs are expressed in rat kidney, GSTα, GSTπ, and GSTμ. Immunolocalization [97] and Western blot analyses in renal tissue and isolated renal proximal and distal tubular cells [98] showed selective localization of GSTα in proximal tubules whereas GSTπ and GSTμ are expressed in the distal nephron. In human kidney, the GST isoenzyme expression pattern is quite different from that in the rat kidney; renal proximal tubular cells express GSTA, GSTP, and GSTM [23,56]. Because of the broad and often overlapping substrate specificities of the different GST isoforms, it is difficult to assess the impact of this difference in expression pattern when extrapolating renal metabolism data from rats to humans.

The other cytoplasmic GST family found in the kidneys is the Zeta-class, which was discovered in the late-1990s using a bioinformatics approach with human expressed sequence tag databases [99–101]. GSTZs are widely distributed in eukaryotes and are identical to maleylacetoacetate isomerase, a key catalyst in tyrosine catabolism. Unlike the other cytoplasmic GSTs, GSTZs lack significant activity towards the prototypical substrate 1-chloro-2,4-dinitrobenzene. An important substrate class is the α-haloacids such as dichloroacetic acid (DCA), which is metabolized to glyoxylic acid. Metabolism of DCA is important because DCA is used in the clinical management of congenital lactic acidosis, is a common drinking water contaminant, and is a metabolite of the environmental contaminant and known human carcinogen TCE [52]. Four polymorphic variants of GSTZ have been described thus far in humans, and these have distinct catalytic activities.

The other family of renal GSTs that is important for drug metabolism are the MAPEG (Membrane Associated Proteins in Eicosanoid and Glutathione metabolism) proteins, which are a unique family of GSTs that share no sequence identity with either the cytoplasmic or mitochondrial GSTs. While a distinctive function includes their involvement in eicosanoid metabolism, MAPEG proteins are also important in drug metabolism. Of the different MAPEG members, MGST1 (microsomal GSH S-transferase 1) seems to function exclusively as a detoxication enzyme whereas MGST2 and MGST3 are involved in both drug metabolism and leukotriene C_4 synthesis [102]. Although the precise role of MAPEG proteins in GSH-dependent bioactivation is unclear, MGSTs have been immunolocalized to several rat tissues, including the kidneys [103], and chemicals such as TCE are readily metabolized to their respective GSH conjugates in the presence of GSH and liver or kidney microsomal fractions from rats or humans [104–106].

Regardless of whether the GSH conjugation reaction occurs within the kidneys themselves or in the liver, the subsequent reactions of the mercapturic acid pathway occur predominantly in the kidneys. The next two steps in the metabolism of GSH conjugates, regardless of whether they are undergoing the classic detoxication pathway to ultimately yield the mercapturate or whether they are being bioactivated, involve successive cleavage of the γ-glutamyl isopeptide and cysteinylglycyl peptide bonds to yield the corresponding cysteine conjugate. These steps are catalyzed by two brush-border membrane enzymes, γ-glutamyltransferase (GGT) and various dipeptidases (DP). Although GGT and DP activities are found on several extrarenal tissues, such as the hepatic canalicular plasma membrane and the jejunal brush-border plasma membrane, their activities are by far the highest on the brush-border plasma membrane of renal proximal tubules [107]. The overall, quantitative significance of these pathways in metabolism and turnover of GSH (and by analogy GSH conjugates) is illustrated by the profound glutathionuria that occurs when GGT activity is inhibited [108].

In the classic mercapturate pathway, cysteine conjugates are subsequently N-acetylated by the microsomal cysteine conjugate N-acetyltransferase (NAT) to yield the mercapturate. For most chemicals, the mercapturates function as highly polar metabolites that are readily excreted in urine. Many mercapturates, however, can be acted on by a deacetylase (or aminoacylase) activity to regenerate the cysteine conjugate. The significance of this for those cysteine conjugates that may also undergo bioactivation (see below), is evident from the observations that N-acetyl-L-cysteine-S-conjugates of nephrotoxic haloalkenes and haloalkanes may be deacetylated and exhibit toxicity in a manner similar to the corresponding cysteine conjugates [109–111].

Cysteine Conjugate β-Lyase and Bioactivation Pathways

Although most chemicals that undergo GSH conjugation and processing to form cysteine conjugates are ultimately metabolized to mercapturates that are excreted in the urine, several classes of chemicals are converted to cysteine conjugates that are substrates for a CCBL activity that results in bioactivation rather than detoxication (Figure 12.4). Substrates are cysteine conjugates of chemicals such as halogenated alkenes and alkanes, which include numerous environmental contaminants, such as the metal degreasing agent TCE [56], the analogue perchloroethylene (Perc), which is used in dry cleaning [112], and chlorofluorocarbons that have been used as refrigerants [113].

CCBL activities are found in both cytoplasm and mitochondria and in numerous tissues besides the kidneys (see [114] for a recent review). In the kidneys, two proteins, each dually localized in the cytoplasm and mitochondria, have been identified as catalyzing CCBL activity. The first is glutamine transaminase K (GTK; EC 2.6.1.64), which exists as a homodimer of 45 kDa subunit molecular weight; the second activity has not been extensively characterized, but has been identified as a high-molecular-weight beta-lyase of 330 kDa molecular weight. Abraham et al. [115,116] have suggested that, at least in mitochondria, this high-molecular-weight form is the primary enzyme catalyzing CCBL activity. Both GTK and the high-molecular-weight CCBL contain pyridoxal-5'-phosphate (PLP) as prosthetic group and can catalyze either a direct beta-elimination to yield a reactive thiolate (Figure 12.5, pathway B) or a transamination

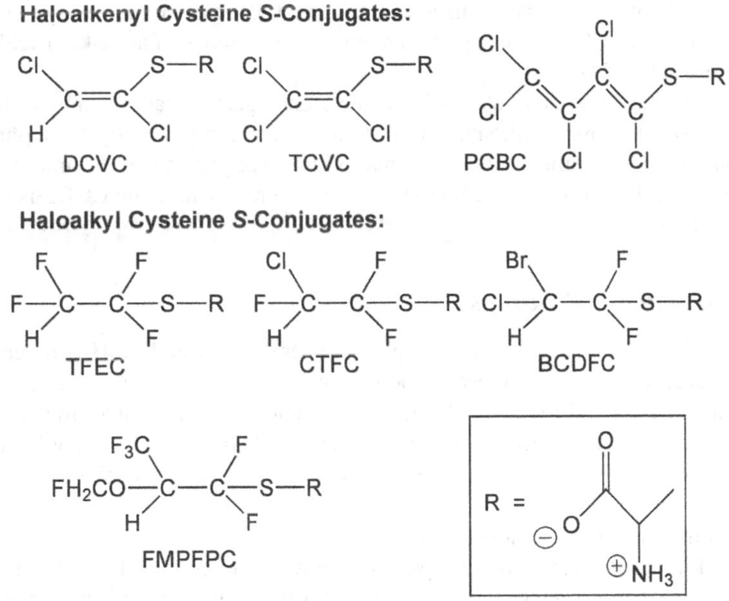

Haloalkenyl Cysteine S-Conjugates:

DCVC   TCVC   PCBC

Haloalkyl Cysteine S-Conjugates:

TFEC   CTFC   BCDFC

FMPFPC

R =

FIGURE 12.4 Structures of selected cysteine conjugates that undergo bioactivation. BCDFC, *S*-(1-bromo-1-chloro-2,2-difluoroethyl)-L-cysteine; CTFC, *S*-(1-chloro-1,2,2-trifluoroethyl)-L-cysteine; DCVC, *S*-(1,2-dichlorovinyl)-L-cysteine; FMPFPC, *S*-(1-fluoromethoxy-1,1,1-trifluoro-3,3-difluoropropyl)-L-cysteine; PCBC, *S*-(1,1,2,3,4-pentachlorobutadienyl)-L-cysteine; TFEC, *S*-(1,1,2,2-tetrafluoroethyl)-L-cysteine; TCVC, *S*-(1,2,2-trichlorovinyl)-L-cysteine.

DCVC   O₂   FMO   DCVSO

Pathway C

E-PLP   E-PLP

Pathway A   Pathway B

Keto acid   Pyruvate + NH₄⁺

Amino acid

DCVMP   DCVSH

chlorothioketene   chlorothionoacetyl chloride

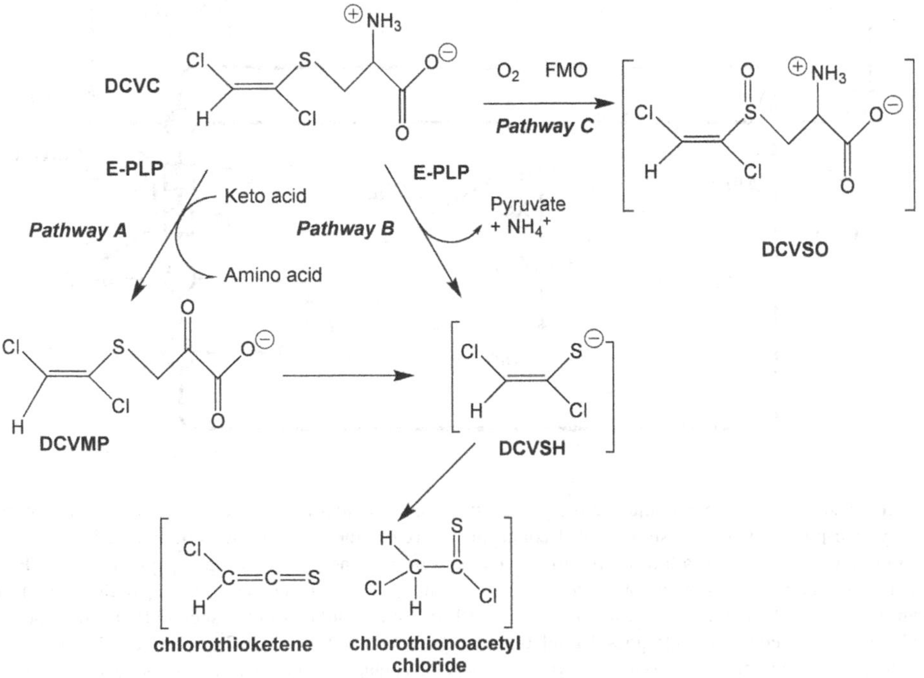

FIGURE 12.5 Bioactivation pathway for DCVC. *S*-(1,2-Dichlorovinyl)-L-cysteine (DCVC) undergoes bioactivation by either the pyridoxal 5′-phosphate (PLP)-containing cysteine conjugate β-lyase, which occurs by either transamination (Pathway A) or beta-elimination (Pathway B), or the flavin-containing monooxygenase (FMO) (Pathway C). Products of the three pathways include *S*-(1,2-dichlorovinyl)-mercaptopropionic acid (DCVMP), *S*-(1,2-dichlorovinyl)-thiol (DCVSH), and DCVC sulfoxide (DCVSO), respectively.

(Figure 12.5, pathway A), which yields an unstable α-keto acid. Because of the ability to undergo a transamination reaction, maximal CCBL activity often requires the presence of an α-keto acid in the reaction mixture as a co-substrate [117,118].

A third potential pathway for bioactivation of cysteine *S*-conjugates is catalyzed by FMO (Figure 12.5, pathway C), as described above. Although most studies on cysteine conjugate nephrotoxicity have focused on the role of CCBL, some studies in human kidney suggest that FMO may have a more significant role than CCBL; the opposite appears to be the case in rats, where the CCBL is more prominent than FMO [22,80,81].

Glutathione Conjugates as Prodrugs

Because of the unique position that the kidneys play in overall GSH and GSH conjugate metabolism, investigators have taken advantage of these properties to synthesize prodrugs that are targeted to the kidneys whereupon they become bioactivated to their therapeutic form. Examples include selenocysteine compounds that are selectively accumulated by the kidneys and converted to selenol compounds [119], *N*-acetyl-γ-glutamyl derivatives that are also selectively accumulated by the kidneys and then metabolized to their active forms [120,121], and various cysteine or GSH conjugates of purine derivatives that are metabolized to antitumor agents within the kidneys [122–126].

An example of taking advantage of the unique properties of transport and metabolism to selectively deliver renal prodrugs to their primary target cell (i.e., the proximal tubules), is illustrated in Figure 12.6. In this study [127], which was an *in vitro* study of transport, metabolism, and toxicity based on the *in vivo*

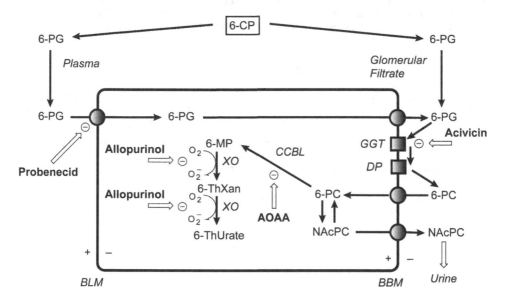

FIGURE 12.6 Handling of a GSH-conjugate prodrug by the renal proximal tubular cell. This scheme summarizes the renal delivery, transport, and metabolism of a GSH-conjugate prodrug by the renal proximal tubular cell. The parent compound, 6-chloropurine (6-CP) was administered to rats and converted to the prodrug 6-purinylglutathione (6-PG). 6-PG undergoes either glomerular filtration or enters the renal periplasmic space, where it can be taken up in the proximal tubular cell by transport across the basolateral plasma membrane (BLM). Intracellular 6-PG is secreted into the tubular lumen where it, along with filtered 6-PG, undergoes degradation by γ-glutamyltransferase (GGT) and dipeptidase (DP) activities on the brush-border plasma membrane (BBM) to yield the cysteine conjugate 6-purinyl-L-cysteine (6-PC). 6-PC is transported into the proximal tubular cell where it can either be converted to the mercapturate, *N*-acetyl-6-purinyl-L-cysteine (NAcPC), or undergo metabolism by the cysteine conjugate β-lyase (CCBL), which generates the chemotherapeutic agent 6-mercaptopurine (6-MP). The NAcPC can either be deacetylated to regenerate 6-PC or transported into the lumen for excretion in the urine. 6-MP can be further metabolized by xanthine oxidase (XO) to generate 6-thioxanthine (6-ThXan) and 6-thiourate (6-ThUrate). The importance of some of these steps was demonstrated by use of selective inhibitors, such as probenecid, allopurinol, acivicin, and aminooxyacetic acid (AOAA).

studies from Elfarra and colleagues [122–126], the importance of each of the three major steps, leading from administration of prodrug to generation of toxicant, was probed by the use of selective inhibitors. Thus, inhibition of uptake of the GSH conjugate prodrug (6-purinylglutathione, 6-PG) was inhibited with probenecid, thereby inhibiting subsequent steps (i.e., metabolism to generate 6-mercaptopurine (6-MP) and toxicity). Probenecid is a well-known inhibitor of organic anion transport and of GSH and GSH S-conjugate transport across the renal basolateral plasma membrane (BLM) [128]. Similar to earlier studies in renal proximal tubular cells to demonstrate the function of each step in TCE bioactivation (reviewed in 45), inhibition of GGT with acivicin or CCBL with AOAA resulted in decreased formation of 6-MP and decreased cytotoxicity. Additionally, inhibition of xanthine oxidase (XO) with allopurinol prevented cytotoxicity, demonstrating that this is the key step in generating the cytotoxic species.

Examples Illustrating Unique Functions of Kidneys in Drug Metabolism

Acetaminophen

Although acetaminophen (APAP) is a widely used analgesic that is considered very safe to use under normal conditions, it can exhibit significant organ toxicity under overdose conditions. Moreover, it is a frequent cause of poisoning due to overdose. The liver is the initial site of damage after APAP overdose and the kidneys are secondary sites due to their significant ability to metabolize APAP to both detoxication and bioactivation products [129], the latter resulting in analgesic nephropathy [130]. The major pathways for metabolism of APAP in either liver or renal cortex (Figure 12.7) show the presence of competing detoxification and bioactivation reactions. Under normal dose conditions (i.e., therapeutic doses), the primary flux of metabolism is generation of glucuronide or sulfate conjugates, which are both readily excreted in urine. Once the capacity of these Phase II enzymes is exceeded as occurs in an acute overdose, however, significant activity with CYP (primarily CYP2E1, but also CYP1A2 and CYP3A4/5 in humans or CYP3A1/2 in rodents) can occur, resulting in formation of a reactive quinoneimine, N-acetyl-p-benzoquinoneimine (NAPQI). Under non-stressed conditions in which ample amounts of GSH are present, NAPQI forms a GSH conjugate, which has generally been considered a detoxification product, leading to formation of a readily excreted mercapturate. When GSH is depleted, however, NAPQI can react with other nucleophiles, such as protein sulfhydryl groups, leading to cell damage and cytotoxicity. APAP may also undergo deacetylation to form p-aminophenol (PAP), which can then be metabolized by similar reactions to produce a reactive quinoneimine [131]. Thus, acute nephrotoxicity due to APAP over-dosage is characterized by tubular necrosis, largely confined to the proximal tubules of the renal cortex and outer stripe of the outer medulla.

Because of the potential for chronic abuse of APAP, renal injury due to long-term exposures to moderate doses is also a problem. The chronic ingestion of APAP can be associated with the so-called analgesic nephropathy, which is characterized by papillary necrosis and interstitial fibrosis. Thus, in contrast to acute overdose, which is associated with damage to the proximal tubules and is associated with CYP-dependent formation of NAPQI and GSH depletion, chronic exposure is due to the one-electron co-oxidation of APAP by PGS in the renal medulla to initially produce a phenoxyl radical, which is further oxidized to yield the reactive NAPQI [132]. This distinct pattern of injury is due to accumulation of APAP in the inner medulla and the presence of PGS in that nephron region.

Cephaloridine

Cephaloridine (CPH), which is a first-generation cephalosporin antibiotic, is limited in its therapeutic efficacy by dose-limiting nephrotoxicity [133]. The CPH molecule possesses two functional groups besides the characteristic beta-lactam ring, giving the molecule three potential sites of bioactivation (Figure 12.8). A thiophene ring on one end of the molecule can undergo CYP-dependent oxidation to yield a reactive epoxide whereas the pyridinium ring on the other end of the molecule is thought to undergo redox cycling similar to paraquat, thereby generating superoxide anions and an oxidative stress. The beta-lactam ring, however, appears to be the primary site at which interactions occur that lead to

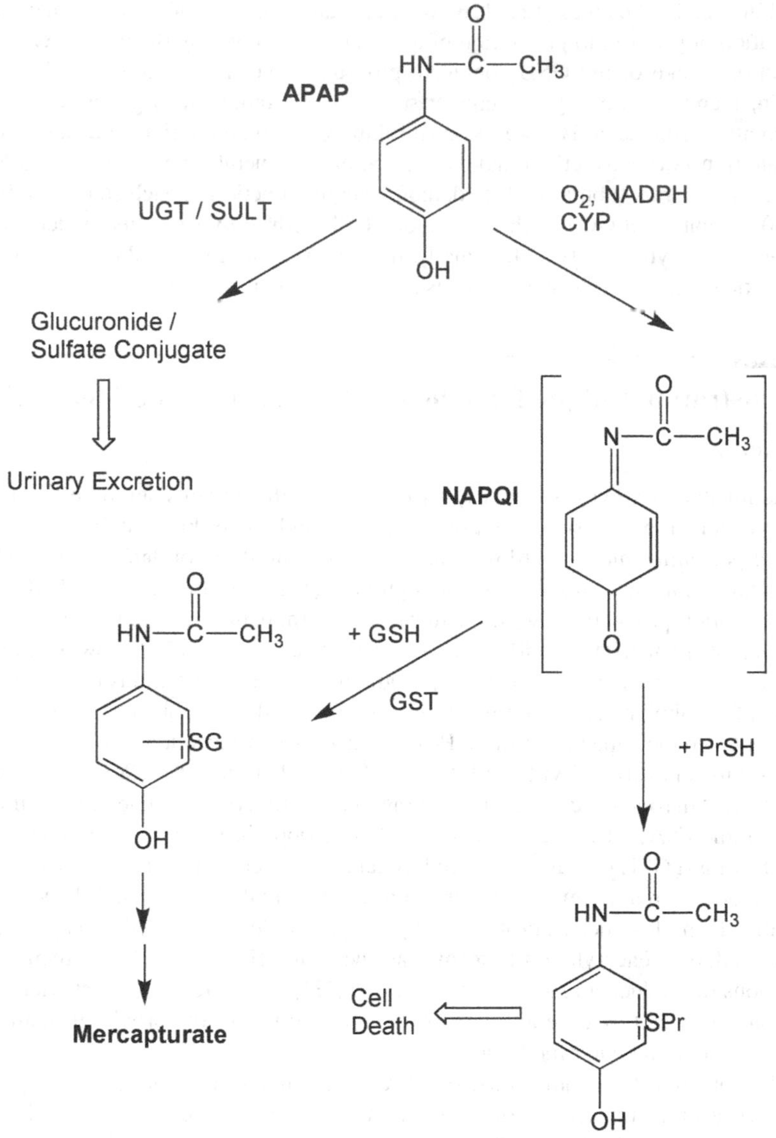

FIGURE 12.7 Metabolism of acetaminophen (APAP). APAP primarily undergoes conjugation by either a UDP-glucuronosyltransferase (UGT) or sulfotransferase (SULT) to form a readily excreted, highly polar product. When these reactions are saturated, APAP may be metabolized by cytochrome P450 (CYP) to form a reactive intermediate, *N*-acetyl-*p*-benzoquinoneimine (NAPQI), which reacts with either GSH via GSH *S*-transferase (GST) catalysis to ultimately form a mercapturate, or with protein sulfhydryl (PrSH) groups. The latter reaction can lead to cytotoxicity.

cytotoxicity. In a series of studies, Tune and colleagues [134–138] showed that the beta-lactam ring can open and selectively form adducts with substrate transporters on the mitochondrial inner membrane, thereby inhibiting mitochondrial function. Similarly, Lash et al. [139] showed that mitochondria are selective targets for CPH and provided additional data suggesting that besides the beta-lactam ring, metabolism at the thiophene ring may also play a significant role in nephrotoxicity [140].

Another point that is critical for CPH-induced nephrotoxicity and that illustrates a general principle that contributes to many forms of drug-induced nephrotoxicity is that CPH is efficiently and selectively transported into proximal tubular cells by organic anion carriers but is poorly secreted, thereby leading to high intracellular concentrations. This accumulated drug is then metabolized by

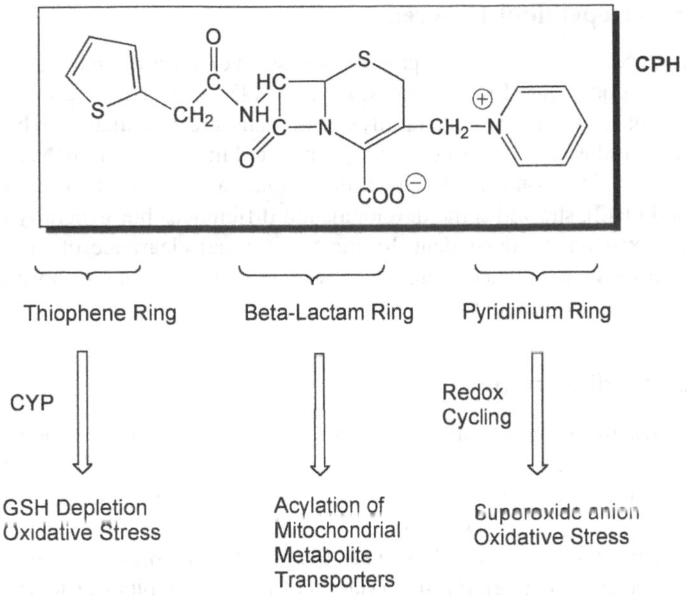

FIGURE 12.8 Structure of cephaloridine (CPH) showing potential sites of bioactivation. CPH has three regions that can be sites of metabolism: (1) a thiophene ring that can undergo cytochrome P450 (CYP)-dependent oxidation; (2) the beta-lactam ring, which may undergo a ring opening reaction that results in acylation of mitochondrial transporter proteins; and (3) a pyridinium ring that may undergo redox cycling to generate superoxide anion.

either CYPs or undergoes non-enzymatic redox cycling or hydrolysis of the beta-lactam ring, thereby leading to the various toxic effects.

Glutathione Conjugates of Trichloroethylene and Perchloroethylene

TCE and Perc provide additional examples of chemicals that are selectively nephrotoxic and whose mode of action takes advantage of some of the unique features of renal proximal tubular function with respect to GSH conjugates. These features include both transport and metabolism, as illustrated in Figure 12.6 for the GSH conjugate prodrugs. For both chemicals, while there can be intrarenal GSH conjugation, most of the GST reaction occurs in the liver, and thus, the GSH conjugate formed is transported out of the liver into bile or plasma [52,54,112]. It eventually reaches the renal circulation as either the GSH conjugate or the cysteine conjugate. The presence of a large array of amino acid and organic anion transporters, primarily in the proximal tubules, enables the kidney to accumulate these chemicals and metabolize them further. It is quite telling that although other tissues have CCBL activity, such as the liver, the kidneys are the predominant, if not sole, target organ [54,112].

Innate Factors that Modify Drug Transport

In this so-called age of personalized medicine, it is clear that pathways for drug transport and metabolism in humans differ amongst individuals, based not only on sex (i.e., hormone-dependent differences), but also age (i.e., developmental differences), lifestyle factors, and genetics. The following brief discussion highlights some key differences in drug transport that may impact the functions of the kidneys in drug disposition. These differences in turn impact both drug efficacy and drug and chemical induced nephrotoxicity. This section also briefly summarizes some of the novel post-translational modifications that selected transporters undergo that impact their function.

Hormones and Sex-Dependent Differences

Sex-dependent differences in mRNA and/or protein expression of several renal plasma membrane transporters have been well-documented in rats and mice [141–145]. For organic anion and organic cation transporters (i.e., members of the SLC22 family), androgens are stimulatory whereas estrogens are inhibitory. In contrast, studies by Groves et al. [146] conducted in rabbits on mRNA and protein expression and function of organic anion transporters 1 and 3 (Oat1 and Oat3) and organic cation transporters 1 and 2 (Oct1 and Oct2), showed some developmental differences but generally no sex differences. Although some data exist on sex-dependent differences in renal clearance of drugs in humans, it is unclear, based on animal studies, whether any of these differences are due to hormonal differences in regulation of renal plasma membrane transporters.

Post-translational Modifications

A number of post-translational modifications in Oats and Octs have been identified, some of which are linked to the hormonal-dependent differences in expression and activity. These modifications can be divided into four mechanisms: (1) glycosylation, (2) phosphorylation, (3) membrane trafficking, and (4) protein-protein interactions [147–149]. Glycosylation has been shown to be required for proper partitioning of various murine and human OATs between the plasma membrane (functional state) and intracellular vesicles (non-functional state). Phosphorylation of mOat1 inhibits transporter function. Protein kinase C, when activated, can enhance the internalization of hOAT1 from the plasma membrane into endosomes, thereby rendering it non-functional. Interactions between various OATs from rodents or humans with various other proteins has also been demonstrated as a short-term regulatory mechanism. These interacting proteins include caveolins, PDZK1 / NHERF1, and ubiquitin.

Genetic Polymorphisms

In recent years, it has become apparent that expression of plasma membrane transporters in humans often varies significantly amongst individuals due to both genetic polymorphisms and single nucleotide polymorphisms. Such variations have been described for most of the major renal plasma membrane transporters, including OAT1 [150–153], OAT3 [151–154], OAT4 [151,155], organic anion transporting polypeptide (OATP) carriers [156–159], the multidrug resistance polypeptide 1 (MRP1) [160] and 4 (MRP4) [161] carriers, and multidrug resistance protein 1 (MDR1; also known as P-glycoprotein) [162,163]. Clear functional effects of many of these polymorphisms, including altered drug efficacy [154,160,163], altered potential for drug-drug interactions and drug-induced toxicity [158,161], and altered drug distribution and pharmacokinetics [154,159,162], have been demonstrated.

Conclusions

The kidneys possess most of the same drug metabolizing enzymes as the much more studied liver. Significant differences exist between tissues, however, in terms of isoenzyme expression, overall amount of enzyme activity, regulation of enzyme expression and activity, and cell type distribution. Hence, for most of the enzymes that are of interest for drug metabolism, the highest levels of expression in the kidneys are found in the proximal tubules. These include enzymes of so-called Phase I metabolism, the CYPs and FMOs, and conjugation enzymes of Phase II metabolism, the UGTs, SULTs, and GSTs. The most notable exception is that of PGS, which is found predominantly in the inner medulla. Another important feature of renal function that correlates with metabolism is transport. Plasma membrane transporters for organic anions and cations are localized predominantly in the proximal tubules as well, and serve to deliver substrates to their sites of metabolism. Significant species differences also exist in the renal expression of several classes of drug metabolism enzymes, making extrapolation from experimental animals to humans very difficult when renal metabolism is involved.

A few selected examples were cited of drugs whose renal metabolism illustrates unique aspects of renal function. For example, the cephalosporin antibiotics (as exemplified by cephaloridine) were discussed as an example of a class of drugs whose nephrotoxicity is enhanced by accumulation in proximal tubular cells due to efficient uptake and poor efflux. Different classes of prodrugs that either possess a selenocysteine, γ-glutamyl, or GSH moiety, were discussed. These prodrugs take advantage of the unique manner in which the kidneys, and in particular, the proximal tubules handle these various *S*-conjugates and GSH-derivatives to effect selective delivery to the proximal tubules. The case of APAP is instructive in showing that distinct patterns of cellular accumulation and metabolism occur, depending on whether exposure is acute or chronic.

REFERENCES

1. Walker LA, Valtin H. Biological importance of nephron heterogeneity. *Annu Rev Physiol* 1982, 44, 203–219.
2. Guder WG, Ross BD. Enzyme distribution along the nephron. *Kidney Int* 1984, 26, 101–111.
3. Lash LH. Use of freshly isolated and primary cultures of proximal tubular and distal tubular cells from rat kidney. In: Zalups RK and Lash LH, eds. *Methods in Renal Toxicology*. Boca Raton, FL: CRC Press, 1996: 189–215.
4. Lash LH. In vitro methods of assessing renal damage. *Toxicol Pathol* 1998, 26, 33–42.
5. Chung SD, Alavi N, Livingston D, Hiller S, Taub M. Characterization of primary rabbit kidney cultures that express proximal tubule functions in a hormonally defined medium. *J Cell Biol* 1982, 95, 118–126.
6. Taub ML, Yang IS, Wang Y. Primary rabbit kidney proximal tubule cell cultures maintain differentiated functions when cultured in a hormonally defined serum-free medium. *In Vitro Cell Dev Biol* 1989, 25, 770–775.
7. Aleo MD, Taub ML, Nickerson PA, Kostyniak PJ. Primary cultures of rabbit renal proximal tubule cells: I. Growth and biochemical characteristics. *In Vitro Cell Dev Biol* 1989, 25, 776–783.
8. Nowak G, Schnellmann RG. Improved culture conditions stimulate gluconeogenesis in primary cultures of renal proximal tubule cells. *Am J Physiol* 1995, 268, C1053–C1061.
9. Blumenthal SS, Lewand DL, Buday MA, Mandel NS, Mandel GS, Kleinman JG. Effect of pH on growth of mouse renal cortical tubule cells in primary culture. *Am J Physiol* 1989, 257, C419–C426.
10. Boogaard PJ, Zoeteweij JP, van Berkel TJC, van't Noordende JM, Mulder GJ, Nagelkerke JF. Primary culture of proximal tubular cells from normal rat kidney as an in vitro model to study mechanisms of nephrotoxicity: Toxicity of nephrotoxicants at low concentrations during prolonged exposure. *Biochem Pharmacol* 1990, 39, 1335–1345.
11. Chen TC, Curthoys NP, Lagenaur CF, Puschett JB. Characterization of primary cell cultures derived from rat renal proximal tubules. *In Vitro Cell Dev Biol* 1989, 25, 714–722.
12. Elliget KA, Trump BF. Primary cultures of normal rat kidney proximal tubule epithelial cells for studies of renal cell injury. *In Vitro Cell Dev Biol* 1991, 27A, 739–748.
13. Hatzinger PB, Stevens JL. Rat kidney proximal tubule cells in defined medium: The roles of cholera toxin, extracellular calcium and serum in cell growth and expression of γ-glutamyltransferase. *In Vitro Cell Dev Biol* 1989, 25, 205–212.
14. Lash LH, Tokarz JJ, Pegouske DM. Susceptibility of primary cultures of proximal tubular and distal tubular cells from rat kidney to chemically induced toxicity. *Toxicology* 1995, 103, 85–103.
15. Miller JH. Restricted growth of rat kidney proximal tubule cells cultured in serum-supplemented and defined media. *J Cell Physiol* 1986, 129, 264–272.
16. Rosenberg MR, Michalopoulos G. Kidney proximal tubular cells isolated by collagenase perfusion grow in defined media in the absence of growth factors. *J Cell Physiol* 1987, 131, 107–113.
17. Sakhrani LM, Badie-Dezfooly B, Trizna W, Mikhail N, Lowe AG, Taub M, Fine LG. Transport and metabolism of glucose by renal proximal tubular cells in primary culture. *Am J Physiol* 1984, 246, F757–F764.
18. Toutain H, Vauclin-Jacques N, Fillastre J-P, Morin J-P. Biochemical, functional, and morphological characterization of a primary culture of rabbit proximal tubule cells. *Exp Cell Res* 1991, 194, 9–18.

19. Pizzonia JH, Gesek FA, Kennedy SM, Coutermarsh BA, Bacskal BJ, Friedman PA. Immunomagnetic separation, primary culture, and characterization of cortical thick ascending limb plus distal convoluted tubule cells from mouse kidney. *In Vitro Cell Dev Biol* 1991, 27A, 409–416.

20. Scott DM, Zierold K, Kinne R. Development of differentiated characteristics in cultured kidney (thick ascending loop of Henle) cells. *Exp Cell Res* 1986, 162, 521–529.

21. Courjault-Gautier F, Chevalier J, Abbou CC, Chopin DK, Toutain HJ. Consecutive use of hormonally defined serum-free media to establish highly differentiated human renal proximal tubule cells in primary culture. *J Am Soc Nephrol* 1995, 5, 1949–1963.

22. Cummings BS, Lash LH. Metabolism and toxicity of trichloroethylene and S-(1,2-dichlorovinyl)-L-cysteine in freshly isolated human proximal tubular cells. *Toxicol Sci* 2000, 53, 458–466.

23. Cummings BS, Lasker JM, Lash LH. Expression of glutathione dependent enzymes and cytochrome P450s in freshly isolated and primary cultures of proximal tubular cells from human kidney. *J Pharmacol Exp Ther* 2000, 293, 677–685.

24. Detrisac CJ, Sens MA, Garvin AJ, Spicer SS, Sens DA. Tissue culture of human kidney epithelial cells of proximal tubule origin. *Kidney Int* 1984, 25, 383–390.

25. Rodilla V, Miles AT, Jenner W, Hawksworth GM. Exposure of cultured human proximal tubular cells to cadmium, mercury, zinc and bismuth: Toxicity and metallothionein induction. *Chem-Biol Interact* 1998, 115, 71–83.

26. Trifillis AL, Regec AL, Trump BF. Isolation, culture and characterization of human renal tubular cells. *J Urol* 1985, 133, 324–329.

27. Van Der Biest I, Nouwen EJ, Van Dromme SA, De Broe ME. Characterization of pure proximal and heterogeneous distal human tubular cells in culture. *Kidney Int* 1994, 45, 85–94.

28. Lash LH. Human proximal tubular cells as an in vitro model for drug screening and mechanistic toxicology. *AltTox Essay* 2012, http://alttox.org/ttrc/toxicity-tests/repeated-dose/way-forward/lash/.

29. Lash LH. Principles and methods for renal toxicology. In: Hayes AW, ed. *Principles and Methods in Toxicology*, 5th Ed. Boca Raton, FL: CRC Press, 2008: 1508–1540.

30. Narayanan K, Schumacher KM, Tasnim F, Kandasamy K, Schumacher A, Ni M, Gao S, Zink D, Ying JY. Human embryonic stem cells differentiate into functional renal proximal tubular-like cells. *Kidney Int* 2013, 83, 593–603.

31. Xia Y, Nivet E, Sancho-Martinez I, Gallegos T, Suzuki K, Okamura D, Wu M-Z, Dubova I, Esteban CR, Montserrat N, Campistol JM, Belmonte JCI. Directed differentiation of human pluripotent cells to ureteric bud kidney progenitor-like cells. *Nat Cell Biol* 2013, 15, 1507–1515.

32. Kang M, Han Y-M. Differentiation of human pluripotent stem cells into nephron progenitor cells in a serum and feeder free system. *PLoS One* 2014, 9, e94888.

33. Lam AQ, Freedman BS, Morizane R, Lerou PH, Valerius MT, Bonventre JV. Rapid and efficient differentiation of human pluripotent stem cells into intermediate mesoderm that forms tubules expressing kidney proximal tubular markers. *J Am Soc Nephrol* 2014, 25, 1211–1225.

34. Takasato M, Er PX, Becroft M, Vanslambrouck JM, Stanley EG, Elefanty AG, Little MH. Directing human embryonic stem cell differentiation towards a renal lineage generates a self-organizing kidney. *Nat Cell Biol* 2014, 16, 118–126.

35. Angelotti ML, Ronconi E, Ballerini L, Peired A, Mazzinghi B, Sagrinati C, Parente E, Gacci M, Carini M, Rotondi M, Fogo AB, Lazzeri E, Lasagni L, Romagnani P. Characterization of renal progenitors committed toward tubular lineage and their regenerative potential in renal tubular injury. *Stem Cells* 2012, 30, 1714–1725.

36. Bi B, Schmitt R, Israilova M, Nishio H, Cantley LG. Stromal cells protect against acute tubular injury via an endocrine effect. *J Am Soc Nephrol* 2007, 18, 2486–2496.

37. Lee P-Y, Chien Y, Chiou G-Y, Lin C-H, Chiou C-H, Tarng D-C. Induced pluripotent stem cells without c-Myc attenuate acute kidney injury via downregulating the signaling of oxidative stress and inflammation in ischemia–reperfusion rats. *Cell Transplant* 2012, 21, 2569–2585.

38. Tiong HY, Huang P, Xiong P, Xiong S, Li Y, Vathsala A, Zink D. Drug-induced nephrotoxicity: Clinical impact and preclinical in vitro models. *Mol Pharmaceutics* 2014, 11, 1933–1948.

39. Berkhin EB, Humphreys MH. Regulation of renal tubular secretion of organic compounds. *Kidney Int* 2001, 59, 17–30.

40. Burckhardt G, Bahn A, Wolff NA. Molecular physiology of renal *p*-aminohippurate secretion. *News Physiol Sci* 2001, 16, 114–118.

41. Hagenbuch B, Peier PJ. Organic anion transporting polypeptides of the OATP/SLC21 family: Phylogenetic classification as OATP/SLCO superfamily, new nomenclature and molecular/functional properties. *Pflugers Arch* 2004, 447, 653–665.

42. Inui K-I, Masuda S, Saito H. Cellular and molecular aspects of drug transport in the kidney. *Kidney Int* 2000, 58, 944–958.

43. Koepsell H, Endou H. The SLC22 drug transporter family. *Pflugers Arch* 2004, 447, 666–676.

44. Lee W, Kim RB. Transporters and renal drug elimination. *Annu Rev Pharmacol Toxicol* 2004, 44, 137–166.

45. Robertson EE, Rankin GO. Human renal organic anion transporters: Characteristics and contributions to drug and drug metabolite excretion. *Pharmacol Ther* 2006, 109, 399–412.

46. Russel FGM, Masereeuw R, van Aubel RAMH. Molecular aspects of renal anionic drug transport. *Annu Rev Physiol* 2002, 64, 563–594.

47. Wright SH, Dantzler WH. Molecular and cellular physiology of renal organic cation and anion transport. *Physiol Rev* 2004, 84, 987–1049.

48. Lock EA, Reed DJ. Renal xenobiotic metabolism. In: Goldstein RS, ed. Comprehensive Series in Toxicology, Vol. 7: Kidney Toxicology. Oxford: Elsevier, 1997, 77–97.

49. Lohr JW, Willsky GR, Acara A. Renal drug metabolism. *Pharmacol Rev* 1998, 50, 107–141.

50. Jones DP, Orrenius S, Jakobson SW. Cytochrome P-450-linked monooxygenase systems in the kidney. In: Gram TE, ed. *Extrahepatic Metabolism of Drugs and Other Foreign Compounds*. New York: Spectrum Publications, 1980, 123–158.

51. Ronis MJJ, Huang J, Longo V, Tindberg N, Ingelman-Sundberg M, Badger TM. Expression and distribution of cytochrome P450 enzymes in male rat kidney: Effects of ethanol, acetone and dietary conditions. *Biochem Pharmacol* 1998, 55, 123–129.

52. Lash LH, Fisher JW, Lipscomb JC, Parker JC. Metabolism of Trichloroethylene. *Environ Health Perspec* 2000, 108 (Suppl. 2), 177–200.

53. NTP (National Toxicology Program). 2016. Report on Carcinogens, Fourteenth Edition.; Research Triangle Park, NC: U.S. Department of Health and Human Services, Public Health Service. http://ntp. niehs.nih.gov/go/roc14/.

54. Lash LH, Parker JC, Scott CS. Modes of action of trichloroethylene for kidney tumorigenesis. *Environ Health Perspec* 2000, 108 (Suppl. 2), 225–240.

55. Cummings BS, Parker JC, Lash LH. Cytochrome P450-dependent metabolism of trichloroethylene in rat kidney. *Toxicol Sci* 2001, 60, 11–19.

56. Lash LH, Putt DA, Cai H. Drug metabolism enzyme expression and activity in primary cultures of human proximal tubular cells. *Toxicology* 2008, 244, 56–65.

57. Lash LH, Putt DA, Huang P, Hueni SE, Parker JC. Modulation of hepatic and renal metabolism and toxicity of trichloroethylene and perchloroethylene by alterations in status of cytochrome P450 and glutathione. *Toxicology* 2007, 235, 11–26.

58. Cummings BS, Zangar RC, Novak RF, Lash LH. Cellular distribution of cytochromes P-450 in the rat kidney. *Drug Metab Dispos* 1999, 27, 542–548.

59. Amet Y, Berthou F, Fournier G, Dréano Y, Bardou L, Cledes J, Ménez J-F. Cytochrome P450 4A and 2E1 expression in human kidney microsomes. *Biochem Pharmacol* 1997, 53, 765–771.

60. Hu JJ, Rhoten WB, Yang CS. Mouse renal cytochrome P450IIE1: Immunocytochemical localization, sex-related differences and regulation by testosterone. *Biochem Pharmacol* 1990, 40, 2597–2602.

61. Bebri K, Boobis AR, Davies DS, Edward RJ. Distribution and induction of CYP3A1 and CYP3A2 in rat liver and extrahepatic tissue. *Biochem Pharmacol* 1995, 50, 2047–2056.

62. Schuetz EG, Schuetz JD, Grogan WM, Naray-Fejes-Toth A, Fejes-Toth G, Raucy J, Guzelian P, Gionela K, Watlington CO. Expression of cytochrome P450 3A in amphibian, rat, and human kidney. *Arch Biochem Biophys* 1992, 294, 206–217.

63. Guengerich FP. Polymorphism of cytochrome P-450 in humans. *Trends Pharmacol Sci* 1989, 10, 107–109.

64. Haener BD, Gorski JC, Vandenbranden M, Wrighton SA, Janardan SK, Watkins PB, Hall SD. Bimodal distribution of renal cytochrome P450 3A activity in humans. *Mol Pharmacol* 1996, 50, 52–59.

65. Ito O, Alonso-Galicia M, Hopp KA, Roman RJ. Localization of cytochrome P-450 4A isoforms along the rat nephron. *Am J Physiol* 1998, 274, F395–F404.

66. Okita JR, Johnson SB, Castle PJ, Dezellem SC, Okita RT. Improved separation and immunodetection of rat cytochrome P450 4A forms in liver and kidney. *Drug Metab Dispos* 1997, 25, 1008–1012.
67. Stec DE, Flasch A, Roman RJ, White JA. Distribution of cytochrome P-450 4A and 4F isoforms along the nephron in mice. *Am J Physiol* 2003, 284, F95–F102.
68. Cashman JR, Zhang J. Human flavin-containing monooxygenases. *Annu Rev Pharmacol Toxicol* 2006, 46, 65–100.
69. Ziegler DM. Recent studies on the structure and function of multisubstrate flavin-containing monooxygenases. *Annu Rev Pharmacol Toxicol* 1993, 33, 179–199.
70. Dolphin CT, Beckett DT, Janmohamed A, Cullingford TE, Smith RL, Shephard EA, Phillips IR. The flavin-containing monooxygenase 2 gene (FMO2) of humans, but not of other primates, encodes a truncated, nonfunctional protein. *J Biol Chem* 1998, 273, 30599–30607
71. Hines RN, Cashman JR, Philpot RM, Williams DE, Ziegler DM. The mammalian flavin-containing monooxygenases: Molecular characterization and regulation of expression. *Toxicol Appl Pharmacol* 1994, 125, 1–6.
72. Koukouritaki SB, Simpson P, Yeung CK, Rettie AE, Hines RN. Human hepatic flavin-containing monooxygenase 1 (FMO1) and 3 (FMO3) developmental expression. *Ped Res* 2002, 51, 236–243.
73. Ripp SL, Itagak IK, Philpot, RM, Elfarra AA. Species and sex differences in expression of flavin-containing monooxygenase form 3 in liver and kidney microsomes. *Drug Metab Dispos* 1999, 27, 46–52.
74. Krause RJ, Lash LH, Elfarra AA. Human kidney flavin-containing monooxygenases and their potential roles in cysteine S-conjugate metabolism and nephrotoxicity. *J Pharmacol Exp Ther* 2003, 304, 185–191.
75. Nishimura M, Naito S. Tissue-specific mRNA expression profiles of human phase I metabolizing enzymes except cytochrome P450 and phase II metabolizing enzymes. *Drug Metab Pharmacokinet* 2006, 21, 357–374.
76. Sausen PJ, Elfarra AA. Cysteine conjugate S-oxidase: Characterization of a novel enzymatic activity in rat hepatic and renal microsomes. *J Biol Chem* 1990, 265, 6139–6145.
77. Sausen PJ, Elfarra AA. Reactivity of cysteine S-conjugates sulfoxides: Formation of S-[1-chloro-2-(S-glutathionyl)vinyl]-L-cysteine sulfoxide by the reaction of S-(1,2-dichlorovinyl)-L-cysteine sulfoxide with glutathione. *Chem Res Toxicol* 1991, 4, 655–660.
78. Sausen PJ, Duescher RJ, Elfarra AA. Further characterization and purification of the flavin-dependent S-benzyl-L-cysteine S-oxidase activities of rat liver and kidney microsomes. *Mol Pharmacol* 1993, 43, 388–396.
79. Elfarra AA, Krause RJ. *S*-(1,2,2-Trichlorovinyl)-L-cysteine sulfoxide, a reactive metabolite of *S*-(1,2,2-trichlorovinyl)-L-cysteine formed in rat liver and kidney microsomes, is a potent nephrotoxicant. *J Pharmacol Exp Ther* 2007, 321, 1095–1101.
80. Lash LH, Sausen PJ, Duescher RJ, Cooley AJ, Elfarra AA. Roles of cysteine conjugate β-lyase and *S*-oxidase in nephrotoxicity: Studies with *S*-(1,2-dichlorovinyl)-L-cysteine and *S*-(1,2-dichlorovinyl)-L-cysteine sulfoxide. *J Pharmacol Exp Ther* 1994, 269, 374–383.
81. Lash LH, Putt DA, Hueni SE, Krause RJ, Elfarra AA. Roles of necrosis, apoptosis, and mitochondrial dysfunction in *S*-(1,2-dichlorovinyl)-L-cysteine sulfoxide-induced cytotoxicity in primary cultures of human renal proximal tubular cells. *J Pharmacol Exp Ther* 2003, 305, 1163–1172.
82. Hao C-M, Breyer MD. Physiologic and pathophysiologic roles of lipid mediators in the kidney. *Kidney Int* 2007, 71, 1105–1115.
83. Nasrallah R, Clark J, Hébert RL. Prostaglandins in the kidney: Developments since Y2K. *Clin Sci* 2007, 113, 297–311.
84. Schlondorff D, Zanger R, Satriano JA, Folkert, VW, Eveloff J. Prostaglandin synthesis by isolated cells from the outer medulla and from the thick ascending loop of Henle of rabbit kidney. *J Pharmacol Exp Ther* 1982, 223, 120–124.
85. Bonventre JV, Nemenoff R. Renal tubular arachidonic acid metabolism. *Kidney Int* 1991, 39, 438–449.
86. Zenser TV, Davis BB. Enzyme systems involved in the formation of reactive metabolites in the renal medulla: Cooxidation via prostaglandin H synthase. *Fund Appl Toxicol* 1984, 4, 922–929.
87. Zenser TV, Cohen SM, Mattammal MB, Wise RW, Rapp NS, Davis BB. Prostaglandin hydroperoxidase catalyzed activation of certain N-substituted aryl renal and bladder carcinogens. *Environ Health Perspec* 1983, 49, 33–41.

88. Wise RW, Zenser TV, Rice JR, Davis BB. Peroxidatic metabolism of benzidine by intact tissue: A prostaglandin H synthase-mediated process. *Carcinogenesis* 1986, 7, 111–115.

89. Zenser TV, Mattammal MB, Davis BB. Cooxidation of benzidine by renal medullary prostaglandin cyclooxygenase. *J Pharmacol Exp Ther* 1979, 211, 460–464.

90. Zenser TV, Mattammal MB, Wise RW, Rice JR, Davis BB. Prostaglandin H synthase-catalyzed activation of benzidine: A model to assess pharmacologic intervention of the initiation of chemical carcinogenesis. *J Pharmacol Exp Ther* 1983, 227, 545–550.

91. Mackenzie PI, Bock KW, Burchell B, Guillemette C, Ikushiro S, Iyanagi T, Miners JO, Owens IS, Nebert DW. Nomenclature update for the mammalian UDP glycosyltransferase (UGT) gene superfamily. *Pharmacogenet Genomics* 2005, 15, 677–685.

92. Shelby MK, Cherrington NJ, Vansell NR, Klaassen CD. Tissue mRNA expression of the rat UDP-glucuronosyltransferase gene family. *Drug Metab Dispos* 2003, 31, 326–333.

93. Wells PG, Mackenzie PI, Chowshury JR, Guillemette C, Gregory PA, Ishii Y, Hansen AJ, Kessler FK, Kim PM, Chowdhury NR, Ritter JK. Glucuronidation and the UDP-glucuronosyltransferases in health and disease. *Drug Metab Dispos* 2004, 32, 281–290.

94. Gamage N, Barnett A, Hempel N, Duggleby RG, Windmill KF, Martin JL, McManus ME. Human sulfotransferases and their role in chemical metabolism. *Toxicol Sci* 2006, 90, 5–22.

95. Lindsay J, Wang LL, Li Y, Zhou SF. Structure, function and polymorphism of human cytosolic sulfotransferases. *Curr Drug Metab* 2008, 9, 99–105.

96. Nowel S, Falany CN. Pharmacogenetics of human cytosolic sulfotransferases. *Oncogene* 2006, 25, 1673–1678.

97. Rozzel B, Hansson H-A, Guthenberg C, Tahir MK, Mannervik B. Glutathione transferases of classes α, μ, and π show selective expression in different regions of rat kidney. *Xenobiotica* 1993, 23, 835–849.

98. Cummings BS, Parker JC, Lash LH. Role of cytochrome P450 and glutathione *S*-transferase α in metabolism and cytotoxicity of trichloroethylene in rat kidney. *Biochem Pharmacol* 2000, 59, 531–543.

99. Board PG, Anders MW. Human glutathione transferase-Zeta. *Methods Enzymol* 2005, 401, 61–77.

100. Board PG, Baker RT, Chelvanayagam G, Jermiin LS. Zeta, a novel class of glutathione transferases in a range of species from plants to humans. *Biochem J* 1997, 328, 929–935.

101. Board PG, Chelvanayagam G, Jermiin LS, Tetlow N, Tzeng HF, Anders MW, Blackburn AC. Identification of novel glutathione transferases and polymorphic variants by expressed sequence tag database analysis. *Drug Metab Dispos* 2001, 29, 544–547.

102. Jakobsson P-J, Morgenstern R, Mancini J, Ford-Hutchinson A, Persson B. Common structural features of MAPEG – a widespread superfamily of membrane associated proteins with highly divergent functions in eicosanoid and glutathione metabolism. *Protein Sci* 1999, 8, 689–692.

103. Otieno MA, Baggs RB, Hayes JD, Anders MW. Immunolocalization of microsomal glutathione *S*-transferases in rat tissues. *Drug Metab Dispos* 1997, 25, 12–20.

104. Lash LH, Lipscomb JC, Putt DA, Parker JC. Glutathione conjugation of trichloroethylene in human liver and kidney: Kinetics and individual variation. *Drug Metab Dispos* 1999, 27, 351–359.

105. Lash LH, Qian W, Putt DA, Jacobs K, Elfarra AA, Krause RJ, Parker JC. Glutathione conjugation of trichloroethylene in rats and mice: Sex-, species-, and tissue-dependent differences. *Drug Metab Dispos* 1998, 26, 12–19.

106. Lash LH, Xu Y, Elfarra AA, Duescher RJ, Parker JC. Glutathione-dependent metabolism of trichloroethylene in isolated liver and kidney cells of rats and its role in mitochondrial and cellular toxicity. *Drug Metab Dispos* 1995, 23, 846–853.

107. Hinchman CA, Ballatori N. Glutathione-degrading capacities of liver and kidney in different species. *Biochem Pharmacol* 1990, 40, 1131–1135.

108. Griffith OW, Meister A. Translocation of intracellular glutathione to membrane-bound γ-glutamyl transpeptidase as a discrete step in the γ-glutamyl cycle: Glutathionuria after inhibition of transpeptidase. *Proc Natl Acad Sci USA* 1979, 76, 268–272.

109. Birner G, Werner M, Rosner E, Mehler C, Dekant W. Biotransformation, excretion, and nephrotoxicity of the hexachlorobutadiene metabolite (E)-N-acetyl-S-(1,2,3,4,4-pentachlorobutadienyl)-L-cysteine sulfoxide. *Chem Res Toxicol* 1998, 11, 750–757.

110. Wolfgang GHI, Gandolfi AJ, Stevens JL, Brendel K. N-Acetyl S-(1,2-dichlorovinyl)-L-cysteine produces a similar toxicity to S-(1,2-dichlorovinyl)-L-cysteine in rabbit renal slices: Differential transport and metabolism. *Toxicol Appl Pharmacol* 1989, 101, 205–219.

111. Zhang G, Stevens JL. Transport and activation of S-(1,2-dichlorovinyl)-L-cysteine and N-acetyl-S-(1,2-dichlorovinyl)-L-cysteine in rat kidney proximal tubules. *Toxicol Appl Pharmacol* 1989, 100, 51–61.

112. Lash LH, Parker JC. Hepatic and renal toxicities associated with perchloroethylene. *Pharmacol Rev* 2001, 53, 177–208.

113. Yin H, Jones JP, Anders MW. Metabolism of 1-fluoro-1,1,2-trichloroethane, 1,2-dichloro-1,1-difluoro-ethane, and 1,1,1-trifluoro-2-chloroethane. *Chem Res Toxicol* 1995, 8, 262–268.

114. Cooper AJL, Pinto JT. Cysteine S-conjugate β-lyases. *Amino Acids* 2006, 30, 1–15.

115. Abraham DG, Patel PP, Cooper AJL. Isolation from rat kidney of a cytosolic high molecular weight cysteine-S-conjugate β-lyase with activity toward leukotriene E_4. *J Biol Chem* 1995, 270, 180–188.

116. Abraham DG, Thomas RJ, Cooper AJL. Glutamine transaminase K is not a major cysteine S-conjugate β-lyase of rat kidney mitochondria: Evidence that a high-molecular weight enzyme fulfills this role. *Mol Pharmacol* 1995, 48, 855–860.

117. Elfarra AA, Lash LH, Anders MW. Alpha-keto acids stimulate rat renal cysteine conjugate β-lyase activity and potentiate the cytotoxicity of S-(1,2-dichlorovinyl)-L-cysteine. *Mol Pharmacol* 1987, 31, 208–212.

118. Stevens JL, Robbins JD, Byrd RA. A purified cysteine conjugate β-lyase from rat kidney cytosol: Requirement for an α-keto acid or an amino acid oxidase for activity and identity with soluble glutamine transaminase K. *J Biol Chem* 1986, 261, 15529–15537.

119. Andreadou I, Menge WMPB, Commandeur JNM, Worthington EA, Vermeulen NPE. Synthesis of novel se-substituted selenocysteine derivatives as potential kidney selective prodrugs of biologically active selenol compounds: Evaluation of kinetics of β-elimination reactions in rat renal cytosol. *J Med Chem* 1996, 39, 2040–2046.

120. Drieman JC, Thijssen HHW, Struyker-Boudier HAJ. Renal selective N-acetyl-γ-glutamyl prodrugs. II. Carrier-mediated transport and intracellular conversion as determinants in the renal selectivity of N-acetyl-γ-glutamyl sulfamethoxazole. *J Pharmacol Exp Ther* 1990, 252, 1255–1260.

121. Drieman JC, Thijssen HHW, Struyker-Boudier HAJ. Renal selective N-acetyl-L-γ-glutamyl prodrugs: Studies on the selectivity of some model prodrugs. *Br J Pharmacol* 1993, 108, 204–208.

122. Elfarra AA, Hwang IY. Targeting of 6-mercaptopurine to the kidneys: Metabolism and kidney-selectivity of S-(6-purinyl)-L-cysteine analogs in rats. *Drug Metab Dispos* 1993, 21, 841–845.

123. Elfarra AA, Duescher RJ, Hwang IY, Sicuri AR, Nelson JA. Targeting 6-thioguanine to the kidney with S-(guanin-6-yl)-L-cysteine. *J Pharmacol Exp Ther* 1995, 274, 1298–1304.

124. Hwang Y, Elfarra AA. Cysteine S-conjugates may act as kidney-selective prodrugs: Formation of 6-mercaptopurine by the renal metabolism of S-(6-purinyl)-L-cysteine. *J Pharmacol Exp Ther* 1989, 251, 448–454.

125. Hwang IY, Elfarra AA. Kidney-selective prodrugs of 6-mercaptopurine: Biochemical basis of kidney selectivity of S-(6-purinyl)-L-cysteine and metabolism of new analogs in rats. *J Pharmacol Exp Ther* 1991, 258, 171–177.

126. Hwang IY, Elfarra AA. Detection and mechanisms of formation of S-(6-purinyl)glutathione and 6-mercaptopurine in rats given 6-chloropurine. *J Pharmacol Exp Ther* 1993, 264, 41–46.

127. Lash LH, Shivnani A, Mai J, Chinnaiyan P, Krause RJ, Elfarra AA. Renal cellular transport, metabolism and cytotoxicity of S-(6-purinyl)glutathione, a prodrug of 6-mercaptopurine, and analogues. *Biochem Pharmacol* 1997, 54, 1341–1349.

128. Lash LH. Role of glutathione transport processes in kidney function. *Toxicol Appl Pharmacol* 2005, 204, 329–342.

129. Newton JF, Braselton WE, Kuo C-H, Kluwe WM, Gemborys MW, Mudge GH, Hook JB. Metabolism of acetaminophen by the isolated perfused kidney. *J Pharmacol Exp Ther* 1982, 221, 76–79.

130. Duggin GG. Mechanisms in the development of analgesic nephropathy. *Kidney Int* 1980, 18, 553–561.

131. Klos C, Koob M, Kramer C, Dekant W. p-Aminophenol nephrotoxicity: Biosynthesis of toxic glutathione conjugates. *Toxicol Appl Pharmacol* 1992, 115, 98–106.

132. West PR, Harman LS, Josephy PD, Mason RP. Acetaminophen: Enzymatic formation of a transient phenoxyl free radical. *Biochem Pharmacol* 1984, 33, 2933–2936.

133. Tune BM. The nephrotoxicity of cephalosporin antibiotics– Structure-activity relationships. *Comments Toxicol* 1986, 1, 145–170.

134. Tune BM, Hsu C-Y. The renal mitochondrial toxicity of cephalosporins: Specificity of the effect on anionic substrate uptake. *J Pharmacol Exp Ther* 1990, 252, 65–69.

135. Tune BM, Hsu C-Y. Effects of nephrotoxic β-lactam antibiotics on the mitochondrial metabolism of monocarboxylic substrates. *J Pharmacol Exp Ther* 1995, 274, 194–199.
136. Tune BM, Hsu C-Y. Toxicity of cephalosporins to fatty acid metabolism in rabbit renal cortical mitochondria. *Biochem Pharmacol* 1995, 49, 727–734.
137. Tune BM, Sibley RK, Hsu C-Y. The mitochondrial respiratory toxicity of cephalosporin antibiotics. An inhibitory effect on substrate uptake. *J Pharmacol Exp Ther* 1988, 245, 1054–1059.
138. Tune BM, Fravert D, Hsu C-Y. Oxidative and mitochondrial toxic effects of cephalosporin antibiotics in the kidney: A comparative study of cephaloridine and cephaloglycin. *Biochem Pharmacol* 1989, 38, 795–802.
139. Lash LH, Tokarz JJ, Woods EB. Renal cell type specificity of cephalosporin-induced cytotoxicity in suspensions of isolated proximal tubular and distal tubular cells. *Toxicology* 1994, 94, 97–118.
140. Lash LH, Tokarz JJ. Oxidative stress and cytotoxicity of 4-(2-thienyl)butyric acid in isolated rat renal proximal tubular and distal tubular cells. *Toxicology* 1995, 103, 167–175.
141. Buist SCN, Cherrington NJ, Choudhuri S, Hartley DP, Klaassen CD. Gender-specific and developmental influences on the expression of rat organic anion transporters. *J Pharmacol Exp Ther* 2002, 301, 145–151.
142. Kobayashi Y, Hirokawa N, Ohshiro N, Sekine T, Sasaki T, Tokuyama S, Endou H, Yamamoto T. Differential gene expression of organic anion transporters in male and female rats. *Biochem Biophys Res Commun* 2002, 290, 482–487.
143. Ljubojevic M, Herak-Kramberger CM, Hagos Y, Bahn A, Endou H, Burckhardt G, van Sabolic I. Rat renal cortical OAT1 and OAT3 exhibit gender differences determined by both androgen stimulation and estrogen inhibition. *Am J Physiol* 2004, 287, F124–F138.
144. Buist SCN, Klaassen CD. Rat and mouse differences in gender-predominant expression of organic anion transporter (Oat1–3; Slc22a6-8) mRNA levels. *Drug Metab Dispos* 2004, 32, 620–625.
145. Breljak D, Brzica H, Sweet DH, Anzai N, Sabolic I. Sex-dependent expression of Oat3 (Slc22a8) and Oat1 (Slc22a6) proteins in murine kidneys. *Am J Physiol* 2013, 304, F1114–F1126.
146. Groves CE, Suhre WB, Cherrington NJ, Wright SH. Sex differences in the mRNA, protein, and functional expression of organic anion transporter (Oat)1, Oat3, and organic cation transporter (Oct) 2 in rabbit renal proximal tubules. *J Pharmacol Exp Ther* 2006, 316, 743–752.
147. Duan P, You G. Short-term regulation of organic anion transporters. *Pharmacol Ther* 2010, 125, 55–61.
148. Wang L, Sweet DW. Renal organic anion transporters (SLC22 family): Expression, regulation, roles in toxicity, and impact on injury and disease. *The AAPS J* 2013, 15, 53–69.
149. Xu D, Wang H, You G. Posttranslational regulation of organic anion transporters by ubiquitination: Known and novel. *Med Res Rev* 2016, 36, 964–979.
150. Fujita T, Brown C, Carlson EJ, Taylor T, de la Cruz M, Johns SJ, Stryke D, Kawamoto M, Fujita K, Castro R, Chen CW, Lin ET, Brett CM, Burchard EG, Ferrin TE, Huang CC, Leabman MK, Giacomini KM. Functional analysis of polymorphisms in the organic anion transporter, SLC22A6 (OAT1). *Pharmacogenet Genomics* 2005, 15, 201–209.
151. Xu G, Bhatnagar V, Wen G, Hamilton BA, Eraly SA, Nigam SK. Analyses of coding region polymorphisms in apical and basolateral human organic anion transporter (OAT) genes [OAT1 (NKT), OAT2, OAT3, OAT4, URAT (RST)]. *Kidney Int* 2005, 68, 1491–1499.
152. Bhatnagar V, Xu G, Hamilton BA, Truong DM, Eraly SA, Wu W, Nigam SK. Analyses of 5′ regulatory region polymorphisms in human SLC22A6 (OAT1) and SLC22A8 (OAT3). *J Hum Genet* 2006, 51, 575–580.
153. Ogasawara K, Terada T, Motohashi H, Asaka J-I, Aoki M, Katsura T, Kamba T, Ogawa O, Inui K-i. Analysis of regulatory polymorphisms in organic ion transporter genes (SLC22A) in the kidney. *J Hum Genet* 2008, 53, 607–614.
154. Yee SW, Nguyen AN, Brown C, Savic RM, Zhang Y, Castro RA, Cropp CD, Choi JH, Singh D, Tahara H, Stocker SL, Huang Y, Brett CM, Giacomini KM. Reduced renal clearance of cefotaxime in Asians with a low-frequency polymorphism of OAT3 (SLC22A8). *J Pharm Sci* 2013, 102, 3451–3457.
155. Zhou F, Zhu L, Cui PH, Church WB, Murray M. Functional characterization of nonsynonymous single nucleotide polymorphisms in the human organic anion transporter 4 (hOAT4). *Br J Pharmacol* 2010, 159, 419–427.
156. König J, Seithel A, Gradh U, Fromm MF. Pharmacogenomics of human OATP transporters. *Naunyn-Schmiedeberg's Arch Pharmacol* 2006, 372, 432–443.

157. Seithel A, Glaeser H, Fromm MF, König J. The functional consequences of genetic variations in transporter genes encoding human organic anion-transporting polypeptide family members. *Expert Opin Drug Metab Toxicol* 2008, 4, 51–64.

158. König J. Uptake transporters of the human OATP family: Molecular characteristics, substrates, their role in drug-drug interactions, and functional consequences of polymorphisms. *Handb Exp Pharmacol* 2011, 201, 1–28.

159. Zhou Y, Yuan J, Li Z, Wang Z, Cheng D, Du Y, Li W, Kan Q, Zhang W. Genetic polymorphisms and function of the organic anion-transporting polypeptide 1A2 and its clinical relevance in drug disposition. *Pharmacology* 2015, 95, 201–208.

160. Conseil G, Cole SPC. Two polymorphic variants of ABCC1 selectively alter drug resistance and inhibitor sensitivity of the multidrug and organic anion transporter multidrug resistance protein 1. *Drug Metab Dispos* 2013, 41, 2187–2196.

161. Likanonsakul S, Suntisuklappon B, Nitiyanontakij R, Prasithsirikul W, Nakayama EE, Shioda T, Sangsajja C. A single-nucleotide polymorphism in ABCC4 is associated with tenofovir-related beta 2-microglobulinuria in Thai patients with HIV-1 infection. *PLoS One* 2016, 25, e0147724.

162. Cascorbi I. P-glycoprotein: Tissue distribution, substrates, and functional consequences of genetic variations. *Handb Exp Pharmacol* 2011, 201, 261–283.

163. Kravljaca M, Perovic V, Pravica V, Brkovic V, Milinkovic M, Lausevic M, Naumovic R. The importance of MDR1 gene polymorphisms for tacrolimus dosage. *Eur J Pharmaceut Sci* 2016, 83, 109–113.

Section III

Technologies to Study Drug Metabolism

13

Mass Spectrometry in Drug Metabolism Research: Principles and Common Practice

Bo Wen

CONTENTS

Introduction

The understanding that drug metabolites often play a critical role in the efficacy and safety profile of drugs has propelled drug metabolism research to become an integral part of pharmaceutical research and development. Drug metabolism (also known as biotransformation) is a biochemical process in which drugs are converted to more hydrophilic species to facilitate their elimination from the body [1]. Most chemicals, including drugs, are transformed in the human body to a wide variety of products by a host of enzymes present mostly intracellularly, though bacteria in the gastrointestinal tract can metabolize some structures. The reactions catalyzed by drug metabolizing enzymes can be categorized into two groups: phase I functionalization and phase II conjugation [2]. Phase I reactions often involve oxidation, reduction, dealkylation, deamination, and hydrolysis, with less frequent reactions including chiral inversion, rearrangement, and dehydration. Many introduce or unmask a functional group (e.g., –OH, –COOH, –NH$_2$, or –SH) within the molecule. Phase II reactions impart the drug or its metabolites with an endogenous molecule such as glucuronic acid, sulfate, amino acids, or glutathione (GSH), which leads in many cases (i.e., methylation and acetylation leads to higher lipophilicity) to an increase in hydrophilicity and a concomitant decrease in the volume of distribution (Vss), resulting in decreased tissue partitioning of the drug. While many of these metabolites are physiologically inactive, some are active either therapeutically or toxicologically. Other undesirable consequences resulting from biotransformation reactions include rapid drug clearance [3] and drug-drug interactions (DDIs) [4].

The role of drug metabolism research in drug discovery and development has significantly expanded over the past decades, from *in vivo* studies mainly performed at the development stage to becoming an integral part of pharmaceutical research, ranging from understanding absorption, distribution, metabolism, and excretion (ADME), flagging active and toxic metabolites, to bridging pharmacokinetic/pharmacodynamic disconnects (Figure 13.1). Early *in vitro* metabolite profiling experiments are designed to evaluate interspecies differences and determine specific metabolic pathways to facilitate prediction of the validity of toxicology and/or efficacy models, determine metabolic "soft spots" leading to unfavorable metabolism or "hot spots" leading to reactive metabolite formation, and aid in development of improved analogs with a maximized likelihood of success and attrition reduction [5]. While the pharmacokinetic properties of a drug candidate are deemed unsuitable, for example, the underlying mechanism is often metabolic instability in either the gastrointestinal tract or the liver leading to overly rapid metabolic clearance and unachievable therapeutic exposures. In the development phase, the goals of drug metabolism studies include the characterization of metabolic pathways and determination of the extent of metabolism and metabolite exposures in laboratory animals and humans in support of safety testing of metabolites (MIST) and clinical DDI studies. Additionally, assessment of the pharmacological activity, toxicity, and DDI potential of metabolites in human circulation is often performed to contribute to understanding of the safety and efficacy profile of the compound, leading to appropriate risk mitigation strategies. An example of the increasing understanding and impact of drug metabolism is the reduced attrition rates due to inappropriate pharmacokinetics and/or bioequivalence [6].

The importance of determination of metabolic profiles has been followed hand-in-hand by the development of analytical tools, in particular mass spectrometry (MS) technologies, necessary to perform this research. Until the late 1980s, metabolite identification by MS was still a major undertaking with insensitive instruments, lengthy isolation of metabolites and tedious sample preparation process. The detection

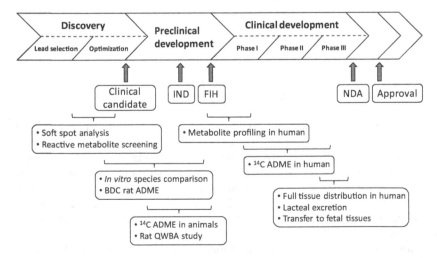

FIGURE 13.1 Schematic representation depicting the role of drug metabolism and disposition studies in discovery and development. BS stands for background subtraction. CSC stands for control sample comparison. ML stands for metabolomics. The three data processing methods require the use of control samples where there are no or significantly lower levels of targeted drug metabolite signals.

and identification of metabolites in biological matrices were complicated by the fact that metabolism often results in a vast array of structurally diverse species at relatively low concentrations (i.e., nM to μM) with a large excess of proteins, lipids, and other endogenous compounds present in the matrices interfering with the detection of drug-related materials. The development of robust, sensitive, and high-performance liquid chromatography (HPLC)-compatible atmospheric pressure electrospray ionization (ESI) sources made it possible to directly couple LC with MS and allowed LC/MS to become the preeminent analytical tool for detection and identification of metabolites. A major recent focus of improvements in early metabolite profiling methods has been increasing the analysis throughput using faster HPLC and faster scanning mass spectrometers, as well as development of integrated profiling methods that allow parent quantification and metabolite profiling in the same run [7]. On the other front, accurate mass-mass spectrometers coupled with mass filters and data-mining techniques have become the cornerstone for the drug metabolism research in recent years. In this chapter, the application, progress, and future perspectives of MS technology in detection and structural characterization of drug metabolites in the discovery and development settings are discussed. The coverage is not intended to be comprehensive, but rather illustrative of key developments to provide an overview of the advance of MS technology and its impact on the drug metabolism research.

Application of Mass Spectrometry in Drug Metabolism

It can be argued that the substantial influence of drug metabolism research on drug discovery and development may have been driven by the advances in analytical tools, in particular MS technology. Over the past decades, MS technology and its applications in drug metabolism research underwent a rapid evolution with two major milestones, namely the emergence of electrospray LC/MS instruments and the development of robust and stable high-resolution mass spectrometry (HRMS) along with data acquisition and data mining tools. Because the analyte is required to be in the gas phase for MS analysis, the ability to introduce liquid directly into the MS by converting solution molecules from the liquid phase to the gas phase is of paramount importance. ESI technology overcame this physical hurdle and made LC/MS into robust instruments with the analytical speed, sensitivity, and selectivity well suited for common drug metabolism studies [8]. On the other front, the development of HRMS instruments enabled the LC/MS platform to collect comprehensive accurate, high resolution mass datasets, distinguish drug metabolite ions from most, if not all, isobaric endogenous species, and determine the elemental composition of metabolite ions and their fragments [9,10]. To date, HRMS-based capabilities have resulted in a paradigm shift in the way metabolite profiling studies are conducted.

Standalone Mass Spectrometry

Prior to the introduction of atmospheric pressure ionization (API) in 1990s, identifying a metabolite by MS in complex biological matrices was a major undertaking. The main obstacle was the lack of an interface that would allow the direct coupling of HPLC with MS. It was common either to isolate the metabolite, usually in microgram quantities because of the relative insensitivity of the instruments, or to derivatize the analyte prior to analysis by gas chromatography (GC)/MS. The ionization techniques, such as electron ionization (EI), chemical ionization (CI), field desorption (FD), and fast atom bombardment (FAB), were operated under a vacuum. These techniques were not readily interfaced with HPLC because removing a vast majority of the liquid solvent without removing the analyte before it entered the ion source under a vacuum was considerably challenging. As a result, standalone MS instruments used for metabolite identification often required microgram quantities of the isolated analyte of interest. In addition, applications were largely limited to samples of highly volatile compounds within low-boiling organic solvents.

Electron and Chemical Ionizations

EI traces its roots to the work of A. J. Dempster [11] a century ago. Solid or liquid samples are introduced into the EI ion source using a direct insertion probe and ionized by bombardment of a stream of high-energy electrons (typically 70 eV). Analyte molecules lose an electron to give a positively charged radical (M$^{+\bullet}$), while some molecules may capture an electron to produce negative ions. In CI, a reagent gas is introduced directly into the EI ion source in addition to the analyte, and the reagent gas produces ions that are essentially nonreactive with the reaction gas but can undergo exoergic ion-molecule reactions with the analyte of interest [12]. Changes in the CI spectra can be obtained using alternative reagent gases. For example, methane and isobutene were commonly used to produce the reagent ions CH_5^+ and $C_4H_9^+$, both of which give a protonated analyte ion MH$^+$ by protein transfer [13,14], whereas ammonia and isobutene can produce ammonium [M+NH$_4$]$^+$ and isobutane [M+C$_4$H$_9$]$^+$ adduct ions, respectively [15]. EI is a "kinetically controlled" ionization process; hence, spectra acquired under standard conditions are reproducible over time and largely independent of the instrument used. Extensive EI mass spectra libraries have been generated and now contain over 270,000 entries (http://www.sisweb. com/software/ms/nist.htm#ei). Despite the well-established utility for structure elucidation purposes of EI MS especially when employed with online GC, thermally-labile metabolites including phase II conjugates are often not stable enough at the elevated temperatures required for vaporization, resulting in a complete cleavage/loss of the molecular ion. For examples, thermal lability and polarity of GSH conjugates limited the success of these techniques to only a few examples [16]. Hence, it is not surprising that "soft ionization" techniques including FD and FAB (or LSIMS) rapidly took preference for the screening of the phase II metabolites.

Field Desorption

FD is considered a forerunner of the "spray" techniques in that it involves the application of a high electric field to a liquid surface resulting in the production of intact molecular ions from nonvolatile samples. The advantage of the "soft ionization" technique was demonstrated by offering molecular weight information of the thioether conjugates of acetaminophen [17]. The molecular ion M$^{+\bullet}$ at m/z 456 of 3-glutathionylacetaminophen was not observed in an EI spectrum, and only a low intensity ion at m/z 411 was observed under CI conditions, corresponding to the loss of formic acid from an MH$^+$ ion. In contrast, the FD mass spectrum exhibited an intense protonated molecular ion [M+H]$^+$ at m/z 457 together with a prominent [M+Na]$^+$ ion at m/z 479 [17]. Additionally, The FD/CID spectrum offered informative product ions that resulted from fragmentation of the acetamido group of the parent drug and of bonds in the cysteinyl and γ-glutamyl residues.

Fast Atom Bombardment

FAB (or LSIMS) is another "soft ionization" technique commonly used in standalone mass spectrometers. A solution of the isolated metabolite in a nonvolatile liquid such as glycerol is loaded onto a metal target and introduced into the ionization source under a vacuum via an airlock, where the target is bombarded with a stream of atoms such as cesium, leading to desorption. Glycerol slows down the evaporation of the sample from the metal target, enabling the acquisition of mass spectra over a reasonable period of time [18]. Because of the relatively high sensitivity and "soft ionization" features, FAB/MS and FAB/MS/MS were well suited for the analysis of polar and thermally labile metabolites [19,20]. Polar metabolites such as glucuronide or sulfate conjugates can be analyzed as the intact species. Analysis of intact glucuronides is critical in the case of amines, because in many instances the conjugates derive from conjugation of the carbamic acids to which the parent amines are transformed via a chemical equilibrium in biological fluids [21,22]. Attempts to hydrolyze such carbamoyl glucuronides prior to isolation will result in decarboxylation of the unstable carbamic acid to yield the free amine, and the conjugate would be misidentified as an *N*-glucuronide. Hence, it is imperative that carbamoyl glucuronides are analyzed as intact to avoid misleading results [23].

Other metabolites including GSH adducts and coenzyme A thioesters are also amenable to the FAB analysis. Characteristic fragmentation of GSH adducts under FAB/MS conditions included the loss of glutamic acid (129 Da) [24], the expulsion of methyl glutamate (143 Da) from the corresponding methyl ester [25], and the elimination of the methyl glycine (89 Da) from the *N*-alkoxycarbonyl methyl ester derivative [24,26]. These characteristic losses were employed to screen for unknown GSH adducts in biological matrices [24]. Coupled with the isotope cluster ("twin ion") technique, a CNL scan at *m/z* 89 selectively revealed the MH⁺ species of unlabeled *S*-(*N*-methylcarbamoyl)glutathione (SMG) and [²H₃]SMG present as biliary metabolites of *N*-methylformamide (NMF) and [²H₃]NMF in mice [26]. Notably, fragmentation patterns of GSH conjugates acquired by FAB over two decades ago were essentially identical to the ones acquired under ESI, the most widely used ionization technique nowadays (Figure 13.2).

Gas Chromatography Mass Spectrometry

Mass spectrometers were first coupled with capillary GC during the 1960s simply because of the requirement for the analyte to be in gas phase prior to MS analysis (Figure 13.3). GC/MS instruments that employed EI or CI sources have been extensively used for quantifying and identifying trace components including drug metabolites in complex biological matrices [27]. GC/MS is most useful for the analysis of organically extractable and non-polar compounds, as well as highly volatile compounds with low vapor pressures that may undergo headspace analysis [28]. Thus, for polar compounds of interest in biological matrices, derivatization is often required to achieve the volatility necessary for GC. Aqueous solutions are treated with derivatization agents to convert the polar analyte to a chemically modified form amendable to organic extraction. Not only does derivatization result in a more volatile compound, this also enhances solvent extractability and MS sensitivity. Derivatization of catechol estrogens with *N*, *O*-bis(trimethylsilyl)trifluoroacetamide (BSTFA) provided both protection for the labile catechols and the volatility required for GC analysis [29]. In addition, the development of multi-dimensional GC/MS offered enhancement of separating capacity suitable for complex biological mixtures [30].

The use of stable isotopes has become commonplace in drug metabolism research [31]. Coupled with stable isotope labeling techniques, GC/MS has proven to be a powerful tool for investigating mechanistic aspects of biotransformation reactions. In an attempt to investigate the bioactivation mechanism of 1,2-dibromo-3-chloropropane (DBCP), GC/MS analysis together with the isotope cluster technique not only facilitated the recognition of the drug-related materials in complex biological matrices but, more importantly, demonstrated that formation of the potent direct-acting mutagen 2-bromoacrolein (2-BA) resulted primarily from the initial oxidation at the C-1 position of DBCP [32].

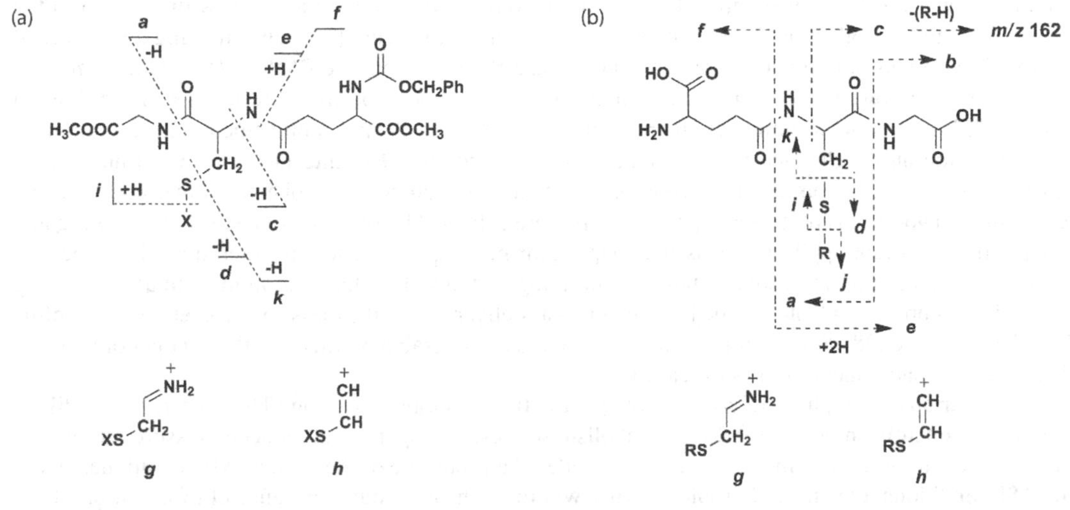

FIGURE 13.2 Characteristic fragmentation of the [M+H]⁺ ions of (a) the N-[(benzoyloxy)-carbonyl] dimethyl ester derivatized GSH conjugates under FAB, and (b) the native GSH conjugates under ESI. (Reproduced from Pearson, P.G. et al., *Anal. Chem.*, 62, 1827–1836, 1990; Wen, B. et al., *Drug Metab. Dispos.*, 37, 1557–1562, 2009. With permission.)

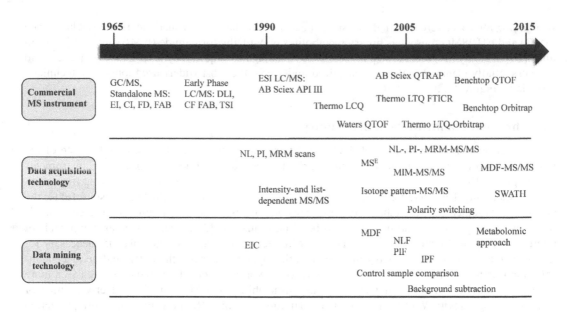

FIGURE 13.3 The advance of mass spectrometry technologies in drug metabolism research.

Liquid Chromatography Mass Spectrometry

Despite its extensive use in drug metabolism studies, GC/MS is limited in the analysis of polar metabolites in aqueous matrices. Derivatization often resulted in excessive components in gas chromatographic analyses yielding additional complexity for identifying the metabolites of interest [33]. From a quantitative perspective, the use of GC/MS for such an analysis requires a minimum extraction efficiency and often a derivatization efficiency, with back-calculations to determine the analyte concentrations within the original sample. These limitations in sample preparation, analysis, and throughput essentially necessitated the development of a robust and stable interface that would allow the direct coupling of HPLC with MS. However, the coupling of HPLC with MS operating under a vacuum proved much more challenging than the coupling of GC and MS. Early examples included the "moving belt" interface in which the mobile phase solution was sprayed onto a continuously looped polyimide belt, with one end in the atmosphere and the other end in the ionization source under a vacuum [34]. The "moving belt" worked well with little loss of chromatographic resolution, and the use of on-line FAB LC/MS with a "moving belt" interface allowed detection of the protonated molecular ions of almitrine and its metabolites in plasma [35]. Direct liquid introduction (DLI) represented a significant improvement with less thermal decomposition and higher sensitivity compared to the "moving belt" interface [36]. Continuous-flow (CF) FAB/MS/MS was used for analysis of drugs such as penicillin G, phentolamine, cocaine, and warfarin, and good sensitivity and reproducibility were achieved by this technique [37]. An exciting and potentially important application was the coupling of mass spectrometers to microdialysis probes for the direct sampling of drugs and metabolites in living systems. The dialysate fluid from an indwelling microdialysis probe implanted in the jugular vein was delivered into the mass spectrometer via an online CF FAB interface [38]. Such online technology offered considerable promise for the conduct of metabolism and pharmacokinetic studies in real time.

Of the various early phase LC/MS couplings, the thermospray ionization (TSI) interface was likely the most frequently employed for drug metabolism studies. TSI operates at reduced pressure rather than under a vacuum or in the atmosphere and is considered a prototype of the current API technique. Under the TSI conditions, the charged droplets shrink within the heated source because of evaporation of the solvent. When the droplet attains a certain diameter, the repulsive forces within the droplet build up, leading to the emission of individual ions, a process known as ion evaporation and columbic explosion [39]. One of the major advantages of TSI over DLI is that LC flow rates up to 1.5 mL/min can be reached with TSI versus 50 µL/min with DLI. A series of cysteine, *N*-acetyl cysteine, and GSH conjugates was successfully analyzed by LC/TSI MS [40], and for most of the compounds, positive ion TSI is more sensitive than negative ion thermospray. Additionally, LC/TSI MS was successfully used for detection and identification of GSH conjugates such as 3-methylindole [41] and propranolol [42].

The ability to introduce an HPLC effluent directly into the MS by converting aqueous polar analytes to gas phase ions is of paramount importance and is dictated by the source from which the HPLC solvent is vaporized and ionized prior to MS analysis. The development of API sources (notably those employing electrospray, ionspray or heated nebulizer interfaces) eventually overcame this physical hurdle, with its capability to operate under atmospheric pressure, readily couple with reverse and normal phase HPLC, and generate intact molecular ions with high sensitivity. On account of their sensitivity, compatibility, applicability, and general ease of operation, a combination of the coupling of LC with MS and the advancement of MS technologies (i.e., development of tandem quadrupole and ion trap mass spectrometers) has propelled LC/MS to the forefront as the preeminent analytical tool for the detection, quantification and structure elucidation of drug-related materials in biological matrices [43].

Scanning Functions

One of the most important uses of MS is the generation and determination of molecular ions of unknown metabolites. Triple quadrupole mass spectrometer-based precursor ion (PI) and neutral loss (NL) scans substantially increased the capability to search for metabolites regardless of their molecular weights based on common or expected fragmentation [44]. This "metabolite mapping" approach was the cornerstone of LC/MS technology for drug metabolite identification in the 1990s (Figure 13.3) and was employed in the detection of unknown oxidative metabolites [45], GSH adducts [46], and glucuronide and sulfate conjugates [47]. On the other hand, MS^n capability on the linear ion trap quadrupole (LTQ), which provides detailed fragmentation information, was another key LC/MS approach utilized for structural elucidation of drug metabolites [48].

Data Acquisition

An intelligent, data-dependent acquisition uses one or two survey scans to trigger the acquisition of MS/MS of targeted metabolites. List-dependent MS^n acquisition on an ion trap instrument was the first practical data-dependent acquisition approach widely employed for metabolite identification [49]. A comprehensive list of predicted molecular ions of metabolites derived from the parent drug is incorporated into its acquisition method, and ions that match the m/z values of predicted metabolites in full scan MS spectra are triggered for "on-the-fly" recording of MS^n spectra. This approach is capable of acquiring full scan MS and MS^n spectral datasets in a single run. Ion trap-based isotope pattern-dependent MS/MS acquisition is another useful acquisition method for both detection of metabolite ions and acquisition of their MS/MS spectra that have distinct isotope patterns. This approach was effectively used for rapid screening of *in vitro* reactive metabolites trapped by stable isotope labeled GSH [50]. Similarly, a combination of isotope pattern-dependent acquisition and polarity switching technique was applied to the detection and structural characterization of GSH adducts using a linear ion trap instrument [51]. The list-dependent MS/MS acquisition in quadrupole time-of-flight (QTOF) instruments enabled the generation of accurate mass MS/MS spectra of predicted metabolites in a single LC/MS run [52].

The use of NL, PI, and multiple reaction monitoring (MRM) as a survey scan to trigger the data-dependent MS/MS acquisition was carried out on the hybrid quadrupole-linear ion trap (QTRAP) instruments, which can function either as a triple quadrupole and/or ion trap within a given scan cycle [53,54]. On account of their high sensitivity, great versatility, and general ease of operation, the NL-, PI-, and MRM-dependent MS/MS approaches using the QTRAP have been widely used for fast profiling of oxidative metabolites and conjugates, offering product ion spectra with structurally informative fragmentation with no low-mass cutoff [55–58]. In the absence of prior knowledge of fragmentation patterns of metabolites, multiple ion monitoring (MIM)-EPI was developed for metabolite profiling and characterization [59,60]. The difference between MIM and MRM is that under MIM, the molecular ions isolated in Q1 pass through Q2 with no fragmentation and are monitored in Q3 of the QTRAP.

The screening and characterization of reactive metabolites using information-dependent acquisition (IDA) scan functions of QTRAP are among the instrument's many applications [55]. Characteristic fragmentation of GSH conjugates has been extensively described above [20,24] and, similar to the CID of peptides, fragmentation of GSH conjugates is mainly a result of cleavage of the peptide backbone of the GSH moiety in the positive mode. For example, GSH conjugates generally undergo a NL of 129 Da (loss of pyroglutamate) to produce e-type fragment ions, which can be readily detected by a CNL scan of 129 Da. However, structurally different classes of GSH conjugates have long been recognized to behave differently upon CID in the positive ion mode, and not all classes of GSH conjugates afford an NL of 129 Da as the primary fragmentation pathway. Many GSH adducts yield doubly charged $[M + 2H]^{2+}$ ions under the positive ion mode, which typically do not fragment by a neutral loss of 129 Da under CID. To overcome this drawback, Dieckhaus et al. demonstrated that a PI scan of m/z 272 (deprotonated γ-glutamyl-dehydroalanyl-glycine) in the negative ion mode provides a broader survey scan for the detection of GSH conjugates of different classes, including benzylic, aromatic, aliphatic, and thioester GSH conjugates [61]. An extension of this methodology incorporates a simultaneous dual negative precursor ion scan for m/z 272 and 254 (the dehydrated form of m/z 272) [62]. With both fragment anions scanned in parallel, this method has achieved a further increase in selectivity. Additionally, a high-throughput screening method was developed using polarity switching technique on a hybrid QTRAP [63]. This method utilized a PI scan of m/z 272 in the negative ion mode for unambiguous detection of GSH adducts, with polarity switching to the positive ion mode for MS/MS acquisition in a single LC/MS run. Several novel reactive metabolites were detected and identified [64–67], and exogenous GSH adducts were distinguished from endogenous GSH conjugates using this polarity switching method when GSH ethyl ester was used as a trapping agent [68]. In humans, GSH conjugates often undergo *in vivo* biotransformation to give rise to N-acetyl-L-cysteine (NAC) adducts (mercapturic acid adducts) [69]. Based on predicted fragmentations, MRM-EPI methods were constructed for detection of both GSH and NAC conjugates [70,71]. Results showed that the MRM-EPI method is well suited for detection of *in vivo* reactive metabolites in complex biological matrices. Whereas MRM-EPI is often chosen as the primary method for detection and characterization of low-level *in vivo* reactive metabolites in complex biological matrices owing to its inherent sensitivity and selectivity, generic approaches such as PI-EPI and NL-EPI are well suited for high-throughput screening of structurally unknown reactive metabolites in a drug discovery setting.

Analytical Strategy

The LC/MS analytical strategies for metabolite identification can be divided into two categories, a single LC/MS platform versus combinations of two or more LC/MS platforms. LC coupled with an ESI triple quadrupole took preference to become the LC/MS platform of choice for drug metabolite identification in the early 1990s; however, limitations of the triple quadrupole-based LC/MS platform included the lack of sensitivity of a full MS scan and the requirement for multiple injections/runs during PI, NL, and product ion scans followed by MS/MS acquisition. The hybrid QTRAP instrument was developed to enable PI-, NL-, and MRM-dependent MS/MS acquisitions, in which PI, NL, and MRM-based survey scans are carried out to trigger the acquisition of both full MS and MS/MS spectra. Because it can function either as a triple quadrupole and/or ion trap within a given scan cycle, QTRAP is well suited for both quantitative and qualitative analysis of drug metabolites. Since its introduction around 2002, the QTRAP has increasingly taken preference as one of the most versatile LC/MS systems in both quantification and structural characterization of drug metabolites as a single LC/MS system. As an alternative, the ion trap-based MS^n analytical strategy was extensively applied for metabolite identification since introduction of the Thermo ion trap mass spectrometer, the LCQ, in the late 1990s. This approach took advantage of its fast MS scanning speed and MS^n acquisition capability. However, since ion trap instruments were not capable of performing NL and PI scans, its utility in detecting low-level, uncommon metabolites with certain fragmentation patterns was limited.

High-Resolution Mass Spectrometry

HRMS generates accurate mass spectral data that provide element composition of the molecular ions or their fragment ions. Since the mid-2000s, significantly improved HRMS instruments including Waters'

QTOF, Thermo Fisher's LTQ-FTICR and LTQ-Orbitrap functioned much better than earlier versions of HRMS in terms of sensitivity, scanning speed, resolution, and stability of mass accuracy (Figure 13.3). Additionally, a new MS^E-based HRMS data acquisition technique [72] and an accurate mass data mining tool namely a mass defect filter (MDF) [73] were developed, enabling HRMS detection of unknown drug metabolites without using PI or NL scans. Cascades of HRMS-based data acquisition and data mining technologies, including isotope-pattern dependent MS/MS acquisition [74], data mining [75], neutral loss filters (NLF) and product ion filters (PIF) [76], and background subtraction algorithms [77–79], were developed and applied to enhance HRMS capabilities in the comprehensive and rapid identification of drug metabolites (Figure 13.4). Since the early 2010s, HRMS has been used as a single, primary LC/MS system in drug metabolism studies. More recently, HRMS-based data acquisition and data mining tools have been increasingly used in metabolite identification and profiling studies, such as metabolic "soft-spot" analysis, reactive metabolite screening, and detection and identification of uncommon metabolites *in vivo*. The emergence and application of HRMS technologies have been summarized previously [9,10,45,80–88].

HRMS-Based Data Acquisition

Accurate mass spectra of drug metabolites can be obtained by HRMS using a targeted product ion scan on each individually detected and/or expected molecular ion. However, this approach typically requires multiple injections because of duty cycle constrains. Since the mid-2000s, multiple data-dependent MS/MS acquisition methods such as list-, isotope pattern-, and mass defect-dependent MS/MS acquisitions and data-independent global fragment generation methods such as MS^E and sequential window acquisition of all theoretical fragment-ion spectra (SWATH) were developed to enhance the capabilities of HRMS in automated acquisition of MS/MS spectra or global fragment ions relevant to metabolites in a single LC/MS injection. Major HRMS-based data acquisition and mining tools for metabolite identification are summarized in Figure 13.4.

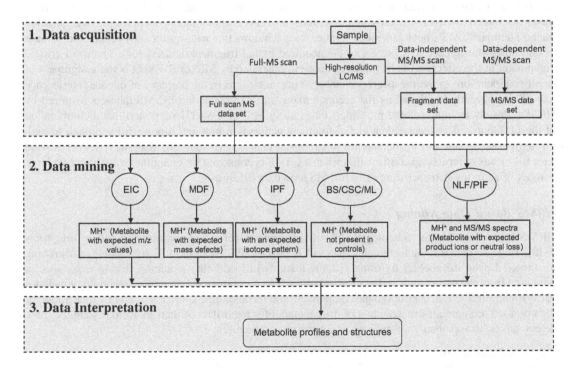

FIGURE 13.4 The general workflow using HRMS technology for drug metabolite detection and identification. (Adapted from Zhu, M. et al., *J. Biol. Chem.*, 2286, 25419–25425, 2011. With permission.)

Data-Dependent MS/MS Acquisition

HRMS-based data-dependent MS/MS acquisition significantly reduces the acquiring of irrelevant MS/MS information. This is simply because of narrower accurate mass windows that can be set around drug metabolites to exclude irrelevant isobaric ions that are otherwise acquired. A single injection with a list-dependent acquisition to obtain MS/MS spectra of expected metabolites along with an intensity-dependent acquisition as a backup to obtain MS/MS spectra for the remaining major ions is a common workflow. Isotope pattern-dependent methods can be effectively applied to trigger MS/MS acquisition of drug metabolites that have a distinct isotope fingerprint [89]. Since HRMS can significantly reduce variability in both the intensity ratio and mass difference, HRMS-based isotope pattern-dependent acquisition is much more effective than a method using low-resolution MS. Mass defect-dependent acquisition is a new data-dependent acquisition method specifically developed for HRMS instruments to trigger MS/MS acquisition of drug metabolites in complex biological matrices [90]. This method imposes one or multiple filters in the mass defect dimension on full scan survey MS spectra to search for ions with matching criteria and trigger acquisition of their MS/MS data. This greatly reduces the possibility of wasting MS duty cycle time on irrelevant ions, while missing metabolite ions of interest. Because of such improved selectivity for drug metabolite ions, a lower intensity threshold may be set to obtain MS/MS spectra for minor drug metabolites. Similar to the polarity switching approach using a hybrid QTRAP described above [63], the selective ion monitoring of *m/z* 272.0888, a characteristic product ion corresponding to deprotonated γ-glutamyl-dehydroalanyl-glycine in the negative ionization mode, was applied as a survey scan to trigger acquisition of accurate mass and multiple MS/MS spectra of GSH conjugates on a Thermo Q Exactive quadrupole orbitrap mass spectrometer [91]. Incorporation of accurate mass PI-dependent data acquisition and fast polarity switching option makes this LC-HRMS platform a sensitive tool for rapid detection and characterization of GSH conjugates.

Data-Independent Global Fragment Acquisition

MS^E acquisition was developed for the QTOF to generate fragments for all of components along with their precursor ions in a single LC-HRMS run [72,92,93]. The global fragment dataset can be utilized for structural characterization and metabolite detection via data mining by NLF or PIF after the fragments are linked to their perspective precursor ions. SWATH is a data-independent fragment acquisition method similar to MS^E, but it has much smaller mass windows that can significantly reduce the number of co-eluted interference ions present in the acquired global fragment datasets [94]. The most critical component in the effective use of fragment datasets generated by MS^E or SWATH is the assignment of small fragment ions to their respective metabolite precursor ions in the presence of intense interference ions. This is greatly facilitated by the accurate mass and high resolution LC/MS datasets acquired by HRMS. Results from metabolite profiling studies using MS^E or SWATH suggested that a combination of the QTOF and data-independent global fragment acquisition provides a powerful approach to high throughput screening of drug metabolites in biological matrices. In addition, MS^E and SWATH provide a useful means of structural confirmation when a QTOF is employed for quantitative analysis of a large number of analytes using accurate mass full MS scan data [95,96].

HRMS-Based Data Mining

HRMS-based data mining technology can be divided into targeted and non-targeted data mining tools [9,10]. Targeted data mining techniques such as EIC, MDF, IPF, NLF, and PIF are capable of searching for targeted drug metabolites by using specific features in metabolite structures and/or mass spectra predicted from the parent drug and/or its metabolites. The non-targeted data mining technology includes background subtraction, control sample comparison, and metabolomic approaches, all of which allow for the unbiased, comprehensive detection of drug metabolites regardless of their molecular weights, mass defect values, isotope pattern, fragmentation patterns or structures.

Targeted Data Mining

MDF is considered as the first data processing technique specially developed for "metabolite mining" from full MS datasets generated from HRMS instruments [73,95,97]. MDF imposes a filter on the residue mass (i.e., the mass defect) dimension in selected mass windows of HRMS datasets. Ions derived from endogenous components in biological matrices are excluded by MDF so that ions corresponding to drug metabolites can be substantially enriched. This is based on the idea that mass defects of metabolites typically fall within a definable window (40–50 mDa) relative to those of the parent drug. Multiple MDFs can be applied to the same full MS dataset across selected mass ranges to retain various classes of drug metabolites, such as glucuronides. The effectiveness of MDF in metabolite identification has been demonstrated [74,86,98–101]. In addition, MDF has been applied to the detection of metabolites of Chinese herbal medicines [102] and designer drugs [103], where multiple xenobiotic components undergo various metabolic pathways to generate large sets of metabolites. It has been suggested that the efficiency of an MDF template is typically better for samples from plasma, bile, and fecal matrices than for samples from urine [104]. Because of its "metabolite-enriching" capabilities, the utility of MDF and its equivalent functions have been widely incorporated into major HRMS data processing software packages.

NLF and PIF are other types of post-acquisition data processing tools specially developed to enable HRMS detection of various unknown drug metabolites. NLF and PIF search for drug metabolites in high resolution MS/MS spectra [76] or fragment datasets [72] based on their fragmentation patterns such as a specific neutral loss or the formation of a certain product ion predicted from the parent drug, a known metabolite of the parent drug or various classes of conjugates of the parent drug. For example, a few unique product ions of triptolide were employed in the PIF process to selectively search for oxidative metabolites of triptolide in rat urine [89]. In a similar manner, NLF targeting a neutral loss of m/z 129.0426, the major and unique fragmentation pathway of GSH adducts, can be effectively applied to detect GSH adduct ions in high resolution MS/MS data [105]. NLF and PIF are well suited for the selective detection of certain types of metabolites and are complimentary to MDF. Both NLF and PIF can be directly applied to processing MS/MS spectral datasets recorded using data-dependent methods such as intensity-, inclusion list-, and isotope-dependent MS/MS acquisition methods, leading to the sensitive and selective detection of minor or trace amounts of metabolites as long as their high resolution MS/MS spectra are acquired. In addition, NLF and PIF can be applied to global fragment ion datasets generated using data-independent acquisition methods such as ion source CID, MS^E, and SWATH. Given the nonspecific nature of the data acquisition, the resultant data acquired by low resolution MS would be of little use because determining the respective precursor ions of fragment ions recorded in the dataset would be difficult. The accurate mass quality of such nonspecific fragmentation data, in combination with the accurate mass molecular ion data typically acquired by HRMS, has made NLF and PIF more effective in such applications [94,106]. Although linking minor fragments to their precursor ions remains challenging, the application of NLF and PIF to processing global fragment ion datasets is a powerful tool in the detection, structural confirmation, and characterization of unknown drug metabolites or other xenobiotics in complex biological samples.

EIC has long been a centerpiece of mass spectrometric data-processing strategies for chromatographically resolving isobaric components. IPF is a method applicable to situations in which drug metabolites exhibit distinct isotope patterns that do not typically exist among endogenous matrix components [9]. Such distinct patterns occur naturally with halogen-containing compounds, stable isotope-labeled drugs and metabolites formed in incubations with stable isotope-labeled trapping agents (e.g., GSH). Although EIC and IPF have been used routinely to find targeted drug metabolite ions in unit-resolution full scan MS datasets, high-resolution LC/MS data-based EIC and IPF can apply a relatively narrower ion extraction window for ion chromatogram generation, which in return enhances both selectivity and sensitivity, resulting in the detection of minor metabolites with minimal false positive signals.

Non-targeted Data Mining

Background subtraction is an effective data processing tool for non-targeted detection of drug metabolites. The concept of background subtraction is not new; however, it is surely a new capability in a practical sense since isobaric ions in high resolution LC/MS data are typically resolved so that background subtraction can be systematically performed on discrete ions in raw MS data. This HRMS-based background subtraction approach is very useful in the fast and comprehensive profiling of both *in vitro* [77] and *in vivo* metabolites [79,107]. The background subtraction process often includes one test sample and one control sample. If populations of sample matrix components significantly differ between the test and control samples or if no good control sample is available to provide adequate matrix component coverage, this approach may not work effectively. Recently, a new "Precise and Thorough Background Subtraction" (PATBS) algorithm was developed for untargeted screening of unknown metabolites to establish a "xenobiotic fingerprint" only present in the patient samples but not in the control samples [108]. Along with targeted data mining tools, unknown metabolites and/or potential toxic xenobiotics present in the patient samples are identified via database search and spectral interpretation. The combination of data-independent acquisition and untargeted background subtraction may have broad applications in the detection and characterization of unknown metabolites/xenobiotics in forensic toxicological analyses and sport enhancement drug screening.

Another useful non-targeted data mining technique is the metabolomic approach [109]. Unlike the data mining tools we have discussed that process HRMS datasets from either two samples (i.e., background subtraction) or one sample (i.e., MDF, NLF, PIF), a metabolomic approach requires two groups of samples, a treated and a non-treated group, each of which requires a minimum of three or four samples; the larger the sample size, the better the data quality. Once accurate mass MS datasets from all of the samples are acquired, individual chromatographic components are determined and compared between the two groups using various statistic analytical tools. Chromatographic components that have significantly higher levels or presented only in the treated samples are either xenobiotic components or endogenous components, whose levels have been elevated as a result of the drug treatment or of being under specific physiological conditions. The metabolomics approach has been extensively applied to studies of perturbations of endogenous small molecules *in vitro* or *in vivo* caused by xenobiotics such as a drug or toxic chemical [110,111]. In addition, a number of applications using this bioanalytical tool have appeared in recent years including identification of new metabolites [112], reactive metabolite screening [113], elucidation of metabolic pathways [114], and identification of metabolic polymorphisms [115].

HRMS-Based Analytical Strategies

The advance of HRMS-based technologies has led to development of new analytical approaches to different types of drug metabolism studies. In general, these new analytical strategies have enabled the detection of unknown metabolites without using NL or PI scans. Waters' QTOF with MS^E acquisition were employed to generate both full HRMS and global fragment datasets, followed by data process using multiple data mining techniques [92,100,116]. As an alternative, Thermo's LTQ-Orbitrap with MDF [95], background subtraction [77,79], and IPF [117] were utilized to perform various types of metabolite identification studies. These HRMS-based workflows have led to a paradigm change in the LC/MS analytical strategy for drug metabolite identification, from the use of multiple LC/MS instruments to the use of a single HRMS instrument [9]. Although a variety of HRMS instruments have been utilized for metabolite identifications studies, data acquisition methods, and data mining tools as the key components of these workflows are the same. Overall, these "all-in-one" workflows can be described as a three-step approach (Figure 13.4): (1) acquire both full scan accurate mass MS and MS/MS or global fragment datasets using either a data-dependent or data-independent method; (2) detect drug metabolite ions and retrieve their MS/MS spectra from recorded datasets using targeted and/or non-targeted data mining tools; (3) identify and characterize metabolite structures based on spectral interpretation.

It is noteworthy to point out that each of these methods has its own advantages and limitations. One should design and apply specific workflows with a selected data acquisition method and typically a combination of several data mining techniques based on the purpose and types of the drug metabolism study. For example, MS^E acquisition followed by data mining is a method of choice for high throughput analysis of metabolic soft spots using a Waters QTOF instrument. On the other front, the use of dynamic background subtraction to acquire both MS and MS/MS datasets followed by EIC, MDF, NLF, and/or PIF-based data mining is a preferred method for the same experiment on an AB Sciex TripleTOF mass spectrometer. Additionally, isotope pattern-dependent acquisition of reactive metabolites trapped by stable isotope labeled GSH using Orbitrap is a good choice for fast and selective analysis of reactive metabolites [74].

For *in vivo* drug metabolism studies, list- or mass defect-dependent MS/MS acquisition would be the method of choice to record MS/MS spectra of predicted or unknown metabolites respectively. MS^E or SWATH would be useful in the structural confirmation of over 50 components when they are subjected to quantitative analysis or screening using full scan MS on an HRMS instrument [118]. On the other front, the flexibility and versatility of HRMS-based data acquisition and data mining tools make it a powerful bioanalytical platform for various types of drug metabolism studies. In particular, the combination of multiple data-mining techniques in tandem, i.e., untargeted background subtraction followed by targeted MDF data processing can be a valuable tool for rapid metabolite profiling of combination drugs in human [119]. Another new HRMS-based strategy is the use of HRMS in profiling, identification, and quantitative estimation of plasma metabolites in humans in early clinical studies to address concerns of metabolite safety testing [75,120,121]. LC/HRMS has been widely used in the metabolomic studies and is the method of choice for determining both xenobiotic metabolite profiles and changes of endogenous component levels as a result of drug treatment. As part of the mechanisms to understand drug-induced toxicity, a recent metabolomic analysis revealed evidence for compromised bile acid homeostasis by a hepatotoxic pyrrolizidine alkaloid [122]. Additionally, HRMS-based online H/D exchange [90], ion mobility technology [123], MS^n acquisition [124], and polarity switching technology [91] provide unique structural information to facilitate metabolite identification.

Current Practice of Metabolite Identification in Drug Discovery and Development

Drug metabolism plays an important role in understanding drug safety and efficacy in preclinical animals and patients. The core activity of detecting and determining the chemical structure of human metabolites has changed little in decades and, in fact, is the starting point for all the other activities in areas such as enzymology, regulation, and genetics. With the advance of the mass spectrometry technology, drug metabolism research has become an integral part of drug discovery and development in pharmaceutical industry (Figure 13.1). Metabolic soft-spot analysis and reactive metabolite screening are often carried out in lead optimization in support of efforts to reduce or minimize metabolic instability and bioactivation, respectively. HRMS-based data-independent (MS^E) or selective data-dependent (isotope pattern) MS/MS acquisition methods are often employed in such studies to enable high throughput analysis. As an alternative, QTRAP-based information-dependent acquisition approaches are effective in both metabolic soft-spot analysis and reactive metabolite screening. *In vitro* metabolism comparison across species and subsequent *in vivo* ADME study in animals provide biochemical basis to support selection of preclinical species for toxicological evaluation, as well as to project human pharmacokinetics in characterization of clinical candidates for drug development. These studies require comprehensive profiling and identification of various classes of drug metabolites in complex biological matrices. Therefore, full scan HRMS data acquisition followed by MDF, EIC, and/or background subtraction data mining is highly recommended for metabolite detection and profiling (Figure 13.4). Radiolabeled *in vivo* ADME studies provide key information on excretion routes, clearance pathways, and exposures of drug-related components in human and animal species. Radiolabel greatly facilitates sensitive detection and quantitation of a dosed drug candidate and its metabolites in biological matrixes so that use of the LC/MS in the radiolabeled studies is mainly for metabolite structural characterization. In contrast, metabolite profiling, structural characterization, and quantitative analysis from nonradiolabeled studies, that is, early clinical studies, are heavily dependent on MS technology. Since circulating metabolites are often at very low abundance, HRMS is a preferred MS platform to fulfil the purpose of such drug metabolism studies [120,121]. The information gathered in these studies can be used to trigger characterization activities for important human metabolites and can potentially be used to prioritize or deprioritize the conduct of the radiolabeled human ADME study.

Conclusion and Future Perspectives

The last several decades have witnessed the advance of MS technologies and its defining impact on drug metabolism research. The evolving role of MS technology in drug metabolism research comes largely with its two major milestones, namely the emergence of commercial LC/MS with API ion sources and the development of HRMS along with data acquisition and data mining technologies. The foremost advantage of HRMS over nominal mass resolution mass spectrometry is the fact that a complete, unbiased metabolism data set can be acquired in a single injection without the requirement to invest upfront resources in method development. To date, the emergence of multitasking workflows to simultaneously acquire accurate mass full MS and MS/MS datasets followed by post acquisition data processing has made HRMS a single and major LC/MS platform for drug metabolite research.

The uptake of the HRMS-based "all-in-one" workflows has led to a period of exponential growth in drug metabolism research in recent years. Metabolite profiling and identification from complex biological matrices are now routinely performed by HRMS with appropriate data acquisition and data mining tools, and results from unlabeled first-in-human studies can be utilized to support the "human first" strategy [121,125]. This accelerated view of human metabolism as a result of advancing MS technologies would continually serve as a main driving force in shaping the direction of drug metabolism research. Over time, however, the goal of drug metabolism studies has remained unchanged, namely answering three fundamental questions: "what is it?", "how much is there?", and "what does it do in the body?". Therefore, further opportunities in drug metabolism may not rely solely on increased MS sensitivity, which now becomes achievable using HRMS-based data acquisition technologies but rather on the application of novel methodologies to contextualize drug metabolite datasets in relation to drug safety and efficacy. The technological advances in xenobiotic metabolomics (also known as pharmacometabolomics) may present such an opportunity for drug metabolism studies [110] as it offers a holistic viewpoint that reflects the dynamic response of a biological system to stimuli such as exogenous metabolites. Thus, the application of metabolomics in drug metabolism research may hold the additional promise of bridging the gap between drug metabolism and drug-induced toxicity [126].

On the other front, the scope of MS applications in drug metabolism research has substantially expanded, from drug metabolites to other xenobiotic metabolites, from exogenous to endogenous components, and from small molecules to proteins. Among them, antibody-drug conjugates [127], covalent drugs [128], and drug-protein adducts [129] represent additional challenges as well as new opportunities in drug metabolism research using MS technologies. Some LC/HRMS technologies primarily developed for metabolite identification, such as MS^E SWATH, data-independent acquisition, and untargeted background subtraction tools, would be very useful in metabolism studies of totally unknown xenobiotics or of combination drugs such as performance-enhancing drugs, Chinese herbal medicines, and environmental contaminants.

More generally, the major advantage of MS technologies may have been its flexibility and versatility that have allowed hybridization with its own and other bioanalytical platforms leading to its broad applications in drug metabolism research. The development of software-assisted mass spectral interpretation for structural elucidation holds the promise to enable full automation of the metabolite identification workflow. The use of a single LC/MS platform for both quantitative and qualitative analysis of the parent drug and its metabolites is expected to improve analytical throughput and productivity. With substantial changes seen in MS technologies, one can ensure that the field of drug metabolism will continue to experience exponential growth in the foreseeable future.

DECLARATION OF INTEREST

The author declares no conflicts of interest.

ABBREVIATIONS

API	atmospheric pressure ionization
CI	chemical ionization
CID	collision induced dissociation
DDI	drug-drug interactions
DLI	direct liquid introduction
EI	electron ionization
EIC	extracted ion chromatography
EPI	enhanced product ion
ESI	electrospray ionization
FAB	fast atom bombardment
FD	field desorption
GC/MS	gas chromatography mass spectrometry
HRMS	high-resolution mass spectrometry
IDA	information dependent acquisition
IPF	isotope pattern filter
LC/MS	liquid chromatography mass spectrometry
LSIMS	liquid secondary ion mass spectrometry
LTQ	linear trap quadrupole
MDF	mass defect filter
MIM	multiple ion monitoring
MIST	metabolite in safety testing
ML	metabolomics
MRM	multiple reaction monitoring
MS/MS	tandem mass spectrometry
NL	neutral loss
NLF	neutral loss filter
P450	cytochrome P450
PI	precursor ion
PIF	product ion filter
QTOF	quadrupole time-of-flight
QTRAP	quadrupole-linear ion trap
SWATH	sequential window acquisition of all theoretical fragment-ion spectra
TCM	traditional Chinese medicine
TSI	thermospray ionization

REFERENCES

1. Parkinson A. Biotransformation of xenobiotics. In: Klaassen CD, editor. *Casarett and Doul's toxicology: The basic science of poisons*. New York: McGraw-Hill. 2001; pp 133–224.
2. Wen B, Nelson SD. Chapter 2. Common biotransformation reactions. In: Lee M, Zhu M, editors. *Mass Spectrometry in Drug Metabolism and Disposition: Basic Principles and Applications*. London, UK: John Wiley & Sons Ltd. 2011; pp 13–41.
3. Laine R. Metabolic stability: Main enzymes involved and best tools to assess it. *Curr Drug Metab* 2008; 9:921–927.
4. Rodrigues AD. Drug–drug interactions, second edition. In: Rodrigues AD, editor. *Drugs and the pharmaceutical sciences*. New York: Informa Healthcare. 2008.
5. Caldwell GW, Yan Z, Tang W, Dasgupta M, Hasting B. ADME optimization and toxicity assessment in early- and late-phase drug discovery. *Curr Top Med Chem* 2009; 9:965–980.

6. Kola I, Landis J. Can the pharmaceutical industry reduce attrition rates? *Nat Rev Drug Discov* 2004; 3:711–715.

7. Bateman KP, Kellmann M, Muenster H, Papp R, Taylor L. Quantitative-qualitative data acquisition using a benchtop Orbitrap mass spectrometer. *J Am Soc Mass Spectrom* 2009; 20:1441–1450.

8. Lee MS, Kerns EH. LC/MS applications in drug development. *Mass Spectrom Rev* 1999; 18:187–279.

9. Zhu M, Zhang H, Humphreys WG. Drug metabolite profiling and identification by high-resolution mass spectrometry. *J Biol Chem* 2011; 2286:25419–25425.

10. Ma S, Chowdhury SK. Data acquisition and data mining techniques for metabolite identification using LC coupled to high-resolution MS. *Bioanalysis* 2013; 5:1285–1297.

11. Dempster AJ. A new method of positive ray analysis. *Phys Rev* 1918; 11:316–325.

12. Munson MSB, Field FH. Chemical ionization mass spectrometry I. General introduction. *J Am Chem Soc* 1966; 88:2621–2630.

13. Garland WA, Trager WF, Nelson SD. Direct (non-chromatographic) quantification of drugs and their metabolites from human plasma utilizing chemical ionization mass spectrometry and stable isotope labeling: Quinidine and lidocaine. *Biomed Mass Spectrom* 1974; 1:124–129.

14. Pohl LR, Nelson SD, Garland WA, Trager WF. The rapid identification of a new metabolite of warfarin via a chemical ionization mass spectrometry ion doublet technique. *Biomed Mass Spectrom* 1975; 2:23–30.

15. Shimizu Y. Adduct ion formation in isobutane chemical ionization of aliphatic olefins. *Mass Spectrosc* 1984; 32:357–364.

16. Nelson SD, Mitchell JR, Pohl LR. Application of Chemical Ionization Ms and the Twin-Ion Technique in the Analysis of Reactive Intermediates in Drug Metabolism. In: Frigerio A, Ghisalberti EL, editors. *Mass Spectrometry in Drug Metabolism*. New York: Plenum. 1977; pp 237–249.

17. Nelson SD, Vaishnav Y, Kambara H, Baillie TA. Comparative electron impact, chemical ionization and field desorption mass spectra of some thioether metabolites of acetaminophen. *Biomed Mass Spectrom* 1981; 8:244–251.

18. Barber M, Bordoli RS, Sedgewick RD, Tyler AN. Fast atom bombardment of solids (F.A.B.): A new ion source for mass spectrometry. *J Chem Soc Chem Commun* 1981; 7:325–327.

19. Haroldsen PE, Reilly MH, Hughes H, Gaskell SJ, Porter CJ. Characterization of glutathione conjugates by fast atom bombardment/tandem mass spectrometry. *Biomed Environ Mass Spectrom* 1988; 15:615–621.

20. Baillie TA, Davis MR. Mass spectrometry in the analysis of glutathione conjugates. *Biol Mass Spectrom* 1993; 22:319–325.

21. Brown SY, Garland WA, Fukuda EK. Isolation and characterization of an unusual glucuronide conjugate of rimantadine. *Drug Metab Dispos* 1990; 18:546–547.

22. Kwok DW, Pillai G, Vaughan R, Axelson JE, McErlane KM. Preparative high-performance liquid chromatography and preparative thin-layer chromatography isolation of tocainide carbamoyl-O-beta-D-glucuronide: Structural characterization by gas chromatography-mass spectrometry and fast atom bombardment-mass spectrometry. *J Pharm Sci* 1990; 79:857–861.

23. Tremaine LM, Stroh JG, Ronfeld RA. Characterization of a carbamic acid ester glucuronide of the secondary amine sertraline. *Drug Metab Dispos* 1989; 17:58–63.

24. Pearson PG, Howald WN, Nelson SD. Screening strategy for the detection of derivatized glutathione conjugates by tandem mass spectrometry. *Anal Chem* 1990; 62:1827–1836.

25. Ballard KD, Raftery MJ, Jaeschke H, Gaskell SJ. Multiple scan modes in the hybrid tandem mass spectrometric screening and characterization of the glutathione conjugate of 2-furamide. *J Am Soc Mass Spectrom* 1991; 2:55–68.

26. Baillie TA, Pearson PG, Rashed MS, Howald WN. The use of mass spectrometry in the study of chemically-reactive drug metabolites. Application of MS/MS and LC/MS to the analysis of glutathione- and related S-linked conjugates of N-methylformamide. *J Pharm Biomed Anal* 1989; 7:1351–1360.

27. De Souza DP. Detection of polar metabolites through the use of gas chromatography-mass spectrometry. *Methods Mol Biol* 2013; 1055:29–37.

28. De Brabander HF, De Wasch K, Impens S, Schilt R, Leloux MS. Gas chromatography–mass spectrometry for residue analysis: Some basic concepts. *Chromatogr Sci Ser* 2001; 86:441–454.

29. Porubek DJ, Nelson SD. A gas chromatographic/mass spectrometric assay for catechol estrogens in microsomal incubations: Comparison with a radiometric assay. *Biomed Environ Mass Spectrom* 1988; 15:157–161.

30. Mondello L, Tranchida PQ, Dugo P, Dugo G. Comprehensive two-dimensional gas chromatography-mass spectrometry: A review. *Mass Spectrom Rev* 2008; 27:101–124.

31. Nelson SD, Trager WF. The use of deuterium isotope effects to probe the active site properties, mechanism of cytochrome P450-catalyzed reactions, and mechanisms of metabolically dependent toxicity. *Drug Metab Dispos* 2003; 31:1481–1498.

32. Omichinski JG, Soderlund EJ, Dybing E, Pearson PG, Nelson SD. Detection and mechanism of formation of the potent direct-acting mutagen 2-bromoacrolein from 1,2-dibromo-3-chloropropane. *Toxicol Appl Pharmacol* 1988; 92:286–294.

33. Streeter AJ, Bjorge SM, Axworthy DB, Nelson SD, Baillie TA. The microsomal metabolism and site of covalent binding to protein of 3'-hydroxyacetanilide, a nonhepatotoxic positional isomer of acetaminophen. *Drug Metab Dispos* 1984; 12:565–576.

34. Scott RPW, Scott CG, Munroe M, Hess J. Interface for on-line liquid chromatography-mass spectroscopy analysis. *J Chromatogr* 1974; 99:395–405.

35. Luijten W, Damien G, Marchand B, Capart J. Analysis of almitrine and its metabolites in plasma using on-line fast atom bombardment liquid chromatography/mass spectrometry. *Biomed Environ Mass Spectrom* 1988; 16:93–97.

36. Henion J, Skrabalak D, Dewey E, Maylin G. Micro LC/MS in drug analysis and metabolism studies. *Drug Metab Rev* 1983; 14:961–1003.

37. Caprioli RM. Bombardment mass spectrometry. *Anal Chem* 1990; 62:477A–485A.

38. Caprioli RM, Lin SN. On-line analysis of penicillin blood levels in the live rat by combined microdialysis/fast-atom bombardment mass spectrometry. *Proc Natl Acad Sci USA* 1990; 87:240–243.

39. Bakhoum SF, Agnes GR. Study of chemistry in droplets with net charge before and after Coulomb explosion: Ion-induced nucleation in solution and implications for ion production in an electrospray. *Anal Chem* 2005; 77:3189–3197.

40. Parker CE, de Wit JS, Smith RW, Gopinathan MB, Hernandez O, Tomer KB, Vestal CH, Sanders JM, Bend JR. Analysis of glutathione conjugates and related compounds by thermospray mass spectrometry. *Biomed Environ Mass Spectrom* 1988; 15:623–633.

41. Nocerini MR, Yost GS, Carlson JR, Liberato DJ, Breeze RG. Structure of the glutathione adduct of activated 3-methylindole indicates that an imine methide is the electrophilic intermediate. *Drug Metab Dispos* 1985; 13:690–694.

42. Sasame HA, Liberato DJ, Gillette JR. The formation of glutathione conjugate derived from propranolol. *Drug Metab Dispos* 1987; 15:349–355.

43. Hop CECA, Prakash C. Metabolite identification by LC–MS: Applications in drug discovery and development. In: Chowdhury SK, editor. *Identification and Quantification of Drugs, Metabolites and Metabolizing Enzymes by LC–MS*. New York: Elsevier. 2005; pp 123–158.

44. Clarke NJ, Rindgen D, Korfmacher WA, Cox KA. Systematic LC/MS metabolite identification in drug discovery. *Anal Chem* 2001; 73:430A–439A.

45. Prakash C, Shaffer CL, Nedderman A. Analytical strategies for identifying drug metabolites. *Mass Spectrom Rev* 2007; 26:340–369.

46. Chen WG, Zhang C, Avery MJ, Fouda HG. Reactive metabolite screen for reducing candidate attrition in drug discovery. *Adv Exp Med Biol* 2001; 500:521–524.

47. Prakash C, Soliman V. Metabolism and excretion of a novel antianxiety drug candidate, CP-93,393, in Long Evans rats. Differentiation of regioisomeric glucuronides by LC/MS/MS. *Drug Metab Dispos* 1997; 25:1288–1297.

48. Taylor EW, Jia W, Bush M, Dollinger GD. Accelerating the drug optimization process: Identification, structure elucidation, and quantification of in vivo metabolites using stable isotopes with LC/MSn and the chemiluminescent nitrogen detector. *Anal Chem* 2002; 74:3232–3238.

49. Anari MR, Sanchez RI, Bakhtiar R, Franklin RB, Baillie TA. Integration of knowledge-based metabolic predictions with liquid chromatography data-dependent tandem mass spectrometry for drug metabolism studies: Application to studies on the biotransformation of indinavir. *Anal Chem* 2004; 76:823–832.

50. Ma L, Wen B, Ruan Q, Zhu M. Rapid screening of glutathione-trapped reactive metabolites by linear ion trap mass spectrometry with isotope pattern-dependent scanning and postacquisition data mining. *Chem Res Toxicol* 2008; 21:1477–1483.

51. Yan Z, Caldwell GW, Maher N. Unbiased high-throughput screening of reactive metabolites on the linear ion trap mass spectrometer using polarity switch and mass tag triggered data-dependent acquisition. *Anal Chem* 2008; 80:6410–6422.

52. Nassar AE, Adams PE. Metabolite characterization in drug discovery utilizing robotic liquid-handling, quadrupole time-of-flight mass spectrometry and in-silico prediction. *Curr Drug Metab* 2003; 4:259–271.

53. Hopfgartner G, Varesio E, Tschäppät V, Grivet C, Bourgogne E, Leuthold LA. Triple quadrupole linear ion trap mass spectrometer for the analysis of small molecules and macromolecules. *J Mass Spectrom* 2004; 39:845–855.

54. King R, Fernandez-Metzler C. The use of Qtrap technology in drug metabolism. *Curr Drug Metab* 2006; 7:541–545.

55. Jian W, Yao M, Wen B, Zhu M. Chapter 15. Use of triple quadrupole–linear ion trap mass spectrometry as a single LC–MS platform in drug metabolism and pharmacokinetics studies. In: Lee M, Zhu M, editors. *Mass Spectrometry in Drug Metabolism and Disposition: Basic Principles and Applications.* London, UK: John Wiley & Sons Ltd. 2011; pp 483–524.

56. Hopfgartner G, Husser C, Zell M. Rapid screening and characterization of drug metabolites using a new quadrupole-linear ion trap mass spectrometer. *J Mass Spectrom* 2003; 38:138–150.

57. Xia YQ, Miller JD, Bakhtiar R, Franklin RB, Liu DQ. Use of a quadrupole linear ion trap mass spectrometer in metabolite identification and bioanalysis. *Rapid Commun Mass Spectrom* 2003; 17:1137–1145.

58. Mauriala T, Chauret N, Oballa R, Nicoll-Griffith DA, Bateman KP. A strategy for identification of drug metabolites from dried blood spots using triple-quadrupole/linear ion trap hybrid mass spectrometry. *Rapid Commun Mass Spectrom* 2005; 19:1984–1992.

59. Yao M, Ma L, Humphreys WG, Zhu M. Rapid screening and characterization of drug metabolites using a multiple ion monitoring-dependent MS/MS acquisition method on a hybrid triple quadrupole-linear ion trap mass spectrometer. *J Mass Spectrom* 2008; 43:1364–1375.

60. Yao M, Ma L, Duchoslav E, Zhu M. Rapid screening and characterization of drug metabolites using multiple ion monitoring dependent product ion scan and postacquisition data mining on a hybrid triple quadrupole-linear ion trap mass spectrometer. *Rapid Commun Mass Spectrom* 2009; 23:1683–1693.

61. Dieckhaus CM, Fernández-Metzler CL, King R, Krolikowski PH, Baillie TA. Negative ion tandem mass spectrometry for the detection of glutathione conjugates. *Chem Res Toxicol* 2005; 18:630–638.

62. Mahajan MK, Evans CA. Dual negative precursor ion scan approach for rapid detection of glutathione conjugates using liquid chromatography/tandem mass spectrometry. *Rapid Commun Mass Spectrom* 2008; 22:1032–1040.

63. Wen B, Ma L, Nelson SD, Zhu M. High-throughput screening and characterization of reactive metabolites using polarity switching of hybrid triple quadrupole linear ion trap mass spectrometry. *Anal Chem* 2008; 80:1788–1799.

64. Wen B, Ma L, Rodrigues AD, Zhu M. Detection of novel reactive metabolites of trazodone: Evidence for CYP2D6-mediated bioactivation of m-chlorophenylpiperazine. *Drug Metab Dispos* 2008; 36:841–850.

65. Wen B, Coe KJ, Rademacher P, Fitch WL, Monshouwer M, Nelson SD. Comparison of in vitro bioactivation of flutamide and its cyano analogue: Evidence for reductive activation by human NADPH:cytochrome P450 reductase. *Chem Res Toxicol* 2008; 21:2393–2406.

66. Wen B, Ma L, Zhu M. Bioactivation of the tricyclic antidepressant amitriptyline and its metabolite nortriptyline to arene oxide intermediates in human liver microsomes and recombinant P450s. *Chem Biol Interact* 2008; 173:59–67.

67. Wen B, Chen Y, Fitch WL. Metabolic activation of nevirapine in human liver microsomes: Dehydrogenation and inactivation of cytochrome P450 3A4. *Drug Metab Dispos* 2009; 37:1557–1562.

68. Wen B, Fitch WL. Screening and characterization of reactive metabolites using glutathione ethyl ester in combination with Q-trap mass spectrometry. *J Mass Spectrom* 2009; 44:90–100.

69. Dickinson DA, Forman HJ. Cellular glutathione and thiols metabolism. *Biochem Pharmacol* 2002; 64:1019–1026.

70. Zheng J, Ma L, Xin B, Olah T, Humphreys WG, Zhu M. Screening and identification of GSH-trapped reactive metabolites using hybrid triple quadrupole linear ion trap mass spectrometry. *Chem Res Toxicol* 2007; 20:757–766.

71. Jian W, Yao M, Zhang D, Zhu M. Rapid detection and characterization of in vitro and urinary N-acetyl-L-cysteine conjugates using quadrupole-linear ion trap mass spectrometry and polarity switching. *Chem Res Toxicol* 2009; 22:1246–1255.

72. Wrona M, Mauriala T, Bateman KP, Mortishire-Smith RJ, O'Connor D. 'All-in-one' analysis for metabolite identification using liquid chromatography/hybrid quadrupole time-of-flight mass spectrometry with collision energy switching. *Rapid Commun Mass Spectrom* 2005; 19:2597–2602.

73. Zhang H, Zhang D, Ray K. A software filter to remove interference ions from drug metabolites in accurate mass liquid chromatography/mass spectrometric analyses. *J Mass Spectrom* 2003; 38:1110–1112.

74. Ruan Q, Zhu M. Investigation of bioactivation of ticlopidine using linear ion trap/orbitrap mass spectrometry and an improved mass defect filtering technique. *Chem Res Toxicol* 2010; 23:909–917.

75. Zhu M, Zhang D, Zhang H, Shyu WC. Integrated strategies for assessment of metabolite exposure in humans during drug development: Analytical challenges and clinical development considerations. *Biopharm Drug Dispos* 2009; 30:163–184.

76. Ruan Q, Peterman S, Szewc MA, Ma L, Cui D, Humphreys WG, Zhu M. An integrated method for metabolite detection and identification using a linear ion trap/Orbitrap mass spectrometer and multiple data processing techniques: Application to indinavir metabolite detection. *J Mass Spectrom* 2008; 43:251–261.

77. Zhang H, Yang Y. An algorithm for thorough background subtraction from high-resolution LC/MS data: Application for detection of glutathione-trapped reactive metabolites. *J Mass Spectrom* 2008; 43:1181–1190.

78. Zhang H, Ma L, He K, Zhu M. An algorithm for thorough background subtraction from high-resolution LC/MS data: Application to the detection of troglitazone metabolites in rat plasma, bile, and urine. *J Mass Spectrom* 2008; 43:1191–1200.

79. Zhu P, Ding W, Tong W, Ghosal A, Alton K, Chowdhury S. A retention-time-shift-tolerant background subtraction and noise reduction algorithm (BgS-NoRA) for extraction of drug metabolites in liquid chromatography/mass spectrometry data from biological matrices. *Rapid Commun Mass Spectrom* 2009; 23:1563–1572.

80. Ma S, Chowdhury SK, Alton KB. Application of mass spectrometry for metabolite identification. *Curr Drug Metab* 2006; 7:503–523.

81. Castro-Perez JM. Current and future trends in the application of HPLC-MS to metabolite-identification studies. *Drug Discov Today* 2007; 12:249–256.

82. Tolonen A, Turpeinen M, Pelkonen O. Liquid chromatography-mass spectrometry in in vitro drug metabolite screening. *Drug Discov Today* 2009; 14:120–133.

83. Zhang Z, Zhu M, Tang W. Metabolite identification and profiling in drug design: Current practice and future directions. *Curr Pharm Des* 2009; 15:2220–2235.

84. Ma S, Zhu M. Recent advances in applications of liquid chromatography-tandem mass spectrometry to the analysis of reactive drug metabolites. *Chem Biol Interact* 2009; 179:25–37.

85. Baillie TA. Approaches to the assessment of stable and chemically reactive drug metabolites in early clinical trials. *Chem Res Toxicol* 2009; 22:263–266.

86. Liang Y, Wang G, Xie L, Sheng L. Recent development in liquid chromatography/mass spectrometry and emerging technologies for metabolite identification. *Curr Drug Metab* 2011; 12:329–344.

87. Xie C, Zhong D, Yu K, Chen X. Recent advances in metabolite identification and quantitative bioanalysis by LC-Q-TOF MS. *Bioanalysis* 2012; 4:937–959.

88. Ma S, Chowdhury SK. Application of LC-high-resolution MS with 'intelligent' data mining tools for screening reactive drug metabolites. *Bioanalysis* 2012; 4:501–510.

89. Du F, Ruan Q, Zhu M, Xing J. Detection and characterization of ticlopidine conjugates in rat bile using high-resolution mass spectrometry: Applications of various data acquisition and processing tools. *J Mass Spectrom* 2013; 48:413–422.

90. Liu T, Du F, Zhu F, Xing J. Metabolite identification of artemether by data-dependent accurate mass spectrometric analysis using an LTQ-Orbitrap hybrid mass spectrometer in combination with the online hydrogen/deuterium exchange technique. *Rapid Commun Mass Spectrom* 2011; 25:3303–3313.

91. Wang Z, Fang Y, Rock D, Ma J. Rapid screening and characterization of glutathione-trapped reactive metabolites using a polarity switch-based approach on a high-resolution quadrupole orbitrap mass spectrometer. *Anal Bioanal Chem* 2018; 410:1595–1606.

92. Mortishire-Smith RJ, O'Connor D, Castro-Perez JM, Kirby J. Accelerated throughput metabolic route screening in early drug discovery using high-resolution liquid chromatography/quadrupole time-of-flight mass spectrometry and automated data analysis. *Rapid Commun Mass Spectrom* 2005; 19:2659–2670.

93. Castro-Perez J, Plumb R, Granger JH, Beattie I, Joncour K, Wright A. Increasing throughput and information content for in vitro drug metabolism experiments using ultra-performance liquid chromatography coupled to a quadrupole time-of-flight mass spectrometer. *Rapid Commun Mass Spectrom* 2005; 19:843–848.

94. Hopfgartner G, Tonoli D, Varesio E. High-resolution mass spectrometry for integrated qualitative and quantitative analysis of pharmaceuticals in biological matrices. *Anal Bioanal Chem* 2012; 402:2587–2596.

95. Zhu M, Ma L, Zhang D, Ray K, Zhao W, Humphreys WG, Skiles G, Sanders M, Zhang H. Detection and characterization of metabolites in biological matrices using mass defect filtering of liquid chromatography/high resolution mass spectrometry data. *Drug Metab Dispos* 2006; 34:1722–1733.

96. Siegel D, Meinema AC, Permentier H, Hopfgartner G, Bischoff R. Integrated quantification and identification of aldehydes and ketones in biological samples. *Anal Chem* 2014; 86:5089–5100.

97. Zhang H, Zhang D, Ray K, Zhu M. Mass defect filter technique and its applications to drug metabolite identification by high-resolution mass spectrometry. *J Mass Spectrom* 2009; 44:999–1016.

98. Mortishire-Smith RJ, Castro-Perez JM, Yu K, Shockcor JP, Goshawk J, Hartshorn MJ, Hill A. Generic dealkylation: A tool for increasing the hit-rate of metabolite rationalization, and automatic customization of mass defect filters. *Rapid Commun Mass Spectrom* 2009; 23:939–948.

99. Zhang D, Cheng PT, Zhang H. Mass defect filtering on high resolution LC/MS data as a methodology for detecting metabolites with unpredictable structures: Identification of oxazole-ring opened metabolites of muraglitazar. *Drug Metab Lett* 2007; 1:287–292.

100. Bateman KP, Castro-Perez J, Wrona M, Shockcor JP, Yu K, Oballa R, Nicoll-Griffith DA. MS^E with mass defect filtering for in vitro and in vivo metabolite identification. *Rapid Commun Mass Spectrom* 2007; 21:1485–1496.

101. Tiller PR, Yu S, Bateman KP, Castro-Perez J, McIntosh IS, Kuo Y, Baillie TA. Fractional mass filtering as a means to assess circulating metabolites in early human clinical studies. *Rapid Commun Mass Spectrom* 2008; 22:3510–3516.

102. Wu C, Zhang H, Wang C, Qin H, Zhu M, Zhang J. An integrated approach for studying exposure, metabolism, and disposition of multiple component herbal medicines using high-resolution mass spectrometry and multiple data processing tools. *Drug Metab Dispos* 2016; 44:800–808.

103. Grabenauer M, Krol WL, Wiley JL, Thomas BF. Analysis of synthetic cannabinoids using high-resolution mass spectrometry and mass defect filtering: Implications for nontargeted screening of designer drugs. *Anal Chem* 2012; 84:5574–5581.

104. Zhang H, Zhu M, Ray KL, Ma L, Zhang D. Mass defect profiles of biological matrices and the general applicability of mass defect filtering for metabolite detection. *Rapid Commun Mass Spectrom* 2008; 22:2082–2088.

105. Barbara JE, Castro-Perez JM. High-resolution chromatography/time-of-flight MSE with in silico data mining is an information-rich approach to reactive metabolite screening. *Rapid Commun Mass Spectrom* 2011; 25:3029–3040.

106. Cuyckens F, Hurkmans R, Castro-Perez JM, Leclercq L, Mortishire-Smith RJ. Extracting metabolite ions out of a matrix background by combined mass defect, neutral loss and isotope filtration. *Rapid Commun Mass Spectrom* 2009; 23:327–332.

107. Zhang H, Patrone L, Kozlosky J, Tomlinson L, Cosma G, Horvath J. Pooled sample strategy in conjunction with high-resolution liquid chromatography-mass spectrometry-based background subtraction to identify toxicological markers in dogs treated with ibipinabant. *Anal Chem* 2010; 82:3834–3839.

108. Chen C, Wohlfarth A, Xu H, Su D, Wang X, Jiang H, Feng Y, Zhu M. Untargeted screening of unknown xenobiotics and potential toxins in plasma of poisoned patients using high-resolution mass spectrometry: Generation of xenobiotic fingerprint using background subtraction. *Anal Chim Acta* 2016; 944:37–43.

109. Johnson CH, Patterson AD, Idle JR, Gonzalez FJ. Xenobiotic metabolomics: Major impact on the metabolome. *Annu Rev Pharmacol Toxicol* 2012; 52:37–56.

110. Fang ZZ, Gonzalez FJ. LC-MS-based metabolomics: An update. *Arch Toxicol* 2014; 88:1491–1502.

111. Patterson AD, Gonzalez FJ, Idle JR. Xenobiotic metabolism: A view through the metabolometer. *Chem Res Toxicol* 2010; 23:851–860.

112. Liu K, Li F, Lu J, Liu S, Dorko K, Xie W, Ma X. Bedaquiline metabolism: Enzymes and novel metabolites. *Drug Metab Dispos* 2014; 42:863–866.

113. Li F, Lu J, Ma X. Profiling the reactive metabolites of xenobiotics using metabolomic technologies. *Chem Res Toxicol* 2011; 24:744–751.

114. Ma X, Chen C, Krausz KW, Idle JR, Gonzalez FJ. A metabolomic perspective of melatonin metabolism in the mouse. *Endocrinology* 2008; 149:1869–1879.

115. Chen C, Gonzalez FJ, Idle JR. LC-MS-based metabolomics in drug metabolism. *Drug Metab Rev* 2007; 39:581–597.

116. Tiller PR, Yu S, Castro-Perez J, Fillgrove KL, Baillie TA. High-throughput, accurate mass liquid chromatography/tandem mass spectrometry on a quadrupole time-of-flight system as a 'first-line' approach for metabolite identification studies. *Rapid Commun Mass Spectrom* 2008; 22:1053–1061.

117. Zhu P, Tong W, Alton K, Chowdhury S. An accurate-mass-based spectral-averaging isotope-pattern-filtering algorithm for extraction of drug metabolites possessing a distinct isotope pattern from LC-MS data. *Anal Chem* 2009; 81:5910–5917.

118. Chindarkar NS, Wakefield MR, Stone JA, Fitzgerald RL. Liquid chromatography high-resolution TOF analysis: Investigation of MSE for broad-spectrum drug screening. *Clin Chem* 2014; 60:1115–1125.

119. Xing J, Zang M, Zhang H, Zhu M. The application of high-resolution mass spectrometry-based data-mining tools in tandem to metabolite profiling of a triple drug combination in humans. *Anal Chim Acta* 2015; 897:34–44.

120. Ma S, Li Z, Lee KJ, Chowdhury SK. Determination of exposure multiples of human metabolites for MIST assessment in preclinical safety species without using reference standards or radiolabeled compounds. *Chem Res Toxicol* 2010; 23:1871–1873.

121. Aubry AF, Christopher LJ, Wang J, Zhu M, Tirucherai G, Arnold ME. Reflecting on a decade of metabolite screening and monitoring. *Bioanalysis* 2014; 6:651–664.

122. Xiong A, Yang F, Fang L, Yang L, He Y, Wan YY, Xu Y et al. Metabolomic and genomic evidence for compromised bile acid homeostasis by senecionine, a hepatotoxic pyrrolizidine alkaloid. *Chem Res Toxicol* 2014; 27:775–786.

123. Shimizu A, Chiba M. Ion mobility spectrometry-mass spectrometry analysis for the site of aromatic hydroxylation. *Drug Metab Dispos* 2013; 41:1295–1299.

124. Meyer GM, Maurer HH. Qualitative metabolism assessment and toxicological detection of xylazine, a veterinary tranquilizer and drug of abuse, in rat and human urine using GC-MS, LC-MSn, and LC-HR-MSn. *Anal Bioanal Chem* 2013; 405:9779–9789.

125. Nedderman AN, Dear GJ, North S, Obach RS, Higton D. From definition to implementation: A cross-industry perspective of past, current and future MIST strategies. *Xenobiotica* 2011; 41:605–622.

126. Wen B. Metabonomics in understanding drug metabolism and toxicity. In: Wienkers L, Korytko P, editors. *Part VII: Role of Metabolism in Toxicology and Pharmacology of "Encyclopedia of Drug Metabolism and Interactions"* Volume 4. London, UK: John Wiley & Sons Ltd. 2012.

127. Shen BQ, Xu K, Liu L, Raab H, Bhakta S, Kenrick M, Parsons-Reponte KL et al. Conjugation site modulates the in vivo stability and therapeutic activity of antibody-drug conjugates. *Nat Biotechnol* 2012; 30:184–189.

128. Singh J, Petter RC, Baillie TA, Whitty A. The resurgence of covalent drugs. *Nat Rev Drug Discov* 2011; 10:307–317.

129. Tailor A, Waddington JC, Meng X, Park BK. Mass spectrometric and functional aspects of drug-protein conjugation. *Chem Res Toxicol* 2016; 29:1912–1935.

14

The Role of NMR as a Qualitative and Quantitative Analytical Technique in Biotransformation Studies

Gregory S. Walker, Raman Sharma, and Shuai Wang

CONTENTS

Introduction

Within the discipline of drug metabolism, the structural elucidation of metabolites can be highly impactful from early discovery through development. Early in the discovery timeline, the structure of a metabolite may have influence on the selection of chemical lead material for progression to development; in later stage development, structural characterization of metabolites is a requirement for drug registration (Iverson and Smith, 2016; Wang and Urban, 2004; Watt et al., 2003). Since the advent of electrospray, mass spectrometry has dominated as the premier analytical technique for structure elucidation of metabolites. This is primarily due to the sensitivity of modern mass spectrometers, which can provide valuable information on the molecular weight, from which the empirical formula may be inferred (Zhang and Mitra, 2012; Zhu et al., 2011). In addition to the empirical formula, MS/MS techniques can lead to the identification of molecular regions that have been modified in a metabolite. While the information gleaned from mass spectrometry data is essential to structural elucidation, it is often not sufficient for unambiguous determination of a metabolite's structure. In these cases, NMR spectroscopy is often the analytical method of choice.

NMR spectroscopy is arguably the quintessential analytical technique for the definitive structural determination of organic compounds, such as drug metabolites (Kwan and Huang, 2008). Even the most basic NMR experiment contains information that can be used to determine the variety and number of atoms within a molecule, as well as their order relative to each other. While the qualitative aspects of NMR spectroscopy are impressive, it is also an essential quantitative analytical tool that, unlike mass spectrometry, requires no authentic material as a reference (Mutlib et al., 2011; Simmler et al., 2014; Walker et al., 2011, 2014). Together the qualitative and quantitative attributes of NMR spectroscopy are very powerful. However, as an analytical technique, NMR has two major short comings: the need for an isolated sample and sensitivity. To avoid the process of direct isolation of metabolites, significant effort has been made in the interfacing of NMR spectrometers to chromatographic separation systems in a manner similar to LC-MS systems (Lindon et al., 2000; Walker et al., 2016; Zhou et al., 2014). For many groups, this has been successful. However, advances in the design of low-volume cryo-probes have provided an effective alternative to online separation/detection schemes (Krunic and Orjala, 2015; Miao et al., 2015; Nagato et al., 2015). In this chapter, all of these advantages as well as the limitations will be discussed in detail.

It is important to distinguish between the classic role of NMR in metabolite identification and metabonomics. Metabonomics, the study of whole systems biology through the quantitation of known and unknown endogenous compounds, is an important concept that frequently uses NMR as its primary analytical tool. There are many excellent reviews of NMR as it relates to metabonomics (Beckonert et al., 2007; Coen et al., 2012; Dona et al., 2016; Robertson et al., 2000, 2011). Although this is an exciting use of NMR, it is not within the scope of this chapter. The text of this chapter will focus on the classic role of NMR in drug metabolism and the structural characterization of pharmaceutical biotransformation products.

NMR as a Qualitative Technique

The qualitative utility of NMR spectroscopy as it pertains to structural elucidation is well known. As stated above, the most basic NMR experiment—the 1D ^{1}H experiment—will contain data that can provide information about the micro-chemical environment through chemical shift values, the number of atoms in a molecule through integration, and the order in which these atoms are arranged though coupling patterns and constants. While this information is very powerful, occasionally resonances overlap or have redundant coupling constants, or there is a need to correlate different types of nuclei within a molecule (correlating specific ^{1}H resonances to specific ^{13}C or ^{15}N resonances). In these situations, the power of 2D NMR can be invoked.

Within the discipline of drug metabolism there are four NMR active nuclei that are relevant; ^{1}H, ^{13}C, ^{15}N, and ^{19}F (Table 14.1). ^{1}H, ^{13}C, and ^{15}N are the most relevant to the structural elucidation of metabolites, while ^{19}F is particularly useful in NMR quantitation of metabolites. The overall sensitivity of each of these nuclei is based on their inherent NMR sensitivity and the percent abundance in the environment. ^{1}H and ^{19}F are "100%" naturally abundant. This abundance enables the collection of direct observed data for both nuclei. Because of the large number of ^{1}H atoms within a typical metabolite, the ^{1}H spectrum is always the first step in the structural elucidation of a metabolite. Conversely, ^{19}F atoms within a pharmaceutical metabolite are typically limited to one to three atoms and, because of the single valence of fluorine, are not critical to the core of the molecule. Hence, the importance of ^{19}F in structural elucidation is also limited. While ^{13}C and ^{15}N have natural abundances of less than 2%, the large numbers of ^{13}C atoms and, the fact that the ^{15}N atoms are often in the core of a molecule, make them particularly useful in structural elucidation. The low natural abundance for these two nuclei precludes the classic direct observed NMR experiment, but chemical shift and other structural information may be easily gleaned through 2D experiments (multiplicity edited HSQC and HMBC, see below).

The physical theory, practical operation, and interpretation of NMR data is complex and beyond the scope of this chapter. Consequently, only a brief description of the most useful experiments and how to interpret the data will be given in this section. For a more detailed understanding of the NMR process there are multiple references targeting varying levels of expertise (Derome, 2013; Ernst et al., 1987). For a better understanding of the practical operation of an NMR instrument, *200 and More NMR Experiments: A Practical Course* by Stefan Berger is an excellent source of information. There are also multiple texts

TABLE 14.1

Properties of Spin ½ Nuclei

Nucleus	NMR Frequency (MHz at 11.75 T)	Natural Abundance (%)	Relative Sensitivity
^{1}H	500	99.98	1.0
^{19}F	470.4	100	0.83
^{13}C	125.7	1.108	0.0159
^{15}N	50.7	0.37	0.00134

that cover the interpretation of 1D and 2D NMR spectra in great depth (Field et al., 2015; Jacobsen, 2016; Simpson, 2011). In this chapter, the interpretation of 1D and 2D NMR spectra will be reviewed through the assignment of the tolbutamide metabolite 4-hydroxytolbutamide. It should be noted that NMR as an analytical technique cannot completely assign the structure of a metabolite alone. It should always be in conjunction with mass spectral data to help establish the molecular weight of the metabolite.

The 1D ^{1}H spectrum of 4-hydroxytolbutamide is contained in Figure 14.1. The three elements that can be gleaned from a 1D ^{1}H spectrum are integrations, chemical shifts, and coupling constants/patterns. The first step in 1D ^{1}H interpretation is defining the relevant hydrogens in the spectrum. Integration values appear below the resonances and are normalized to the resonance at 7.5 ppm (two hydrogens from the 13/14 positions) (Figure 14.1). The total number of hydrogens observed in the 1D ^{1}H spectrum is 15 hydrogens. The total number of expected hydrogens is 18; thus, the hydrogen count is different by three hydrogens. Because the sample was dissolved in deutero methanol, exchangeable hydrogens will not be observable. Thus, the hydrogen of the alcohol and the two NHs of the urea moiety are not present in the spectrum. The methyl group of the butyl side chain is easily recognized based on the integration of three hydrogens. All of the other resonances have integration values that indicate two hydrogens per resonance. Chemical shift is measured in ppm from a base frequency that is defined as zero. A generally agreed upon distinction between aromatic resonances and aliphatic resonances is 6 ppm, resonances with chemical shifts greater than 6 ppm are generally considered aromatic while those that are lower are considered aliphatic. In the case of 4-hydroxytolbutamide, there are two resonances that integrate to a total of four hydrogens. This is consistent with the aromatic hydrogens of the 4-hydroxytolbutamide. In the aliphatic portion of the molecule, there are five resonances. Based on chemical shift and integration, four resonances may be assigned to the butyl chain; 3.10 ppm (2Hs), 1.40 ppm (2Hs), 1.25 ppm (2Hs) and 0.89 ppm (3Hs). The fifth resonance, because of its chemical shift at 4.72 ppm, is assigned as the C9 methylene (CH$_2$OH). Coupling patterns and coupling constants (which are measured in Hertz) can be extremely useful in the interpretation of 1D ^{1}H NMR. There is one simple rule for coupling patterns: the (n+1) rule. The (n+1) rule is an empirical rule used to predict the multiplicity and splitting pattern of 1D ^{1}H resonances (Derome, 2013). This rule states that if a given hydrogen is coupled to n number of nuclei that are equivalent, the multiplicity of the observed resonance is n+1. In the ^{1}H spectrum

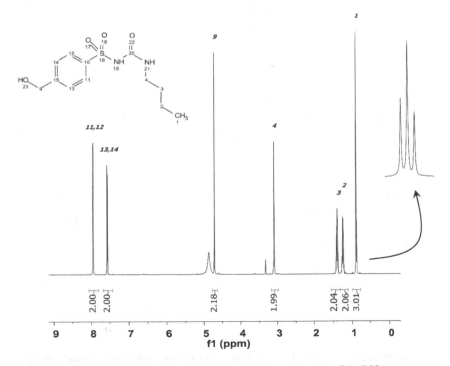

FIGURE 14.1 The 1D ^{1}H spectrum of 4-hydroxytolbutamide, Inset is an expansion of the 0.89 ppm resonance.

of 4-hydroxytolbutamide, the resonance at 0.89 ppm, which based on integration was assigned as the terminal methyl (and is adjacent to a single methylene with equivalent hydrogens), should be a triplet (Figure 14.1). For the same reasons the resonance at 3.10 ppm also appears as a triplet. This resonance may then be assigned as C4 of the butyl side chain. Of the remaining two aliphatic resonances, 1.40 and 1.25 ppm, chemical shift arguments can be made about their assignments, but definitive assignments cannot be made without the use of 2D NMR, specifically ^{1}H-^{1}H COSY.

    ^{1}H-^{1}H COSY data sets correlate hydrogens that are two, three and sometimes four bonds distant from each other. In a ^{1}H-^{1}H COSY spectrum the off axis cross peaks indicate a correlation between the two ^{1}H resonances. In the case of 4-hydroxytolbutamide, the aliphatic portion of the ^{1}H-^{1}H COSY spectra contains cross peaks from the 0.89 ppm resonance to the 1.25 ppm resonance then to the 1.40 ppm resonance and finally to the 3.10 ppm resonance (Figure 14.2a). In this case, integration and coupling patterns had established the 0.89 ppm resonance as the terminal methyl of the butyl side chain. Using this as a starting point the ^{1}H-^{1}H COSY data demonstrates correlation to the 1.25 ppm resonance and is assigned as the methylenes of C2. The remaining resonance at 1.40 ppm, which has ^{1}H-^{1}H COSY correlations to both the 1.25 ppm resonance and the 3.10 ppm resonance may then be assigned as the methylenes of C3. It should also be noted that the 4.72 ppm resonance, which was assigned as the C9 methylene (CH$_2$OH) based on integration, and chemical shift has no correlation to any other resonance, which is consistent with the previous assignment.

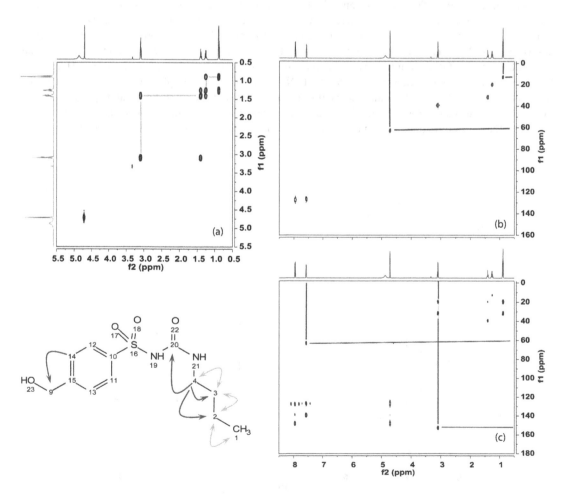

FIGURE 14.2 (a) Aliphatic portion of the ^{1}H-^{1}H COSY spectra of 4-hydroxytolbutamide (b) multiplicity edited ^{1}H-^{13}C HSQC spectrum of 4-hydroxytolbutamide (c) ^{1}H-^{13}C HMBC spectrum of 4-hydroxytolbutamide.

On occasion, for a complete structural elucidation of a metabolite, it is useful to not only know the chemical shift of the hydrogens in a molecule, but also the chemical shifts of the carbon atoms. This can be a challenge in isolated metabolites because the small amount of material that is available precludes a 1D direct observed ^{13}C acquisition. In cases such as these, the much more sensitive heteronuclear 2D experiments ^{1}H-^{13}C HSQC and ^{1}H-^{13}C HMBC must be used to establish the carbon chemical shifts. ^{1}H-^{13}C HSQC data correlates the chemical shifts of hydrogens to the chemical shifts of carbons that are directly bonded to them. ^{1}H-^{13}C HMBC data correlates the chemical shifts of hydrogens to the chemical shifts of carbons that are two or three bonds remote from the hydrogen of interest (Bax and Summers, 1986). Using these two data sets, ^{1}H-^{13}C HSQC and ^{1}H-^{13}C HMBC, together the carbon backbone of a metabolite can be assigned.

There are several ^{1}H-^{13}C HSQC experiments that can be performed. One that is particularly useful is the multiplicity edited ^{1}H-^{13}C HSQC (Boyer et al., 2003). In this experiment, methines and methyls can be distinguished from methylenes based on the "phase" of the cross peak. In this context, phase refers to the magnitude, positive or negative, of the cross peak. In the case of 4-hydroxytolbutamide, the multiplicity edited ^{1}H-^{13}C HSQC data correlates the ^{1}H resonance at 0.89 ppm to a ^{13}C resonance with chemical shift of 12.6 ppm (Figure 14.2b). Additionally, this data set also demonstrates the ^{1}H 0.89 ppm/^{13}C 12.6 ppm cross peak to have the same phase as the aromatic resonances. Because methines and methyls in this experiment have the same phase, this further supports the assignment of the 0.89 ppm resonance as the terminal methyl of the butyl moiety. More important than the terminal methyl is the resonance at 4.72 ppm, which was previously assigned as the C9 methylene (CH$_2$OH). The multiplicity edited ^{1}H-^{13}C HSQC correlates the ^{1}H resonance at 4.72 ppm with a ^{13}C resonance at 63.0 ppm with a phase that is consistent with a methylene, adding further evidence of the assignment of this resonance as the C9 (CH$_2$OH).

Once the chemical shifts of the directly attached hydrogens are correlated with their respective carbon chemical shifts, the ^{1}H-^{13}C HMBC experiment becomes very useful in the structural assignment of a metabolite. The ^{1}H-^{13}C HMBC experiment correlates the ^{1}H chemical shifts to carbon chemical shifts that are two or three bonds away from the hydrogen. This allows correlations to be established that skip over hetero atoms or quaternary atoms. In the case of the example molecule 4-hydroxytolbutamide, the presence of the carbonyl (C20) can be verified with ^{1}H-^{13}C HMBC data (Figure 14.2c). In the ^{1}H-^{13}C HMBC spectrum, the ^{1}H resonance at 3.1 ppm has correlations to three ^{13}C chemical shifts, 19.5, 31.9, and 152.7 ppm. With the ^{1}H-^{13}C HSQC data the 19.5 and 31.9 ppm cross peaks can be assigned as the ^{1}Hs from C2 and C3 respectively. The 152.7 ppm cross peak, based on its chemical shift and bond distance from the ^{1}Hs of C4, can only be assigned to the C20 carbonyl. While the identification of the carbonyl resonance in this particular metabolite is not critical to the overall structural elucidation, this example demonstrates the power of a ^{1}H-^{13}C HMBC data to "skip" over hetero atoms and allow the assignment of the carbon backbone of a small molecule. A second example of the utility of an ^{1}H-^{13}C HMBC is directly related to the structural assignment of a 4-hydroxytolbutamide. There are two aromatic resonances observed in the 1D ^{1}H spectrum, 7.57 and 7.96 ppm. From all previous data (1D ^{1}H, ^{1}H-^{1}H COSY and ^{1}H-^{13}C HSQC) these resonances cannot be definitively differentiated. In the ^{1}H-^{13}C HMBC data set, only the 7.57 ppm resonance contains a cross peak with a carbon chemical shift of 62.3 ppm. The 62.3 ppm resonance was previously assigned as the C9 methylene (CH$_2$OH), because of the ^{1}H chemical shift, the ^{1}H multiplicity and the carbon chemical shift established from the ^{1}H-^{13}C HSQC. Because of the ^{1}H-^{13}C HMBC cross peak with the 62.3 ppm carbon resonance, the 7.57 ppm ^{1}H resonances are assigned as the C13/C14 hydrogens and by inference the 7.96 ppm resonances are assigned as the C11/C12 hydrogens.

NMR as a Quantitative Technique

qNMR is most frequently used for the assessment of purity of a synthetic compound (Pauli et al., 2014). This is usually accomplished by replicate accurate weighings of the material being assayed followed by volumetric addition of solvent to the individual weighings and then qNMR analysis in which the concentrations of the quantitatively prepared solutions are determined. There are a variety of ways to execute qNMR analyses that are described below. This concentration is then compared to the theoretical concentration that could be achieved, as determined by the accurate weighings, and the percent purity is established. Analytical standards can then be prepared from this original solid material with a purity correction factor applied to correct for the impurities.

In drug metabolism studies, metabolites are isolated in the tens of μg range making quantitative weighings not feasible. As an alternative to the gravimetric method described above several groups have simply reconstituted the isolated metabolite in deuterated solvent, determined the concentration of the metabolite via qNMR and this solution used as a quantitative standard for a variety of assays related to drug metabolism and pharmacology.

In an appropriately acquired 1D NMR spectrum the response of an individual nuclei is independent of the molecule that it is contained within. Hence, the response of an NMR system to a nanomole of anomeric hydrogens for an isolated glucuronide metabolite will be the same as the response from a nanomole of hydrogens from benzoic acid. To further clarify this concept, ^{1}H spectra were acquired for six separate structurally diverse compounds from six separate weighings in separate samples. The six samples ranged in concentration from 0.1 to 32 mM (this range covers the concentrations of most isolated metabolites). Each spectrum was integrated, and the raw integration number normalized to the number of hydrogens for that resonance. A varied set of resonances were selected for inclusion in the concentration response plot varying in both bond type and chemotype. The resulting response concentration curve demonstrates strong linearity over the range of interest (Figure 14.3). The practical implications of this plot are that an isolated unknown metabolite can be quantified using known compounds. Once quantified these isolated metabolites can then be used as a standard in a variety of assays including bioanalytical concentration time profiles, pharmacological potency, or many other metabolism-based assays. The advantage of this system, over having a metabolite chemically synthesized is time. Metabolites can often be difficult to chemically synthesize and may even require separate synthetic schemes from the parent compound. Alternatively, small amounts of metabolites (low μg) may be biologically generated through a variety of *in vitro* methods, the products isolated, structurally characterized by MS and NMR, and quantitated in a few days.

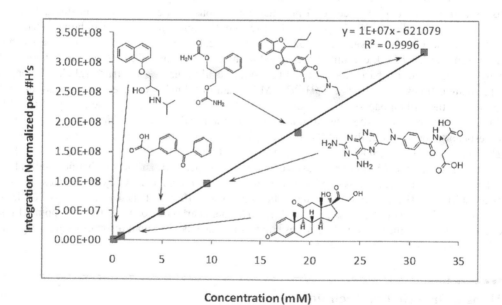

FIGURE 14.3 ^{1}H NMR concentration versus response curve of six chemically distinct molecules at various concentrations integrated and normalized to the appropriate number of hydrogens. Individual samples were prepared in DMSO-d6. Data were acquired on a Bruker 600 MHz NMR system with 1.7 mm TCI cryoprobe. The system was controlled, and the data processed using Topspin 3.2. Forty transients were acquired for each spectrum with a total recycle time of 10 s between the transients. (Reproduced with permission from EMAGRES.)

Beyond the quantitation of isolated metabolites, qNMR has been used to quantitate complex mixtures in a variety of settings. Most relevant to the drug metabolism scientists are the studies that have focused on the assessment of systemic exposure in human clinical trials. This can be done by semi-preparative HPLC fractionation of plasma samples followed by qNMR assessment of all fractions using ^{1}H resonances for quantitation (Dear et al., 2008). While this method has proven effective in certain cases, the potential of endogenous compounds interfering with resonances needed for quantitation does exist. If the compound of interest has a fluorine atom within the molecule, ^{19}F NMR is an attractive alternative. qNMR using ^{19}F has been used in both determining mass balance and plasma exposure (Mutlib et al., 2012).

Metabolites can be quantitated by NMR by two general methods: internal standard addition and external standard. The internal standard method is performed by adding a known quantity of an internal standard to your sample and calculating the concentration of the unknown based on the response and concentration of the internal standard. This method is perhaps the classic method for the determination of purity in a medicinal chemistry setting. However, it does have several disadvantages. The internal standard must be soluble in the solvent of choice for the analyte. Additionally, the internal standard must have no interference from resonances of the sample in order to obtain clean integration. And lastly, the addition of an internal standard to a sample detracts from the purity of the sample. In the case of determining a metabolite concentration, the added internal standard must be considered in all future assays that use that isolated material. In an effort to avoid the addition of an internal standard, some laboratories have used the residual deuterated solvent signal as an internal standard (Mutlib et al., 2011). While this approach avoids the addition of a potentially interfering compound to the isolated samples it also has drawbacks of its own. First the concentration of the residual protio solvent must be determined in a given lot. This can be easily done with the external standard method described above. However, the manufacturers of deuterated solvents guarantee only minimum concentrations of residual protio solvent. There are certainly lot to lot variations that necessitate determining the concentration of the residual protio solvent in every lot. The greatest disadvantage of this approach is the potential of interference with the residual solvent line. If there is another resonance, either from the metabolite or from an endogenous impurity due to the isolation, which interferes with the residual solvent signal, accurate quantitation will not be possible in that sample.

There are three general methods for qNMR that can be considered external standard methods; ERETIC (Electronic Reference To access *In vivo* Concentrations), aSICCO (artificial signal insertion for calculation of concentration observed)/QUANTUS (quantification by artificial signal) and the pure external standard method (Akoka et al., 1999; Farrant et al., 2010; Pauli et al., 2014; Walker et al., 2011). In the original ERETIC method, through the use of a second NMR coil, an internal standard signal was imparted on the FID of the metabolite as it was being acquired. Once the FID was transformed, the artificial signal could be used as an internal standard. This method had the advantage of being able to select the frequency and magnitude of the internal standard signal and hence avoid the problems mentioned earlier. However, not all spectrometers were equipped with the appropriate hardware to do this and this method requires a special pulse sequence. The aSICCO method relies on the post-acquisition insertion of a mathematically generated internal signal into the ^{1}H spectrum of the metabolite. This method avoids all of the challenges of a chemical internal standard and the requirement for special hardware as in the case of ERETIC quantitation. Certainly, the easiest approach to implement is the external standard method. In this method, a qualified external standard 1D ^{1}H spectrum is acquired, and the resonances of interest are integrated and calibrated to determine a response factor based on number of hydrogens. Once this is done a similarly acquired ^{1}H spectrum of the metabolite can have the concentration calculated by applying the previously determined response factor.

Sensitivity

One of the challenges of using NMR for drug metabolism studies is determining how much isolated metabolite is needed to solve the structural question at hand. This question is complicated by several drug metabolism and NMR limitations. From the drug metabolism point of view the question is complicated by the fact that the metabolites are always at relatively low abundance (low μM) and are always contained in a complicated biological mixture. *In vivo* sources for metabolites (urine, plasma and fecal extracts) tend to be more complicated by both the large variety and high concentrations of endogenous compounds present in these matrixes. *In vitro* sources for metabolites such as hepatocytes or microsomes tend to be a cleaner source for metabolite isolation but may not contain the metabolite of interest that has been observed in an *in vivo* system. From the NMR perspective, the question of sensitivity is complicated by the nature of the metabolite. Simple aromatic oxidations of a phenyl ring can be easily identified by 1D ¹H spectrum (Hutzler et al., 2004) while complicated rearrangements need more elegant NMR experiments (HSQC, HMBC or NOE), which in turn require larger amounts of material (Hong et al., 2010). Because of the aforementioned reasons, defining exactly how much material is needed to solve the structure of a metabolite is a difficult task.

As stated earlier, NMR has a long history of being utilized for both qualitative and quantitative analysis and it has been extremely useful in many facets of both drug discovery and development (Holzgrabe et al., 2005). One of the major limitations of NMR is its lack of sensitivity when compared to other spectroscopic techniques, specifically mass spectrometry. Mass spectrometry sensitivity, although highly dependent on the molecule being analyzed, may be in the femtomole range, while from a practical point of view ¹H NMR sensitivity tends to be in the nanomole range depending on the equipment used and the time available for data acquisition. The evaluation of the sensitivity of NMR as an analytical technique is confounded by the fact that signal to noise in an NMR spectrum increases by a factor of $\sqrt{2}$ for every doubling of the number of scans; the more time you spend acquiring data, the greater the signal to noise. Therefore, if you perform multi-pulse experiments and the experiments last several days, the sensitivity may be very high for a given system. The practical limitations of typically acquired direct observed ¹H experiments are in the range of minutes to hours. The absolute sensitivity of NMR with a standard from a serial dilution, has been reported to be in the sub-microgram range for ¹H-NMR (Hilton and Martin, 2010). However, for the analysis of a metabolite from a drug metabolism study the instrumental sensitivity may not be the limiting factor. The ability to interpret the spectra may be limited by the relative purity of the isolation.

The NMR analysis of metabolites requires isolation of the metabolite of interest from a complex matrix to obtain an interpretable spectrum. This may be done in-line, as in the case of LC-NMR systems, or it may be done as a separate process off-line. In either case the ultimate sensitivity of the ¹H spectrum may be limited by impurities from endogenous material from the matrix, impurities from the isolation process or impurities from the deuterated solvent. Thus, the sample preparation is the important first step for successful analysis of drug metabolites using NMR. In order to probe the practical limits of NMR sensitivity as it pertains to metabolite characterization and quantitation, a series of experiments were performed to analyze metabolites from *in vitro* microsomal incubations.

Human liver microsomes are one of the most extensively used tools for *in vitro* drug metabolism studies. To test the limits of qualitative and quantitative NMR from a drug metabolism environment, several different compound classes and corresponding metabolites were selected: tolbutamide, 4-hydroxytolbutamide, clozapine, clozapine N-oxide, estradiol, estradiol-17-glucuronide, and N-nitrobenzyl-glutathione. Human liver microsome incubates were augmented with drug and corresponding metabolite without the addition of NADPH. Parallel control experiments were performed with compound incubations containing only compounds in HPLC water.

Initially all compounds were incubated at 20 μM (80 nmole) and 4 μM (16 nmole) in a 4 mL solution. These concentrations were selected in order to mimic typical microsomal incubations designed for the isolation of metabolites for structural characterization by NMR. After 1 h at 37°C, the incubations were quenched with 2× volumes of acetonitrile and centrifuged at 2500 rpm to obtain the supernatant. These supernatant solutions were spun a second time at 40,000 g for 30 min and decanted. The acetonitrile in the resulting supernatant was removed by vacuum centrifugation. The solution was then transferred to a graduated cylinder, mixed with 0.1% formic acid to a total volume of 50 mL and directly applied onto a Varian Polaris C18 column (4.6 × 250 mm; 5 mm particle size) through a Jasco HPLC pump at a flow rate of 0.8 mL/min. After application of the initial solution, another 10 mL of 0.1% formic acid was pumped onto the column to ensure that the HPLC lines were cleared of the supernatant. Immediately after the loading, the column was transferred to a Thermo-Fisher HPLC-MS system containing Surveyor quaternary HPLC, Surveyor PDA detector and LTQ mass spectrometer and with a previously established LC program to separate out the compound and its metabolite. The instrument was connected with a Gilson FC-204 fraction collector and the HPLC fractions taken continuously throughout the program with 1 min per tube acquisition. Fractions were then analyzed with the LC-MS to confirm the fractions containing compounds of interest, which were pooled and evaporated to dryness for NMR analysis (Walker et al., 2014).

The samples were prepared in a dry argon atmosphere glove box to further remove water from the sample. The samples were then dissolved in 40 μl of DMSO-d6 "100%" and placed in a 1.7 mm NMR tube. NMR spectra were recorded on a Bruker 600 MHz Avance II controlled by Topspin V3.2 and equipped with a 1.7 mm TCI Cryo probe. 1D spectra were recorded using 40 transients and an approximate sweep width of 8400 Hz and a total recycle time of approximately 7 s. The 2D data were recorded using the standard pulse sequences provided by Bruker. Post-acquisition data processing was performed with either Topspin V3.2 or MestReNova V8.1. ^1H and ^{13}C spectra were referenced using DMSO-d6 (^1H $\delta = 2.50$ ppm relative to TMS, $\delta = 0.00$, ^{13}C $\delta = 39.50$ ppm relative to TMS, $\delta = 0.00$). Concentrations were determined using the ERETIC2 software within Brukers Topspin software. The obtained spectrums of the isolated materials were compared with compound standards that were prepared gravimetrically before use in DMSO-d6.

To test the robustness and reproducibility of the sample preparation process, HLM and water control samples were quantitated for respective compounds by qNMR and the percent recovery calculated. From the initial concentrations in the incubations (20 μM or 80 nmole and 4 μM or 16 nmole) assuming a 100% recovery, final concentrations in the NMR tube would be 2 mM and 0.4 mM respectively for all compounds. Clozapine N-oxide was found to convert to clozapine during the isolation process, hence these values are not included in the summary statistics (Temesi et al., 2013). The range of recovery for all other compounds is from 41% to 97% with a median recovery of 83% (Table 14.2). The percent recovery appeared to be independent of concentration of analyte, but the water control samples tended to have higher percent recoveries than HLM isolates, with a water median recovery of 87.5%, and an HLM median recovery of 79.5%. These values indicate that the loss of material during the isolation accounts for approximately 60% of the total loss in an HLM isolation while presumed protein binding accounts for 40% of the total loss. Several isolates were repeated either in duplicate or triplicate on separate days to evaluate the consistency of isolation. The relative standard deviations of these recoveries ranged from 1% to 25%. These results indicated recoveries that were greater than expected and reproducibility that was acceptable for qualitative isolations.

To evaluate the qualitative limits of this isolation process, a series of 1D and 2D NMR experiments were performed on the 0.4 mM (16 nmole) estradiol-17-glucuronide HLM isolate. The ^1H-NMR spectrum of the

TABLE 14.2

Percentage Recovery of LC-MS Fractionations from *In Vitro* Incubations

Matrix	Water		HLM		
Conc. (final in 40 μl)	2 mM	0.4 mM	2 mM	0.4 mM	0.125 mM
Tolbutamide	85%	96%	82% ± 6 n = 3	94% ± 13 n = 3	
4-hydroxy-tolbutamide	96%	90%	91% ± 3 n = 3	77% ± 20 n = 3	
Estradiol	80%	97% ± 1 n = 2	87% ± 7 n = 2	53%	
Estradiol-17-glucuronide	81%	93% ± 4 n = 2	88% ± 3 n = 2	77%	91%
Clozapine	69%	53%	71%	84% ± 5 n = 2	
Nitro-benzyl GSH	93%	72%	67%	41%	

Data were Acquired on a Bruker 600 MHz NMR System with 1.7 mm TCI Cryoprobe. The System was Controlled and the Data Processed using Topspin V3.2. Concentrations were Determined using Bruker ERETIC2 Software Contained in Topspin

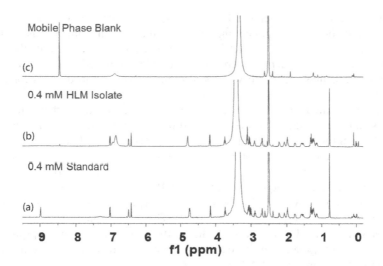

FIGURE 14.4 ¹H-NMR comparison of mobile phase blank, estradiol-17-glucuronide from 0.4 mM HLM isolate, and 0.4 mM standard. Data were acquired on a Bruker 600 MHz NMR system with 1.7 mm TCI cryoprobe. The system was controlled, and the data processed using Topspin 3.2. Forty transients were acquired for each spectrum with a total recycle time of 10 s between the transients.

0.4 mM HLM isolate showed comparable signal to noise levels with the 0.4 mM standard (Figure 14.4). Beyond the signal to noise of the HLM isolated sample, the resonances of the estradiol-17-glucuronide are unobstructed by resonances from the isolation process, enabling the interpretation of the resonances of the glucuronide. Additionally, the 0.4 mM estradiol-17-glucuronide HLM sample was also analyzed by 2D COSY, ¹H-¹³C multiplicity edited HSQC and ¹H-¹³C HMBC and compared to a 70 mM standard (Figure 14.5). The COSY and ¹H-¹³C multiplicity edited HSQC data sets of the 0.4 mM HLM estradiol-17-glucuronide isolate contain all of the qualitatively important cross peaks observed in the 70 mM standard. The ¹H-¹³C HMBC data sets of the 0.4 mM HLM estradiol-17-glucuronide isolate contain fewer and less intense cross peaks than the 70 mM standard, but there is still sufficient data to confirm the presence of a glucuronide and discriminate the site of attachment as the 17 position. Based on this data, a 0.5 mM solution would be the recommended minimum concentration for a successful metabolite ¹H-¹³C HMBC. Hence, when designing an incubation experiment for the isolation of metabolites, initial concentration, projected turnover and final NMR volume should be adjusted to result in a final isolate concentration of 0.5 mM assuming including a 35% loss on isolation.

In many cases, an ¹H-¹³C HMBC is not necessary for the structural determination of a metabolite. To establish the limits of material needed in these situations, the 1D and 2D COSY and multiplicity edited HSQC data sets were acquired on an isolate of 0.125 mM estradiol-17-glucuronide. Examination of the 1D ¹H of the 0.125 mM estradiol-17-glucuronide spectra demonstrates the need for cleaner isolations, particularly in the 3 to 0.5 ppm region of the spectra (Figure 14.6). While the resonances of the estradiol-17-glucuronide are clearly present, the resonances of the impurities from the isolation process are now nearing the same magnitude. The difficulties in interpretation of spectra at this level can be somewhat mitigated by the acquisition of 2D data. While this sample was not sufficient for an HMBC, the data from the COSY and the ¹H-¹³C multiplicity edited HSQC data clearly contained all of the cross peaks of a much more concentrated sample.

The above data suggests that with NMR instrumentation that is commercially available and routinely found within the pharmaceutical industry, NMR characterization of metabolites is eminently possible. As NMR technology develops and instrumentation becomes more sensitive, NMR characterization of metabolites will become a routine part of drug discovery within the pharmaceutical industry.

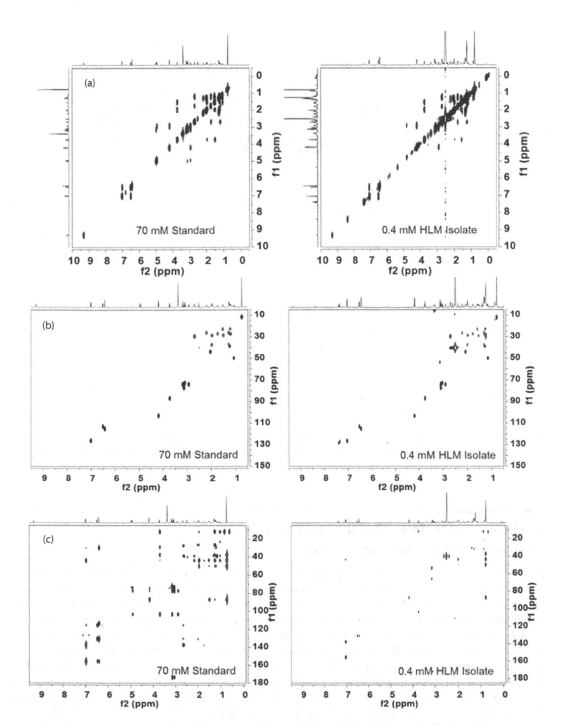

FIGURE 14.5 (a) ^{1}H-^{1}H COSY, (b) ^{1}H-^{13}C HSQC, and (c) ^{1}H-^{13}C HMBC spectrum comparison between 70 and 0.4 mM estradiol-17-glucuronide standards. The 70 mM sample spectrums were acquired for 0.25 h for each experiment and 0.4 mM sample was acquire 2.5 h (COSY), 3.75 h (HSQC) and 7.75 h (HMBC).

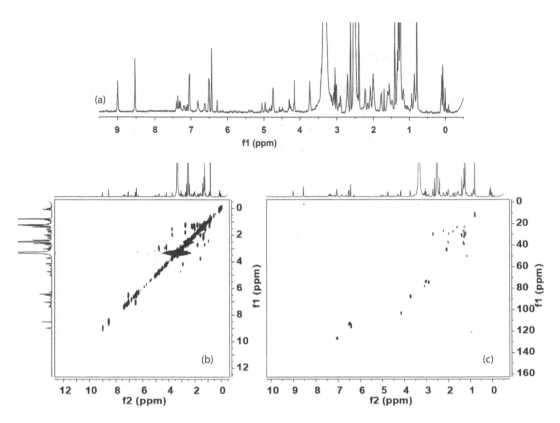

FIGURE 14.6 ^{1}H-NMR, ^{1}H-^{1}H COSY, and ^{1}H-^{13}C HSQC spectrums of 0.125 mM estradiol-17-glucuronide HLM isolate (from 5 μM incubation in a 1 mL HLM solution). 2D data were acquired for 2.5 h (^{1}H-^{1}H COSY) and 8 h (^{1}H-^{13}C HSQC).

Application of Different NMR Experiments in Metabolite Structural Characterization

From the early stages of discovery through the late stages of drug development, there are numerous examples throughout the literature demonstrating the use of NMR in drug metabolism applications. At the discovery (pre-candidate) stage, structural elucidation of metabolites is often performed to aid in chemistry design (i.e., circumventing metabolic "hot spots" for reducing clearance or removing reactive metabolite liabilities). Once the site of metabolism is determined, structural modifications can be made (often in iterative fashion) to eliminate or reduce the associated liability. Additionally, the concentration of an isolated metabolite may be determined using one of the methods described in the previous sections and further tested in a relevant pharmacological assay or used as a standard in bioanalytical measurements. In the clinical stages of drug development, major human metabolites not predicted from pre-clinical studies can be isolated from the relevant matrix (urine, plasma, etc.) and characterized. This becomes particularly important when the metabolite is human unique or expected to possess pharmacological activity (Yu et al., 2010) (U.S. Department of Health and Human Services 2016, ICH M(R2) 2010).

The types of NMR experiments typically used in metabolite measurement and characterization generally depend on the types of problems being addressed and the amount/purity of the metabolite(s) being isolated. Four basic experiments: 1D ^{1}H experiment, 2D correlation spectroscopy (COSY), multiplicity edited heteronuclear single quantum coherence (HSQC) and heteronuclear multiple bond correlation (HMBC) are generally performed to yield a full structural characterization.

While the full suite of NMR experiments is generally desirable for unambiguous structural assignments, in specific situations, a 1D experiment alone may suffice. A case example comes from the metabolite of T-5, a selective cyclic GMP phosphodiesterase-5 inhibitor (Li et al., 2014). T-5 was found to be a selective marker for CYP3A5 activity through its formation of a mono-hydroxylated metabolite (T-5). In order to identify the site of hydroxylation, the T-5 metabolite was generated from T-5 using recombinant CYP3A5. A comparison of the aromatic portion of the ¹H spectra of T-5 against the T-5 metabolite reveals that the aromatic resonances (H1, H5, H19, H20, H21, H29, H30, H31, and H32) present in T-5 are also present and relatively unmodified in the T-5 metabolite (Figure 14.7). The aromatic resonances corresponding to H38-H41 in T-5 have shifted dramatically in the T-5 metabolite. Although shifted, the resonances retained similar multiplicity (doublet for H38 and H39 and triplet for H41) to T-5. Furthermore, integration of ¹H spectra for both T-5 and the isolated T-5 metabolite revealed the same number of hydrogens in both parent and metabolite. The only rational explanation consistent with the mass of the metabolite was the formation of an N-Oxide on the pyridine nitrogen of T-5. While other 2D data (COSY, HSQC and HMBC experiments) were also collected for both T-5 and the T-5N-Oxide, the initial structural assignment of the N-Oxide was made from 1D data alone.

Compound A is a kynurenine aminotransferase inhibitor with a hydroxamic acid motif. A glucuronide conjugate of Compound A was successfully prepared by incubating Compound A with human liver microsomes and cofactors to support glucuronidation reactions (Walker et al., 2014). The isolated metabolite confirmed the presence of a glucuronide peak via observation of anomeric ¹H and ¹³C resonances (δ 5.04, 109.6, doublet, ¹H, J = 7.9 Hz) (Figure 14.8). There are two sites available in Compound A for glucuronidation: the amine nitrogen and the alcoholic oxygen of the hydroxamic acid.

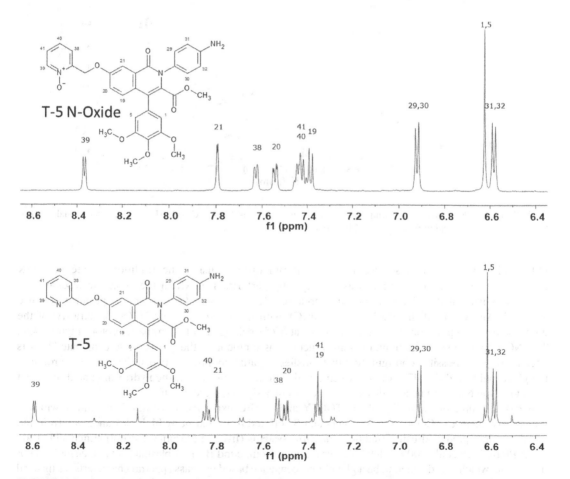

FIGURE 14.7 Aromatic portion of the ¹H spectrum of T-5 *N*-oxide (top) and T-5 (bottom).

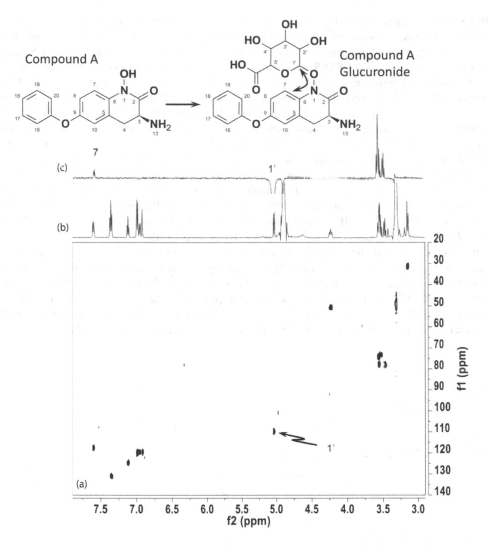

FIGURE 14.8 NMR spectra of Compound A glucuronide. (a) ^{1}H-^{13}C HSQC. (b) ^{1}H. (c) One-dimensional Nuclear Overhauser Effect excitation frequency at δ5.03 (H1′).

Differentiation between these two positions proved difficult using the traditional suite of NMR experiments. An NOE experiment was subsequently performed in which the anomeric resonance at δ 5.04 was irradiated yielding a nuclear overhauser effect response to an aromatic proton resonance at δ 7.51. An overlay of the 1D NOE spectra (C), with ^{1}H spectra (B) and HSQC spectra (A) of the glucuronide conjugate, confirmed the resonance at δ 7.51 belonged to H7 aromatic proton (Figure 14.8). The NOE data allowed the unambiguous structural assignment of the glucuronide conjugate. This is because the only possible configuration that satisfies a spatial coupling between the anomeric proton of the glucuronide and the H7 proton is when the glucuronide is placed on the hydroxamic acid. In select situations, the NOE can be a highly diagnostic tool in assigning regiochemistry.

A case example of the utility of the TOCSY and HMBC experiments comes from studies with the glucokinase activator, Compound B. Compound B suffered from unusually high clearance *in vivo* in rat, which was not predicted using traditional *in vitro* systems (liver microsomes/cytosol) (Litchfield et al., 2010; Pfefferkorn et al., 2009). Metabolite profiling of Compound B in rat plasma revealed a single major metabolite, which was deemed to be a glutathione conjugate based on mass spectral characteristics (neutral loss of 129 corresponding to gamma glutamic acid). The mass of the unusual GSH conjugate suggested loss

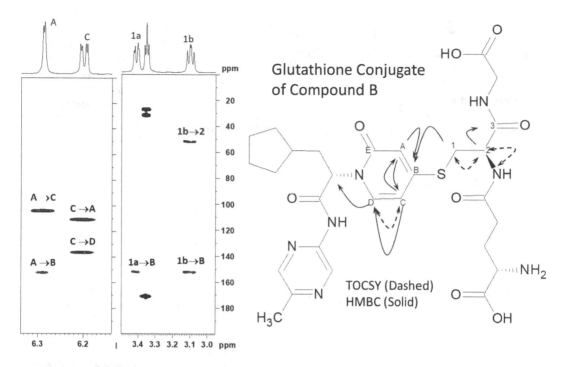

FIGURE 14.9 HMBC and TOCSY correlations for glutathione conjugate of Compound B.

of the methyl sulfone portion of the molecule followed by conjugation to glutathione. Interestingly, incubation of Compound B in rat liver microsomes supplemented with GSH also revealed that the formation of the glutathione conjugate was not dependent on NADPH. Isolation of the GSH conjugate from rat hepatocytes allowed structural elucidation by NMR which confirmed the site of conjugation and the mechanism involved in its formation. TOCSY and HMBC cross peaks helped to assign the identities of position 1 and position B (Figure 14.9), while an HMBC cross peak from the methylene resonances 1a and 1b adjacent to the sulfur atom into carbon B of the pyridone ring suggested that glutathione had reacted in a non-enzymatic Michael addition through nucleophilic attack at carbon B followed by subsequent elimination of the methyl sulfone to yield the GSH conjugate (Figure 14.10). Design strategies to minimize both the clearance and reactive functional group involved replacing the methyl sulfone with less facile leaving groups that were resistant to metabolism (CF_3, CNH_2O, etc.) and changing regiochemistry of substitutions on the pyridone ring to avoid reactivity. Subsequent analogs of Compound B retained favorable pharmacological attributes while exhibiting significantly reduced clearance values and reactive liabilities.

The utility of the HMBC experiment is well demonstrated for the hepatic microsomal triglyceride transfer protein (MTP) inhibitor JTT-130, a prodrug for treatment of dyslipidemia and related metabolic disorders (Ryder et al., 2012). As a prodrug, the expected route of biotransformation is illustrated in Figure 14.11, whereby JTT-130 is expected to be hydrolyzed by carboxyesterase enzymes in the liver to an inactive carboxylic acid metabolite [1] and the corresponding alcohol [2]. This metabolic reaction, if performed in $H_2^{18}O$, would be expected to yield [1] with ^{18}O incorporated into the acid group. Incubation with JTT-130 in liver microsomes supplemented with $H_2^{18}O$ did result in the formation of [1] but did not result in incorporation of the ^{18}O label into the carboxylic acid as anticipated. Furthermore, the corresponding alcohol [2] was not detected in the human liver microsomal incubations. Instead, a different metabolite with an unexpected mass was detected. This metabolite was subsequently isolated in an attempt to determine its structure and potentially shed light on the hydrolysis mechanism in formation of [1]. ^1H NMR analysis of the metabolite indicated that the isolate contained five aromatic resonances, two olefinic resonances (labeled D in Figure 14.12), and a complete absence of aliphatic resonances. Multiplicity edited HSQC and HMBC NMR spectra positively identified two olefinic protons proximal to a carbonyl carbon and an aromatic ring, which is consistent with the structure of atropic acid

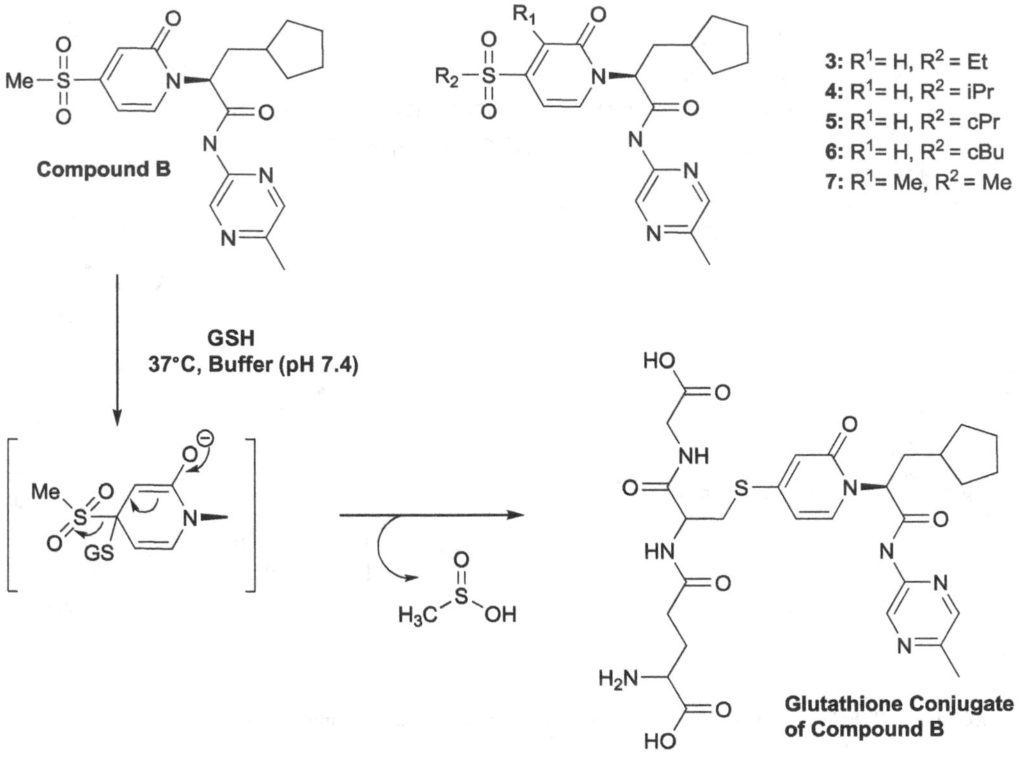

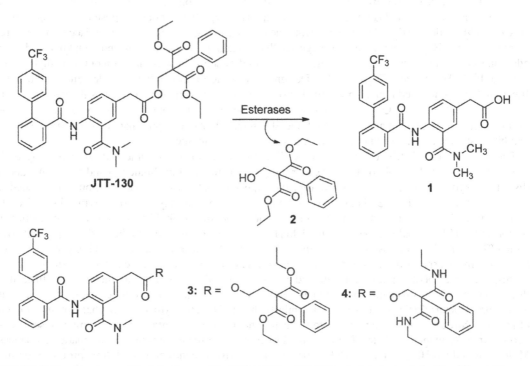

FIGURE 14.10   Structure of Compound B and proposed mechanism for formation of glutathione conjugate.

FIGURE 14.11   Structures of the intestine-specific MTP inhibitor JTT-130 and related ester derivatives [3] and [4].

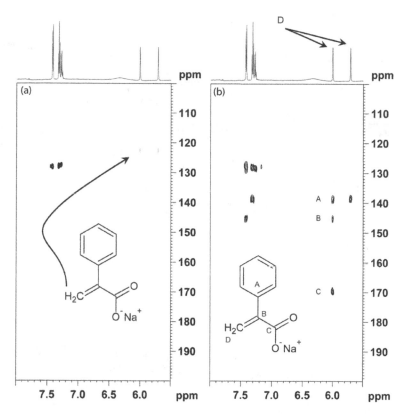

FIGURE 14.12 Expanded aromatic region of the (a) ^{1}H–^{13}C multiplicity edited HSQC and (b) HMBC spectra of unknown metabolite of JTT-130.

(Figure 14.12). Unambiguous confirmation of the structure was obtained via comparison of the NMR characteristics of the isolated metabolite with a commercially available atropic acid standard (data not shown). The characterization of this metabolite enabled a rationalization of the mechanism behind its formation (Figure 14.13): an initial hydrolysis of one of the pendant malonate ethyl ester groups followed by decarboxylative elimination to yield the carboxylic acid metabolite [1]. The mechanism was further substantiated by the fact that a similar analog [3], which possessed an additional methylene group, did not undergo the same decarboxylative elimination as observed with JTT-130.

Beyond metabolite structural characterization and quantitative determinations of metabolite concentrations, NMR is often used to determine the kinetics of chemical reactions. An important example of this is the measurement of migration rates of acyl glucuronides, which have been linked to toxicity in a certain class of non-steroidal anti-inflammatory drugs. Compounds that are glucuronidated on carboxylic acids with minimal substitution on the carbon α to the acid group are particularly susceptible to this phenomenon (Bailey and Dickinson, 2003). The pronounced difference in toxicity profiles between Ibuprofen and Ibufenac has been attributed to the differences in the migration rate of the acyl glucuronide metabolite formed in both compounds (Castillo and Smith, 1995). Drugs that have migration rates with a $T_{1/2}$ of less than 1.5 hours have either been withdrawn from the market or received black box warnings (Figure 14.14). An example of this is found with Compound C, a CRTh2 antagonist for treatment of asthma, which possessed a carboxylic acid unsubstituted at the α position that formed an acyl glucuronide. The glucuronide was found to migrate very rapidly as judged by its quick degradation *in vitro*. Due to the rapid rate of migration a half-life could not be accurately measured by LC/MS due to the length of time required to run the sample. Through a simple 1D proton measurement of the anomeric resonance of the glucuronide, a half-life of 0.2 h was easily calculated in D_2O buffered at pH 7.4 (Figure 14.15). Since the projected human dose of Compound C was rather high at >100 mg,

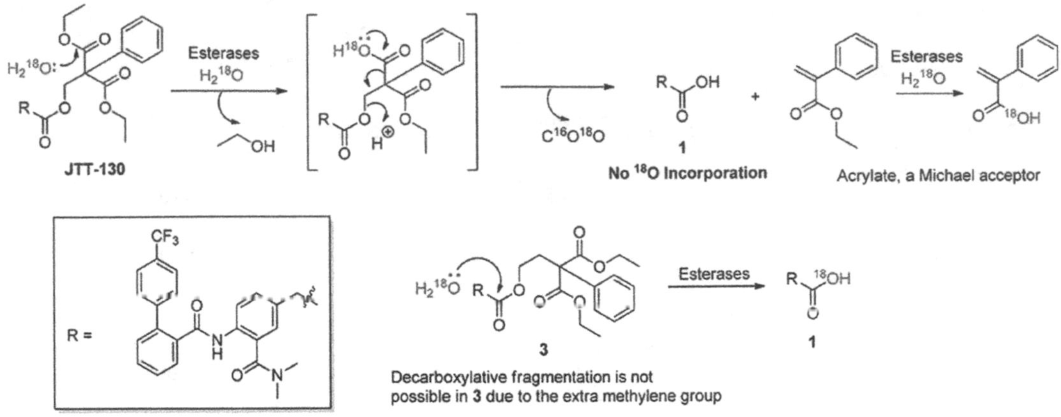

FIGURE 14.13 Suggested hydrolysis mechanism in formation of **[1]** and atropic acid from JTT-130 and hydrolysis mechanism for JTT-130 analog **[3]**.

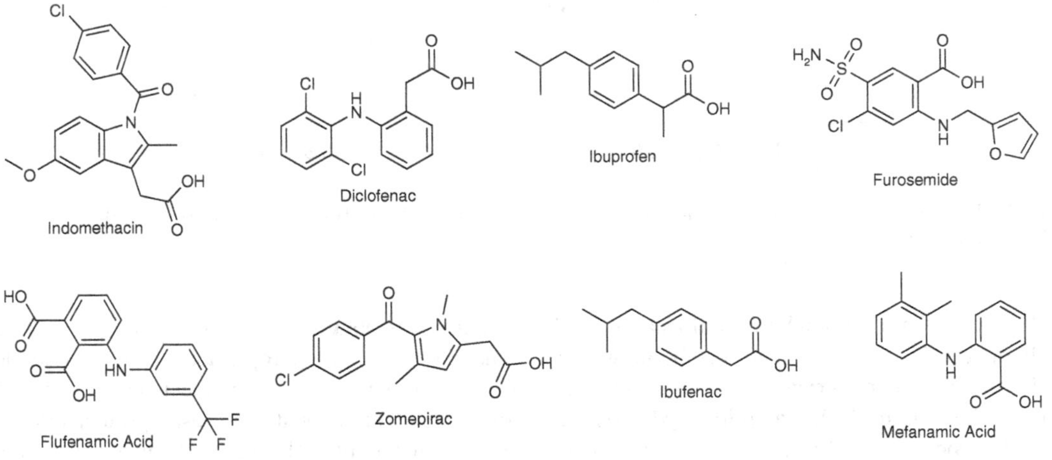

	Literature half-life (h)	NMR determined half-life (h)
Diclofenac	0.5	0.6
Zomepirac	0.6	0.5
Ibufenac	1.1	1.1
Indomethacin	1.5	1.4
Ibuprofen	3.3	4.6
Furosemide	3.6	5.3
Flufenamic Acid	7	10
Mefanamic Acid	22	17

Compounds with $t_{1/2}$ of less than 1.5 h have either been withdrawn from the market or have been issued black box warnings

FIGURE 14.14 List of nonsteroidal inflammatory drugs (NSAID'S) and rates of acyl migration calculated by measuring NMR half-life.

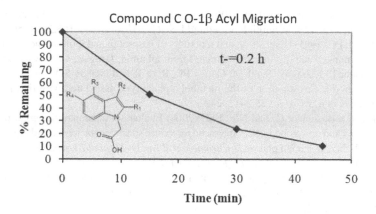

FIGURE 14.15 Half-life determination of Compound C via disappearance of the anomeric ^1H resonance.

coupled with the fact that glucuronidation was the major metabolic pathway, it was decided to terminate this compound and others in the series possessing α unsubstituted carboxylic acid structural motifs and move on to different chemical matter.

Conclusions

The role of NMR in the drug metabolism setting has changed significantly over the last twenty years. Historically in the DMPK environment, NMR was reserved almost exclusively for situations in development where complete structural elucidation of a metabolite was a regulatory requirement. Advances in NMR instrument design and the development of *in vitro* metabolite generation systems, which decreased the amount of material required for structural characterization of metabolites, helped move the utility of NMR from development to a more routine discovery tool. As the sample requirements continue to decrease, the potential for the structural elucidation of metabolites via NMR will have a greater influence on candidate selection as compounds move from discovery to development. Together with the rediscovery of the importance of qNMR and an increase in its ease of use these isolated, characterized and quantitated samples will have increasing value in the future. Concomitant with these impacts in discovery, the increase in sensitivity will also enhance our ability to characterize human unique metabolites in drug development as well as more effectively address regulatory issues such as Metabolites In Safety Testing (MIST) (U.S. Department of Health and Human Services Food and Drug Administration Center for Drug Evaluation and Research, CDER).

REFERENCES

Akoka S, Barantin L and Trierweiler M (1999) Concentration measurement by proton NMR using the ERETIC method. *Anal Chem* **71**:2554–2557.

Bailey MJ and Dickinson RG (2003) Acyl glucuronide reactivity in perspective: Biological consequences. *Chem-Biol Interact* **145**:117–137.

Bax A and Summers MF (1986) Proton and carbon-13 assignments from sensitivity-enhanced detection of heteronuclear multiple-bond connectivity by 2D multiple quantum NMR. *J Am Chem Soc* **108**:2093–2094.

Beckonert O, Keun HC, Ebbels TMD, Bundy J, Holmes E, Lindon JC and Nicholson JK (2007) Metabolic profiling, metabolomic and metabonomic procedures for NMR spectroscopy of urine, plasma, serum and tissue extracts. *Nat Protocols* **2**:2692–2703.

Boyer RD, Johnson R and Krishnamurthy K (2003) Compensation of refocusing inefficiency with synchronized inversion sweep (CRISIS) in multiplicity-edited HSQC. *J Magn Reson* **165**:253–259.

Castillo M and Smith PC (1995) Disposition and reactivity of ibuprofen and ibufenac acyl glucuronides in-vivo in the rhesus-monkey and in-vitro with human serum-albumin. *Drug Metab and Dispos* **23**:566–572.

Coen M, Rademacher PM, Zou W, Scott M, Ganey PE, Roth R and Nelson SD (2012) Comparative NMR-based metabonomic investigation of the metabolic phenotype associated with tienilic acid and tienilic acid isomer. *Chem Res Toxicol* **25**:2412–2422.

Dear GJ, Roberts AD, Beaumont C, and North SE (2008) Evaluation of preparative high performance liquid chromatography and cryoprobe-nuclear magnetic resonance spectroscopy for the early quantitative estimation of drug metabolites in human plasma. *J Chromatogr B Analyt Technol Biomed Life Sci* **876**:182–190.

Derome AE (2013)*Modern NMR Techniques for Chemistry Research*, Elsevier.

Dona AC, Kyriakides M, Scott F, Shephard EA, Varshavi D, Veselkov K and Everett JR (2016) A guide to the identification of metabolites in NMR-based metabonomics/metabolomics experiments. *Comput Struct Biotechnol J* **14**:135–153.

Ernst RR, Bodenhausen G and Wokaun A (1987) *Principles of Nuclear Magnetic Resonance in One and Two Dimensions*, Clarendon Press Oxford.

Farrant RD, Hollerton JC, Lynn SM, Provera S, Sidebottom PJ and Upton RJ (2010) NMR quantification using an artificial signal. *Magn Reson Chem* **48**:753–762.

Field LD, Li HL and Magill AM (2015) *Organic Structures from 2D NMR Spectra, Instructor's Guide and Solutions Manual*, John Wiley & Sons.

Hilton BD and Martin GE (2010) Investigation of the experimental limits of small-sample heteronuclear 2D NMR. *J Nat Prod* **73**:1465–1469.

Holzgrabe U, Deubner R and Schollmayer C (2005) Quantitative NMR spectroscopy—Applications in drug analysis. *J Pharmaceut Biomed* **38**:806–812.

Hong H, Caceres-Cortes J, Su H, Huang X, Roongta V, Bonacorsi Jr S, Hong Y, Tian Y, Iyer RA and Humphreys WG (2010) Mechanistic studies on a P450-mediated rearrangement of BMS-690514: Conversion of a pyrrolotriazine to a hydroxypyridotriazine†. *Chem Res Toxicol* **24**:125–134.

Hutzler JM, Steenwyk RC, Smith EB, Walker GS and Wienkers LC (2004) Mechanism-based inactivation of cytochrome P450 2D6 by 1-[(2-ethyl-4-methyl-1H-imidazol-5-yl)methyl]- 4-[4-(trifluoromethyl)-2-pyridinyl] piperazine: Kinetic characterization and evidence for apoprotein adduction. *Chem Res Toxicol* **17**:174–184.

ICH (2010) Guidance on nonclinical safety studies for the conduct of human clinical trials and marketing for pharmaceuticals M3 (R2) http://www.ich.org/products/guidelines/safety/safety-single/article/guidance-on-nonclinical-safety-studies-for-the-conduct-of-human-clinical-trials-and-marketing-author.html.

Iverson SL and Smith DA (2016) *Metabolite Safety in Drug Development*, Wiley Blackwell, Chichester, UK.

Jacobsen NE (2016) *NMR Data Interpretation Explained: Understanding 1D and 2D NMR Spectra of Organic Compounds and Natural Products*, John Wiley & Sons.

Krunic A and Orjala J (2015) Application of high-field NMR spectroscopy for characterization and quantitation of submilligram quantities of isolated natural products. *Magn Reson Chem* **53**:1043–1050.

Kwan EE and Huang SG (2008) Structural elucidation with NMR spectroscopy: Practical strategies for organic chemists. *Eur J Org Chem* **2008**:2671–2688.

Li XH, Jeso V, Heyward S, Walker GS, Sharma R, Micalizio GC and Cameron MD (2014) Characterization of T-5 N-oxide formation as the first highly selective measure of CYP3A5 activity. *Drug Metab Dispos* **42**:334–342.

Lindon JC, Nicholson JK and Wilson ID (2000) Directly coupled HPLC-NMR and HPLC-NMR-MS in pharmaceutical research and development. *J Chromatogr B* **748**:233–258.

Litchfield J, Sharma R, Atkinson K, Filipski KJ, Wright SW, Pfefferkorn JA, Tan BJ, Kosa RE, Stevens B, Tu MH and Kalgutkar AS (2010) Intrinsic electrophilicity of the 4-methylsulfonyl-2-pyridone scaffold in glucokinase activators: Role of glutathione-S-transferases and *in vivo* quantitation of a glutathione conjugate in rats. *Bioorg Med Chem Lett* **20**:6262–6267.

Miao Z, Jin M, Liu X, Guo W, Jin X, Liu H and Wang Y (2015) The application of HPLC and microprobe NMR spectroscopy in the identification of metabolites in complex biological matrices. *Anal Bioanal Chem* **407**:3405–3416.

Mutlib A, Espina R, Atherton J, Wang J, Talaat R, Scatina J, Chandrasekaran A. (2012) Alternate strategies to obtain mass balance without the use of radiolabeled compounds: Application of quantitative fluorine (19F) nuclear magnetic resonance (NMR) spectroscopy in metabolism studies. *Chem Res Toxicol.* **25**:572–583.

Mutlib A, Espina R, Vishwanathan K, Babalola K, Chen Z, Dehnhardt C, Venkatesan A, Mansour T, Chaudhary I, Talaat R and Scatina J (2011) Application of quantitative NMR in pharmacological evaluation of biologically generated metabolites: Implications in drug discovery. *Drug Metab Dispos* **39**:106–116.

Nagato EG, Lankadurai BP, Soong R, Simpson AJ and Simpson MJ (2015) Development of an NMR microprobe procedure for high-throughput environmental metabolomics of Daphnia magna. *Magne Reson Chem* **53**:745–753.

Pauli GF, Chen S-N, Simmler C, Lankin DC, Gödecke T, Jaki BU, Friesen JB, McAlpine JB and Napolitano JG (2014) Importance of purity evaluation and the potential of quantitative 1H NMR as a purity assay. *J Med Chem* **57**:9220–9231.

Pfefferkorn JA, Lou JH, Minich ML, Filipski KJ, He MY, Zhou R, Ahmed S et al. (2009) Pyridones as glucokinase activators: Identification of a unique metabolic liability of the 4-sulfonyl-2-pyridone heterocycle. *Bioorg Med Chem Lett* **19**:3247–3252.

Robertson DG, Reily MD, Sigler RE, Wells DF, Paterson DA and Braden TK (2000) Metabonomics: Evaluation of nuclear magnetic resonance (NMR) and pattern recognition technology for rapid *in vivo* screening of liver and kidney toxicants. *Toxicol Sci* **57**:326–337.

Robertson DG, Watkins PB and Reily MD (2011) Metabolomics in toxicology: Preclinical and clinical applications. *Toxicol Sci* **120**:S146–S170.

Ryder T, Walker GS, Goosen TC, Ruggeri RB, Conn EL, Rocke BN, Lapham K, Steppan CM, Hepworth D and Kalgutkar AS (2012) Insights into the novel hydrolytic mechanism of a Diethyl 2-Phenyl-2-(2-arylacetoxy)methyl malonate ester-based microsomal triglyceride transfer protein (MTP) inhibitor. *Chem Res Toxicol* **25**:2138–2152.

Simmler C, Napolitano JG, McAlpine JB, Chen SN and Pauli GF (2014) Universal quantitative NMR analysis of complex natural samples. *Curr Opin Biotech* **25**:51–59.

Simpson JH (2011) *Organic Structure Determination using 2-D NMR Spectroscopy: A Problem-Based Approach*, Academic Press.

Temesi D. John S, Warren K, and Samuel D (2013) The stability of amitriptyline N-oxide and clozapine N-oxide on treated and untreated dry blood spot cards. *J Pharmaceut Biomed* **76**:164–168.

U.S. Department of Health and Human Services Food and Drug Administration Center for Drug Evaluation and Research, CDER) 2016, https://www.fda.gov/downloads/Drugs/.../Guidances/ucm079266.pdf.

Walker GS, Bauman JN, Ryder TF, Smith EB, Spracklin DK and Obach RS (2014) Biosynthesis of drug metabolites and quantitation using NMR spectroscopy for use in pharmacologic and drug metabolism studies. *Drug Metab Dispos* **42**:1627–1639.

Walker GS, Ryder TF, Sharma R, Smith EB and Freund A (2011) Validation of isolated metabolites from drug metabolism studies as analytical standards by quantitative NMR. *Drug Metab Dispos* **39**:433–440.

Walker LR, Hoyt DW, Walker SM, Ward JK, Nicora CD and Bingol K (2016) Unambiguous metabolite identification in high-throughput metabolomics by hybrid 1D H-1 NMR/ESI MS1 approach. *Magn Reson Chem* **54**:998–1003.

Wang J and Urban L (2004) The impact of early ADME profiling on drug discovery and development strategy. *Drug Discov World* **5**:73–86.

Watt AP, Mortishire-Smith RJ, Gerhard U and Thomas SR (2003) Metabolite identification in drug discovery. *Curr Opin Drug Disc* **6**:57–65.

Yu H, Bischoff D and Tweedie D (2010) Challenges and solutions to metabolites in safety testing: Impact of the international conference on harmonization M3 (R2) guidance. *Expert Opin Drug Met* **6**:1539–1549.

Zhang Z and Mitra K (2012) Application of accurate mass spectrometry for metabolite identification, in *ADME-Enabling Technologies in Drug Design and Development* pp 317–330, John Wiley & Sons, Inc.

Zhou YT, Liao QF, Lin MN, Deng XJ, Zhang PT, Yao MC, Zhang L and Xie ZY (2014) Combination of H-1 NMR- and GC-MS-based metabonomics to study on the toxicity of coptidis rhizome in rats. *PLoS One* **9**:12.

Zhu M, Zhang H and Humphreys WG (2011) Drug metabolite profiling and identification by high-resolution mass spectrometry. *J Biol Chem* **286**:25419–25425.

15

In Vitro *Metabolism: Subcellular Fractions*

Michael A. Mohutsy

CONTENTS

Introduction

The *in vitro* study of xenobiotic metabolism in the pharmaceutical industry has routinely been used to help evaluate properties of new molecular entities and help optimize these properties to allow for evaluation of the pharmacologic target in animal models, along with safe dosing in humans. Subcellular fractions, abundant, commercially available, and often well-characterized before purchase, are the most often used *in vitro* tools to predict both *in vivo* clearance and the potential for drug interactions via enzyme inhibition. *In vitro* studies not only allow for evaluation to predict drug properties in human, but also decrease the use of animals in drug discovery and development.

The previous version of this chapter, "Subcellular Fractions," concentrated on the various methods for the preparation, characterization, storage, and special considerations necessary for extrahepatic fractions. With the exception of the characterization, the science concerning these "situations" has not evolved to any great extent since the previous publication of this chapter in 2007. The characterization of the fractions, however, has advanced dramatically with the development and implementation of more advanced mass spectrometry methods to quantify individual drug metabolizing enzymes. This improved characterization along with specific examples of the utility of subcellular fractions since the last publication of this book will be the focus of the present chapter.

Subcellular Systems

Overview

The *in vitro* metabolism models are often broadly separated into subcellular fractions and whole cell models, including isolated primary cells, tissue slices, and cell lines. Subcellular fractions can be isolated from virtually any available tissue from any available species. While the different species/tissue/fraction possibilities are very extensive, the subcellular fractions used most often in early drug discovery are those encompassing the most common preclinical pharmacology/toxicology species (mouse, rat, dog, and monkey) along with human, the organ that is the most responsible for drug metabolism (liver), and the subcellular fraction containing the enzyme systems most predominantly involved in drug metabolism (microsomes).

The xenobiotic and endobiotic metabolizing enzymes are usually localized to specific organelles within the cell. Through the process of isolating these various organelles a highly concentrated enzyme source, relatively free of enzymes found in other organelles and without sufficient levels of cofactors necessary for enzymatic activity. Thus, through appropriate selection of subcellular fraction, cofactors, and other incubation conditions, enzymes can be evaluated in enzyme phenotyping (Table 14.1). The predominant enzymes involved in drug metabolism are predominantly found in the endoplasmic reticulum (ER), including the P450s, UGTs, and some hydrolytic enzymes. The P450s and the UGTs both require cofactors, NADPH and UDPGA, respectively, while other enzymes found in the ER, hydrolases (carboxylesterase 1 and 2, epoxide hydrolase), and reductases, for example, do not require addition of cofactor for enzymatic activity. With the liver being the predominant organ responsible for the metabolism of drugs and the P450s and UGTs responsible for greater than 75% of the metabolism of drugs cleared through metabolism approved between 2006 and 2015 (Cerny 2016), it is of no surprise that liver microsomes are the most commonly used subcellular fraction for use in *in vitro* metabolism studies. Other enzymes found in the ER have been extensively studied including the Flavin Containing Monooxygenases (FMOs), though they have been relatively unimportant in the overall metabolism of drugs.

Advantages of subcellular fractions are the commercial availability of fractions from a variety of tissues and a large number of species and a flexibility of incubation conditions. Incubation conditions such as cofactors added, buffer type, pH of buffer, and temperature of reaction can be altered to optimize or minimize specific enzymatic reactions. Disadvantages of subcellular fractions include lability of some enzymes during preparation and loss of specific intracellular environment that may be necessary for the enzyme function. The lack of membrane/transporters can lead to lower or higher concentrations at the site of metabolism, which may result in an over- or under-estimation of the contribution of the particular metabolic pathway.

While the liver is most often the predominant drug metabolizing organ, depending on the specific enzyme and xenobiotic, other organs may also be important for metabolism: for example, UGT1A7, 1A8, and 1A10 are expressed predominantly in the gastrointestinal tract and other enzymes predominantly in the kidney and GI tract; membrane dipeptidase involved in the hydrolysis of penicillin is found predominantly in the intestine and kidney (Table 15.1).

Review of Protocols for Preparation

Isolation of multiple subcellular fractions requires disruption of the cell by homogenization, then differential centrifugation of the homogenate (possible due to differences in density and size of particles), and followed by resuspension of the pellet or isolation of a soluble fraction (Figure 15.1). Very few advances in the isolation of fractions have taken place since the last edition. With that in mind, a quick overview of the different isolation conditions with a focus on factors that can influence *in vitro* drug metabolism is included.

TABLE 15.1

Major Oxidation/Reduction Enzymes

Enzyme	Reaction	Cofactor	Location
Cytochromes P450	Oxidation Reduction	NADPH	Endoplasmic reticulum
Hydrolases (Esterases and Amidases, Epoxide Hydrolase)	Oxidation (Hydrolysis)		Cytosol Endoplasmic reticulum
Reductases (Aldo keto reductases and Carbonyl reductases)	Reduction	NAD, NADP	Cytosol Endoplasmic reticulum
Aldehyde Oxidase	Oxidation		Cytosol
Flavin containing monooxygenases	Oxidation	NADPH	Endoplasmic reticulum
Alcohol or aldehyde dehydrogenases			
UDP-glucuronysyltransferases	Transferase	UDPGA	Endoplasmic reticulum
Sulfotransferases	Transferase	PAPS	Cytosol
Methyltransferases	Transferase	SAM	Endoplasmic reticulum Cytosol
N-acetyltransferase	Transferase	Acetyl-CoA	Cytosol
Glutathione S-transferase	Transferase	GSH	Cytosol Endoplasmic reticulum

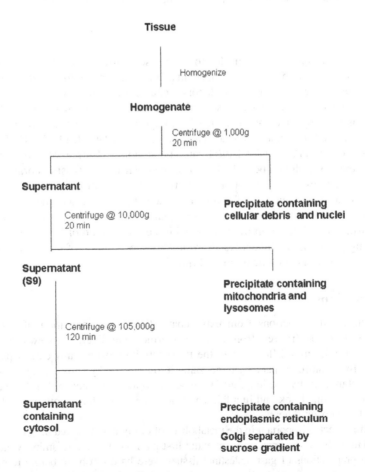

FIGURE 15.1   Generalized subcellular fractionation scheme.

Preparation of microsomes was suggested to be performed using livers from fasted animals to prevent contamination with glycogen particles in one of the earliest published protocols (Siekevitz 1962). The authors also believed that different procedures may be necessary for different organs. The choice of procedure often leads the choice between high recovery and high impurity, or lower recovery and higher purity, of a specific fraction and will often be determined by the ultimate use of the subcellular fraction.

Important considerations required for successful subcellular fractionation from any organ or species include the use of optimal conditions throughout the procedure. Additions to the preparation protocol include using the serine protease/esterase inhibitor, phenylmethylsulfonylfluorine (PMSF), in the homogenization buffer and the chelating agent-antioxidant ethylenediaminetetraacetic acid (EDTA), thiol-protecting agent dithiothreitol, and the antioxidant butylated hydroxytoluene as additives in the microsomal buffer to retard lipid peroxidation and protein degradation. Sometimes when a second high speed centrifugation step is performed, a pyrophosphate buffer to remove hemoglobin and nucleic acids from the microsomal or subcellular fraction preparation is used (Guengerich 1994). High concentrations of PMSF during microsome isolation can limit the utility of the subcellular fraction to study enzymes such as carboxylesterases along with other serine hydrolases.

With their importance as drug metabolizing enzymes, the cytochromes P450 are probably the most-studied system found in liver microsomal fractions. Since the quantification of P450s involves spectral measurements, early work also suggested that using Ringers solution to wash microsomes was necessary to remove hemoglobin that would interfere with the spectral measurements (Garfinkel 1958). The effect of washing rat hepatic microsomes with sucrose solutions, with or without EDTA, has also been evaluated using xenobiotic metabolism as a marker (Powis and Boobis 1975). EDTA prevented the decrease in metabolism of some substrates after washing with sucrose alone, stimulating metabolism of other substrates.

Storage

Subcellular fractions are especially useful due to their ease of use and their ability to be frozen and easily stored. One of the strengths of the use subcellular fractions for *in vitro* metabolism studies are the ability to use fractions prepared from the same donors over a period of many years, even a decade or more. The ability to use subcellular fractions over several years was rigorously tested in 1996. In this evaluation, the effects of freezing, thawing, and time in storage (up to 2 years at −80°C) of human liver microsomes was examined. The results indicated no change in CYP1A2, CYP2A6, CYP2C9, CYP2C19, CYP2D6, CYP2E1, CYP3A4/5, or CYP4A9/11 catalytic activities (Pearce, McIntyre et al. 1996). The starting quality of the tissue should be as high as possible to ensure successful storage of human livers and the subcellular fractions prepared from them. In the early years of drug metabolism research with human liver, tissue quality was questionable, as demonstrated by enzyme activities (Powis, Jardine et al. 1988, Chapman, Christensen et al. 1993). The overall quality and availability of human tissue available for drug metabolism research has improved, along with the preparation of large batches of subcellular fractions containing greater than 100 donors allowing for the evaluation of *in vitro* metabolism parameters using the same material over long periods of time.

Extrahepatic Fractions

When isolating subcellular fractions from extrahepatic tissue, sedimentation of ER into the final 100,000g pellet will often be different from what is performed with liver. A review of the differences in preparation of microsomes and differences in the P450 activities from many extrahepatic microsomal fractions obtained from multiple species can be found in the review by Burke and Orrenius (Burke and Orrenius 1979). Metabolism by the lung, gut, kidney, and brain were covered in Chapters 11 through 14 of the 2nd edition of this book and in a fairly recent review (Gundert-Remy et al. 2014). Very brief highlights will only be covered here.

The gastrointestinal tract is important in the metabolism of orally administered drugs, due to the localization of enzymes within the tissue, increasing potential first-pass metabolism (Kaminsky and Zhang 2003). Stable microsomal preparations of gastrointestinal tissues were hard to obtain before researchers demonstrated that the addition of a trypsin inhibitor from soybean and glycerol (20%) in isotonic potassium chloride could stabilize enzymatic activity (Stohs et al. 1976). The addition of a protease inhibitor is a common procedure when isolating microsomes from intestinal tissue, with the non-specific serine protease inhibitor PMSF commonly used. Whether intestinal microsomes are isolated using an elution method or via manual scraping of the tissue (Kolars et al. 1994, Paine et al. 1997, Madani et al. 1999), if PMSF is added at some point in the preparation of microsomes and any serine protease activities such as the carboxylesterases should be expected to be minimized or potentially not present at all. While the method of intestinal microsomes isolation does not appear to influence the affinity of the CYP3A4, V_{max} values varied greatly, with a 10-fold greater V_{max} with microsomes isolated from eluted enterocytes compared to microsomes from mucosal scraping (Galetin and Houston 2006). The portion of intestine from where the microsomes were isolated also will influence the activity of the fraction. Greater amounts of CYP3A4 were found when microsomes were isolated from proximal rather than distal intestinal sections (Paine et al. 1997). This can result in very high variability when enzyme activities are reported with different preparations of intestinal microsomes.

The kidney is particularly complex organ from which to isolate subcellular fractions since the tissue will contain multiple localized cell types. The subcellular fractions must be isolated from the cell types involved in drug metabolism (e.g., proximal tubule cells) in order to provide meaningful data on cell specific metabolism. While P450 metabolism has been shown to be a mere fraction of that observed in the liver (Litterst et al. 1975), other enzymes such as UGT1A6, UGT1A9, and UGT2B7 (Fallon et al. 2013) and hydrolysis enzymes, such as membrane dipeptidase (Kropp et al. 1982) involved in antibiotic metabolism, are found in fairly high levels in the kidney.

Very little recent information on drug metabolism by the lung has been reported, with a review focusing on the different drug metabolizing enzymes found in the lung is a good resource (Zhang et al. 2006). Lung P450 activities are much lower than in liver however, the lung does contain several preferentially expressed P450 forms including CYP1A1, 1B1, 2A13, 2F1, 2S1, and 4B1. The lung will metabolize drugs that enter the organ via inhalation and have also been shown to metabolize compounds that enter the lung through systemic circulation (Borlak et al. 2005).

Metabolism with subcellular fractions isolated from brain, heart, epidermis, and other tissues has been covered in the second edition of this book along with several comprehensive reviews and more recent studies (Sarkar 1992, Meyer, Gehlhaus et al. 2007, Ravindranath and Strobel 2013, Manevski et al. 2015, Oliveira et al. 2016). The reader is prompted to reference these sources for more information on these organs with less extensive metabolic capacity.

Characterization of Subcellular Fractions

As expounded upon in the first and second editions of "Subcellular Fractions," the characterization of the fractions often involves the determination of total protein and catalytic activities across a variety enzymes in each fraction and tissue homogenate. In addition to these common measures of subcellular fractions, quantification of specific proteins had been performed using western blotting. Western blotting is a relatively high cost, labor intensive method that would only allow for a relatively small number of proteins in a subcellular fraction. In the second edition, the various phenotypic enzymatic reactions used in the characterization of the preparations and to determine contamination by other subcellular fractions was discussed. The table and references are included here (Table 15.2).

Much of the recent work with subcellular fractions has been aimed at the mass spectrometry based absolute quantification of enzymes and the potential to scale up the activity of the particular enzyme in the subcellular fraction to the whole organ. The ability to accurately measure the absolute quantity of drug metabolizing enzymes has been the topic of several recent reviews (Al Feteisi et al. 2015, Bhatt and Prasad 2017) with caveats on the various proteomic methodologies employed. The authors mention the "significant technical challenges" and the need to "thoroughly address the critical variables" that could influence the ultimate results. "Quantitative proteomics research requires specialist practical skills and there is a pressing need to dedicate more effort and investment to training personnel in this area. Large-scale multicenter collaborations are also needed to standardize quantitative strategies in order to improve physiologically based pharmacokinetic models." This section will focus on the reports of the quantification of the important drug metabolizing enzymes (Cerny 2016) along with the more recent global proteomic quantification of a wide range of liver proteins.

TABLE 15.2

Selected Enzyme Markers of Subcellular Fractions

Subcellular Location	Marker	References
Microsomal	Glucose-6-phosphate	Powis and Boobis (1975)
	Cytochrome c reductase	Masters (1967)
Cytosol	Lactate dehydrogenase	Bergmeyer (1974)
	Glutathione S-transferase	Habig, Pabst et al. (1974)
	Alcohol dehydrogenase	Wynne, Wood et al. (1992)
Lysosomal	Acid phosphatase	Drexler and Gignac (1994)
	β-glucuronidase	Lombardo, Caimi et al. (1980)
	N-Acetyl-β-glucuronidase	Lombardo, Caimi et al. (1980)
Mitochondrial	Succinic INT reductase	Pennington (1961)
	Cytochrome c oxidase	Wikstrom (1977)
	Succinate dehydrogenase	Gutman (1978)
	Xanthine oxidase	Hille and Nishino (1995)
	Glutamate dehydrogenase	Schmidt (1974)
	Monoamine oxidase	Schnaitman, Erwin et al. (1967)
Golgi	Galactosyltransferase	Baxter and Durham (1979)
Peroxisomes	Catalase	Chance and Herbert (1950)
Plasma membrane	Alkaline phosphatase	Emmelot, Bos et al. (1964)
	Alkaline phosphodiesterase	Emmelot, Bos et al. (1964)

Cytochromes P450

The absolute quantification of cytochromes P450s have been reported for many years by many different laboratories throughout the world. One of the first published reports compared the amount of CYP3A enzymes in microsomes to both immunoquantified proteins (CYP3A4 and CYP3A5) and to CYP activity including midazolam-1'hydroxylation (CYP3A4/5) testosterone-6β-hydroxylation (CYP3A4), itraconazole-6-hydroxylation (CYP3A4), and Vincristine M1 formation (CYP3A5) (Wang et al. 2008). A very strong correlation was seen between mass spectrometry-based quantification and immunoquantification ($r^2 \geq 0.87$) and mass spectrometry quantification and activities ($r^2 \geq 0.88$). While a good correlation was seen between mass spec and immunoblot quantification, the absolute values in pmol/mg of microsome protein were ~50% lower using the mass spectrometry derived method. A very wide range of values for CYP3A4 were also seen with the individual microsome CYP3A4 range of 9 to 322 pmol/mg microsome protein.

The quantification of a large number of P450 enzymes including CYP1A2, CYP2A6, CYP2B6, CYP2C8, CYP2C9 CYP2C19, CYP2D6, CYP2E1, and CYP3A4 was also subsequently reported (Kawakami, Ohtsuki et al. 2011). The authors showed high variability in several of the enzymes studied including CYP1A2, CYP2C19, and CYP3A4 and, somewhat surprisingly, showed CYP2C9 to be the most abundant enzyme in human liver microsomes. No correlations between enzyme activities or immunoblotting were reported.

UDP-glucuronysyltransferases

The initial study to look at the UGT enzymes using a mass spectrometry-based approach quantified UGT1A1 and UGT1A6 in 10 individual human liver microsomes (Fallon et al. 2008). Here the authors showed good correlation between western blot (% intensity) and quantities of UGT1A1 measured by mass spectrometry ($r^2 = 0.988$); however, the UGT1A6 had a much poorer correlation possibly due to a lower specificity of the UGT1A6 antibody or the low concentrations of UGT1A6 relative to the quantification curve. UGT1A1 was also quantified in human intestinal microsomes, though UGT1A6 was below the limit of quantification. This first study showed the potential of mass spectrometry to quantify many more UGT1A enzymes and led to a more extensive evaluation of subcellular fractions from intestine, liver, and kidney (Harbourt et al. 2012).

A recent manuscript went beyond simple quantification of the UGT enzymes and attempted to correlate the protein abundance measured using two different methodologies, a mass spectrometry method using a stable isotope labeled (SIL) peptide as a standard and a quantitative concatamer (QConCAT) (Achour, Al Feteisi et al. 2017). Very little correlation was seen between the two methodologies with only UGT1A1 showing a strong correlation between the two mass spectrometry methods. Quantitative UGT measurements generally gave a lower quantity of protein and in a narrower range than the QConCAT method and mass spectrometry methods. The SIL method showed moderate to strong correlations with enzymatic activities for UGT1A1, UGT1A3, UGT1A4, UGT1A6, UGT1A9, UGT2B7, and UGT2B15. The QConcat showed only moderate correlation with UGT1A1, UGT1A3, and UGT2B7 and poor correlation with activity for all other UGTs tested. As stated by the authors, "quantitative proteomic data should be validated against catalytic activity whenever possible." This should be kept in mind when evaluating the numerous studies that have attempted to quantify drug metabolizing enzymes in subcellular fractions without correlating to activity.

P450s and UGTs

With the successful quantification of proteins using mass spectrometric methods many groups have publishing studies quantifying both the P450s and the UGTs in individual subcellular fractions. Laboratories have also begun to quantify enzymes in subcellular fractions obtained from livers from donors with diseased livers. A few examples of quantification of both enzyme systems will be presented.

One of the first studies to look at both the P450s and UGTs showed that many enzymes including CYP2C9, CYP2E1, CYP3A4, CYP2A6, UGT1A6, UGT2B7, UGT2B15, and P450 reductase were abundantly expressed in human liver microsomes (Ohtsuki et al. 2012). The authors correlated quantified proteins with enzyme activity (CYP only) and mRNA levels and showed that CYP3A4, CYP2B6, and CYP2C8 protein amounts were each highly correlated with both enzyme activity and mRNA expression levels, whereas for other P450s, CYP1A2, CYP2C8, CYP2C9, CYP2C19, CYP2D6, CYP2E1, and CYP4A11 the protein expression levels were better correlated with the enzyme activities than the mRNA expression levels were (Ohtsuki et al. 2012).

Quantification of P450 and UGT enzymes was performed in human intestinal microsomes from two donors (Akazawa et al. 2018). A very large difference between two human intestinal donors with the expression of the intestinal P450 enzymes higher in one sample. UGT1A1, UGT1A6, UGT2B7, and UGT2B17 enzymes were also only found in that same donor. While UGT2B17 was found in both donors, the same donor also had much higher UGT2B17 levels. Care must be taken when extrapolating information from a very small number of individual donor microsomes, especially with the differences of age, sex, and disease state between the two donors.

A study to compare P450 and UGT enzymes from microsomes prepared from human hepatocellular cariconama along with pericarcinomatous tissue and commercial purchased microsomes, showed the ability to quantify enzymes from disease tissue (Yan et al. 2015). Similar expression of CYP1A2, CYP2A6, CYP2B6, CYP2C8, CYP2C9, CYP2C19, CYP2D, CYP2E1, CYP3A4/3A43, CYP3A43, UGT1A1, UGT1A6, UGT1A4, UGT1A9, and UGT2B7 were observed from reference microsomes and pooled human liver microsomes prepared from pericarcinomatous tissues of 15 donors, and pooled human liver microsomes prepared from tumor tissues of 15 donors. Amounts of UGT1A6 were greater in the tumor tissue microsomes, though the difference was not statistically all other enzymes were statistically significantly lower, with the exception of CYP2C19 and UGT1A9. These enzymes were lower, but the differences were not statistically significant.

Aldehyde Oxidase

A single report of the absolute quantification of aldehyde oxidase (AO) showed about a 2-fold batch-to-batch variation in the content of AO content with different pooled human liver cytosol preparations (Barr et al. 2013). A modest correlation with the quantity of protein and the oxidation of DACA was observed. The authors also showed that heterologously expressed AO enzyme was substantially less active per pmol than the cytosolic enzyme.

Carboxylesterase

Quantification of the carboxylesterase 1 in human liver S9 fractions was reported using a targeted absolute quantitative mass spectrometry method (Wang, Liang et al. 2016). The authors looked for only CE1 even though both carboxylesterase 1 and 2 are found in the liver. The amount of CE1 found in 24 different liver S9 samples showed variability in the pmol CE1 per mg of S9 protein with a range of 42.0 to 477.9 pmol/mg S9 and a mean of 176.1 pmol/mg S9. As is common in many of the absolute quantification studies, no attempts were made to correlate the quantity of enzyme with enzyme activity.

A much more extensive evaluation was performed looking at both CE1 and CE2 in liver and distribution between microsome and cytosol (Boberg et al. 2017). The ontogenies of the enzymes were also determined by quantifying the amounts of protein in subcellular fractions from neonates to adults. The amount of CE1 found in adult cytosol and microsomes was 556.5 and 1664.4 pmol/mg respectively. CE2 in adult microsomes only had an abundance of 174.1 pmol/mg, showing the preponderance of CE1 in the liver. Good correlation between CE1 and CE2 was observed suggesting both proteins are regulated through a common mechanism. CE1 abundance in microsomes increased approximately 5-fold in adults compared with neonates, while the cytosolic enzyme increased approximately 3-fold between the samples. In addition to the absolute quantification of the enzymes in the various subcellular fractions, the authors also compared the activities of the pediatric and adult samples and showed 2.4 fold greater formation rate of oseltamivir carboxylate from oseltamivir in the adult samples.

The amounts of CE1 between the two studies stated above are evidence of the large differences in protein abundances that can reported between labs. The mean value of CE1 in the S9 reported by Wang et al. of 174 pmol/ mg S9 was much less than a calculated 833.4 pmol/mg assuming S9 consists of 20% microsomal protein and 75% cytosolic protein (Jia and Liu 2007).

Global Proteomics Quantification of Drug Metabolizing Enzymes

The use of global proteomic approaches allow is the ability to quantify other proteins that are not normally studied using targeted approaches. A recent paper using ion mobility mass spectrometry to quantify the drug metabolism enzymes P450s and UGTs showed good correlation with previous targeted quantification data (Achour et al. 2017). While a common drug metabolizing enzyme, carboxyesterase 1 was the overall highest abundant enzyme in the human liver microsomes, and the most abundant P450, CYP3A4, was the 44th most abundant protein in the microsomes, demonstrating the relatively low abundance of these enzymes compared to some of the other enzymes found in microsomes. As has been reported previously, preparation of microsomes do not lead to a pure, isolated endoplasmic reticulum but rather to a more concentrated organelle with cytosol, mitochondria, nuclei, and plasma membrane present along with secreted proteins. This was exemplified with the second, fifth, and eighth most abundant proteins in the human liver microsomes being Cytoplasmic actin 1, ATP synthase subunit b, and Haptoglobin, cytosolic, mitochondrial, and secreted proteins respectively. The most abundant protein involved in CYP metabolism is not actually one of the CYP drug metabolizing enzymes but the associated protein Cytochrome b5. A fairly large variability in many of these most abundant proteins in microsomes can lead to vastly different amounts of the drug metabolizing enzymes when values such as intrinsic clearance are reported in units normalized to mg total human liver microsome protein. The authors state, "We suggest that protein concentrations used in pharmacokinetic predictions and scaling to *in vivo* clinical situations (physiologically based pharmacokinetics and *in vitro-in vivo* extrapolation) should be referenced instead to tissue mass." At the same time, the demonstration of a correlation of quantified proteins with activity also should be implemented. In another recent report, the authors took flash frozen liver homogenates fractionated by differential centrifugation and quantified the proteins in these fraction using a global proteomic quantification, or "total protein approach." (Wiśniewski et al. 2016) While the centrifugation steps did differ from traditional isolation steps for microsomes used in the study of drug metabolism, the results were surprising. The authors isolated 6 different fractions labeled A through H with fraction A being centrifugation of the homogenate at 1000×g for 10 minutes, fraction B 2000×g for 10 minutes, fraction C 5000×g for 10 minutes, fraction D 10000×g for 10 minutes, fraction E 21000×g for 60 minutes, corresponding to microsomes used in drug metabolism experiments, and fraction F was the cytosol. The largest amount of the total homogenate protein was found in Fraction A the initial 1000×g precipitate with over 60% of the total protein found in this fraction. Cytosol was the fraction with the second highest percentage of the protein at 19.1% of average total protein. The putative microsomal fraction on the other hand made up a modest 4.3% of the total average protein. A surprising result from the study that important drug metabolizing enzymes P450s and UGTs found in the endoplasmic reticulum were found throughout the various subcellular fractions isolated. In fact, greater than 50% of the total CYP1A2 and UGT1A1 protein was found in Fraction A 1000×g, the fraction associated with nuclei. The study shows the potential for issues with recovery of expected proteins when isolating subcellular fraction and the potential for contamination from different organelles.

Use of Subcellular Systems

Metabolite Identification

While with the increased availability, higher quality, and decreased price of primary hepatocytes, whole cell models are now much more commonly used as initial models for identifying metabolites than when the second edition of this book was published. Microsomes supplemented with NADPH or a NADPH regenerating system, however, continue to be an appropriate model for initial Metabolite ID. This is due to the fact that despite the introduction of microsomal screening as an initial tier in drug discovery, the metabolism of most small molecule drugs approved by the FDA continues to be through CYP enzymes. Microsomes, though most associated with P450s, do contain other enzymes such as FMOs, carboxylesterases, and others. Incubation conditions are important to optimize for the enzyme systems that one needs to be operative. FMO has the same subcellular location, microsomes, and cofactor. FMO is often thought to be equally active as P450s in NADPH-supplemented microsomal incubations. Heat inactivation in the absence of NADPH has been shown however to decrease the amount of FMO activity in microsomes. This is often performed by incubating the microsomes at 45°C for 1–5 minutes. Including NADPH in the preincubation step or limiting the amount of preincubation time will allow for optimal FMO activity. The second most common enzyme system involved in drug metabolism is the UGTs. While the second edition stated that the UGT2B7 isoform was found to have very little activity in microsomes, advances in the understanding of the enzyme system and the potential for free fatty acids explains this lack of activity. Inclusion of bovine serum albumin (BSA) in the incubations will bind the free fatty acids allowing for greatly increased activity (Manevski et al. 2011). The advantage of no cellular membrane in subcellular fractions allows for a higher concentration of substrate molecule at the site of metabolism than can likely be achieved in a whole cell model.

Advances in the ability to determine the metabolic stability along with the identification of the metabolic soft spots have been reported since the last edition (Paiva, Klakouski et al. 2017). The development of an integrated qualitative/quantitative approach with advanced UHPLC-mass spec methodology and automated identification of potential metabolites (Bateman et al. 2009, Bonn et al. 2010, Zelesky et al. 2013, Zhu et al. 2014).

Species Comparisons of Xenobiotic Metabolism

The wide availability, ease of use, and relatively low cost of subcellular fractions has made them useful as a first-tier tool to compare metabolism between species. The use of *in vitro* subcellular fractions allows for a much more extensive evaluation of species differences in metabolism than can be performed with *in vivo* metabolism studies. Subcellular fractions are a very useful tool to study the species differences in metabolism early in drug discovery and development to begin to determine metabolite coverage in preclinical toxicology studies. This is especially important with the necessity to test metabolites for safety in accordance with the FDAs guidance on "Metabolites in Safety Testing." Numerous reports of drug metabolism studies between many different species have been published including studies comparing numerous enzyme-specific oxidation and conjugation activities in human, dog, and cynomolgus and rhesus monkey microsomes and cytosol (Stevens et al. 1993, Sharer et al. 1995, Emoto et al. 2013).

Much of the more recent work on species differences has dealt with non-hepatic subcellular fractions and non-P450 non-UGT enzymes. Characterization of species differences in intestinal metabolism of CYP3A substrates between rats and dogs (Kadono et al. 2014), intestinal glucuronidation between rats, dogs, monkeys, and humans (Furukawa et al. 2014), hepatic and intestinal metabolism of 43 CYP metabolized compounds between humans and rats or dogs (Nishimuta et al. 2013), and intestinal metabolism between monkeys and humans (Takahashi et al. 2009, Nishimuta et al. 2011). Much work has been done concerning the species differences in hydrolytic activities between the subcellular fractions of different species including carboxylesterase and arylacetamide deacetylase between dogs and humans (Yoshida et al. 2018), carboxylesterase 2 in human and cynomolgus monkey intestinal microsomes (Igawa et al. 2016), hydrolysis by plasma, intestinal, renal, and liver enzymes in human, rat, dog, and monkey (Nishimuta et al. 2014), carboxymethylenebutenolidase and CES1 in cytosols and microsomes of mice, rats, monkeys, dogs, and humans (Ishizuka et al. 2013), and arylacetamide deacetylase activities in liver microsomes between human, rats, and mouse (Kobayashi et al. 2012). Species differences (most often in rate or extent of formation) are observed in metabolism of drugs by virtually all enzyme systems using subcellular fractions. For example, species differences were observed for sulfoxidation of 4-hydroxypropranolol (Narimatsu et al. 2001), glucuronidation of propofol (Mukai et al. 2015), N-acetyltransferase metabolism of a selective androgen receptor modulator (Gao et al. 2006) and numerous others.

Xenobiotic Activation

Activation of xenobiotics to potential reactive species using subcellular fractions are commonly performed laboratory experiments (Bauman et al. 2009, Usui et al. 2009). In addition, S9 fraction from arochlor induced rats is used to activate xenobiotics prior to testing for mutagenicity to a salmonella strain in the classic Ames mutagenicity (McCann et al. 1975).

Comparisons of carcinogen activation by hepatic microsomes from different species have been highly useful in explaining differential susceptibility to xenobiotic agents. For example, *N*-hydroxylation of the food-borne carcinogen 2-amino-l-methyl-6-phenylimidazo[4,5-*b*]pyridine (PhIP) is considerably higher in human, rather than in rat and mouse *in vitro*. The ability to detoxify PhIP by 4-hydroxylation is high in rats and mice, while humans have little of this activity (Gao et al. 2006). The activation of xenobiotics by subcellular fractions will also be covered more extensively elsewhere in the book.

In Vitro Model Comparisons from Multiple Organs

Studies comparing the *in vitro* metabolism by subcellular fractions from multiple organs are usually limited to the liver and intestine for P450 enzymes and liver intestine and kidney for the UGT enzymes due to the limited expression of these enzymes in other tissues. A variety of hydrolase enzymes on the other hand are expressed throughout the body and studies with wider arrays tissue subcellular fractions should be conducted. One such study compared hydrolase activities from tissue homogenates (of rat liver, lung, skin, and blood), mitochondria, nuclei, microsomes, and cytosol from these tissues and found to be highest in liver and plasma (McCracken et al. 1993). Additionally, prodrug hydrolysis was analyzed using liver, kidney, and intestine S9 along with plasma from a variety of preclinical species along with humans (Nishimuta et al. 2014).

In Vitro-In Vivo Pharmacokinetic Predictions

A significant research effort has gone into using *in vitro* microsomal data to quantitatively predict human P450 inhibitory potential and pharmacokinetics parameters such as clearance for new drug entities. Thus, *in vitro* microsomal models of drug metabolism and P450 inhibition have been incorporated into the drug-development paradigm from early discovery into the development stages. *In vitro* microsomal assays in early discovery are primarily focused around identification of metabolic liabilities of compounds using high throughput absorption metabolism distribution excretion (ADME) screening with a goal of reducing these liabilities with structural modification. To predict *in vivo* exposure and help choose compounds with a good chance to demonstrate pharmacology, the microsomal assays are performed with subcellular fractions from preclinical species. As clinical candidates are identified, in-depth *in vitro* analyses of the candidate's potential to cause drug-drug interactions and their metabolic fate are performed with human microsomes following guidelines set by regulatory agencies resulting in an assessment of possible metabolic liabilities, which are further examined in the clinic (EMA 2012, FDA 2017). Often slimmed down versions of enzyme inhibition assays will be run in a screening mode early in drug discovery process (Foti et al. 2010).

P450 Inhibition

Definitive *in vitro* studies with human liver microsomes evaluate the potential for a new chemical entity (NCE) to inhibit the metabolism of co-administered drugs, which could lead to serious side effects. Varying concentrations of both probe substrates of each of the P450s and the NCE are incubated with human liver microsomes. The K_i or IC_{50} of reversible inhibition are calculated using the resultant inhibition profile. A quick static estimation of the inhibition potential uses the *in vitro* parameter above with the maximal expected unbound concentration of inhibitor in human plasma ($I_{max,u}$) to determine a R1 value for liver and R1,gut (FDA 2017). The R1 value is calculated as $1+(I_{max,u}/K_i)$ and R1,gut calculated as $1 + (Igut/K_i)$. Igut is calculated as dose/250 mL. If the R1 value is ≥ 1.02 and/or R1,gut ≥ 11 the interaction should be evaluated further using a mechanistic model or even with a clinical drug interaction study. Time-dependent inhibition or mechanism-based inhibition can be similarly evaluated following preincubation of the NCE with human liver microsomes and NADPH prior to incubations with probe P450 substrates to calculate kinetic parameters K_I and k_{inact} (Grimm et al. 2009). An R2 value for a static evaluation of time dependent inhibition R2 = (kobs + kdeg)/kdeg, where kobs = $(k_{inact} \times 50 \times I_{max,u})/$ $(K_I + 50 \times I_{max,u})$ and kdeg = the apparent first-order degradation rate constant of the affected enzyme. An R2 value ≥ 1.25 will necessitate the further evaluation of the drug interaction potential (FDA 2017).

Prediction of Exposure and Pharmacokinetic Variability of New Chemical Entities

In vitro studies are performed to predict drug exposure in the human population and to understand the metabolic basis of variability in exposure and the potential to be a victim of drug-drug interactions (reaction phenotyping). Though the use of primary hepatocytes to predict a compound's clearance is becoming more common, *in vitro* microsomal techniques are very useful to predict clearance when oxidative metabolism and/or direct glucuronidation are the primary clearance routes. Human *in vitro* intrinsic clearance ($Cl_{int,h,in vitro}$), an estimate of *in vivo* intrinsic hepatic clearance ($Cl_{int,h,in vivo}$), can be determined using liver microsomes either through a determination of K_m and V_{max} of the metabolic pathways responsible for clearance or through examination of the rate of loss (k_{loss}) of compound (Obach, Baxter et al. 1997). Using physiologically-based scaling factors, $Cl_{int,h,in vitro}$ is scaled to $Cl_{int,h,in vivo}$. ($Cl_{int,h,in vivo}=Cl_{int,h,in vitro}$(mL/min/mg protein)* mg microsomal protein per gram of liver*gram of liver per kg body weight). The $Cl_{int,h,in vivo}$ is then scaled to total hepatic Cl_h most often by using the well-stirred model in which hepatic blood flow (Q_h) plasma protein binding (fu_p), microsomal protein binding (fu_{mic}), and blood/plasma (R_B) partitioning terms are included.

$$Cl_h = \frac{\dfrac{Cl_{int,h,in vitro}}{fu_{mic}} * Qh * \left(\dfrac{fu_p}{R_B}\right)}{Q_h + \left(\dfrac{Cl_{int,h,in vitro}}{fu_{mic}} * \left(\dfrac{fu_p}{R_B}\right)\right)} \qquad (15.1)$$

The resultant predictions of clearance exhibit a 2-3-fold prediction error and a systemic underprediction bias, which has been corrected by some groups with an empirical scaling factor (Ito and Houston 2005). In a recent commentary on the prediction of clearance using microsomes, the authors state that the mechanistic scaling methodology tends to underpredict clearance by 2.8 fold in humans and 2.3 fold in rats (Wood, Houston et al. 2017). The trend of increased underprediction with increasing *in vivo* intrinsic clearance is seen with microsomes in both humans and rats. These data, with the uncertainty around the prediction, can be used with other preclinical data to calculate efficacious or safe first human doses prior to human dosing for hepatically cleared drugs.

Summary and Conclusion

Subcellular fractions can be isolated from many different cell types, organs, and species and stored for a number of years at −80°C while retaining their enzymatic activity similar to fresh tissue. To ensure that a subcellular fraction is relatively pure, some form of characterization should be performed to ensure the isolated fraction is essentially from a single organelle. Characterization techniques include mass spectrometry-based protein quantification, immunochemical techniques, and should include enzyme activities. Microsomes are clearly the most widely used subcellular fraction for *in vitro* drug metabolism studies, and the liver is the most extensively studied organ. While a trend toward the underprediction of clearance by microsomes has been reported there is a reasonable *in vitro-in vivo* extrapolation of xenobiotic metabolism. While use of cytosol may be necessary if a compound undergoes metabolism mediated by enzymes found outside of the endoplasmic reticulum fraction, the availability of high-quality cryopreserved hepatocytes make the whole cell system a good choice for these studies. For compounds that undergo metabolism by several different enzyme systems different cofactors at appropriate concentrations need to be added. This may also be a situation where a whole-cell system may be more favorable.

The use of subcellular fractions to determine differences in metabolism between species is a useful tool to help in the choice of preclinical species in toxicology studies with coverage of prominent metabolites in humans. When human tissue is available the formation of a phenotyped bank is possible. While the utility of phenotyped bank is somewhat diminished with the availability of heterologously expressed enzymes it is still of value for early definition of metabolic routes and rates of formation for new drugs. A sufficiently large bank of subcellular fractions may also allow for an estimation of the variability in metabolism that may be present in the patient population. Subcellular fractions are also useful to predict hepatic clearance, which can be used to help choose first human dose and for enzyme phenotyping to determine the potential for a new drug to be a victim of drug-drug interactions. The P450 inhibition liability of a new chemical entity is determined using human liver microsomes, and this data may prevent the need for a clinical drug interaction study.

In conclusion, subcellular systems when supplemented with the required cofactors are a representation of only part of the whole cell and allows the scientist to control the enzyme system studied making this system extremely powerful. However, the need to take into account the regulatory effects of cell–cell contact-communication, the heterogeneous cellular nature of many organs, or the interplay between different enzymes and transporters require a whole cell system. These considerations aside, it is clear that subcellular fractions have many useful roles in the pharmaceutical industry.

ACKNOWLEDGEMENT

The author wishes to thank Jukka Mäenpää and Sean Ekins for their contributions to the initial version and Steve Wrighton and Barb Ring for their contributions to the second version.

REFERENCES

Achour, B., H. Al Feteisi, F. Lanucara, A. Rostami-Hodjegan and J. Barber (2017). "Global proteomic analysis of human liver microsomes: Rapid characterization and quantification of hepatic drug-metabolizing enzymes." *Drug Metab Dispos* **45**(6): 666–675.

Akazawa, T., Y. Uchida, E. Miyauchi, M. Tachikawa, S. Ohtsuki and T. Terasaki (2018). "High expression of UGT1A1/1A6 in monkey small intestine: Comparison of protein expression levels of cytochromes P450, UDP-glucuronosyltransferases, and transporters in small intestine of cynomolgus monkey and human." *Mol Pharm* **15**(1): 127–140.

Al Feteisi, H., B. Achour, A. Rostami-Hodjegan and J. Barber (2015). "Translational value of liquid chroma-tography coupled with tandem mass spectrometry-based quantitative proteomics for *in vitro-in vivo* extrapolation of drug metabolism and transport and considerations in selecting appropriate techniques." *Expert Opin Drug Metab Toxicol* **11**(9): 1357–1369.

Barr, J. T., J. P. Jones, C. A. Joswig-Jones and D. A. Rock (2013). "Absolute quantification of aldehyde oxidase protein in human liver using liquid chromatography-tandem mass spectrometry." *Mol Pharm* **10**(10): 3842–3849.

Bateman, K. P., M. Kellmann, H. Muenster, R. Papp and L. Taylor (2009). "Quantitative-qualitative data acquisition using a benchtop Orbitrap mass spectrometer." *J Am Soc Mass Spectrom* **20**(8): 1441–1450.

Bauman, J. N., J. M. Kelly, S. Tripathy, S. X. Zhao, W. W. Lam, A. S. Kalgutkar and R. S. Obach (2009). "Can *in vitro* metabolism-dependent covalent binding data distinguish hepatotoxic from nonhepato-toxic drugs? An analysis using human hepatocytes and liver S-9 fraction." *Chem Res Toxicol* **22**(2): 332–340.

Baxter, A. and J. P. Durham (1979). "A rapid, sensitive disk assay for the determination of glycoprotein glyco-syltransferases." *Anal Biochem* **98**(1): 95–101.

Bergmeyer, H. U. and E. Bernt (1974). Lactate dehydrogenase. *Methods of Enzymatic Analysis*. Bergmeyer, H. U. (Ed.), New York, Academic Press, pp. 574–579.

Bhatt, D. K. and B. Prasad (2017). "Critical Issues and Optimized Practices in Quantification of Protein abun-dance level to determine interindividual variability in DMET proteins by LC-MS/MS proteomics." *Clin Pharmacol Ther* **103**: 619–630.

Boberg, M., M. Vrana, A. Mehrotra, R. E. Pearce, A. Gaedigk, D. K. Bhatt, J. S. Leeder and B. Prasad (2017). "Age-dependent absolute abundance of hepatic carboxylesterases (CES1 and CES2) by LC-MS/MS proteomics: Application to PBPK modeling of oseltamivir *in vivo* pharmacokinetics in infants." *Drug Metab Dispos* **45**(2): 216–223.

Bonn, B., C. Leandersson, F. Fontaine and I. Zamora (2010). "Enhanced metabolite identification with MS(E) and a semi-automated software for structural elucidation." *Rapid Commun Mass Spectrom* **24**(21): 3127–3138.

Borlak, J., M. Blickwede, T. Hansen, W. Koch, M. Walles and K. Levsen (2005). "Metabolism of verapamil in cultures of rat alveolar epithelial cells and pharmacokinetics after administration by intravenous and inhalation routes." *Drug Metab Dispos* **33**(8): 1108–1114.

Burke, M. D. and S. Orrenius (1979). "Isolation and comparison of endoplasmic reticulum membranes and their mixed function oxidase activities from mammalian extrahepatic tissues." *Pharmacol Ther* **7**(3): 549–599.

Cerny, M. A. (2016). "Prevalence of non-cytochrome P450-mediated metabolism in food and drug adminis-tration-approved oral and intravenous drugs: 2006–2015." *Drug Metab Dispos* **44**(8): 1246–1252.

Chance, B. and D. Herbert (1950). "The enzymesubstrate compounds of bacterial catalase and peroxides." *Biochem J* **46**(4): 402–414.

Chapman, D. E., T. A. Christensen, S. R. Michener et al. (1993). Xenobiotic metabolism studies with human liver. In: Jeffery E. H (ed.), *Human Drug Metabolism from Molecular Biology to Man*. Boca Raton, FL, CRC Press.

Drexler, H. G. and S. M. Gignac (1994). "Characterization and expression of tartrate-resistant acid phospha-tase (TRAP) in hematopoietic cells." *Leukemia* **8**(3): 359–368.

EMA (2012). "Guideline on the investigation of drug interactions." from http://www.ema.europa.eu/docs/en_GB/document_library/Scientific_guideline/2012/07/WC500129606.pdf.

Emmelot, P., C. J. Bos, E. L. Benedetti and P. Ruemke (1964). "Studies on plasma membranes. I. Chemical composition and enzyme content of plasma membranes isolated from rat liver." *Biochim Biophys Acta* **90**: 126–145.

Emoto, C., N. Yoda, Y. Uno, K. Iwasaki, K. Umehara, E. Kashiyama and H. Yamazaki (2013). "Comparison of p450 enzymes between cynomolgus monkeys and humans: p450 identities, protein contents, kinetic parameters, and potential for inhibitory profiles." *Curr Drug Metab* **14**(2): 239–252.

Fallon, J. K., D. E. Harbourt, S. H. Maleki, F. K. Kessler, J. K. Ritter and P. C. Smith (2008). "Absolute quan-tification of human uridine-diphosphate glucuronosyl transferase (UGT) enzyme isoforms 1A1 and 1A6 by tandem LC-MS." *Drug Metab Lett* **2**(3): 210–222.

Fallon, J. K., H. Neubert, T. C. Goosen and P. C. Smith (2013). "Targeted precise quantification of 12 human recombinant uridine-diphosphate glucuronosyl transferase 1A and 2B isoforms using nano-ultra-high-performance liquid chromatography/tandem mass spectrometry with selected reaction monitoring." *Drug Metab Dispos* **41**(12): 2076–2080.

FDA (2017). "*In Vitro* Metabolism and Transporter Mediated Drug-Drug Interaction Studies Guidance for Industry." from https://www.fda.gov/downloads/Drugs/GuidanceComplianceRegulatoryInformation/Guidances/UCM581965.pdf.

Foti, R. S., L. C. Wienkers and J. L. Wahlstrom (2010). "Application of cytochrome P450 drug interaction screening in drug discovery." *Comb Chem High Throughput Screen* **13**(2): 145–158.

Furukawa, T., Y. Naritomi, K. Tetsuka, F. Nakamori, H. Moriguchi, K. Yamano, S. Terashita, K. Tabata and T. Teramura (2014). "Species differences in intestinal glucuronidation activities between humans, rats, dogs and monkeys." *Xenobiotica* **44**(3): 205–216.

Galetin, A. and J. B. Houston (2006). "Intestinal and hepatic metabolic activity of five cytochrome P450 enzymes: Impact on prediction of first-pass metabolism." *J Pharmacol Exp Ther* **318**(3): 1220–1229.

Gao, W., J. S. Johnston, D. D. Miller and J. T. Dalton (2006). "Interspecies differences in pharmacokinetics and metabolism of S-3-(4-acetylamino-phenoxy)-2-hydroxy-2-methyl-N-(4-nitro-3-trifluoromethylphenyl)-propionamide: the role of N-acetyltransferase." *Drug Metab Dispos* **34**(2): 254–260.

Garfinkel, D. (1958). "Studies on pig liver microsomes. I. Enzymic and pigment composition of different microsomal fractions." *Arch Biochem Biophys* **77**(2): 493–509.

Grimm, S. W., H. J. Einolf, S. D. Hall, K. He, H. K. Lim, K. H. Ling, C. Lu et al. (2009). "The conduct of *in vitro* studies to address time-dependent inhibition of drug-metabolizing enzymes: A perspective of the pharmaceutical research and manufacturers of America." *Drug Metab Dispos* **37**(7): 1355–1370.

Guengerich, F. (1994). Analysis and characterisation of enzymes. In: Hayes A. W (ed.) *Principles and Methods of Toxicology*. New York, Raven Press.

Gundert-Remy, U., U. Bernauer, B. Blomeke, B. Doring, E. Fabian, C. Goebel, S. Hessel et al. (2014). "Extrahepatic metabolism at the body's internal-external interfaces." *Drug Metab Rev* **46**(3): 291–324.

Gutman, M. (1978). "Modulation of mitochondrial succinate dehydrogenase activity, mechanism and function." *Mol Cell Biochem* **20**(1): 41–60.

Habig, W. H., M. J. Pabst and W. B. Jakoby (1974). "Glutathione S-transferases. The first enzymatic step in mercapturic acid formation." *J Biol Chem* **249**(22): 7130–7139.

Harbourt, D. E., J. K. Fallon, S. Ito, T. Baba, J. K. Ritter, G. L. Glish and P. C. Smith (2012). "Quantification of human uridine-diphosphate glucuronosyl transferase 1A isoforms in liver, intestine, and kidney using nanobore liquid chromatography-tandem mass spectrometry." *Anal Chem* **84**(1): 98–105.

Hille, R. and T. Nishino (1995). "Flavoprotein structure and mechanism. 4. Xanthine oxidase and xanthine dehydrogenase." *FASEB J* **9**(11): 995–1003.

Igawa, Y., S. Fujiwara, K. Ohura, T. Hirokawa, Y. Nishizawa, S. Uehara, Y. Uno and T. Imai (2016). "Differences in intestinal hydrolytic activities between cynomolgus monkeys and humans: Evaluation of substrate specificities using recombinant carboxylesterase 2 isozymes." *Mol Pharm* **13**(9): 3176–3186.

Ishizuka, T., Y. Yoshigae, N. Murayama and T. Izumi (2013). "Different hydrolases involved in bioactivation of prodrug-type angiotensin receptor blockers: Carboxymethylenebutenolidase and carboxylesterase 1." *Drug Metab Dispos* **41**(11): 1888–1895.

Ito, K. and J. B. Houston (2005). "Prediction of human drug clearance from *in vitro* and preclinical data using physiologically based and empirical approaches." *Pharm Res* **22**(1): 103–112.

Jia, L. and X. Liu (2007). "The conduct of drug metabolism studies considered good practice (II): *In vitro* experiments." *Curr Drug Metab* **8**(8): 822–829.

Kadono, K., A. Koakutsu, Y. Naritomi, S. Terashita, K. Tabata and T. Teramura (2014). "Comparison of intestinal metabolism of CYP3A substrates between rats and humans: Application of portal-systemic concentration difference method." *Xenobiotica* **44**(6): 511–521.

Kaminsky, L. S. and Q. Y. Zhang (2003). "The small intestine as a xenobiotic-metabolizing organ." *Drug Metab Dispos* **31**(12): 1520–1525.

Kawakami, H., S. Ohtsuki, J. Kamiie, T. Suzuki, T. Abe and T. Terasaki (2011). "Simultaneous absolute quantification of 11 cytochrome P450 isoforms in human liver microsomes by liquid chromatography tandem mass spectrometry with in silico target peptide selection." *J Pharm Sci* **100**(1): 341–352.

Kobayashi, Y., T. Fukami, A. Nakajima, A. Watanabe, M. Nakajima and T. Yokoi (2012). "Species differences in tissue distribution and enzyme activities of arylacetamide deacetylase in human, rat, and mouse." *Drug Metab Dispos* 40(4): 671–679.

Kolars, J. C., K. S. Lown, P. Schmiedlin-Ren, M. Ghosh, C. Fang, S. A. Wrighton, R. M. Merion and P. B. Watkins (1994). "CYP3A gene expression in human gut epithelium." *Pharmacogenetics* 4(5): 247–259.

Kropp, H., J. G. Sundelof, R. Hajdu and F. M. Kahan (1982). "Metabolism of thienamycin and related carbapenem antibiotics by the renal dipeptidase, dehydropeptidase." *Antimicrob Agents Chemother* 22(1): 62–70.

Litterst, C. L., E. G. Mimnaugh, R. L. Reagan and T. E. Gram (1975). "Comparison of *in vitro* drug metabolism by lung, liver, and kidney of several common laboratory species." *Drug Metab Dispos* 3(4): 259–265.

Lombardo, A., L. Caimi, S. Marchesini, G. C. Goi and G. Tettamanti (1980). "Enzymes of lysosomal origin in human plasma and serum: Assay conditions and parameters influencing the assay." *Clin Chim Acta* 108(3): 337–346.

Madani, S., M. F. Paine, L. Lewis, K. E. Thummel and D. D. Shen (1999). "Comparison of CYP2D6 content and metoprolol oxidation between microsomes isolated from human livers and small intestines." *Pharm Res* 16(8): 1199–1205.

Manevski, N., P. S. Moreolo, J. Yli-Kauhaluoma and M. Finel (2011). "Bovine serum albumin decreases Km values of human UDP-glucuronosyltransferases 1A9 and 2B7 and increases Vmax values of UGT1A9." *Drug Metab Dispos* 39(11): 2117–2129.

Manevski, N., P. Swart, K. K. Balavenkatraman, B. Bertschi, G. Camenisch, O. Kretz, H. Schiller et al. (2015). "Phase II metabolism in human skin: Skin explants show full coverage for glucuronidation, sulfation, N-acetylation, catechol methylation, and glutathione conjugation." *Drug Metab Dispos* 43(1): 126–139.

Masters, Jr B. S., Williams, Js C. H. and Kamin, H. (1967). "The preparation and properties of microsomal NADPH-cytochrome c reductase from pig liver." *Methods Enzymol* 10: 565–573.

McCann, J., E. Choi, E. Yamasaki and B. N. Ames (1975). "Detection of carcinogens as mutagens in the Salmonella/microsome test: Assay of 300 chemicals." *Proc Natl Acad Sci USA* 72(12): 5135–5139.

McCracken, N. W., P. G. Blain and F. M. Williams (1993). "Nature and role of xenobiotic metabolizing esterases in rat liver, lung, skin and blood." *Biochem Pharmacol* 45(1): 31–36.

Meyer, R. P., M. Gehlhaus, R. Knoth and B. Volk (2007). "Expression and function of cytochrome p450 in brain drug metabolism." *Curr Drug Metab* 8(4): 297–306.

Mukai, M., T. Isobe, K. Okada, M. Murata, M. Shigeyama and N. Hanioka (2015). "Species and sex differences in propofol glucuronidation in liver microsomes of humans, monkeys, rats and mice." *Pharmazie* 70(7): 466–470.

Narimatsu, S., N. Kobayashi, K. Asaoka, Y. Masubuchi, T. Horie, M. Hosokawa, T. Ishikawa et al. (2001). "High-performance liquid chromatographic analysis of the sulfation of 4-hydroxypropranolol enantiomers by monkey liver cytosol." *Chirality* 13(3): 140–147.

Nishimuta, H., J. B. Houston and A. Galetin (2014). "Hepatic, intestinal, renal, and plasma hydrolysis of prodrugs in human, cynomolgus monkey, dog, and rat: Implications for *in vitro-in vivo* extrapolation of clearance of prodrugs." *Drug Metab Dispos* 42(9): 1522–1531.

Nishimuta, H., K. Sato, Y. Mizuki, M. Yabuki and S. Komuro (2011). "Species differences in intestinal metabolic activities of cytochrome P450 isoforms between cynomolgus monkeys and humans." *Drug Metab Pharmacokinet* 26(3): 300–306.

Nishimuta, H., T. Nakagawa, N. Nomura and M. Yabuki (2013). "Species differences in hepatic and intestinal metabolic activities for 43 human cytochrome P450 substrates between humans and rats or dogs." *Xenobiotica* 43(11): 948–955.

Obach, R. S., J. G. Baxter, T. E. Liston, B. M. Silber, B. C. Jones, F. MacIntyre, D. J. Rance and P. Wastall (1997). "The prediction of human pharmacokinetic parameters from preclinical and *in vitro* metabolism data." *J Pharmacol Exp Ther* 283(1): 46–58.

Ohtsuki, S., O. Schaefer, H. Kawakami, T. Inoue, S. Liehner, A. Saito, N. Ishiguro, W. Kishimoto, E. Ludwig-Schwellinger, T. Ebner and T. Terasaki (2012). "Simultaneous absolute protein quantification of transporters, cytochromes P450, and UDP-glucuronosyltransferases as a novel approach for the characterization of individual human liver: Comparison with mRNA levels and activities." *Drug Metab Dispos* 40(1): 83–92.

Oliveira, P., A. Fortuna, G. Alves and A. Falcao (2016). "Drug-metabolizing enzymes and efflux transporters in nasal epithelium: Influence on the bioavailability of intranasally administered drugs." *Curr Drug Metab* **17**(7): 628–647.

Paine, M. F., M. Khalighi, J. M. Fisher, D. D. Shen, K. L. Kunze, C. L. Marsh, J. D. Perkins and K. E. Thummel (1997). "Characterization of interintestinal and intraintestinal variations in human CYP3A– dependent metabolism." *J Pharmacol Exp Ther* **283**(3): 1552–1562.

Paiva, A. A., C. Klakouski, S. Li, B. M. Johnson, Y. Z. Shu, J. Josephs, T. Zvyaga, I. Zamora and W. Z. Shou (2017). "Development, optimization and implementation of a centralized metabolic soft spot assay." *Bioanalysis* **9**(7): 541–552.

Pearce, R. E., C. J. McIntyre, A. Madan, U. Sanzgiri, A. J. Draper, P. L. Bullock, D. C. Cook, L. A. Burton, J. Latham, C. Nevins and A. Parkinson (1996). "Effects of freezing, thawing, and storing human liver microsomes on cytochrome P450 activity." *Arch Biochem Biophys* **331**(2): 145–169.

Pennington, R. J. (1961). "Biochemistry of dystrophic muscle. Mitochondrial succinate-tetrazolium reductase and adenosine triphosphatase." *Biochem J* **80**: 649–654.

Powis, G. and A. R. Boobis (1975). "Effect of washing the hepatic microsomal fraction in sucrose solutions and in sucrose solution containing EDTA upon the metabolism of foreign compounds." *Biochem Pharmacol* **24**(19): 1771–1776.

Powis, G., I. Jardine, R. Van Dyke, R. Weinshilboum, D. Moore, T. Wilke, W. Rhodes, R. Nelson, L. Benson and C. Szumlanski (1988). "Foreign compound metabolism studies with human liver obtained as surgical waste. Relation to donor characteristics and effects of tissue storage." *Drug Metab Dispos* **16**(4): 582–589.

Ravindranath, V. and H. W. Strobel (2013). "Cytochrome P450-mediated metabolism in brain: Functional roles and their implications." *Expert Opin Drug Metab Toxicol* **9**(5): 551–558.

Sarkar, M. A. (1992). "Drug metabolism in the nasal mucosa." *Pharm Res* **9**(1): 1–9.

Schmidt, E. (1974). Glutamate dehydrogenase. *Methods of Enzymatic Analysis*. B. HU. New York, Academic Press, pp. 650–656.

Schnaitman, C., V. G. Erwin and J. W. Greenawalt (1967). "The submitochondrial localization of monoamine oxidase. An enzymatic marker for the outer membrane of rat liver mitochondria." *J Cell Biol* **32**(3): 719–735.

Sharer, J. E., L. A. Shipley, M. R. Vandenbranden, S. N. Binkley and S. A. Wrighton (1995). "Comparisons of phase I and phase II *in vitro* hepatic enzyme activities of human, dog, rhesus monkey, and cynomolgus monkey." *Drug Metab Dispos* **23**(11): 1231–1241.

Siekevitz, P. (1962). "Preparation of microsomes and submicrosomal fractions: Mammalian." *Methods Enzymolgy* **5**: 61–68.

Stevens, J. C., L. A. Shipley, J. R. Cashman, M. Vandenbranden and S. A. Wrighton (1993). "Comparison of human and rhesus monkey *in vitro* phase I and phase II hepatic drug metabolism activities." *Drug Metab Dispos* **21**(5): 753–760.

Stohs, S. J., R. C. Grafstrom, M. D. Burke, P. W. Moldeus and S. G. Orrenius (1976). "The isolation of rat intestinal microsomes with stable cytochrome P-450 and their metabolism of benzo(alpha) pyrene." *Arch Biochem Biophys* **177**(1): 105–116.

Takahashi, M., T. Washio, N. Suzuki, K. Igeta and S. Yamashita (2009). "The species differences of intestinal drug absorption and first-pass metabolism between cynomolgus monkeys and humans." *J Pharm Sci* **98**(11): 4343–4353.

Usui, T., M. Mise, T. Hashizume, M. Yabuki and S. Komuro (2009). "Evaluation of the potential for drug-induced liver injury based on *in vitro* covalent binding to human liver proteins." *Drug Metab Dispos* **37**(12): 2383–2392.

Wang, M. Z., J. Q. Wu, J. B. Dennison, A. S. Bridges, S. D. Hall, S. Kornbluth, R. R. Tidwell et al. (2008). "A gel-free MS-based quantitative proteomic approach accurately measures cytochrome P450 protein concentrations in human liver microsomes." *Proteomics* **8**(20): 4186–4196.

Wang, X., Y. Liang, L. Liu, J. Shi and H. J. Zhu (2016). "Targeted absolute quantitative proteomics with SILAC internal standards and unlabeled full-length protein calibrators (TAQSI)." *Rapid Commun Mass Spectrom* **30**(5): 553–561.

Wikstrom, M. K. (1977). "Proton pump coupled to cytochrome c oxidase in mitochondria." *Nature* **266**(5599): 271–273.

Wiśniewski, J. R., C. Wegler, P. Artursson (2016). "Subcellular fractionation of human liver reveals limits in global proteomic quantification from isolated fractions." *Anal Biochem.* **15**(509): 82–88.

Wood, F. L., J. B. Houston and D. Hallifax (2017). "Clearance prediction methodology needs fundamental improvement: Trends common to rat and human hepatocytes/microsomes and implications for experimental methodology." *Drug Metab Dispos* **45**(11): 1178–1188.

Wynne, H. A., P. Wood, B. Herd, P. Wright, M. D. Rawlins and O. F. James (1992). "The association of age with the activity of alcohol dehydrogenase in human liver." *Age Ageing* **21**(6): 417–420.

Yan, T., S. Gao, X. Peng, J. Shi, C. Xie, Q. Li, L. Lu, Y. Wang, F. Zhou, Z. Liu and M. Hu (2015). "Significantly decreased and more variable expression of major CYPs and UGTs in liver microsomes prepared from HBV-positive human hepatocellular carcinoma and matched pericarcinomatous tissues determined using an isotope label-free UPLC-MS/MS method." *Pharm Res* **32**(3): 1141–1157.

Yoshida, T., T. Fukami, T. Kurokawa, S. Gotoh, A. Oda and M. Nakajima (2018). "Difference in substrate specificity of carboxylesterase and arylacetamide deacetylase between dogs and humans." *Eur J Pharm Sci* **111**: 167–176.

Zelesky, V., R. Schneider, J. Janiszewski, I. Zamora, J. Ferguson and M. Troutman (2013). "Software automation tools for increased throughput metabolic soft-spot identification in early drug discovery." *Bioanalysis* **5**(10): 1165–1179.

Zhang, J. Y., Y. Wang and C. Prakash (2006). "Xenobiotic-metabolizing enzymes in human lung." *Curr Drug Metab* **7**(8): 939–948.

Zhu, X., Y. Chen and R. Subramanian (2014). "Comparison of information-dependent acquisition, SWATH, and MS(All) techniques in metabolite identification study employing ultrahigh-performance liquid chromatography-quadrupole time-of-flight mass spectrometry." *Anal Chem* **86**(2): 1202–1209.

16

Drug Interaction Studies in the Drug Development Process: Studies In Vitro

R. Scott Obach and Kimberly Lapham

CONTENTS

Introduction: *In Vitro* Inhibition in Drug Development

Determination of the potential effects of new molecules on the activities of drug metabolizing enzymes *in vitro* can be useful in several areas of drug research. The data can serve as an indicator of whether a new compound could cause pharmacokinetic-based drug-drug interactions. In early research, such assays can be conducted using high-throughput approaches to accommodate the large numbers of compounds synthesized and tested for pharmacological activity (Figure 16.1). To be fit-for-purpose (i.e., development

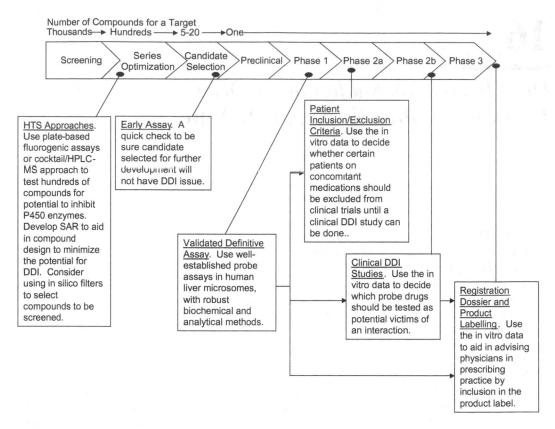

FIGURE 16.1 Strategy for placement of *in vitro* inhibition studies in the drug discovery and development processes.

of structure-activity relationships, driving compound design), these assays require high capacity and sacrifice some aspects of assay performance to allow for this capacity. Miniaturized methods that use fluorogenic substrates and plate reader platforms[1] or cocktail methods (in which multiple substrates are mixed and the assays done simultaneously[2] are well suited for these needs.

The focus of this chapter is on *in vitro* methods used during the latter development phase of drug research (Figure 16.1). The purposes of the *in vitro* inhibition data gathered during this phase are for (a) determining which drug metabolizing enzymes are unaffected by the drug candidate, (b) planning a clinical drug-drug interaction strategy (i.e., which, if any, drug interactions should be anticipated and explored in clinical studies), and (c) product labeling used to advise prescribing physicians whether certain drug combinations should be avoided. Because conclusions are drawn from these *in vitro* data regarding the potential safety of human study subjects and patients and potentially forgoing clinical drug-drug interaction (DDI) studies, it is of utmost importance that the data is unassailable—there is no room for error. Thus, unlike the aforementioned assay approaches appropriate for early drug research, *in vitro* inhibition studies done in support of compounds in the development phase must be done with a high degree of accuracy and no chance of false negative results. While it has not been mandated from government drug regulatory agencies that such assays be done under the guidance of Good Laboratory Practices, some have suggested that this be considered.[3] Since the publication of the previous edition of this book, some of the government drug regulatory agencies have issued guidance or draft guidance documents that include descriptions of the conduct of *in vitro* DDI studies and their interpretation.[4] The description of methods and approaches in this chapter are consistent with the expectations of these agencies.

This chapter describes the assays used for testing new compounds as inhibitors of drug metabolizing enzymes during the later phases of drug research and how the data can be used in drug development. It will not cover the aforementioned high throughput methods applied in early drug research and readers are directed to other reviews of that topic.[5] Also, this chapter addresses the testing of new drugs as potential "perpetrators" or "precipitants" of drug interactions. Focus on new compounds as "victims" or "objects" of drug interactions using *in vitro* data that aim to identify the enzyme(s) involved in the metabolism of a new drug is in Chapter 15 in this volume.

Elements of Assay Design and Performance

Biochemical Elements

The possible sources of drug metabolizing enzymes for determination of enzyme kinetics and inhibition data include pure enzymes, enzymes expressed in heterologous systems from recombinant DNA, tissue subcellular fractions, or whole cell assays. Pros and cons can be derived for each of these systems. The focus of this chapter will be on the most frequently used system (liver microsomes) to address the potential for DDI with the most important drug metabolizing enzyme systems (cytochrome P450s and UGTs).

The collection of accurate *in vitro* inhibition data requires that fundamentally sound enzyme kinetic practices be employed. To ensure this, reaction characteristics must be well defined. The most important experimental variables for drug metabolism reactions are substrate concentration, incubation time, and protein concentration. Other important parameters such as temperature, pH, and buffer strength are usually set to match or mimic *in vivo* conditions. It should be noted that a temperature of 37°C and neutral pH are routinely used as standard since these are appropriate for human liver). However, there is variability around buffers used. Effects of different buffers and concentrations on drug metabolizing enzymes have been noted.[6] The incubation time needs to be long enough such that adequate product is formed for precise quantitation but it also must be within a linear range so that reaction velocities are accurate. Likewise, the protein concentration must be high enough to permit formation of an adequate amount of product to be measured but must not be so high as to consume too much substrate or show a non-linear relationship between reaction velocity and protein concentration. An initial experiment is required in which product formation is measured at multiple time points in incubations containing different concentrations of enzyme source. A lack of velocity linearity with time can arise from two sources: autoinactivation of the enzyme or too much substrate depletion. The substrate concentration chosen for this determination of linearity should be the lowest one anticipated to be used in substrate saturation experiments. A depiction of a linearity experiment is illustrated in Figure 16.2a. From this experiment, an incubation time and protein concentration can be selected for all subsequent experiments using the reaction and enzyme source. The lowest protein concentration that still yields adequate product formation should be selected. The use of high microsomal protein concentrations have been demonstrated to cause an alteration of inhibition constants for highly lipophilic drugs due to nonspecific binding.[7] The incubation time used can be the longest one feasible that is still linear (i.e. the reaction velocity does not fall below 95% of what is measured using earlier incubation time points) (Figure 16.2b). The linear formation of metabolite with increasing microsomal protein concentration should be verified at the chosen incubation time Figure 16.2c. When the enzyme source is changed (e.g., one lot of liver microsomes to another, from liver microsomes to heterologously expressed recombinant enzymes, etc.), this linearity determination must be re-done.

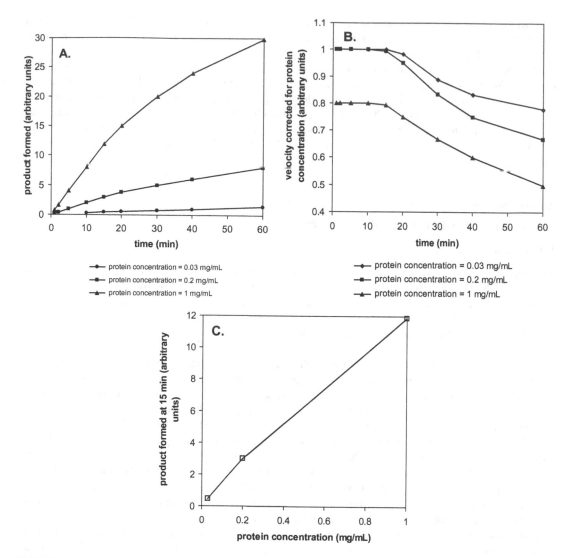

FIGURE 16.2 Demonstration of linearity of enzymatic reactions. In plot A, the product formed is measured over incubation time at three different protein concentrations. The limit of detection in this example is 0.25, so the incubation conducted at 0.03 mg/mL has too low a protein concentration because 95% inhibition would yield an amount of product that would be below the lower limit of quantitation (LLOQ) of the assay. In plot B, the data from plot A are converted to velocity values to determine the longest incubation time for which linearity is demonstrated. In this example, a maximum incubation time of 15 min should not be exceeded. In plot C, the velocity at 15 min is plotted versus the protein concentration, which shows that the reaction is linear for the 0.03 and 0.2 mg/mL concentrations but not the 1 mg/mL concentration. Therefore, a protein concentration of 0.2 mg/mL should not be exceeded.

After appropriate incubation conditions are established, a substrate saturation experiment is conducted to establish the enzyme kinetic parameters for the reaction in that system. The kinetic parameters, especially K_M, should be within a range of those reported in the scientific literature. The enzyme kinetic behavior for drug metabolism reactions may not follow the simple hyperbolic relationship defined by the basic Michaelis-Menten equation (Figure 16.3a and b). Other common kinetic phenomena include activation kinetics (i.e., Hill equation), substrate inhibition kinetics, or two-enzyme kinetics (Figure 16.3c–h). The kinetic behavior can be diagnosed using linearized plots of the data (e.g., Eadie-Hofstee plots), and the data fit using non-linear regression and statistical criteria, such as the Aikake Information Criteria, to select the most appropriate fit of the data.

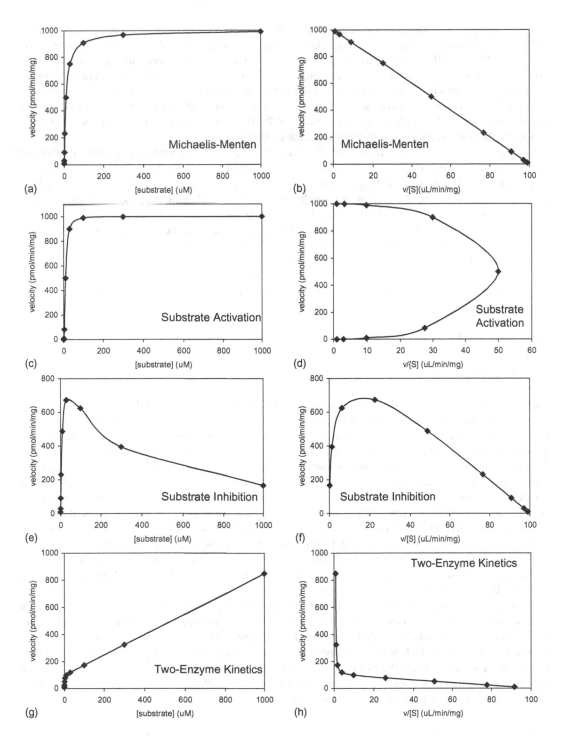

FIGURE 16.3 Four common enzyme kinetic models for cytochrome P450 and UGT catalyzed reactions in human liver microsomes. Left side (a, c, e, and g): substrate saturation curves; Right side (b, d, f, and h): Eadie-Hofstee transformed plots of the data on the left.

There is a special technical nuance regarding UGT incubations and the use of bovine serum albumin (BSA) as an additive to incubations. Drug glucuronidation kinetics for 3 of the 7 major hepatic UGTs (e.g., 1A9, 2B7, and 2B15) tend to underestimate *in vivo* rates. The addition of fatty acid free BSA significantly enhances enzyme activity thereby improving *in vivo* clearance correlations.[8] The mechanism by which BSA works is debatable; however, the result is a decrease in the $K_{m,u}$ with the potential for an increase in V_{max} depending on the substrate. Given that inclusion of 2% BSA improves *in vitro-in vivo* extrapolations (IVIVE) for clearance, the inclusion of 2% BSA could impact DDI predictions as demonstrated by the improved fluconazole-zidovudine interaction prediction.[9]

Binding of the test inhibitor to BSA is always a concern—especially for acidic compounds. Performing incubations in the presence and absence of BSA offers a window into whether BSA binding is preventing IC_{50} estimations. If a measurable IC_{50} is obtained in the absence of BSA but not in the presence of BSA then the inhibitor may need to be tested at higher concentrations. If limited aqueous solubility is also an issue, then the amount of BSA in the incubation can be decreased but it must be kept in mind that this could result in an underestimation of inhibitor potency. In the same vein, the apparent IC_{50} and the unbound IC_{50} could be dramatically different; therefore, measuring the free fraction of a test compound under the incubation conditions is needed before data can be interpreted.

The enzyme kinetic data are subsequently used to select the most appropriate substrate concentrations for routine testing of new compounds as inhibitors of drug metabolizing enzymes. A three-step testing paradigm of:

(a) Single inhibitor concentration
(b) IC_{50} determination
(c) K_i determination

can be resource sparing, yet still provide data needed for decision making in drug development. Initial testing should be done at a single concentration of test compound, using a substrate concentration at or below K_M, such that the large number of compounds that will show no effect can be adequately addressed with minimal yet appropriate resources (i.e., single concentration of test compound). For those compounds that demonstrate some degree of inhibition, a follow up in rapid succession can be done to measure IC_{50}, again using a substrate concentration at or below K_M. (If $[S] = K_M$, then it can be inferred that $IC_{50} = 2X K_i$ for a competitive inhibitor). The utility of such an approach is described in the Interpretation section below. Later on, a K_i can be determined using multiple substrate and inhibitor concentrations that will define the enzyme kinetic mechanism of inhibition. However, whether a compound is a competitive, noncompetitive, or uncompetitive inhibitor is not known to impact decision making around the potential for clinical relevance for DDI.

Testing whether a new compound can cause time-dependent inhibition is also important, as some of the most important clinical DDI are caused by drugs that are mechanism-based inactivators. This is particularly true for P450 enzymes but not so much for UGTs. Initial experiments in which the test compound is incubated with enzyme and cofactors in the absence of substrate, followed by addition of the substrate, or dilution into an incubation mixture containing substrate, can be done to detect whether a new compound is a time-dependent inhibitor. Follow-up experiments for those compounds demonstrating this activity can include the measurement of inactivation parameters k_{inact} and K_I (the maximum inactivation rate constant and the inactivator concentration that provides half of this rate), which can be used in prediction of DDI. However, specifics around the conduct of these experiments are described in Chapter 19 and will not be discussed in detail here.

Analytical Elements

High quality *in vitro* inhibition data requires not only sound enzyme kinetic practice but also robust quantitative methods to analyze the incubation samples. In this case, the assay is designed to quantitate the product of the reaction. Almost all standard assays used in the drug development phase utilize a chromatographic separation step in-line with either ultraviolet/visible (UV/VIS), fluorescence, or mass spectrometric (MS) detectors. While the early assays for P450 and UGT enzymes commonly used the two former techniques, current assays typically use tandem quadrupole MS/MS instrumentation using selected reaction monitoring. The sensitivity and specificity of this approach makes it the preferred standard for simple, robust assays.[10]

For *in vitro* samples, the sample work-up needed prior to sample analysis is generally simple, as compared to procedures usually required for other more complex biological matrices. For UV/VIS and fluorescence detection-based methods, some sample work up may be required in order to remove interfering endogenous materials or to concentrate the sample for effective detection. Samples will have required termination of the reaction, which is usually done by addition of miscible organic solvent, acid, or base. For more robust assays, a suitable internal standard will be added to account for intersample variability in analyte recovery and HPLC injector variability. Internal standards for UV/VIS and fluorescence methods should be structural analogues of the analytes that behave similarly throughout the sample processing technique, have similar detection properties, and are adequately resolved from the analyte (as well as the substrate) on HPLC. For MS detection, internal standards that are identical to the analyte except that at least three atoms are replaced with stable isotopes (i.e., ^{2}H, ^{13}C, or ^{15}N) to allow for an isotopic dilution approach to quantitation, and this is ideal when such materials are available. Liquid and solid-phase extraction techniques are typical for UV/VIS and fluorescence methods. For MS detection, filtration, or centrifugation of the samples is all that is needed so that protein, which can clog HPLC columns, is removed.

There are several standard criteria that must be met for an acceptable analytical method. These are:

(a) Assay Interferences Eliminated. The method used, typically HPLC, should be free of interferences from the matrix. In the case of *in vitro* assays, the matrix is usually a terminated incubation mixture containing a source of enzyme (e.g., liver microsomes), buffer, and other cofactors, and compared to most biological matrices this is fairly clean. To avoid problems, the analyte needs to be eluted from the column at a retention time that is after the time that the void volume elutes since this time is where most potential interferences will elute (i.e., absorbing materials for UV/VIS detection or ion suppressing materials for MS detection.) Thus, control samples in which the *in vitro* matrix lacking analyte should be run.

(b) Definition of a Standard Curve Range. The lower limit of quantitation LLOQ should be such that an uninhibited reaction should yield an amount of product that is 20-fold greater than the LLOQ; thus, allowing for the accurate determination of up to 95% inhibition. The upper limit of quantitation (ULOQ) should be high enough that the concentration of product formed does not exceed the ULOQ when the substrate incubations are done at saturating conditions (e.g., at [S] $\geq$ 9X K_M). The standard curve should contain a blank and at least four other points residing between LLOQ and ULOQ.

(c) Quality Control (QC) Standards. Separately prepared quality control standards at concentrations within the standard curve range should be analyzed and measured in each assay run, and the measured concentrations should be within −25% of the nominal value for the run to be considered acceptable.

(d) Stability of Standards and Stock Solutions. In most cases, the analytes (metabolites) for these assays are valuable materials and for cost and convenience it is advantageous to prepare stock solutions from which standard curve and quality control samples can be made, and to store these solutions for extended periods (e.g., months). Therefore, conditions under which such solutions can be stored (e.g., solution strength, solvent, temperature) need to be established and stock solutions that exceed this expiry need to be discarded and prepared fresh. The initial potency of standard solid materials needs to be established; if purchased from a vendor, this should be provided as part of the analytical specifications datasheet. Furthermore, storage stability of the standard solid materials needs to be established, using standard analytical methods (e.g., HPLC-UV). The solid material may need to be stored in a dry box containing desiccant or may have temperature requirements for storage.

In addition to these analytical assay characteristics, there are a couple aspects that are unique to *in vitro* incubation mixtures for DDI:

(e) Interference by the Test Compound. In rare instances, the compound being tested can share detection features of the analyte (i.e., absorbance in the same wavelength range for UV/VIS assays; same ions for MS assays) or interfere with the analyte response (i.e., coelution with the analyte and suppression of its signal in MS). This could yield misleading results such that the inhibition by a compound could be overlooked or a compound could be concluded to be an inhibitor when it is not. Therefore, the test compound at the highest concentration tested should be added to a QC sample to ensure that the QC response is minimally affected.

(f) Interference by Contamination in the Substrate. For some assays, the substrate material can contain the product (analyte) as a trace contaminant. This is particularly common for P450 reactions in which the reaction is one where some low level of spontaneous oxidation is energetically favorable (e.g., N-dealkylations; aromatizations). Since good enzyme kinetic practice demands that substrate turnover is kept to a minimum, even a very small level of impurity of the substrate by the product can confound inhibition assays. This needs to be tested when characterizing the assay and should be monitored in assay runs by including injection of the unincubated substrate at the highest concentration used. When unavoidable, a correction for this contamination can be applied, but this represents another source of variability that can confound an assay.

Individual Enzymes and Substrates: Cytochrome P450

Among the many drug metabolizing enzymes that could be potentially inhibited by new drugs, the ones of greatest focus are the cytochrome P450s followed by the UDP-glucuronosyltransferase enzymes. It is an expectation that the effects of new agents on these enzymes be studied and included in the government regulatory agency registration dossiers.[4]

The ideal reactions to use as probes for P450 activities will have the following characteristics: (a) selectivity for one enzyme, (b) high reaction rate, (c) readily available substrate, metabolite standard, and internal standard for the metabolite from common commercial suppliers at reasonable costs, (d) preferably has one metabolite product with unique spectral properties, (e) metabolite has high responsivity and selectivity in UV, fluorescence, or MS detectors, (f) substrate, metabolite, and internal standard possess stability as dry materials and in concentrated stock solutions, (g) substrate has high solubility in aqueous solution, (h) substrate is easy to handle (does not bind non-specifically to lab ware or microsomes), (i) materials are not DEA controlled substances, and (j) materials possess safety characteristics for routine use in the lab. None of the P450 or UGT probe substrates possess all of these properties, but the most important attribute is selectivity for one enzyme, and other attributes are sacrificed to varying extents to ensure that selectivity meets the needs of the analysis. The substrates and reactions described in the following sections are depicted in Figures 16.4 and 16.5, and listed in Table 16.1.

Cytochrome P4501A2

CYP1A2 is responsible for the clearance of numerous drugs. For clinical DDI, the most studied drugs that have a high dependence on CYP1A2 for clearance are theophylline and caffeine. Theophylline has a fairly low therapeutic index and some notable DDI arising from CYP1A2 inhibition were observed when enoxacin was prescribed to patients with bacterial infection who were already on chronic theophylline regimens to control asthma.[11] However, theophylline clearance is partially mediated by renal secretion, limiting the maximum DDI to about 5-fold, whereas caffeine has a much greater dependence on CYP1A2 for clearance.[12] Two other drugs have been noted to have very high dependence on CYP1A2 for clearance: tizanidine and ramelteon.[13]

The main *in vitro* assay to test for CYP1A2 inhibition in drug development is the phenacetin O-deethylase assay. The assay offers the advantage that the metabolite, acetaminophen, is readily available, inexpensive, and chemically stable. The earlier HPLC assays for measuring phenacetin O-deethylase activity in human liver microsomes involved the use of UV detection.[14] These have been adapted for MS detection, and preparation of stable isotope labeled acetaminophen is facile, to provide a robust assay.[10b,10c] Also, a radiometric assay was described, in which [^{14}C-ethyl]phenacetin was used as substrate and the radioactive acetaldehyde quantitated after separation from the unreacted substrate.[15] Phenacetin *O*-deethylation demonstrates linearity out to relatively long incubation times, allowing for the use of lower protein concentrations to still yield enough product formation for measurement. Interestingly, a wide range of K_M values have been reported for phenacetin *O*-deethylase, emphasizing the need that individual laboratories should determine their own enzyme kinetic parameters before conducting inhibition studies. Other enzymes besides CYP1A2 have been shown to catalyze phenacetin *O*-deethylase, but with high K_M values,[16] it is important that assays testing for CYP1A2 inhibition keep substrate concentrations within an appropriate range (i.e., <200 µM).

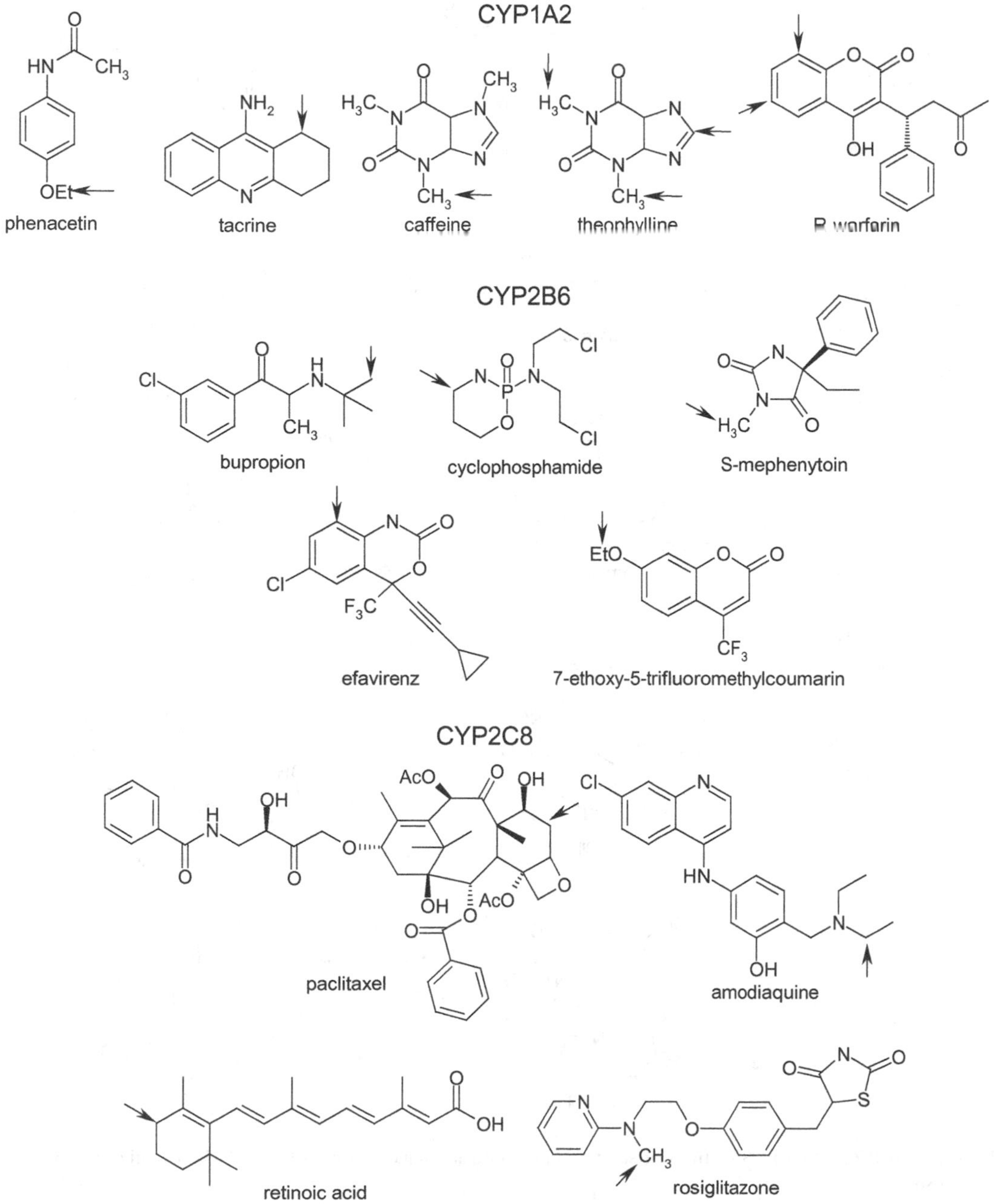

FIGURE 16.4   Structures of substrates used in measurement of cytochrome P450 activities and sites of metabolism.

(Continued)

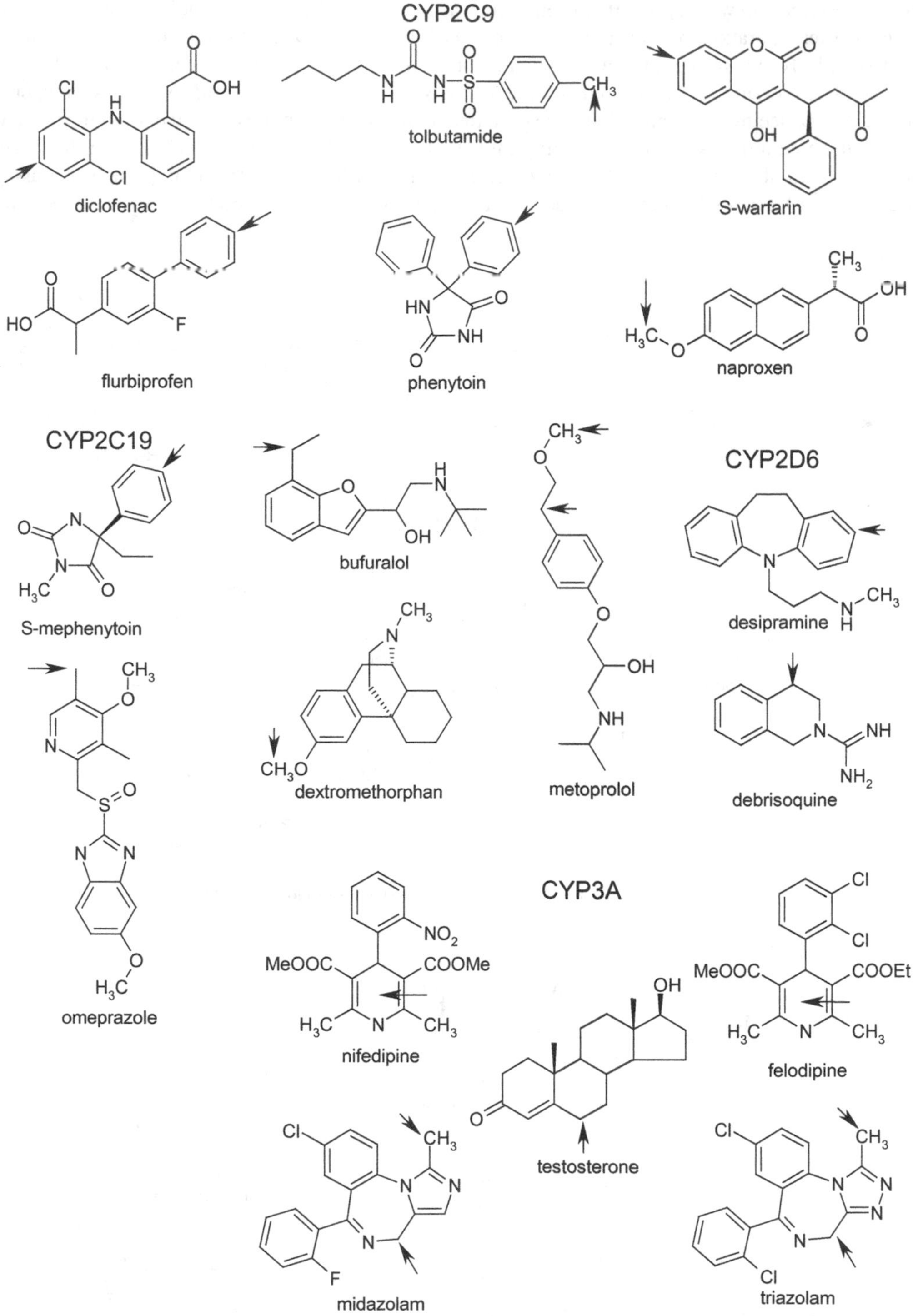

FIGURE 16.4 (Continued)   Structures of substrates used in measurement of cytochrome P450 activities and sites of
metabolism.   (*Continued*)

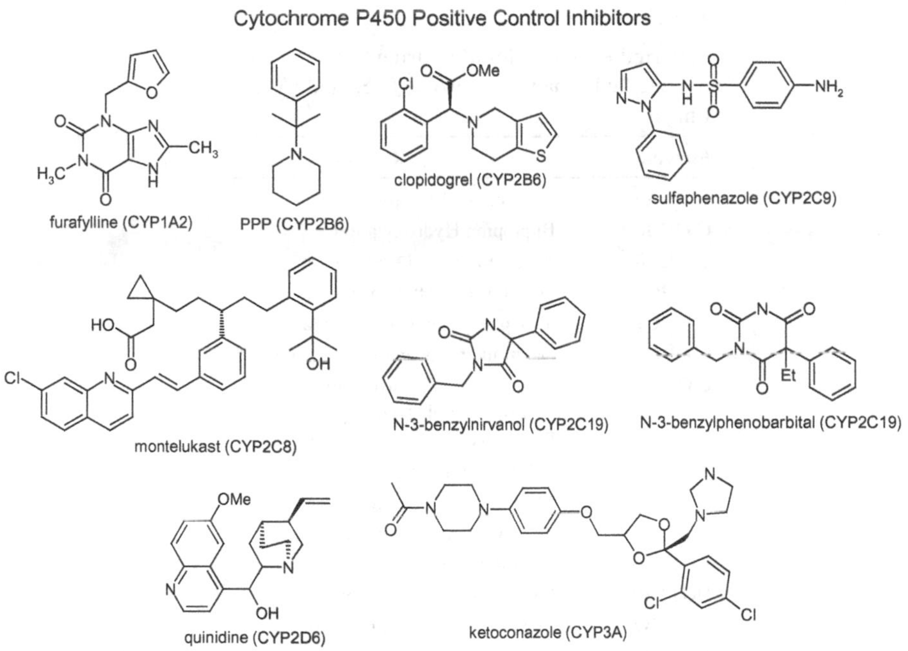

Cytochrome P450 Positive Control Inhibitors

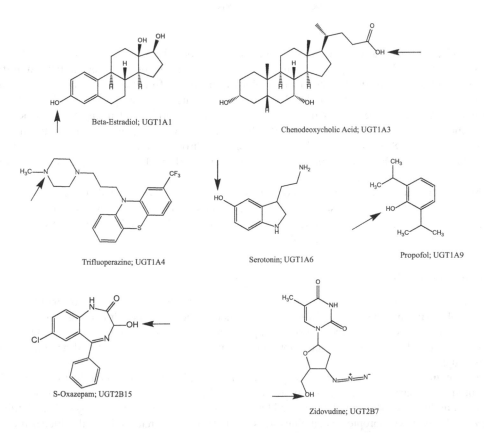

furafylline (CYP1A2)

PPP (CYP2B6)

clopidogrel (CYP2B6)

sulfaphenazole (CYP2C9)

montelukast (CYP2C8)

N-3-benzylnirvanol (CYP2C19)

N-3-benzylphenobarbital (CYP2C19)

quinidine (CYP2D6)

ketoconazole (CYP3A)

FIGURE 16.4 (Continued) Structures of substrates used in measurement of cytochrome P450 activities and sites of metabolism.

Beta-Estradiol; UGT1A1

Chenodeoxycholic Acid; UGT1A3

Trifluoperazine; UGT1A4

Serotonin; UGT1A6

Propofol; UGT1A9

S-Oxazepam; UGT2B15

Zidovudine; UGT2B7

FIGURE 16.5 Structures of substrates used in measurement of UGT activities and sites of conjugation.

TABLE 16.1

Preferred Reactions for Measuring Catalytic Activity
of Specific Human Cytochrome P450 and UGT
Enzymes

Enzyme	Reaction
CYP1A2	Phenacetin *O*-Deethylation
CYP2B6	Bupropion Hydroxylation
CYP2C8	Amodiaquine *N*-Deethylation
CYP2C9	Diclofenac 4′-Hydroxylation
CYP2C19	*S*-Mephenytoin 4′-Hydroxylation
CYP2D6	Dextromethorphan *O*-Demethylation
CYP3A[a]	Midazolam 1′-Hydroxylation
	Testosterone 6β-Hydroxylation
	Felodipine Dehydrogenation
UGT1A1	β-Estradiol 3-Glucuronidation
UGT1A3	Chenodeoxycholic Acid 24-Glucuronidation
UGT1A4	Trifluoperazine *N*-Glucuronidation
UGT1A6	Serotonin *O*-Glucuronidation
UGT1A9	Propofol Glucuronidation
UGT2B7	Zidovudine 5′-Glucuronidation
UGT2B15	*S*-Oxazepam Glucuronidation

[a] Due to substrate heterogeneity, more than one catalytic activity
is required to measure CYP3A activity. The degree of selectivity
of these reactions for CYP3A4 versus CYP3A5 is variable.

CYP1A2 activity has also been assayed using other reactions. Tacrine is hydroxylated to four regioi-someric products,[17] the major product being the 1-hydroxytacrine isomer. To accurately quantify this activity, 1-hydroxytacrine must be chromatographically separated from the 2-, 4-, and 7-hydroxytacrine minor products. While theophylline has been a commonly used *in vivo* probe for CYP1A2 activity, its use as an *in vitro* probe is limited by the very slow turnover to its *N*-demethylated products. Other less frequently used reactions for CYP1A2 have been caffeine *N*-demethylation to paraxanthine[14,18] and (R)-warfarin 6- and 8-hydroxylation,[19] which also require chromatographic resolution of other isomeric metabolites. Many of the assays used for CYP1A2 have cross-talk with CYP1A1, although expression of the latter in liver is very low.

Inhibitors that can be used as positive controls for CYP1A2 inhibition include furafylline and fluvox-amine. The former is a mechanism-based inactivator and should be incubated prior to addition of the substrate.[20] The latter is a potent reversible inhibitor[21] that also has activity against CYP2C19. Others inactivators include zileuton and rofecoxib.[22]

Cytochrome P4502B6

Relative to the other P450s discussed in this chapter, CYP2B6 is of generally lower importance in drug metabolism but it has been gaining in importance in recent years.[23] It is important in the bioactivation of the cytotoxic anticancer agent cyclophosphamide.[24] It has also been shown to be involved in the clearance of efavirenz and a contributing enzyme in the clearance of sertraline and buproprion among others.[7,25]

A commonly used *in vitro* probe reaction specific for CYP2B6 is bupropion hydroxylation. While bupropion is primarily cleared *in vivo* by reduction of the ketone,[26] the hydroxylation reaction on the t-butyl group has been shown to be mediated by CYP2B6 *in vitro*[27] and affected by CYP2B6 inhibitors *in vivo*.[28] The hydroxybupropion metabolite forms a stable six-membered cyclic ketal, which is likely what is detected on HPLC. The early HPLC-UV assays utilized a low wavelength to detect hydroxybupropion;

greater selectivity was afforded by the use of MS detection and stable isotope labeled hydroxybupropion is now commercially available for use as an internal standard.

Other assays that have been used to measure CYP2B6 activity have included cyclophosphamide 4-hydroxylation,[29] *S*-mephenytoin *N*-demethylation,[30] efavirenz 8-hydroxylation,[31] and 7-ethoxytrifluoromethylcoumarin *O*-deethylase.[32] The former three are HPLC-UV assays and the latter a plate-based method using fluorescence detection. The mephenytoin *N*-demethylation reaction suffers from the fact that CYP2B6 is a high K_M component and that CYP2C9 also catalyzes the reaction with a lower K_M; thus, requiring great care in selection of appropriate substrate concentrations. Inhibitors used as positive controls have included thioTEPA, clopidogrel, methylphenethyl piperidine ("PPP"), and orphenadrine. The latter is a reversible inhibitor with low potency and selectivity,[33] while the former three are mechanism-based inactivators.[34] Clopidogrel can be challenging to use because the ester group in it can be readily hydrolyzed and the resulting acid does not appear to inactivate, while thiotepa is not selective for CYP2B6.[34c]

Cytochrome P4502C8

While there are not many DDIs caused by inhibition of CYP2C8, there have been a few notable ones, including the inhibition of clearance of cerivastatin, repaglinide, and montelukast by gemfibrozil.[35] The mechanism of DDIs caused by gemfibrozil is mediated by inactivation by the gemfibrozil glucuronide metabolite and part of the effect on hepatic transport mechanisms.[36] The acyl glucuronide metabolite of clopidogrel has also been shown to be a mechanism-based inactivator of CYP2C8 and is putatively responsible for *in vivo* drug interactions with repaglinide.[37] It is possible that CYP2C8, by virtue of binding large anionic compounds, may be sensitive to inhibition by glucuronide conjugates. While 10 years ago the importance of CYP2C8 was just emerging, it is now considered an important enzyme that should be examined for the potential for new chemicals and drugs to affect it.

In early assays, CYP2C8 activity has been measured *in vitro* using paclitaxel 6α-hydroxylase or retinoic acid 4-hydroxylase activities.[38a–d] However, the cost of reagents for paclitaxel (drug, metabolite) and challenges in handling for retinoic acid reagents (instability), along with the discovery that CYP2C8 was the predominant enzyme in the catalysis of the *N*-deethylation of the antimalarial agent amodiquine has led to the adoption of the latter activity as a facile CYP2C8 marker activity.[39] The initial report utilized an HPLC-UV assay and this has been converted to a MS-based assay.[10b] Rosiglitazone *N*-demethylation has also been shown to be catalyzed by CYP2C8. However, this reaction also has a significant contribution by CYP2C9 making it a less optimal marker activity.[40] The most potent *in vitro* inhibitor of CYP2C8 is montelukast, with a potency in the nM range, with the caveat that the apparent potency is dependent on protein concentration used as montelukast demonstrates non-specific binding[41] and is also a substrate of CYP2C8.[42] Montelukast 36-hydroxylation was shown to be a CYP2C8 selective reaction.[43] Trimethoprim has also been shown to selectively inhibit CYP2C8 although with much lower potency.[44] Quercetin has also been used but is not specific for CYP2C8.[41]

Cytochrome P4502C9

CYP2C9 is one of the most important of the human P450s in DDI since it metabolizes hundreds of drugs, and in some instances its contribution to the clearance of some drugs predominates to a large enough extent that inhibition of the enzyme *in vivo* can result in substantial DDI.[45] The CYP2C9 substrate of greatest clinical concern is warfarin, since CYP2C9 catalyzed 7-hydroxylation contributes around 90% of the clearance of the pharmacologically potent *S*-isomer. Other drugs cleared by CYP2C9 include many NSAIDs and agents involved in regulation of glucose in diabetic patients, and there are many other classes of drugs to which CYP2C9 plays a contributory role in the clearance of some members of these classes (e.g., benzodiazepine anxiolytic agents, antidepressants, etc.).

The three most commonly used assays to measure CYP2C9 activity in *in vitro* inhibition studies are diclofenac 4′-hydroxylase, tolbutamide methyl hydroxylase, and (S)-warfarin 7-hydroxylase. Diclofenac 4′-hydroxylation is an easy assay to conduct since the rate is very high relative to other P450 assays. In the past, the challenge was obtaining suitable authentic standard for the 4′-hydroxy metabolite, and the material was expensive; however, biosynthetic methods have been developed that can yield gram quantities and have reduced the cost.[46] Early methods used HPLC-UV,[47] while later the assay was adapted for MS based detection.[10b,10c] Tolbutamide hydroxylase has also been used as a CYP2C9 marker activity, with early HPLC-UV assays and later on MS-based assays.[10b,48] A portion of this activity can be attributed to CYP2C19.[49] (S)-Warfarin 7-hydroxylase is selective for CYP2C9; however, use of this substrate in human liver microsomes requires that the regioisomeric metabolites (e.g., 6- and 8-hydroxywarfarin) be chromatographically resolved.[50] Other assays that have been used for CYP2C9 include flurbiprofen 4′-hydroxylase,[50b] naproxen O-demethylase,[51] and phenytoin p-hydroxylase,[52] although care must be taken when using naproxen or phenytoin since other P450 enzymes can contribute to metabolism of these substrates.[53] There has been evidence obtained that suggests that inhibitors of CYP2C9 will have different effects on different CYP2C9 reactions and different genetic variants of the enzyme.[52,54] The activities of a large panel of CYP2C9 inhibitors showed that there appear to be at least three classes of substrate for CYP2C9: S-warfarin as one class, flurbiprofen as a second, and a third that has diclofenac, tolbutamide, and phenytoin. For example, indomethacin inhibited CYP2C9 warfarin 7-hydroxylase activity with a potency (K_i) of 0.66 μM while inhibiting tolbutamide or diclofenac hydroxylase activities at 14 μM and inhibiting flurbiprofen hydroxylase at 53 μM. Such different potency values would lead to different conclusions to be made regarding the potential importance of the finding. There was no pattern regarding which activity would be most potently inhibited and some inhibitors demonstrated activities that did not depend on the specific substrate used, so for new compounds it presently cannot be predicted which substrate activity will be most potently inhibited. Furthermore, the carrier solvent can have an effect on the metabolism of some substrates but not others.[52] As a positive control inhibitor, sulfaphenazole has been shown to be selective[55] and consistently used and even the recent data regarding substrate classes have not altered the usefulness of this compound as a suitable, selective, positive control inhibitor. Tienilic acid is also a suitably selective mechanism-based inactivator of CYP2C9.[56]

Cytochrome P4502C19

CYP2C19 has been the focus of considerable attention over the years although there are actually very few drugs that have this enzyme as a large enough contributor to clearance that substantial DDI can be observed by inhibiting this enzyme. The 4′-hydroxylation of (S)-mephenytoin and the use of metabolite/parent ratios in urine have been the most studied experimental endpoints to measure CYP2C19 activity *in vivo* (for both enzyme activity and effects of genotype polymorphisms.[57] However, mephenytoin is not a therapeutically used drug. Omeprazole metabolism, specifically the hydroxylation of the methyl group on the 5-position of the pyridine ring, is a CYP2C19 selective activity and omeprazole demonstrates marked differences in pharmacokinetics in CYP2C19 extensive and poor metabolizers.[58]

The most frequently used assay for CYP2C19 is S-mephenytoin 4′-hydroxylase. Analysis of 4′-hydroxymephenytoin originated as an HPLC-UV method but has since been converted to a MS-based method as well as a tritium release approach.[10b,10c,59] The assay suffers from a slow turnover rate and possesses challenges in detection of the product as it neither absorbs UV light particularly strongly nor at long wavelengths. It also does not strongly ionize in HPLC-MS as compared to other P450 products. Fortunately, the CYP2C19 mephenytoin 4′-hydroxylase activity appears to be linear out to long (relative to other P450s) incubation times (e.g., >40 min) and the substrate does not bind to microsomes so that higher enzyme concentrations can be used compared to other activities. The only other activity widely used to measure CYP2C19 activity is omeprazole 5-hydroxylase. Selective positive control inhibitors for CYP2C19 are rare. Benzyl substituted nirvanol and phenobarbital have shown to be selective inhibitors for CYP2C19.[60] Ticlopidine had been reported to inactivate CYP2C19 but it also significantly affects other P450s,[34b,60b,61] and fluvoxamine is a potent reversible inhibitor, which also affects CYP1A2.

Cytochrome P4502D6

One of the most important drug metabolizing enzymes is CYP2D6. Compared to the other P450 enzymes, CYP2D6 tends to have a high affinity for many of its substrates and inhibitors and is frequently involved as an underlying mechanism for DDI. It is involved in the metabolism of many basic amine containing compounds including neuroleptics, antidepressants, and cardiovascular agents. Testing new experimental drugs for their potential to inhibit CYP2D6 is important because of the number of drugs cleared by this enzyme. However, it is noteworthy that many drugs that are cleared primarily by CYP2D6 have relatively large therapeutic indices because of the naturally occurring genetic polymorphisms that result in such a wide range of enzyme activities across the population. If a CYP2D6 cleared compound were to have a low therapeutic index, it would very challenging to use in clinical practice because the same dose level would be ineffective in many patients and toxic to many others.

While there are many possible selective substrates that could be used to measure CYP2D6 activity,[62] the most commonly used ones have been bufuralol 1'-hydroxylase, dextromethorphan *O*-demethylase, debrisoquine 4-hydroxlase,[63] and other activities have included metoprolol (both *O*-demethylation and α-hydroxylation[64]) desipramine 2-hydroxylation,[65] and sparteine dehydrogenation.[66] Bufuralol 1'-hydroxylase was originally run as an HPLC assay with fluorescence detection since the benzofuran ring system is highly fluorescent. The activity is almost exclusively dependent on CYP2D6, especially at concentrations <10 μM. Some contribution by CYP2C19, particularly when stereochemical considerations are made, is evident at higher concentrations,[66–67] but racemic bufuralol can be used reliably at an appropriate concentration range (<100 μM). Debrisoquine 4-hydroxylation has also been used as a selective probe activity for CYP2D6 using GC-MS methods.[68]

Dextromethorphan *O*-demethylase has been a widely utilized CYP2D6 probe substrate and possesses the advantage compared to bufuralol and debrisoquine activities that this probe is also used easily in clinical studies. Neither bufuralol or debrisoquine are available clinically in the USA. The dextrorphan/dextromethorphan urinary ratio has been a common CYP2D6 phenotyping tool in humans provided that urinary pH is not aberrant.[69] Likewise, the conversion of dextromethorphan to dextrorphan has been a commonly employed assay to measure the potential for new drugs to inhibit CYP2D6, with early assays employing HPLC with fluorescence detection[63] or radiometric detection using [*O*-methyl^{14}C]dextromethorphan as substrate[70] and later assays using mass spectrometric detection.[10b,10c] Dextromethorphan can also be *N*-demethylated to methoxymorphinan by CYP3A so care needs to be taken to resolve these two demethylated metabolites by HPLC and trace quantities of the *N*-desmethyl metabolite can be present as a contaminant in commercial samples of dextromethorphan. Otherwise, this assay is a robust and facile method for making this measurement. There are several compounds that could be potentially used as positive control inhibitors; however, the most regularly used one is quinidine.

Cytochrome P4503A

CYP3A poses the greatest complexities when attempting to measure the potential effect of a new drug as an inhibitor. First, the term "CYP3A" refers to two closely related enzymes CYP3A4 and CYP3A5, which have some subtle differences with regard to substrate and inhibitor specificities[71]; (see below). CYP3A5 possesses a common genetic polymorphism, with possession of two copies of genes coding for functional enzyme highly dependent on the ethnicity of the population.[72] Second, CYP3A4 is present in both liver and intestine, and both of these tissues plays a substantial role in the pharmacokinetics and DDI for CYP3A cleared drugs (reviewed in Galetin et al., 2007). Third, CYP3A, more often than other P450s, demonstrates atypical enzyme kinetic behaviors, including autoactivation, substrate inhibition kinetics, and heterotropic activation. These can be affected by cytochrome b_5 as well as buffer and Mg_{2+}.[73] Finally, CYP3A4 appears to possess different substrate classes (like CYP2C9 above) such that a new drug can show inhibition against some substrates but not others.[74] The *in vivo* relevance of these various phenomena is not known.

Assays to measure the effect on CYP3A in liver microsomes essentially measure the effect on CYP3A4 and 3A5 simultaneously. In liver microsome samples *pooled* from multiple individual donors, the amount of CYP3A4 should exceed the amount of CYP3A5 and dominate the activity; however, in individual samples the opposite can be true. With the observation of different effects of inhibitors on different activities, measurement of the effect of new drugs on CYP3A involves the operation of three different assays. One substrate class is well-represented by imidazobenzodiazepine drugs (e.g., midazolam, triazolam, etc.), a second by dihydropyridine calcium channel blockers (e.g., nifedipine, felodipine), and a third by steroids and macrolide antibiotics (e.g., testosterone, erythromycin, etc.). The three most commonly used assays are midazolam 1'-hydroxylase, testosterone 6β-hydroxylase, and nifedipine dehydrogenase.

Midazolam is metabolized at two positions by both CYP3A4 and 3A5: the 1'-methyl group and the 4-position on the diazepine ring. The 1'-hydroxylase assay is more commonly used. Measurement of the 4-hydroxymidazolam product can be challenging because the product demonstrates some instability. Midazolam also demonstrates time-dependent inhibition,[75] forcing the use of relatively quick incubation times (i.e., <5 min). Substrate inhibition kinetics are observed for midazolam 1'-hydroxylation, which requires that additional substrate concentrations be used when determining K_M values.[10b]

Testosterone is hydroxylated at several positions by several P450 enzymes; however, the hydroxylation at the 6-position in the β orientation predominates and is catalyzed by CYP3A4. Early assays utilized long HPLC-UV runs developed for rat metabolism experiments to permit resolution of the many hydroxytestosterone regioisomers[76]; optimization of the assay chromatography has resulted in more rapid HPLC-MS assays.[10b]

The third class of substrate represented by the dihydropyridine calcium channel blockers is the one that more often demonstrates the outlier behavior compared to the other two; with test compounds either inhibiting the other two and not affecting the dihydrpyridine metabolic activity (e.g., cyclosporine); or potently inhibiting the nifedipine dehydrogenation and affecting the others much less (e.g., haloperidol).[77] The use of nifedipine can be particularly challenging because of the instability of this compound with visible light. Felodipine does not have this problem to the same degree. In both cases, since dihydropyridines can spontaneously oxidize in air, obtaining substrates that are free of the metabolites is challenging. This requires the use of corrections for formation of dehydrogenated products in control incubations in which NADPH is not included.

To discern CYP3A4 and 3A5, a couple specific reactions have been shown to be catalyzed more efficiently by the latter enzyme than the former. Vincristine dehydrogenation to form an imine was observed to be catalyzed by CYP3A5 and not 3A4;[71d] however, this metabolite is difficult to synthesize and not commercially available. A discontinued phosphodiesterase-5 inhibitor was shown to undergo a pyridine *N*-oxidation reaction that was specifically catalyzed by CYP3A5, while other reactions on this compound were catalyzed by CYP3A4.[78] Unfortunately, this metabolite is also not commercially available. Some other substrates such as atazanavir appear to be better metabolized by CYP3A5 but not to the extent that they are selective.[79] Thus, the search continues for a selective CYP3A5 reaction that is easily employed in the lab.

Despite these complexities with CYP3A assays and substrates, ketoconazole can serve adequately as a positive control inhibitor. Ketoconazole is a potent inhibitor that binds by forming a tight ligand interaction with the heme iron and the imidazole and does not appear to be influenced by substrate. When CYP3A inhibition is observed in pooled human liver microsomes, it is advisable to test the effect on CYP3A4 and 3A5 separately. This can be accomplished by using recombinant enzymes, or by testing in liver microsome samples from different individual donors in which the amounts of CYP3A4 and 3A5 show considerable differences. Some CYP3A inhibitors such as TAO can be more potent for CYP3A4 than CYP3A5. Cyp3cide was recently described as a selective mechanism-based inactivator of CYP3A4 and a procedure for its use in assigning a relative CYP3A4 versus 3A5 contribution to metabolism using liver microsomes from CYP3A5 * 1 donors has been described.[80]

Individual Enzymes and Substrates: UDP Glucuronosyltransferases

UDP-Glucuronosyltransferase 1A1

Of the top 200 drugs that undergo glucuroniation as a clearance mechanism, UGT1A1 catalyzes reactions for 15% of them.[81] The most clinically studied UGT1A1 substrate is SN-38, the active metabolite of irinotecan. Co-administration of irinotecan with UGT1A1 inhibitors sorafenib[82] and lopinavir-ritonavir combination[83] have resulted in increased SN-38 plasma concentrations and in some cases given rise to adverse events such as diarrhea and neutropenia. UGT1A1 also catalyzes glucuronidation of the endogenous substrate bilirubin. When UGT1A1 enzyme activity is reduced, the unconjugated bilirubin levels can elevate resulting in jaundice. An increase in plasma bilirubin levels has been observed following indinavir administration,[84] which was attributed to direct inhibition of UGT1A1.[85] Following co-administration of atazanavir and the UGT1A1 substrate raltegravir,[86] mean bilirubin levels increased 200% and raltegravir pharmacokinetics increased.[87] Overall, the relative importance of UGT1A1 in drug metabolism merits investigation of the potential for new compounds to inhibit this enzyme.

The most common UGT1A1 substrate utilized *in vitro* is β-estradiol (ES). In human liver microsomes, ES is conjugated almost exclusively by UGT1A1 to form β-estradiol-3-glucuronide (ES3-G). ES3-G formation is characterized by atypical kinetics and is best fit using the Hill equation. Recombinant human UGTs 1A3, 1A8, and 1A10 also catalyze the formation of ES3-G;[88] however, quantitative targeted absolute proteomics (QTAP) by LC-MS/MS has demonstrated that UGT1A1 is significantly more abundant in the liver compared to UGT1A3,[89] and UGTs 1A8 and 1A10 are negligible in the liver, confirming ES as a suitable hepatic UGT1A1 substrate.

Alternative UGT1A1 probe substrates include bilirubin, SN-38, and etoposide. Bilirubin and its glucuronide metabolites can be challenging assays due to instability and non-specific binding.[90] SN-38 has low solubility and the stability of SN-38 in solution is questionable beyond a day.[91] Etoposide is glucuronidated almost exclusively by UGT1A1 with potential minor involvement from UGT1A3 and UGT1A8.[92]

Atazanavir is a well-documented inhibitor of UGT1A1 and is referred to in the FDA DDI guidance document as a potential clinical perpetrator of drug interactions.[4b] The IC_{50} value in human liver microsomes is 2.5 µM with the caveat that it also inhibits recombinant UGT1A3 and UGT1A4 catalytic activity with IC_{50} values of 7.9 and 21 µM, respectively.[93] Erlotinib inhibits UGT1A1 with an IC_{50} value of 4.19 µM in HLM.[94] However, it also inhibits UGT1A9 and UGT2B7 but to a lesser extent.[94]

UDP-Glucuronosyltransferase 1A3

UGT1A3 contributes to the metabolism of approximately 9% of the top 200 prescribed drugs that undergo glucuronidation-mediated clearance[81]; however, it seems none are truly selective for UGT1A3.

The most commonly used probe substrate for UGT1A3 is the bile acid chenodeoxycholic acid (CDCA) that undergoes conjugation to form CDCA-24-glucuronide.[95] CDCA-24 glucuronide formation kinetics in HLM result in a K_m value of 10.6 µM. Incubations in recombinant systems indicate CDCA-24 glucuronide is also catalyzed to a minor extent by UGTs 1A1 and 2B7;[96] however, UGT2B7 may be involved to a greater extent in the presence of BSA. Montelukast acyl-β-D-glucuronide is reportedly generated predominately by UGT1A3 based on kinetic analysis in HLM and experiments in recombinant UGT enzymes[97] with the potential for minor contribution from hepatic UGTs 1A1, 1A6, 1A9 as well as UGT1A7 and 1A8. The formation kinetics in HLM resulted in K_m values ranging from 0.9 to 1.72 µM and V_{max} values of 101–207 pmol/min/mg protein. The glucuronide metabolites for both CDCA and montelukast are commercially available.

Based on data generated in recombinant UGT1A3, additional probe substrates proposed for use *in vitro* includes 26,26,26,27,27-F6-1α,23S,25-trihydroxyvitamin D3,[98] R-lorazepam,[99] fimasartan,[100] telmisartan,[101] zolasartan,[102] desacetylcinobufagin-16-*O*-glucuronide[103] norursodeoxycholic acid-23-glucuronide,[104] and lithocholic acid and hyodeoxycholic acid.[105] However, the selectivity of these potential substrates should be further evaluated in human liver microsomes prior to their use.

Deoxyschizandrin[106] and pentacyclic triterpenoid-13 and -14,[107] components of herbals used in traditional Chinese medicine, have demonstrated potent inhibition of UGT1A3 in recombinant systems, but further testing in human liver microsomes and commercial availability is needed before having broader utility.

UDP-Glucuronosyltransferase 1A4

UGT1A4 is a common isoform involved in the glucuronidation of drugs and is second only to UGT2B7.[81] UGT1A4 catalyzes *N*-glucuronidation of amines,[108] such as lamotrigine, and azole containing compounds,[109] such as anastrozole,[110] but it's also capable of *O*-glucuronidation.[103,111] Given the preference for *N*-glucuronidation and the link between the number of nitrogens in a compound and lipophilicity, it is common for UGT1A4 to be involved in the conjugation of many antifungal and neurotherapeutic agents.

Clinically relevant DDIs associated with inhibition of UGT1A4 are minimal in frequency and severity. When asenapine, an antipsychotic agent that undergoes *N*-glucuronidation, was co-administered with valproate, asenapine-*N*-glucuronide $AUC_{0-\infty}$ and C_{max} were reduced 7.4- and 6.6-fold, respectively, but valproate did not significantly affect the pharmacokinetics of asenapine itself.[112] Probenecid resulted in statistically significant increases in olanzapine AUC_{0-24} (1.26-fold) and C_{max} (1.2-fold), but the increases were not clinically relevant.[113]

The UGT1A4 probe reaction routinely monitored *in vitro* is trifluoperazine *N*-glucuronidation.[114] The selectivity of this probe has been demonstrated across a panel of recombinant UGTs[108a,114] and confirmed in HLM with the selective UGT1A4 inhibitor hecogenin.[114] Trifluoperazine-*N*-glucuronidation $K_{m,u}$ in human liver microsomes decreased from 11 to 4.1 µM in the presence of 2% BSA suggesting fatty-acids released from the microsomal membrane have a minor but measurable effect on UGT1A4 enzyme activity.[6b] Trifluoperazine, trifluoperazine *N*-glucuronide and trifluoperazine-d3 *N*-glucuronide metabolite are all commercially available.

Other potential reactions reported to be selective for UGT1A4 catalytic activity include desacetylcinobufagin (DACB) 3β-*O*-glucuronide,[103] olanzapine-10'-*N*-glucuronide,[115] anastrozole-*N*-glucuronide[110] imipramine-*N*-glucuronide,[116] asenapine-*N*-glucuronide,[117] and 1-hydroxymidazolam–*N*-glucuronide and 4-hydroxymidazolam-*O*-glucuronide.[111] 3β-*O*-glucuronidation of DACB was shown to be selective reaction for UGT1A4 mediated *O*-glucuronidation in recombinant enzymes and glucuronide formation was significantly inhibited by hecogenin in HLM.[103] Olanzapine-10'-*N*-glucuronide and 4'-*N*-glucuronide were only formed by UGT1A4; however, 4'-*N*-glucuronide formation is very low in HLM and 10'-*N*-glucuronide is not available commercially.[115b] Asenapine-*N*-glucuronide was generalized as primarily a UGT1A4 mediated reaction, but the full panel of UGT isoforms has not been investigated.[117] Anastrozole-*N*-glucuronide was catalyzed predominately by UGT1A4 with minor contribution from UGTs 1A3 and 2B7.[110] BSA was not incorporated in the reactions; accordingly, it is possible the contribution from UGT2B7 is underestimated. Imipramine-*N*-glucuronide was only formed in recombinant UGT1A4; however, UGTs 2B4, 2B10, and 2B17 were not investigated. Additionally, imipramine-*N*-glucuronidation exhibited bi-phasic kinetics in human liver microsomes suggesting an additional UGT enzyme could be catalyzing glucuronidation.[116] 4'-Hydroxymidazolam-*O*-glucuronide and 1-hydroxymidazolam-*N*-glucuronide are reported as selective UGT1A4 mediated reactions; however, both exhibit sigmoidal kinetics with hill coefficients of 1.2 and 1.6, respectively. Analytically, the 1- and 4-hydroxy metabolites must be separated from each other.[111]

The most commonly used positive control is hecogenin, a highly selective inhibitor of UGT1A4 with an IC_{50} of 1.5 µM in human liver microsomes.[114] Finasteride has also been reported as a selective inhibitor in human liver microsomes with an IC_{50} of 11.5 µM.[118]

UDP-Glucuronosyltransferase 1A6

UGT1A6 is known for catalyzing the conjugation of non-bulky phenol molecules and primary amines.[108c] Although there are few drugs that undergo UGT1A6 mediated conjugation as the primary clearance mechanism, investigating the potential for a new chemical entity to inhibit this enzyme is of utmost importance given that it catalyzes the conjugation of important molecules such as acetaminophen, endogenous substrates like serotonin, and potential carcinogens related to hydroxylated polycyclic aryl hydrocarbons.

In vitro the most commonly monitored UGT1A6 reaction is serotonin-*O*-glucuronidase. The K_m value typically ranges from 5.2 to 8.8 mM in human liver microsomes.[119] Other potential reactions that could be monitored include 4-hydroxindole-*O*-glucuronidation,[120] 1-naphthol-*O*-glucuronidation,[121] 4-nitrophenyl-*O*-glucuronidation,[122] 5-hydroxytryptophol-*O*-glucuronidation,[123] and deferiprone 3-*O*-glucuronidation.[124] The K_m values are typically in the mM range suggesting UGT1A6 substrates have low affinity for the enzyme.[108c,125]

Oblongifolin C, a polycyclin polyprenylated acylphloroglucinol isolated from Garcinia plants, has demonstrated superior inhibition potency in recombinant UGT1A6 relative to the other major hepatic UGT enzymes with a competitive K_i value was 3.49 µM.[126] The superoxide of rose bengal, a xanthene dye, is a potent inhibitor of UGT1A6 (0.035 µM) in HLM when the oxygen species is formed under a yellow light;[127] however, further evaluation regarding selectivity is needed. In general, a commercially available, selective UGT1A6 inhibitor has not been fully characterized hence non-selective positive controls such as 1-napthol and troglitizone[96] are used in these assays.

UDP-Glucuronosyltransferase 1A9

Few clinical DDI studies have been conducted for UGT1A9 substrates (e.g., R- and S-morinidazole, canagliflozin, and dapagliflozin). Neither C_{max} nor AUC_{0-t} for morinidazole N^+-glucuronides demonstrated clinically significant changes when co-administered with ketoconazole.[128] Although modest changes in AUC and/or clearance were reported for canagliflozin and dapagliflozin, the changes were not considered clinically relevant.[129] To date, dapagliflozin demonstrated the largest UGT1A9 inhibitory DDI; co-administration of dapagliflozin with mefenamic acid to healthy volunteers resulted in a 51% increase in AUC.

Propofol[99,130] and mycophenolic acid[131] are highly selective and commonly used UGT1A9 enzyme assays. In HLM, previously reported K_m values for propofol ranged from 64 to 280 μM[6b,130,132] in the absence of BSA and in the presence of BSA the total K_m ranged from 16 to 46 μM.[6b,132] Mycophenolic acid K_m in the absence of BSA was 77 μM.[133] Individual kinetic parameters for mycophenolic acid in the presence of BSA have not been published. Additional potential selective UGT1A9 reactions include phenylbutazone-C-glucuronidation,[134] sulfinpyrazone-C-glucuronidation,[135] dapagliflozin-O-glucuronidation,[136] entacaptone-glucuronidation,[137] and psoralidin-3-O-glucuronidation;[138] however, the marker metabolites are not commercially available.

Common UGT1A9 inhibitors include mefenamic acid and niflumic acid. Mefenamic acid is potent against UGT1A9 but it appears to be equally potent against UGT2B7 in recombinant UGTs. Glucuronide formation was inhibited in recombinant UGT1A9 and UGT2B7 97% and 93%, respectively, at a concentration of 50 μM.[6b] Niflumic acid is a mixed mechanism inhibitor of propofol glucuronidation in HLM, with Ki values ranging from 0.1 to 0.4 μM. It also inhibits UGT1A1, but K_i values differ by 35-fold.[139]

UDP-Glucuronosyltransferase 2B7

UGT2B7 is one of the most important human conjugating enzymes given that UGT2B7 catalyzed the glucuronidation of 35% of the top 200 compounds that have glucuronidation as a clearance mechanism.[81] Additionally, UGT2B7 is the most abundant UGT enzyme in the liver compared to others[140] and is prevalent in kidney second only to UGT1A9.[141] Clinical DDI studies with zidovudine as the probe substrate have demonstrated relevant interactions with a variety of co-administered drugs. Probenecid,[142] valproic acid,[143] fluconazole,[144] methadone and atovaquone[145] are a few examples that have all resulted in 1.3- to 2-fold increase in zidovudine AUC corresponding to a decrease in clearance.

UGT2B7 activity is commonly measured *in vitro* using zidovudine-5'-glucuronidation activity.[6b,99,146] Similar to the UGT1A9 activity assay, UGT2B7 activity in human liver microsomes should be conducted in the presence of BSA. The $K_{m,u}$ for zidovudine-5'-glucuronidation in HLM decreases from 420 to 100 μM in the presence of 2% BSA[6b] without significant effect on V_{max} suggesting BSA increases the apparent substrate affinity (Figure 16.6). Zidovudine, zidovudine-5'-glucuronide and [$^{13}C_6$]zidovudine-5'-glucuronide are readily available for purchase from commercial vendors.

Other potential probe substrates for measuring UGT2B7 enzyme activity include morphine, epirubicin, denopamine, and 6α- and 21α-hydroxyprogesterone,[147] but they all are potentially problematic. Both morphine 3- and 6-glucuronide are catalyzed predominately by UGT2B7;[148] however, morphine is a Schedule II-controlled substance. Epirubicin glucuronidation demonstrated good correlation with morphine 3- and 6-glucuronidation in human liver microsomes;[149] however, UGT2B4 activity was not assessed. Further evaluation is needed since UGT2B7 and UGT2B4 exhibit overlapping substrate specificity.[150] Denopamine glucurondation was inhibited by diclofenac,[151] a known UGT2B7 substrate but a non-selective inhibitor;[152] thus, further evaluation is needed. Finally, glucuronide metabolite standards are not readily available for purchase for epirubicin, denopamine nor 6α- or 21α-hydroxyprogesterone.

16β-Phenyllongifolol has been reported as a potent and selective inhibitor of UGT2B7 but not commercially available. The IC_{50} is 91 nM in HLM in the absence of BSA.[153] In the presence of 2% BSA, the selectivity and potency is maintained.[154] Other inhibitors used *in vitro* including quinidine, diclofenac, and fluconazole are non-selective for UGT2B7.[9,96,114,152a,155]

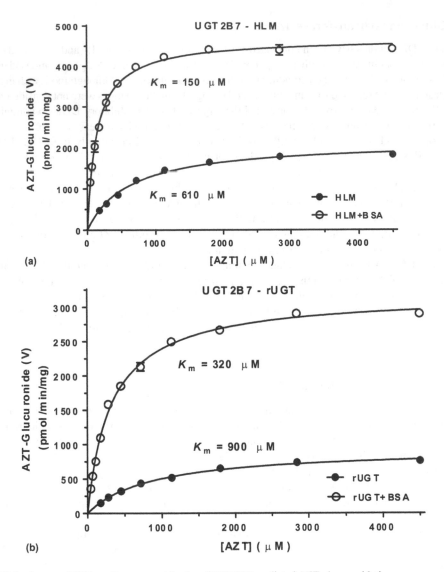

FIGURE 16.6 Impact of BSA on the enzyme kinetics of UGT2B7 mediated AZT glucuronidation.

UDP-Glucuronosyltransferase 2B15

There are few examples of DDIs resulting from the co-adminstration of UGT2B15 substrates with inhibitors. The co-administration of probenecid with the UGT2B7/2B15 substrate lorazepam resulted in a prolonged lorazepam half-life, an approximately 2-fold decrease in clearance, and a reduction in the formation of the ether glucuronide metabolite.[156] Valproate had a similar effect on lorazepam pharmacokinetics. This interaction resulted in a 20% increase in lorazepam AUC and 31% increase in the trough plasma concentrations albeit no pharmacodynamic changes were observed.[157]

The only reported selective probe substrate for UGT2B15 is oxazepam. Oxazepam is a racemic mixture of R- and S-diastereomers. S-Oxazepam glucuronidation is selective for UGT2B15, whereas R-oxazepam glucuronidation is catalyzed by UGTs 1A9 and 2B7.[158] The K_m for S-oxazepam glucuronidation in HLM ranged from 43 to 60 µM, similar to the apparent K_m in recombinant UGT2B15. The V_{max} values ranged from 267 to 325 pmol/min/mg. This reaction is the most challenging of all the UGTs mentioned. The incubation time is longer since the formation rate of S-oxazepam glucuronide is low. The separation of R- and S-glucuronides can be analytically challenging requiring a longer HPLC run time.

Finally, oxazepam is a schedule IV-controlled substance requiring special handling. Oxazepam and the (R/S)-oxazepam glucuronide mixture are available commercially.

Given that UGT2B15 enzyme activity was enhanced 2-fold in the presence of 0.1% BSA using 17α-estradiol (17-glucuronide) as the probe substrate[88,159] UGT2B15 inhibition assessments in the presence of BSA should be considered.

Other potential probe substrates include, 4-hydroxy-3-methoxymethamphetamine (HMMA),[160] bisphenol A,[161] and 5-hydroxyrofecoxib.[162] 5-Hydroxyrofecoxib is not desirable because it is light sensitive. Bisphenol A conjugation is catalyzed by UGTs 1A3, 2B4, and 2B7 in addition to 2B15 and HMMA metabolite is not commercially available.

A selective positive control inhibitor for UGT2B15 has yet to be identified. Typically, non-selective inhibitors such as valproic acid are used. At 5 mM concentration, valproic acid inhibits UGT2B7 enzyme activity 54% and UGT2B15 enzyme activity 36%–59%.[163]

Interpretation of Inhibition Data in Drug Development

Collection of *in vitro* data on the ability of experimental drugs to inhibit drug metabolizing enzymes is important to drug development because the information is used both in the design of clinical DDI studies and in determining enzymes requiring no further evaluation. Through the extensive amount of research conducted on P450 enzymes and their role in drug metabolism over the years, there is enough confidence to utilize *in vitro* information to make predictions of DDI without necessarily requiring that clinical DDI studies be run. In the drug development phase, *in vitro* inhibition data collected using the definitive methods described above need to be available before patients in phase 2 and 3 studies are dosed with the new compound. Without this information, patient recruitment may need to be limited to exclude patients on concomitant medications, because it would not be known whether the new compound could affect the clearance of the concomitant drugs. (Note that in some target indications, such as cancer, phase 1 study subjects are also patients on other medications, so the *in vitro* data should be gathered before administration of the new compound.) Two approaches to utilizing *in vitro* inhibition data for the drug metabolizing enzymes to predict DDI are described below.

Prediction of DDI

Although some of the fundamental principles describing the relationship between inhibitory potency and magnitude of DDI have been available for over three decades, the use of these relationships to predict DDI has only been reduced to practice over the past fifteen years or so.

Static Models. Predicting *in vivo* DDI from *in vitro* inhibition data begins with the Rowland-Matin equation[164] that describes the relationship between the magnitude of the DDI for a hepatically cleared orally administered drug and the inhibitory potency:

$$\text{Fold change in exposure} = \frac{CL_{po,control}}{CL_{po,inhibited}} = \frac{AUC_{inhibited}}{AUC_{control}} = \frac{1}{\dfrac{f_{CLh,CYP}}{\left(1 + \dfrac{[I]_{hepatic}}{K_i}\right)} + (1 - f_{CLh,CYP})}$$

$AUC_{inhibited}$ and $AUC_{control}$ are the exposure values to the affected drug in the presence and absence of the inhibiting drug respectively and $CL_{po,inhibited}$ and $CL_{po,control}$ are the oral clearance values for the affected drug in the presence and absence of the inhibiting drug, respectively. K_i is the inhibitory potency of the inhibiting drug against the enzyme that clears the affected drug and $[I]_{hepatic}$ is the intrahepatic concentration of the inhibiting drug that is available to bind to the enzyme. The value f_{CLh}, is the fraction of the affected drug that is cleared by the enzyme in the liver that is inhibited. The value of f_{CLh}, is important and provides a ceiling on the magnitude of the interaction; when this parameter is ignored the predictions of DDI will almost always be overestimated. For example, if f_{CLh}, is 0.5, then no matter how extensively the

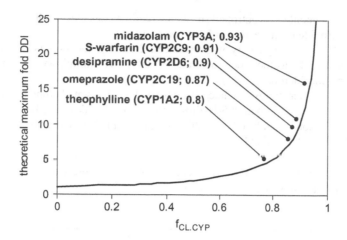

FIGURE 16.7 Theoretical maximum magnitude of a drug interaction versus the fraction of the victim drug cleared by the affected enzyme.

affected enzyme is inhibited, the largest interaction can be 2-fold. For f_{CLh}, values of 0.8 and above, larger interactions can theoretically be observed (Figure 16.7). Values of f_{CLh}, for victim drugs in which high confidence can be placed are not commonly available and estimates of these can be made from EM/PM pharmacokinetic studies (for CYP2C9, 2C19, and 2D6 cleared drugs) or from combining *in vitro* reaction phenotyping data with radiolabel ADME studies in humans. (Some examples of these are in Figure 16.7.) The value for K_i is the value measured from the *in vitro* study. In the case where just an IC_{50} is measured, competitive inhibition can be assumed, and the value converted to a K_i using the Cheng-Prusoff equation[165]:

$$K_i = \frac{IC_{50}}{1 + \dfrac{[S]}{K_M}}$$

(If the incubations are run at $[S] = K_M$ then $K_i = 0.5 \times IC_{50}$). These values refer to free values, assuming that all of the inhibitor in the *in vitro* incubation is free in solution to bind the enzyme. In some cases, this may not be true, especially for lipophilic cationic compounds that are known to bind non-specifically to phospholipid membranes in microsomes. In those instances, the free fraction of the inhibitor should be measured using mock incubation conditions.[7] The value for $[I]_{hep}$ represents an *in vivo* concentration that is unmeasurable and must be estimated. An assumption that unbound inhibitor concentrations in the plasma are equal to those in the liver is needed and that only unbound inhibitor can bind the enzyme (consistent with the free drug hypothesis). For this, the inhibitor must be able to freely diffuse across the cell membrane and there can be no active transport processes altering the ratio of free inhibitor concentration inside and outside the cell from a value of unity. Clearly, there are some drugs for which this assumption will not be valid, and there are *in vitro* methods available to better understand whether new compounds are substrates for hepatic transporters. Finally, for liver, the concentrations occurring during absorption can be profoundly greater than those in the systemic circulation. To deal with this factor, the value used for $[I]_{hep}$ is estimated from the following equation[166]:

$$[I]_{hepatic} = f_u \cdot \left(C_{max} + \frac{Dose \cdot F_{abs} \cdot k_{abs}}{Q_h} \right)$$

in which F_{abs} and k_{abs} are estimates of the fraction absorbed and the absorption rate constant for the inhibitor, respectively, C_{max} is the systemic maximum concentration of inhibitor, f_u is the unbound fraction of the inhibitor in plasma, and Q_h is hepatic blood flow (~21 mL/min/kg body weight). (If the blood/plasma ratio for the inhibitor is substantially different from unity, f_u will need to be corrected for this factor.) For drugs that inhibit hepatic enzymes, this approach predicts the magnitude of DDI with mean fold-error of 1.7X for victim drugs that are affected by 2-fold or more.[77]

For CYP3A, an additional consideration for the effect on the intestinal extraction during first-pass must also be considered. A similar equation is used to account for this:

$$\frac{AUC_{inhibited}}{AUC_{control}} = \frac{1}{\dfrac{f_{CLh,CYP3A}}{\left(1 + \dfrac{[I]_{hepatic}}{K_i}\right)} + (1 - f_{CLh,CYP3A})} \cdot \frac{1}{F_g + (1 - F_g) \cdot \left(\dfrac{1}{1 + \dfrac{[I]_{gut}}{K_i}}\right)}$$

The first term is the same and accounts for the effect on hepatic CYP3A. The second term addresses the effect in the intestine during first pass. The parameter F_g is the fraction of the victim drug that ordinarily evades first-pass extraction by the intestine in the control state. It can be estimated from the CYP3A4 *in vitro* intrinsic clearance combined with the knowledge of the ratio of CYP3A4 in the liver and the intestine (approximately 100:1[167]), the free fraction in plasma of the victim drug, and the *in vivo* oral clearance (assuming complete absorption). Or it can be obtained for drugs for which a pharmacokinetic study was done with liver transplant patients during the anhepatic phase of the procedure (e.g., midazolam; cyclosporine).[168] In many cases, the value of F_g can drive the prediction of DDI because the $[I]_{gut}/K_i$ ratio will be very high.[169] $[I]_{gut}$ is the concentration of the inhibitor in the intestinal enterocytes. It is estimated from:

$$[I]_{gut} = \frac{Dose \cdot F_{abs} \cdot k_{abs}}{Q_g}$$

in which Q_g is the intestinal flow (ca. 3.5 mL/min/kg body weight). Using this equation, the mean-fold error for CYP3A inhibitors that caused at least a 2-fold increase in a CYP3A cleared compound was 1.87.[77]

This sort of approach requires application of a static situation with the system fully at equilibrium. Thus, it uses some simplifications, and recently more sophisticated software packages have been developed based on this fundamental physiological approach that can better model the dynamic situation that occurs *in vivo*.

For time-dependent inhibitors, equations similar in structure can be used to make predictions of DDI, but with *in vitro* inactivation parameters (K_I and k_{inact}) in place of reversible K_i values and inclusion of *in vivo* degradation rate constants for the enzymes[71c,170]:

$$\frac{AUC_{inhibited}}{AUC_{control}} = \frac{1}{\dfrac{f_{CLh,CYP}}{\left(1 + \dfrac{k_{inact} \cdot [I]_{hepatic}}{k_{deg(CYP)} \cdot ([I]_{hepatic} + K_I)}\right)} + (1 - f_{CLh,CYP})}$$

is for hepatic enzymes and:

$$\frac{AUC_{inhibited}}{AUC_{control}} = \frac{1}{\dfrac{f_{CLh,CYP3A}}{\left(1 + \dfrac{k_{inact} \cdot [I]_{hepatic}}{k_{deg(CYP3A,hepatic)} \cdot ([I]_{hepatic} + K_I)}\right)} + (1 - f_{CLh,CYP3A})} \cdot$$

$$\frac{1}{F_g + (1 - F_g) \cdot \left(\dfrac{1}{1 + \dfrac{k_{inact} \cdot [I]_{gut}}{k_{deg(CYP3A,gut)} \cdot ([I]_{gut} + K_I)}}\right)}$$

for CYP3A that also incorporates the effect in the intestine. The other parameters are as described above. Values for *in vivo* degradation rate constants for P450 enzymes can be estimated from clinical inactivation and induction data.[77] Half-lives of 39, 51, 36, and 24 hours have been estimated for CYP1A2, CYP2D6, hepatic CYP3A4, and intestinal CYP3A4, respectively. Data needed to calculate these values for the other important P450 enzymes are not available, but since the values for the hepatic enzymes are fairly similar to each other, it might be assumed that degradation half-lives for CYP2B6, 2C8, 2C9, and 2C19 may be in the same range. The value for intestinal CYP3A4 is similar to the half-life for enterocytes, which are constantly sloughing off and being replenished. In general, this approach tends to over-predict the magnitude of DDI, even when using unbound systemic C_{max} for the value for $[I]_{hep}$.

Dynamic Models

While static models of DDI prediction from *in vitro* data offer a simple and conceptual approach, over the past several years the use of more sophisticated dynamic models has increased. The same underlying principles are used for dynamic models as for static models; however, the changes in concentration of the inhibitor *in vivo* are accounted for, rather than using a single concentration (like C_{max} or C_{avg}). Also, dynamic models attempt to simulate changes in the entire plasma concentration vs time curve, rather than simply predicting a change in the overall AUC. Commercial software programs are available that can carry out dynamic PBPK modeling of DDI, as well as include interindividual variability and simulation of DDI studies. These approaches can be very helpful in design of *in vivo* DDI studies (e.g., deciding on dose level, timing of dose, number of subjects, need for inclusion of special populations, etc.) Also, if some clinical DDI data exist, the model parameters can be adjusted to better simulate the C vs t profile of that study to account for unknown factors—also referred to as a "top-down" modeling approach. This in turn empowers the predictions of DDIs for the effect of a new drug on other drugs. PBPK modeling of DDI has become a prevalent practice that is even described in guidance documents from governmental drug regulatory agencies (FDA, 2012).

The Rank-Order Approach

A more cautious approach to using *in vitro* inhibition data to predict clinical DDI is the use of the "rank order" approach, in which at least one clinical DDI study is run irrespective of the potency of the K_i values.[171] Since the prediction methods described above require acceptance of some assumptions and estimates for input parameters (e.g., $[I]_{hep}$) the fundamental assumption underlying the rank order approach is that the drugs most likely to be subject to the largest DDI will be the ones cleared by the P450 enzyme most potently inhibited *in vitro*. A clinical DDI study for a new compound as a potential perpetrator of an interaction would be run using a good probe substrate for the most potently inhibited P450 *in vitro* (i.e., $f_{CL,CYP} >0.85$). If that study shows that no interaction occurs (i.e., <2-fold increase in AUC), then it can be assumed that there will be no interaction for drugs cleared by the other less potently inhibited P450 enzymes, and this conclusion can be claimed in the product labeling. It must be assured that a probe substrate with a very high $f_{CL,CYP}$ value is the one selected for the clinical DDI study. Some cautions using this approach must be exhibited:

(a) Applying the rank order approach for a new drug that reversibly inhibits one enzyme but irreversibly inactivates a second enzyme should not be done. Reversible and irreversible inhibitors cannot be compared since the irreversible effect also depends on k_{inact}.

(b) Applying the approach for CYP3A4 should be done cautiously. A new compound that inhibits CYP3A less potently than another P450 may show an interaction with a CYP3A cleared probe and not a probe for the other enzyme, if the CYP3A probe has a high intestinal extraction.

(c) The approach assumes that there is not a metabolite of the drug that affects the activity of a different CYP enzyme than the parent.

However, if used thoughtfully and with an understanding the fundamentals behind the mechanisms of DDI, the rank-order approach can be an effective method to leverage *in vitro* inhibition data to gain an understanding of DDI potential for a new compound without having to empirically run multiple clinical studies. A test of this approach using retrospective data yielded a favorable outcome, with only a very small percentage of DDI being missed, and even of those the magnitude of the interaction was just over 2X. No major DDI were missed.[171b]

Conclusions

Our understanding of the P450 enzymes involved in drug metabolism coupled with pharmacokinetic theory and physiological underpinnings has led us to an era of possessing an ability to fully leverage *in vitro* inhibition data to reliably predict clinical DDI. This provides a great advantage to clinical DDI strategies that can be mechanistically based rather than the empirical approaches that needed to be used in the past. *In vitro* experimental approaches to P450 and UGT inhibition studies have matured to the point that they have become a routine part of drug discovery and development. In early drug discovery research, the experimental approaches have been modified to high-throughput platforms that can accommodate the thousands of new chemical entities synthesized for each new pharmacological target. In the drug development phase, the assays have become such a routine part of the safety characterization process such that it is not unreasonable to place particular expectations around assay characteristics and robustness.[3b,4b,172] The more recent advances have shown that *in vitro* data, properly obtained, can be used for predicting the magnitude of DDI in the clinic and can also be used in lieu of conducting clinical DDI studies when it is shown that there is no inhibition. This provides a boost to the efficiency of an already costly drug development process and will ensure that medications get to patients with the information required to prescribe them safely in combination with other medications as needed.

REFERENCES

1. (a) Crespi, C. L., Higher-throughput screening with human cytochromes P450. *Current Opinion in Drug Discovery & Development* **1999**, *2* (1), 15–19; (b) Crespi, C. L., Miller, V. P., Penman, B. W., Microtiter plate assays for inhibition of human, drug-metabolizing cytochromes P450. *Analytical Biochemistry* **1997**, *248* (1), 188–190.
2. (a) Bu, H. Z., Magis, L., Knuth, K., Teitelbaum, P., High-throughput cytochrome P450 (CYP) inhibition screening via cassette probe-dosing strategy. I. Development of direct injection/on-line guard cartridge extraction/tandem mass spectrometry for the simultaneous detection of CYP probe substrates and their metabolites. *Rapid Communications in Mass Spectrometry: RCM* **2000**, *14* (17), 1619–1624; (b) Dierks, E. A., Stams, K. R., Lim, H. K., Cornelius, G., Zhang, H., Ball, S. E., A method for the simultaneous evaluation of the activities of seven major human drug-metabolizing cytochrome P450s using an *in vitro* cocktail of probe substrates and fast gradient liquid chromatography tandem mass spectrometry. *Drug Metabolism and Disposition: The Biological Fate of Chemicals* **2001**, *29* (1), 23–29; (c) Testino, S. A., Jr., Patonay, G., High-throughput inhibition screening of major human cytochrome P450 enzymes using an *in vitro* cocktail and liquid chromatography-tandem mass spectrometry. *Journal of Pharmaceutical and Biomedical Analysis* **2003**, *30* (5), 1459–1467; (d) Turpeinen, M., Uusitalo, J., Jalonen, J., Pelkonen, O., Multiple P450 substrates in a single run: Rapid and comprehensive *in vitro* interaction assay. *European Journal of Pharmaceutical Sciences: Official Journal of the European Federation for Pharmaceutical Sciences* **2005**, *24* (1), 123–132; (e) Di, L., Kerns, E. H., Li, S. Q., Carter, G. T., Comparison of cytochrome P450 inhibition assays for drug discovery using human liver microsomes with LC-MS, rhCYP450 isozymes with fluorescence, and double cocktail with LC-MS. *International Journal of Pharmaceutics* **2007**, *335* (1–2), 1–11; (f) Smith, D., Sadagopan, N., Zientek, M., Reddy, A., Cohen, L., Analytical approaches to determine cytochrome P450 inhibitory potential of new chemical entities in drug discovery. *Journal of Chromatography. B, Analytical Technologies*

in the Biomedical and Life Sciences **2007**, *850* (1–2), 455–463; (g) Dixit, V., Hariparsad, N., Desai, P., Unadkat, J. D., *In vitro* LC-MS cocktail assays to simultaneously determine human cytochrome P450 activities. *Biopharmaceutics & Drug Disposition* **2007**, *28* (5), 257–262.

3. (a) Bajpai, M., Esmay, J. D., *In vitro* studies in drug discovery and development: An analysis of study objectives and application of good laboratory practices (GLP). *Drug Metabolism Reviews* **2002**, *34* (4), 679–689; (b) Tucker, G. T., Houston, J. B., Huang, S. M., Optimizing drug development: Strategies to assess drug metabolism/transporter interaction potential—toward a consensus. *Pharmaceutical Research* **2001**, *18* (8), 1071–1080.

4. (a) EMA, *Guideline on the Investigation of Drug Interactions*. Health, E. M. A. S. M., Ed. London, United Kingdom, 2012; (b) FDA, Guidance for Industry: Drug Interactions Studies—Study Design, Data Analysis, Implication for Dosing, and Labeling Recommendations. U.S. Department of Health and Human Services, F. A. D. A., Center for Drug Evaluation and Research, Ed. FDA Maryland: 2012; (c) PMDA, *Drug Interaction Guideline for Drug Development and Labeling Recommendations* (Draft for Public Comment). Agency, P. a. M. D., Ed. Japan, 2014.

5. Zlokarnik, G., Grootenhuis, P. D., Watson, J. B., High throughput P450 inhibition screens in early drug discovery. *Drug Discovery Today* **2005**, *10* (21), 1443–1450.

6. (a) Hutzler, J. M., Powers, F. J., Wynalda, M. A., Wienkers, L. C., Effect of carbonate anion on cytochrome P450 2D6-mediated metabolism *in vitro*: The potential role of multiple oxygenating species. *Archives of Biochemistry and Biophysics* **2003**, *417* (2), 165–75; (b) Walsky, R. L., Bauman, J. N., Bourcier, K., Giddens, G., Lapham, K., Negahban, A., Ryder, T. F., Obach, R. S., Hyland, R., Goosen, T. C., Optimized assays for human UDP-glucuronosyltransferase (UGT) activities: Altered alamethicin concentration and utility to screen for UGT inhibitors. *Drug Metabolism and Disposition: The Biological Fate of Chemicals* **2012**, *40* (5), 1051–1065.

7. Margolis, J. M., Obach, R. S., Impact of nonspecific binding to microsomes and phospholipid on the inhibition of cytochrome P4502D6: implications for relating *in vitro* inhibition data to *in vivo* drug interactions. *Drug Metabolism and Disposition: The Biological Fate of Chemicals* **2003**, *31* (5), 606–611.

8. (a) Kilford, P. J., Stringer, R., Sohal, B., Houston, J. B., Galetin, A., Prediction of drug clearance by glucuronidation from *in vitro* data: Use of combined cytochrome P450 and UDP-glucuronosyltransferase cofactors in alamethicin-activated human liver microsomes. *Drug Metabolism and Disposition: The Biological Fate of Chemicals* **2009**, *37* (1), 82–89; (b) Gill, K. L., Houston, J. B., Galetin, A., Characterization of *in vitro* glucuronidation clearance of a range of drugs in human kidney microsomes: Comparison with liver and intestinal glucuronidation and impact of albumin. *Drug Metabolism and Disposition: The Biological Fate of Chemicals* **2012**, *40* (4), 825–835.

9. Uchaipichat, V., Winner, L. K., Mackenzie, P. I., Elliot, D. J., Williams, J. A., Miners, J. O., Quantitative prediction of *in vivo* inhibitory interactions involving glucuronidated drugs from *in vitro* data: The effect of fluconazole on zidovudine glucuronidation. *British Journal of Clinical Pharmacology* **2006**, *61* (4), 427–439.

10. (a) Ayrton, J., Plumb, R., Leavens, W. J., Mallett, D., Dickins, M., Dear, G. J., Application of a generic fast gradient liquid chromatography tandem mass spectrometry method for the analysis of cytochrome P450 probe substrates. *Rapid Communications in Mass Spectrometry: RCM* **1998**, *12* (5), 217–224; (b) Walsky, R. L., Obach, R. S., Validated assays for human cytochrome P450 activities. *Drug Metabolism and Disposition: The Biological Fate of Chemicals* **2004**, *32* (6), 647–660; (c) Yao, M., Zhu, M., Sinz, M. W., Zhang, H., Humphreys, W. G., Rodrigues, A. D., Dai, R., Development and full validation of six inhibition assays for five major cytochrome P450 enzymes in human liver microsomes using an automated 96-well microplate incubation format and LC-MS/MS analysis. *Journal of Pharmaceutical and Biomedical Analysis* **2007**, *44* (1), 211–223.

11. Wijnands, W. J., Vree, T. B., van Herwaarden, C. L., The influence of quinolone derivatives on theophylline clearance. *British Journal of Clinical Pharmacology* **1986**, *22* (6), 677–683.

12. Culm-Merdek, K. E., von Moltke, L. L., Harmatz, J. S., Greenblatt, D. J., Fluvoxamine impairs single-dose caffeine clearance without altering caffeine pharmacodynamics. *British Journal of Clinical Pharmacology* **2005**, *60* (5), 486–493.

13. (a) Granfors, M. T., Backman, J. T., Neuvonen, M., Ahonen, J., Neuvonen, P. J., Fluvoxamine drastically increases concentrations and effects of tizanidine: A potentially hazardous interaction. *Clinical Pharmacology and Therapeutics* **2004**, *75* (4), 331–341; (b) Obach, R. S., Ryder, T. F., Metabolism of

ramelteon in human liver microsomes and correlation with the effect of fluvoxamine on ramelteon pharmacokinetics. *Drug Metabolism and Disposition: The Biological Fate of Chemicals* **2010**, *38* (8), 1381–1391.

14. Butler, M. A., Iwasaki, M., Guengerich, F. P., Kadlubar, F. F., Human cytochrome P-450PA (P-450IA2), the phenacetin *O*-deethylase, is primarily responsible for the hepatic 3-demethylation of caffeine and *N*-oxidation of carcinogenic arylamines. *Proceedings of the National Academy of Sciences of the United States of America* **1989**, *86* (20), 7696–7700.

15. Rodrigues, A. D., Surber, B. W., Yao, Y., Wong, S. L., Roberts, E. M., [*O*-ethyl 14C]phenacetin *O*-deethylase activity in human liver microsomes. *Drug Metabolism and Disposition: The Biological Fate of Chemicals* **1997**, *25* (9), 1097–1100.

16. (a) Venkatakrishnan, K., von Moltke, L. L., Greenblatt, D. J., Human cytochromes P450 mediating phenacetin *O*-deethylation *in vitro*: Validation of the high affinity component as an index of CYP1A2 activity. *Journal of Pharmaceutical Sciences* **1998**, *87* (12), 1502–1507; (b) Kobayashi, K., Nakajima, M., Oshima, K., Shimada, N., Yokoi, T., Chiba, K., Involvement of CYP2E1 as A low-affinity enzyme in phenacetin *O*-deethylation in human liver microsomes. *Drug Metabolism and Disposition: The Biological Fate of Chemicals* **1999**, *27* (8), 860–865.

17. Spaldin, V., Madden, S., Adams, D. A., Edwards, R. J., Davies, D. S., Park, B. K., Determination of human hepatic cytochrome P4501A2 activity *in vitro* use of tacrine as an isoenzyme-specific probe. *Drug Metabolism and Disposition: The Biological Fate of Chemicals* **1995**, *23* (9), 929–934.

18. Berthou, F., Flinois, J. P., Ratanasavanh, D., Beaune, P., Riche, C., Guillouzo, A., Evidence for the involvement of several cytochromes P-450 in the first steps of caffeine metabolism by human liver microsomes. *Drug Metabolism and Disposition: The Biological Fate of Chemicals* **1991**, *19* (3), 561–567.

19. Kaminsky, L. S.; Zhang, Z. Y., Human P450 metabolism of warfarin. *Pharmacology & Therapeutics* **1997**, *73* (1), 67–74.

20. (a) Kunze, K. L., Trager, W. F., Isoform-selective mechanism-based inhibition of human cytochrome P450 1A2 by furafylline. *Chemical Research in Toxicology* **1993**, *6* (5), 649–656; (b) Clarke, S. E., Ayrton, A. D., Chenery, R. J., Characterization of the inhibition of P4501A2 by furafylline. *Xenobiotica; the Fate of Foreign Compounds in Biological Systems* **1994**, *24* (6), 517–526.

21. (a) Brosen, K., Skjelbo, E., Rasmussen, B. B., Poulsen, H. E., Loft, S., Fluvoxamine is a potent inhibitor of cytochrome P4501A2. *Biochemical Pharmacology* **1993**, *45* (6), 1211–1214; (b) Jensen, K. G., Poulsen, H. E., Doehmer, J., Loft, S., Kinetics and inhibition by fluvoxamine of phenacetin *O*-deethylation in V79 cells expressing human CYP1A2. *Pharmacology & Toxicology* **1995**, *76* (4), 286–288.

22. (a) Lu, P., Schrag, M. L., Slaughter, D. E., Raab, C. E., Shou, M., Rodrigues, A. D., Mechanism-based inhibition of human liver microsomal cytochrome P450 1A2 by zileuton, a 5-lipoxygenase inhibitor. *Drug Metabolism and Disposition: The Biological Fate of Chemicals* **2003**, *31* (11), 1352–1360; (b) Karjalainen, M. J., Neuvonen, P. J., Backman, J. T., Rofecoxib is a potent, metabolism-dependent inhibitor of CYP1A2: Implications for *in vitro* prediction of drug interactions. *Drug Metabolism and Disposition: The Biological Fate of Chemicals* **2006**, *34* (12), 2091–2096.

23. (a) Zanger, U. M., Klein, K., Saussele, T., Blievernicht, J., Hofmann, M. H., Schwab, M., Polymorphic CYP2B6: Molecular mechanisms and emerging clinical significance. *Pharmacogenomics* **2007**, *8* (7), 743–759; (b) Turpeinen, M., Raunio, H., Pelkonen, O., The functional role of CYP2B6 in human drug metabolism: Substrates and inhibitors *in vitro*, *in vivo* and *in silico*. *Current Drug Metabolism* **2006**, *7* (7), 705–714.

24. Xie, H. J., Yasar, U., Lundgren, S., Griskevicius, L., Terelius, Y., Hassan, M., Rane, A., Role of polymorphic human CYP2B6 in cyclophosphamide bioactivation. *The Pharmacogenomics Journal* **2003**, *3* (1), 53–61.

25. (a) Desta, Z., Saussele, T., Ward, B., Blievernicht, J., Li, L., Klein, K., Flockhart, D. A., Zanger, U. M., Impact of CYP2B6 polymorphism on hepatic efavirenz metabolism *in vitro*. *Pharmacogenomics* **2007**, *8* (6), 547–558; (b) Obach, R. S., Cox, L. M., Tremaine, L. M., Sertraline is metabolized by multiple cytochrome P450 enzymes, monoamine oxidases, and glucuronyl transferases in human: an *in vitro* study. *Drug Metabolism and Disposition: The Biological Fate of Chemicals* **2005**, *33* (2), 262–270; (c) Kobayashi, K., Ishizuka, T., Shimada, N., Yoshimura, Y., Kamijima, K., Chiba, K., Sertraline *N*-demethylation is catalyzed by multiple isoforms of human cytochrome P-450 *in vitro*. *Drug Metabolism and Disposition: The Biological Fate of Chemicals* **1999**, *27* (7), 763–766; (d) Turpeinen,

M., Nieminen, R., Juntunen, T., Taavitsainen, P., Raunio, H., Pelkonen, O., Selective inhibition of CYP2B6-catalyzed bupropion hydroxylation in human liver microsomes *in vitro*. *Drug Metabolism and Disposition: The Biological Fate of Chemicals* **2004**, *32* (6), 626–631.

26. Schroeder, D. H., Metabolism and kinetics of bupropion. *The Journal of Clinical Psychiatry* **1983**, *44* (5 Pt 2), 79–81.

27. (a) Hesse, L. M., Venkatakrishnan, K., Court, M. H., von Moltke, L. L., Duan, S. X., Shader, R. I., Greenblatt, D. J., CYP2B6 mediates the *in vitro* hydroxylation of bupropion: Potential drug interactions with other anti-depressants. *Drug Metabolism and Disposition: The Biological Fate of Chemicals* **2000**, *28* (10), 1176–1183; (b) Faucette, S. R., Hawke, R. L., Lecluyse, E. L.,; Shord, S. S., Yan, B., Laethem, R. M., Lindley, C. M., Validation of bupropion hydroxylation as a selective marker of human cytochrome P450 2B6 catalytic activity. *Drug Metabolism and Disposition: The Biological Fate of Chemicals* **2000**, *28* (10), 1222–1230.

28. Turpeinen, M., Tolonen, A., Uusitalo, J., Jalonen, J., Pelkonen, O., Laine, K., Effect of clopidogrel and ticlopidine on cytochrome P450 2B6 activity as measured by bupropion hydroxylation. *Clinical Pharmacology and Therapeutics* **2005**, *77* (6), 553–559.

29. Chang, T. K., Weber, G. F., Crespi, C. L., Waxman, D. J., Differential activation of cyclophosphamide and ifosfamide by cytochromes P-450 2B and 3A in human liver microsomes. *Cancer Research* **1993**, *53* (23), 5629–5637.

30. Heyn, H., White, R. B., Stevens, J. C., Catalytic role of cytochrome P4502B6 in the *N*-demethylation of *S*-mephenytoin. *Drug Metabolism and Disposition: The Biological Fate of Chemicals* **1996**, *24* (9), 948–954.

31. Ward, B. A., Gorski, J. C., Jones, D. R., Hall, S. D., Flockhart, D. A., Desta, Z., The cytochrome P450 2B6 (CYP2B6) is the main catalyst of efavirenz primary and secondary metabolism: Iplication for HIV/AIDS therapy and utility of efavirenz as a substrate marker of CYP2B6 catalytic activity. *The Journal of Pharmacology and Experimental Therapeutics* **2003**, *306* (1), 287–300.

32. Chang, T. K., Crespi, C. L., Waxman, D. J., Determination of CYP2B6 component of 7-ethoxy-4-trifluoromethylcoumarin *O*-deethylation activity in human liver microsomes. *Methods in Molecular Biology* **2006**, *320*, 97–102.

33. Guo, Z., Raeissi, S., White, R. B., Stevens, J. C., Orphenadrine and methimazole inhibit multiple cytochrome P450 enzymes in human liver microsomes. *Drug Metabolism and Disposition: The Biological Fate of Chemicals* **1997**, *25* (3), 390–393.

34. (a) Rae, J. M., Soukhova, N. V., Flockhart, D. A., Desta, Z., Triethylenethiophosphoramide is a specific inhibitor of cytochrome P450 2B6: Implications for cyclophosphamide metabolism. *Drug Metabolism and Disposition: The Biological Fate of Chemicals* **2002**, *30* (5), 525–530; (b) Richter, T., Murdter, T. E., Heinkele, G., Pleiss, J., Tatzel, S., Schwab, M., Eichelbaum, M., Zanger, U. M., Potent mechanism-based inhibition of human CYP2B6 by clopidogrel and ticlopidine. *The Journal of Pharmacology and Experimental Therapeutics* **2004**, *308* (1), 189–197; (c) Walsky, R. L., Obach, R. S., A comparison of 2-phenyl-2-(1-piperidinyl)propane (ppp), 1,1′,1″-phosphinothioylidynetrisaziridine (thioTEPA), clopidogrel, and ticlopidine as selective inactivators of human cytochrome P450 2B6. *Drug Metabolism and Disposition: The Biological Fate of Chemicals* **2007**, *35* (11), 2053–2059; (d) Obach, R. S., Walsky, R. L., Venkatakrishnan, K., Mechanism-based inactivation of human cytochrome p450 enzymes and the prediction of drug-drug interactions. *Drug Metabolism and Disposition: The Biological Fate of Chemicals* **2007**, *35* (2), 246–255.

35. (a) Niemi, M., Backman, J. T., Neuvonen, M., Neuvonen, P. J., Effects of gemfibrozil, itraconazole, and their combination on the pharmacokinetics and pharmacodynamics of repaglinide: Potentially hazardous interaction between gemfibrozil and repaglinide. *Diabetologia* **2003**, *46* (3), 347–351; (b) Backman, J. T., Kyrklund, C., Neuvonen, M., Neuvonen, P. J., Gemfibrozil greatly increases plasma concentrations of cerivastatin. *Clinical Pharmacology and Therapeutics* **2002**, *72* (6), 685–691.

36. (a) Shitara, Y., Hirano, M., Sato, H., Sugiyama, Y., Gemfibrozil and its glucuronide inhibit the organic anion transporting polypeptide 2 (OATP2/OATP1B1:SLC21A6)-mediated hepatic uptake and CYP2C8-mediated metabolism of cerivastatin: Analysis of the mechanism of the clinically relevant drug-drug interaction between cerivastatin and gemfibrozil. *The Journal of Pharmacology and Experimental Therapeutics* **2004**, *311* (1), 228–236; (b) Ogilvie, B. W., Zhang, D., Li, W., Rodrigues, A. D., Gipson, A. E., Holsapple, J., Toren, P., Parkinson, A., Glucuronidation converts gemfibrozil to a potent, metabolism-dependent inhibitor of CYP2C8: Implications for drug-drug interactions. *Drug Metabolism and Disposition: The Biological Fate of Chemicals* **2006**, *34* (1), 191–197.

37. Tornio, A., Filppula, A. M., Kailari, O., Neuvonen, M., Nyronen, T. H., Tapaninen, T., Neuvonen, P. J., Niemi, M., Backman, J. T., Glucuronidation converts clopidogrel to a strong time-dependent inhibitor of CYP2C8: A phase II metabolite as a perpetrator of drug-drug interactions. *Clinical Pharmacology and Therapeutics* **2014**, *96* (4), 498–507.

38. (a) Walle, T., Assays of CYP2C8- and CYP3A4-mediated metabolism of taxol *in vivo* and *in vitro*. *Methods in Enzymology* **1996**, *272*, 145–151; (b) Desai, P. B., Duan, J. Z., Zhu, Y. W., Kouzi, S., Human liver microsomal metabolism of paclitaxel and drug interactions. *European Journal of Drug Metabolism and Pharmacokinetics* **1998**, *23* (3), 417–424; (c) Fujino, H., Yamada, I., Shimada, S., Yoneda, M., Simultaneous determination of taxol and its metabolites in microsomal samples by a simple thin-layer chromatography radioactivity assay—inhibitory effect of NK-104, a new inhibitor of HMG-CoA reductase. *Journal of Chromatography. B, Biomedical Sciences and Applications* **2001**, *757* (1), 143–150; (d) Nadin, L., Murray, M., Participation of CYP2C8 in retinoic acid 4-hydroxylation in human hepatic microsomes. *Biochemical Pharmacology* **1999**, *58* (7), 1201–1208.

39. Li, X. Q., Bjorkman, A., Andersson, T. B., Ridderstrom, M., Masimirembwa, C. M., Amodiaquine clearance and its metabolism to *N*-desethylamodiaquine is mediated by CYP2C8: A new high affinity and turnover enzyme-specific probe substrate. *The Journal of Pharmacology and Experimental Therapeutics* **2002**, *300* (2), 399–407.

40. Baldwin, S. J., Clarke, S. E., Chenery, R. J., Characterization of the cytochrome P450 enzymes involved in the *in vitro* metabolism of rosiglitazone. *British Journal of Clinical Pharmacology* **1999**, *48* (3), 424–432.

41. Walsky, R. L., Obach, R. S., Gaman, E. A., Gleeson, J. P., Proctor, W. R., Selective inhibition of human cytochrome P4502C8 by montelukast. *Drug Metabolism and Disposition: The Biological Fate of Chemicals* **2005**, *33* (3), 413–418.

42. Filppula, A. M., Laitila, J., Neuvonen, P. J., Backman, J. T., Reevaluation of the microsomal metabolism of montelukast: Major contribution by CYP2C8 at clinically relevant concentrations. *Drug Metabolism and Disposition: The Biological Fate of Chemicals* **2011**, *39* (5), 904–9011.

43. VandenBrink, B. M., Foti, R. S., Rock, D. A., Wienkers, L. C., Wahlstrom, J. L., Evaluation of CYP2C8 inhibition *in vitro*: Utility of montelukast as a selective CYP2C8 probe substrate. *Drug Metabolism and Disposition: The Biological Fate of Chemicals* **2011**, *39* (9), 1546–1554.

44. Wen, X., Wang, J. S., Backman, J. T., Laitila, J., Neuvonen, P. J., Trimethoprim and sulfamethoxazole are selective inhibitors of CYP2C8 and CYP2C9, respectively. *Drug Metabolism and Disposition: The Biological Fate of Chemicals* **2002**, *30* (6), 631–635.

45. Rettie, A. E., Jones, J. P., Clinical and toxicological relevance of CYP2C9: Drug-drug interactions and pharmacogenetics. *Annual Review of Pharmacology and Toxicology* **2005**, *45*, 477–494.

46. Webster, R., Pacey, M., Winchester, T., Johnson, P., Jezequel, S., Microbial oxidative metabolism of diclofenac: Production of 4′-hydroxydiclofenac using Epiccocum nigrum IMI354292. *Applied Microbiology and Biotechnology* **1998**, *49* (4), 371–376.

47. (a) Leemann, T., Transon, C., Dayer, P., Cytochrome P450TB (CYP2C): A major monooxygenase catalyzing diclofenac 4′-hydroxylation in human liver. *Life Sciences* **1993**, *52* (1), 29–34; (b) Crespi, C. L., Chang, T. K., Waxman, D. J., Determination of CYP2C9-catalyzed diclofenac 4′-hydroxylation by high-performance liquid chromatography. *Methods in Molecular Biology* **1998**, *107*, 129–133.

48. Miners, J. O., Birkett, D. J., Use of tolbutamide as a substrate probe for human hepatic cytochrome P450 2C9. *Methods in Enzymology* **1996**, *272*, 139–145.

49. (a) Lasker, J. M., Wester, M. R., Aramsombatdee, E., Raucy, J. L., Characterization of CYP2C19 and CYP2C9 from human liver: Respective roles in microsomal tolbutamide, *S*-mephenytoin, and omeprazole hydroxylations. *Archives of Biochemistry and Biophysics* **1998**, *353* (1), 16–28; (b) Wester, M. R., Lasker, J. M., Johnson, E. F., Raucy, J. L., CYP2C19 participates in tolbutamide hydroxylation by human liver microsomes. *Drug Metabolism and Disposition: The Biological Fate of Chemicals* **2000**, *28* (3), 354–359.

50. (a) Fasco, M. J., Piper, L. J., Kaminsky, L. S., Biochemical applications of a quantitative high-pressure liquid chromatographic assay of warfarin and its metabolites. *Journal of Chromatography* **1977**, *131*, 365–373; (b) Hutzler, J. M., Hauer, M. J., Tracy, T. S., Dapsone activation of CYP2C9-mediated metabolism: Evidence for activation of multiple substrates and a two-site model. *Drug Metabolism and Disposition: The Biological Fate of Chemicals* **2001**, *29* (7), 1029–1034.

51. (a) Zhang, Z. Y., King, B. M., Wong, Y. N., Quantitative liquid chromatography/mass spectrometry/mass spectrometry warfarin assay for *in vitro* cytochrome P450 studies. *Analytical Biochemistry* **2001**, *298* (1), 40–49; (b) Rodrigues, A. D., Kukulka, M. J., Roberts, E. M., Ouellet, D., Rodgers, T. R.,

[*O*-methyl 14C]naproxen *O*-demethylase activity in human liver microsomes: Evidence for the involvement of cytochrome P4501A2 and P4502C9/10. *Drug Metabolism and Disposition: The Biological Fate of Chemicals* **1996**, *24* (1), 126–136; (c) Miners, J. O., Coulter, S., Tukey, R. H., Veronese, M. E., Birkett, D. J., Cytochromes P450, 1A2, and 2C9 are responsible for the human hepatic *O*-demethylation of R- and *S*-naproxen. *Biochemical Pharmacology* **1996**, *51* (8), 1003–1008.

52. Tang, C., Shou, M., Rodrigues, A. D., Substrate-dependent effect of acetonitrile on human liver microsomal cytochrome P450 2C9 (CYP2C9) activity. *Drug Metabolism and Disposition: The Biological Fate of Chemicals* **2000**, *28* (5), 567–572.

53. Giancarlo, G. M., Venkatakrishnan, K., Granda, B. W., von Moltke, L. L., Greenblatt, D. J., Relative contributions of CYP2C9 and 2C19 to phenytoin 4-hydroxylation *in vitro*: Inhibition by sulfaphenazole, omeprazole, and ticlopidine. *European Journal of Clinical Pharmacology* **2001**, *57* (1), 31–36.

54. Kumar, V., Wahlstrom, J. L., Rock, D. A., Warren, C. J., Gorman, L. A., Tracy, T. S., CYP2C9 inhibition: Impact of probe selection and pharmacogenetics on *in vitro* inhibition profiles. *Drug Metabolism and Disposition: The Biological Fate of Chemicals* **2006**, *34* (12), 1966–1975.

55. Newton, D. J., Wang, R. W., Lu, A. Y., Cytochrome P450 inhibitors. Evaluation of specificities in the *in vitro* metabolism of therapeutic agents by human liver microsomes. *Drug Metabolism and Disposition: The Biological Fate of Chemicals* **1995**, *23* (1), 154–158.

56. Hutzler, J. M., Balogh, L. M., Zientek, M., Kumar, V., Tracy, T. S., Mechanism-based inactivation of cytochrome P450 2C9 by tienilic acid and (+/-)-suprofen: A comparison of kinetics and probe substrate selection. *Drug Metabolism and Disposition: The Biological Fate of Chemicals* **2009**, *37* (1), 59–65.

57. (a) Shimada, T., Shea, J. P., Guengerich, F. P., A convenient assay for mephenytoin 4-hydroxylase activity of human liver microsomal cytochrome P-450. *Analytical Biochemistry* **1985**, *147* (1), 174–179; (b) Ward, S. A., Goto, F., Nakamura, K., Jacqz, E., Wilkinson, G. R., Branch, R. A., *S*-mephenytoin 4-hydroxylase is inherited as an autosomal-recessive trait in Japanese families. *Clinical Pharmacology and Therapeutics* **1987**, *42* (1), 96–99.

58. Furuta, T., Shirai, N., Sugimoto, M., Nakamura, A., Hishida, A., Ishizaki, T., Influence of CYP2C19 pharmacogenetic polymorphism on proton pump inhibitor-based therapies. *Drug Metabolism and Pharmacokinetics* **2005**, *20* (3), 153–167.

59. (a) Chiba, K., Manabe, K., Kobayashi, K., Takayama, Y., Tani, M., Ishizaki, T., Development and preliminary application of a simple assay of *S*-mephenytoin 4-hydroxylase activity in human liver microsomes. *European Journal of Clinical Pharmacology* **1993**, *44* (6), 559–562; (b) Di Marco, A., Cellucci, A., Chaudhary, A., Fonsi, M., Laufer, R., High-throughput radiometric CYP2C19 inhibition assay using tritiated (S)-mephenytoin. *Drug Metabolism and Disposition: The Biological Fate of Chemicals* **2007**, *35* (10), 1737–1743.

60. (a) Suzuki, H., Kneller, M. B., Haining, R. L., Trager, W. F., Rettie, A. E., (+)-*N*-3-Benzyl-nirvanol and (-)-*N*-3-benzyl-phenobarbital: New potent and selective *in vitro* inhibitors of CYP2C19. *Drug Metabolism and Disposition: The Biological Fate of Chemicals* **2002**, *30* (3), 235–239; (b) Cai, X., Wang, R. W., Edom, R. W., Evans, D. C., Shou, M., Rodrigues, A. D., Liu, W., Dean, D. C., Baillie, T. A., Validation of (-)-*N*-3-benzyl-phenobarbital as a selective inhibitor of CYP2C19 in human liver microsomes. *Drug Metabolism and Disposition: The Biological Fate of Chemicals* **2004**, *32* (6), 584–586.

61. (a) Donahue, S. R., Flockhart, D. A., Abernethy, D. R., Ko, J. W., Ticlopidine inhibition of phenytoin metabolism mediated by potent inhibition of CYP2C19. *Clinical Pharmacology and Therapeutics* **1997**, *62* (5), 572–577; (b) Mankowski, D. C., The role of CYP2C19 in the metabolism of (+/-) bufuralol, the prototypic substrate of CYP2D6. *Drug Metabolism and Disposition: The Biological Fate of Chemicals* **1999**, *27* (9), 1024–1028.

62. Zanger, U. M., Raimundo, S., Eichelbaum, M., Cytochrome P450 2D6: Overview and update on pharmacology, genetics, biochemistry. *Naunyn-Schmiedeberg's Archives of Pharmacology* **2004**, *369* (1), 23–37.

63. Kronbach, T., Mathys, D., Gut, J., Catin, T., Meyer, U. A., High-performance liquid chromatographic assays for bufuralol 1'-hydroxylase, debrisoquine 4-hydroxylase, and dextromethorphan *O*-demethylase in microsomes and purified cytochrome P-450 isozymes of human liver. *Analytical Biochemistry* **1987**, *162* (1), 24–32.

64. Belpaire, F. M., Wijnant, P., Temmerman, A., Rasmussen, B. B., Brosen, K., The oxidative metabolism of metoprolol in human liver microsomes: Inhibition by the selective serotonin reuptake inhibitors. *European Journal of Clinical Pharmacology* **1998**, *54* (3), 261–264.

65. Henthorn, T. K., Spina, E., Dumont, E., von Bahr, C., *In vitro* inhibition of a polymorphic human liver P-450 isozyme by narcotic analgesics. *Anesthesiology* **1989**, *70* (2), 339–342.

66. Dayer, P., Gasser, R., Gut, J., Kronbach, T., Robertz, G. M., Eichelbaum, M., Meyer, U. A., Characterization of a common genetic defect of cytochrome P-450 function (debrisoquine-sparteine type polymorphism)-increased Michaelis is Constant (Km) and loss of stereoselectivity of bufuralol 1'-hydroxylation in poor metabolizers. *Biochemical and Biophysical Research Communications* **1984**, *125* (1), 374–380.

67. Narimatsu, S., Takemi, C., Tsuzuki, D., Kataoka, H., Yamamoto, S., Shimada, N., Suzuki, S., Satoh, T., Meyer, U. A., Gonzalez, F. J., Stereoselective metabolism of bufuralol racemate and enantiomers in human liver microsomes. *The Journal of Pharmacology and Experimental Therapeutics* **2002**, *303* (1), 172–178.

68. Boobis, A. R., Murray, S., Kahn, G. C., Robertz, G. M., Davies, D. S., Substrate specificity of the form of cytochrome P-450 catalyzing the 4-hydroxylation of debrisoquine in man. *Molecular Pharmacology* **1983**, *23* (2), 474–4781.

69. Ozdemir, M., Crewe, K. H., Tucker, G. T., Rostami-Hodjegan, A., Assessment of *in vivo* CYP2D6 activity: Differential sensitivity of commonly used probes to urine pH. *Journal of Clinical Pharmacology* **2004**, *44* (12), 1398–1404.

70. Rodrigues, A. D., Kukulka, M. J., Surber, B. W., Thomas, S. B., Uchic, J. T., Rotert, G. A., Michel, G., Thome-Kromer, B., Machinist, J. M., Measurement of liver microsomal cytochrome p450 (CYP2D6) activity using [O-methyl-14C]dextromethorphan. *Analytical Biochemistry* **1994**, *219* (2), 309–320.

71. (a) Gorski, J. C., Hall, S. D., Jones, D. R., VandenBranden, M., Wrighton, S. A., Regioselective biotransformation of midazolam by members of the human cytochrome P450 3A (CYP3A) subfamily. *Biochemical Pharmacology* **1994**, *47* (9), 1643–1653; (b) Gibbs, M. A., Thummel, K. E., Shen, D. D., Kunze, K. L., Inhibition of cytochrome P-450 3A (CYP3A) in human intestinal and liver microsomes: comparison of Ki values and impact of CYP3A5 expression. *Drug Metabolism and Disposition: The Biological Fate of Chemicals* **1999**, *27* (2), 180–187; (c) Wang, Y. H., Jones, D. R., Hall, S. D., Differential mechanism-based inhibition of CYP3A4 and CYP3A5 by verapamil. *Drug Metabolism and Disposition: The Biological Fate of Chemicals* **2005**, *33* (5), 664–671; (d) Dennison, J. B., Kulanthaivel, P., Barbuch, R. J., Renbarger, J. L., Ehlhardt, W. J., Hall, S. D., Selective metabolism of vincristine *in vitro* by CYP3A5. *Drug Metabolism and Disposition: The Biological Fate of Chemicals* **2006**, *34* (8), 1317–1327; (e) Pearson, J. T., Wahlstrom, J. L., Dickmann, L. J., Kumar, S., Halpert, J. R., Wienkers, L. C., Foti, R. S., Rock, D. A., Differential time-dependent inactivation of P450 3A4 and P450 3A5 by raloxifene: A key role for C239 in quenching reactive intermediates. *Chemical Research in Toxicology* **2007**, *20* (12), 1778–1786.

72. Xie, H. G., Wood, A. J., Kim, R. B., Stein, C. M., Wilkinson, G. R., Genetic variability in CYP3A5 and its possible consequences. *Pharmacogenomics* **2004**, *5* (3), 243–272.

73. (a) Maenpaa, J., Hall, S. D., Ring, B. J., Strom, S. C., Wrighton, S. A., Human cytochrome P450 3A (CYP3A) mediated midazolam metabolism: The effect of assay conditions and regioselective stimulation by alpha-naphthoflavone, terfenadine and testosterone. *Pharmacogenetics* **1998**, *8* (2), 137–155; (b) Yamazaki, H., Nakajima, M., Nakamura, M., Asahi, S., Shimada, N., Gillam, E. M., Guengerich, F. P., Shimada, T., Yokoi, T., Enhancement of cytochrome P-450 3A4 catalytic activities by cytochrome b(5) in bacterial membranes. *Drug Metabolism and Disposition: The Biological Fate of Chemicals* **1999**, *27* (9), 999–1004; (c) Schrag, M. L., Wienkers, L. C., Topological alteration of the CYP3A4 active site by the divalent cation Mg(2+). *Drug Metabolism and Disposition: The Biological Fate of Chemicals* **2000**, *28* (10), 1198–1201; (d) Yamaori, S., Yamazaki, H., Suzuki, A., Yamada, A., Tani, H., Kamidate, T., Fujita, K., Kamataki, T., Effects of cytochrome b(5) on drug oxidation activities of human cytochrome P450 (CYP) 3As: Similarity of CYP3A5 with CYP3A4 but not CYP3A7. *Biochemical Pharmacology* **2003**, *66* (12), 2333–2340; (e) Jushchyshyn, M. I., Hutzler, J. M., Schrag, M. L., Wienkers, L. C., Catalytic turnover of pyrene by CYP3A4: Evidence that cytochrome b5 directly induces positive cooperativity. *Archives of Biochemistry and Biophysics* **2005**, *438* (1), 21–28.

74. Kenworthy, K. E., Bloomer, J. C., Clarke, S. E., Houston, J. B., CYP3A4 drug interactions: Correlation of 10 *in vitro* probe substrates. *British Journal of Clinical Pharmacology* **1999**, *48* (5), 716–727.

75. Khan, K. K., He, Y. Q., Domanski, T. L., Halpert, J. R., Midazolam oxidation by cytochrome P450 3A4 and active-site mutants: An evaluation of multiple binding sites and of the metabolic pathway that leads to enzyme inactivation. *Molecular Pharmacology* **2002**, *61* (3), 495–506.

76. Sonderfan, A. J., Arlotto, M. P., Dutton, D. R., McMillen, S. K., Parkinson, A., Regulation of testosterone hydroxylation by rat liver microsomal cytochrome P-450. *Archives of Biochemistry and Biophysics* **1987**, *255* (1), 27–41.

77. Obach, R. S., Walsky, R. L., Venkatakrishnan, K., Gaman, E. A., Houston, J. B., Tremaine, L. M., The utility of *in vitro* cytochrome P450 inhibition data in the prediction of drug-drug interactions. *The Journal of Pharmacology and Experimental Therapeutics* **2006**, *316* (1), 336–348.

78. Li, X., Jeso, V., Heyward, S., Walker, G. S., Sharma, R., Micalizio, G. C., Cameron, M. D., Characterization of T-5 *N*-oxide formation as the first highly selective measure of CYP3A5 activity. *Drug Metabolism and Disposition: The Biological Fate of Chemicals* **2014**, *42* (3), 334–342.

79. Wempe, M. F., Anderson, P. L., Atazanavir metabolism according to CYP3A5 status: An *in vitro-in vivo* assessment. *Drug Metabolism and Disposition: The Biological Fate of Chemicals* **2011**, *39* (3), 522–527.

80. (a) Walsky, R. L., Obach, R. S., Hyland, R., Kang, P., Zhou, S., West, M., Geoghegan, K. F. et al., Selective mechanism-based inactivation of CYP3A4 by CYP3cide (PF-04981517) and its utility as an *in vitro* tool for delineating the relative roles of CYP3A4 versus CYP3A5 in the metabolism of drugs. *Drug Metabolism and Disposition: The Biological Fate of Chemicals* **2012**, *40* (9), 1686–1697; (b) Tseng, E., Walsky, R. L., Luzietti, R. A., Jr., Harris, J. J., Kosa, R. E., Goosen, T. C., Zientek, M. A., Obach, R. S., Relative contributions of cytochrome CYP3A4 versus CYP3A5 for CYP3A-cleared drugs assessed *in vitro* using a CYP3A4-selective inactivator (CYP3cide). *Drug Metabolism and Disposition: The Biological Fate of Chemicals* **2014**, *42* (7), 1163–1173.

81. Williams, J. A., Hyland, R., Jones, B. C., Smith, D. A., Hurst, S., Goosen, T. C., Peterkin, V., Koup, J. R., Ball, S. E., Drug-drug interactions for UDP-glucuronosyltransferase substrates: A pharmacokinetic explanation for typically observed low exposure (AUCi/AUC) ratios. *Drug Metabolism and Disposition: The Biological Fate of Chemicals* **2004**, *32* (11), 1201–1208.

82. Mross, K., Steinbild, S., Baas, F., Gmehling, D., Radtke, M., Voliotis, D., Brendel, E., Christensen, O., Unger, C., Results from an *in vitro* and a clinical/pharmacological phase I study with the combination irinotecan and sorafenib. *European Journal of Cancer* **2007**, *43* (1), 55–63.

83. Corona, G., Vaccher, E., Sandron, S., Sartor, I., Tirelli, U., Innocenti, F., Toffoli, G., Lopinavir-ritonavir dramatically affects the pharmacokinetics of irinotecan in HIV patients with Kaposi's sarcoma. *Clinical Pharmacology and Therapeutics* **2008**, *83* (4), 601–606.

84. Merck, Patient Information about Crixivan for HIV Infection. 1997.

85. Zucker, S. D., Qin, X., Rouster, S. D., Yu, F., Green, R. M., Keshavan, P., Feinberg, J., Sherman, K. E., Mechanism of indinavir-induced hyperbilirubinemia. *Proceedings of the National Academy of Sciences of the United States of America* **2001**, *98* (22), 12671–12676.

86. Kassahun, K., McIntosh, I., Cui, D., Hreniuk, D., Merschman, S., Lasseter, K., Azrolan, N., Iwamoto, M., Wagner, J. A., Wenning, L. A., Metabolism and disposition in humans of raltegravir (MK-0518), an anti-AIDS drug targeting the human immunodeficiency virus 1 integrase enzyme. *Drug Metabolism and Disposition: The Biological Fate of Chemicals* **2007**, *35* (9), 1657–1663.

87. Krishna, R., East, L., Larson, P., Valiathan, C., Deschamps, K., Luk, J. A., Bethel-Brown, C., Manthos, H., Brejda, J., Gartner, M., Atazanavir increases the plasma concentrations of 1200 mg raltegravir dose. *Biopharmaceutics & Drug Disposition* **2016**, *37* (9), 533–541.

88. Itaaho, K., Mackenzie, P. I., Ikushiro, S., Miners, J. O., Finel, M., The configuration of the 17-hydroxy group variably influences the glucuronidation of beta-estradiol and epiestradiol by human UDP-glucuronosyltransferases. *Drug Metabolism and Disposition: The Biological Fate of Chemicals* **2008**, *36* (11), 2307–2315.

89. Fallon, J. K., Neubert, H., Hyland, R., Goosen, T. C., Smith, P. C., Targeted quantitative proteomics for the analysis of 14 UGT1As and -2Bs in human liver using NanoUPLC-MS/MS with selected reaction monitoring. *Journal of Proteome Research* **2013**, *12* (10), 4402–4413.

90. Ma, G., Lin, J., Cai, W., Tan, B., Xiang, X., Zhang, Y., Zhang, P., Simultaneous determination of bilirubin and its glucuronides in liver microsomes and recombinant UGT1A1 enzyme incubation systems by HPLC method and its application to bilirubin glucuronidation studies. *Journal of Pharmaceutical and Biomedical Analysis* **2014**, *92*, 149–159.

91. Zhang, J. A., Xuan, T., Parmar, M., Ma, L., Ugwu, S., Ali, S., Ahmad, I., Development and characterization of a novel liposome-based formulation of SN-38. *International Journal of Pharmaceutics* **2004**, *270* (1–2), 93–107.

92. (a) Wen, Z., Tallman, M. N., Ali, S. Y., Smith, P. C., UDP-glucuronosyltransferase 1A1 is the principal enzyme responsible for etoposide glucuronidation in human liver and intestinal microsomes: structural characterization of phenolic and alcoholic glucuronides of etoposide and estimation of enzyme kinetics. *Drug Metabolism and Disposition: The Biological Fate of Chemicals* **2007**, *35* (3), 371–380; (b) Watanabe, Y., Nakajima, M., Ohashi, N., Kume, T., Yokoi, T., Glucuronidation of etoposide in human liver microsomes is specifically catalyzed by UDP-glucuronosyltransferase 1A1. *Drug Metabolism and Disposition: The Biological Fate of Chemicals* **2003**, *31* (5), 589–595.

93. Zhang, D., Chando, T. J., Everett, D. W., Patten, C. J., Dehal, S. S., Humphreys, W. G., *In vitro* inhibition of UDP glucuronosyltransferases by atazanavir and other HIV protease inhibitors and the relationship of this property to *in vivo* bilirubin glucuronidation. *Drug Metabolism and Disposition: The Biological Fate of Chemicals* **2005**, *33* (11), 1729–1739.

94. Liu, Y., Ramirez, J., House, L., Ratain, M. J., Comparison of the drug-drug interactions potential of erlotinib and gefitinib via inhibition of UDP-glucuronosyltransferases. *Drug Metabolism and Disposition: The Biological Fate of Chemicals* **2010**, *38* (1), 32–39.

95. Trottier, J., Verreault, M., Grepper, S., Monte, D., Belanger, J., Kaeding, J., Caron, P., Inaba, T. T., Barbier, O., Human UDP-glucuronosyltransferase (UGT)1A3 enzyme conjugates chenodeoxycholic acid in the liver. *Hepatology* **2006**, *44* (5), 1158–1170.

96. Seo, K. A., Kim, H. J., Jeong, E. S., Abdalla, N., Choi, C. S., Kim, D. H., Shin, J. G., *In vitro* assay of six UDP-glucuronosyltransferase isoforms in human liver microsomes, using cocktails of probe substrates and liquid chromatography-tandem mass spectrometry. *Drug Metabolism and Disposition: The Biological Fate of Chemicals* **2014**, *42* (11), 1803–1810.

97. Cardoso Jde, O., Oliveira, R. V., Lu, J. B., Desta, Z., *In Vitro* Metabolism of montelukast by cytochrome P450s and UDP-glucuronosyltransferases. *Drug Metabolism and Disposition: The Biological Fate of Chemicals* **2015**, *43* (12), 1905–1916.

98. Kasai, N., Sakaki, T., Shinkyo, R., Ikushiro, S., Iyanagi, T., Ohta, M., Inouye, K., Metabolism of 26,26,26,27,27,27-F6-1 alpha,23S,25-trihydroxyvitamin D3 by human UDP-glucuronosyltransferase 1A3. *Drug Metabolism and Disposition: The Biological Fate of Chemicals* **2005**, *33* (1), 102–107.

99. Court, M. H., Isoform-selective probe substrates for *in vitro* studies of human UDP-glucuronosyltransferases. *Methods in Enzymology* **2005**, *400*, 104–116.

100. Jeong, E. S., Kim, Y. W., Kim, H. J., Shin, H. J., Shin, J. G., Kim, K. H., Chi, Y. H., Paik, S. H., Kim, D. H., Glucuronidation of fimasartan, a new angiotensin receptor antagonist, is mainly mediated by UGT1A3. *Xenobiotica, the Fate of Foreign Compounds in Biological Systems* **2015**, *45* (1), 10–18.

101. Yamada, A., Maeda, K., Ishiguro, N., Tsuda, Y., Igarashi, T., Ebner, T., Roth, W., Ikushiro, S., Sugiyama, Y., The impact of pharmacogenetics of metabolic enzymes and transporters on the pharmacokinetics of telmisartan in healthy volunteers. *Pharmacogenetics and Genomics* **2011**, *21* (9), 523–530.

102. Alonen, A., Finel, M., Kostiainen, R., The human UDP-glucuronosyltransferase UGT1A3 is highly selective towards N2 in the tetrazole ring of losartan, candesartan, and zolarsartan. *Biochemical Pharmacology* **2008**, *76* (6), 763–772.

103. Jiang, L., Liang, S. C., Wang, C., Ge, G. B., Huo, X. K., Qi, X. Y., Deng, S., Liu, K. X., Ma, X. C., Identifying and applying a highly selective probe to simultaneously determine the *O*-glucuronidation activity of human UGT1A3 and UGT1A4. *Scientific Reports* **2015**, *5*, 9627.

104. Trottier, J., El Husseini, D., Perreault, M., Paquet, S., Caron, P., Bourassa, S. et al., The human UGT1A3 enzyme conjugates norursodeoxycholic acid into a C23-ester glucuronide in the liver. *The Journal of Biological Chemistry* **2010**, *285* (2), 1113–1121.

105. Gall, W. E., Zawada, G., Mojarrabi, B., Tephly, T. R., Green, M. D., Coffman, B. L., Mackenzie, P. I., Radominska-Pandya, A., Differential glucuronidation of bile acids, androgens and estrogens by human UGT1A3 and 2B7. *The Journal of Steroid Biochemistry and Molecular Biology* **1999**, *70* (1–3), 101–108.

106. Liu, C., Cao, Y. F., Fang, Z. Z., Zhang, Y. Y., Hu, C. M., Sun, X. Y., Huang, T., Zeng, J., Fan, X. R., Mo, H., Strong inhibition of deoxyschizandrin and schisantherin A toward UDP-glucuronosyltransferase (UGT) 1A3 indicating UGT inhibition-based herb-drug interaction. *Fitoterapia* **2012**, *83* (8), 1415–1419.

107. Liu, D., Li, S., Qi, J. Q., Meng, D. L., Cao, Y. F., The inhibitory effects of nor-oleanane triterpenoid saponins from Stauntonia brachyanthera towards UDP-glucuronosyltransferases. *Fitoterapia* **2016**, *112*, 56–64.

108. (a) Kubota, T., Lewis, B. C., Elliot, D. J., Mackenzie, P. I., Miners, J. O., Critical roles of residues 36 and 40 in the phenol and tertiary amine aglycone substrate selectivities of UDP-glucuronosyltransferases 1A3 and 1A4. *Molecular Pharmacology* **2007**, *72* (4), 1054–1062; (b) Green, M. D., King, C. D., Mojarrabi, B., Mackenzie, P. I., Tephly, T. R., Glucuronidation of amines and other xenobiotics catalyzed by expressed human UDP-glucuronosyltransferase 1A3. *Drug Metabolism and Disposition: The Biological Fate of Chemicals* **1998**, *26* (6), 507–512; (c) Tukey, R. H., Strassburg, C. P., Human UDP-glucuronosyltransferases: Metabolism, expression, and disease. *Annual Review of Pharmacology and Toxicology* **2000**, *40*, 581–616.

109. Bourcier, K., Hyland, R., Kempshall, S., Jones, R., Maximilien, J., Irvine, N., Jones, B., Investigation into UDP-glucuronosyltransferase (UGT) enzyme kinetics of imidazole- and triazole-containing antifungal drugs in human liver microsomes and recombinant UGT enzymes. *Drug Metabolism and Disposition: The Biological Fate of Chemicals* **2010**, *38* (6), 923–929.

110. Kamdem, L. K., Liu, Y., Stearns, V., Kadlubar, S. A., Ramirez, J., Jeter, S., Shahverdi, K. et al., *In vitro* and *in vivo* oxidative metabolism and glucuronidation of anastrozole. *British Journal of Clinical Pharmacology* **2010**, *70* (6), 854–869.

111. Seo, K. A., Bae, S. K., Choi, Y. K., Choi, C. S., Liu, K. H., Shin, J. G., Metabolism of 1'- and 4-hydroxymidazolam by glucuronide conjugation is largely mediated by UDP-glucuronosyltransferases 1A4, 2B4, and 2B7. *Drug Metabolism and Disposition: The Biological Fate of Chemicals* **2010**, *38* (11), 2007–2013.

112. Gerrits, M. G., de Greef, R., Dogterom, P., Peeters, P. A., Valproate reduces the glucuronidation of asenapine without affecting asenapine plasma concentrations. *Journal of Clinical Pharmacology* **2012**, *52* (5), 757–765.

113. Markowitz, J. S., Devane, C. L., Liston, H. L., Boulton, D. W., Risch, S. C., The effects of probenecid on the disposition of risperidone and olanzapine in healthy volunteers. *Clinical Pharmacology and Therapeutics* **2002**, *71* (1), 30–38.

114. Uchaipichat, V., Mackenzie, P. I., Elliot, D. J., Miners, J. O., Selectivity of substrate (trifluoperazine) and inhibitor (amitriptyline, androsterone, canrenoic acid, hecogenin, phenylbutazone, quinidine, quinine, and sulfinpyrazone) "probes" for human udp-glucuronosyltransferases. *Drug Metabolism and Disposition: The Biological Fate of Chemicals* **2006**, *34* (3), 449–456.

115. (a) Linnet, K., Glucuronidation of olanzapine by cDNA-expressed human UDP-glucuronosyltransferases and human liver microsomes. *Human Psychopharmacology* **2002**, *17* (5), 233–238, (b) Korprasertthaworn, P., Polasek, T. M., Sorich, M. J., McLachlan, A. J., Miners, J. O., Tucker, G. T., Rowland, A., *In Vitro* Characterization of the human liver microsomal kinetics and reaction phenotyping of olanzapine metabolism. *Drug Metabolism and Disposition: The Biological Fate of Chemicals* **2015**, *43* (11), 1806–1814.

116. Nakajima, M., Tanaka, E., Kobayashi, T., Ohashi, N., Kume, T., Yokoi, T., Imipramine N-glucuronidation in human liver microsomes: Biphasic kinetics and characterization of UDP-glucuronosyltransferase isoforms. *Drug Metabolism and Disposition: The Biological Fate of Chemicals* **2002**, *30* (6), 636–642.

117. Citrome, L., Asenapine review, part I: Chemistry, receptor affinity profile, pharmacokinetics and metabolism. *Expert Opinion on Drug Metabolism & Toxicology* **2014**, *10* (6), 893–903.

118. Lee, S. J., Park, J. B., Kim, D., Bae, S. H., Chin, Y. W., Oh, E., Bae, S. K., *In vitro* selective inhibition of human UDP-glucuronosyltransferase (UGT) 1A4 by finasteride, and prediction of *in vivo* drug-drug interactions. *Toxicology Letters* **2015**, *232* (2), 458–465.

119. (a) Krishnaswamy, S., Duan, S. X., Von Moltke, L. L., Greenblatt, D. J., Court, M. H., Validation of serotonin (5-hydroxtryptamine) as an *in vitro* substrate probe for human UDP-glucuronosyltransferase (UGT) 1A6. *Drug Metabolism and Disposition: The Biological Fate of Chemicals* **2003**, *31* (1), 133–139; (b) Sakakibara, Y., Katoh, M., Kawayanagi, T., Nadai, M., Species and tissue differences in serotonin glucuronidation. *Xenobiotica, The Fate of Foreign Compounds in Biological Systems* **2015**, 1–7.

120. Manevski, N., Kurkela, M., Hoglund, C., Mauriala, T., Court, M. H., Yli-Kauhaluoma, J., Finel, M., Glucuronidation of psilocin and 4-hydroxyindole by the human UDP-glucuronosyltransferases. *Drug Metabolism and Disposition: The Biological Fate of Chemicals* **2010**, *38* (3), 386–395.

121. (a) Harding, D., Fournel-Gigleux, S., Jackson, M. R., Burchell, B., Cloning and substrate specificity of a human phenol UDP-glucuronosyltransferase expressed in COS-7 cells. *Proceedings of the National Academy of Sciences of the United States of America* **1988**, *85* (22), 8381–8385; (b) Ebner, T., Remmel, R. P., Burchell, B., Human bilirubin UDP-glucuronosyltransferase catalyzes the glucuronidation of ethinylestradiol. *Molecular Pharmacology* **1993**, *43* (4), 649–654.

122. Hanioka, N., Jinno, H., Tanaka-Kagawa, T., Nishimura, T., Ando, M., Determination of UDP-glucuronosyltransferase UGT1A6 activity in human and rat liver microsomes by HPLC with UV detection. *Journal of Pharmaceutical and Biomedical Analysis* **2001**, *25* (1), 65–75.

123. Krishnaswamy, S., Hao, Q., Von Moltke, L. L., Greenblatt, D. J., Court, M. H., Evaluation of 5-hydroxytryptophol and other endogenous serotonin (5-hydroxytryptamine) analogs as substrates for UDP-glucuronosyltransferase 1A6. *Drug Metabolism and Disposition: The Biological Fate of Chemicals* **2004**, *32* (8), 862–869.

124. Benoit-Biancamano, M. O., Connelly, J., Villeneuve, L., Caron, P., Guillemette, C., Deferiprone glucuronidation by human tissues and recombinant UDP glucuronosyltransferase 1A6: An *in vitro* investigation of genetic and splice variants. *Drug Metabolism and Disposition: The Biological Fate of Chemicals* **2009**, *37* (2), 322–329.

125. (a) Li, Q., Lamb, G., Tukey, R. H., Characterization of the UDP-glucuronosyltransferase 1A locus in lagomorphs: Evidence for duplication of the UGT1A6 gene. *Molecular Pharmacology* **2000**, *58* (1), 89–97; (b) Tephly, T. R., Burchell, B., UDP-glucuronosyltransferases: A family of detoxifying enzymes. *Trends in Pharmacological Sciences* **1990**, *11* (7), 276–279.

126. Gao, C., Shi, R., Wang, T., Tan, H., Xu, H., Ma, Y., Interaction between oblongifolin C and UDP-glucuronosyltransferase isoforms in human liver and intestine microsomes. *Xenobiotica; the Fate of Foreign Compounds in Biological Systems* **2015**, *45* (7), 578–585.

127. Kazmi, F., Haupt, L. J., Horkman, J. R., Smith, B. D., Buckley, D. B., Wachter, E. A., Singer, J. M., *In vitro* inhibition of human liver cytochrome P450 (CYP) and UDP-glucuronosyltransferase (UGT) enzymes by rose bengal: System-dependent effects on inhibitory potential. *Xenobiotica; the Fate of Foreign Compounds in Biological Systems* **2014**, *44* (7), 606–614.

128. Pang, X., Zhang, Y., Gao, R., Zhong, K., Zhong, D., Chen, X., Effects of rifampin and ketoconazole on pharmacokinetics of morinidazole in healthy chinese subjects. *Antimicrobial Agents and Chemotherapy* **2014**, *58* (10), 5987–5993.

129. (a) Devineni, D., Vaccaro, N., Murphy, J., Curtin, C., Mamidi, R. N., Weiner, S., Wang, S. S. et al., Effects of rifampin, cyclosporine A, and probenecid on the pharmacokinetic profile of canagliflozin, a sodium glucose co-transporter 2 inhibitor, in healthy participants. *International Journal of Clinical Pharmacology and Therapeutics* **2015**, *53* (2), 115–128; (b) Kasichayanula, S., Liu, X., Griffen, S. C., Lacreta, F. P., Boulton, D. W., Effects of rifampin and mefenamic acid on the pharmacokinetics and pharmacodynamics of dapagliflozin. *Diabetes, Obesity & Metabolism* **2013**, *15* (3), 280–283.

130. Soars, M. G., Petullo, D. M., Eckstein, J. A., Kasper, S. C., Wrighton, S. A., An assessment of udp-glucuronosyltransferase induction using primary human hepatocytes. *Drug Metabolism and Disposition: The Biological Fate of Chemicals* **2004**, *32* (1), 140–148.

131. (a) Bernard, O., Guillemette, C., The main role of UGT1A9 in the hepatic metabolism of mycophenolic acid and the effects of naturally occurring variants. *Drug Metabolism and Disposition: The Biological Fate of Chemicals* **2004**, *32* (8), 775–778; (b) Picard, N., Ratanasavanh, D., Premaud, A., Le Meur, Y., Marquet, P., Identification of the UDP-glucuronosyltransferase isoforms involved in mycophenolic acid phase II metabolism. *Drug Metabolism and Disposition: The Biological Fate of Chemicals* **2005**, *33* (1), 139–146.

132. Rowland, A., Knights, K. M., Mackenzie, P. I., Miners, J. O., The "albumin effect" and drug glucuronidation: Bovine serum albumin and fatty acid-free human serum albumin enhance the glucuronidation of UDP-glucuronosyltransferase (UGT) 1A9 substrates but not UGT1A1 and UGT1A6 activities. *Drug Metabolism and Disposition: The Biological Fate of Chemicals* **2008**, *36* (6), 1056–1062.

133. Miles, K. K., Stern, S. T., Smith, P. C., Kessler, F. K., Ali, S., Ritter, J. K., An investigation of human and rat liver microsomal mycophenolic acid glucuronidation: Evidence for a principal role of UGT1A enzymes and species differences in UGT1A specificity. *Drug Metabolism and Disposition: The Biological Fate of Chemicals* **2005**, *33* (10), 1513–1520.

134. Nishiyama, T., Kobori, T., Arai, K., Ogura, K., Ohnuma, T., Ishii, K., Hayashi, K., Hiratsuka, A., Identification of human UDP-glucuronosyltransferase isoform(s) responsible for the C-glucuronidation of phenylbutazone. *Archives of Biochemistry and Biophysics* **2006**, *454* (1), 72–79.

135. Kerdpin, O., Elliot, D. J., Mackenzie, P. I., Miners, J. O., Sulfinpyrazone C-glucuronidation is catalyzed selectively by human UDP-glucuronosyltransferase 1A9. *Drug Metabolism and Disposition: The Biological Fate of Chemicals* **2006**, *34* (12), 1950–1953.

136. Yao, M., Cao K, Zhang D, Rodriques D, Humphreys WG, Zhu M. In *Identification of the Human UDP-glucuronosyltransferase Enyzme(s) Involved in Glucuronidation of Dapagliflozin.*, America Association of Pharmaceutical Scintists, Los Angeles, CA, November 8–12, 2009.

137. Lautala, P., Ethell, B. T., Taskinen, J., Burchell, B., The specificity of glucuronidation of entacapone and tolcapone by recombinant human UDP-glucuronosyltransferases. *Drug Metabolism and Disposition: The Biological Fate of Chemicals* **2000**, *28* (11), 1385–1389.

138. Sun, H., Ma, Z., Lu, D., Wu, B., Regio- and isoform-specific glucuronidation of psoralidin: Evaluation of 3-o-glucuronidation as a functional marker for UGT1A9. *Journal of Pharmaceutical Sciences* **2015**, *104* (7), 2369–2377.

139. Miners, J. O., Bowalgaha, K., Elliot, D. J., Baranczewski, P., Knights, K. M., Characterization of niflumic acid as a selective inhibitor of human liver microsomal UDP-glucuronosyltransferase 1A9: Application to the reaction phenotyping of acetaminophen glucuronidation. *Drug Metabolism and Disposition: The Biological Fate of Chemicals* **2011**, *39* (4), 644–652.

140. Margaillan, G., Rouleau, M., Klein, K., Fallon, J. K., Caron, P., Villeneuve, L., Smith, P. C., Zanger, U. M., Guillemette, C., Multiplexed targeted quantitative proteomics predicts hepatic glucuronidation potential. *Drug Metabolism and Disposition: The Biological Fate of Chemicals* **2015**, *43* (9), 1331–1335.

141. Margaillan, G., Rouleau, M., Fallon, J. K., Caron, P., Villeneuve, L., Turcotte, V., Smith, P. C., Joy, M. S., Guillemette, C., Quantitative profiling of human renal UDP-glucuronosyltransferases and glucuronidation activity: A comparison of normal and tumoral kidney tissues. *Drug Metabolism and Disposition: The Biological Fate of Chemicals* **2015**, *43* (4), 611–619.

142. (a) Hedaya, M. A., Elmquist, W. F., Sawchuk, R. J., Probenecid inhibits the metabolic and renal clearances of zidovudine (AZT) in human volunteers. *Pharmaceutical Research* **1990**, *7* (4), 411–4117; (b) de Miranda, P., Good, S. S., Yarchoan, R., Thomas, R. V., Blum, M. R., Myers, C. E., Broder, S., Alteration of zidovudine pharmacokinetics by probenecid in patients with AIDS or AIDS-related complex. *Clinical Pharmacology and Therapeutics* **1989**, *46* (5), 494–500; (c) Kornhauser, D. M., Petty, B. G., Hendrix, C. W., Woods, A. S., Nerhood, L. J., Bartlett, J. G., Lietman, P. S., Probenecid and zidovudine metabolism. *Lancet* **1989**, *2* (8661), 473–475.

143. Lertora, J. J., Rege, A. B., Greenspan, D. L., Akula, S., George, W. J., Hyslop, N. E., Jr., Agrawal, K. C., Pharmacokinetic interaction between zidovudine and valproic acid in patients infected with human immunodeficiency virus. *Clinical Pharmacology and Therapeutics* **1994**, *56* (3), 272–278.

144. Sahai, J., Gallicano, K., Pakuts, A., Cameron, D. W., Effect of fluconazole on zidovudine pharmacokinetics in patients infected with human immunodeficiency virus. *The Journal of Infectious Diseases* **1994**, *169* (5), 1103–1107.

145. Lee, B. L., Tauber, M. G., Sadler, B., Goldstein, D., Chambers, H. F., Atovaquone inhibits the glucuronidation and increases the plasma concentrations of zidovudine. *Clinical Pharmacology and Therapeutics* **1996**, *59* (1), 14–21.

146. Barbier, O., Turgeon, D., Girard, C., Green, M. D., Tephly, T. R., Hum, D. W., Belanger, A., 3′-azido-3′-deoxythimidine (AZT) is glucuronidated by human UDP-glucuronosyltransferase 2B7 (UGT2B7). *Drug Metabolism and Disposition: The Biological Fate of Chemicals* **2000**, *28* (5), 497–502.

147. Bowalgaha, K., Elliot, D. J., Mackenzie, P. I., Knights, K. M., Miners, J. O., The glucuronidation of Delta4-3-Keto C19- and C21-hydroxysteroids by human liver microsomal and recombinant UDP-glucuronosyltransferases (UGTs): 6alpha- and 21-hydroxyprogesterone are selective substrates for UGT2B7. *Drug Metabolism and Disposition: The Biological Fate of Chemicals* **2007**, *35* (3), 363–370.

148. (a) Court, M. H., Krishnaswamy, S., Hao, Q., Duan, S. X., Patten, C. J., Von Moltke, L. L.; Greenblatt, D. J., Evaluation of 3′-azido-3′-deoxythymidine, morphine, and codeine as probe substrates for UDP-glucuronosyltransferase 2B7 (UGT2B7) in human liver microsomes: Specificity and influence of the UGT2B7 * 2 polymorphism. *Drug Metabolism and Disposition: The Biological Fate of Chemicals* **2003**, *31* (9), 1125–1133; (b) Coffman, B. L., Rios, G. R., King, C. D., Tephly, T. R., Human UGT2B7 catalyzes morphine glucuronidation. *Drug Metabolism and Disposition: The Biological Fate of Chemicals* **1997**, *25* (1), 1–4.

149. Innocenti, F., Iyer, L., Ramirez, J., Green, M. D., Ratain, M. J., Epirubicin glucuronidation is catalyzed by human UDP-glucuronosyltransferase 2B7. *Drug Metabolism and Disposition: The Biological Fate of Chemicals* **2001**, *29* (5), 686–692.

150. Barre, L., Fournel-Gigleux, S., Finel, M., Netter, P., Magdalou, J., Ouzzine, M., Substrate specificity of the human UDP-glucuronosyltransferase UGT2B4 and UGT2B7. Identification of a critical aromatic amino acid residue at position 33. *The FEBS Journal* **2007**, *274* (5), 1256–1264.

151. Kaji, H., Kume, T., Regioselective glucuronidation of denopamine: Marked species differences and identification of human udp-glucuronosyltransferase isoform. *Drug Metabolism and Disposition: The Biological Fate of Chemicals* **2005**, *33* (3), 403–412.

152. (a) Donato, M. T., Montero, S., Castell, J. V., Gomez-Lechon, M. J., Lahoz, A., Validated assay for studying activity profiles of human liver UGTs after drug exposure: Inhibition and induction studies. *Analytical and Bioanalytical Chemistry* **2010**, *396* (6), 2251–2263; (b) Uchaipichat, V., Mackenzie, P. I., Guo, X. H., Gardner-Stephen, D., Galetin, A., Houston, J. B., Miners, J. O., Human udp-glucuronosyltransferases: isoform selectivity and kinetics of 4-methylumbelliferone and 1-naphthol glucuronidation, effects of organic solvents, and inhibition by diclofenac and probenecid. *Drug Metabolism and Disposition: The Biological Fate of Chemicals* **2004**, *32* (4), 413–423.

153. Bichlmaier, I., Kurkela, M., Joshi, T., Siiskonen, A., Ruffer, T., Lang, H., Finel, M., Yli-Kauhaluoma, J., Potent inhibitors of the human UDP-glucuronosyltransferase 2B7 derived from the sesquiterpenoid alcohol longifolol. *ChemMedChem* **2007**, *2* (6), 881–889.

154. Lapham, K., Bauman, J. N., Walsky, R. L., Niosi, M., Orozco, C. C., Bourcier, K., Giddens, G., Obach, R. S., Hyland, R., Goosen, T. C., Digoxin and tranilast identified as novel isoform-selective inhibitors of human UDP glucuronosyltransferase 1A9 (UGT1A9) activity. In *18th North American International Society of Xenobiotics*, Drug Metabolism Review: 2012, Vol. 44.

155. Ghosal, A., Hapangama, N., Yuan, Y., Achanfuo-Yeboah, J., Iannucci, R., Chowdhury, S., Alton, K., Patrick, J. E., Zbaida, S., Identification of human UDP-glucuronosyltransferase enzyme(s) responsible for the glucuronidation of ezetimibe (Zetia). *Drug Metabolism and Disposition: The Biological Fate of Chemicals* **2004**, *32* (3), 314–320.

156. Abernethy, D. R., Greenblatt, D. J., Ameer, B., Shader, R. I., Probenecid impairment of acetaminophen and lorazepam clearance: Direct inhibition of ether glucuronide formation. *The Journal of Pharmacology and Experimental Therapeutics* **1985**, *234* (2), 345–349.

157. Samara, E. E., Granneman, R. G., Witt, G. F., Cavanaugh, J. H., Effect of valproate on the pharmacokinetics and pharmacodynamics of lorazepam. *Journal of Clinical Pharmacology* **1997**, *37* (5), 442–450.

158. Court, M. H., Duan, S. X., Guillemette, C., Journault, K., Krishnaswamy, S., Von Moltke, L. L., Greenblatt, D. J., Stereoselective conjugation of oxazepam by human UDP-glucuronosyltransferases (UGTs): S-oxazepam is glucuronidated by UGT2B15, while R-oxazepam is glucuronidated by UGT2B7 and UGT1A9. *Drug Metabolism and Disposition: The Biological Fate of Chemicals* **2002**, *30* (11), 1257–1265.

159. Manevski, N., Troberg, J., Svaluto-Moreolo, P., Dziedzic, K., Yli-Kauhaluoma, J., Finel, M., Albumin stimulates the activity of the human UDP-glucuronosyltransferases 1A7, 1A8, 1A10, 2A1, and 2B15, but the effects are enzyme and substrate dependent. *PloS one* **2013**, *8* (1), e54767.

160. (a) Gradinaru, J., Romand, S., Geiser, L., Carrupt, P. A., Spaggiari, D., Rudaz, S., Inhibition screening method of microsomal UGTs using the cocktail approach. *European Journal of Pharmaceutical Sciences: Official Journal of the European Federation for Pharmaceutical Sciences* **2015**, *71*, 35–45; (b) Shoda, T., Fukuhara, K., Goda, Y., Okuda, H., 4-Hydroxy-3-methoxymethamphetamine glucuronide as a phase II metabolite of 3,4-methylenedioxymethamphetamine: Enzyme-assisted synthesis and involvement of human hepatic uridine 5′-diphosphate-glucuronosyltransferase 2B15 in the glucuronidation. *Chemical & Pharmaceutical Bulletin* **2009**, *57* (5), 472–475.

161. Hanioka, N., Naito, T., Narimatsu, S., Human UDP-glucuronosyltransferase isoforms involved in bisphenol A glucuronidation. *Chemosphere* **2008**, *74* (1), 33–36.

162. Zhang, J. Y., Zhan, J., Cook, C. S., Ings, R. M., Breau, A. P., Involvement of human UGT2B7 and 2B15 in rofecoxib metabolism. *Drug Metabolism and Disposition: The Biological Fate of Chemicals* **2003**, *31* (5), 652–658.

163. Ethell, B. T., Anderson, G. D., Burchell, B., The effect of valproic acid on drug and steroid glucuronidation by expressed human UDP-glucuronosyltransferases. *Biochemical Pharmacology* **2003**, *65* (9), 1441–1449.

164. Rowland, M., Matin, S. B., Kinetics of drug-drug interactions. *Journal of Pharmacokinetics and Biopharmaceutics* **1973**, *1* (6), 553–567.

165. Cheng, Y., Prusoff, W. H., Relationship between the inhibition constant (K1) and the concentration of inhibitor which causes 50 per cent inhibition (I50) of an enzymatic reaction. *Biochemical Pharmacology* **1973**, *22* (23), 3099–3108.

166. Kanamitsu, S., Ito, K., Sugiyama, Y., Quantitative prediction of *in vivo* drug-drug interactions from *in vitro* data based on physiological pharmacokinetics: Use of maximum unbound concentration of inhibitor at the inlet to the liver. *Pharmaceutical Research* **2000**, *17* (3), 336–343.

167. Shen, D. D., Kunze, K. L., Thummel, K. E., Enzyme-catalyzed processes of first-pass hepatic and intestinal drug extraction. *Advanced Drug Delivery Reviews* **1997**, *27* (2–3), 99–127.

168. (a) Paine, M. F., Shen, D. D., Kunze, K. L., Perkins, J. D., Marsh, C. L., McVicar, J. P., Barr, D. M., Gillies, B. S., Thummel, K. E., First-pass metabolism of midazolam by the human intestine. *Clinical Pharmacology and Therapeutics* **1996**, *60* (1), 14–24; (b) Kolars, J. C., Awni, W. M., Merion, R. M., Watkins, P. B., First-pass metabolism of cyclosporin by the gut. *Lancet* **1991**, *338* (8781), 1488–1490.

169. Galetin, A., Hinton, L. K., Burt, H., Obach, R. S., Houston, J. B., Maximal inhibition of intestinal first-pass metabolism as a pragmatic indicator of intestinal contribution to the drug-drug interactions for CYP3A4 cleared drugs. *Current Drug Metabolism* **2007**, *8* (7), 685–693.

170. Rostami-Hodjegan, A., Tucker, G., "*In silico*" simulations to assess the "*in vivo*" consequences of "*in vitro*" metabolic drug-drug interactions. *Drug Discovery Today. Technologies* **2004**, *1* (4), 441–448.

171. (a) Huang, S. M., Lesko, L. J., Williams, R. L., Assessment of the quality and quantity of drug-drug interaction studies in recent NDA submissions: Study design and data analysis issues. *Journal of Clinical Pharmacology* **1999**, *39* (10), 1006–1014; (b) Obach, R. S., Walsky, R. L., Venkatakrishnan, K., Houston, J. B., Tremaine, L. M., *In vitro* cytochrome P450 inhibition data and the prediction of drug-drug interactions: Qualitative relationships, quantitative predictions, and the rank-order approach. *Clinical Pharmacology and Therapeutics* **2005**, *78* (6), 582–592; (c) Rodrigues, A. D., Prioritization of clinical drug interaction studies using *in vitro* cytochrome P450 data: Proposed refinement and expansion of the "rank order" approach. *Drug Metabolism Letters* **2007**, *1* (1), 31–35.

172. Bjornsson, T. D., Callaghan, J. T., Einolf, H. J., Fischer, V., Gan, L., Grimm, S., Kao, J. et al., Manufacturers of America Drug Metabolism/Clinical Pharmacology Technical Working, G., Evaluation, F. D. A. C. F. D., Research, The conduct of *in vitro* and *in vivo* drug-drug interaction studies: A pharmaceutical research and manufacturers of America (PhRMA) perspective. *Drug Metabolism and Disposition: The Biological Fate of Chemicals* **2003**, *31* (7), 815–832.

17

Enzyme Induction Studies in Drug Discovery and Development

Joshua G. Dekeyser and Jan L. Wahlstrom

CONTENTS

Introduction

Changes in the expression of absorption, distribution, metabolism and excretion (ADME) genes can impact the pharmacokinetics (PK) of many small molecule drugs. Regulation of the expression of these genes can occur at the level of transcription, translation, mRNA stability, and protein stability. The most common and well-studied of these is altered transcription through the activation of a trio of receptors the aryl hydrocarbon receptor (AHR), the constitutive androstane receptor (CAR), and the pregnane X receptor (PXR). Activation of these receptors leads to an increase in transcription of their target genes (Table 17.1) and increased protein concentrations in the cell. In the case of enzyme induction, the most common consequence is a decrease in exposure of drugs that are substrates of

TABLE 17.1

Target ADME Genes and Prototypical Activators of the Xenobiotic Receptors

Xenobiotic Receptor	Human ADME Genes Regulated				Prototypical Activators	References
	Phase 1	Phase 2	Transporters			
			Efflux	Uptake		
AHR	CYP1A1, CYP1A2, CYP1B1	UGT1A1, UGT1A3, UGT1A4, UGT1A6, UGT1A7, UGT1A8, UGT1A10, UGT2B4	MRP3, MRP4, BCRP	None identified	Dioxin, omeprazole, 3-methylcholanthrene, beta napthoflavone	2–11
CAR	CYP2A6, CYP2B6, CYP3A4, CYP2C8, CYP2C9, CYP2C19	UGT1A1, UGT2B7, SULT1A1	Pgp, MRP2, BCRP	None identified	Phenobarbital, phenytoin, carbamazepine, efavirenz, nevirapine, CITCO	4,6,12–19
PXR	CYP2A6, CYP2B6, CYP2C8, CYP2C9, CYP2C19, CYP3A4, CYP3A7	UGT1A1, UGT1A3, UGT1A4, SULT2A1	Pgp, MRP2, MRP3, BCRP	OATP1A2	Rifampicin, hyperforin, bosentan, ritonavir, simvastatin, reserpine, nicardipine, terbinafine, tamoxifen, troglitazone, RU486, cyclophosphamide	6,13,15–18,20–27

the induced enzyme. Induction of transporters can result in an increase or decrease in absorption for uptake and efflux transporters, respectively, and may also alter the intracellular concentrations of their substrates. Most commonly, the site of this response is in the liver and GI tract, but response at the lungs and blood brain barrier are also important for understanding systemic ADME implications. AHR is expressed ubiquitously, while expression of CAR and PXR is generally restricted to the liver and GI tract.[1] For the purposes of this chapter, the term "xenobiotic receptors" will refer to AHR, CAR, and PXR. Other receptors will be discussed but their role in regulating ADME genes is limited compared to the xenobiotic receptors.

The focus of this chapter will be to provide a broad understanding of the process of induction as well as other phenomenon related to the change in expression levels of ADME genes. There will be an emphasis on how this field is applied to the drug discovery and development process. The bulk of the content will focus on induction through changes in gene transcription since this is the most common mechanism for clinically relevant events. Non-transcriptional induction and gene suppression will be discussed in less detail. Generally speaking, the impact of induction leads to a decrease in exposure of victim substrates that can lead to a loss of efficacy or an increase in the formation of a toxic metabolite; the goal of the ADME scientist is ultimately to assess this risk and ensure patient safety.

Inducible Genes

Phase I

The Phase I oxidation enzymes play an important role in drug metabolism. The two major families of phase I enzymes are the cytochromes P450 (CYPs) and flavin-monooxygenases (FMOs). Through their activity on substrates, these enzymes function to deactivate pharmacologic molecules by increasing their hydrophilicity and clearance. The FMOs are generally not thought to be inducible by xenobiotics,[28] although some recent reports suggest induction by AHR in mouse liver.[29,30] The CYPs have a much larger role in drug metabolism compared to the FMOs and many of the CYP enzymes are inducible. In humans, CYP1A2, CYP2A6, CYP2B6, CYP2C8, CYP2C9, CYP2C19, CYP2D6, CYP2E1, CYP3A4, and CYP3A5 have been the most widely implicated in drug metabolism; although emerging CYPs such as CYP2J2 have garnered attention due to the identification of a number of known drugs as substrates for this enzyme.[31] Of these, all but CYP2D6 are known to be inducible, and only CYP2E1 has been shown to be induced by a non-transcriptional mechanism.[32] In the case of CYP2J2, the evidence for its potential to be induced is limited with a modest 1.8-fold increase noted in human primary cardiomyocytes after treatment with rosiglitazone.[33]

Phase II

The phase II conjugation enzymes: UDP-glucuronosyltransferases (UGTs), glutathione S-transferases (GSTs), N-acetyltransferases, methyltransferases, and sulfotransferases (SULTs) work by conjugating a functional group to their substrates. All of these enzymes are known to be inducible to varying degrees.[34–38] The human UDP-glucuronosyltransferase 1A (UGT1A) gene is probably the most relevant to drug metabolism, and transcriptional regulation of this gene is complex.[6] The nine different UGT1A isoforms (UGT1A1, 1A3, 1A4, 1A5, 1A6, 1A7, 1A8, 1A9, and 1A10) are derived by splicing a unique first exon to 4 common exons and a shared 3′-UTR (untranslated region). The promoter region immediately upstream of the first exon provides the genetic context for differential gene expression and regulation by transcription factors. Further regulation occurs at the level of mRNA stability with repression of UGT1A1 protein expression by miRNA 491-3p having been demonstrated.[39] Since the 9 isoforms share a common 3′-UTR, it seems likely that all isoforms will undergo similar regulation at the mRNA level. In light of these complexities, it is not surprising that evidence suggests UGT mRNA levels may poorly correlate with protein levels in tissues,[40] and researchers should use caution when trying to extrapolate between any single endpoint of UGT1A expression.

Transporters

Induction of both efflux and uptake transporters has been demonstrated in the GI tract and liver.[41–43] It has also been suggested to occur at the blood brain barrier, but further investigation of this and its potential ramifications for drug distribution to the brain is warranted.[44] P-glycoprotein (Pgp/MDR1a) can transport a large number of structurally diverse molecules across cell membranes. A clinical trial investigating the effects of rifampicin (600 mg/day for 10 days) on single-dose pharmacokinetics of digoxin (1mg PO and IV) found an approximately 30% decrease in AUC for oral digoxin versus about a 15% decrease in AUC after IV administration. The AUC of orally administered digoxin correlated with Pgp expression in patient biopsies. These results led to the conclusion that induction of Pgp by rifampicin leads to significant decreases in plasma concentrations of orally administered digoxin.[45] A similar result was found for talinolol,[46] which, like digoxin, has little metabolic clearance. Taken together, these results suggest the potential for clinical DDIs due to induction of transporters when victim drugs are highly cleared by transport mechanisms; however, it is difficult to assess how important this effect is for compounds that have metabolism as an additional route of clearance since many enzymes are also targets for inducers. Furthermore, with the exception of Pgp, there is a dearth of validated substrates for transporters important to drug development.

Mechanisms of ADME Gene Regulation

Transcriptional Induction

The regulation of transcription is a complex process, and here we will only provide a highly simplified overview on the process to orient the reader. The most important thing for the ADME scientist to keep in mind is that receptor activation is the first step in a time-dependent process that generally involves, receptor translocation, DNA binding, increased mRNA transcription, increased protein translation, and ultimately increased enzyme activity. For a deeper dive into the regulation of gene transcription, the reader is referred to a number of reviews on the topic.[47–49]

The transcription of genes is a tightly controlled system that involves multiple modes of regulation. First is the structure of chromatin, controlled by the acetylation and deacetylation of histones, which leads to the loosening and tightening of chromatin structure, respectively. This allows greater or lesser access to the RNA holoenzyme, a conglomerate of protein machinery made up of RNA polymerase II and other proteins. Transcription factors (trans-acting elements), such as the xenobiotic receptors, bind to specific DNA sequences (cis-acting elements) in the promoter region of target genes where they recruit coactivators that can alter the chromatin structure and recruit the holoenzyme, increasing the rate of transcription. These cis-acting elements are often referred to as response elements (REs), the most pertinent REs for the induction of ADME genes are the phenobarbital response element (PBREM),[12] the xenobiotic response element (XREM),[50] and the antioxidant response element (ARE).[51] These are most commonly associated with CAR, PXR, and AHR, respectively, although there is promiscuity in the receptors that can bind specific Res, and the upstream regulatory region of a gene can have multiple REs. Conversely, corepressors can be recruited to the promoter region of a gene to increase chromatin packing, restrict holoenzyme access, and decrease transcription.

Non-Transcriptional Induction (CYP2E1)

Induction can also occur through non-transcriptional mechanisms such as protein stabilization, as is the case for CYP2E1. Alcohol, acetone, and isoniazid induce CYP2E1 by stabilizing the protein, which effectively increases the half-life of the enzyme.[52] CYP2E1 is known to metabolize acetaminophen into a toxic metabolite and, therefore, induction of CYP2E1 has important implications in hepatotoxicity.[53]

CYP Suppression

Recently, there has been growing focus on the potential for suppression of CYPs; defined as a decrease in CYP expression or activity that is not caused by enzyme inhibition. Clinical evidence suggests that elevated levels of cytokines that are found in autoimmune diseases may cause reduced CYP activity in the liver and increased exposure of drugs that rely on CYP mediated clearance in this patient population compared to healthy patients. A clinical study of 12 rheumatoid arthritis patients, who were being treated with the anti-IL6 antibody tocilizumab, found that reversal of the suppression occurred upon treatment and lead to an increased exposure of simvastatin in the study.[54] A number of studies have investigated the *in vitro* effects of cytokine treatment on CYP expression in hepatocytes.[55–57] Much of that work was summarized in a 2013 White Paper, which concluded that cytokine-mediated DDIs observed with anti-inflammatory therapeutic proteins cannot currently be predicted using *in vitro* data.[58]

Species Differences in Induction

Although the general function and target gene specificity of the xenobiotic receptors is conserved across species, the ligand binding profiles of CAR and PXR vary significantly. The reason for this may be supported by the "plant-animal warfare" hypothesis proposed by Nebert and Gonzalez.[59] The hypothesis states that species differences in drug metabolism arise from the constant battle of plants evolving new toxins to discourage their consumption, and animals continually evolving the enzyme systems that metabolize these toxins so that they can continue to use them as a source of food. Thereby as speciation occurs and diets change, the metabolic machinery of that species evolves to accommodate the specific diet. This hypothesis may be particularly relevant to CAR and PXR, which demonstrate positive evolution. Specific amino acid residues within their ligand binding pockets are more likely to see nonsynonymous mutations across species than what would be expected if there were a negative evolutionary pressure favoring conservation of amino acid sequence. This suggests that natural selection is favoring sequence diversity in the ligand binding pockets of CAR and PXR, presumably to allow for relatively rapid adaptation to important ligands.[60] For these reasons, most pre-clinical induction work in drug discovery focuses on understanding induction in human models.

Transcription Factors Involved in the Regulation of ADME Genes

AHR

The aryl hydrocarbon receptor (AHR) is a member of the basic helix-loop-helix per-arnt-sim family of transcription factors. It has been known for almost 50 years that the enzymes responsible for the hydroxylation of aryl hydrocarbons are inducible.[5,61] Initial reports suggested that it was responsible for regulating genetic pathways related to dioxin toxicity. These findings were later confirmed when AHR was cloned and ligand binding and transcriptional activity studies were conducted. Inactive AHR is sequestered in the cytoplasm where it is bound to heat shock protein 90 (HSP90) and the hepatitis B virus X-associated protein (XAP2). Upon binding, ligand translocates to the nucleus where it heterodimerizes with the AHR nuclear translocator protein (ARNT) and transcribes its target genes.[62] Additionally, it has been demonstrated that AHR is rapidly degraded in the nucleus after becoming active with the bulk of the transcription factor undergoing proteolysis through the ubiquitin proteasomal pathway within 30 minutes. This tightly linked control over AHR transcriptional activation and proteasomal degradation provides a negative feedback loop on the system.[63]

The Nuclear Receptors

The nuclear receptor (NR) family of transcription factors includes 47, 48, and 49 different genes in rat, human, and mouse, respectively, that share a modular domain structure.[64] They are involved in regulating numerous physiological processes including steroidogenesis, reproduction and development, circadian and basal metabolic functions, lipid metabolism, energy homeostasis, and bile acid and xenobiotic metabolism.[1,65] CAR and PXR are the most widely associated with xenobiotic metabolism, although others are implicated as indicated at the end of this section.

The human constitutive androstane receptor (hCAR) was initially cloned as MB67 in 1994. The initial report determined it to be an orphan nuclear receptor that could constitutively activated subset of retinoic acid response elements.[66] Shortly thereafter, the mouse orthologue (mCAR) was cloned and MB67 was renamed hCAR, the constitutive activity of both receptors was found to be dependent on the presence of the c-terminal AF-2 transcriptional activation motif.[67] Few CAR specific ligands have been identified. The most specific CAR ligand to date is CITCO, which was developed specifically to target CAR by GSK.[14] The X-ray crystal structure showed that the constitutive activity is due to a single turn Helix X that restricts the movement of the AF-2 helix, favoring the active state.[68]

In the inactive state, CAR is sequestered in the cytoplasm bound to the cytoplasmic CAR retention protein (CCRP) and HSP90.[69] Activation of the receptor can occur through direct binding of the receptor or through indirect mechanisms that are not yet fully elucidated but are believed to involve phosphorylation of the receptor by protein phosphatase 2A (PP2A).[70,71] Both direct and indirect activation leads to translocation of the receptor to the nucleus where it can bind to the promoter region of its target genes and activate transcription.

The human CAR gene undergoes alternative splicing leading, and over 20 different hCAR transcripts have been identified.[72] Two of these alternatively spliced transcripts hCAR2 and hCAR3 have been studied extensively *in vitro* and were found to have lost the constitutive activity of wild-type CAR (aka hCAR1) instead acting in the more typical ligand dependent fashion. Initial investigations into CAR3 suggested that its ligand binding profile closer mirrored that of CAR1. Contrarily, CAR2 has been shown to have a unique ligand binding profile demonstrating distinct yet overlapping ligand specificity.[73–80] The clinical significance of these splice variants is not known.

The human pregnane X receptor gene was initially cloned in 2002 and was determined to be an orphan nuclear receptor. The importance of this receptor was recognized almost immediately when it was found to be responsible for the induction of CYP3A4, a phenomenon long known to have significant implications in drug development but for which the mechanism was previously unknown.[81–84] PXR has a large flexible ligand binding pocket, which allows for broad ligand specificity leading to a diverse array of identified ligands.[85–88] It is notable that two of the gene targets of PXR, CYP3A4, and Pgp, are also highly promiscuous proteins involved in the metabolism and excretion of xenobiotics. Together they present a potent defense against potentially toxic xenobiotics and, at times, a difficult barrier to drug development.

The subcellular localization of PXR is not as well established as it is for CAR. In mouse, it has been demonstrated to be sequestered in the cytoplasm by CCRP and HSP90, in the same manner as CAR.[89] Cytoplasmic sequestration has yet to be established for human and there are indications that unliganded PXR resides in the nucleus.[90] Functionally speaking, the cellular localization of PXR may not be as important as it is for CAR, since PXR is not known to demonstrate activity in the absence of ligand and, unlike CAR, ligand binding is the primary activating event, not nuclear translocation. However, if human PXR does reside primarily in the nucleus, it could act as a gene silencer by remaining bound to its REs and corepressors to its target genes.[91]

Both transcriptional and post-transcriptional regulation of PXR are known to occur. Another nuclear receptor, hepatocyte nuclear factor 4α (HNF4A), has been shown to transactivate the PXR gene through a DR1 response element.[92] Binding of micro-RNA 148a to the 3′UTR of PXR decreases protein levels of the receptor and also decreases basal CYP3A4 levels as well as the magnitude of CYP3A4 induction in response to rifampicin.[93] It has also been proposed that SUMOylation and ubiquitylation of PXR can lead to degradation by the proteasome and direct the response in liver to xenobiotic or inflammatory stress.[94–96]

Cross-talk between CAR and PXR is well documented, both in the genes that they regulate and their ligand specificity.[13] Although there are well-established PXR specific ligands, such as rifampicin, hyperforin, bosentan, and ritonavir, this is not the case for CAR. Even CITCO, the most specific CAR ligand, has been shown to activate PXR at concentrations approximately 50-fold higher than those that demonstrate CAR selectivity.[14] Functionally speaking, this can make it very difficult to ascribe a particular inducer to an individual receptor.

A number of other nuclear receptors have also been implicated in the regulation of ADME genes. This includes the glucocorticoid receptor (GR), the peroxisome proliferator-activated receptors (PPARs), the farnesoid X receptor (FXR), the liver X receptor (LXR), and the small hetero dimer partner (SHP). The direct relationships can be difficult to assess due to the hierarchical nature of transcription factors. For example, GR activation has been shown to increase PXR expression *in vitro* an observation suggests that increased CYP3A4 expression by GR activators may be at least be in part due to increases PXR expression.[97] The PPARs have been shown to regulate CYP4A11 and a number of SULTs.[98–100] FXR induces the bile salt export pump (BSEP) in response the bile salt chenodeoxycholic acid[101] as well as OATP1B.[43] LXR is activated by cholesterol and increases the transcription of CYP7A1 and SULT1E1.[102,103] SHP is unique amongst nuclear receptors in that it lacks a DNA binding domain but is still able to heterodimerize with other nuclear receptors and inhibit their transcriptional activity.[104] Expression of SHP is induced by FXR and represses expression of CYP7A1.[105] The importance of SHP for drug metabolism remains to be established; however, the mechanism of this nuclear receptor highlights the complexity of the nuclear receptor transcriptional network.

NRF2

The nuclear factor (erythroid-derived 2)-like 2 (NRF2) is a basic leucine zipper (bZIP) transcription factor that protects against oxidative damage by regulating the expression of antioxidant proteins. First described in 1994, NRF2 was found to be ubiquitously expressed and showed strong transcriptional stimulation of β-globin genes.[106] NRF2 has been implicated in the regulation of many phase II enzymes including the UGTs, GSTs, NAD(P)H:quinone oxidoreductase, and aldehyde dehydrogenase.[6,107–109] Recent evidence suggests interplay between NRF2 and AHR.[110,111] Cross-talk between these receptors in their regulation of ADME genes may serve to further complicate mechanistic understanding of induction processes. The importance of NRF2 to the field of drug metabolism is still emerging, and further work is necessary to understand the clinical significance of these findings.

Preclinical Assessment of Induction

There are a number of *in vitro* and *in vivo* tools available for preclinical investigations aiming to determine whether or not a drug candidate will be an inducer *in vivo*. These range from relatively simple biochemical binding assays to complex transgenic animal models. A typical work flow for the evaluation of induction is to start with simple binding or reporter assays that can be set up in very high throughput assays followed by more robust assays using highly differentiated hepatocyte cell lines or, more commonly, primary hepatocytes. Data from these assays may be integrated into various mathematical models discussed later. A number of *in vivo* models also exist that have been engineered to better reflect human biology. The following sections will discuss the technical aspects of each of these assays as well as data interpretations and pros and cons of each.

Binding Assays

Biochemical ligand binding assays can be employed to determine if a chemical of interest binds to a specific receptor. Typically, this receptor is purified and then incubated with radiolabeled ligand. These assays can have very high throughput and be cost effective; however, they are limited to only providing information about binding, no information as to whether or not that binding leads to activation is gained. By running the assay as a displacement assay, one can assess whether or not binding is to the ligand binding pocket or another region of the protein.[112]

Reporter Assays

Reporter assays are one of the most common *in vitro* methods employed to determine activation of a specific receptor. In general, there are three components to these assays, a cell line, a plasmid containing the reporter gene and a plasmid containing the receptor of interest. Typical promoters include b-galactosidase and luciferase. Luciferase has become the reporter of choice due to its ease of use and low cost. By altering the promoter proximal to the reporter gene, a number of aspects of transactivation can be studied. Typically, the promoter region consists of the mammalian TATA box common to all genes and response elements specific to the gene of interest such as the PBREM, XREM, or ARE for CYP2B6, CYP3A4, and CYP1A2, respectively.[113–115]

PXR reporter assays have been validated and are useful in detecting potential CYP3A4 inducers.[27] On the other hand, a validated CAR assay has proven elusive. In transfected cell lines, CAR spontaneously translocates to the nucleus where it constitutively activates the reporter gene.[116] Efforts have been made to address this by using inverse agonists to lower constitutive activity, using known ligand activated splice variants instead of wild-type CAR[75,78,117] and by introducing specific mutations to remove constitutive activity.[118] Importantly, none of these alternative CAR reporter assays are able to detect indirect activation of the receptor like what is observed with phenobarbital and differences in ligands between the CAR isoforms has been observed.[73,74,117]

Another reporter assay that has utility in the study of nuclear receptors is the galactose-responsive transcription factor 4 (GAL4) system. The structure of the nuclear receptors allows for DNA binding domain (DBD) and the ligand binding domain (LBD) to function independently of one another. This observation has led researchers to fuse the LBD of nuclear receptors to the DBD of the yeast GAL4 gene. This system allows for the use of a single reporter construct containing the GAL4 promoter region to test activation of all the nuclear receptors by ligands.[119]

Cell Lines

A number of immortalized cell lines can be used to study various induction pathways without transfecting in any exogenous genes. The most common are the liver derived HepG2, Fa2N4, and HepaRG and the intestinal line LS174T. HepG2 cells retain a functional AHR pathway and can be used to assess activation of AHR by compounds by assessing changes in CYP1A; however, very little metabolic activity is retained in these cells and neither CAR nor PXR has been demonstrated to be functional. Fa2N4 cells retain more hepatocyte functions than HepG2 but lack CAR functionality.[120] The most recent hepatocyte cell line to garner attention in the field is the HepaRG line.[121] The parental line is a bipotent progenitor cell that can be driven to differentiate into two phenotypes in culture, biliary-epithelial like cells and hepatocyte-like cells. After differentiation, the resulting co-culture has been shown to respond to activators of all three major xenobiotic receptors, AHR, CAR, and PXR. The biggest downside to the HepaRG line is that the differentiation process is long and requires considerable expertise. However, differentiated cells are available commercially in cryopreserved vials and may offer some advantages over primary hepatocytes in terms of cost and data consistency since the supply of cells is theoretically infinite.

Primary Hepatocytes

Primary hepatocytes that have been isolated from human livers have long been considered the gold standard for *in vitro* studies investigating CYP induction and are the only *in vitro* model for which regulatory agencies currently accept *in vitro* data. CYP induction by the prototypical inducers phenobarbital and 3-methlycholanthrene using primary cultures of hepatocytes was first demonstrated in 1976.[4] Methods were refined and standardized over the following decades and the use of cultured hepatocytes has become common practice in the field. However, the need for freshly isolated cells meant that availability (particularly for human cells) was low and variability was high. This issue has been largely resolved with the development of robust cryopreservation techniques allowing for the creation of large cryopreserved lots of cells from a single donor. These lots can be qualified and maintained for use over periods of time. In culture, these cells retain the metabolic functions and induction pathways of hepatocytes *in vivo*. Typically, they are cultured in monolayer on collagen I coated plates or, in sandwich culture, by adding an overlay of matrigel or similar basement matrix.

After being allowed to attach to the plate and adapt to the culture conditions for a short period (typically a day or two), investigational drugs are added for a period of 24–72 hours after which the cells are washed, and probe substrates are added to measure rates of metabolite formation by inducible enzymes. Cells can also be lysed and mRNA quantified as a direct measurement of increased transcription.[122] The use of mRNA has gained favor recently due to a possible increase in sensitivity and lack of false negatives arising from compounds that are both inhibitors and inducers of enzymes.[123]

In Vivo Models

Due to the evolutionary divergence of the xenobiotic receptors, the use of animal models has questionable value regarding predictions of outcomes in humans. For questions that require the use of a whole organism, there are a few engineered rodent models that aim to recapitulate the human xenobiotic receptor functionality. Two mouse models of interest are the chimeric mouse in which mouse hepatocytes are largely replaced with human hepatocytes resulting in a chimeric animal with liver metabolic functions that are much more representative of the human condition, including induction.[124] The second is a transgenic model in which the mouse CAR and PXR genes have been removed and replaced with the full length human orthologues. These mice have been shown to generate functional CAR and PXR (as well as known splice variants) and to respond to prototypical activators of the human receptors.[125] Finally, recent advances in the engineering of knock-out (KO) animals has led to viable rat KO models, which are now commercially available for all the xenobiotic receptors as well as many other ADME genes.

Preclinical Regulatory Guidance

The FDA, EMA, and PMDA all issue regularly updated guidance on the use of preclinical induction data to support IND filings. These guidelines are available on the regulatory agencies websites and provide suggestions on study design and interpretation as well as decision trees to help investigators determine the likelihood of an investigational new drug to cause induction in the clinic.

Predictive Models of Induction

A number of models have been proposed and used in attempts to make quantitative predictions regarding clinical effects of induction. These include basic models, mechanistic/static models, and physiologically based pharmacokinetic (PBPK) modeling. The basic and mechanistic static models are mathematical equations, which allow for an assessment of clinical risk based on *in vitro* measurements of the EC_{50} and E_{max} values for induction as well as the expected clinical concentration of the inducer. The basic model assesses the risk of induction alone, whereas the mechanistic static model incorporates the effects of reversible inhibition, time-depending inhibition and induction.[126] Correlation approaches such as the relative induction score (RIS) are also used to assess the risk of clinical induction.[127,128] All of the above models assume worst-case scenarios for factors such as rate of dissolution and absorption in the gut as well as an assumption of a static maximal concentration in the system. More recently PBPK has emerged as a model that allows for much greater flexibility in the input parameters.[129–131]

PBPK modeling and simulation incorporates demographic, genetic, anatomical, physiological, and drug-specific parameters to predict drug concentration-time profiles.[132] PBPK may be used to simulate the effects of DDIs in a dynamic manner by allowing the victim and perpetrator concentrations and effects to vary over time; this approach more accurately represents the clinical situation than basic and static models, which assume constant and maximal exposure to an inducer.[130] Other advantages of DDI simulation using PBPK approaches include the ability to stagger victim and perpetrator dosing, quantitative prediction of expected inter-individual variability, dynamic alteration of the fraction metabolized (f_m) due to induction throughout the simulation, and the possibility to integrate multiple DDI mechanisms (reversible inhibition, mechanism-based inactivation, induction and transporter-mediated DDI) simultaneously into the same simulation.[133] Appropriate calibration of induction characteristics to the clinical situation, when known, have been demonstrated to improve the accuracy of induction predictions using PBPK.[129,131]

Regardless of the type of modeling used, key questions to be considered when implementing DDI modeling and simulation include: How accurate is our current estimation of f_m for a victim drug? Does induction in the gut need to be considered (CYP3A4)? Are major metabolites observed *in vitro* or *in vivo*, and do they exhibit contributory DDI characteristics? Are multiple mechanisms of DDI ("complex DDI") involved? Obtaining successively higher quality *in vitro* and *in vivo* information throughout pre-clinical and clinical development enables more accurate prediction of induction-based DDIs.[134]

Induction in the Clinical Setting

Based on the results of *in vitro* experiments and modeling using basic or mechanistic models, a clinical induction DDI study may be run. The first consideration is whether this study will use the drug under development as a perpetrator or victim of induction. If the drug is a perpetrator of induction, *in vitro* and multiple-dose first-in-human data will indicate whether it induces its own metabolism (autoinduction) in the event that the drug is cleared by the same drug metabolizing enzymes that it induces. Other considerations for design of a clinical induction study include: Will the study be run in healthy volunteers or patients? Should the study subjects be characterized for drug metabolizing enzyme genotype or phenotype? Will the study employ a crossover design? What is the dose regimen? What is the timing of the inducer dosing relative to the victim drug dose? Do the inducer, victim, or both need to be dosed to steady state? What concomitant medications, dietary constituents (i.e., grapefruit juice or herbal supplements such as St. John's Wort), or other environmental factors (i.e., smoking) may require exclusion from the study? Will measuring metabolites provide useful information on the enzyme pathways involved with induction? Careful consideration of these factors will allow for appropriate design of the induction study and prioritize patient safety.

The magnitude of the observed induction effect is dependent upon characteristics of both the victim and perpetrator drugs.[135] For clinical DDI studies, sensitive substrates (drugs that achieve a 5-fold or greater change in the area under the plasma concentration-time curve [AUC] when concomitantly administered with a known inhibitor or inducer of a specific drug elimination pathway) are generally selected as the victim in order to fully characterize the magnitude of the DDI. The inducing drug is then characterized as a strong ($\geq$5-fold reduction in victim AUC), moderate ($\geq$2 and <5-fold reduction in victim AUC), or weak ($\geq$1.25 and <2-fold reduction in victim AUC) inducer based on the magnitude of change observed with the victim drug (FDA, EMA, and Japanese regulatory guidance). Other commonly co-administered drugs may be tested as victims of induction if their major mechanism of clearance is inducible by the perpetrator drug, particularly if the victim has a narrow therapeutic range with high potential for the loss of efficacy.

Often multiple potential DDI mechanisms exist for drugs, and this can lead to unexpected clinical results. For example, induction studies using rifampicin as the perpetrator have led to counterintuitive results in the clinic when the victim drug is given intravenously.[136,137] In one study, 600 mg of rifampicin given orally for 5 days prior to IV dosing of romidepsin resulted in 80% and 60% increases in AUC and Cmax, respectively. This result is likely due to inhibition of active liver uptake transporters OATP1B1 and OATP1B3 by rifampicin[138,139] and brings into question the utility of rifampicin as an inducer for studies where the victim is known to require uptake transporters for liver exposure.[136] Another example is ritonavir known to be both a potent inducer and time-dependent inhibitor of CYP3A4.[140,141] In the clinic, ritonavir presents as an inhibitor of CYP3A4, markedly increasing exposures of CYP3A4 substrates such as midazolam and simvastatin.[142,143] This latter case demonstrates why it is important to not view *in vitro* data in isolation; particularly as the induction field moves towards mRNA as the preferred *in vitro* endpoint.

Summary

Induction of ADME genes is well recognized for its importance in altering the exposure of substrates of the induced enzyme; leading to loss of efficacy and, in some cases, toxicity. Over the past two decades, a molecular understanding of this process has emerged with the xenobiotic receptors having a primary role. Our understanding of CYP3A4 induction through PXR has made enormous progress during this time with quantitative predictions of clinical effect from *in vitro* data now being possible. It is important for the field to continue to extend our predictive capabilities to include the other inducible CYPs, phase II enzymes and transporters. The ability to incorporate a mechanistic understanding of induction, along with similar learnings from our colleagues in other areas of ADME science, into complex, dynamic models, such as PBPK, will in time allow for greatly enhanced predictions of clinical outcomes in humans and further reduce reliance on animal models. Even with the promise held by these models, it is still and will remain the job of the ADME scientist to understand the available tools (*in vitro*, *in vivo*, and *in silico*) and the limitations of each so that the appropriate questions are being asked to properly inform models, develop appropriate clinical trial design and ensure patient safety.

REFERENCES

1. Bookout AL, Jeong Y, Downes M, Yu RT, Evans RM, Mangelsdorf DJ. Anatomical profiling of nuclear receptor expression reveals a hierarchical transcriptional network. *Cell.* 2006;126(4):789–799.
2. Gotovdorj T, Lee E, Lim Y et al. 2,3,7,8-Tetrachlorodibenzo-p-dioxin induced cell-specific drug transporters with acquired cisplatin resistance in cisplatin sensitive cancer cells. *Journal of Korean Medical Science.* 2014;29(9):1188–1198.
3. Xu S, Weerachayaphorn J, Cai SY, Soroka CJ, Boyer JL. Aryl hydrocarbon receptor and NF-E2-related factor 2 are key regulators of human MRP4 expression. *American Journal of Physiology Gastrointestinal and Liver Physiology.* 2010;299(1):G126–G135.
4. Michalopoulos G, Sattler CA, Sattler GL, Pitot HC. Cytochrome P-450 induction by phenobarbital and 3-methylcholanthrene in primary cultures of hepatocytes. *Science.* 1976;193(4256):907–909.
5. Nebert DW, Gelboin HV. Substrate-inducible microsomal aryl hydroxylase in mammalian cell culture. I. Assay and properties of induced enzyme. *The Journal of Biological Chemistry.* 1968;243(23):6242–6249.

6. Hu DG, Meech R, McKinnon RA, Mackenzie PI. Transcriptional regulation of human UDP-glucuronosyltransferase genes. *Drug Metabolism Reviews.* 2014;46(4):421–458.

7. Cheng X, Maher J, Dieter MZ, Klaassen CD. Regulation of mouse organic anion-transporting polypeptides (Oatps) in liver by prototypical microsomal enzyme inducers that activate distinct transcription factor pathways. *Drug Metabolism and Disposition: The Biological Fate of Chemicals.* 2005;33(9):1276–1282.

8. Patel RD, Hollingshead BD, Omiecinski CJ, Perdew GH. Aryl-hydrocarbon receptor activation regulates constitutive androstane receptor levels in murine and human liver. *Hepatology.* 2007;46(1):209–218.

9. Beischlag TV, Luis Morales J, Hollingshead BD, Perdew GH. The aryl hydrocarbon receptor complex and the control of gene expression. *Critical Reviews in Eukaryotic Gene Expression.* 2008;18(3):207–250.

10. Harper PA, Prokipcak RD, Bush LE, Golas CL, Okey AB. Detection and characterization of the Ah receptor for 2,3,7,8-tetrachlorodibenzo-p-dioxin in the human colon adenocarcinoma cell line LS180. *Archives of Biochemistry and Biophysics.* 1991;290(1):27–36.

11. Le Vee M, Jouan E, Stieger B, Lecureur V, Fardel O. Regulation of human hepatic drug transporter activity and expression by diesel exhaust particle extract. *PLoS One.* 2015;10(3):e0121232.

12. Honkakoski P, Negishi M. Regulatory DNA elements of phenobarbital-responsive cytochrome P450 CYP2B genes. *Journal of Biochemical and Molecular Toxicology.* 1998;12(1):3–9.

13. Faucette SR, Zhang TC, Moore R et al. Relative activation of human pregnane X receptor versus constitutive androstane receptor defines distinct classes of CYP2B6 and CYP3A4 inducers. *The Journal of Pharmacology and Experimental Therapeutics.* 2007;320(1):72–80.

14. Maglich JM, Parks DJ, Moore LB et al. Identification of a novel human constitutive androstane receptor (CAR) agonist and its use in the identification of CAR target genes. *The Journal of Biological Chemistry.* 2003;278(19):17277–17283.

15. Kast HR, Goodwin B, Tarr PT et al. Regulation of multidrug resistance-associated protein 2 (ABCC2) by the nuclear receptors pregnane X receptor, farnesoid X-activated receptor, and constitutive androstane receptor. *The Journal of Biological Chemistry.* 2002;277(4):2908–2915.

16. Guo GL, Choudhuri S, Klaassen CD. Induction profile of rat organic anion transporting polypeptide 2 (oatp2) by prototypical drug-metabolizing enzyme inducers that activate gene expression through ligand-activated transcription factor pathways. *The Journal of Pharmacology and Experimental Therapeutics.* 2002;300(1):206–212.

17. Stedman CA, Liddle C, Coulter SA et al. Nuclear receptors constitutive androstane receptor and pregnane X receptor ameliorate cholestatic liver injury. *Proceedings of the National Academy of Sciences of the United States of America.* 2005;102(6):2063–2068.

18. Jigorel E, Le Vee M, Boursier-Neyret C, Parmentier Y, Fardel O. Differential regulation of sinusoidal and canalicular hepatic drug transporter expression by xenobiotics activating drug-sensing receptors in primary human hepatocytes. *Drug Metabolism and Disposition: The Biological Fate of Chemicals.* 2006;34(10):1756–1763.

19. Qatanani M, Zhang J, Moore DD. Role of the constitutive androstane receptor in xenobiotic-induced thyroid hormone metabolism. *Endocrinology.* 2005;146(3):995–1002.

20. Jones SA, Moore LB, Shenk JL et al. The pregnane X receptor: A promiscuous xenobiotic receptor that has diverged during evolution. *Molecular Endocrinology.* 2000;14(1):27–39.

21. Goodwin B, Moore LB, Stoltz CM, McKee DD, Kliewer SA. Regulation of the human CYP2B6 gene by the nuclear pregnane X receptor. *Molecular Pharmacology.* 2001;60(3):427–431.

22. Teng S, Jekerle V, Piquette-Miller M. Induction of ABCC3 (MRP3) by pregnane X receptor activators. *Drug Metabolism and Disposition: The Biological Fate of Chemicals.* 2003;31(11):1296–1299.

23. Harmsen S, Meijerman I, Febus CL, Maas-Bakker RF, Beijnen JH, Schellens JH. PXR-mediated induction of P-glycoprotein by anticancer drugs in a human colon adenocarcinoma-derived cell line. *Cancer Chemotherapy and Pharmacology.* 2010;66(4):765–771.

24. Meyer zu Schwabedissen HE, Tirona RG, Yip CS, Ho RH, Kim RB. Interplay between the nuclear receptor pregnane X receptor and the uptake transporter organic anion transporter polypeptide 1A2 selectively enhances estrogen effects in breast cancer. *Cancer Research.* 2008;68(22):9338–9347.

25. Shukla SJ, Sakamuru S, Huang R et al. Identification of clinically used drugs that activate pregnane X receptors. *Drug Metabolism and Disposition: The Biological Fate of Chemicals.* 2011;39(1):151–159.

26. Moore LB, Maglich JM, McKee DD et al. Pregnane X receptor (PXR), constitutive androstane receptor (CAR), and benzoate X receptor (BXR) define three pharmacologically distinct classes of nuclear receptors. *Molecular Endocrinology.* 2002;16(5):977–986.

27. Sinz M, Kim S, Zhu Z et al. Evaluation of 170 xenobiotics as transactivators of human pregnane X receptor (hPXR) and correlation to known CYP3A4 drug interactions. *Current Drug Metabolism.* 2006;7(4):375–388.

28. Krueger SK, Williams DE. Mammalian flavin-containing monooxygenases: Structure/function, genetic polymorphisms and role in drug metabolism. *Pharmacology & Therapeutics.* 2005;106(3):357–387.

29. Celius T, Roblin S, Harper PA et al. Aryl hydrocarbon receptor-dependent induction of flavin-containing monooxygenase mRNAs in mouse liver. *Drug Metabolism and Disposition: The Biological Fate of Chemicals.* 2008;36(12):2499–2505.

30. Celius T, Pansoy A, Matthews J et al. Flavin-containing monooxygenase-3: Induction by 3-methylcholanthrene and complex regulation by xenobiotic chemicals in hepatoma cells and mouse liver. *Toxicology and Applied Pharmacology.* 2010;247(1):60–69.

31. Lee CA, Neul D, Clouser-Roche A et al. Identification of novel substrates for human cytochrome P450 2J2. *Drug Metabolism and Disposition: The Biological Fate of Chemicals.* 2010;38(2):347–356.

32. Burk O, Koch I, Raucy J et al. The induction of cytochrome P450 3A5 (CYP3A5) in the human liver and intestine is mediated by the xenobiotic sensors pregnane X receptor (PXR) and constitutively activated receptor (CAR). *The Journal of Biological Chemistry.* 2004;279(37):38379–38385.

33. Evangelista EA, Kaspera R, Mokadam NA, Jones JP, 3rd, Totah RA. Activity, inhibition, and induction of cytochrome P450 2J2 in adult human primary cardiomyocytes. *Drug Metabolism and Disposition: The Biological Fate of Chemicals.* 2013;41(12):2087–2094.

34. Butcher NJ, Tetlow NL, Cheung C, Broadhurst GM, Minchin RF. Induction of human arylamine N-acetyltransferase type I by androgens in human prostate cancer cells. *Cancer Research.* 2007;67(1):85–92.

35. Ishii Y, Takami A, Tsuruda K, Kurogi A, Yamada H, Oguri K. Induction of two UDP-glucuronosyltransferase isoforms sensitive to phenobarbital that are involved in morphine glucuronidation: Production of isoform-selective antipeptide antibodies toward UGT1.1r and UGT2B1. *Drug Metabolism and Disposition: The Biological Fate of Chemicals.* 1997;25(2):163–167.

36. Hayes JD, Chanas SA, Henderson CJ et al. The Nrf2 transcription factor contributes both to the basal expression of glutathione S-transferases in mouse liver and to their induction by the chemopreventive synthetic antioxidants, butylated hydroxyanisole and ethoxyquin. *Biochemical Society Transactions.* 2000;28(2):33–41.

37. Wong DL, Siddall BJ, Ebert SN, Bell RA, Her S. Phenylethanolamine N-methyltransferase gene expression: Synergistic activation by Egr-1, AP-2 and the glucocorticoid receptor. *Brain Research Molecular Brain Research.* 1998;61(1–2):154–161.

38. Echchgadda I, Song CS, Oh T, Ahmed M, De La Cruz IJ, Chatterjee B. The xenobiotic-sensing nuclear receptors pregnane X receptor, constitutive androstane receptor, and orphan nuclear receptor hepatocyte nuclear factor 4alpha in the regulation of human steroid-/bile acid-sulfotransferase. *Molecular Endocrinology.* 2007;21(9):2099–2111.

39. Dluzen DF, Sun D, Salzberg AC et al. Regulation of UDP-glucuronosyltransferase 1A1 expression and activity by microRNA 491-3p. *The Journal of Pharmacology and Experimental Therapeutics.* 2014;348(3):465–477.

40. Izukawa T, Nakajima M, Fujiwara R et al. Quantitative analysis of UDP-glucuronosyltransferase (UGT) 1A and UGT2B expression levels in human livers. *Drug Metabolism and Disposition: The Biological Fate of Chemicals.* 2009;37(8):1759–1768.

41. Harmsen S, Meijerman I, Maas-Bakker RF, Beijnen JH, Schellens JH. PXR-mediated P-glycoprotein induction by small molecule tyrosine kinase inhibitors. *European Journal of Pharmaceutical Sciences: Official Journal of the European Federation for Pharmaceutical Sciences.* 2013;48(4–5):644–649.

42. Guo GL, Staudinger J, Ogura K, Klaassen CD. Induction of rat organic anion transporting polypeptide 2 by pregnenolone-16alpha-carbonitrile is via interaction with pregnane X receptor. *Molecular Pharmacology.* 2002;61(4):832–839.

43. Meyer Zu Schwabedissen HE, Bottcher K, Chaudhry A, Kroemer HK, Schuetz EG, Kim RB. Liver X receptor alpha and farnesoid X receptor are major transcriptional regulators of OATP1B1. *Hepatology.* 2010;52(5):1797–1807.

44. Loscher W, Potschka H. Role of drug efflux transporters in the brain for drug disposition and treatment of brain diseases. *Progress in Neurobiology.* 2005;76(1):22–76.

45. Greiner B, Eichelbaum M, Fritz P et al. The role of intestinal P-glycoprotein in the interaction of digoxin and rifampin. *The Journal of Clinical Investigation.* 1999;104(2):147–153.

46. Westphal K, Weinbrenner A, Zschiesche M et al. Induction of P-glycoprotein by rifampin increases intestinal secretion of talinolol in human beings: A new type of drug/drug interaction. *Clinical Pharmacology and Therapeutics.* 2000;68(4):345–355.

47. Shandilya J, Roberts SG. The transcription cycle in eukaryotes: From productive initiation to RNA polymerase II recycling. *Biochimica et Biophysica Acta.* 2012;1819(5):391–400.

48. Lee TI, Young RA. Transcription of eukaryotic protein-coding genes. *Annual Review of Genetics.* 2000;34:77–137.

49. Nikolov DB, Burley SK. RNA polymerase II transcription initiation: A structural view. *Proceedings of the National Academy of Sciences of the United States of America.* 1997;94(1):15–22.

50. Bertilsson G, Berkenstam A, Blomquist P. Functionally conserved xenobiotic responsive enhancer in cytochrome P450 3A7. *Biochemical and Biophysical Research Communications.* 2001;280(1):139–144.

51. Rushmore TH, King RG, Paulson KE, Pickett CB. Regulation of glutathione S-transferase Ya subunit gene expression: Identification of a unique xenobiotic-responsive element controlling inducible expression by planar aromatic compounds. *Proceedings of the National Academy of Sciences of the United States of America.* 1990;87(10):3826–3830.

52. Song BJ, Veech RL, Park SS, Gelboin HV, Gonzalez FJ. Induction of rat hepatic N-nitrosodimethylamine demethylase by acetone is due to protein stabilization. *The Journal of Biological Chemistry.* 1989;264(6):3568–3572.

53. Lu Y, Cederbaum AI. CYP2E1 and oxidative liver injury by alcohol. *Free Radical Biology & Medicine.* 2008;44(5):723–738.

54. Schmitt C, Kuhn B, Zhang X, Kivitz AJ, Grange S. Disease-drug-drug interaction involving tocilizumab and simvastatin in patients with rheumatoid arthritis. *Clinical Pharmacology and Therapeutics.* 2011;89(5):735–740.

55. Dickmann LJ, McBride HJ, Patel SK, Miner K, Wienkers LC, Slatter JG. Murine collagen antibody induced arthritis (CAIA) and primary mouse hepatocyte culture as models to study cytochrome P450 suppression. *Biochemical Pharmacology.* 2012;83(12):1682–1689.

56. Dickmann LJ, Patel SK, Rock DA, Wienkers LC, Slatter JG. Effects of interleukin-6 (IL-6) and an anti-IL-6 monoclonal antibody on drug-metabolizing enzymes in human hepatocyte culture. *Drug Metabolism and Disposition: The Biological Fate of Chemicals.* 2011;39(8):1415–1422.

57. Dickmann LJ, Patel SK, Wienkers LC, Slatter JG. Effects of interleukin 1beta (IL-1beta) and IL-1beta/interleukin 6 (IL-6) combinations on drug metabolizing enzymes in human hepatocyte culture. *Current Drug Metabolism.* 2012;13(7):930–937.

58. Evers R, Dallas S, Dickmann LJ et al. Critical review of preclinical approaches to investigate cytochrome p450-mediated therapeutic protein drug-drug interactions and recommendations for best practices: A white paper. *Drug Metabolism and Disposition: The Biological Fate of Chemicals.* 2013;41(9):1598–1609.

59. Gonzalez FJ, Nebert DW. Evolution of the P450 gene superfamily: Animal-plant 'warfare', molecular drive and human genetic differences in drug oxidation. *Trends in Denetics: TIG.* 1990;6(6):182–186.

60. Reschly EJ, Krasowski MD. Evolution and function of the NR1I nuclear hormone receptor subfamily (VDR, PXR, and CAR) with respect to metabolism of xenobiotics and endogenous compounds. *Current Drug Metabolism.* 2006;7(4):349–365.

61. Nebert DW, Gelboin HV. Substrate-inducible microsomal aryl hydroxylase in mammalian cell culture. II. Cellular responses during enzyme induction. *The Journal of Biological Chemistry.* 1968;243(23):6250–6261.

62. Ramadoss P, Marcus C, Perdew GH. Role of the aryl hydrocarbon receptor in drug metabolism. *Expert Opinion on Drug Metabolism & Toxicology.* 2005;1(1):9–21.

63. Davarinos NA, Pollenz RS. Aryl hydrocarbon receptor imported into the nucleus following ligand binding is rapidly degraded via the cytoplasmic proteasome following nuclear export. *The Journal of Biological Chemistry.* 1999;274(40):28708–28715.

64. Gronemeyer H, Gustafsson JA, Laudet V. Principles for modulation of the nuclear receptor superfamily. *Nature Reviews Drug Discovery.* 2004;3(11):950–964.

65. Yang X, Downes M, Yu RT et al. Nuclear receptor expression links the circadian clock to metabolism. *Cell.* 2006;126(4):801–810.

66. Baes M, Gulick T, Choi HS, Martinoli MG, Simha D, Moore DD. A new orphan member of the nuclear hormone receptor superfamily that interacts with a subset of retinoic acid response elements. *Molecular and Cellular Biology.* 1994;14(3):1544–1552.
67. Choi HS, Chung M, Tzameli I et al. Differential transactivation by two isoforms of the orphan nuclear hormone receptor CAR. *The Journal of Biological Chemistry.* 1997;272(38):23565–23571.
68. Xu RX, Lambert MH, Wisely BB et al. A structural basis for constitutive activity in the human CAR/RXRalpha heterodimer. *Molecular Cell.* 2004;16(6):919–928.
69. Kobayashi K, Sueyoshi T, Inoue K, Moore R, Negishi M. Cytoplasmic accumulation of the nuclear receptor CAR by a tetratricopeptide repeat protein in HepG2 cells. *Molecular Pharmacology.* 2003;64(5):1069–1075.
70. Sidhu JS, Omiecinski CJ. An okadaic acid-sensitive pathway involved in the phenobarbital-mediated induction of CYP2B gene expression in primary rat hepatocyte cultures. *The Journal of Pharmacology and Experimental Therapeutics.* 1997;282(2):1122–1129.
71. Pustylnyak VO, Gulyaeva LF, Lyakhovich VV. CAR expression and inducibility of CYP2B genes in liver of rats treated with PB-like inducers. *Toxicology.* 2005;216(2–3):147–153.
72. Lamba JK, Lamba V, Yasuda K et al. Expression of constitutive androstane receptor splice variants in human tissues and their functional consequences. *The Journal of Pharmacology and Experimental Therapeutics.* 2004;311(2):811–821.
73. DeKeyser JG, Stagliano MC, Auerbach SS, Prabhu KS, Jones AD, Omiecinski CJ. Di(2-ethylhexyl) phthalate is a highly potent agonist for the human constitutive androstane receptor splice variant CAR2. *Molecular Pharmacology.* 2009;75(5):1005–1013.
74. DeKeyser JG, Laurenzana EM, Peterson EC, Chen T, Omiecinski CJ. Selective phthalate activation of naturally occurring human constitutive androstane receptor splice variants and the pregnane X receptor. *Toxicological Sciences: An Official Journal of The Society of Toxicology.* 2011;120(2):381–391.
75. Auerbach SS, Ramsden R, Stoner MA, Verlinde C, Hassett C, Omiecinski CJ. Alternatively spliced isoforms of the human constitutive androstane receptor. *Nucleic Acids Research.* 2003;31(12):3194–3207.
76. Savkur RS, Wu Y, Bramlett KS et al. Alternative splicing within the ligand binding domain of the human constitutive androstane receptor. *Molecular Genetics and Metabolism.* 2003;80(1–2):216–226.
77. Jinno H, Tanaka-Kagawa T, Hanioka N et al. Identification of novel alternative splice variants of human constitutive androstane receptor and characterization of their expression in the liver. *Molecular Pharmacology.* 2004;65(3):496–502.
78. Auerbach SS, Dekeyser JG, Stoner MA, Omiecinski CJ. CAR2 displays unique ligand binding and RXRalpha heterodimerization characteristics. *Drug Metabolism and Disposition: The Biological Fate of Chemicals.* 2007;35(3):428–439.
79. Lau AJ, Yang G, Chang TK. Isoform-selective activation of human constitutive androstane receptor by Ginkgo biloba extract: Functional analysis of the SV23, SV24, and SV25 splice variants. *The Journal of Pharmacology and Experimental Therapeutics.* 2011;339(2):704–715.
80. Sharma D, Lau AJ, Sherman MA, Chang TK. Differential activation of human constitutive androstane receptor and its SV23 and SV24 splice variants by rilpivirine and etravirine. *British Journal of Pharmacology.* 2015;172(5):1263–1276.
81. Bertilsson G, Heidrich J, Svensson K et al. Identification of a human nuclear receptor defines a new signaling pathway for CYP3A induction. *Proceedings of the National Academy of Sciences of the United States of America.* 1998;95(21):12208–12213.
82. Kliewer SA, Moore JT, Wade L et al. An orphan nuclear receptor activated by pregnanes defines a novel steroid signaling pathway. *Cell.* 1998;92(1):73–82.
83. Lehmann JM, McKee DD, Watson MA, Willson TM, Moore JT, Kliewer SA. The human orphan nuclear receptor PXR is activated by compounds that regulate CYP3A4 gene expression and cause drug interactions. *The Journal of Clinical Investigation.* 1998;102(5):1016–1023.
84. Blumberg B, Sabbagh W, Jr., Juguilon H et al. SXR, a novel steroid and xenobiotic-sensing nuclear receptor. *Genes & Development.* 1998;12(20):3195–3205.
85. Watkins RE, Davis-Searles PR, Lambert MH, Redinbo MR. Coactivator binding promotes the specific interaction between ligand and the pregnane X receptor. *Journal of Molecular Biology.* 2003;331(4):815–828.
86. Watkins RE, Maglich JM, Moore LB et al. 2.1 A crystal structure of human PXR in complex with the St. John's wort compound hyperforin. *Biochemistry.* 2003;42(6):1430–1438.

87. Watkins RE, Wisely GB, Moore LB et al. The human nuclear xenobiotic receptor PXR: Structural determinants of directed promiscuity. *Science*. 2001;292(5525):2329–2333.

88. Chrencik JE, Orans J, Moore LB et al. Structural disorder in the complex of human pregnane X receptor and the macrolide antibiotic rifampicin. *Molecular Endocrinology*. 2005;19(5):1125–1134.

89. Squires EJ, Sueyoshi T, Negishi M. Cytoplasmic localization of pregnane X receptor and ligand-dependent nuclear translocation in mouse liver. *The Journal of Biological Chemistry*. 2004;279(47):49307–49314.

90. Saradhi M, Sengupta A, Mukhopadhyay G, Tyagi RK. Pregnane and Xenobiotic Receptor (PXR/SXR) resides predominantly in the nuclear compartment of the interphase cell and associates with the condensed chromosomes during mitosis. *Biochimica et Biophysica Acta*. 2005;1746(2):85–94.

91. Wang YM, Ong SS, Chai SC, Chen T. Role of CAR and PXR in xenobiotic sensing and metabolism. *Expert Opinion on Drug Metabolism & Toxicology*. 2012;8(7):803–817.

92. Iwazaki N, Kobayashi K, Morimoto K et al. Involvement of hepatocyte nuclear factor 4 alpha in transcriptional regulation of the human pregnane X receptor gene in the human liver. *Drug Metabolism and Pharmacokinetics*. 2008;23(1):59–66.

93. Takagi S, Nakajima M, Mohri T, Yokoi T. Post-transcriptional regulation of human pregnane X receptor by micro-RNA affects the expression of cytochrome P450 3A4. *The Journal of Biological Chemistry*. 2008;283(15):9674–9680.

94. Cui W, Sun M, Galeva N, Williams TD, Azuma Y, Staudinger JL. Sumoylation and ubiquitylation circuitry controls pregnane X receptor biology in hepatocytes. *Drug Metabolism and Disposition: The Biological Fate of Chemicals*. 2015;43(9):1316–1325.

95. Hu G, Xu C, Staudinger JL. Pregnane X receptor is SUMOylated to repress the inflammatory response. *The Journal of Pharmacology and Experimental Therapeutics*. 2010;335(2):342–350.

96. Rana R, Coulter S, Kinyamu H, Goldstein JA. RBCK1, an E3 ubiquitin ligase, interacts with and ubiquinates the human pregnane X receptor. *Drug Metabolism and Disposition: The Biological Fate of Chemicals*. 2013;41(2):398–405.

97. Pascussi JM, Drocourt L, Fabre JM, Maurel P, Vilarem MJ. Dexamethasone induces pregnane X receptor and retinoid X receptor-alpha expression in human hepatocytes: Synergistic increase of CYP3A4 induction by pregnane X receptor activators. *Molecular Pharmacology*. 2000;58(2):361–372.

98. Runge-Morris M, Kocarek TA, Falany CN. Regulation of the cytosolic sulfotransferases by nuclear receptors. *Drug Metabolism Reviews*. 2013;45(1):15–33.

99. Raucy JL, Lasker J, Ozaki K, Zoleta V. Regulation of CYP2E1 by ethanol and palmitic acid and CYP4A11 by clofibrate in primary cultures of human hepatocytes. *Toxicological Sciences: An Official Journal of the Society of Toxicology*. 2004;79(2):233–241.

100. Waxman DJ. Role of metabolism in the activation of dehydroepiandrosterone as a peroxisome proliferator. *The Journal of Endocrinology*. 1996;150 Suppl:S129–S147.

101. Plass JR, Mol O, Heegsma J et al. Farnesoid X receptor and bile salts are involved in transcriptional regulation of the gene encoding the human bile salt export pump. *Hepatology*. 2002;35(3):589–596.

102. Gupta S, Pandak WM, Hylemon PB. LXR alpha is the dominant regulator of CYP7A1 transcription. *Biochemical and Biophysical Research Communications*. 2002;293(1):338–343.

103. Gong H, Guo P, Zhai Y et al. Estrogen deprivation and inhibition of breast cancer growth *in vivo* through activation of the orphan nuclear receptor liver X receptor. *Molecular Endocrinology*. 2007;21(8):1781–1790.

104. Seol W, Choi HS, Moore DD. An orphan nuclear hormone receptor that lacks a DNA binding domain and heterodimerizes with other receptors. *Science*. 1996;272(5266):1336–1339.

105. Lu TT, Makishima M, Repa JJ et al. Molecular basis for feedback regulation of bile acid synthesis by nuclear receptors. *Molecular Cell*. 2000;6(3):507–515.

106. Moi P, Chan K, Asunis I, Cao A, Kan YW. Isolation of NF-E2-related factor 2 (Nrf2), a NF-E2-like basic leucine zipper transcriptional activator that binds to the tandem NF-E2/AP1 repeat of the beta-globin locus control region. *Proceedings of the National Academy of Sciences of the United States of America*. 1994;91(21):9926–9930.

107. Gorrini C, Harris IS, Mak TW. Modulation of oxidative stress as an anticancer strategy. *Nature Reviews Drug Discovery*. 2013;12(12):931–947.

108. Thimmulappa RK, Mai KH, Srisuma S, Kensler TW, Yamamoto M, Biswal S. Identification of Nrf2-regulated genes induced by the chemopreventive agent sulforaphane by oligonucleotide microarray. *Cancer Research*. 2002;62(18):5196–5203.

109. Buckley DB, Klaassen CD. Induction of mouse UDP-glucuronosyltransferase mRNA expression in liver and intestine by activators of aryl-hydrocarbon receptor, constitutive androstane receptor, pregnane X receptor, peroxisome proliferator-activated receptor alpha, and nuclear factor erythroid 2-related factor 2. *Drug Metabolism and Disposition: The Biological Fate of Chemicals.* 2009;37(4):847–856.

110. Zhang S, Patel A, Moorthy B, Shivanna B. Omeprazole induces NAD(P)H quinone oxidoreductase 1 via aryl hydrocarbon receptor-independent mechanisms: Role of the transcription factor nuclear factor erythroid 2-related factor 2. *Biochemical and Biophysical Research Communications.* 2015;467(2):282–287.

111. Wakabayashi N, Slocum SL, Skoko JJ, Shin S, Kensler TW. When NRF2 talks, who's listening? *Antioxidants & Redox Signaling.* 2010;13(11):1649–1663.

112. Raucy JL, Lasker JM. Current *in vitro* high throughput screening approaches to assess nuclear receptor activation. *Current Drug Metabolism.* 2010;11(9):806–814.

113. Moore JT, Kliewer SA. Use of the nuclear receptor PXR to predict drug interactions. *Toxicology.* 2000;153(1–3):1–10.

114. Honkakoski P, Zelko I, Sueyoshi T, Negishi M. The nuclear orphan receptor CAR-retinoid X receptor heterodimer activates the phenobarbital-responsive enhancer module of the CYP2B gene. *Molecular and Cellular Biology.* 1998;18(10):5652–5658.

115. Sogawa K, Iwabuchi K, Abe H, Fujii-Kuriyama Y. Transcriptional activation domains of the Ah receptor and Ah receptor nuclear translocator. *Journal of Cancer Research and Clinical Oncology.* 1995;121(9–10):612–620.

116. Kobayashi K, Hashimoto M, Honkakoski P, Negishi M. Regulation of gene expression by CAR: An update. *Archives of Toxicology.* 2015;89(7):1045–1055.

117. Dring AM, Anderson LE, Qamar S, Stoner MA. Rational quantitative structure-activity relationship (RQSAR) screen for PXR and CAR isoform-specific nuclear receptor ligands. *Chemico-Biological Interactions.* 2010;188(3):512–525.

118. Hosseinpour F, Moore R, Negishi M, Sueyoshi T. Serine 202 regulates the nuclear translocation of constitutive active/androstane receptor. *Molecular Pharmacology.* 2006;69(4):1095–1102.

119. Elliott DA, Brand AH. The GAL4 system: A versatile system for the expression of genes. *Methods in Molecular Biology.* 2008;420:79–95.

120. Hariparsad N, Carr BA, Evers R, Chu X. Comparison of immortalized Fa2N-4 cells and human hepatocytes as *in vitro* models for cytochrome P450 induction. *Drug Metabolism and Disposition: The Biological Fate of Chemicals.* 2008;36(6):1046–1055.

121. Gripon P, Rumin S, Urban S et al. Infection of a human hepatoma cell line by hepatitis B virus. *Proceedings of the National Academy of Sciences of the United States of America.* 2002;99(24):15655–15660.

122. Lecluyse EL, Alexandre E. Isolation and culture of primary hepatocytes from resected human liver tissue. *Methods in Molecular Biology.* 2010;640:57–82.

123. Fahmi OA, Kish M, Boldt S, Obach RS. Cytochrome P450 3A4 mRNA is a more reliable marker than CYP3A4 activity for detecting pregnane X receptor-activated induction of drug-metabolizing enzymes. *Drug Metabolism and Disposition: The Biological Fate of Chemicals.* 2010;38(9):1605–1611.

124. Kakuni M, Yamasaki C, Tachibana A, Yoshizane Y, Ishida Y, Tateno C. Chimeric mice with humanized livers: A unique tool for *in vivo* and *in vitro* enzyme induction studies. *International Journal of Molecular Sciences.* 2014;15(1):58–74.

125. Scheer N, Ross J, Rode A et al. A novel panel of mouse models to evaluate the role of human pregnane X receptor and constitutive androstane receptor in drug response. *The Journal of Clinical Investigation.* 2008;118(9):3228–3239.

126. Fahmi OA, Hurst S, Plowchalk D et al. Comparison of different algorithms for predicting clinical drug-drug interactions, based on the use of CYP3A4 *in vitro* data: Predictions of compounds as precipitants of interaction. *Drug Metabolism and Disposition: The Biological Fate of Chemicals.* 2009;37(8):1658–1666.

127. Fahmi OA, Boldt S, Kish M, Obach RS, Tremaine LM. Prediction of drug-drug interactions from *in vitro* induction data: Application of the relative induction score approach using cryopreserved human hepatocytes. *Drug Metabolism and Disposition: The Biological Fate of Chemicals.* 2008;36(9):1971–1974.

128. Ripp SL, Mills JB, Fahmi OA et al. Use of immortalized human hepatocytes to predict the magnitude of clinical drug-drug interactions caused by CYP3A4 induction. *Drug Metabolism and Disposition: The Biological Fate of Chemicals.* 2006;34(10):1742–1748.

129. Wagner C, Pan Y, Hsu V, Sinha V, Zhao P. Predicting the effect of CYP3A inducers on the pharmacokinetics of substrate drugs using physiologically based pharmacokinetic (PBPK) modeling: An analysis of PBPK submissions to the US FDA. *Clinical Pharmacokinetics.* 2016;55(4):475–483.

130. Einolf HJ, Chen L, Fahmi OA et al. Evaluation of various static and dynamic modeling methods to predict clinical CYP3A induction using *in vitro* CYP3A4 mRNA induction data. *Clinical Pharmacology and Therapeutics.* 2014;95(2):179–188.

131. Xu Y, Zhou Y, Hayashi M, Shou M, Skiles GL. Simulation of clinical drug-drug interactions from hepatocyte CYP3A4 induction data and its potential utility in trial designs. *Drug Metabolism and Disposition: The Biological Fate of Chemicals.* 2011;39(7):1139–1148.

132. Jamei M, Marciniak S, Feng K, Barnett A, Tucker G, Rostami-Hodjegan A. The simcyp population-based ADME simulator. *Expert Opinion on Drug Metabolism & Toxicology.* 2009;5(2):211–223.

133. Huang F, Allen L, Huang DB et al. Evaluation of steady-state pharmacokinetic interactions between ritonavir-boosted BILR 355, a non-nucleoside reverse transcriptase inhibitor, and lamivudine/zidovudine in healthy subjects. *Journal of Clinical Pharmacy and Therapeutics.* 2012;37(1):81–88.

134. Bohnert T, Patel A, Templeton I et al. Evaluation of a new molecular entity as a victim of metabolic drug-drug interactions-an industry perspective. *Drug Metabolism and Disposition: The Biological Fate of Chemicals.* 2016;44(8):1399–1423.

135. Wahlstrom JL, Rock DA, Slatter JG, Wienkers LC. Advances in predicting CYP-mediated drug interactions in the drug discovery setting. *Expert Opinion on Drug Discovery.* 2006;1(7):677–691.

136. Laille E, Patel M, Jones SF et al. Evaluation of CYP3A-mediated drug-drug interactions with romidepsin in patients with advanced cancer. *Journal of Clinical Pharmacology.* 2015;55(12):1378–1385.

137. Sarantopoulos J, Mita AC, Wade JL et al. Phase I study of cabazitaxel plus cisplatin in patients with advanced solid tumors: Study to evaluate the impact of cytochrome P450 3A inhibitors (aprepitant, ketoconazole) or inducers (rifampin) on the pharmacokinetics of cabazitaxel. *Cancer Chemotherapy and Pharmacology.* 2014;74(6):1113–1124.

138. Vavricka SR, Van Montfoort J, Ha HR, Meier PJ, Fattinger K. Interactions of rifamycin SV and rifampicin with organic anion uptake systems of human liver. *Hepatology.* 2002;36(1):164–172.

139. Fattinger K, Cattori V, Hagenbuch B, Meier PJ, Stieger B. Rifamycin SV and rifampicin exhibit differential inhibition of the hepatic rat organic anion transporting polypeptides, Oatp1 and Oatp2. *Hepatology.* 2000;32(1):82–86.

140. Rock BM, Hengel SM, Rock DA, Wienkers LC, Kunze KL. Characterization of ritonavir-mediated inactivation of cytochrome P450 3A4. *Molecular Pharmacology.* 2014;86(6):665–674.

141. Luo G, Cunningham M, Kim S et al. CYP3A4 induction by drugs: Correlation between a pregnane X receptor reporter gene assay and CYP3A4 expression in human hepatocytes. *Drug Metabolism and Disposition: The Biological Fate of Chemicals.* 2002;30(7):795–804.

142. Greenblatt DJ, Peters DE, Oleson LE et al. Inhibition of oral midazolam clearance by boosting doses of ritonavir, and by 4,4-dimethyl-benziso-(2H)-selenazine (ALT-2074), an experimental catalytic mimic of glutathione oxidase. *British Journal of Clinical Pharmacology.* 2009;68(6):920–927.

143. Fichtenbaum CJ, Gerber JG, Rosenkranz SL et al. Pharmacokinetic interactions between protease inhibitors and statins in HIV seronegative volunteers: ACTG Study A5047. *Aids.* 2002;16(4):569–577.

18

Transporters in Drug Discovery and Development

Yaofeng Cheng and Yurong Lai

CONTENTS

Introduction

Systemic exposure of a drug is determined by the pharmacokinetic (PK) properties including absorption, distribution, metabolism, and elimination (ADME). Often, an efficacious drug relies on adequate drug levels distributed to the target tissues for a desired period of time to regulate the pathway of disease.[1] Over the last two decades, pharmaceutical industries have been focusing to develop *in vitro* tools using hepatocytes or liver microsome to select the compounds that are metabolically stable and have optimal half-lives to fit at least once a day dosing regimen. Surprisingly, metabolic stable compounds often result in unpredictable drug elimination *in vivo*, due to the involvement of drug transporters. While drug clearance via CYP P450 metabolizing enzymes have been well-characterized,[2] membrane transporters involve in drug pharmacokinetics and disposition are increasingly scrutinized for their contribution to the suboptimal PK and organ distribution and the undesired safety or efficacy outcomes. As a result, the impact of transporters on patient safety and efficacy become critical considerations in drug discovery and development, mainly to assess drug distribution to the target or off-target organs and to minimize the potential drug-drug interactions (DDIs).

Membrane transporters are expressed in a variety of organs in the body such as the liver, brain, intestine, and kidney, and play a pivotal role in the absorption, distribution, clearance, and elimination of many drugs and their metabolites. Currently, more than 400 membrane transporter genes have been discovered and are categorized into two distinct superfamilies, the solute carrier (SLC) and ATP-binding cassette (ABC) families. As our knowledge has expanded, increasing numbers of membrane transporters are found to interact with drugs and the movement of endogenous compounds within or between the organs. Alteration of these transporter functions or protein expressions can significantly change the ADME of a drug, leading to the changes of drug or endogenous compound exposure in plasma and/or organs, subsequently transporter-mediated drug interactions.[3,4] Inhibition of transporter function can significantly change the drug clearance and disposition of other drugs that are substrates of those transporters. The interactions can, therefore, disturb the tolerability and safety profiles of therapeutic agents. Consequently, regulatory agencies require investigating the role of several major drug transporters in drug discovery and development and assessing the potential risk of clinical drug-drug interactions. Currently OATP1B1/1B3 (*SLCO1B1/SLCO1B3*), P-glycoprotein (P-gp, *ABCB1*), breast cancer resistance protein (BCRP, *ABCG1*), organic anion transporter (OAT1/3, *SLC22A6/22A8*), organic cation transporter (OCT1/2, *SLC22A1/SLC22A2*), multidrug and toxin extrusion proteins (MATE1/2k, *SLC47A1/SLC47A2*), multidrug resistance protein 2 (MRP2, *ABCC2*), and bile salt export pump (BSEP, *ABCB11*) are routinely characterized in drug discovery and development (https://www.fda.gov/downloads/Drugs/GuidanceComplianceRegulatoryInformation/Guidances/UCM581965.pdf; http://www.ema.europa.eu/docs/en_GB/document_library/Scientific_guideline/2012/07/WC500129606.pdf). These transporters are well-investigated and considered to have significant roles in drug biology and disposition as demonstrated in reported DDIs, drug responses, and drug related toxicities.[5-7]

Studies of drug interactions with transporters are primarily conducted by monitoring the changes of pharmacokinetics in the plasma (unexpected changes of systemic exposure). However, drug transporters regulating drug disposition to specific organs can read to the asymmetric tissue distribution. Since organ exposure is often the determinant of drug efficacy or safety, clinical adverse effects (AEs) of new drugs involving the modulation of drug transporter functions or protein expressions in special population have become important considerations in drug development. In addition to transporter roles in drug disposition, membrane transporters have increasingly been studied as pharmacological targets for disease treatment.[9] For example, utilization of liver-specific uptake transporter OATPs to target hepatic HMG-CoA reductase[8] has been a viable approach for liver specific efficacy while minimizing exposures in other organs, e.g., muscles of statin drugs. Sodium-glucose cotransporter 2 (SGLT2; SLC5A2) has been the target to control blood glucose level for the treatment of type II diabetes.[10] The potentiators or correctors of cystic fibrosis transmembrane conductance regulator (CFTR; ABCC7) are used for the treatment of cystic fibrosis.[11] On the other hand, inhibitor of the thiamine transporter (hTHTR2, SLC19A3), e.g., Fedratinib, may limit thiamine absorption in gastrointestinal tract, resulting in Wernicke's encephalopathy due to the thiamine deficiency.[12]

The clinical significance of the drug transporters are demonstrated by the alternation of drug pharmacokinetics and/or clinical responses by investigating transporter genetic polymorphism and DDI with inhibitors of the transporter. However, the tissue exposure is not regularly monitored in clinical trial and the systemic exposure in plasma also does not represent the tissue concentrations.[13] Regardless of the importance of the transporter role on drug elimination and disposition, tools for characterizing transporter interactions are much less advanced than those for metabolizing enzymes. *In vitro* to *in vivo* extrapolation to predict potential transporter interactions remains significant challenging. To this end, transporter basic and applied research publications over the past decade have demonstrated the importance of transporters in drug disposition, DDI, and drug-related organ toxicity.[14,15] The chapter reconnoitres the role of transporters in ADME, genetic polymorphisms and PK variability, organ toxicity, drug clearance and DDIs, as well as giving a concise overview of *in vitro* tools to assess transporter interaction in drug discovery and development. Relevant examples are provided throughout the text with references of comprehensive reviews on drug transporters.

Role of Transporters in ADME

The therapeutic effect and the adverse events of a drug are strongly associated with the number of molecules presented at the reaction sites, which in most cases is proportional to the systemic blood exposure. As the main carrier to facilitate molecules to cross cell plasma membranes, transporters have a critical role in the determination of drug pharmacokinetics.

Absorption

Absorption is the procedure that a drug reaches systemic circulation from the site of administration. Intravascular administration does not involve the absorption phase as the drug is introduced directly into blood. However, the extent of absorption can greatly affect the blood exposure of a drug in other administration routes, particularly for orally-dosed drugs. Following an oral administration, drugs can be absorbed at any segment of the gastrointestinal tract including the stomach, small intestine, and large intestine. The amount of drug absorbed at each section is determined by the physicochemical properties of a drug molecule, dosing formulation, and subject physiology. Most of the time, the majority of the oral dose will be absorbed from the small intestine because of the large absorption surface area and the rich expression of various membrane transporters.

No matter the dose formulation (tablet, capsule, solution, etc.), the orally taken drug needs to be in a soluble form in order to be absorbed into the circulation system. There are multiple pathways that the dissolved molecules can permeate through the epithelium layer in the GI track, including paracellular transport, passive diffusion, and protein mediated transportation. Paracellular transport transfers substances through the intercellular space between the epithelial cells. Water is primarily absorbed through this pathway. Ions, sugars, and small hydrophilic ionized drugs (<200 Da) can also be absorbed by paracellular transport when the concentrations above the capacity of their transport carriers (Figure 18.1). Both passive diffusion and protein mediated transportation belong to transcellular process that moves solutes through a live cell. Passive diffusion does not need energy input and the movement of molecular substances is driven predominantly by the concentration gradient. Usually hydrophobic compounds with a neutral charge can penetrate the lipid bilayers with passive diffusion. Hydrophilic molecules and ionized drugs in general require the assistance of transport proteins to permeate cell membrane (Figure 18.1).

Many transporters have been identified in the epithelial cells of GI track and found to significantly impact the drug absorption. On the luminal membrane of enterocytes, uptake transporters like OATP2B1, PETP1, ASBT, and MCT1 can assist the absorption from gut lumen into cells (Figure 18.2). Meanwhile, efflux transporters on the luminal membrane including P-gp, BCRP, and MRP2 can pump the intracellular drugs back to the gut.[4,16,17] Example drugs transported by these membrane proteins are listed in

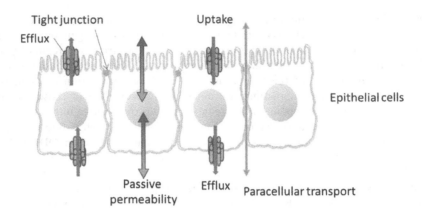

FIGURE 18.1 Paracelluar and transcellular transport.

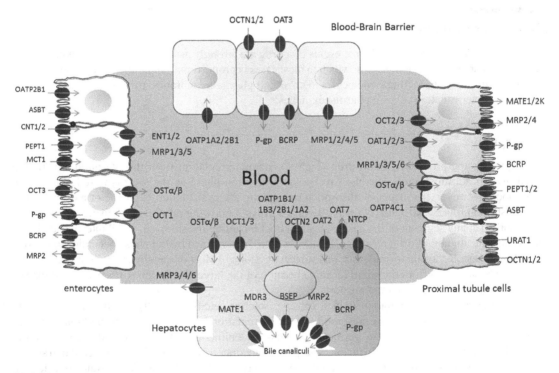

FIGURE 18.2 Transporter expressions in major organs.

Table 18.1. Therefore, drugs could have a boosted absorption for the substrates of uptake transporters. In contrast, a decreased fraction of oral absorption could occur with drugs transported by luminal efflux transporters. In the case that P-gp activity was induced by rifampin, digoxin plasma concentrations was substantially reduced after oral administration.[18] In contrast, coadministration of P-gp inhibitor, quinidine causes a considerable increase digoxin absorption and plasma exposure.[19]

The completion of the absorption procedure requires an extra step that intracellular drug molecules penetrate the basolateral membrane of GI epithelial cells in order to reach blood circulation. The presence of OCT1, OSTα/β, and MPR3 has been confirmed on the basolateral membrane of gut cells.[4] The functions of these transporters are also characterized in *in vitro* assays, and many drugs are found to be substrates (Table 18.1). However, the clinical significance of the basolateral transporter on drug absorption is still not well characterized.

TABLE 18.1
Tissue Localization and Example Substrates/Inhibitors of Drug Transporters

| Transporter | Tissue Expression | Membrane Localization | Substrates | | Inhibitors |
			Endogenous	Exogenous	
ABC					
P-gp	Intestine	Apical (luminal)	Opioid peptides	Digoxin	
	Liver	Apical (canalicular)	Oxidized lipids	Vinblastine	Quinidine
	Kidney	Apical (brush border)	Steroid metabolites	Verapamil	Cyclosporine A
	Brain	Apical (capillary)	Bilirubin	Talinolol tacrolimus	Ketoconazole
	Placenta	Apical (capillary)			
BCRP	Intestine	Apical (luminal)		Topotecan	Cyclosporine A
	Liver	Apical (canalicular)	Estrone 3-sulfate	Prazosin	KO143
	Kidney	Apical (brush border)		SN-38	GF120918
	Brain	Apical (capillary)		Glyburide	
	Placenta	Apical (capillary)		Vinblastine	
MRP2	Intestine	Apical (luminal)	Bilirubin	Indomethacin	MK-571
	Liver Intestine	Apical (canalicular)	Sulfates Porphyrins	Telmisartan	Cyclosporine A
	Kidney	Apical (brush border)	Glutathione conjugates		
	Brain	Basolateral (capillary)	Bile acids		
MRP3	Liver Intestine	Basolateral (sinusoidal)	Estradiol-17β-glucuronide	Fexofenadine	Indomethacin
			Bile acids leukotriene C4	Methotrexate	
	Kidney	Basolateral	cAMP	Adefovir	
MRP4	Liver	Basolateral (sinusoidal)	DHEAS prostaglandin	Methotrexate	Indomethacin
	Kidney	Basolateral			sildenafil
	Brain	Apical (capillary)		Topotecan	
BSEP	Liver	Apical (canalicular)	Bile acids	—	Cyclosporine A
					Rifampicin
					Glibenclamide
					Glyburide

(Continued)

TABLE 18.1 (*Continued*)

Tissue Localization and Example Substrates/Inhibitors of Drug Transporters

Transporter	Tissue Expression	Membrane Localization	Substrates Endogenous	Substrates Exogenous	Inhibitors
SLC					
OATP1B1	Liver	Basolateral (sinusoidal)	Thyroid hormones (T4 and T3) prostaglandin E2 Coproporphyrin 1/3 Estrone 3-sulfate Estradiol-17β-glucuronide	Statins Valsartan	Cyclosporine A Rifampin Bromosulfophthalein
OATP1B3	Liver	Basolateral (sinusoidal)	Thyroid hormones Leukotriene C4 Coproporphyrin 1/3	Statins Valsartan	Cyclosporine A Rifampin Bromosulfophthalein
OATP2B1	Liver Intestine Brain	Basolateral (sinusoidal) Apical (capillary)	Estrone 3-sulfate	Statins Bromosulfophthalein	Rifampin Bromosulfophthalein
OCT1	Intestine Liver Kidney	Basolateral Basolateral (sinusoidal) Basolateral	Prostaglandin E2	Metformin Acyclovir	Quinidine Cimetidine Verapamil
OCT2	Kidney	Basolateral	Acetylcholine Dopamine Epinephrine Prostaglandin E2	Metformin Ranitidine Cimetidine	Quinine Cimetidine
OCT3	Intestine Liver Kidney	Apical (luminal) Basolateral (sinusoidal) Basolateral	Epinephrine Histamine	Metformin Ranitidine Cimetidine	Cimetidine Verapamil
MATE1	Liver Kidney	Apical (canalicular) Apical (Brush border)	Creatinine Thiamine	Metformin Acyclovir	Quinidine Cimetidine
MATE2-K	Kidney	Apical (Brush border)	Creatinine thiamine	Metformin	Cimetidine Pyrimethamine

(Continued)

TABLE 18.1 (Continued)

Tissue Localization and Example Substrates/Inhibitors of Drug Transporters

Transporter	Tissue Expression	Membrane Localization	Substrates — Endogenous	Substrates — Exogenous	Inhibitors
OAT1	Kidney	Basolateral	Prostaglandin E2, Uric acid	Adefovir, Raltegravir, Olmesartan, Furosemide	Probenecid, Raltegravir, Diclofenac
OAT2	Liver	Basolateral (sinusoidal)	cAMP	Ganciclovir	Indomethacine, Bromsulphthalein, Probenecid
OAT3	Kidney	Basolateral	Uric acid	Acyclovir	Probenecid
	Liver	Basolateral (sinusoidal)	Homovanillic acid	Bumetanide	
	Kidney	Basolateral	Prostaglandins	Rosuvastatin	
	Brain	Basolateral	Uric acid	Furosemide	
ASBT	Intestine	Apical (luminal)	Bile acids	Benzothiazepine	GSK2330672
	Kidney	Apical (Brush border)		Ursodiol	SC-435
PEPT1	Intestine	Apical (luminal)	di- and tripeptides	Valacyclovir	Sartans
	Kidney	Apical (Brush border)		Prodrug with amino fatty acids	
MCT1	Intestine	Apical (luminal)	L-lactate, Pyruvate	—	AR-C155858
OSTα/β	Intestine	Basolateral	Bile acids	—	Probenecid, Indomethacin, Bromosulfophthalein
	Liver	Basolateral (sinusoidal)	Steroids		
	Kidney	Basolateral	Estrone-3-sulfate		
NTCP	Liver	Basolateral (sinusoidal)	Bile acid	Atorvastatin	Cyclosporine A, Rifamycin
URAT1	Kidney	Apical (brush border)	Uric acid	—	Probenecid, Furosemide

The absorbed drug will be carried by portal vein to hepatic sinusoids and distributed to liver first before entering the systemic circulation. Nutrition, drugs, and toxicants in the sinusoids will be extracted by liver cells, primarily by hepatocytes. Hepatocytes are the predominant cell type in the liver, contributing to approximately 70%–85% of liver mass. One of the critical functions of hepatocytes is to extract, detoxify, biotransform, and excretion of endogenous and exogenous substances. Drugs can enter into hepatocytes by either passive diffusion or transporter mediated uptake. Many uptake transporters have been found to express on the sinusoid membrane of hepatocytes, including OATP1B1, OATP1B3, OATP2B1, OCT1, OAT2, and NTCP (Figure 18.2). Meanwhile, efflux transporters on sinusoid membrane, such as MRP3/4/6, can pump the intrahepatic molecules back to blood (Figure 18.2). Drugs escaped from liver extraction will flow into systemic circulation and complete the absorption phase. Liver extraction, together with the physical barrier of the gut wall and gut metabolism, builds a very effective protection mechanism for the body in order to reduce the exposure of exogenous toxicants, named the first-pass effect.

Distribution and Excretion

Systemic available drugs from oral absorption or intravascular injection will be circulated to each organ of the body following blood flow and then distributed to extravascular fluids and intracellular spaces. The whole procedure is called distribution. The extent of distribution of a drug among tissues can be affected by the physical chemical properties of drug molecules and the physiology of the organ. The former includes compound protein binding, passive permeability, and blood to plasma ratio. Drug with high plasma protein binding and high blood to plasma ratio are less likely to be distributed to tissues. Blood flow is a key driver for drug distribution to specific organ. For example, a drug is easily distributed in highly perfused organs such as the liver, heart, and kidney, and only small amount is allocated to less perfused tissues like fat.

Distribution of compounds to intracellular compartments is correlated to the compound passive permeability and the activity of membrane transporters. So far, most research on drug transporters is focused on two organs, liver and kidney, not only because they are critical for drug distribution and metabolism, but they are the two major players for drug excretion. Transporter functions on blood–brain barrier are also heavily studied because drug delivery into CNS is the key for many neurological diseases.

Liver is the largest organ in the body and receives approximately 25% of total cardiac output from hepatic artery and portal vein. As described above, transporters expressed on the sinusoidal (basolateral) membrane can facilitate the drug molecules into hepatocytes. Therefore, drug distribution to liver can be affected by the transporter function, to impact the volume of distribution.[20] For example, the volume distribution of atorvastatin was decreased 94% in healthy subjects co-dosed with rifampin.[21] Polymorphism of OATP1B1 (SLCO1B1 c.521CC) reduced the volume distribution of atorvastatin and rosuvastatin by 58% and 51%, respectively.[22] Once in the hepatocyte, drugs are biotransformed to metabolites by phase I and phase II liver enzymes. The drug or its metabolites can be either pumped back to plasma by sinusoidal efflux transporters or excreted into bile by transporters expressed on canalicular (apical) membrane. Both ABC transporters (P-gp, BCRP, MRP2, MDR3, and BSEP) and SLC transporter (MATE1) are found on the canalicular membrane of hepatocytes (Figure 18.2). These transporters are important for drug biliary secretion.

The kidney is the other major organ for drug distribution and excretion. Approximately 20% of cardiac output goes to the kidney. Drug molecules from renal arteries will flow into afferent arterioles, then the unbound drug will be partially filtrated through glomeruli. After filtration, the blood moves through a small network of venules that exchange nutrition with the functional unit of kidney, named nephron. Proximal tubule cells (PTC) form the first segment of nephron lumen and express variety of transporters. On the basolateral membrane, OAT1, OAT2, OAT3, OCT2, and OATP4C1 are known to uptake many drugs from blood into PTC (Figure 18.2). Efflux transporters, MRP2/4, MATE1/2-K, and P-gp, on the apical membrane can pump drugs into urinary lumen. URAT1 and PEPT1/2 are recycling transporters on apical membrane, which reabsorb the substances from urine back to PTC (Figure 18.2). URAT1 mediates the reabsorption of uric acid from the glomerular filtration, thereby playing a key role in uric acid homeostasis. OCTN1/2 and OAT4 are also expressed on the apical membrane but they are bidirectional transporters. The significance of URAT1, PEPT1/2, OCTN1/2, and OAT4 on drug excretion and reabsorption are not well studied yet.

Blood–brain barrier (BBB) is a protection barrier formed by brain endothelial cells, astrocytes and membrane transporters expressed on endothelial cells. The major function of BBB is to separate blood flow from extracellular fluid in the central nervous system. Tight junctions between brain endothelial cells prevent the paracellular permeability of almost all large molecules and small molecules.[23] Transporters expressed on apical membrane (facing blood) such as P-gp, BCRP, and MPR4/5 can limit the penetration of lipophilic compounds by effluxing them back to blood (Figure 18.2). Uptake transporters OATP1A2 and OATP2B1 are also expressed on the apical membrane and reports have shown that these transporters can enhance the brain exposure of certain therapeutic agents (Figure 18.2). The expression of other transporters, such as OCTN2 on basolateral membrane (facing brain), are also reported (Figure 18.2), but the clinical impact of these transporters on drug distribution is still not well investigated. Overall, drug distribution to brain is very limited and delivering drugs to specific regions of the brain is a major challenge to treatment of most brain diseases.

The distribution of drug molecules to other organs is generally assumed to be perfusion limited, in which passive permeability is the predominant factor for intracellular distribution. However, the expression of transporters has been reported for almost every tissue. For example, the expression of OATP2B1 is a key modulator in skeletal muscles for statin exposure and toxicity.[24] Little has been done to understand how transporters can alter the distribution in tissues other than in the liver, kidney, and brain.

Metabolism

Transporters do not directly involve drug biotransformation. Transporters are often the facilitators for drug molecules to penetrate through cell membrane and make available for metabolism in cell cytosol. Therefore, the interplay of transporters and metabolic enzymes are important for drug ADME. Liver is the principle organ in the body for drug metabolism, which produces a variety of metabolic enzymes. Reduced hepatic uptake can limit the drug entering hepatocytes, resulting in reduced metabolism. Transporters expressed on kidney can also impact drug metabolism as several CYP and UGT isoforms are expressed in proximal tubule cells.[25,26]

Transporters are also important for the distribution and elimination of drug metabolites. Metabolites formed in hepatocytes can either be excreted into bile or pumped back sinusoidal. Either of the pathways requires the assistance of membrane transporters, especially for hydrophilic metabolites. The conjugated metabolites from phase II metabolism are usually hydrophilic and have low passive permeability. MRP2 on the canaliculi membrane is known to transport glucuronide conjugates, and MRP3/4 can efflux them back to extrahepatic space. In disease conditions where transporter function is altered, the pharmacokinetics of metabolites can also be changed. For example, the conjugated bilirubin in blood is increased in patients with Rotor syndrome, with whom the function of OATP1B1 and OATP1B3 is completed lost and hepatic uptake of conjugated bilirubin is reduced.

Transporter-Mediated Drug Clearance and Extended Clearance Classification System (ECCS)

Transporter Role in Drug Clearance

Hepatic drug elimination is involved in multiple processes: drugs entering into the hepatocyte via passive diffusion or specific transporter proteins, phase I or II drug metabolism in the hepatocytes, and biliary secretion into bile by canalicular transporters.[27,28] When passive diffusion of a drug is low, transporter mediated hepatic uptake can be the rate determining step, which acts as "gatekeeper" functions of the drug to assess the metabolic enzymes and/or biliary elimination and, therefore, affects drug pharmacokinetics (PK) and liver concentration.[29] OAT2, NTCP, OATP1B1/1B3, OCT1 are selectively expressed in the liver[30,31] and play a key role in hepatic drug disposition and elimination. OATP substrates include a large number of widely prescribed drugs, such as HMG-coenzyme A reductase inhibitors (statins), antibiotics, protease inhibitors, and anticancer drugs.[32–36] Transporter-mediated active hepatic uptake results in higher liver exposure, which is beneficial to the efficacy of statins. On the other hand, inhibition of active hepatic transport can prevent a drug reaching the liver and, therefore, cause the increased systemic exposure.[21,37,38] For example, cerivastatin is a substrate of OATP transporters and metabolized by CYP2C8 and 3A4.[39] A 3.8-fold increase of the area under the plasma concentration-time curve (AUC) of cerivastatin is observed in kidney transplant recipients with co-treatment of cyclosporine A, a potent OATP inhibitor,[40] while only a 1.15- to 1.27-fold increase of cerivastatin AUC in healthy subjects with co-treatment of itraconazole, a potent CYP inhibitor.[41,42] The results indicate that OATP-mediated active hepatic uptake is the key contributor to the DDIs with cyclosporine A.[43] Similarly, pravastatin is metabolically stable and mainly eliminated equivalent between renal and non-renal routes (i.e., biliary excretion). A 10-fold change in pravastatin AUC is observed by cyclosporine treatment.[44]

Transporters expressed on the canalicular membrane of hepatocytes are important in biliary excretion of drugs and their metabolites. For example, topotecan and cimetidine are transported into bile by BCRP.[45] MRP2 contributes to the biliary excretion of endogenous chemicals, such as conjugated bilirubin, and many structurally diverse xenobiotics and their metabolites.[46–50] While the physiological role of BSEP is to secrete bile salts to the bile duct and maintain the normal bile flow, inhibition of BSEP have been found to associate with cholestatic liver injury.[51] In fact, troglitazone and its sulfate metabolite inhibit BSEP and the inhibition possibly contributes to the hepatotoxicity of troglitazone, resulting in the withdrawal of the drug from the market.[52,53]

The kidney is another important excretory organ for many clinical drugs and their metabolites.[54,55] Glomerular filtration, tubular secretion, and reabsorption are three determinants for urinary elimination. OATs, OCTs, and MATEs expressed on the renal proximal tubular cells play key roles in active renal secretion (Figure 18.2). Basal uptake transporter-mediated uptakes can increase drug accumulation in the proximal tubular cells resulting in drug-related nephrotoxicity.[56] Therefore, inhibition of renal transporters can reduce the active renal secretion, leading to increased systemic drug exposure and/or altered drug exposure in the proximal tubule cells. For example, probenecid inhibits OAT function and increases the systemic exposure of penicillin and cephalosporin antibiotics.[57,58] Similar to renal OATs, DDI can also be attributed by OCT inhibition. For example, the renal clearance of metformin is reduced by inhibition of OCT2 activity.[59–62]

Estimation of *In Vivo* Hepatic Clearance

Under the condition of "well-stirred" that a drug is rapidly and homogenously equilibrated between the plasma and liver, hepatic drug clearance in the blood ($CL_{h,b}$) is defined by a function of the hepatic blood flow (Q_h), the intrinsic metabolic clearance in the liver (CL_{int}), and the unbound fraction of the drug ($f_{u,b}$) (Equation 18.1). The intrinsic metabolic clearance (CL_{int}) can be estimated from *in vitro* systems such as human liver microsomes, hepatocytes, or recombinant CYP enzymes. Since the well-stirred model is based on the assumptions that the drug concentration is homogeneous throughout the liver, the equation can be further derived into the parallel-tube model or dispersion model to account for concentration changes during the drug passing through the liver, using complex mathematic equations to model the pattern of drug mixing within the liver. However, only minor difference is observed between the models for the prediction of *in vivo* hepatic clearance,[63] the well-stirred model remains the most often used, due to the simpler mathematical equation with similar predictive power.

$$CL_{h,b} = \frac{Q_h * f_{u,b} * CL_{int}}{Q_h * + f_{u,b} * CL_{int}} \quad (18.1)$$

Extended Clearance Concept and the Drug Classification System

It is now generally accepted that drug transporters on hepatic sinusoidal membrane can regulate the rate of a drug entering into hepatocyte and serve as the determinants of the drug elimination. It is true even for the drugs that ultimately undergo metabolism and/or biliary excretion in the liver. In contrast to the rapid-equilibrium between the blood and throughout the liver, extended clearance concept was introduced to catch up the hepatic uptake-determined clearance.[64] Therefore, a mathematic equation (Equation 18.2) is developed to elucidate the contribution of transporter-mediated uptake to the overall drug clearance.[64] The concept has been further validated in different groups for the application to define the rate-determining step in hepatic clearance.[43,65–70] Using the mathematical equations as shown below, transporter-mediated sinusoidal uptake (PS_{influx}), basal (sinusoidal) efflux (PS_{efflux}), intrinsic metabolic and/or biliary clearances (here $CL_{int} = CL_{bile} + CL_{met}$), and passive diffusion (PS_{pd}) are incorporated in the equation to compute the transporter contribution to the overall drug clearance[71] (Equation 18.2). Based on the equation, the model can predict pharmacokinetic variations due to transporter inhibition (transporter DDIs) and pharmacogenomics for the compounds that are not predicted by well-stirred model using metabolic parameters.[72,73]

$$CL_{h,\ total} = \frac{Q_h * f_{u,b} * \left(PS_{influx} + PS_{pd}\right) * CL_{int}}{Q_h * \left(PS_{efflux} + PS_{pd} + CL_{int}\right) + f_{u,b} * \left(PS_{influx} + PS_{pd}\right) * CL_{int}} \tag{18.2}$$

Extended Clearance Classification System (ECCS)

When dosed orally, intrinsic properties such as solubility, ionization, and permeability are important factors determining fraction absorbed (Fa) of a drug. Accordingly, Biopharmaceutics Classification System (BCS) for correlating *in vitro* dissolution and *in vivo* bioavailability has been introduced to place a drug in one of four categories depending on its solubility and permeability.[74] The BCS categories include: Class 1, high solubility-high permeability molecules; Class 2, high permeability-low solubility molecules; Class 3, low permeability-high solubility molecules; and Class 4, low permeability-low solubility molecules (Figure 18.3).[74] The BCS is used to aid in the regulation of post-approval changes (https://www.fda.gov/RegulatoryInformation/Guidances/default.htm). Possibility to skip *in vivo* bioequivalence and bioavailability can be granted by the US Food and Drug Administration (FDA) for drugs that are in the category with absorption potential, e.g., BCS Class I compounds with rapid dissolution rate (https://www.fda.gov/RegulatoryInformation/Guidances/default.htm).

In 2005, Wu and Benet[75] replaced the permeability in the BCS with extensive and poor metabolism and formed the Biopharmaceutics Drug Disposition Classification System or BDDCS. The BDDCS is applied to predict *in vivo* major route of elimination, disposition, and subsequently potential drug-drug interactions of a drug. Accordingly, the major route of elimination of highly permeable molecules,

Class 1	Class 2	Class 1	Class 2
High solubility High permeability	Low solubility High permeability	High solubility Extensive metabolism Transporter effects are minimal	Low solubility Extensive metabolism Transporter effects can be significant
Class 3	Class 4	Class 3	Class 4
High solubility Low permeability	Low solubility Low permeability	High solubility Poor metabolism Transporter effects can be significant	Low solubility Poor metabolism Transporter effects can be significant
Biopharmaceutics classification system (BCS)		Biopharmaceutics Drug Disposition Classification System (BDDCS)	

FIGURE 18.3 Biopharmaceutics classification system (BCS) and Biopharmaceutics Drug Disposition Classification System (BDDCS).

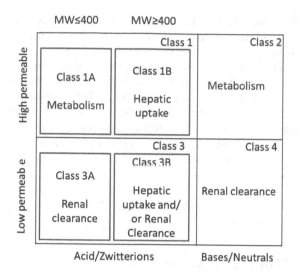

FIGURE 18.4   Extended Clearance Classification System (ECCS).

e.g., in BDDCS class 1 and class 2, is metabolism (≥70%), while the poorly permeable molecules, e.g., in BDDCS Class 3 and 4 are mainly eliminated from renal and/or biliary excretion of unchanged drugs. Therefore, as shown in the Figure 18.3, transporter effects on drug disposition and elimination can be minimal for molecules in the class 1 of the BDDCS, while the transporter effects can be significant for the molecules in the class 2, 3, and 4[76–78] (Figure 18.3).

Recently, on the basis of investigating the corrections between physiochemical properties of a drug and its clearance, Varma and colleagues proposed a framework of Extended Clearance Classification System (ECCS) (Figure 18.4).[79] The ECCS is applied to define *in vivo* rate-determining clearance processes based on *in vitro* drug passive permeability and physiochemical properties, e.g., ionization.[79] As illustrated in Figure 18.4, the ECCS assigns drugs into six classes. Class 1A drugs, the molecules with low molecular weight, high permeability and ionization state of acids and zwitterions, are predominantly cleared through metabolism; Class 1B drugs, the molecules with high molecular weight and permeability and the ionization state of acids and zwitterions, are predominantly cleared by transporter-mediated hepatic uptake; Class 2 drugs, the molecules with high permeability and ionization state of bases and/ or neutrals, are predominantly cleared by metabolic enzymes; Class 3A drugs, the molecules with low molecular weight, low permeability and ionization state of acids and zwitterions, are mainly eliminated by renal clearance mechanism; Class 3B drugs, the molecules with high molecular weight, low permeability and ionization state of acids and zwitterions are predominantly cleared by hepatic uptake or renal secretion; and Class 4 drugs, the molecules with low permeability and ionization state of bases and neutrals are mainly eliminated through renal clearance.[78,79] The framework of ECCS can be useful in understanding the predominant drug clearance mechanism for design of new molecules in early drug discovery stage using minimal experimental and physiochemical properties. The classification can, therefore, guide to further characterize the most likely pharmacokinetics attributes for the late stage compound development.[79,81]

Transporter Genetic Polymorphisms and PK Variability

Variability on drug pharmacokinetics is a leading cause for weakened efficacy or unwanted adverse effects for many drugs. As described in the above section, transporters play an important role in drug absorption, distribution, metabolism, and excretion. Therefore, it is reasonable to believe that altered transporter activity will have an impact on the pharmacokinetic and pharmacodynamics of a therapeutic agent. Genetic polymorphisms can cause alteration on the sequence and structure of a transporter and, therefore, lead to malfunctioned protein. Transporter genetic polymorphisms were first documented from subjects with noticeable clinical syndromes. For example, subjects developed type 2 progressive intrahepatic cholestasis (PFIC2) are carrying mutations on gene ABCB11 that encodes BSEP protein.[82,83] Rotor syndrome is a result of genetic deficiency of both OATP1B1 and AOTP1B3.[84] As the development of gene sequencing technology and the prevalent research on human genome, more and more polymorphisms are identified in drug transporters that are found to alter drug ADME in clinical studies.

P-gp/MDR1

P-gp is the earliest identified and is also the most studied drug transporter so far.[85] It is an ABC transporter excreting drugs from enterocytes into gut lumen in small and large intestine, from hepatocytes to bile in liver, and from proximal tubules cells to urine in kidney. The first two SNPs identified in P-gp were 2677G>T in exon 21 and 2995G>A in exon 24.[86] Nearly 40,000 genetic variations are detected in P-gp based on NCBI database search, of which a few hundred are occurring at the coding region. It has to be noted that SNPs at both coding and noncoding regions can affect transporter activity. For example, SNP (4036A>G) in the 3' untranslated (30-UTR) non-coding region is reported to increase different pharmacokinetic parameters of efavirenz in HIV patients.[87]

Majority of the current observed variants in P-gp are at low frequencies (<0.01) and only a few of these rare SNPs have been characterized in *in vitro* systems. The most studied variants are 1236C>T, 3435C>T, and 2677G>T/A, in which the former two are synonymous mutation with no amino acid substitution. 2677G>T/A is a nonsynonymous variant, and alanine is replaced by serine or threonine in the intracellular region of P-gp. However, the synonymous SNPs may affect the mRNA stability or translating speed, resulting in incorrectly folded transporter protein.[88,89] These three variants are closely linked and usually screened together in the haplotype analysis. The haplotypes CGC (1236C, 2677G, and 3435C) and TTT (1236T, 2677T, and 3435T) were reported in many populations (Table 18.2).[90,91] It was observed that the two synonymous SNPs can derive from the linkage disequilibrium with the missense variant 2677G>T/A.[92,93]

The frequency of SNPs in P-gp is greatly variable among racial populations. The 3435T allele has prevalence rates of 0.17–0.27 in African populations, and 0.41–57 in Asians and Caucasians.[94] The 1236C allele is a minor allele in Asian populations and 1236T is the minor allele in African populations. The frequency of 2677T is common in Caucasian subjects (0.46), but 2677A is very rare, with a prevalence of 0.02.[95] Compared to the C-G-C haplotype, The T-T-T variant occurs significantly less frequent in African populations than in Caucasians and is the most common haplotype in Asians.[90, 91, 93] The different frequency of SNPs is one of the causes leading to interethnic variance in the pharmacokinetics of P-gp substrate drugs.

The impact of P-gp SNPs on drug disposition has been reported in many studies. However, the outcomes are quite controversial from clinical studies. Digoxin is a gold standard substrate for P-gp and is commonly used in *in vitro* and clinical studies to assess P-gp function. In some reports, the maximum plasma concentration was reached earlier and also higher in subjects with 2677G>T/A or 3435C>T, as compared to people with WT P-gp following an oral dose of digoxin in healthy subjects.[96–98] However, no changes in PK or opposite results were obtained in other clinical studies with the same variant and same ethnic groups.[99,100] These questionable results are also observed for other drugs, such as fexofenadine, tacrolimus, and cyclosporine.[90, 101–105] Again, a PET imaging study demonstrated that the brain level of [^{11}C]verapamil, another model P-gp substrate, is not different between haplotype C-G-C and T-T-T.[106] The underlying mechanism for these controversial observations is still not clear.

BCRP

BCRP is another ABC transporter, which is usually expressed in parallel with P-gp in intestine, liver, kidney, and BBB. Numerous SNPs have been found in BCRP gene. The two well-known nonsynonymous polymorphisms are 34G>A and 421C>A, in which valine and glutamine are replaced by methionine and lysine, respectively (Table 18.2). The frequency of 421C>A SNP is very high in Asian populations (0.30–0.34), common in Caucasian (0.11), and very low in African populations (<0.05).[107,108] For 34G>A,

TABLE 18.2

Impact of Commonly Observed Transporter Polymorphisms on Function and Drug Pharmacokinetics

	Variant or Haplotype	Effect	Functional Change	Clinical Impact
P-gp	1236C>T	Synonymous		
	3435C>T	Synonymous	↓	↑ BA, AUC, Ctrough
	2677G>T/A	893Ala>Ser/Thr	↓	↑ AUC, Ctrough
	C-G-C>T-T-T	—	↓	↑ AUC, Ctrough
BCRP	34G>A	12Val>Met		
	421C>A	141Gln>Lys	↓	↑ BA, AUC
	376C>T	126Gln> stop codon	↓	
	G-C-C > G-C-A/ A-C-C/ G-T-C			
MRP2	−24C>T	Promotor		
	1249G>A	417Val>Ile		
	C3972T	synonymous		
OATP1B1	388A>G	130Asn>Asp	↑, ↔	
	521T>C	174Val>Ala	↓, ↔	
	−11187G>A	Promotor	↓	↓ AUC; ↑ CL
	*1a>1*b		↑	↓ AUC; ↑ CL
	*1a>*5		↓	↑ AUC; ↓ CL
	*1a> *15		↓	↑ AUC; ↓ CL
OATP1B3	334T>G	112Ser>Ala	↔	No Change
	699G>A	233Met>Ile	↔, ↓	No Change
	1564G>T	522Gly>Cys	↓	No Change
	IVS12-5676A>G	3'UTR		Mixed change
OCT2	808G>T	270Ala>Ser	↓	↓ CL
	−66T>C	5'UTR	↓	No Change
OAT1	1361G>A	454Arg>Gln		No Change
OATP3	723T>A	Synonymous		No Change
	1166C>T	389Ala>Val		No Change

the frequency is high in Japanese but low in Caucasian and African. Another SNP for BCRP is 376C>T, leading to an early stop codon, which is extremely rare. Haplotype analysis of these 3 SNPs revealed 4 haplotypes G-C-C, G-C-A, A-C-C, and G-T-C with frequencies of 46%, 35%, 18%, and 1%, respectively, in Japanese.[108]

The expression level of BCRP were decreased in the presence of SNP 421C>A as evaluated in *in vitro* system.[109] Therefore, it is expecting that BCRP substrate drug will have reduced clearance from liver and kidney and increased bioavailability from intestine. This expectation is supported by clinical observations that uric acid, a nature BCRP substrate, is higher in subject carrying 421C>A.[110] Following an IV administration, the plasma exposure of diflomotecan was increased 3 folds in patients with heterozygous 421A as compared to the homozygous 421C WT.[111] The bioavailability of topotecan was increased 1.34 fold in two heterozygous 421A subjects.[112] However, no significant changes in pharmacokinetics are also reported for diflomotecan oral dose and other drugs.[107,111]

MRP2

MRP2 is known from Dubin-Johnson syndrome, a disorder characterized by conjugated hyperbili-rubinaemia and accumulation of dark pigments in the liver. Genetic modification of MRP2 from missense mutation, nonsense mutation, splice site mutation, and deletion mutation are reported to be associated with Dubin-Johnson syndrome.[113–115] Several common SNPs were reported for MRP2, including C-24T (promoter), 1249G>A (417Val>Ile), and C3972T (synonymous) (Table 18.2). However, little is known regarding the occurring frequency in different populations and the impact on drug disposition.

OATP1B1 and OATP1B3

OATP1B1 and OATP1B3 are two SLC transporters specifically expressed on the sinusoidal membrane of hepatocytes, contributing to liver uptake of many therapeutic drugs. The two transporters share 80% of amino acid and have a great overlap for substrates. A variety of genetic variants has been identified in OATP1B1.[116,117] The two commonly occurring ones are 388A>G (130Asn>Asp) and 521T>C (174Val>Ala). One SNP located in the promoter region of OATP1B1 (g.-11187G>A) is tightly linked with 521T>C.[118] Major Haplotypes in humans are as follow: *1a (130Asn, 174Val), *1b (130Asp, 174Val), *5 (130Asn, 174Ala), *15 (130Asp, 174Ala), and *17 (-11187G>A, 130Asp174Ala) (Table 18.2). The distribution of OATP1B1 genetic variants is closely related to geographical regions. In general, the East Asian population has high frequency of OATP1B1 * 1b (~63%) and *15 (~12%) but very low *5 haplotype. The haplotype *1b is also very high in Sub-Saharan Africa (77%), while *5 and *15 are extremely low. In North America, the frequency of *1b and *15 are approximately 39% and 24%, respectively.[119]

Both OATP1B1 * 5 and *15 are conferred with reduced transporter capability. In cells transfected with either, a variant is reported with a decreased uptake probe substrate as compared to the WT.[34,120,121] More than 20 clinical studies have been conducted by various groups to investigate the impact of OATP1B1 * 5 and *15 haplotype (Table 18.2). The conclusion is similar to that of drugs known to be a OATP1B1 substrate with an increased plasma exposure and reduced hepatic clearance in subjects carrying OATP1B1 * 5 or *15. For example, as shown in Figure 18.5, the plasma exposure of pravastatin is increased in subjects with heterozygous or homozygous OATP1B1 * 5.[122] Although controversial results have been reported, OATP1B1 * 1b, in general, is believed to increase the transporter activity, which will enhance hepatic uptake and decrease plasma exposure.

Similar to OATP1B1, a great number of SNPs are also reported for OATP1B3, including 334T>G (112Ser>Ala), 699G>A (233Met>Ile), 1564G>T (522Gly>Cys), and IVS12-5676A>G (3'UTR) (Table 18.2).[123–125] However, the function of these variants is not comprehensively studied as compared to OATP1B1. In the limited reported clinical studies, the 3 nonsynonymous SNPs demonstrated no impact on the pharmacokinetics of OATP1B3 substrate, docetaxel.[126–128] Controversial results have been reported for IVS12-5676A>G in the pharmacokinetic profile of telmisartan.[129,130]

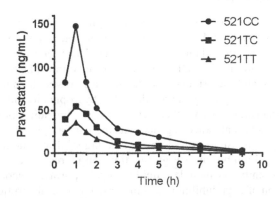

FIGURE 18.5 The plasma exposure of pravastatin in subjects with OATP1B1 polymorphism. Polymorphisms of OATP1B1 on the plasma concentration of pravastatin following a signal oral dose (40 mg). (Adapted from Niemi, M. et al., *Clin. Pharmacol. Ther.*, 80, 356–366, 2006.)

OCT2 and MATE1/MATE-2K

OCT2 is predominately expressed on the basolateral membrane to uptake drugs into proximal tubule cells, and MATE1 and MATE-2K are expressed on the apical membrane to export drugs to urine in human kidney (Figure 18.2). The genetic polymorphisms have been screened, and several non-synonymous SNPs are identified for all 3 transporters.[131,132] The allele frequency is relatively low for all polymorphisms, except for a SNP located at 5'UTR on MATE1.[34] The OCT2-MATE1/MATE-2K is a major channel for renal secretion of metformin. As thus, genetic variations of either OCT2 or MATE1/2K transporter genes may affect the renal clearance of metformin. In a clinical study conducted in Chinese population, OCT2 808G>T polymorphism is associated with a reduced metformin renal clearance (Table 18.2).[133] However, metformin plasma concentrations and apparent plasma clearance were not changed in hetero-zygous carriers of the MATE1 and MATE2-K variants.[134]

OAT1 and OAT3

Both OAT1 and OAT3 are substantially expressed on the basolateral membrane of proximal tubules. A list of SNPs is reported for these two transporters, but the overall frequency is very low in all popula-tions. In two separated clinical studies, neither OAT1 1361G>A nor OAT3 723T>A and 1166C>T dem-onstrated any impact on renal clearance of tested substrate (Table 18.2).[135,136]

Naturally occurring genetic polymorphism is a good resource to understand the function of transport-ers in humans. The accumulation of the knowledge can guide the pharmaceutical companies to develop drugs with improved efficacy and less adverse effects. The above discussed transporters are only a few of the whole transporter family, which have demonstrated clinical significance on drug pharmacokinetics and been nominated by multiple health authorities to investigate their role in drug discovery and devel-opment. As described, numerous genetic polymorphisms have been identified for drug transporters, but the impact on functions is still not well understood. It is even more challenge to explore the influence clinically. First of all, highly selective probe substrates are not available. Many drugs are substrates of multiple transporters so that single genetic variant may not lead to a change in plasma concentration. Second, transporters expressed on the apical membrane in liver and kidney is more likely to affect the tissue concentration, and the impact in most case will not be reflected in plasma drug pharmacokinetics. In addition, subject enrollment is difficult especially for low occurring variant. The condition of the studied subjects can be varied from many aspects such as disease status, living habit, and co-medications. All these can lead to interindividual variability on studied drug PK. This may explain the controversial results reported from different groups.

Transporters Involved DDIs

During the past decades, efforts by the pharmaceutical industry have been made to examine and de-risk DDIs potentials during drug discovery and development. Inhibition of drug transporters can affect both drug pharmacokinetics and pharmacodynamics. The reviews of transporter-mediated DDI are well-documented in the literature.[137] Of the many reported clinical DDI studies, P-glycoprotein[138] is clearly the most studied, and the original finding and basic research continues to have strong ties with clinical oncology.[139,140] Many drugs, particularly the hydrophobic and cationic molecules, have been identified as P-gp substrates across therapeutics classes including protease inhibitors, immu-nosuppressants, beta-blockers, anticancer agents, and the cardiac glycoside digoxin.[141,142] For oral administered drugs, P-gp expression in the luminal membrane of the enterocyte plays an important role in drug absorption, and inhibition of P-gp function can increase the exposure of drugs that are substrates of P-gp. P-gp inhibitors include quinidine, cyclosporine, itraconazole, and clarithromy-cin[143] and coadministration of P-gp inhibitors can increase the drug absorption in the gastrointestinal track. For example, increased bioavailability and decreased renal secretion of digoxin were observed when coadministration with P-gp inhibitor quinidine.[143,144] P-gp also serve as an efflux pump on blood–brain barrier (BBB) and has the highest relevance of all transporters for drug transport across

BBB for many xenobiotics (Figure 18.2). Functional activities of P-gp on BBB is testified using positron emission tomography scanning with [11C]verapamil.[145,146] Inhibition of P-gp function on BBB causes respiratory depression in healthy volunteers, which is undesirable effects of loperamide.[147] As such, P-gp was the first transporter being included in the FDA guidance in 2006 due to the apparent clinically relevant DDIs reported. Metabolic stable P-gp substrates such as digoxin, dabigatran etexilate, and fexofenadine are listed as probe substrates to investigate clinical DDIs with P-gp inhibitors in EMA guidance (http://www.ema.europa.eu/docs/en_GB/document_library/Scientific_guideline/2012/07/WC500129606.pdf).

In addition to P-gp, BCRP is also expressed on apical membrane of enterocytes to limit drug absorption. Many drugs such as statins (e.g., rosuvastatin) and antineoplastic agents (e.g., mitoxantrone, topotecan, gefitinib, imatinib) are identified as substrates of BCRP.[148,149] The altered disposition of atorvastatin and rosuvastatin in the subjects with BCRP 421C>A polymorphism in the ABCG2 gene that causes a reduced activity of BCRP provides the evidence of BCRP role on drug absorption in human.[150–152] Therefore, inhibition of BCRP can alter disposition of BCRP substrates.[152]

OATP1B1, OATP1B3 and OATP2B1 are expressed in the liver and are important uptake transporters for drug disposition and hepatic clearance. Many drugs have been identified as substrates and/or inhibitors for the OATP transporters. Interactions with OATP mediated hepatic transport can cause significant PK changes, not only for drugs that are metabolic stable, e.g., pravastatin,[153] also for many compounds that are metabolized by phase I and/or II enzymes, e.g., bosentan.[154] Although considerable differences in the affinity to drug metabolizing enzymes and uptake/efflux transporters are noted for statins, the evidence for OATPs' role on DDIs is mostly documented for statins. For example, fluvastatin is metabolized by CYP2C9 and atorvastatin and simvastatin by CYP3A4, whereas metabolic clearance plays a minor role for pitavastatin, rosuvastatin and pravastatin.[155,156] The systemic exposures of cerivastatin and atorvastatin were significantly increased by coadministration of OATP inhibitor gemfibrozil and cyclosporine, respectively.[157,158] AUCs of OATP substrate cerivastatin and repaglinide were increased about 4-fold and 3.4-fold increased respectively by cyclosporine A.[157,159] Rifampicin is a potent OATP1B inhibitor and cause increased systemic exposure of its substrates bosentan and repaglinide.[21,160] Clinical DDI studies have shown that CYP3A4 inhibitors clarithromycin and itraconazole can only modestly increase the plasma exposure, e.g., AUC of repaglinide.[161] The large drug interaction of repaglinide was detected when co-dosed with gemfibrozil,[161] likely due to inhibition of both OATP1B1 and CYP2C8 by gemfibrozil and its glucuronide metabolite.[162] In addition, elevation of repaglinide plasma levels in subjects with the OATP1B1 521CC genotype with reduced OATP1B1 activities demonstrates the importance of OATP1B1-mediated hepatic uptake for repaglinide elimination. As aforementioned, circulating metabolites can also be OATP inhibitors and cause significant DDIs. Glucuronide metabolite of gemfibrozil is more potent inhibitor of OATP1B than its parent gemfibrozil and account for the DDIs with a number of statins.[39,163]

Although members of the OAT family are present in various tissues in the body, the inhibition of OAT functions mainly attribute to the DDIs for drugs eliminated from urine. OAT1 and OAT3 are expressed on the basolateral membrane of the proximal renal tubular cells and facilitate the basolateral uptake of anionic drugs into proximal renal tubular cells.[164] OATs operate as an organic anion/alpha-ketoglutarate exchanger to transport many anionic drugs including antibiotics, antivirals or H2-receptor, and endogenous compounds.[165,166] The antivirals acyclovir and cidofovir are OAT1 substrates,[167,168] whereas the antibiotic benzylpenicillin is a well-characterized substrate of OAT3. Diuretic reagent furosemide is transported by both OAT1 and OAT3.[169] Probenecid is an inhibitor for both OAT1 and OAT3 used for characterizing clinical DDIs mediated OAT inhibition.[170,171] Furosemide is mainly eliminated by active renal excretion of the unchanged drug. Coadministration of probenecid increased plasma exposure of OAT substrate furosemide,[172] or methotrexate.[173]

OCT2 and MATE1/MATE2K are expressed on the basalateral and luminal membrane of renal proximal tubule cells, respectively, and mediate the uptake and efflux of their substrate from the blood into the urine. The transporters play an important role in the renal tubular secretion for basic drugs.[132,174] OCT and MATE commonly share their substrate specificity such as cimetidine and metformin.[175,176] Inhibition of OCT and/or MATE activity can cause DDIs for organic cation drugs that are secreted from urine. Cimetidine, an inhibitor for both OCT and MATE, decreased renal clearance and increased the systemic exposure of the antiarrhythmic drug procainamide in healthy volunteers.[177] Similarly, coadministration of cimetidine increased the systemic exposure of metformin and decreased its renal clearance in healthy subjects.[178] Studies from other research group revealed that a single oral dose of 50 mg of pyrimethamine, an potent inhibitor of MATE, reduced the renal clearance of the anti-diabetic metformin in healthy volunteers.[179] Pyrimethamine also reduced the renal secretion of the endogenous metabolite N-methylnicotinamide (NMN),[180] suggesting that NMN can be an endogenous probe for evaluation of DDIs involving MATE inhibition.[181] Similar to OAT transporters, inhibition of OCT uptake can also reduce the drug exposure in proximal tubule cells and provide protective effects prevent renal damage. For example, coadministration of cimetidine protects mice from nephrotoxicity of cisplatin, which is attributed to the inhibition of OCT-mediated accumulation of cisplatin in proximal renal tubule cells.[182,183]

Transporter Roles in Toxicity

Transporters play a pivotal role in transporting many fundamental physiological substances.[184] Transporter-mediated active uptake can cause drug accumulation in a target organ to an unsafe level, or disruption of transport pathways may lead to serious drug-induced toxicities including liver cho-lestasis, cardiac myopathy, and nephrotoxicity. In the kidney, basolaterally expressed transporters such as OAT1, OAT3, and OCT2 and apically expressed MATE1 and MATE2-K in the proximal tubule play an important role in renal secretion of a drug and its metabolites. As such, the kidney is often a target organ of drug toxicity. For example, antivirals (e.g., acyclic nucleoside phosphonates), antibiot-ics (e.g., β-lactams), and chemotherapeutic agents (e.g., methotrexate and cisplatin) can accumulate in the proximal tubule and cause direct cellular toxicity.[185-187] The mechanism of OAT-mediated cidofo-vir uptake has led to the clinical use of the OAT inhibitor probenecid to reduce the accumulation in the proximal tubule cells and, therefore, greatly reduce the incidence of renal adverse events.[188] The neph-rotoxicity of cisplatin is a basal transporter OCT2 and apical efflux transporter MATE substrates.[189,190] Coadministration of MATE inhibitors ondansetron or vandetanib can cause cisplatin accumulation in the kidney resulting in enhanced toxicity either in mice or transfected cell lines.[191,192]

Bile acids are produced from cholesterol in the liver and undergo enterohepatic recycling to aid in the absorption of lipids and nutrients.[193,194] In the gut, bile acids are absorbed by apical sodium dependent bile salt transporter (ASBT). In the liver, bile salts are taken up predominantly by NTCP[195,196] and pumped out into the bile via into the bile mediated by BSEP.[197,198] BSEP function can be inhibited by many drugs such as troglitazone, bosentan, rifampicin, erythromycin estolate, and glibenclamide. Inhibition of BSEP function can cause the accumulation of bile salts in the liver and is found to correlate with liver liabilities in humans.[51] Antidiabetic drug troglitazone and anti-depressant drug nefazodone were withdrawn from the market due to severe liver injury, and they both inhibit taurocholate transport mediated by BSEP.[52,53,199,200] Inhibition of BSEP by troglitazone may contribute to the drug induced liver injury observed in clinic. Therefore, evaluation of BSEP is recommended in the drug discovery and development to screen out the compounds with potential risk of liver cholestasis.[201]

Hepatic transporter expressions are sensitive to the regulation of transcription factors and nuclear receptors or disease conditions.[202] In addition, the expression of BSEP is highly regulated by bile acid receptor, the heterodimer of farnesoid X receptor (FXR) and retinoid X receptor alpha (RXR).[203-205] For example, acetaminophen overdose can upregulate the expression of basolateral efflux transporters (MRP4 and MPR5) and canalicular efflux transporters (BCRP and P-glycoprotein).[203] The transporter upregula-tion could be a protective mechanism from liver injury. In cholestatic patients, down-regulation of NTCP and OAPTs and upregulation of basolateral efflux transporters (MRP3 and MPR4) are reported,[207] which can limit the excessive bile salts exposure in hepatocytes. Disruption of the transporter regulations may change and disable the adaptive response of the liver to the drug-induced liver injury, leading to a greater risk of toxicities.

Tools to Assess Transporter Interaction in Drug Discovery and Development

A variety of tools have been developed to access transporter functions in drug discovery and development. The *in vitro* systems include cell lines, membrane vesicles, and primary cells. The function of transporters can also be studied in animals and humans by applying specific inhibitors. Gene KO animal model or humans with nature occurring genetic polymorphisms are also used to explore the transporter functions *in vivo*.

Passive Permeability with PAMPA, Caco-2, and MDCK

Passive permeability of a drug candidate is usually determined in discovery stage. Although a transporter is not involved in this process, measurement of passive permeability can be used to explore the oral absorption potential and to predict the distribution and elimination of a drug candidate. The relative contribution of passive permeability against transporter mediated cell membrane penetration can be important for drug ADME in special populations or in patients taking multiple drugs.

Two systems are commonly used in pharmaceutical industry to determine the permeability of substances, parallel artificial membrane permeability assay (PAMPA) and cell lines forming monolayer with low paracellular permeability. The membrane layer in both systems will divide the incubation buffer to two separated spaces and prevent the free movement of chemicals. In PAMPA assays, the permeation is measured using a lipid-infused artificial membrane. Caco-2 and MDCK are the two widely used cell lines, which can form a tight monolayer with the differentiation of apical and basolateral cell membrane, when cultured on permeable membrane inserts (Figure 18.6). Caco-2 is a cell line derived from human epithelial colorectal adenocarcinoma cells. After culture, Caco-2 cells can form a monolayer similar to small intestine: tight junction, microvilli, and metabolic enzymes and drug transporters (Figure 18.6). MDCK cell line was derived from canine kidney, which can also form a monolayer with tight junction. The expression of canine transporters is observed in the original MDCK cells. Recently, genetically engineered MDCK cells with no P-gp/ BCRP are usually used to determine passive permeability.[208]

The integrity of the cell monolayer can be measured by transepithelial electrical resistance or TEER value and paracellular flux of a low-permeability compound (e.g., inulin, mannitol, or Lucifer yellow). For both systems, the compound is loaded to the buffer in the "donor" compartment at the beginning, and no drug is presented in the buffer in the "acceptor" compartment. The buffer presented in each side can be the same or different to mimic various *in vivo* scenarios. The test drug is first loaded to one side of the cell monolayer, either in the apical (A) compartment or the basolateral (B) compartment. At predetermined time points, the amount of drug appearing in the other side of cell monolayer will be quantified. The apparent permeability (Papp) is calculated for both A to B (A-B) and B to A (B-A) using Equation 18.3. For PAMPA assay and MDCK cells, the permeability is usually tested in one direction (A to B), in which a compound is dosed in compartment facing the apical side (only for MDCK cells).

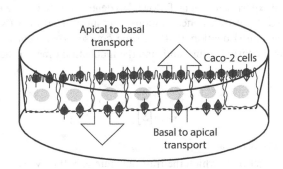

FIGURE 18.6 Bidirection transport in cell monolayers cultured on permeable membrane inserts.

For Caco-2 assay, drug is dosed on both sides separately to determine A to B and B to A permeability. An efflux ratio (P_{B-A}/P_{A-B}) greater than 2 indicates the tested compound is a substrate for efflux transporters such as P-gp and/or BCRP.

$$Papp = \frac{dQ}{dt} * \frac{1}{A*C_0} \tag{18.3}$$

where A is the membrane surface area, C_0 is the donor drug concentration at t = 0, and dQ/dt is the amount of drug transported within a given period.

Bidirectional transporter assay is usually conducted to study efflux transporters such as P-gp and BCRP. Similar to the Caco-2 assays, MDCK or LLC-PK1 cells expressing the interested transporter are cultured on a permeable membrane insert to form a tight cell monolayer (Figure 18.6). An efflux ratio greater than 2 generally suggests substrate potential. The inhibition of a drug molecule can also be determined with the bidirectional transporter assay. The efflux ratio of a probe substrate is determined and the decreased efflux ratio in the presence of the test compound indicates the inhibitory effect. The efflux transporter kinetics for substrate and inhibitor measurement can be determined in a similar rationale to the uptake transporters as described above. The parameters of Km and IC50/Ki can be calculated using Equations 18.2 and 18.3, respectively, by fitting efflux ratio concentration curve.

Cell Lines with Overexpressed Transporters

Cells expressing a single transporter of interest are used to phenotype whether a drug molecule is a substrate or inhibitor of this transporter. This system can also be used to determine the substrate affinity (Km) and inhibition potency (IC_{50} or Ki). HEK293, CHO, and MDCK cells are commonly used as host cells for expressing uptake transporters. MDCK and LLC-PK1 cells can form tight polarized cell monolayers with apical and basolateral differentiation, and are used for the expression of efflux transporters on the apical membrane. Oocytes from Xenopus laevis were widely used historically for expression transporters but have stopped these days in the drug discovery and development. The major concern is that transport results obtained from oocytes are not always able to translate to those generated in mammalian cells.

Uptake Transporter Evaluation

For uptake transporters like OATP, OCT, and OAT, the substrate determination is carried out by incubating the drug molecules with cells expressing individual transporter. The assay can be conducted with cells attached to multiple well cell culture plates or in suspension. The accumulation of the compound significantly higher (generally>2 fold) in transporter-expressing cells than in nontransfected, or empty vector transfected cells, indicates that the tested compound is a substrate. Substrate potential can be further confirmed by comparing the intracellular drug amount in the absence and presence of a known inhibitor. A more profound experiment can be followed to determine the uptake kinetics. The uptake rate is measured at a wide range of substrate concentrations. The substrate affinity (Km) can be modeled with the Michaelis-Menten equation (Equation 18.4). A time course assessment is necessary to determine the linear uptake range for the tested compound, and the incubation time for the kinetic study should be within this linear phase.

$$v = \frac{V_{max}*[S]}{K_m +[S]} + P_{dif}*[S] \tag{18.4}$$

V_{max}: the maximum transporter rate

K_m: the substrate concentration at which the transport rate is half of Vmax

[S]: substrate concentration

P_{dif}: passive diffusion

Linear uptake range should also be established for the probe substrate (Table 18.1) in order to test whether a drug molecule is an inhibitor of the interested transporter. The intracellular accumulation of the probe substrate should be measured in the presence and absence of the test compound. A decreased probe substrate uptake suggested inhibitory effect. The IC_{50} parameter, the concentration of an inhibitor that inhibits 50% transport activity, can be derived from the concentration inhibition curve, in which the probe substrate uptake is measured with increasing concentrations of the tested compound. In this case where the inhibition is competitive, the inhibition constant K_i can be calculated using the Cheng-Prusoff equation (Equation 18.5).

$$K_i = \frac{IC_{50}}{1 + \frac{[s]}{K_m}}$$ (18.5)

K_i: inhibition constant

IC_{50}: the concentration of the inhibitor that inhibits 50% transport activity

[S]: probe substrate concentration

$[K_m]$: concentration of probe substrate at which the transport rate is half of V_{max}

Membrane Vesicles

The other most commonly used *in vitro* model to study efflux transporter is the inside-out membrane vesicle assay. Membrane vesicles are usually prepared from crude membranous of insect *Spodoptera frugiperda* (sf9 or sf21) or mammalian cells genetically modified to overexpress the interested protein. Membrane vesicles containing major efflux transporters such as P-gp, BCRP, MPR2/3/4, and BSEP are commercially available.

The inside-out membrane vesicle assay can be conducted either by direct measurement of intravesicular drug uptake or by indirect ATPase assay (Figure 18.7). The method for direct uptake assay in membrane vesicles is similar to the cell-based uptake transporter assay. Briefly, the test compound is incubated with membrane vesicles, and then intravesicular accumulation is measured at designated time. However, unlike the cell-based assay that can generate ATP, external ATP must be added in the membrane vesicle assays to provide energy for the function of ABC transporters. In order to avoid false positive result from passive diffusion and specific/nonspecific binding, a control experiment with AMP is

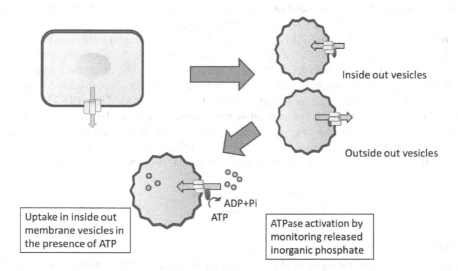

FIGURE 18.7 ATPase and uptake assays in membrane vesicles.

usually conducted in parallel. A significant difference between the ATP and AMP treatments suggests the test compound as a substrate. This assay is also suitable for inhibition experiments, as well as kinetic studies to determine K_m and IC_{50}/K_i.

Activation of ABC transporters by interacting with substrate requires the hydrolysis of ATP by ATPase, which will release inorganic phosphate. Therefore, the transporter activity in membrane vesicles can be determined indirectly by measuring released inorganic phosphate in the incubation buffer, named ATPase assay. In this assay, membrane vesicles are incubated with ATP and the test compound. The reaction is then stopped by adding 12% sodium dodecyl sulfate, and the released inorganic phosphate is quantified by a colorimetric assay.

Hepatocytes in Suspension

Freshly isolated and cryopreserved hepatocytes are known to maintain the uptake transporter activity when incubated in the suspension setup and, therefore, are commonly used in the evaluation of hepatic drug uptake. Hepatocytes are first suspended in ice-cold hanks balanced salt solution (HBSS) to minimize cell degradation. Prior to the experiment, suspension hepatocytes are warmed to 37°C and then an equal volume of HBSS containing the tested compound (pre-warmed to 37°C) is added to initiate the uptake. At predetermined time points, the incubation is terminated by rapidly separating the cells from the incubation buffer using a rapid filtration approach with a cell harvester or centrifugation through a layer of mineral oil. The amount of drug presenting in the cells is quantified to calculate the uptake. Uptake rate or clearance can be derived from the initial linear curve. To separate transporter mediated uptake from passive diffusion, a parallel study is usually conducted at 4°C to determine passive permeability in hepatocytes. The assumption is that transporter activity is halted at 4°C. However, the fluidity of the buffer and cell membrane can be affected at low temperature so that the passive diffusion obtained at 4°C may not represent the value at 37°C. Selective inhibitor can also be applied to determine the contribution of individual transporter for overall hepatic uptake. The concentration of inhibitor should be optimized due to the great overlap of inhibition.

Sandwich Cultured Hepatocytes (SCH)

When cultured in a collagen-hepatocyte-collagen format, hepatocytes are able to form tight junctions among individual cells to generate sealed pockets similar to bile canalicular (Figure 18.8). The uptake and efflux transporters will be trafficked to basolateral or canalicular membrane as in the native distribution. Therefore, the recovered canalicular structure in SCH can be used to study drug biliary excretion. Detailed protocols for hepatocyte isolation and preparation of SCH cultures have been reported previously. Ready-to-use SCH plates are also commercially available.

For biliary excretion study, the SCH is pre-incubated with two different buffers in parallel: standard HBSS buffer containing Ca^{2+} and Ca^{2+}-free HBSS buffer (Figure 18.8). Ca^{2+} is the modulator for tight junction formation among hepatocytes. With the removal of Ca^{2+} in the incubation system, tight junctions will break, and the canalicular contents are released. Following a short period of preincubation (~10 min), cells are incubated with the tested compound prepared in standard HBSS buffer containing Ca^{2+} for up to 30 minutes. At the end of incubation, the reaction was stopped by washing with an ice-cold buffer and then cells are lyzed for drug quantitation. The amount of drug excreted into the canalicular pocket is determined by the difference between the Ca^{2+} buffer and Ca^{2+}-free buffer. The biliary excretion index (BEI), a parameter to evaluate canalicular excretion, is calculated as shown in Equation 18.6.

$$BEI = \frac{(Amount_{+Ca^{2+}} - Amount_{-Ca^{2+}})}{Amount_{+Ca^{2+}}} * 100\% \tag{18.6}$$

BEI: biliary excretion index

$Amount_{+Ca^{2+}}$: Amount of drug in SCH preincubated with standard HBSS buffer containing Ca^{2+}

$Amount_{-Ca^{2+}}$: Amount of drug in SCH preincubated with Ca^{2+}-free HBSS buffer

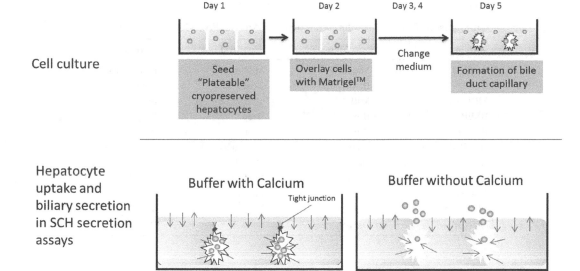

FIGURE 18.8 Hepatic uptake and biliary secretion in sandwich cultured hepatocytes (SCH).

Other *In Vitro* Models

In addition to the common assays described above, other *in vitro* models are occasionally used to address specific issues in drug discovery and development. To test the low permeable compound in the bidirectional transport assay, double transporter transfected cell model is developed to facilitate the hydrophilic compound uptake in the basolateral membrane. For example, LLC-PK1 or HeLa cells co-transfected with NTCP and BSEP demonstrate great application to investigate bile salt excretion and drug interactions with BSEP.

Due to the native expression of efflux transporter P-gp and BCRP, Caco-2 assay can also be used for substrate confirmation for these two transporters. An efflux ratio greater than 2 indicates the active transport of the tested compound through either P-gp or BCRP. A following Caco-2 assay can then be conducted with the inclusion of verapamil and fumitremorgin as the specific inhibitor for P-gp and BCRP, respectively. Decreased efflux ratio in the presence of inhibitor suggests that the compound is a substrate. Usually, a second assay with membrane vesicles or transporter overexpressed cells is needed to confirm the Caco-2 results.

In additional to hepatocytes, other primary cells are also developed to understand the complicated interplay between multiple transporters and enzymes in physiological relevant systems. Renal proximal tubule cell (PTC) monolayer is an *in vitro* model developed to study transporter mediated drug excretion, DDIs, and nephrotoxicity in kidney. An organ-on-a-chip model is built with continuously perfused chambers inhabited by living cells arranged to simulate tissue- and organ-level physiology.[209] A more complexed system is the integration of multiple organ-on-a-chip devices to mimic the interplay among different organs in the body.

Animal Model

The well-known human transporters are also identified in the preclinical animal models. The comparison of the transporter orthologues from mouse, rat, monkey, and humans are summarized in Table 18.3. Prior to the clinical investigations in humans, animal models are commonly used to evaluate the significance of transporters in drug ADME.

The impact of efflux transporters on the drug oral absorption can be studied in animals with two different approaches. Multiple ascending doses can be orally administered. A greater than dose proportional increase in systemic plasma exposure (AUC) suggests that the drug is most likely a substrate

TABLE 18.3

Comparison of the Transporter Orthologues in Mouse, Rat, Monkey, and Human

Human	Mouse	Rat	Monkey
P-gp (MDR1)	Mdr1a/1b	Mdr1a/1b	P-gp (Mdr1)
BCRP	Bcrp	Bcrp	Bcrp
MRP2/3/4	MRP2/3/4	MRP2/3/4	MRP2/3/4
BSEP	Bsep	Bsep	Bsep
PEPT1/2	Pept2	Pept1	Pept1/2
OATP1B1/1B3/2B1	Oatp1b2/1a1/1a4	Oatp1b2/1a1/1a4	Oatp1B1/1B3
OAT1/3	Oat1/3	Oat1/3	Oat1/3
OCT1/2/3	Oct1/2/3	Oct1/2/3	Oct1/2/3
MATE1	Mate1	Mate1	MATE1
MATE2-K	Mate2	Mate2	MATE2-K
OSTα/β	Ostα/β	Ostα/β	OSTα/β

for intestinal efflux transporters. A high dose is believed to saturate the efflux capacity and, therefore, increase the fraction of absorption in a nonlinear pattern. The other approach is to coadminister P-gp or BCRP inhibitor to check the plasma exposure change. In both methods, caution should be taken to interpret the data as systemic AUC change can also be contributed from saturation clearance from high dose and transporter inhibition from other tissue. Direct evidence is to evaluate the drug exposure in portal vein. Coadministration of selective inhibitors can also be applied to study transporter function in other organs such as in liver, kidney, and brain.

The other direction is to study transporter function in transporter deficient animal models, either from nature loss or genetic modified. To date, the genetic KO mouse model is available for major transporters. The KO rat model is also developed and commercial available for selected transporter. By removing the specific transporter, these animal models are believed to be most straightforward tool to study transporter function *in vivo*. Promising results have been reported for many transporter KO animal models. For example, the brain concentration of digoxin, a typical substrate for P-gp, was significantly increased in mdr1a KO mouse.[210,211] The plasma concentration of rosuvastatin was significantly increased in Oatp KO mice.[212,213]

There are still many considerations of using animal models. Due to the great overlap in inhibitor specificity across transporters, the observed PK alteration is usually a result contributed from many transporter inhibitions. For example, cyclosporine is potent inhibitor to many transporters, including P-gp, BCRP, MRP, and OATP. Rifampin is commonly used as an inhibitor *in vivo* to evaluate OATP DDI. However, rifampin also demonstrates inhibition against P-gp and MRP2. In addition, compensatory mechanisms through gene regulations of other transporters are also reported in KO animals. More importantly, species differences exist in regards to the transporter roles in drug ADME and toxicity. For example, Human with BSEP polymorphisms can develop progressive familiar intrahepatic cholestasis type 2 (PFIC-2), a progressive cholestasis typically leading to hepatic failure, but BSEP KO mouse and rat have much less consequences.[82,83,214,215] Rodents are able to tolerate drugs that cause severe clinical toxicity. Therefore, preclinical to clinical translation should be carefully evaluated.

Clinical Studies

Transporter functions in humans are commonly investigated through DDI studies in drug clinical development. In addition, the role of transporter in drug ADME can also be evaluated in subjects carrying SNPs. As summarized above, the genetic variance has been observed for many drug transporters. Due to the low frequency of SNPs for many transporters, it is very challenging and costly to enroll enough subjects for one clinical study. This methodology is not routinely used in clinical investigation of new chemical entities.

Characterizing Transporter Interaction in Drug Discovery and Development

The first consideration in characterizing transporter interactions is to select the most appropriate assay. Cells with overexpressed transporter of interest are good to phenotype whether a drug molecule is a substrate or inhibitor of a specific transporter, as well as to determine the kinetic parameters. This assay is particularly good for uptake transporters such as OATP, OCT, and OAT. It can be challenging sometimes for low permeable compounds in the bidirectional assay with cells overexpressing efflux transporters (Table 18.4). The slow penetration of basolateral membrane can misinform the efflux activity. Membrane vesicle assay is a more straightforward tool for efflux transporter phenotyping. The caveat is that it is an artificial system lacking of cellular components, which may contain key cofactors required for ABC transporter activity. For example, reduced glutathione should be supplied in the membrane vesicle assays to evaluate the function of MRP family.[216–218] Application of hepatocytes in either suspension or sandwich cultured format allows to assess overall drug disposition by multiple drug transporter and metabolic enzymes in a physiologically relevant system. Due to the great overlap in inhibitor specificity across transporters, *in vitro* assay using hepatocytes is not a suitable system for determining transporter substrate specificity. The advantages, limitations and applications of each assay are summarized in Table 18.4.

TABLE 18.4

Advantages, Limitations, and Applications of *In Vitro* Assays

Assay Format	Advantages	Limitations	Applications
Caco-2 MDCK	• High throughput • Commercially available	• Long culture time for Caco-2 • Endogenous transporter activity	• Passive permeability measurement • P-gp or BCRP substrate/inhibition pre-evaluation • Screening in early drug discovery
Cell lines with overexpressed individual transporter	• High transporter expression and activity • Single transporter system • High throughput • Commercially available	• Endogenous transporter activity • Bidirectional cell assay not compatible with low permeable compound • Transporter expression varies	• Substrate or inhibitor confirmation • Transporter kinetics (K_m and IC_{50}) • SNP and mutation characterization • Screening in early drug discovery
Membrane vesicles	• High transporter expression and activity • Compatible with cytotoxic compounds • Good with low permeability compounds • High throughput • Commercially available	• Endogenous transporter activity • Artificial system lacking physiological relevance • Need to optimize cofactors	• Substrate or inhibitor confirmation • Transporter kinetics (K_m and IC_{50}) • Screening in early drug discovery
Hepatocytes in suspension	• Physiological relevant • Hepatic uptake form multiple transporters • Cross species comparison • Pooled hepatocytes to avoid individual variability	• Hepatocyte preparation from liver • No canalicular structure • Reduced transporter and enzyme activity • Low throughput	• Hepatic uptake • Active uptake versus passive diffusion
Sandwich cultured hepatocytes	• Physiological relevant • Hepatic uptake, metabolism, and biliary simultaneously • Cross species comparison • Commercial available	• Complicated and time consuming • Need high quality hepatocytes • Inter individual variability • Limited throughput	• Hepatic uptake • Biliary clearance • Drug liver disposition • Drug-induced cholestasis investigation

Control group should always be properly designed in the *in vitro* assays and the inclusion of positive and negative controls is critical for accurate interpretation of the generated data. The proper function of a transporter can be confirmed by the transport of a probe substrate. A prototypical inhibitor can also be included in inhibition experiment. Evaluated of a negative control compound is also important to prevent a false positive readout. The inclusion of these control compounds allows data comparison from separate experiments and different labs. Due to expression of endogenous transporters in transfected cells, nontransfected parental (wild-type) cells or cells transfected with empty vector (mock-transfected) should be also evaluated as the control comparison to determine passive diffusion and nonspecific membrane binding. In the membrane vesicle assays, ATP is substitute with AMP to determine the activity from uninterested transporter.

Experiment conditions and procedures should be optimized in all *in vitro* assays in order to generate meaningful and consistence data. Consistent procedures should be maintained to minimize experimental variability such as cell seeding numbers, cell growing period, dosing solution preparation, and incubation time and temperature. The incubation is usually carried out at 37°C. The amount of organic solvent should be kept less than <1% at the final concentration in the cell based assay to avoid cytotoxicity. Albumin or other specimens can be added in the incubation buffer to improve solubility and to reduce nonspecific binding, but free fraction of the compound should be incorporated in the data analysis. In the assays to confirm substrate or inhibitor, multiple concentrations should be tested to avoid false results. Prior to a kinetic experiment, a variety of incubation times should be evaluated to determine a time period of linear response.

REFERENCES

1. Morgan, P., Van Der Graaf, P. H., Arrowsmith, J., Feltner, D. E., Drummond, K. S., Wegner, C. D.,Street, S. D. Can the flow of medicines be improved? Fundamental pharmacokinetic and pharmacological principles toward improving Phase II survival. *Drug Discov. Today* **2012**, *17*, (9–10), 419–424.
2. Bachmann, K. A. R., J.B., Wrighton, S.A. Cytochrome P450 and its place in drug discovery and development. In *Drug Metabolizing Enzymes*, Lee, J. O., S.R., Fisher, M.B., Ed. Marcel Dikker: New York, 2003; pp. 311–332.
3. Hillgren, K. M., Keppler, D., Zur, A. A., Giacomini, K. M., Stieger, B., Cass, C. E., Zhang, L. International Transporter, C. Emerging transporters of clinical importance: An update from the international transporter consortium. *Clin. Pharmacol. Ther.* **2013**, *94*, (1), 52–63.
4. International Transporter, C., Giacomini, K. M., Huang, S. M., Tweedie, D. J., Benet, L. Z., Brouwer, K. L., Chu, X. et al. Membrane transporters in drug development. *Nat. Rev. Drug Discov.* **2010**, *9*, (3), 215–236.
5. Arya, V., Kiser, J. J. Role of Transporters in drug development. *J. Clin. Pharmacol.* **2016**, *56*, (Suppl 7), S7–S10.
6. Benadiba, M., Maor, Y. Importance of ABC transporters in drug development. *Curr. Pharm. Des.* **2016**, *22*, (38), 5817–5829.
7. Liu, H., Sahi, J. Role of hepatic drug transporters in drug development. *J. Clin. Pharmacol.* **2016**, *56*, (Suppl 7), S11–S22.
8. Pfefferkorn, J. A., Litchfield, J., Hutchings, R., Cheng, X. M., Larsen, S. D., Auerbach, B., Bush, M. R. et al. Discovery of novel hepatoselective HMG-CoA reductase inhibitors for treating hypercholesterolemia: A bench-to-bedside case study on tissue selective drug distribution. *Bioorg. Med. Chem. Lett.* **2011**, *21*, (9), 2725–2731.
9. Lin, L., Yee, S. W., Kim, R. B., Giacomini, K. M. SLC transporters as therapeutic targets: Emerging opportunities. *Nat. Rev. Drug Discov.* **2015**, *14*, (8), 543–560.
10. Jabbour, S. A., Whaley, J. M., Tirmenstein, M., Poucher, S. M., Reilly, T. P., Boulton, D. W., Saye, J., List, J. F., Parikh, S. Targeting renal glucose reabsorption for the treatment of type 2 diabetes mellitus using the SGLT2 inhibitor dapagliflozin. *Postgrad. Med.* **2012**, *124*, (4), 62–73.
11. Haggie, P. M., Phuan, P. W., Tan, J. A., Xu, H., Avramescu, R. G., Perdomo, D., Zlock, L. et al. Correctors and potentiators rescue function of the truncated W1282X-cystic fibrosis transmembrane regulator (CFTR) translation product. *J. Biol. Chem.* **2017**, *292*, (3), 771–785.

12. Zhang, Q., Zhang, Y., Diamond, S., Boer, J., Harris, J. J., Li, Y., Rupar, M. et al. The Janus kinase 2 inhibitor fedratinib inhibits thiamine uptake: A putative mechanism for the onset of Wernicke's encephalopathy. *Drug Metab. Dispos.* **2014**, *42*, (10), 1656–1662.

13. Kusuhara, H., Sugiyama, Y. *In vitro-in vivo* extrapolation of transporter-mediated clearance in the liver and kidney. *Drug Metab. Pharmacokinet.* **2009**, *24*, (1), 37–52.

14. Shitara, Y., Horie, T., Sugiyama, Y. Transporters as a determinant of drug clearance and tissue distribution. *Eur. J. Pharm. Sci.* **2006**, *27*, (5), 425–446.

15. Calcagno, A. M., Kim, I. W., Wu, C. P., Shukla, S., Ambudkar, S. V. ABC drug transporters as molecular targets for the prevention of multidrug resistance and drug-drug interactions. *Curr. Drug. Deliv.* **2007**, *4*, (4), 324–333.

16. Estudante, M., Morais, J. G., Soveral, G., Benet, L. Z. Intestinal drug transporters: An overview. *Adv. Drug Deliv. Rev.* **2013**, *65*, (10), 1340–1356.

17. Katsura, T., Inui, K. Intestinal absorption of drugs mediated by drug transporters: Mechanisms and regulation. *Drug Metab. Pharmacokinet.* **2003**, *18*, (1), 1–15.

18. Greiner, B., Eichelbaum, M., Fritz, P., Kreichgauer, H. P., von Richter, O., Zundler, J., Kroemer, H. K. The role of intestinal P-glycoprotein in the interaction of digoxin and rifampin. *J. Clin. Invest.* **1999**, *104*, (2), 147–153.

19. Igel, S., Drescher, S., Murdter, T., Hofmann, U., Heinkele, G., Tegude, H., Glaeser, H. et al. Increased absorption of digoxin from the human jejunum due to inhibition of intestinal transporter-mediated efflux. *Clin. Pharmacokinet.* **2007**, *46*, (9), 777–785.

20. Grover, A., Benet, L. Z. Effects of drug transporters on volume of distribution. *AAPS J.* **2009**, *11*, (2), 250–261.

21. Lau, Y. Y., Huang, Y., Frassetto, L., Benet, L. Z. Effect of OATP1B transporter inhibition on the pharmacokinetics of atorvastatin in healthy volunteers. *Clin. Pharmacol. Ther.* **2007**, *81*, (2), 194–204.

22. Pasanen, M. K., Fredrikson, H., Neuvonen, P. J., Niemi, M. Different effects of SLCO1B1 polymorphism on the pharmacokinetics of atorvastatin and rosuvastatin. *Clin. Pharmacol. Ther.* **2007**, *82*, (6), 726–733.

23. Daneman, R., Prat, A. The blood-brain barrier. *Cold Spring Harb. Perspect. Biol.* **2015**, *7*, (1), a020412.

24. Knauer, M. J., Urquhart, B. L., Meyer zu Schwabedissen, H. E., Schwarz, U. I., Lemke, C. J., Leake, B. F., Kim, R. B., Tirona, R. G. Human skeletal muscle drug transporters determine local exposure and toxicity of statins. *Circ. Res.* **2010**, *106*, (2), 297–306.

25. Knights, K. M., Rowland, A., Miners, J. O. Renal drug metabolism in humans: The potential for drug-endobiotic interactions involving cytochrome P450 (CYP) and UDP-glucuronosyltransferase (UGT). *Br J. Clin. Pharmacol.* **2013**, *76*, (4), 587–602.

26. Lohr, J. W., Willsky, G. R., Acara, M. A. Renal drug metabolism. *Pharmacol Rev* **1998**, *50*, (1), 107–141.

27. Ishikawa, T. The ATP-dependent glutathione S-conjugate export pump. *Trends Biochem. Sci.* **1992**, *17*, (11), 463–48.

28. Morrow, C. S., Smitherman, P. K., Townsend, A. J. Role of multidrug-resistance protein 2 in glutathione S-transferase P1-1-mediated resistance to 4-nitroquinoline 1-oxide toxicities in HepG2 cells. *Mol. Carcinog.* **2000**, *29*, (3), 170–178.

29. Hagenbuch, B., Meier, P. J. Organic anion transporting polypeptides of the OATP/SLC21 family: Phylogenetic classification as OATP/ SLCO superfamily, new nomenclature and molecular/functional properties. *Pflugers Arch.* **2004**, *447*, (5), 653–665.

30. Tamai, I., Ogihara, T., Takanaga, H., Maeda, H., Tsuji, A. Anion antiport mechanism is involved in transport of lactic acid across intestinal epithelial brush-border membrane. *Biochim. Biophys. Acta* **2000**, *1468*, (1–2), 285–292.

31. Konig, J., Cui, Y., Nies, A. T., Keppler, D. A novel human organic anion transporting polypeptide localized to the basolateral hepatocyte membrane. *Am. J. Physiol. Gastrointest. Liver Physiol.* **2000**, *278*, (1), G156–G164.

32. Hsiang, B., Zhu, Y., Wang, Z., Wu, Y., Sasseville, V., Yang, W. P., Kirchgessner, T. G. A novel human hepatic organic anion transporting polypeptide (OATP2). Identification of a liver-specific human organic anion transporting polypeptide and identification of rat and human hydroxymethylglutaryl-CoA reductase inhibitor transporters. *J. Biol. Chem.* **1999**, *274*, (52), 37161–37168.

33. Kopplow, K., Letschert, K., Konig, J., Walter, B., Keppler, D. Human hepatobiliary transport of organic anions analyzed by quadruple-transfected cells. *Mol. Pharmacol.* **2005**, *68*, (4), 1031–1038.

34. Ho, R. H., Tirona, R. G., Leake, B. F., Glaeser, H., Lee, W., Lemke, C. J., Wang, Y., Kim, R. B. Drug and bile acid transporters in rosuvastatin hepatic uptake: Function, expression, and pharmacogenetics. *Gastroenterology* **2006**, *130*, (6), 1793–1806.

35. Nezasa, K., Higaki, K., Takeuchi, M., Nakano, M., Koike, M. Uptake of rosuvastatin by isolated rat hepatocytes: Comparison with pravastatin. *Xenobiotica* **2003**, *33*, (4), 379–388.

36. Hirano, M., Maeda, K., Shitara, Y., Sugiyama, Y. Contribution of OATP2 (OATP1B1) and OATP8 (OATP1B3) to the hepatic uptake of pitavastatin in humans. *J. Pharmacol. Exp. Ther.* **2004**, *311*, (1), 139–146.

37. Poirier, A., Funk, C., Lave, T., Noe, J. New strategies to address drug-drug interactions involving OATPs. *Curr. Opin. Drug Discov. Devel.* **2007**, *10*, (1), 74–83.

38. Smith, N. F., Figg, W. D., Sparreboom, A. Role of the liver-specific transporters OATP1B1 and OATP1B3 in governing drug elimination. *Expert Opin. Drug Metab. Toxicol.* **2005**, *1*, (3), 429–445.

39. Shitara, Y., Hirano, M., Sato, H., Sugiyama, Y. Gemfibrozil and its glucuronide inhibit the organic anion transporting polypeptide 2 (OATP2/OATP1B1:SLC21A6)-mediated hepatic uptake and CYP2C8-mediated metabolism of cerivastatin: Analysis of the mechanism of the clinically relevant drug-drug interaction between cerivastatin and gemfibrozil. *J. Pharmacol. Exp. Ther.* **2004**, *311*, (1), 228–236.

40. Muck, W., Mai, I., Fritsche, L., Ochmann, K., Rohde, G., Unger, S., Johne, A. et al. Increase in cerivastatin systemic exposure after single and multiple dosing in cyclosporine-treated kidney transplant recipients. *Clin. Pharmacol. Ther.* **1999**, *65*, (3), 251–261.

41. Kantola, T., Kivisto, K. T., Neuvonen, P. J. Effect of itraconazole on cerivastatin pharmacokinetics. *Eur. J. Clin. Pharmacol.* **1999**, *54*, (11), 851–855.

42. Mazzu, A. L., Lasseter, K. C., Shamblen, E. C., Agarwal, V., Lettieri, J., Sundaresen, P. Itraconazole alters the pharmacokinetics of atorvastatin to a greater extent than either cerivastatin or pravastatin. *Clin. Pharmacol. Ther.* **2000**, *68*, (4), 391–400.

43. Shitara, Y., Sugiyama, Y. Pharmacokinetic and pharmacodynamic alterations of 3-hydroxy-3-methylglutaryl coenzyme A (HMG-CoA) reductase inhibitors: Drug-drug interactions and interindividual differences in transporter and metabolic enzyme functions. *Pharmacol. Ther.* **2006**, *112*, (1), 71–105.

44. Vuletic, S., Riekse, R. G., Marcovina, S. M., Peskind, E. R., Hazzard, W. R., Albers, J. J. Statins of different brain penetrability differentially affect CSF PLTP activity. *Dement. Geriatr. Cogn. Disord.* **2006**, *22*, (5–6), 392–398.

45. Merino, G., van Herwaarden, A. E., Wagenaar, E., Jonker, J. W., Schinkel, A. H. Sex-dependent expression and activity of the ATP-binding cassette transporter breast cancer resistance protein (BCRP/ABCG2) in liver. *Mol. Pharmacol.* **2005**, *67*, (5), 1765–1771.

46. Paulusma, C. C., van Geer, M. A., Evers, R., Heijn, M., Ottenhoff, R., Borst, P., Oude Elferink, R. P. Canalicular multispecific organic anion transporter/multidrug resistance protein 2 mediates low-affinity transport of reduced glutathione. *Biochem. J.* **1999**, *338 (Pt 2)*, 393–401.

47. Keppler, D., Arias, I. M. Hepatic canalicular membrane. Introduction: Transport across the hepatocyte canalicular membrane. *FASEB J.* **1997**, *11*, (1), 15–18.

48. Ito, K., Suzuki, H., Hirohashi, T., Kume, K., Shimizu, T., Sugiyama, Y. Functional analysis of a canalicular multispecific organic anion transporter cloned from rat liver. *J. Biol. Chem.* **1998**, *273*, (3), 1684–1688.

49. Konig, J., Nies, A. T., Cui, Y., Leier, I., Keppler, D. Conjugate export pumps of the multidrug resistance protein (MRP) family: Localization, substrate specificity, and MRP2-mediated drug resistance. *Biochim. Biophys. Acta* **1999**, *1461*, (2), 377–394.

50. Kusuhara, H., Sugiyama, Y. Role of transporters in the tissue-selective distribution and elimination of drugs: Transporters in the liver, small intestine, brain and kidney. *J. Control. Release* **2002**, *78*, (1–3), 43–54.

51. Morgan, R. E., Trauner, M., van Staden, C. J., Lee, P. H., Ramachandran, B., Eschenberg, M., Afshari, C. A., Qualls, C. W., Jr., Lightfoot-Dunn, R., Hamadeh, H. K. Interference with bile salt export pump function is a susceptibility factor for human liver injury in drug development. *Toxicol. Sci.* **2010**, *118*, (2), 485–500.

52. Funk, C., Pantze, M., Jehle, L., Ponelle, C., Scheuermann, G., Lazendic, M., Gasser, R. Troglitazone-induced intrahepatic cholestasis by an interference with the hepatobiliary export of bile acids in male and female rats. Correlation with the gender difference in troglitazone sulfate formation and the inhibition of the canalicular bile salt export pump (Bsep) by troglitazone and troglitazone sulfate. *Toxicology* **2001**, *167*, (1), 83–98.

53. Funk, C., Ponelle, C., Scheuermann, G., Pantze, M. Cholestatic potential of troglitazone as a possible factor contributing to troglitazone-induced hepatotoxicity: *In vivo* and *in vitro* interaction at the canalicular bile salt export pump (Bsep) in the rat. *Mol. Pharmacol.* **2001**, *59*, (3), 627–635.

54. Lee, W., Kim, R. B. Transporters and renal drug elimination. *Annu. Rev. Pharmacol. Toxicol.* **2004**, *44*, 137–166.

55. Wright, S. H., Dantzler, W. H. Molecular and cellular physiology of renal organic cation and anion transport. *Physiol. Rev.* **2004**, *84*, (3), 987–1049.

56. Izzedine, H., Launay-Vacher, V., Deray, G. Renal tubular transporters and antiviral drugs: An update. *AIDS* **2005**, *19*, (5), 455–462.

57. Sircar, I., Gudmundsson, K. S., Martin, R., Liang, J., Nomura, S., Jayakumar, H., Teegarden, B. R. et al. Synthesis and SAR of N benzoyl-L-biphenylalanine derivatives: Discovery of TR-14035, a dual alpha(4) beta(7)/alpha(4)beta(1) integrin antagonist. *Bioorg. Med. Chem.* **2002**, *10*, (6), 2051–2066.

58. Mischler, T. W., Sugerman, A. A., Willard, D. A., Brannick, L. J., Neiss, E. S. Influence of probenecid and food on the bioavailability of cephradine in normal male subjects. *J. Clin. Pharmacol.* **1974**, *14*, (11-12), 604–611.

59. Dresser, M. J., Xiao, G., Leabman, M. K., Gray, A. T., Giacomini, K. M. Interactions of n-tetraalkylammonium compounds and biguanides with a human renal organic cation transporter (hOCT2). *Pharm. Res.* **2002**, *19*, (8), 1244–1247.

60. Kimura, N., Masuda, S., Tanihara, Y., Ueo, H., Okuda, M., Katsura, T., Inui, K. Metformin is a superior substrate for renal organic cation transporter OCT2 rather than hepatic OCT1. *Drug Metab. Pharmacokinet.* **2005**, *20*, (5), 379–386.

61. Somogyi, A. Renal transport of drugs: Specificity and molecular mechanisms. *Clin. Exp. Pharmacol. Physiol.* **1996**, *23*, (10–11), 986–989.

62. Somogyi, A., Muirhead, M. Pharmacokinetic interactions of cimetidine 1987. *Clin. Pharmacokinet.* **1987**, *12*, (5), 321–366.

63. Ito, K., Houston, J. B. Comparison of the use of liver models for predicting drug clearance using *in vitro* kinetic data from hepatic microsomes and isolated hepatocytes. *Pharm. Res.* **2004**, *21*, (5), 785–792.

64. Sirianni, G. L., Pang, K. S. Organ clearance concepts: New perspectives on old principles. *J. Pharmacokinet. Biopharm.* **1997**, *25*, (4), 449–470.

65. Poirier, A., Cascais, A. C., Funk, C., Lave, T. Prediction of pharmacokinetic profile of valsartan in humans based on *in vitro* uptake-transport data. *Chem. Biodivers.* **2009**, *6*, (11), 1975–1987.

66. Watanabe, T., Maeda, K., Kondo, T., Nakayama, H., Horita, S., Kusuhara, H., Sugiyama, Y. Prediction of the hepatic and renal clearance of transporter substrates in rats using *in vitro* uptake experiments. *Drug Metab. Dispos.* **2009**, *37*, (7), 1471–1479.

67. Jones, H. M., Chan, P. L., van der Graaf, P. H., Webster, R. Use of modelling and simulation techniques to support decision making on the progression of PF-04878691, a TLR7 agonist being developed for hepatitis C. *Br. J. Clin. Pharmacol.* **2012**, *73*, (1), 77–92.

68. Patilea-Vrana, G., Unadkat, J. D. Transport versus metabolism: What determines the pharmacokinetics and pharmacodynamics of drugs? Insights from the extended clearance model. *Clin. Pharmacol. Ther.* **2016**, *100*, (5), 413–418.

69. Jamei, M., Bajot, F., Neuhoff, S., Barter, Z., Yang, J., Rostami-Hodjegan, A., Rowland-Yeo, K. A mechanistic framework for *in vitro-in vivo* extrapolation of liver membrane transporters: Prediction of drug-drug interaction between rosuvastatin and cyclosporine. *Clin. Pharmacokinet.* **2014**, *53*, (1), 73–87.

70. Mathialagan, S., Piotrowski, M. A., Tess, D. A., Feng, B., Litchfield, J., Varma, M. V. Quantitative prediction of human renal clearance and drug-drug interactions of organic anion transporter substrates using *in vitro* transport data: A relative activity factor approach. *Drug Metab. Dispos.* **2017**, *45*, (4), 409–417.

71. Liu, L., Pang, K. S. The roles of transporters and enzymes in hepatic drug processing. *Drug Metab. Dispos.* **2005**, *33*, (1), 1–9.

72. Watanabe, T., Kusuhara, H., Maeda, K., Kanamaru, H., Saito, Y., Hu, Z., Sugiyama, Y. Investigation of the rate-determining process in the hepatic elimination of HMG-CoA reductase inhibitors in rats and humans. *Drug Metab. Dispos.* **2010**, *38*, (2), 215–222.

73. Varma, M. V., Bi, Y. A., Kimoto, E., Lin, J. Quantitative prediction of transporter- and enzyme-mediated clinical drug-drug interactions of organic anion-transporting polypeptide 1B1 substrates using a mechanistic net-effect model. *J. Pharmacol. Exp. Ther.* **2014**, *351*, (1), 214–223.

74. Amidon, G. L., Lennernas, H., Shah, V. P., Crison, J. R. A theoretical basis for a biopharmaceutic drug classification: The correlation of *in vitro* drug product dissolution and *in vivo* bioavailability. *Pharm. Res.* **1995**, *12*, (3), 413–420.

75. Wu, C. Y., Benet, L. Z. Predicting drug disposition via application of BCS: Transport/absorption/ elimination interplay and development of a biopharmaceutics drug disposition classification system. *Pharm. Res.* **2005**, *22*, (1), 11–23.

76. Benet, L. Z. The drug transporter-metabolism alliance: Uncovering and defining the interplay. *Mol. Pharm.* **2009**, *6*, (6), 1631–1643.

77. Benet, L. Z. Predicting drug disposition via application of a biopharmaceutics drug disposition classification system. *Basic Clin. Pharmacol. Toxicol.* **2010**, *106*, (3), 162–167.

78. Benet, L. Z. The role of BCS (biopharmaceutics classification system) and BDDCS (biopharmaceutics drug disposition classification system) in drug development. *J. Pharm. Sci.* **2013**, *102*, (1), 34–42.

79. Varma, M. V., Steyn, S. J., Allerton, C., El-Kattan, A. F. Predicting clearance mechanism in drug discovery: Extended clearance classification system (ECCS). *Pharm. Res.* **2015**, *32*, (12), 3785–3802.

80. El-Kattan, A. F., Varma, M. V., Steyn, S. J., Scott, D. O., Maurer, T. S., Bergman, A. Projecting ADME behavior and drug-drug interactions in early discovery and development: Application of the extended clearance classification system. *Pharm. Res.* **2016**, *33*, (12), 3021–3030.

81. El-Kattan, A. F., Varma, M. V. S. Navigating transporter sciences in pharmacokinetics characterization using the extended clearance classification system. *Drug Metab. Dispos.* **2018**, *46*, (5), 729–739.

82. Strautnieks, S. S., Bull, L. N., Knisely, A. S., Kocoshis, S. A., Dahl, N., Arnell, H., Sokal, E. et al. A gene encoding a liver-specific ABC transporter is mutated in progressive familial intrahepatic cholestasis. *Nat. Genet.* **1998**, *20*, (3), 233–238.

83. Strautnieks, S. S., Byrne, J. A., Pawlikowska, L., Cebecauerova, D., Rayner, A., Dutton, L., Meier, Y. et al. Severe bile salt export pump deficiency: 82 different ABCB11 mutations in 109 families. *Gastroenterology* **2008**, *134*, (4), 1203–12014.

84. van de Steeg, E., Stranecky, V., Hartmannova, H., Noskova, L., Hrebicek, M., Wagenaar, E., van Esch, A. et al. Complete OATP1B1 and OATP1B3 deficiency causes human Rotor syndrome by interrupting conjugated bilirubin reuptake into the liver. *J. Clin. Invest.* **2012**, *122*, (2), 519–528.

85. Juliano, R. L., Ling, V. A surface glycoprotein modulating drug permeability in Chinese hamster ovary cell mutants. *Biochim. Biophys. Acta* **1976**, *455*, (1), 152–162.

86. Mickley, L. A., Lee, J. S., Weng, Z., Zhan, Z., Alvarez, M., Wilson, W., Bates, S. E., Fojo, T. Genetic polymorphism in MDR-1: A tool for examining allelic expression in normal cells, unselected and drug-selected cell lines, and human tumors. *Blood* **1998**, *91*, (5), 1749–1756.

87. Swart, M., Ren, Y., Smith, P., Dandara, C. ABCB1 4036A>G and 1236C>T polymorphisms affect plasma efavirenz levels in South African HIV/AIDS patients. *Front. Genet.* **2012**, *3*, 236.

88. Fung, K. L., Pan, J., Ohnuma, S., Lund, P. E., Pixley, J. N., Kimchi-Sarfaty, C., Ambudkar, S. V., Gottesman, M. M. MDR1 synonymous polymorphisms alter transporter specificity and protein stability in a stable epithelial monolayer. *Cancer Res.* **2014**, *74*, (2), 598–608.

89. Wang, D., Johnson, A. D., Papp, A. C., Kroetz, D. L., Sadee, W. Multidrug resistance polypeptide 1 (MDR1, ABCB1) variant 3435C>T affects mRNA stability. *Pharmacogenet. Genomics* **2005**, *15*, (10), 693–704.

90. Kim, R. B., Leake, B. F., Choo, E. F., Dresser, G. K., Kubba, S. V., Schwarz, U. I., Taylor, A. et al. Identification of functionally variant MDR1 alleles among European Americans and African Americans. *Clin. Pharmacol. Ther.* **2001**, *70*, (2), 189–199.

91. Kroetz, D. L., Pauli-Magnus, C., Hodges, L. M., Huang, C. C., Kawamoto, M., Johns, S. J., Stryke, D. et al. Pharmacogenetics of membrane transporters, I. Sequence diversity and haplotype structure in the human ABCB1 (MDR1, multidrug resistance transporter) gene. *Pharmacogenetics* **2003**, *13*, (8), 481–494.

92. Horinouchi, M., Sakaeda, T., Nakamura, T., Morita, Y., Tamura, T., Aoyama, N., Kasuga, M., Okumura, K. Significant genetic linkage of MDR1 polymorphisms at positions 3435 and 2677: Functional relevance to pharmacokinetics of digoxin. *Pharm. Res.* **2002**, *19*, (10), 1581–1585.

93. Tang, K., Ngoi, S. M., Gwee, P. C., Chua, J. M., Lee, E. J., Chong, S. S., Lee, C. G. Distinct haplotype profiles and strong linkage disequilibrium at the MDR1 multidrug transporter gene locus in three ethnic Asian populations. *Pharmacogenetics* **2002**, *12*, (6), 437–450.

94. Ameyaw, M. M., Regateiro, F., Li, T., Liu, X., Tariq, M., Mobarek, A., Thornton, N. et al. MDR1 pharmacogenetics: Frequency of the C3435T mutation in exon 26 is significantly influenced by ethnicity. *Pharmacogenetics* **2001**, *11*, (3), 217–221.

95. Cascorbi, I., Gerloff, T., Johne, A., Meisel, C., Hoffmeyer, S., Schwab, M., Schaeffeler, E., Eichelbaum, M., Brinkmann, U., Roots, I. Frequency of single nucleotide polymorphisms in the P-glycoprotein drug transporter MDR1 gene in white subjects. *Clin. Pharmacol. Ther.* **2001**, *69*, (3), 169–174.

96. Hoffmeyer, S., Burk, O., von Richter, O., Arnold, H. P., Brockmoller, J., Johne, A., Cascorbi, I. et al. Functional polymorphisms of the human multidrug-resistance gene: Multiple sequence variations and correlation of one allele with P-glycoprotein expression and activity *in vivo. Proc. Natl. Acad. Sci. USA* **2000**, *97*, (7), 3473–3478.

97. Kurata, Y., Ieiri, I., Kimura, M., Morita, T., Irie, S., Urae, A., Ohdo, S. et al. Role of human MDR1 gene polymorphism in bioavailability and interaction of digoxin, a substrate of P-glycoprotein. *Clin. Pharmacol. Ther.* **2002**, *72*, (2), 209–219.

98. Verstuyft, C., Schwab, M., Schaeffeler, E., Kerb, R., Brinkmann, U., Jaillon, P., Funck-Brentano, C., Becquemont, L. Digoxin pharmacokinetics and MDR1 genetic polymorphisms. *Eur. J. Clin. Pharmacol.* **2003**, *58*, (12), 809–812.

99. Gerloff, T., Schaefer, M., Johne, A., Oselin, K., Meisel, C., Cascorbi, I., Roots, I. MDR1 genotypes do not influence the absorption of a single oral dose of 1 mg digoxin in healthy white males. *Br. J. Clin. Pharmacol.* **2002**, *54*, (6), 610–616.

100. Sakaeda, T., Nakamura, T., Horinouchi, M., Kakumoto, M., Ohmoto, N., Sakai, T., Morita, Y. et al. MDR1 genotype-related pharmacokinetics of digoxin after single oral administration in healthy Japanese subjects. *Pharm. Res.* **2001**, *18*, (10), 1400–1404.

101. Drescher, S., Schaeffeler, E., Hitzl, M., Hofmann, U., Schwab, M., Brinkmann, U., Eichelbaum, M., Fromm, M. F. MDR1 gene polymorphisms and disposition of the P-glycoprotein substrate fexofenadine. *Br. J. Clin. Pharmacol.* **2002**, *53*, (5), 526–534.

102. Haufroid, V., Mourad, M., Van Kerckhove, V., Wawrzyniak, J., De Meyer, M., Eddour, D. C., Malaise, J., Lison, D., Squifflet, J. P., Wallemacq, P. The effect of CYP3A5 and MDR1 (ABCB1) polymorphisms on cyclosporine and tacrolimus dose requirements and trough blood levels in stable renal transplant patients. *Pharmacogenetics* **2004**, *14*, (3), 147–154.

103. Macphee, I. A., Fredericks, S., Tai, T., Syrris, P., Carter, N. D., Johnston, A., Goldberg, L., Holt, D. W. Tacrolimus pharmacogenetics: polymorphisms associated with expression of cytochrome p4503A5 and P-glycoprotein correlate with dose requirement. *Transplantation* **2002**, *74*, (11), 1486–1489.

104. von Ahsen, N., Richter, M., Grupp, C., Ringe, B., Oellerich, M., Armstrong, V. W. No influence of the MDR-1 C3435T polymorphism or a CYP3A4 promoter polymorphism (CYP3A4-V allele) on dose-adjusted cyclosporin A trough concentrations or rejection incidence in stable renal transplant recipients. *Clin. Chem.* **2001**, *47*, (6), 1048–1052.

105. Yates, C. R., Zhang, W., Song, P., Li, S., Gaber, A. O., Kotb, M., Honaker, M. R., Alloway, R. R., Meibohm, B. The effect of CYP3A5 and MDR1 polymorphic expression on cyclosporine oral disposition in renal transplant patients. *J. Clin. Pharmacol.* **2003**, *43*, (6), 555–564.

106. Brunner, M., Langer, O., Sunder-Plassmann, R., Dobrozemsky, G., Muller, U., Wadsak, W., Krcal, A. et al. Influence of functional haplotypes in the drug transporter gene ABCB1 on central nervous system drug distribution in humans. *Clin. Pharmacol. Ther.* **2005**, *78*, (2), 182–190.

107. de Jong, F. A., Marsh, S., Mathijssen, R. H., King, C., Verweij, J., Sparreboom, A., McLeod, H. L. ABCG2 pharmacogenetics: Ethnic differences in allele frequency and assessment of influence on irinotecan disposition. *Clin. Cancer. Res.* **2004**, *10*, (17), 5889–5894.

108. Kobayashi, D., Ieiri, I., Hirota, T., Takane, H., Maegawa, S., Kigawa, J., Suzuki, H. et al. Functional assessment of ABCG2 (BCRP) gene polymorphisms to protein expression in human placenta. *Drug Metab. Dispos.* **2005**, *33*, (1), 94–101.

109. Kondo, C., Suzuki, H., Itoda, M., Ozawa, S., Sawada, J., Kobayashi, D., Ieiri, I., Mine, K., Ohtsubo, K., Sugiyama, Y. Functional analysis of SNPs variants of BCRP/ABCG2. *Pharm. Res.* **2004**, *21*, (10), 1895–1903.

110. Matsuo, H., Takada, T., Ichida, K., Nakamura, T., Nakayama, A., Ikebuchi, Y., Ito, K. et al. Common defects of ABCG2, a high-capacity urate exporter, cause gout: A function-based genetic analysis in a Japanese population. *Sci. Transl. Med.* **2009**, *1*, (5), 5ra11.

111. Sparreboom, A., Gelderblom, H., Marsh, S., Ahluwalia, R., Obach, R., Principe, P., Twelves, C., Verweij, J., McLeod, H. L. Diflomotecan pharmacokinetics in relation to ABCG2 421C>A genotype. *Clin. Pharmacol. Ther.* **2004**, *76*, (1), 38–44.

112. Sparreboom, A., Loos, W. J., Burger, H., Sissung, T. M., Verweij, J., Figg, W. D., Nooter, K., Gelderblom, H. Effect of ABCG2 genotype on the oral bioavailability of topotecan. *Cancer Biol. Ther.* **2005**, *4*, (6), 650–658.

113. Kajihara, S., Hisatomi, A., Mizuta, T., Hara, T., Ozaki, I., Wada, I., Yamamoto, K. A splice mutation in the human canalicular multispecific organic anion transporter gene causes Dubin-Johnson syndrome. *Biochem. Biophys. Res. Commun.* **1998**, *253*, (2), 454–457.

114. Keitel, V., Kartenbeck, J., Nies, A. T., Spring, H., Brom, M., Keppler, D. Impaired protein maturation of the conjugate export pump multidrug resistance protein 2 as a consequence of a deletion mutation in Dubin-Johnson syndrome. *Hepatology* **2000**, *32*, (6), 1317–1328.

115. Tsujii, H., Konig, J., Rost, D., Stockel, B., Leuschner, U., Keppler, D. Exon-intron organization of the human multidrug-resistance protein 2 (MRP2) gene mutated in Dubin-Johnson syndrome. *Gastroenterology* **1999**, *117*, (3), 653–660.

116. Nakanishi, T., Tamai, I. Genetic polymorphisms of OATP transporters and their impact on intestinal absorption and hepatic disposition of drugs. *Drug Metab. Pharmacokinet.* **2012**, *27*, (1), 106–121.

117. Niemi, M., Pasanen, M. K., Neuvonen, P. J. Organic anion transporting polypeptide 1B1: A genetically polymorphic transporter of major importance for hepatic drug uptake. *Pharmacol. Rev.* **2011**, *63*, (1), 157–181.

118. Niemi, M., Schaeffeler, E., Lang, T., Fromm, M. F., Neuvonen, M., Kyrklund, C., Backman, J. T. et al. High plasma pravastatin concentrations are associated with single nucleotide polymorphisms and haplotypes of organic anion transporting polypeptide-C (OATP-C, SLCO1B1). *Pharmacogenetics* **2004**, *14*, (7), 429–440.

119. Pasanen, M. K., Neuvonen, P. J., Niemi, M. Global analysis of genetic variation in SLCO1B1. *Pharmacogenomics* **2008**, *9*, (1), 19–33.

120. Katz, D. A., Carr, R., Grimm, D. R., Xiong, H., Holley-Shanks, R., Mueller, T., Leake, B. et al. . Organic anion transporting polypeptide 1B1 activity classified by SLCO1B1 genotype influences atrasentan pharmacokinetics. *Clin. Pharmacol. Ther.* **2006**, *79*, (3), 186–196.

121. Tirona, R. G., Leake, B. F., Merino, G., Kim, R. B. Polymorphisms in OATP-C: Identification of multiple allelic variants associated with altered transport activity among European- and African-Americans. *J. Biol. Chem.* **2001**, *276*, (38), 35669–35675.

122. Niemi, M., Pasanen, M. K., Neuvonen, P. J. SLCO1B1 polymorphism and sex affect the pharmacokinetics of pravastatin but not fluvastatin. *Clin. Pharmacol. Ther.* **2006**, *80*, (4), 356–366.

123. Laitinen, A., Niemi, M. Frequencies of single-nucleotide polymorphisms of SLCO1A2, SLCO1B3 and SLCO2B1 genes in a Finnish population. *Basic Clin. Pharmacol. Toxicol.* **2011**, *108*, (1), 9–13.

124. Letschert, K., Keppler, D., Konig, J. Mutations in the SLCO1B3 gene affecting the substrate specificity of the hepatocellular uptake transporter OATP1B3 (OATP8). *Pharmacogenetics* **2004**, *14*, (7), 441–452.

125. Schwarz, U. I., Meyer zu Schwabedissen, H. E., Tirona, R. G., Suzuki, A., Leake, B. F., Mokrab, Y., Mizuguchi, K., Ho, R. H., Kim, R. B. Identification of novel functional organic anion-transporting polypeptide 1B3 polymorphisms and assessment of substrate specificity. *Pharmacogenet. Genomics* **2011**, *21*, (3), 103–114.

126. Baker, S. D., Verweij, J., Cusatis, G. A., van Schaik, R. H., Marsh, S., Orwick, S. J., Franke, R. M. et al. Pharmacogenetic pathway analysis of docetaxel elimination. *Clin. Pharmacol. Ther.* **2009**, *85*, (2), 155–163.

127. Chew, S. C., Singh, O., Chen, X., Ramasamy, R. D., Kulkarni, T., Lee, E. J., Tan, E. H., Lim, W. T., Chowbay, B. The effects of CYP3A4, CYP3A5, ABCB1, ABCC2, ABCG2 and SLCO1B3 single nucleotide polymorphisms on the pharmacokinetics and pharmacodynamics of docetaxel in nasopharyngeal carcinoma patients. *Cancer Chemother. Pharmacol.* **2011**, *67*, (6), 1471–1478.

128. Smith, N. F., Marsh, S., Scott-Horton, T. J., Hamada, A., Mielke, S., Mross, K., Figg, W. D., Verweij, J., McLeod, H. L., Sparreboom, A. Variants in the SLCO1B3 gene: Interethnic distribution and association with paclitaxel pharmacokinetics. *Clin. Pharmacol. Ther.* **2007**, *81*, (1), 76–82.

129. Ieiri, I., Nishimura, C., Maeda, K., Sasaki, T., Kimura, M., Chiyoda, T., Hirota, T. et al. Pharmacokinetic and pharmacogenomic profiles of telmisartan after the oral microdose and therapeutic dose. *Pharmacogenet. Genomics* **2011**, *21*, (8), 495–505.

130. Yamada, A., Maeda, K., Ishiguro, N., Tsuda, Y., Igarashi, T., Ebner, T., Roth, W., Ikushiro, S., Sugiyama, Y. The impact of pharmacogenetics of metabolic enzymes and transporters on the pharmacokinetics of telmisartan in healthy volunteers. *Pharmacogenet. Genomics* **2011**, *21*, (9), 523–530.

131. Leabman, M. K., Huang, C. C., Kawamoto, M., Johns, S. J., Stryke, D., Ferrin, T. E., DeYoung, J. et al. Pharmacogenetics of membrane transporters, I. polymorphisms in a human kidney xenobiotic transporter, OCT2, exhibit altered function. *Pharmacogenetics* **2002**, *12*, (5), 395–405.

132. Yonezawa, A., Inui, K. Importance of the multidrug and toxin extrusion MATE/SLC47A family to pharmacokinetics, pharmacodynamics/toxicodynamics and pharmacogenomics. *Br. J. Pharmacol.* **2011**, *164*, (7), 1817–1825.

133. Wang, Z. J., Yin, O. Q., Tomlinson, B., Chow, M. S. OCT2 polymorphisms and *in-vivo* renal functional consequence: Studies with metformin and cimetidine. *Pharmacogenet. Genomics* **2008**, *18*, (7), 637–645.

134. Toyama, K., Yonezawa, A., Tsuda, M., Masuda, S., Yano, I., Terada, T., Osawa, R. et al. Heterozygous variants of multidrug and toxin extrusions (MATE1 and MATE2-K) have little influence on the disposition of metformin in diabetic patients. *Pharmacogenet. Genomics* **2010**, *20*, (2), 135–138.

135. Fujita, T., Brown, C., Carlson, E. J., Taylor, T., de la Cruz, M., Johns, S. J., Stryke, D. et al. Functional analysis of polymorphisms in the organic anion transporter, SLC22A6 (OAT1). *Pharmacogenet. Genomics* **2005**, *15*, (4), 201–209.

136. Nishizato, Y., Ieiri, I., Suzuki, H., Kimura, M., Kawabata, K., Hirota, T., Takane, H. et al. Polymorphisms of OATP-C (SLC21A6) and OAT3 (SLC22A8) genes: Consequences for pravastatin pharmacokinetics. *Clin. Pharmacol. Ther.* **2003**, *73*, (6), 554–565.

137. Muller, F., Fromm, M. F. Transporter-mediated drug-drug interactions. *Pharmacogenomics* **2011**, *12*, (7), 1017–1037.

138. Ueda, K., Cornwell, M. M., Gottesman, M. M., Pastan, I., Roninson, I. B., Ling, V., Riordan, J. R. The mdr1 gene, responsible for multidrug-resistance, codes for P-glycoprotein. *Biochem. Biophys. Res. Commun.* **1986**, *141*, (3), 956–962.

139. Lockhart, A. C., Tirona, R. G., Kim, R. B. Pharmacogenetics of ATP-binding cassette transporters in cancer and chemotherapy. *Mol. Cancer Ther.* **2003**, *2*, (7), 685–698.

140. Lum, B. L., Gosland, M. P., Kaubisch, S., Sikic, B. I. Molecular targets in oncology: Implications of the multidrug resistance gene. *Pharmacotherapy* **1993**, *13*, (2), 88–109.

141. Cascorbi, I. P-glycoprotein: Tissue distribution, substrates, and functional consequences of genetic variations. *Handb. Exp. Pharmacol.* **2011**, *201*, 261–283.

142. Giacomini, K. M., Huang, S. M., Tweedie, D. J., Benet, L. Z., Brouwer, K. L., Chu, X., Dahlin, A. et al. Membrane transporters in drug development. *Nat. Rev. Drug Discov.* **2010**, *9*, (3), 215–236.

143. Fenner, K. S., Troutman, M. D., Kempshall, S., Cook, J. A., Ware, J. A., Smith, D. A., Lee, C. A. Drug-drug interactions mediated through P-glycoprotein: Clinical relevance and *in vitro-in vivo* correlation using digoxin as a probe drug. *Clin. Pharmacol. Ther.* **2009**, *85*, (2), 173–181.

144. Hager, W. D., Fenster, P., Mayersohn, M., Perrier, D., Graves, P., Marcus, F. I., Goldman, S. Digoxin-quinidine interaction Pharmacokinetic evaluation. *N. Engl. J. Med.* **1979**, *300*, (22), 1238–1241.

145. Ke, A. B., Eyal, S., Chung, F. S., Link, J. M., Mankoff, D. A., Muzi, M., Unadkat, J. D. Modeling cyclosporine A inhibition of the distribution of a P-glycoprotein PET ligand, 11C-verapamil, into the maternal brain and fetal liver of the pregnant nonhuman primate: impact of tissue blood flow and site of inhibition. *J. Nucl. Med.* **2013**, *54*, (3), 437–446.

146. Hsiao, P., Sasongko, L., Link, J. M., Mankoff, D. A., Muzi, M., Collier, A. C., Unadkat, J. D. Verapamil P-glycoprotein transport across the rat blood-brain barrier: Cyclosporine, a concentration inhibition analysis, and comparison with human data. *J. Pharmacol. Exp. Ther.* **2006**, *317*, (2), 704–710.

147. Sadeque, A. J., Wandel, C., He, H., Shah, S., Wood, A. J. Increased drug delivery to the brain by P-glycoprotein inhibition. *Clin. Pharmacol. Ther.* **2000**, *68*, (3), 231–237.

148. Poguntke, M., Hazai, E., Fromm, M. F., Zolk, O. Drug transport by breast cancer resistance protein. *Expert Opin. Drug Metab. Toxicol.* **2010**, *6*, (11), 1363–1384.

149. Meyer zu Schwabedissen, H. E., Kroemer, H. K. *In vitro* and *in vivo* evidence for the importance of breast cancer resistance protein transporters (BCRP/MXR/ABCP/ABCG2). *Handb. Exp. Pharmacol.* **2011**, *201*, (201), 325–371.

150. Zhang, Y., Zhou, G., Wang, H., Zhang, X., Wei, F., Cai, Y., Yin, D. Transcriptional upregulation of breast cancer resistance protein by 17beta-estradiol in ERalpha-positive MCF-7 breast cancer cells. *Oncology* **2006**, *71*, (5-6), 446–455.

151. Keskitalo, J. E., Zolk, O., Fromm, M. F., Kurkinen, K. J., Neuvonen, P. J., Niemi, M. ABCG2 polymorphism markedly affects the pharmacokinetics of atorvastatin and rosuvastatin. *Clin. Pharmacol. Ther.* **2009**, *86*, (2), 197–203.

152. Neuvonen, P. J. Drug interactions with HMG-CoA reductase inhibitors (statins): The importance of CYP enzymes, transporters and pharmacogenetics. *Curr. Opin. Investig. Drugs.* **2010**, *11*, (3), 323–332.

153. Christians, U., Jacobsen, W., Floren, L. C. Metabolism and drug interactions of 3-hydroxy-3-methylglutaryl coenzyme A reductase inhibitors in transplant patients: Are the statins mechanistically similar? *Pharmacol. Ther.* **1998**, *80*, (1), 1–34.

154. Treiber, A., Schneiter, R., Hausler, S., Stieger, B. Bosentan is a substrate of human OATP1B1 and OATP1B3: Inhibition of hepatic uptake as the common mechanism of its interactions with cyclosporin A, rifampicin, and sildenafil. *Drug Metab. Dispos.* **2007**, *35*, (8), 1400–1407.

155. Neuvonen, P. J., Backman, J. T., Niemi, M. Pharmacokinetic comparison of the potential over-the-counter statins simvastatin, lovastatin, fluvastatin and pravastatin. *Clin. Pharmacokinet.* **2008**, *47*, (7), 463–474.

156. Elsby, R., Hilgendorf, C., Fenner, K. Understanding the critical disposition pathways of statins to assess drug-drug interaction risk during drug development: it's not just about OATP1B1. *Clin. Pharmacol. Ther.* **2012**, *92*, (5), 584–598.

157. Shitara, Y., Hirano, M., Adachi, Y., Itoh, T., Sato, H., Sugiyama, Y. *In vitro* and *in vivo* correlation of the inhibitory effect of cyclosporin A on the transporter-mediated hepatic uptake of cerivastatin in rats. *Drug Metab. Dispos.* **2004**, *32*, (12), 1468–1475.

158. Lemahieu, W. P., Hermann, M., Asberg, A., Verbeke, K., Holdaas, H., Vanrenterghem, Y., Maes, B. D. Combined therapy with atorvastatin and calcineurin inhibitors: no interactions with tacrolimus. *Am. J. Transplant.* **2005**, *5*, (9), 2236–2243.

159. Kajosaari, L. I., Niemi, M., Neuvonen, M., Laitila, J., Neuvonen, P. J., Backman, J. T. Cyclosporine markedly raises the plasma concentrations of repaglinide. *Clin. Pharmacol. Ther.* **2005**, *78*, (4), 388–399.

160. Hirano, M., Maeda, K., Shitara, Y., Sugiyama, Y. Drug-drug interaction between pitavastatin and various drugs via OATP1B1. *Drug Metab. Dispos.* **2006**, *34*, (7), 1229–1236.

161. Gan, J., Chen, W., Shen, H., Gao, L., Hong, Y., Tian, Y., Li, W. et al. Repaglinide-gemfibrozil drug interaction: Inhibition of repaglinide glucuronidation as a potential additional contributing mechanism. *Br. J. Clin. Pharmacol.* **2010**, *70*, (6), 870–880.

162. Varma, M. V., El-Kattan, A. F. Transporter-enzyme interplay: Deconvoluting effects of hepatic transporters and enzymes on drug disposition using static and dynamic mechanistic models. *J. Clin. Pharmacol.* **2016**, *56*, (Suppl 7), S99–S109.

163. Kalliokoski, A., Backman, J. T., Kurkinen, K. J., Neuvonen, P. J., Niemi, M. Effects of gemfibrozil and atorvastatin on the pharmacokinetics of repaglinide in relation to SLCO1B1 polymorphism. *Clin. Pharmacol. Ther.* **2008**, *84*, (4), 488–496.

164. Lepist, E. I., Ray, A. S. Renal drug-drug interactions: What we have learned and where we are going. *Expert Opin. Drug Metab. Toxicol.* **2012**, *8*, (4), 433–448.

165. Burckhardt, G., Burckhardt, B. C. *In vitro* and *in vivo* evidence of the importance of organic anion transporters (OATs) in drug therapy. *Handb. Exp. Pharmacol.* **2011**, *201*, (201), 29–104.

166. VanWert, A. L., Gionfriddo, M. R., Sweet, D. H. Organic anion transporters: Discovery, pharmacology, regulation and roles in pathophysiology. *Biopharm. Drug Dispos.* **2010**, *31*, (1), 1–71.

167. Cihlar, T., Ho, E. S., Lin, D. C., Mulato, A. S. Human renal organic anion transporter 1 (hOAT1) and its role in the nephrotoxicity of antiviral nucleotide analogs. *Nucleos. Nucleot. Nucl. Acids.* **2001**, *20*, (4–7), 641–648.

168. Cihlar, T., Ho, E. S. Fluorescence-based assay for the interaction of small molecules with the human renal organic anion transporter 1. *Anal. Biochem.* **2000**, *283*, (1), 49–55.

169. Hasannejad, H., Takeda, M., Taki, K., Shin, H. J., Babu, E., Jutabha, P., Khamdang, S. et al. Interactions of human organic anion transporters with diuretics. *J. Pharmacol. Exp. Ther.* **2004**, *308*, (3), 1021–1029.

170. Robbins, N., Koch, S. E., Tranter, M., Rubinstein, J. The history and future of probenecid. *Cardiovasc. Toxicol.* **2012**, *12*, (1), 1–9.

171. Nozaki, Y., Kusuhara, H., Kondo, T., Hasegawa, M., Shiroyanagi, Y., Nakazawa, H., Okano, T., Sugiyama, Y. Characterization of the uptake of organic anion transporter (OAT) 1 and OAT3 substrates by human kidney slices. *J. Pharmacol. Exp. Ther.* **2007**, *321*, (1), 362–369.

172. Vree, T. B., van den Biggelaar-Martea, M., Verwey-van Wissen, C. P. Probenecid inhibits the renal clearance of frusemide and its acyl glucuronide. *Br. J. Clin. Pharmacol.* **1995**, *39*, (6), 692–695.

173. Lilly, M. B., Omura, G. A. Clinical pharmacology of oral intermediate-dose methotrexate with or without probenecid. *Cancer Chemother. Pharmacol.* **1985**, *15*, (3), 220–222.

174. Yonezawa, A., Inui, K. Organic cation transporter OCT/SLC22A and H(+)/organic cation antiporter MATE/SLC47A are key molecules for nephrotoxicity of platinum agents. *Biochem. Pharmacol.* **2011**, *81*, (5), 563–568.

175. Damme, K., Nies, A. T., Schaeffeler, E., Schwab, M. Mammalian MATE (SLC47A) transport proteins: Impact on efflux of endogenous substrates and xenobiotics. *Drug Metab. Rev.* **2011**, *43*, (4), 499–523.

176. Nies, A. T., Koepsell, H., Damme, K., Schwab, M. Organic cation transporters (OCTs, MATEs), *in vitro* and *in vivo* evidence for the importance in drug therapy. *Handb. Exp. Pharmacol.* **2011**, (201), 105–167.

177. Somogyi, A., Heinzow, B. Cimetidine reduces procainamide elimination. *N. Engl. J. Med.* **1982**, *307*, (17), 1080.

178. Somogyi, A., Stockley, C., Keal, J., Rolan, P., Bochner, F. Reduction of metformin renal tubular secretion by cimetidine in man. *Br. J. Clin. Pharmacol.* **1987**, *23*, (5), 545–551.

179. Kusuhara, H., Ito, S., Kumagai, Y., Jiang, M., Shiroshita, T., Moriyama, Y., Inoue, K., Yuasa, H., Sugiyama, Y. Effects of a MATE protein inhibitor, pyrimethamine, on the renal elimination of metformin at oral microdose and at therapeutic dose in healthy subjects. *Clin. Pharmacol. Ther.* **2011**, *89*, (6), 837–844.

180. Ito, S., Kusuhara, H., Kumagai, Y., Moriyama, Y., Inoue, K., Kondo, T., Nakayama, H. et al. *N*-Methylnicotinamide is an endogenous probe for evaluation of drug-drug interactions involving multidrug and toxin extrusions (MATE1 and MATE2-K). *Clin. Pharmacol. Ther.* **2012**, *92*, (5), 635–641.

181. Muller, F., Sharma, A., Konig, J., Fromm, M. F. Biomarkers for *in vivo* assessment of transporter function. *Pharmacol. Rev.* **2018**, *70*, (2), 246–277.

182. Franke, R. M., Sparreboom, A. Drug transporters: Recent advances and therapeutic applications. *Clin. Pharmacol. Ther.* **2010**, *87*, (1), 3–7.

183. Ciarimboli, G., Deuster, D., Knief, A., Sperling, M., Holtkamp, M., Edemir, B., Pavenstadt, H. et al. Organic cation transporter 2 mediates cisplatin-induced oto- and nephrotoxicity and is a target for protective interventions. *Am. J. Pathol.* **2010**, *176*, (3), 1169–1180.

184. Lai, Y., Hsiao, P. Beyond the ITC White paper: Emerging sciences in drug transporters and opportunities for drug development. *Curr. Pharm. Des.* **2014**, *20*, (10), 1577–1594.

185. Lee, W. K., Wolff, N. A., Thevenod, F. Organic cation transporters: Physiology, toxicology and special focus on ethidium as a novel substrate. *Curr. Drug Metab.* **2009**, *10*, (6), 617–631.

186. Hagos, Y., Wolff, N. A. Assessment of the role of renal organic anion transporters in drug-induced nephrotoxicity. *Toxins (Basel)* **2010**, *2*, (8), 2055–2082.

187. Ciarimboli, G. Membrane transporters as mediators of cisplatin side-effects. *Anticancer Res.* **2014**, *34*, (1), 547–550.

188. Cundy, K. C., Petty, B. G., Flaherty, J., Fisher, P. E., Polis, M. A., Wachsman, M., Lietman, P. S., Lalezari, J. P., Hitchcock, M. J., Jaffe, H. S. Clinical pharmacokinetics of cidofovir in human immunodeficiency virus-infected patients. *Antimicrob. Agents Chemother.* **1995**, *39*, (6), 1247–1252.

189. Yonezawa, A., Masuda, S., Yokoo, S., Katsura, T., Inui, K. Cisplatin and oxaliplatin, but not carboplatin and nedaplatin, are substrates for human organic cation transporters (SLC22A1-3 and multidrug and toxin extrusion family). *J. Pharmacol. Exp. Ther.* **2006**, *319*, (2), 879–886.

190. Filipski, K. K., Loos, W. J., Verweij, J., Sparreboom, A. Interaction of Cisplatin with the human organic cation transporter 2. *Clin. Cancer Res.* **2008**, *14*, (12), 3875–3880.

191. Li, Q., Guo, D., Dong, Z., Zhang, W., Zhang, L., Huang, S. M., Polli, J. E., Shu, Y. Ondansetron can enhance cisplatin-induced nephrotoxicity via inhibition of multiple toxin and extrusion proteins (MATEs). *Toxicol. Appl. Pharmacol.* **2013**, *273*, (1), 100–109.

192. Shen, H., Yang, Z., Zhao, W., Zhang, Y., Rodrigues, A. D. Assessment of vandetanib as an inhibitor of various human renal transporters: inhibition of multidrug and toxin extrusion as a possible mechanism leading to decreased cisplatin and creatinine clearance. *Drug Metab. Dispos.* **2013**, *41*, (12), 2095–2103.

193. Chiang, J. Y. Regulation of bile acid synthesis: Pathways, nuclear receptors, and mechanisms. *J. Hepatol.* **2004**, *40*, (3), 539–551.

194. Pai, R., French, D., Ma, N., Hotzel, K., Plise, E., Salphati, L., Setchell, K. D. et al. Antibody-mediated inhibition of fibroblast growth factor 19 results in increased bile acids synthesis and ileal malabsorption of bile acids in cynomolgus monkeys. *Toxicol. Sci.* **2012**, *126*, (2), 446–456.
195. Dawson, P. A., Lan, T., Rao, A. Bile acid transporters. *J. Lipid Res.* **2009**, *50*, (12), 2340–2357.
196. Hagenbuch, B., Dawson, P. The sodium bile salt cotransport family SLC10. *Pflugers Arch.* **2004**, *447*, (5), 566–570.
197. Stieger, B. The role of the sodium-taurocholate cotransporting polypeptide (NTCP) and of the bile salt export pump (BSEP) in physiology and pathophysiology of bile formation. *Handb. Exp. Pharmacol.* **2011**, *201*, 205–259.
198. Stieger, B., Meier, Y., Meier, P. J, The bile salt export pump. *Pflugers Arch.* **2007**, *453*, (5), 611–620.
199. Stieger, B., Fattinger, K., Madon, J., Kullak-Ublick, G. A., Meier, P. J. Drug- and estrogen-induced cholestasis through inhibition of the hepatocellular bile salt export pump (Bsep) of rat liver. *Gastroenterology* **2000**, *118*, (2), 422–430.
200. Bolder, U., Trang, N. V., Hagey, L. R., Schteingart, C. D., Ton-Nu, H. T., Cerre, C., Elferink, R. P., Hofmann, A. F. Sulindac is excreted into bile by a canalicular bile salt pump and undergoes a cholehepatic circulation in rats. *Gastroenterology* **1999**, *117*, (4), 962–971.
201. Sakurai, A., Kurata, A., Onishi, Y., Hirano, H., Ishikawa, T. Prediction of drug-induced intrahepatic cholestasis: *In vitro* screening and QSAR analysis of drugs inhibiting the human bile salt export pump. *Expert Opin. Drug Saf.* **2007**, *6*, (1), 71–86.
202. Gandhi, A., Moorthy, B., Ghose, R. Drug disposition in pathophysiological conditions. *Curr. Drug Metab.* **2012**, *13*, (9), 1327–1344.
203. Makishima, M., Okamoto, A. Y., Repa, J. J., Tu, H., Learned, R. M., Luk, A., Hull, M. V., Lustig, K. D., Mangelsdorf, D. J., Shan, B. Identification of a nuclear receptor for bile acids. *Science* **1999**, *284*, (5418), 1362–1365.
204. Parks, D. J., Blanchard, S. G., Bledsoe, R. K., Chandra, G., Consler, T. G., Kliewer, S. A., Stimmel, J. B. et al. Bile acids: Natural ligands for an orphan nuclear receptor. *Science* **1999**, *284*, (5418), 1365–1368.
205. Wang, H., Chen, J., Hollister, K., Sowers, L. C., Forman, B. M. Endogenous bile acids are ligands for the nuclear receptor FXR/BAR. *Mol. Cell* **1999**, *3*, (5), 543–553.
206. Barnes, S. N., Aleksunes, L. M., Augustine, L., Scheffer, G. L., Goedken, M. J., Jakowski, A. B., Pruimboom-Brees, I. M., Cherrington, N. J., Manautou, J. E. Induction of hepatobiliary efflux transporters in acetaminophen-induced acute liver failure cases. *Drug Metab. Dispos.* **2007**, *35*, (10), 1963–1969.
207. Clarke, J. D., Hardwick, R. N., Lake, A. D., Canet, M. J., Cherrington, N. J. Experimental nonalcoholic steatohepatitis increases exposure to simvastatin hydroxy Acid by decreasing hepatic organic anion transporting polypeptide expression. *J. Pharmacol. Exp. Ther.* **2014**, *348*, (3), 452–458.
208. Karlgren, M., Simoff, I., Backlund, M., Wegler, C., Keiser, M., Handin, N., Muller, J. et al. A CRISPR-Cas9 generated MDCK cell line expressing human MDR1 without endogenous canine MDR1 (cABCB1): An improved tool for drug efflux studies. *J. Pharm. Sci.* **2017**, *106*, (9), 2909–2913.
209. Bhatia, S. N., Ingber, D. E. Microfluidic organs-on-chips. *Nat. Biotechnol.* **2014**, *32*, (8), 760–772.
210. Schinkel, A. H., Wagenaar, E., van Deemter, L., Mol, C. A., Borst, P. Absence of the mdr1a P-Glycoprotein in mice affects tissue distribution and pharmacokinetics of dexamethasone, digoxin, and cyclosporin A. *J. Clin. Invest.* **1995**, *96*, (4), 1698–1705.
211. Kawahara, M., Sakata, A., Miyashita, T., Tamai, I., Tsuji, A. Physiologically based pharmacokinetics of digoxin in mdr1a knockout mice. *J. Pharm. Sci.* **1999**, *88*, (12), 1281–1287.
212. Shen, H., Dai, J., Liu, T., Cheng, Y., Chen, W., Freeden, C., Zhang, Y., Humphreys, W. G., Marathe, P., Lai, Y. Coproporphyrins I and III as functional markers of OATP1B activity: *In vitro* and *in vivo* evaluation in preclinical species. *J. Pharmacol. Exp. Ther.* **2016**, *357*, (2), 382–393.
213. Iusuf, D., van Esch, A., Hobbs, M., Taylor, M., Kenworthy, K. E., van de Steeg, E., Wagenaar, E., Schinkel, A. H. Murine Oatp1a/1b uptake transporters control rosuvastatin systemic exposure without affecting its apparent liver exposure. *Mol. Pharmacol.* **2013**, *83*, (5), 919–929.
214. Wang, R., Salem, M., Yousef, I. M., Tuchweber, B., Lam, P., Childs, S. J., Helgason, C. D., Ackerley, C., Phillips, M. J., Ling, V. Targeted inactivation of sister of P-glycoprotein gene (spgp) in mice results in nonprogressive but persistent intrahepatic cholestasis. *Proc. Natl. Acad. Sci. U. S. A.* **2001**, *98*, (4), 2011–2016.

215. Cheng, Y., Freeden, C., Zhang, Y., Abraham, P., Shen, H., Wescott, D., Humphreys, W. G., Gan, J., Lai, Y. Biliary excretion of pravastatin and taurocholate in rats with bile salt export pump (Bsep) impairment. *Biopharm. Drug Dispos.* **2016**, *37*, (5), 276–286.
216. Bakos, E., Evers, R., Sinko, E., Varadi, A., Borst, P., Sarkadi, B. Interactions of the human multidrug resistance proteins MRP1 and MRP2 with organic anions. *Mol. Pharmacol.* **2000**, *57*, (4), 760–768.
217. Loe, D. W., Deeley, R. G., Cole, S. P. Characterization of vincristine transport by the M(r) 190,000 multidrug resistance protein (MRP): Evidence for cotransport with reduced glutathione. *Cancer Res.* **1998**, *58*, (22), 5130–5136.
218. Rius, M., Nies, A. T., Hummel-Eisenbeiss, J., Jedlitschky, G., Keppler, D. Cotransport of reduced glutathione with bile salts by MRP4 (ABCC4) localized to the basolateral hepatocyte membrane. *Hepatology* **2003**, *38*, (2), 374–384.

19

Experimental Characterization of Cytochrome P450 Mechanism-Based Inhibition

Dan Rock, Michael Schrag, and Larry C. Wienkers

CONTENTS

Introduction

Oxidative metabolism mediated by the superfamily of heme enzymes known as the cytochromes P450 represents an important elimination pathway for the majority of drugs prescribed today [1]. In general, the enzymes catalyze the oxidative metabolism of a wide range of drugs and endogenous compounds to yield products (e.g., metabolites) that are usually more hydrophilic through the addition of a polar functional group, which may then serve as a reactive site for conjugating enzymes to enhance the rate of clearance and excretion of the products further by the addition of a yet more polar moiety [1]. For the most part, cytochrome P450–mediated reactions are typically considered to reflect detoxification pathways of xenobiotics as the hydrophilic metabolites are rapidly excreted from the body. In some instances, however, P450 metabolism results in the formation of reactive intermediates that can react with cellular macromolecules, such as DNA, RNA, and proteins, and lead to toxicity [2]. Given the chemical nature of these reactive intermediates, it is not surprising then that the same enzymes responsible for their formation are also susceptible to modification by these bioactivated species [3]. Compounds that are transformed by the P450 enzymes into reactive intermediates, which then react with active-site moieties leading to inactivation of the enzyme, are referred to as mechanism-based inactivators [4].

    Cytochrome P450 mechanism-based inhibitors (MBIs) have been identified across multiple therapeutic areas including antiarrhythmics (e.g., amiodarone [5]), antibacterials (e.g., clarithromycin [6] and troleandomycin [7]), antidepressants (e.g., fluoxetine [8] and paroxetine [9]), anti-HIV agents (e.g., rito-navir [10] and delavirdine [11]), antihypertensives (e.g., diltiazem [12] and verapamil [13]), nonsteroidal anti-inflamatory drugs (NSAIDs) (suprofen [14] and zileuton [15]), steroids/receptor modulators (e.g., gestodene [16] and raloxifene [17]), methylenedioxymethamphetamine ((MDMA) [18]), and oncology drugs (e.g., tamoxifen [19] and irinotecan [20]). In addition, P450 MBIs can be found in environmental sources such as illicit drugs (e.g., phencyclidine (PCP) [21] and various dietary constituents (e.g., berga-mottin [22], resveratrol [23], and 8-methoxypsoralen [24]). Consistent with the concepts outlined previ-ously for a reversible inhibitor, the severity of the observed drug-drug interactions (DDIs) encountered with P450 MBIs is primarily dependent on two factors: (i) the number of relevant clearance pathways associated with the victim drug's clearance and (ii) how well the increase in victim drug concentration is tolerated by the system [25]. In response to the observed safety risks associated with P450 inhibition (reversible or irreversible), global regulatory agencies now require a robust understanding of the potential for drug inhibition of P450 enzymes for any new drug application [26].

MBIs are a class of enzyme inhibitors, which contain a latent functional group that is by itself chemically unreactive, but can become activated to a highly reactive intermediate upon metabolism [27]. The activated species then binds irreversibly to the enzyme-active site and thereby inactivates the enzyme.

Given that the reactive groups present within the active site of the enzyme are nucleophiles (such as hydroxyl or sulfhydryl groups), irreversible inhibition via covalent addition of reactive species to the enzymes requires that the reactive species be some form of electrophilic moiety. For many enzymes, the formation of a reactive species (using the catalytic mechanism of the enzyme) falls into a few distinct cat-egories, such as the generation of Michael acceptors, haloalkyl derivatives, and rearrangements leading to an acyl-enzyme intermediate (e.g., proteases). For P450 MBIs, several structural moieties can serve as latent chemical groups associated with enzyme activation (Figure 19.1).

Criteria for Cytochrome P450 Mechanism-Based Inhibition

Characterization of MBIs follows intuitive kinetic and chemical criteria [28,29]. In short, an MBI is required to be a substrate, where physical binding to the enzyme-active site precedes catalysis. The interaction between substrate and enzyme needs to reflect a binding equilibrium followed by first-order chemical process leading to inactivation. To this end, as inhibitor concentration is increased, a greater fraction of the total enzyme will be occupied with inhibitor and the saturation of enzyme with inhibitor will be consistent with the kinetic specificity of the initial binding step. In addition, if covalent modifica-tion of the enzyme is a mechanism-based process, which proceeds via adduct formation to a key amino acid residue within the enzyme-active site, the chemical stoichiometry of modification should be unity (1:1 adduct/enzyme ratio) [30].

Today there exist well-defined criteria to assess whether a substrate is a P450 mechanism-based inac-tivator. Briefly, the inhibition must include the following:

1. The loss of enzyme activity must exhibit time dependence.
2. Enzyme inactivation should exhibit saturation kinetics with respect to the concentration of the inhibitor.
3. The inactivation occurs in a catalytically competent system (e.g., necessary cofactors are pres-ent and metabolism is occurring).
4. The enzyme should be protected from inactivation upon co-incubation with a competitive substrate/inhibitor.
5. Lack of suppression of inactivation by reactive intermediate scavengers.
6. The inactivation should be irreversible, and activity should not return upon dialysis or gel filtration.
7. Following inactivation, it should be possible to demonstrate a 1:1 stoichiometry of inactivator to enzyme molecule inactivated.

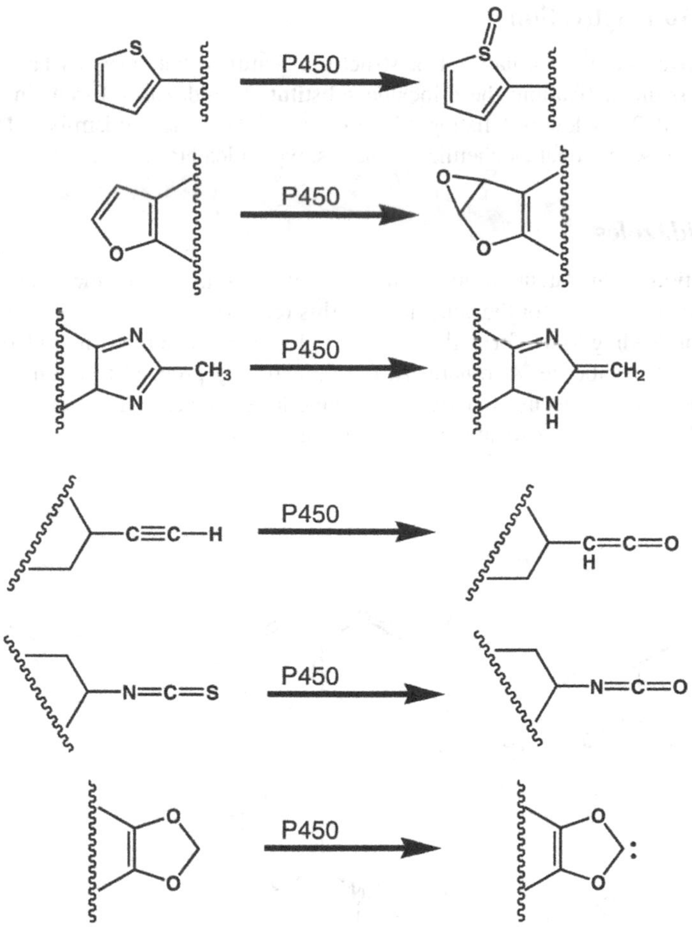

FIGURE 19.1   A listing of common P450 bioactivation reactions.

Interestingly, while metabolic intermediates (MIs) associated with many P450 MBIs are quite reactive, the rate of P450 enzyme inactivation for many MBIs is quite slow. The apparent discrepancy between the robust chemical reactivity of the activated species and the rate of enzyme inactivation is a reflection of the multiple metabolic pathways typically associated with P450 substrates. For non-P450 MBIs, the mechanism of enzyme inactivation takes advantage of a highly ordered catalytic mechanism between substrate and enzyme. As stated earlier, P450 enzymes have large active sites, which allow for multiple substrate orientations and, thus, are susceptible to multiple oxidative reactions [31]. A second feature that adds to the complexity of understanding P450 mechanism-based inhibition is the fact that in some cases the underlying mechanism of enzyme inactivation for one P450 enzyme does not extrapolate to a different P450 enzyme. For instance, while there are only subtle sequence differences between P450 3A4 and P450 3A5 (e.g., these enzymes share >95% amino acid homology), there are profound differences in susceptibility to mechanism-based inhibition by raloxifene [32].

Characterization of Cytochrome P450 Mechanism-Based Inhibition

In general, there are three types of P450 enzyme mechanism-based inactivators, which can be refined into two classes: irreversible MBIs, inhibitors, which, upon activation, bind covalently to the apoprotein or cause destruction of the prosthetic heme group; and pseudo-irreversible MBIs, inhibitors, which, upon activation, coordinate with the heme iron.

Irreversible P450 Inactivation

As mentioned above, there are a handful of structural features that serve as latent chemical groups associated with enzyme activation; these include substituted imidazoles, furan rings, thiophenes, and acetylenes (Figure 19.2). Below is a listing of the types of P450 mechanism-based inhibition and the chemistry associated with the latent chemical moieties, which lead to irreversible enzyme inactivation.

Substituted Imidazoles

Putative bioactivation of this latent group requires formation of an imidazomethide, as the electrophilic species [33]. The mechanism(s) for the generation of this reactive species involves initial P450-mediated electron abstraction leading to the formation of a radical intermediate that can undergo oxygen rebound to form the hydroxyl metabolite. Alternatively, the radical may proceed through a second electron or hydrogen atom abstraction to form a reactive imidazomethide species, which can adduct to nucleophilic sites within the P450 enzyme-active site or react with water [34].

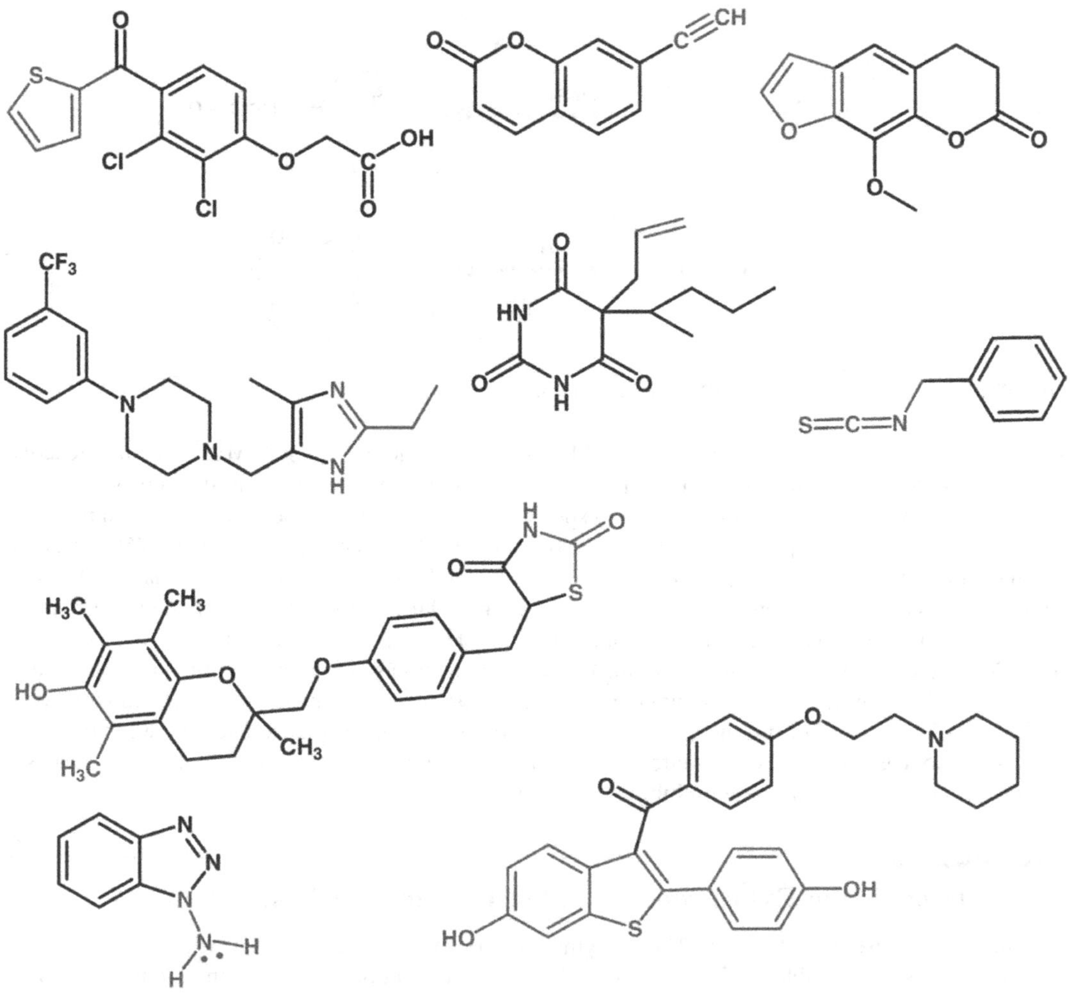

FIGURE 19.2   Known cytochrome P450 mechanism-based inhibitors with highlighted latent chemistry groups.

Furans

Furans are electron-rich aromatic groups that are readily oxidized by P450 enzymes to form electrophilic species, which have been linked to drug-related toxicities [35] as well as serve as MBIs [36]. The current hypothesis regarding P450-mediated bioactivation of furan rings involves epoxide formation that could either be deactivated via hydrolysis to yield the diol [37] or react irreversibly with the P450 enzyme either through direct adduction of the epoxide or through an intramolecular rearrangement of the epoxide to form an α, β-unsaturated carbonyl, which serves as a Michael acceptor for protein adduction [38].

Thiophenes

Currently, the cytochrome P450–mediated bioactivation of thiophene-containing drugs is thought to proceed via two possible mechanisms. The first mechanism proceeds via P450 oxidation of the thiophene sulfur atom leading to formation of a reactive thiophene-S-oxide intermediate. The thiophene-S-oxide is susceptible to a Michael-type addition with nucleophilic amino acids within the P450-active site [39]. The second mechanism stems from a P450-mediated oxidation of the thiophene ring to form a reactive thiophene epoxide metabolite, which may react directly with the P450 enzyme [40]. Alternatively, the epoxide in a mechanism analogous to furan bioactivation generates a cis-2-butene-1,4 dialdehyde reactive intermediate. In this instance, the thioketo-α, β-unsaturated aldehyde serves as the electrophilic intermediate that covalently binds to P450 enzyme [14].

Acetylenes

Many compounds containing an acetylenic group have been shown to be mechanism-based inactivators of P450 enzymes [41]. For this functional moiety, two mechanisms for the inactivation of P450 have been described in detail [42]. In this mechanism (Figure 19.2), the transfer of the oxygen from the activated oxygen intermediate of the P450 to the terminal carbon of the acetylene results in an intermediate that is able to rearrange via a 1,2 shift of the terminal hydrogen to the vicinal carbon to generate a ketene. The reactive ketene species produced by this rearrangement can then be hydrolyzed to produce the carboxylic acid product, or it can acylate nucleophilic residues within the P450-active site and inactivate the protein. Alternatively, the transfer of the oxygen from the P450-activated oxygen intermediate to the internal carbon of the acetylene would generate a reactive intermediate that leads to heme alkylation.

As discussed above, modification of the P450 apoprotein by reactive species typically involves covalent binding to an active-site nucleophilic amino acid residue such as lysine, serine, threonine, tyrosine, or cysteine [17,43,44]. In contrast, the chemistry associated with modification of the heme moiety by a MBI is more complex. There are two potential mechanisms of cytochrome P450 self-inactivation during catalytic turnover that can be considered. The first is via the formation of active substrate intermediates that are capable of covalently modifying the heme. Direct heme adduction has been demonstrated for many compounds [45]. For example, norethisterone, a steroid with an ethynyl substitution, diminishes the drug-metabolizing activity of the liver via a time- and dose-dependent inactivation of cytochrome P450 both *in vitro* and *in vivo* [46]. For this type of inactivation, P450 heme loss occurs only in the presence of NADPH and oxygen and can be inhibited by carbon monoxide [47]. Additional experimental evidence that implicates P450 oxidation as a requisite in heme destruction is the presence of a green-brown pigment [48].

The second mechanism is postulated to arise from the uncoupled cytochrome P450–catalyzed monooxygenase reactions. Specifically, the mechanism involves formation of hydrogen peroxide (H_2O_2) within the enzyme-active site, which interacts with the enzyme associated Fe^{2+}, thereby generating hydroxyl radicals that ultimately bleach the heme. This mechanism operates unlike enzymatic degradation, which specifically attacks the α-methene bridge, as reactive oxygen species are able to randomly attack all the carbon methene bridges of the tetrapyrrole rings, producing various pyrrole products in addition to releasing iron [49]. For example, it was found that H_2O_2-mediated P450 self-inactivation during benzphetamine oxidation is accompanied by heme degradation [50]. In this instance, the P450 heme modification involves heme release from the enzyme because of H_2O_2 formation within the P450 enzyme-active site via the peroxycomplex decay. The inactivation of cytochrome P450 by H_2O_2 is distinct from heme destruction via adduct formation as the destruction of heme does not mediate cytochrome P420 formation [51].

Characterization of Irreversible MBIs

Cytochrome P450 apoprotein adducts are characterized by the covalent labeling of a bioactivated drug reacting with a surrounding P450 active-site nucleophile. Typically, the drug-P450 adducts represent a mechanism of P450 inactivation and reduces the metabolic capacity of the adducted protein. When feasible, characterizing the chemical composition of the resultant adducts provides detailed information required to eliminate the structural motif responsible for inactivation from future chemical leads. Techniques that facilitate the speed and detail of the analysis of the chemical mechanism leading to adduct formation may readily reduce cost and time that it takes to develop novel therapeutics.

Radiolabel drug provides a quantitative tool to rapidly assess irreversible binding of protein and locate peptides that have radiolabel drug incorporated, and serves as a tool to determine binding stoichiometry [2]. Covalent-binding assays often serve as a part of the final safety assessment for a lead compound prior to development [2,52,53]. The strategies for covalent binding in drug discovery and the imposed limits will be reviewed in subsequent chapters. Irreversible–covalent binding experiments do not distinguish adduction of the P450 versus other hepatic proteins, without further isolation of the protein adduct sample from the *in vitro* incubation with additional techniques such as separation by HPLC-size exclusion chromatography or gel electrophoresis [41,54–56].

The use of mass spectrometry to elucidate P450-drug adducts is an attractive approach given its ability to yield molecular weight changes to the protein as a result of the drug adduct and simultaneously provides the adduct stoichiometry and proof of irreversibility of the drug-P450 complex [17,57,58]. Adducts to several of the major hepatic P450s have been observed using intact protein mass spectrometry and will be briefly reviewed. Figure 19.3 illustrates an example of P450 3A4 incubated with the MBI raloxifene [17]. The protein envelop of P450 3A4 dominates the chromatogram; however, at lower abundance, a new envelop representing a new protein entity is observed. The new species is right-shifted from the native protein envelop. Deconvulation of the protein envelope reveals two species present in the chromatogram. The smaller envelop corresponds to the 472-Da adducted P450 3A4 implicating the

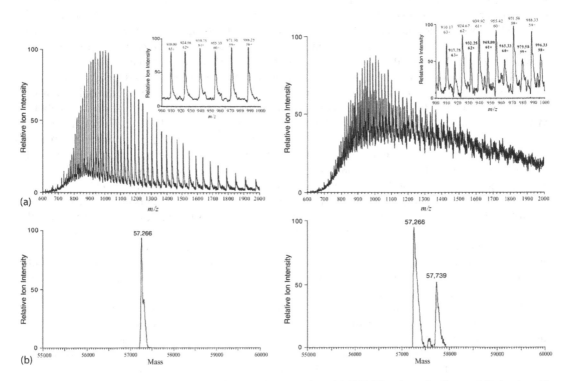

FIGURE 19.3 ESI-MS spectrum of P450 3A4 (a) control incubation with NADPH and no raloxifene and (b) incubated in the presence of raloxifene. Deconvoluted mass is consistent with parent mass of raloxifene.

reactive diquinone methide of raloxifene as the reactive intermediate responsible P450 3A4 inactivation. Glutathione adducts of raloxifene include m/z of 779, 795, and 1050. Without protein mass spectrometry of the P450 3A4–adduct it would be impossible to know which reactive species inactivates P450 3A4. This information could be used to generate raloxifene analogs void of the capacity to form the diquinone methide, as was observed with the close analog arzoxifene [59].

Adducts with P450 3A4 and 3A5 have also been observed with 17α-ethynyl estradiol (EE). Using mass spectrometry which aided in the elucidation of the mechanism of MBI formation [60,61]. With P450 3A5, the inactivation by EE was also dependent on the presence of cytochrome b5. This example also provides a unique case where inactivation was well characterized to implicate that the inactivation occurs through both heme and apoprotein adduction presumably through the formation of a 17α-oxirene-related reactive metabolite that partitions the oxygen between the internal and terminal carbons of the ethynyl group dictating the mode of inactivation.

Tienilic acid is an MBI of P450 2C9 [39,62]. When tienilic acid is incubated with P450 2C9, two tienilic acid adducts are observed (Figure 19.4a), whereas in the presence of glutathione, the adduct formation is reduced to a 1:1 stoichiometry (Figure 19.4b). This indicates that in addition to MBI, the reactive metabolite(s) from tienilic acid can adduct with an alternate amino acid of the enzyme that is not associated with MBI. The mass spectral chromatogram indicates the formation of both apo adducts arising from the oxidation of tienilic acid. Two mechanisms were proposed: (i) direct sulfur oxidation where, upon covalent adduction, the oxidation does not dehydrate and (ii) through a thiophene epoxide, which could undergo nucleophilic ring opening. Both mechanisms could result in the observed P450 2C9 adduct of tienilic acid shown in Figure 19.4. Interestingly, despite the direct evidence for apoprotein adduction, CO difference spectra indicate a loss of >60% of the P-450, which has been a technique used to implicate heme adducts by P450. This brings into question the use of CO binding as a diagnostic to differentiate heme adducts from apo adducts.

1-[(2-ethyl-4-methyl-1H-imidazol-5-yl)methyl]-4-[4-(trifluoromethyl)-2-pyridinyl] piperazine (EMTPP) was demonstrated to produce an adduct with P450 2D6 by mass spectrometry [34]. The mass difference from the unlabeled P450 was 353 Da, consistent with addition of the parent compound (Figure 19.5). Metabolism data from NMR and CID mass spectrometry complimented the protein adduct mass spectrometry data in showing that adduct formation potentially resulted from multiple oxidations of the drug to form a dehydrated methide of EMTPP, similar to that proposed for 3-methylindole [63]. The EMTPP-P450 2D6 example illustrates the challenges with identifying the nature of MBI and the potential resolution limitations of intact protein mass spectrometry when trying to identify the molecular entity responsible for inactivation.

At present, most laboratory instruments cannot distinguish a difference of 2 Da for proteins >50 kDa (resolution ¼ 100,000 Da). This becomes especially difficult with the increasing level of heterogeneity observed in P450 enzymes after *in vitro* incubations. This has been well documented by Bateman et al., who illustrated the effect of incubation time on the quality of the P450 3A4 protein envelope and the difficulty that arises with protein deconvolution from heterogeneous samples [57]. Several factors can be employed to minimize sample degradation, including short incubation times, limiting oxygen to the incubation sample or using subsaturating amounts of NADPH, and through the addition of reactive oxygen scavenger to reduce protein oxidation (superoxide dismutase and catalase). The latter point, protein oxidation, highlights a potential pitfall of protein mass spectrometry for determining the MBI precursor because of the potential for misinterpretation of mass differences upon adduct formation. Despite the theoretical possibility, no examples of direct P450 oxidation have been described. Overall, the detection of intact P450-protein adducts has been met with variable success and, on the basis of the limited number of protein adducts identified to this point, may indicate a number of factors that contribute to the success of protein adduct detection, such as the composition of the chemical moiety undergoing bioactivation and the kinetics of its formation.

The resolution limitations of intact protein mass spectrometry can be circumvented by proteolytic digestion of the adducted protein [64,65]. This added step has the potential to provide greater detail with respect to the structural composition of the protein adduct and the chemistry resulting in the irreversible binding of the drug to the protein. The adducted peptide is easily tracked through the numerous steps of isolation and purification by the use of radiolabel. Through CID spectral characterization, analytical

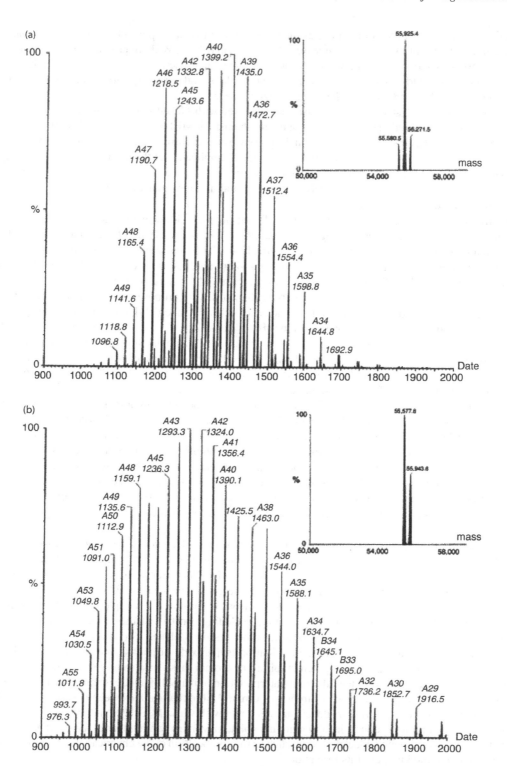

FIGURE 19.4   ESI-MS spectrum of P450 2C9 (a) after incubation with NADPH and tienilic acid and (b) incubated with NADPH tienilic acid and glutathione. Deconvoluted mass is consistent with single oxidized product of tienilic acid responsible for adduct formation.

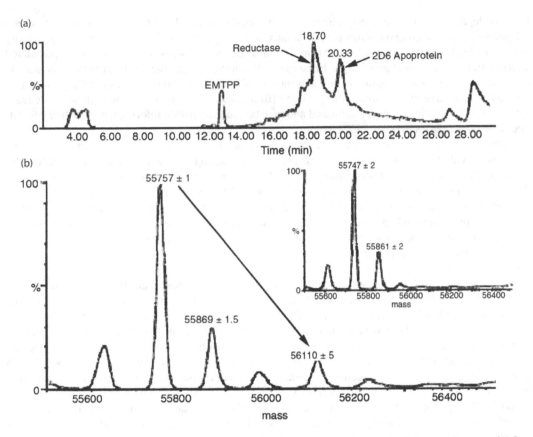

FIGURE 19.5   (a) Representative chromatogram illustrating separation of components (reductase and apoprotein) from an incubation containing recombinant P450 2D6. (b) Deconvoluted mass spectrum of EMTPP-inactivated P450 2D6 illustrating an EMTPP adduct with a mass shift consistent with the mass of EMTPP. Inset shows the absence of this additional mass in control incubations (-NADPH). Abbreviation: EMTPP, 1-[(2-ethyl-4-methyl-1H-imidazol-5-yl)methyl]-4[4-(trifluoromethyl)-2-pyridinyl]piperazine.

digests of the protein adduct also provide an opportunity to unambiguously identify the adducted amino acid residue The ability to elucidate the covalently bound drug adducts of P450 enzymes is filled with technical challenges stemming from the difficulty in isolating the membrane-associated enzymes themselves and from the innate difficulty in obtaining sufficient sequence coverage from the digests necessary to characterize the location and nature of MBI adduct [66]. Cytochrome P450 2C9 adducts with tienilic acid were identified as mentioned above with intact protein mass spectrometry. Subsequent tryptic digests were used to identify the site of adduction but failed to yield the location of the drug adduct [67]. The lack of adduct was attributed to the potential instability of the covalent linkage. This phenomenon is not specific to P450 2C9 and tienilic acid. For example, L-754,394 was found to be an MBI of P450 3A4 observable by intact protein mass spectrometry, but upon digestion, no adduct was identified [66].

The difficulty in observing direct structural information from peptide adducts has lead several investigators to probe various P450-active sites for nucleophilic residues susceptible to covalent adduction by electophilic species. Tools including photoaffinity labeling [68,69], alkylation with xenobiotic linked to biotin [70], and direct alkylation of purified P450 with reactive electrophiles like iodoacetamide [17] have been investigated. In combination with the nucleophilicity of active-site amino acid residues, these tools provide a focal point for locating drug-P450 adducts and may simplify data mining by narrowing in on specific "soft spots" of the P450, which favor adduction by MBI.

Photoaffinity labels have long been used to probe enzyme structure function of cytosolic and transmembrane proteins [71,72]. The use of photoaffinity probes in P450 labeling has also been explored. Initial efforts were performed with 1-(4-azidophenyl) imidazole with soluble, bacterial P450cam [73].

Recently, lapachenole was selected to investigate the alkylation of P450 3A4 [69]. The photoactivation of lapachenole produced two distinct peptide adducts at Cys98 and Cys468. Cys98 is in close proximity to the B-B' loop region, which is located near the substrate recognition site 1 (SRS-1) and is postulated to form part of the access channel to the heme iron [74]. On the basis of the crystal structure, the second adducted species, Cys468, appears to be a solvent-accessible cysteine on the exterior of the protein and, thus, less informative with regard to prospective MBI adducts. The ability of these tools to locate reactive nucleophilic residues is well established and may be used to provide information regarding solvent-accessible nucleophiles in other P450 enzymes.

Alternatively, the use of biotin-linked electrophiles holds promise for use in identifying key enzyme electrophiles with the added benefit of having a selective isolation tool when combined with streptavidin for isolation. Proof of concept was explored by linking biotin with raloxifene and subsequently used to illustrate binding of the activated raloxifene moiety to Cys47 of GST P1-1 [70]. When employed against a dexamethasone-treated preparation of rat liver microsomes, five adducts were identified, none of which, however, corresponded to P450. This capture and isolation technique illustrates how labeling of an MBI with biotin can be accomplished without inhibiting its bioactivation; therefore, this technique could be amenable to isolating adducted P450 enzymes from catalytically active systems such as reconstituted enzymes or insect membrane preparations.

Direct alkylation with reactive electrophiles offers the simplest method in an attempt to locate solvent-accessible nucleophilic amino acid residues. A diverse set of electrophilic reagents can be utilized to label both the soft and hard protein nucleophiles. The use of maleimide as a soft electrophile to covalently label cysteines has long been used in protein biochemistry. With respect to P450 enzymes, maleimide has a detrimental effect on the integrity of the protein and results in inactive protein after labeling occurs [75]. Iodoactemide (IA) derivatives are also commonly used and have a variety of chemistries linked to them including fluorescent tags, biotin for capturing, and spintrapping reagents (www.invitrogen.com). Interestingly, in P450 3A4, the use of IA or PIA resulted in single stoichiometric reactions when run for one hour [17]. Upon digestion with proteinase K, the alkylated residue was identified by LC-MS/MS as Cys239. Upon analysis of the crystal structure of P450 3A4 (www.rcsb.org, 1TQN.pdb), Cys239 resides between the G and G' helices and may serve a perfect hook for electrophilic residues as they egress the active site of P450 3A4. Surprisingly, the label of P450 3A4 by photoaffinity label lapachenole and that of IA provide unique sites of reactivity. Further, investigation of the regioselectivity differences between these electrophilic agents may help to determine if the reactive metabolic species produce structural alteration of the enzyme leading to unique accessibility to the different protein nucleophiles or if the reactivities of Cys239 and Cys98 differ in their microenvironments (pKa) within the P450 such that their inherent nucleophilic properties differ substantially so as to favor unique electrophiles.

Detailed characterization of the amino acid residues involved in protein adduct formation requires protein digestion for analysis. The use of different digesting reagents can provide a unique series of fragments, which may help to visualize the adducted protein. Cyanogen bromide is a chemical agent used to digest proteins and produces large peptide fragments. Given the size of fragments generated, this agent typically works well when interfaced with a MALDI-TOF instrument, but is limited because of the lack of MS/MS capabilities. Lysyl endopeptidase also generates rather large fragments as this protease cleaves at the c-terminus of lysine residues. Lysyl endopeptidase digestions are also very amenable to TOF technology given their large molecular weights and the generation of limited protein fragments of the protein to be searched. Trypsin digests are most commonly employed and serve to digest proteins at the c-terminus of lysine and arginine residues. The fragments produced from trypsin are very suitable for LC-MS/MS using a variety of mass spectrometry platforms largely because of their tendency to carry $[M+2H]^{+2}$ since the end caps are both capable of carrying a charge. Recently, proteinase K has been used to exploit its lack of discrimination in protein cleavage sites to generate small peptide fragments [17]. When separating a proteinase K–digested sample on a reverse phase column, the bulk of peptides elute quickly, with the more hydrophobic drug-based adduct retaining on the column, providing easy identification of the adducted peptide. This is not the case with larger peptides, where the physical properties of the drug have minimal impact on the chromatographic properties of the peptide adduct. In addition, the use of proteinase K should improve ionization efficiencies by reduced hydrophobic aggregation and less ion suppression from the reduced number of coeluting peptides. The tools described for identifying active-site nucleophiles provide a focal point for future studies aimed at locating drug-based peptide adducts and should ultimately lead to our improved ability to generate high-quality structural data in a more timely fashion.

Pseudo-Irreversible P450 Inactivation

These classes of MBI represent molecules that are transformed by P450 enzymes into MI products, which are able to coordinate with the heme iron. The interaction between MI product and heme iron is extremely strong, however, not covalent, as the MI/heme complex can be displaced under extreme experimental conditions (e.g., potassium ferricyanide), consequently, the inactivation is described as pseudo-irreversible.

Methylenedioxy Compounds

The effects of methylenedioxyphenyl (MDP) compounds on P450 may be traced back to early observations that sesame oil could synergize the effects of the insecticide pyrethrum. Early investigators noted that "the inhibition of biological oxidation of methyl parathion and of aldrin to dieldrin leads to the speculation that pyrethrin may also be detoxified by biological oxidations and that the synergism produced by pyrethrins and synergists may be due to the inhibition of such oxidation." This initial suggestion by Hodgson and Casida was followed by the observation that both piperonyl butoxide and sesamex inhibited the oxidation of *N, N*-dimethyl-p-nitro-phenyl carbamate and the corresponding diethyl compound in rat microsomes [76,77]. MDP compounds are not only inhibitors of oxidation but they are also P450 substrates. Metabolism of piperonyl butoxide has been studied extensively and *in vivo* mouse studies have demonstrated that the methylene bridge carbon is metabolized to carbon dioxide [78,79]. *In vitro* it has also been shown that the bridge carbon is metabolized to carbon monoxide and formate [80]. Moreover, the cleavage of the methylenedioxy ring to yield catechol metabolites was also documented for 6-nitro-3,4-methlyenedioxybenzene [79] and 1,2,5,6-tetrachloro-3,4-methlenedioxybenzene [81].

The contemporary view of MDP compounds is that the class is characterized by metabolism-dependent noncompetitive inhibition. Clearly, the extent of observed noncompetitive inhibition depends on the compound being metabolized, and so MDP compounds as a whole will contain examples of a variety of inhibition types. However, early studies involving metabolism and inhibition of MDP compounds contained conflicting reports of both competitive and noncompetitive inhibition. In a review by Hodgson and Philpot, it was noted that in many of these studies, nicotinamide was added to *in vitro* incubations because it was thought to be a requirement for microsomal reactions (inhibition of pyridine nucleotidase) [80]. Schenkman et al. reported that nicotinamide was not required and that, furthermore, it was an inhibitor of several oxidative reactions [82]. Thus, the inclusion of nicotinamide in early experiments may have been a confounding influence on data interpretation. As an alternative explanation, Franklin showed that when piperonyl butoxide was incubated with microsomes (plus NADPH), the inhibition of N-demethylation of ethylmorphine was at first competitive but then was noncompetitive after the formation of an observable complex. The complex that was formed is now known as a MI complex. This complex has been shown to be formed in a manner that is dependent on time, NADPH, and oxygen, consistent with the requirement of cytochrome P450 oxidation to uncover the latent ability of MDP compounds to complex with the heme [83].

The method used to detect MI complex formation is difference spectroscopy and the Soret region of absorbance (blue wavelength) is the region of interest. When the iron of P450 is in the reduced state (ferrous), these complexes show absorbance maxima similar to those of well-documented ligands such as carbon monoxide (450 nm) and ethylisocyanate (455 nm) [84,85]. MI complexes from a number of MDP compounds are characterized by an absorbance maximum at both 455 and 427 nm [83]. The intensity of these peaks depends on both pH and the substrate involved. In the ferric state, the absorbance maximum is found at a single absorption spectrum of 437–438 nm [83,84]. It is an interesting observation that when an MDP compound is administered *in vivo*, the resulting *in vitro* ferrous spectra are often not observed until after the addition of a reducing agent such as dithionate. Not only can reducing agents help visualize the complex, but the 455-nm absorbance is resistant to oxidative agents such as potassium ferricyanide. When added, potassium ferricyanide will diminish the 455-nm absorbance, but subsequent addition of dithionite will regenerate the peak [86]. It is also worth noting that the ferric state is less stable, and some ligands can be displaced by incubation with lipophilic compounds, with the subsequent regeneration of P450 activity [41]. In contrast, the ferrous state is unaffected by such incubations, but it can be dissociated by irradiation at 400–500 nm as shown by Ullrich and Schnabel [42].

In early studies, the nature of the mechanism leading to MI complex formation was the subject of much speculation. Several mechanisms were proposed, which involved either carbocation [87], free radical, [42] or carbanion intermediates. Using fluorine as a model, Ullrich and Schnabel produced a convincing argument for the binding of carbanions to P450 [42]. In this instance, the authors noted that when fluorine was added to NADPH-supplemented microsomes from phenobarbitol-treated rats, a difference spectrum was produced with an absorbance at 446 nm. It was then observed that neither anaerobic conditions nor the addition of NADH under aerobic conditions could reproduce the absorbance at 446 nm. This suggested to the investigators that a mono-oxidation product of fluorine was responsible for complex formation, although incubating known oxidative metabolites with microsomes could not reproduce the effect (fluorenol and fluorenonone). In addition, the incubation time used in this experiment was very short, only 10–20 seconds, so it was not likely that enough time had passed for the accumulation of significant amounts of oxidation products to potentially complex with the enzyme.

Fluorine is a very simple structure, and the methylene bridge is the most likely moiety to form a reactive species. Moreover, one chemical feature of this group is the acidity of its hydrogens (pKa value of 22 in aprotic solutions) [42]. Ullrich and Schnabel noted that the dissociation of this proton yielded a species with increased resonance and it had an absorption maximum at 373 nm [42]. When they examined the difference spectra of a reduced microsomal suspension after incubation of fluorene with NADPH, a peak at 374 nm was observed, which they postulated was due to a species similar to the fluorine anion. The free electron pair of the fluorine could potentially interact with the ferrous iron in the same way as carbon monoxide or ethylisocyanide. Thus, in principle, the binding of fluorene or MDP compounds would be similar to carbon monoxide, and consequently, one might expect that a photodissociation of the complex with light could be achieved. As noted above, these investigators were able to partially decrease the inhibition of ethylmorphine demethylation caused by piperonyl butoxide by irradiation with highintensity light between 400 and 500 nm. This experiment provided evidence for the ligand binding nature of piperonyl butoxide. The only questions remaining were what "monooxidation" product of fluorene (or piperonyl butoxide) was involved and how that gave rise to MI complex formation.

Although the evidence for a carbanion presented by Ullrich and Schnabel is compelling, the exact mechanism by which cytochrome P450 would produce this species is not clear. An additional mechanism proposed by Ullrich and Schnabel showed that a carbene could be produced from MDP compounds by hydroxylation of the methylene bridge followed by elimination of water (Figure 19.6) [88]. Like the carbanion proposed above, the carbene would also have free electrons available for coordination to the heme. The metabolism of the methylene bridge to form a carbene is most consistent with the data reported in the literature. For example, it has been shown that when the methylene group hydrogens are substituted with methyl groups, there is an almost complete loss in P450 complex formation [81]. In addition, a deuterium isotope effect of similar magnitude has been reported for both the formation rate of carbon monoxide *in vitro* and attenuation of *in vivo* insecticide effects [89]. These observations coupled with the fact that MDP compounds labeled with isotopes have shown that carbon monoxide derives directly from the methylene carbon indicates that the reaction appears to involve the cleavage of the C-H bond with the subsequent formation of a species that can then complex with cytochrome P450, or the form of a variety of oxidative metabolites.

In Figure 19.6, two pathways are shown that could result in carbene formation. In the first pathway (path A), initial hydrogen abstraction leaves a carbon-centered radical on the methylene bridge, which (without oxygen rebound), if oxidized further, will yield a cationic species that can then deprotenate to form a carbene. The second pathway involves the elimination of water after hydroxylation of the methylene bridge, which could then directly form a carbene (path B). However, it is likely that the elimination of water in this mechanism is more complex and may involve cationic intermediates such as an oxonium ion, which, upon further deprotenation, could yield a carbene [90]. As an example of how metabolites

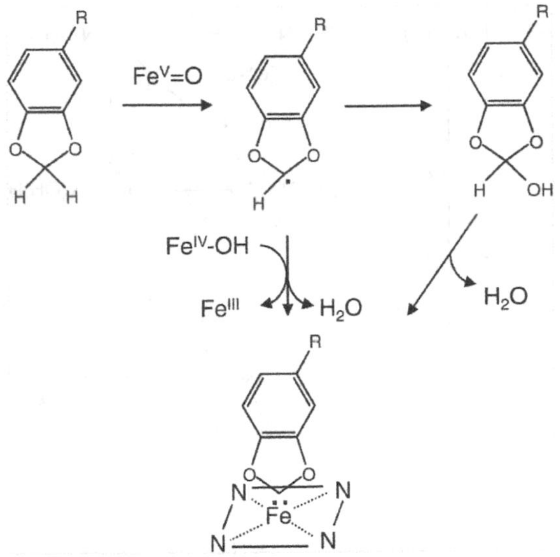

FIGURE 19.6 Proposed mechanism for the formation of a metabolic intermediate complex from the metabolism of methylenedioxy compounds.

could arise from this mechanism, one possibility is the rearrangement of the methylenic hydroxyl-MDP intermediate to 2-hydroxyphenylformate and hydrolysis to the subsequent catechol and carbon monoxide or formate metabolites [91].

Amine Compounds

In the 1950s, a number of reports were published that showed that a new compound, diehtylamono-ethyl-2,2,-diphenylvalerate HCl (SKF 525-A), potentiated the pharmacology of drugs such as methodone and morphine [92], some hypnotic drugs, [93] and nervous system stimulants such as amphetamine [94]. Like the observation of Hodgson and Casida regarding MDP compounds and their mode of action on insecticides, the potentiating effect of SKF 525-A was reported to result from decreased biotransformation of these drugs and, therefore, decreased clearance [95,96]. Castro and Sasame observed that irreversible inhibition of drug metabolism occurred when microsomes were preincubated *in vitro* with (i) NADPH, (ii) SKF 525-A, and (iii) oxygen [97]. Further studies with this compound and others showed not only that MDP compounds could form an observable MI complex but also that SKF 525-A [98] and benzphetamine [99] could yield absorption bands in the 455-nm region. One moiety that was common to many of these compounds including SKF 525-A was a substituted amine. It is now generally understood that substituted amines must first be dealkylated to primary amines before heme coordination can take place (Figure 19.7a). It was also found that an MI complex could be formed from hyroxylamines or by reduction of some nitroalkanes [100]. These observations suggested that a species intermediate to a hydroxylamine and the nitro-oxidation state was involved in P450 complex formation. Consequently, it was proposed and widely accepted that a nitrosoalkane was the iron ligand producing the 455 nm-absorbing complex (Figure 19.7a). In iron-porphyrin model studies, a crystal structure between a nitroso ligand in a tetraphenylporphyrin-iron complex showed that the nitroso ligand was bound to the iron by its nitrogen atom and that the resulting bond was very stable (e.g., could not be displaced by strong ligands such as carbon monoxide) [101].

In general, MI complexes derived from amines differ from those formed from MDP compounds. The wavelength that characterizes the absorbance maxima for amine complexes is in a wider range than that observed for MDP compounds (446–455 nm). One of the primary differences between MDP-P450 complexes and amine-P450 complexes is their instability in the ferric state. When potassium ferricyanide is added to an *in vitro* incubation, the ferrous 455-nm peak of the nitroso complex is diminished presumably as the complex is shifted to the ferric state. However, the 455-nm peak cannot be regenerated by the addition

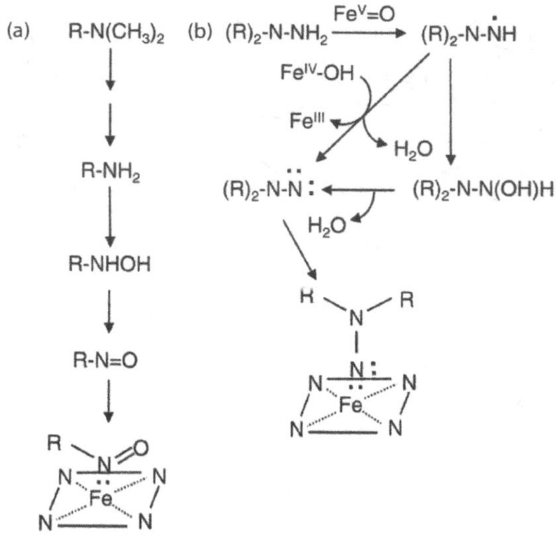

FIGURE 19.7   Proposed pathways for formation of metabolic intermediate complexes from oxidation of (a) amines and (b) hydrazines.

of dithionite, as can be observed with MDP complexes [98]. It is also worth noting that some complexes are unstable in the presence of dithionite and it appears that many aryl amines yield complexes that are characterized by this instability [102]. Finally, in contrast to MDP compounds, when amine-containing compounds form complexes *in vivo*, they are immediately observed in the resulting microsomes without the addition of dithionite [98], thus showing that *in vivo* nitroso complexes stabilize P450 in the ferrous state.

Hydrazines

The incubation of microsomes with 1,1-disubstituted hydrazines in the presence of NADPH and oxygen reveals a spectral complex that can be observed in the Soret region with a maximum at 438 nm and a minimum at 414 nm (ferric state). Under anaerobic conditions, the minimum shifts to 407 nm and the maxima shifts to 449 nm (ferrous state). It has also been shown that to produce an observable complex, hydrazines should be 1,1-disubstituted and cannot be monosubstituted or 1,2-disubstituted [103]. An exception to this rule is some acyl hydrazines such as isoniazid (INH). INH was introduced as a drug in the 1950s and has been reported to decrease the clearance of several other drugs including phenytoin [104]. When INH is incubated with microsomes, NADPH, and oxygen, a complex is formed that has an absorption maximum at 449 nm (ferrous state) [105]. This result is in contrast with the 1,1-disubstituted hydrazine spectrum that is visualized in the ferric state. In addition, when potassium ferricyanide is added, the complex dissociates demonstrate that the INH complex is stable only in the ferrous form, similar to the nitroso complexes discussed *vida supra* [106].

It has been proposed that INH and 1,1-disubstituted hydrazines can be metabolized to a nitrene, which can then coordinate with cytochrome P450 both *in vivo* and *in vitro* (Figure 19.7b) [103]. Studies with porphyrin systems indicate that the nitrene formed coordinates with the iron via the terminal nitrogen [103,105]. It is likely that both acyl hydrazines and 1,1-disubstituted hydrazines are oxidized in a stepwise fashion by cytochrome P450 to produce an aminonitrene-iron complex as shown in Figure 19.7b.

Kinetics of Cytochrome P450 Mechanism-Based Inhibition

The structural and functional characterization to this point has been focused on the structural identification and characterization employed to develop the most appropriate clinical candidate. If MBI persists in the lead candidate, the potential impact on the exposure of other medications is required to clearly define the clinical limitations of the therapeutic agent including defining drugs susceptible to drug interaction upon coadministration of the MBI, defining at-risk patient population (e.g., age or pharmacogenetics), and the duration of treatment (acute or chronic) to properly context all the potential safety concerns. This requires the combination of much of the data already accumulated including the K_I and k_{inact}, with the endogenous enzyme degradation rate to describe the extent of drug interaction that could result on the basis of irreversible inhibition kinetics. Additional information regarding the expected metabolism and disposition of the substrate responsible for producing irreversible inhibitor will typically serve to increase the predictive power of the estimated changes expected in AUC and includes an understanding of the overall metabolic pathway, potential for gut metabolism, and the existence of multiple inactivation pathways including those produced from metabolites may also be incorporated in an attempt to refine *in vivo* extrapolations. Furthermore, when possible, the fraction of total hepatic metabolism due to the affected P450 should be considered for improved predictability of the magnitude of the drug interaction [107].

When a cytochrome P450 enzyme converts a nonreactive molecule into a species that is reactive, there are several general outcomes. The reactive species can be released as some form of product (where it can potentially react with water) or react with the P450 apoprotein structure or the active-site heme moiety.

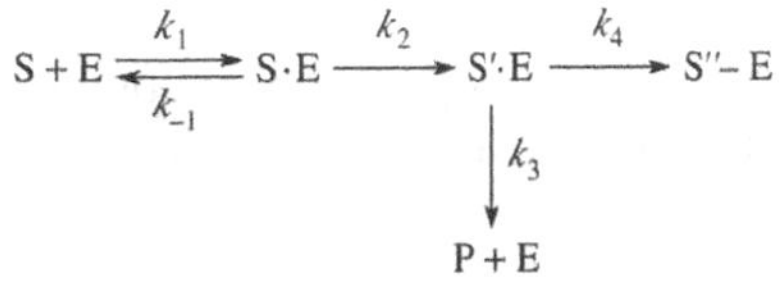

$$S + E \underset{k_{-1}}{\overset{k_1}{\rightleftharpoons}} S{\cdot}E \overset{k_2}{\longrightarrow} S'{\cdot}E \overset{k_4}{\longrightarrow} S''{-}E$$
$$\downarrow k_3$$
$$P + E$$

The above scheme illustrates the possible outcomes by depicting two separate pathways described by the rate constants k_4 and k_3. Subsequent to the formation of a reactive species (S'-E), the substrate is shown forming product (P) or reacting with the enzyme (S''-E). These two pathways and associated rate constants are the basis for an important descriptive parameter in mechanism-based inactivation—the partition ratio. This term was introduced by Walsh in an effort to describe the number of inactivator molecules released as product versus those that reacted with the enzyme to form an inactivated complex [108]. It is apparent that very efficient enzyme inactivators would lead to very little product formation and greater enzyme inactivation, and the converse would be true for inefficient inactivation. Therefore, efficient enzyme inactivation would be described by a low partition ratio (k_3/k_4). The most efficient inactivation would produce no product and only inactivated enzyme and be characterized by a partition ratio of zero. No molecules have been described to inactivate P450 with a partition ratio of 0, however, a Merck compound L-754,394 has been reported to have a partition ratio for P450 3A4 of approximately 1.34 [109].

Another important parameter is k_{inact}, which is the rate of inactivation. If one examines scheme 1, it is tempting to conclude that k_{inact} and k_2 are the same. However, this is not the case. The term k_{inact} is more complex and is comprised of rate constants k_2, k_3, and k_4, and only under specific conditions (i.e., $k_2 << k_4$, k_3 is very slow or equal to zero), k_{inact} ¼ k_2 [109]. Early work of Kitz and Wilson and subsequent derivations of Jung and Metcalf provide the following expression, which relates active enzyme concentration to k_{inact}.

$$\frac{d[E]_t}{dt} = \frac{-k_{inact}[I]}{K_I + [I]}[E]_t \tag{19.1}$$

where $[E]_t$ is the concentration of active enzyme at time t, K_I is the concentration of inhibitor at which half-maximal inactivation occurs, and I is the concentration of inhibitor [110,111]. Experimentally, k_{inact} and K_I are most often determined from a dilution assay where aliquots of enzyme incubated with inhibitor in a primary incubation are then transferred at different time intervals to a secondary incubation that contains a reporter substrate (i.e., testosterone for P450 3A4). To reflect this type of experiment, the relationship in Eq. 19.1 can be integrated.

$$\frac{[E]}{[E]_{total}} = e^{\frac{-k_{inact}[I]t}{K_I + [I]}} \tag{19.2}$$

or

$$\ln\frac{[E]}{[E]_{total}} = \frac{-k_{inact}[I]t}{K_I + [I]} \tag{19.3}$$

In the experiment described above, the aliquots from a primary incubation are taken at various time points, and the amount of enzyme activity remaining (e.g., fractional activity) is reported in the secondary incubation by a reporter substrate. This data is then plotted on a semilogarithmic plot as the natural log of fractional activity versus time (Figure 19.8). When the reporter substrate is at a concentration of approximately 5 its k_m value, then the velocity of product formation is approximated by

$$Vel \approx V_{max}$$

or

$$Vel \approx [E]k_{cat}$$

Therefore, under these conditions, the velocity of product formation is proportional to the enzyme concentration, atnd the natural log of fractional activity is essentially given by Eq. 19.3. The slope of this data is then given by

$$\frac{-k_{inact}[I]}{K_I + [I]} \tag{19.4}$$

This is a hyperbolic relationship similar to the familiar Michaelis-Menten kinetics where the "velocity" of inactivation or k_{obs} is equal to

$$k_{obs} = \frac{k_{inact}[I]}{k_I + [I]} \tag{19.5}$$

Therefore, when the absolute value of the slopes from the experimental data shown in Figure 19.8 are plotted versus inhibitor concentration, the resulting graph should obey a hyperbolic relationship as shown in Figure 19.9. As such, this data is akin to Michaelis-Menten kinetics, and the resulting parameters (K_I and k_{inact}) may be determined in a manner that is analogous to the parameter determination for standard hyperbolic enzyme kinetics. Before the advent of computers, this was most easily achieved through linear transformation, but today the slope data from Eq. 19.3 (or slopes of the experimental data in

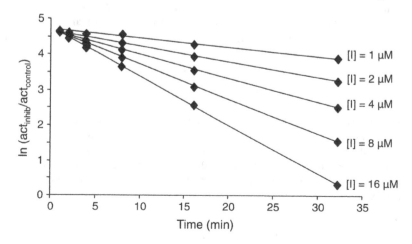

FIGURE 19.8   Slopes of the natural log of fractional activity yield k_{obs} values for varying concentrations of inhibitor.

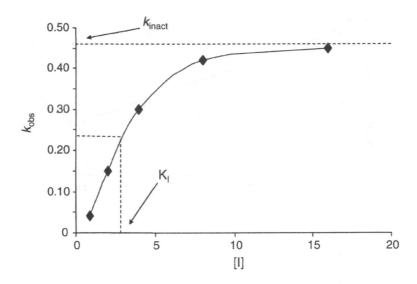

FIGURE 19.9   Determination of k_{inact} and K_I from a plot of k_{obs} versus inhibitor concentration.

Figure 19.9) can be fitted to a hyperbolic curve by any number of commercially available programs, and the values of K_I and k_{inact} can be readily determined.

Examination of Eq. 19.3 suggests that the rate of inactivation for a given inhibitor concentration should be linear with time (Figure 19.10a). However, this may not be the case, and it is often observed that the data becomes nonlinear with time (Figure 19.10b). One explanation for this nonlinearity is that significant inhibitor depletion may have occurred in the primary incubation prior to dilution into the secondary-reporter assay. It is apparent from examination of the relationship in Eq. 19.3 that no change in the inhibitor concentration is assumed. Therefore, assay conditions that minimize inhibitor depletion should be used. These conditions can include shorter assay time or a reduction in the temperature of the assay to slow down inhibitor metabolism [58].

As an alternative, it may also be possible that several mechanisms of inactivation are occurring simultaneously and that the passage of time serves to unmask the slower rate of inactivation. The result would be apparent nonlinearity in the data similar to inhibitor depletion. In such cases of nonlinearity, it is the best practice to take the slope of early time points to determine parameters such as K_I and k_{inact} (Figure 19.10b).

Experimentally, determination of the partition ratio can be accomplished in two ways. The first method is by titration; the use of this method involves increasing amounts of inhibitor that is added to a known, fixed amount of enzyme, and the reaction is allowed to go to completion [50]. The enzyme is then dialyzed, or diluted sufficiently in a secondary reaction with a reporter substrate, and a plot is constructed of remaining enzyme activity versus moles of inhibitor divided by moles of enzyme (see Figure 19.11). Theoretically, this plot should yield a straight line. However, in practice, this does not often occur, and the data must be extrapolated to the *x*-axis, which gives the ratio of inhibitor to enzyme needed for complete inactivation of enzyme activity. When extrapolation to the *x*-axis is performed, the intersection of the line and the axis yields the turnover number. It is important to note that this number or ratio includes the amount of inhibitor required to inactivate the enzyme, and if one assumes a 1:1 stoichiometry, then the partition ratio is the turnover number minus one.

A second and more direct method involves determination of the molar amount of products formed from reaction of the inhibitor with P450 and an assessment of the amount of P450 enzyme inactivated. This may be accomplished in several ways. In microsomes a high concentration of inhibitor can be used along with an appropriate incubation period to insure complete inactivation of the enzyme. The resulting decrease in the carbon monoxide–binding spectrum can be used to quantitate the amount of enzyme inactivated. Once this value is established, a separate incubation containing enzyme and inhibitor is assayed with the dilution method, and this can be used to estimate the molar amount of enzyme inactivated. In the same incubation, product formation of the reaction is then measured (or inhibitor depletion is measured), and the ratio of

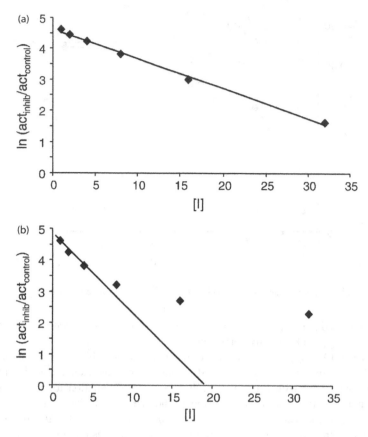

FIGURE 19.10 Determining kobs where (a) inactivation is linear with time and (b) inactivation is non-linear with time possibly due to significant inhibitor depletion.

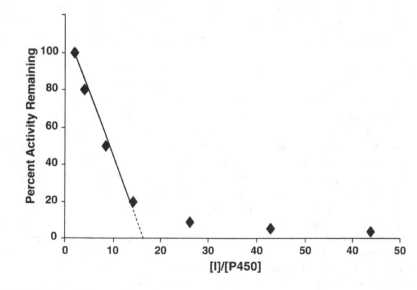

FIGURE 19.11 Estimation of the partition ratio.

product formed versus enzyme inactivated directly yields the partition ratio. Alternatively, the experiment can be performed with expressed enzyme, which has the advantage of containing only one P450, and in this case, the confounding influences of other P450 enzymes on carbon monoxide binding and inhibitor metabolism are not present. These methods were used by Kunze and Trager to estimate the partition ratio of furafylline for P450 1A2 inactivation [33]. The obvious drawback to this approach is that it is necessary to have a method to quantitate all of the products formed (radio label or synthetic standards). Therefore, in the absence of a radiolabel or metabolite standard(s), the titration method is often used to estimate the partition ratio.

Predicting *In Vivo* Cytochrome P450 Mechanism-Based Inhibition

The accurate *in vivo* extrapolation of irreversible (MBI) inhibition based on *in vitro* DDI data requires two key elements; the ability to differentiate reversible from irreversible inhibition (MBI) and, thereafter, to correctly express the impact of the irreversible mechanisms *in vivo*. In practice, MBI is the result of a chemical transformation of an inhibitor to an intermediate that irreversibly binds to and inactivates the P450 prior to exiting the active site [112]. The impact of this mechanism is distinct from competitive inhibition. Foremost, when a competitive inhibitor is eliminated, the potential for a drug interaction is gone, whereas for MBI, the potential persists well after the compound has been eliminated [113]. This relates to the second difference, which is that the MBI perturbs the steady-state levels of the P450 it inactivates and levels recover only with the natural synthesis rate within the organism [114]. Numerous mechanistic models have been developed to describe this relationship [115–117].

The synergy between in silico and experimental data is enabled by the ability to approximate the expected clinical impact on AUC based on *in vitro* DDI data [118]. The most visible program Simcyp has gained popularity amongst pharmaceutical companies and the FDA (www.simcyp.com). The underlying drug interaction predictions are based on the equations described by Brown et al. [119,120]. The *in vivo* extrapolations can be determined from a variety of *in vitro* systems including human liver microsomes (HLMs), hepatocytes, or recombinant P450 (rP450). The relative activities of the latter system often vary kinetically from HLM and hepatocytes and, therefore, need to be corrected with the use of scaling factors. The intersystem extrapolation factor (ISEF) is used to normalize *in vitro* data generated from rP450s [121]. Simcyp also has the unique ability to represent the patient-variable response to drugs in clinical trials by using Monte Carlo simulations to vary patient demographics, genetics, and physiology to introduce "typical" population variance [122]. Within Simcyp, inhibition and induction parameters can be included with the intrinsic clearance for a given compound to predict its *in vivo* exposure. One area of interest regarding the predictive capacity of Simcyp is the consistent overprediction of the Rss (AUC change due to the addition of inhibitor) for inhibitors that proceed through mechanism-based inhibition. This overprediction could be due to variability in the k_{degrad} rate constants reported for various P450 isoforms. Most commonly, the data from *in vitro* human hepatocytes as well as the data generated from rats *in vivo* are used despite their disparate half-lives, 14–44 hours, respectively. Experimental evidence suggests the homeostasis of a hepatocyte is disrupted precluding the accurate half-life determination of P450 enzymes within *in vitro* experiments [114], while the rat determined values clearly have limited human physiological relevance. Despite the k_{degrad} being an attractive target for potential error in Rss estimates, it must be tempered with the potential error associated with the additional *in vitro* measurements that are used in predicting the *in vivo* clearance; thus, any combination of inaccurate *in vitro* data could skew the Rss predictions. As computational tools like Simcyp become more commonly used for predicting DDI, the predictive limitations will be more readily identified, leading to improved strategies for *in vitro* to *in vivo* predictions of drug pharmacokinetics and possible MBI-based DDIs.

Conclusion

Mechanism-based inhibition of cytochrome P450 enzyme activity is an important factor in clinically relevant DDIs. Over the past 30 years, our knowledge of the structure and associated chemistry of P450 mechanism-based inhibition has increased immensely. Our ability to elucidate the nature of MBI and potentially avoid key structural drug features in drug candidate selection. Moreover, the magnitude of P450 MBI is now predictable in a manner that patient risk for serious DDIs is minimized.

REFERENCES

1. Wienkers LC, Heath TG. Predicting *in vivo* drug interactions from *in vitro* drug discovery data. *Nat Rev Drug Discov* 2005; 4:825–833.
2. Evans DC, Watt AP, Nicoll-Griffith DA, Baillie TA. Drug-protein adducts: An industry perspective on minimizing the potential for drug bioactivation in drug discovery and development. *Chem Res Toxicol* 2004; 17.3–16.
3. Kent UM, Juschyshyn MI, Hollenberg PF. Mechanism-based inactivators as probes of cytochrome P450 structure and function. *Curr Drug Metab* 2001; 2:215–243.
4. Kalgutkar AS, Obach RS, Maurer TS. Mechanism-based inactivation of cytochrome P450 enzymes: Chemical mechanisms, structure-activity relationships and relationship to clinical drug-drug interactions and idiosyncratic adverse drug reactions. *Curr Drug Metab* 2007; 8:407–447.
5. Polasek TM, Elliot DJ, Lewis BC, Miners JO. Mechanism-based inactivation of human cytochrome P4502C8 by drugs *in vitro*. *J Pharmacol Exp Ther* 2004; 311:996–1007.
6. Ito K, Ogihara K, Kanamitsu S, Itoh T. Prediction of the *in vivo* interaction between midazolam and macrolides based on *in vitro* studies using human liver microsomes. *Drug Metab Dispos* 2003; 31:945–954.
7. Yamazaki H, Shimada T. Comparative studies of *in vitro* inhibition of cytochrome P450 3A4dependent testosterone 6beta-hydroxylation by roxithromycin and its metabolites, troleandomycin, and erythromycin. *Drug Metab Dispos* 1998; 26:1053–1057.
8. Murray M, Murray K. Mechanism-based inhibition of CYP activities in rat liver by fluoxetine and structurally similar alkylamines. *Xenobiotica* 2003; 33:973–987.
9. Hara Y, Nakajima M, Miyamoto KI, Yokoi T. Inhibitory effects of psychotropic drugs onmexiletine metabolism in human liver microsomes: Prediction of *in vivo* drug interactions. *Xenobiotica* 2005; 35:549–560.
10. von Moltke LL, Durol AL, Duan SX, Greenblatt DJ. Potent mechanism-based inhibition of human CYP3A *in vitro* by amprenavir and ritonavir: Comparison with ketoconazole. *Eur J Clin Pharmacol* 2000; 56:259–261.
11. Voorman RL, Maio SM, Payne NA, Zhao Z, Koeplinger KA, Wang X. Microsomal metabolism of delavirdine: Evidence for mechanism-based inactivation of human cytochrome P450 3A. *J Pharmacol Exp Ther* 1998; 287:381–388.
12. Jones DR, Gorski JC, Hamman MA, Mayhew BS, Rider S, Hall SD. Diltiazem inhibition of cytochrome P-450 3A activity is due to metabolite intermediate complex formation. *J Pharmacol Exp Ther* 1999; 290:1116–1125.
13. Wang YH, Jones DR, Hall SD. Differential mechanism-based inhibition of CYP3A4 andCYP3A5 by verapamil. *Drug Metab Dispos* 2005; 33:664–671.
14. O'Donnell JP, Dalvie DK, Kalgutkar AS, Obach RS. Mechanism-based inactivation of human recombinant P450 2C9 by the nonsteroidal anti-inflammatory drug suprofen. *Drug Metab Dispos* 2003; 31:1369–1377.
15. Lu P, Schrag ML, Slaughter DE, Raab CE, Shou M, Rodrigues AD. Mechanism-based inhibition of human liver microsomal cytochrome P450 1A2 by zileuton, a 5-lipoxygenase inhibitor. *Drug Metab Dispos* 2003; 31:1352–1360.
16. Guengerich FP. Mechanism-based inactivation of human liver microsomal cytochrome P-450 IIIA4 by gestodene. *Chem Res Toxicol* 1990; 3:363–371.
17. Baer BR, Wienkers LC, Rock DA. Time-dependent inactivation of P450 3A4 by raloxifene: Identification of Cys239 as the site of apoprotein alkylation. *Chem Res Toxicol* 2007; 20:954–964.
18. Van LM, Swales J, Hammond C, Wilson C, Hargreaves JA, Rostami-Hodjegan A. Kinetics of the time-dependent inactivation of CYP2D6 in cryopreserved human hepatocytes by methylenedioxymethamphetamine (MDMA). *Eur J Pharm Sci* 2007; 31:53–61.
19. Zhao XJ, Jones DR, Wang YH, Grimm SW, Hall SD. Reversible and irreversible inhibition ofCYP3A enzymes by tamoxifen and metabolites. *Xenobiotica* 2002; 32:863–878.

20. Hanioka N, Ozawa S, Jinno H,,o M, Saito Y, Sawada J. Human liver UDP-glucuronosyltransferase isoforms involved in the glucuronidation of 7-ethyl-10-hydroxycamptothecin. *Xenobiotica* 2001; 31: 687–699.

21. Crowley JR, Hollenberg PF. Mechanism-based inactivation of rat liver cytochrome P4502B1 byphencyclidine and its oxidative product, the iminium ion. *Drug Metab Dispos* 1995; 23:786–793.

22. He K, Iyer KR, Hayes RN, Sinz MW, Woolf TF, Hollenberg PF. Inactivation of cytochrome P450 3A4 by bergamottin, a component of grapefruit juice. *Chem Res Toxicol* 1998; 11:252–259.

23. Chan WK, Delucchi AB. Resveratrol, a red wine constituent, is a mechanism-based inactivator of cytochrome P450 3A4. *Life Sci* 2000; 67:3103–3112.

24. Koenigs LL, Trager WF. Mechanism-based inactivation of cytochrome P450 2B1 by8-methoxypsoralen and several other furanocoumarins. *Biochemistry* 1998; 37:13184–13193.

25. Bertz RJ, Granneman GR. Use of *in vitro* and *in vivo* data to estimate the likelihood of metabolic pharmacokinetic interactions. *Clin Pharmacokinet* 1997; 32:210–258.

26. Bjornsson TD, Callaghan JT, Einolf HJ, Fischer V, Gan L, Grimm S, Kao J et al. The conduct of *in vitro* and *in vivo* drug-drug interaction studies: A PhRMA perspective. *J Clin Pharmacol* 2003; 43:443–469.

27. Walsh CT. Suicide substrates, mechanism-based enzyme inactivators: Recent developments. *Annu Rev Biochem* 1984; 53:493–535.

28. Shannon P, Marcotte P, Coppersmith S, Walsh C. Studies with mechanism-based inactivators of lysine epsilon-transaminase from Achromobacter liquidum. *Biochemistry* 1979; 18:3917–3920.

29. Walsh C. Suicide substrates: Mechanism-based inactivators of specific target enzymes. *MolBiol Biochem Biophys* 1980; 32:62–77.

30. Wang EA, Kallen R, Walsh C. Mechanism-based inactivation of serine transhydroxymethylases by D-fluoroalanine and related amino acids. *J Biol Chem* 1981; 256:6917–6926.

31. Desta Z, Ward BA, Soukhova NV, Flockhart DA. Comprehensive evaluation of tamoxifen sequential biotransformation by the human cytochrome P450 system *in vitro*: Prominent roles for CYP3A and CYP2D6. *J Pharmacol Exp Ther* 2004; 310:1062–1075.

32. Pearson JT, Wahlstrom JL, Dickmann LJ, Kumar S, Halpert JR, Wienkers LC, Foti RS, Rock DA. Differential time-dependent inactivation of P450 3A4 and P450 3A5 by raloxifene: A key role for C239 in quenching reactive intermediates. *Chem Res Toxicol* 2007; 20:1778–1786.

33. Kunze KL, Trager WF. Isoform-selective mechanism-based inhibition of human cytochromeP450 1A2 by furafylline. *Chem Res Toxicol* 1993; 6:649–656.

34. Hutzler JM, Steenwyk RC, Smith EB, Walker GS, Wienkers LC. Mechanism-based inactivation of cytochrome P450 2D6 by 1-[(2-ethyl-4-methyl-1H-imidazol-5-yl)methyl]-4[4-(trifluoromethyl)-2-pyridinyl]-piperazine: Kinetic characterization and evidence for apoprotein adduction. *Chem Res Toxicol* 2004; 17:174–184.

35. Kouzi SA, McMurtry RJ, Nelson SD. Hepatotoxicity of germander (Teucrium chamaedrys L.) and one of its constituent neoclerodane diterpenes teucrin A in the mouse. *Chem Res Toxicol* 1994; 7:850–856.

36. Sahali-Sahly Y, Balani SK, Lin JH, Baillie TA. *In vitro* studies on the metabolic activation of the furanopyridine L-754,394, a highly potent and selective mechanism-based inhibitor of cytochrome P450 3A4. *Chem Res Toxicol* 1996; 9:1007–1012.

37. Khojasteh-Bakht SC, Chen W, Koenigs LL, Peter RM, Nelson SD. Metabolism of (R)-(þ)pulegone and (R)-(þ)-menthofuran by human liver cytochrome P-450s: Evidence for formation of a furan epoxide. *Drug Metab Dispos* 1999; 27:574–580.

38. Chen LJ, Hecht SS, Peterson LA. Characterization of amino acid and glutathione adducts ofcis-2-butene-1,4-dial, a reactive metabolite of furan. *Chem Res Toxicol* 1997; 10:866–874.

39. Lopez-Garcia MP, Dansette PM, Mansuy D. Thiophene derivatives as new mechanism-based inhibitors of cytochromes P-450: Inactivation of yeast-expressed human liver cytochrome P450 2C9 by tienilic acid. *Biochemistry* 1994; 33:166–175.

40. Dansette PM, Bertho G, Mansuy D. First evidence that cytochrome P450 may catalyze both S-oxidation and epoxidation of thiophene derivatives. *Biochem Biophys Res Commun* 2005; 338:450–455.

41. Dickins M, Elcombe CR, Moloney SJ, Netter KJ, Bridges JW. Further studies on the dissociation of the isosafrole metabolite-cytochrome P-450 complex. *Biochem Pharmacol* 1979; 28:231–238.

42. Ullrich V, Schnabel KH. Formation and binding of carbanions by cytochrome P-450 of livermicrosomes. *Drug Metab Dispos* 1973; 1:176–183.

43. Lin HL, Hollenberg PF. The inactivation of cytochrome P450 3A5 by 17alphaethynylestradiol is cytochrome b5-dependent: Metabolic activation of the ethynyl moiety leads to the formation of glutathione conjugates, a heme adduct, and covalent binding to the apoprotein. *J Pharmacol Exp Ther* 2007; 321:276–287.

44. Yukinaga H, Takami T, Shioyama SH, Tozuka Z, Masumoto H, Okazaki O, Sudo K. Identification of cytochrome P450 3A4 modification site with reactive metabolite using linear ion trap-Fourier transform mass spectrometry. *Chem Res Toxicol* 2007; 20:1373–1378.

45. Ortiz de Montellano PR, Kunze KL, Yost GS, Mico BA. Self-catalyzed destruction of cytochrome P-450: Covalent binding of ethynyl sterols to prosthetic heme. *Proc Natl Acad Sci USA* 1979; 76:746–749.

46. Reilly PE, Gomi RJ, Mason SR. Mechanism-based inhibition of rat liver microsomal diazepam C3 hydroxylase by mifepristone associated with loss of spectrally detectable cytochrome P450. *Chem Biol Interact* 1999; 118:39–49.

47. De Matteis F, Sparks RG. Iron-dependent loss of liver cytochrome P-450 haem *in vivo* and *in vitro*. *FEBS Lett* 1973; 29:141–144.

48. Correia MA, Farrell GC, Olson S, Wong JS, Schmid R, Ortiz de Montellano PR, Beilan HS, Kunze KL, Mico BA. Cytochrome P-450 heme moiety. The specific target in drug-induced heme alkylation. *J Biol Chem* 1981; 256:5466–5470.

49. Karuzina II and Archakov AI. The oxidative inactivation of cytochrome P450 inmonooxygenase reactions. *Free Radic Biol Med* 1994; 16:73–97.

50. Karuzina II, Zgoda VG, Kuznetsova GP, Samenkova NF, Archakov AI. Heme and apoprotein modification of cytochrome P450 2B4 during its oxidative inactivation in monooxygenase reconstituted system. *Free Radic Biol Med* 1999; 26:620–632.

51. Barr DP, Mason RP. Mechanism of radical production from the reaction of cytochrome c with organic hydroperoxides. An ESR spin trapping investigation. *J Biol Chem* 1995; 270: 12709–12716.

52. Baillie TA. Future of toxicology-metabolic activation and drug design: Challenges and opportunities in chemical toxicology. *Chem Res Toxicol* 2006; 19:889–893.

53. Williams DP, Antoine DJ, Butler PJ, Jones R, Randle L, Payne A, Howard M, Gardner I, Blagg J, Park BK. The metabolism and toxicity of furosemide in the Wistar rat and CD-1 mouse: A chemical and biochemical definition of the toxicophore. *J Pharmacol Exp Ther* 2007; 322:1208–1220.

54. Buckpitt AR, Bahnson LS, Franklin RB. Hepatic and pulmonary microsomal metabolism of naphthalene to glutathione adducts: Factors affecting the relative rates of conjugate formation. *J Pharmacol Exp Ther* 1984; 231:291–300.

55. Buckpitt AR, Warren DL. Evidence for hepatic formation, export and covalent binding of reactive naphthalene metabolites in extrahepatic tissues *in vivo*. *J Pharmacol Exp Ther* 1983; 225:8–16.

56. Kent UM, Bend JR, Chamberlin BA, Gage DA, Hollenberg PF. Mechanism-based inactivation of cytochrome P450 2B1 by *N*-benzyl-1-aminobenzotriazole. *Chem Res Toxicol* 1997; 10:600–608.

57. Bateman KP, Baker J, Wilke M, Lee J, Leriche T, Seto C, Day S, Chauret N, Ouellet M, Nicoll-Griffith DA. Detection of covalent adducts to cytochrome P450 3A4 using liquid chromatography mass spectrometry. *Chem Res Toxicol* 2004; 17:1356–1361.

58. Regal KA, Schrag ML, Kent UM, Wienkers LC, Hollenberg PF. Mechanism-based inactivation of cytochrome P450 2B1 by 7-ethynylcoumarin: Verification of apo-P450 adduction by electrospray ion trap mass spectrometry. *Chem Res Toxicol* 2000; 13:262–270.

59. Liu H, Liu J, van Breemen RB, Thatcher GR, Bolton JL. Bioactivation of the selective estrogen receptor modulator desmethylated arzoxifene to quinoids: 4'-fluoro substitution prevents quinoid formation. *Chem Res Toxicol* 2005; 18:162–173.

60. Kent UM, Lin HL, Mills DE, Regal KA, Hollenberg PF. Identification of 17-alphaethynylestradiol-modified active site peptides and glutathione conjugates formed during metabolism and inactivation of P450s 2B1 and 2B6. *Chem Res Toxicol* 2006; 19:279–287.

61. Kent UM, Mills DE, Rajnarayanan RV, Alworth WL, Hollenberg PF. Effect of 17-alphaethynylestradiol on activities of cytochrome P450 2B (P450 2B) enzymes: Characterization of inactivation of P450s 2B1 and 2B6 and identification of metabolites. *J Pharmacol Exp Ther* 2002; 300:549–558.

62. Melet A, Assrir N, Jean P, Pilar Lopez-Garcia M, Marques-Soares C, Jaouen M, Dansette PM, Sari MA, Mansuy D. Substrate selectivity of human cytochrome P450 2C9: Importance of residues 476, 365, and 114 in recognition of diclofenac and sulfaphenazole and in mechanism based inactivation by tienilic acid. *Arch Biochem Biophys* 2003; 409:80–91.

63. Skiles GL, Yost GS. Mechanistic studies on the cytochrome P450-catalyzed dehydrogenation of 3-methylindole. *Chem Res Toxicol* 1996; 9:291–297.
64. Dooley GP, Prenni JE, Prentiss PL, Cranmer BK, Andersen ME, Tessari JD. Identification of a novel hemoglobin adduct in Sprague Dawley rats exposed to atrazine. *Chem Res Toxicol* 2006; 19:692–700.
65. Guengerich FP, Arneson KO, Williams KM, Deng Z, Harris TM. Reaction of aflatoxin B(1) oxidation products with lysine. *Chem Res Toxicol* 2002; 15:780–792.
66. Lightning LK, Jones JP, Friedberg T, Pritchard MP, Shou M, Rushmore TH, Trager WF.Mechanism-based inactivation of cytochrome P450 3A4 by L-754,394. *Biochemistry* 2000; 39:4276–4287.
67. Koenigs LL, Peter RM, Hunter AP, Haining RL, Rettie AE, Friedberg T, Pritchard MP, Shou M, Rushmore TH, Trager WF. Electrospray ionization mass spectrometric analysis of intact cytochrome P450: Identification of tienilic acid adducts to P450 2C9. *Biochemistry* 1999; 38:2312–2319.
68. Wen B, Lampe JN, Roberts AG, Atkins WM, David Rodrigues A, Nelson SD. Cysteine 98 inCYP3A4 contributes to conformational integrity required for P450 interaction with CYP reductase. *Arch Biochem Biophys* 2006; 454:42–54.
69. Gartner CA, Wen B, Wan J, Becker RS, Jones G, 2nd, Gygi SP, Nelson SD. Photochromic agents as tools for protein structure study: Lapachenole is a photoaffinity ligand of cytochrome P450 3A4. *Biochemistry* 2005; 44:1846–1855.
70. Liu J, Li Q, Yang X, van Breemen RB, Bolton JL, Thatcher GR. Analysis of protein covalent modification by xenobiotics using a covert oxidatively activated tag: Raloxifene proof-of principle study. *Chem Res Toxicol* 2005; 18:1485–1496.
71. Wang J, Bauman S, Colman RF. Photoaffinity labeling of rat liver glutathione S-transferase,4-4, by glutathionyl S-[4-(succinimidyl)-benzophenone]. *Biochemistry* 1998; 37:15671–15679.
72. Tessier S, Boivin S, Aubin J, Lampron P, Detheux M, Fournier A. Transmembrane domain V of the endothelin-A receptor is a binding domain of ETA-selective TTA-386-derived photoprobes. *Biochemistry* 2005; 44:7844–7854.
73. Swanson RA, Dus KM. Specific covalent labeling of cytochrome P-450CAM with 1-(4azidophenyl)imidazole, an inhibitor-derived photoaffinity probe for P-450 heme proteins. *J Biol Chem* 1979; 254:7238–7246.
74. Williams PA, Cosme J, Vinkovic DM, Ward A, Angove HC, Day PJ, Vonrhein C, Tickle IJ, Jhoti H. Crystal structures of human cytochrome P450 3A4 bound to metyrapone and progesterone. *Science* 2004; 305:683–686.
75. Paul H, Illing A, Netter KJ. The effects of sulphydryl reagents on the binding and mixed function oxidation of hexobarbital in rat hepatic microsomes. *Xenobiotica* 1975; 5:1–15.
76. Hodgson E, Casida JE. Biological oxidation of *N, N*-dialkyl carbamates. *Biochim BiophysActa* 1960; 42:184–186.
77. Hodgson E, Casida JE. Metabolism of *N:N*-dialkyl carbamates and related compounds by rat liver. *Biochem Pharmacol* 1961; 8:179–191.
78. Casida JE, Engel JL, Essac EG, Kamienski FX and Kuwatsuka S. Methylene-C14dioxyphenyl compounds: Metabolism in relation to their synergistic action. *Science* 1966; 153:1130–1133.
79. Kamienski FX, Casida JE. Importance of demethylenation in the metabolism *in vivo* and in *vitro* of methylenedioxyphenyl synergists and related compounds in mammals. *Biochem Pharmacol* 1970; 19:91–112.
80. Hodgson E, Philpot RM. Interaction of methylenedioxyphenyl (1,3-benzodioxole) compounds with enzymes and their effects on mammals. *Drug Metab Rev* 1974; 3:231–301.
81. Wilkinson GR, Way EL. Sub-microgram estimation of morphine in biological fluids by gas liquid chromatography. *Biochem Pharmacol* 1969; 18:1435–1439.
82. Schenkman JB, Ball JA, Estabrook RW. On the use of nicotinamide in assays for microsomal mixed-function oxidase activity. *Biochem Pharmacol* 1967; 16:1071–1081.
83. Casida JE. Mixed-function oxidase involvement in the biochemistry of insecticide synergists. *J Agric Food Chem* 1970; 18:753–772.
84. Franklin MR. The enzymic formation of methylenedioxyphenyl derivative exhibiting anisocyanide-like spectrum with reduced cytochrome P-450 in hepatic microsomes. *Xenobiotica* 1971; 1:581–591.
85. Philpot RM, Hodgson E. A cytochrome P-450-piperonyl butoxide spectrum similar to that produced by ethyl isocyanide. *Life Sci* II 1971; 10:503–512.

86. Philpot RM, Hodgson E. The production and modification of cytochrome P-450 difference spectra by *in vivo* administration of methylenedioxyphenyl compounds. *Chem Biol Interact* 1972; 4:185–194.

87. Hansch C. The use of homolytic, steric, and hydrophobic constants in a structure-activity study of 1,3-benzodioxole synergists. *J Med Chem 1968*; 11:920–924.

88. Ullrich V, Schnabel KH. Formation and ligand binding of the fluorenyl carbanion by hepatic cytochrome P-450. *Arch Biochem Biophys* 1973; 159:240–248.

89. Yu LS, Wilkinson CF, Anders MW. Generation of carbon monoxide during the microsomal metabolism of methylenedioxyphenyl compounds. *Biochem Pharmacol* 1980; 29:1113–1122.

90. Anders MW, Sunram JM, Wilkinson CF. Mechanism of the metabolism of 1,3-benzodioxolesto carbon monoxide. *Biochem Pharmacol* 1984; 33:577–580.

91. Dahl AR, Brezinski DA. Inhibition of rabbit nasal and hepatic cytochrome P-450-dependenthexamethylphosphoramide (HMPA) N-demethylase by methylenedioxyphenyl compounds. *Biochem Pharmacol* 1985; 34:631–636.

92. Cook L, Navis G, Fellows EJ. Enhancement of the action of certain analgetic drugs by beta diethylaminoethyl diphenyl-propylacetate hydrochloride. *J Pharmacol Exp Ther* 1954; 112:473–479.

93. Cook L, Macko E, Fellows EJ. The effect of beta-diethylaminoethyldiphenyl-propylacetatehydrochloride on the action of a series of barbiturates and C.N.S. depressants. *J Pharmacol Exp Ther* 1954; 112:382–386.

94. Jonsson KH, Lindeke B. Cytochrome P-455 nm complex formation in the metabolism of phenylalkylamines. XII. Enantioselectivity and temperature dependence in microsomes and reconstituted cytochrome P-450 systems from rat liver. *Chirality* 1992; 4:469–477.

95. Axelrod J, Reichenthal J, Brodie BB. Mechanism of the potentiating action of betadiethylaminoethyl diphenylpropylacetate. *J Pharmacol Exp Ther* 1954; 112:49–54.

96. Cooper JR, Axelrod J, Brodie BB. Inhibitory effects of beta-diethylaminoethyl diphenylpropylacetate on a variety of drug metabolic pathways *in vitro*. *J Pharmacol Exp Ther* 1954; 112:55–63.

97. Castro JA, Sasame HA, Sussman H, Gillette JR. Diverse effects of SKF 525-A and antioxidants on carbon tetrachloride-induced changes in liver microsomal P-450 content and ethyl morphine metabolism. *Life Sci* 1968; 7:129–136.

98. Schenkman JB, Wilson BJ, Cinti DL. Dimethylaminoethyl 2,2-diphenylvalerate HCl (SKF525-A)– *in vivo* and *in vitro* effects of metabolism by rat liver microsomes–formation of an oxygenated complex. *Biochem Pharmacol* 1972; 21:2373–2383.

99. Werringloer J, Estabrook RW. Evidence for an inhibitory product-cytochrome P-450 complex generated during benzphetamine metabolism by liver microsomes. *Life Sci* 1973; 13:1319–1330.

100. Mansuy D, Beaune P, Chottard JC, Bartoli JF, Gans P. The nature of the "455 nm absorbing complex" formed during the cytochrome P450 dependent oxidative metabolism of amphetamine. *Biochem Pharmacol* 1976; 25:609–612.

101. Franklin MR. The influence of cytochrome P-450 induction on the metabolic formation of455-NM complexes from amphetamines. *Drug Metab Dispos* 1974; 2:321–326.

102. Mansuy D, Rouer E, Bacot C, Gans P, Chottard JC, Leroux JP. Interaction of aliphaticN-hydroxylamines with microsomal cytochrome P450: Nature of the different derived complexes and inhibitory effects on monoxygenases activities. *Biochem Pharmacol* 1978; 27:1129–1137.

103. Hines RN, Prough RA. The characterization of an inhibitory complex formed with cytochromeP-450 and a metabolite of 1,1-disubstituted hydrazines. *J Pharmacol Exp Ther* 1980; 214:80–86.

104. Kutt H, Brennan R, Dehejia H, Verebely K. Diphenylhydantoin intoxication. A complication of isoniazid therapy. *Am Rev Respir Dis* 1970; 101:377–384.

105. Muakkassah SF, Yang WC. Mechanism of the inhibitory action of phenelzine on microsomal drug metabolism. *J Pharmacol Exp Ther* 1981; 219:147–155.

106. Muakkassah SF, Bidlack WR, Yang WC. Reversal of the effects of isoniazid on hepaticcyto chrome P-450 by potassium ferricyanide. *Biochem Pharmacol* 1982; 31:249–251.

107. Wang YH, Jones DR, Hall SD. Prediction of cytochrome P450 3A inhibition by verapamilenantiomers and their metabolites. *Drug Metab Dispos* 2004; 32:259–266.

108. Walsh C, Cromartie T, Marcotte P, Spencer R. Suicide substrates for flavoprotein enzymes. *Methods Enzymol* 1978; 53:437–448.

109. Chiba M, Nishime JA, Lin JH. Potent and selective inactivation of human liver microsomal cytochrome P-450 isoforms by L-754,394, an investigational human immune deficiency virus protease inhibitor. *J Pharmacol Exp Ther* 1995; 275:1527–1534.

110. Jung MJ, Metcalf BW. Catalytic inhibition of gamma-aminobutyric acid—Alpha-ketoglutarate transaminase of bacterial origin by 4-aminohex-5-ynoic acid, a substrate analog. *Biochem Biophys Res Commun* 1975; 67:301–306.
111. Kitz R, Wilson IB. Esters of methane sulfonic acid as irreversible inhibitors of acetylcholinesterase. *J Biol Chem* 1962; 237:3245–3249.
112. Silverman RB. Mechanism-based enzyme inactivators. *Methods Enzymol* 1995; 249:240–283.
113. Waley SG. Kinetics of suicide substrates. Practical procedures for determining parameters. *Biochem J* 1985; 227:843–849.
114. Correia MA. Cytochrome P450 turnover. *Methods Enzymol* 1991; 206:315–325.
115. Waley SG. Kinetics of suicide substrates. *Biochem J* 1980; 185:771–773.
116. Funaki T, Takanohashi Y, Fukazawa H, Kuruma I. Estimation of kinetic parameters in the inactivation of an enzyme by a suicide substrate. *Biochim Biophys Acta* 1991; 1078:43–46.
117. Mayhew BS, Jones DR, Hall SD. An *in vitro* model for predicting *in vivo* inhibition of cytochrome P450 3A4 by metabolic intermediate complex formation. *Drug Metab Dispos* 2000; 28:1031–1037.
118. Rostami-Hodjegan A, Tucker GT. "*In silico*" simulations to assess the "*in vivo*" consequences of "*in vitro*" metabolic drug-drug interactions. *Drug Discov Today Technol* 2004; 1:441–448.
119. Brown HS, Galetin A, Hallifax D, Houston JB. Prediction of *in vivo* drug-drug interactions from *in vitro* data: Factors affecting prototypic drug-drug interactions involving CYP2C9, CYP2D6 and CYP3A4. *Clin Pharmacokinet* 2006; 45:1035–1050.
120. Brown HS, Ito K, Galetin A, Houston JB. Prediction of *in vivo* drug-drug interactions from *invitro* data: Impact of incorporating parallel pathways of drug elimination and inhibitor absorption rate constant. *Br J Clin Pharmacol* 2005; 60:508–518.
121. Proctor NJ, Tucker GT, Rostami-Hodjegan A. Predicting drug clearance from recombinantly expressed CYPs: Intersystem extrapolation factors. *Xenobiotica* 2004; 34:151–178.
122. Howgate EM, Rowland Yeo K, Proctor NJ, Tucker GT, Rostami-Hodjegan A. Prediction of *in vivo* drug clearance from *in vitro* data. I: Impact of inter-individual variability. *Xenobiotica* 2006; 36:473–497.

Section IV

Applications of Metabolism Studies in Drug Discovery and Development

20

Clinical Drug Metabolism

Kirk R. Henne, George R. Tonn, and Bradley K. Wong

CONTENTS

Introduction

Advances in the mechanistic knowledge of drug metabolism enzymology are enabling the early-stage understanding of clearance pathways that can be applied in designing clinical pharmacology programs. Clinical drug metabolism studies provide definitive characterization of the metabolic fate of drug candidates. Frequently, the human absorption, distribution, metabolism, and excretion (ADME) study will be the only clinical study of a New Chemical Entity (NCE) designed specifically to characterize metabolism and disposition. In addition to fulfilling a regulatory requirement for registration of a new drug, a main purpose of these studies is to support qualitative extrapolation of the preclinical animal toxicology results to humans by demonstrating that the metabolites formed by humans are formed also by animals. Until recently, clinical drug metabolism studies have been conducted late in the development timeline; however, a changed regulatory environment and improvements in technology are driving the early conduct of human ADME studies. With the current generation of mass spectrometry instrumentation, it is now possible to routinely profile major metabolites in the earliest first-in-human studies without being limited by method sensitivity. Accelerator mass spectrometry is emerging as an enabling technology for assessing mass balance with very low doses of radioactivity, with potential application in very early, if not the earliest, human trials. This chapter focuses on clinical drug metabolism studies using labeled or unlabeled materials to assess disposition pathways and excretion routes of development-stage candidates.

Evolving Regulatory Environment and Clinical Drug Metabolism

The US Food and Drug Administration (FDA) recently (November 2016) issued a revision of an industry guidance *Safety Testing of Drug Metabolites* that may impact the timing and conduct of human ADME studies (http://www.fda.gov/cder/guidance/index.htm). The FDA guidance defines conditions in which a metabolite will need to undergo additional toxicity evaluation. The regulatory impetus behind it is to understand the specific contribution of metabolites to the toxicity of an investigational drug. The guidance defines a quantitatively "disproportionate metabolite" that may be subject to separate toxicology studies involving administration of the metabolite itself. A key difference in the revised guidance is that it defines disproportionate metabolites as those with steady-state systemic exposure in humans that exceeds 10% of the total drug-related exposure, while the original 2008 version defined these as 10% of parent drug exposure. The guidance provides additional decision criteria for requiring toxicity testing—if the steady-state metabolite exposure in animal studies does not approximate the corresponding exposure in humans, then nonclinical toxicology testing will be needed (Figure 20.1). The type of toxicology studies that are recommended include those conducted for parent drug: general toxicity, genotoxicity, embryo-fetal development, and carcinogenicity. A disproportionate metabolite whose exposure in animals is equal to or higher than in humans would not require further testing to be considered qualified, in-line with current practice. A change from historical practice is that the decision criteria within the guidance does not consider the pharmacological activity of the metabolite, recognizing the potential for toxicities that are mediated by off-target actions of the NCE. It does recognize that separate toxicity testing of certain types of metabolites (ether glucuronides and some phase 2 conjugates) does not add to the understanding of the risk associated with the parent drug. The guidance does not apply to cancer therapies where different risk-benefit considerations apply. In addition, the revised guidance indicates that the requisite data can be modified on a case-by-case basis for NCEs that address serious life-threatening

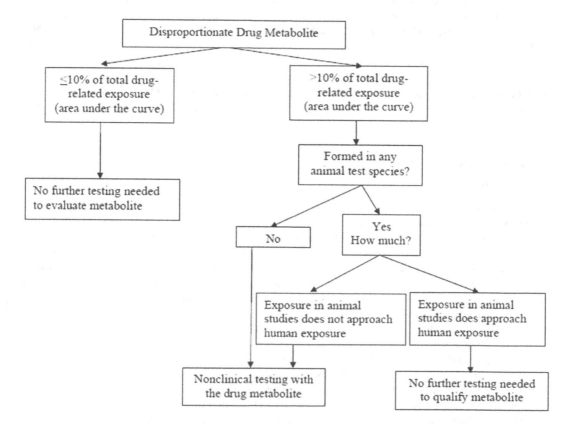

FIGURE 20.1   A decision tree flow diagram from FDA Guidance (2016) *Safety Testing of Drug Metabolites.*

diseases (ALS, stroke, HIV) or provide major beneficial therapeutic advances for unmet medical needs. It should be noted that updated FDA guidelines regarding metabolite safety are generally consistent with those published by other regulatory authorities, namely EMA via ICH guideline M3(R2) (http://www. ema.europa.eu/ema/). Overall, a consequence of implementation of FDA and EMA regulatory guidance is that earlier and more detailed characterization of metabolite exposure in toxicology studies and humans is required.

Extrapolating the toxicological significance of synthetic metabolites to risk assessments of parent drug is complicated by the potential kinetic differences in the behavior of the metabolite after administration of the parent drug and the metabolite itself (Prueksaritanont et al. 2006). Physical properties (e.g., lipophilicity), metabolizing enzyme distribution, and effects of transporters can result in substantially different metabolite concentrations in tissue despite the same systemic exposure. The biological complexity associated with separate administration of metabolites is illustrated by the case of simvastatin, which is administered in its inactive lactone form and undergoes enzymatic and chemical hydrolysis *in vivo* to the pharmacologically active acid metabolite (Prueksaritanont et al. 2006). Administration of the lactone form produces concentrations of the acid metabolite in brain and muscle that are two- to three-fold higher than those achieved after giving the acid itself. This different metabolite pharmacokinetic behavior is attributable to the greater passive permeability and absence of P-gp-mediated efflux, which increases availability of the precursor lactone (Hochman et al. 2004). Interestingly, despite the substantially differing tissue exposures, administration of simvastatin lactone and acid metabolite results in comparable plasma concentrations of the acid metabolite. The evolving regulatory environment that requires the interpretation of metabolite toxicology studies will benefit from research in metabolite pharmacokinetics, animal models of human drug metabolism, and bioanalytical methodology (Espina et al. 2009; Powley et al. 2009; Gao and Obach 2011; Martin et al. 2016).

Impact of FDA Guidance for Industry *Safety Testing of Drug Metabolites* on Clinical Drug Metabolism Studies

Implementation of the FDA *Safety Testing of Drug Metabolites* guidance will affect the timing of preclinical and clinical ADME studies because the potential need for additional toxicology studies of metabolites could delay timelines and require the commitment of additional sponsor resources (Baillie et al. 2002; Smith and Obach 2006). Minimizing the risk of late identification of a disproportionate metabolite would include a full preclinical characterization of metabolites by knowledgeable scientists using modern technologies. These studies will need to be completed well in advance of the initiation of registration-enabling toxicology studies. As the guidance dictates that the metabolite toxicology studies should be conducted to GLP standards, synthetic metabolite material would have to be qualified and bioanalytical methods validated with defined storage conditions for maintaining metabolite integrity (which may differ from those for parent drug). Another implication is that sufficient time must be allowed for follow-up studies that could be required for a proper scientific perspective of the metabolite toxicity evaluations (Prueksaritanont et al. 2006). Assessing total drug-related exposure can be readily achieved with radiolabeleled compounds; however, non-isotopic methods based upon NMR and mass spectrometry can provide fit-for-purpose information before availability of positive clinical data that justifies the investment in radiosynthesis (Espina et al. 2009; Vishwanathan et al. 2009; Gao and Obach 2011). The use of low-dose radioactivity regimens and accelerator mass spectrometric detection to characterize human metabolism and total drug-related exposure during Phase 1 multiple dose studies is one possible means to obtaining steady-state drug metabolism information at the earliest stages of clinical development. As with other issues encountered during the registration process, discussions between the sponsor and agency are a means of arriving at scientific- and technical-based resolution.

Rationale for Conducting Clinical Drug Metabolism Studies Early in the Drug Development Timeline

Changes in regulatory requirements along with significant advances in the molecular understanding of the enzymology related to drug metabolism provide a strong rationale for conducting human drug metabolism studies early in the NCE development timeline. Commercially available, well-characterized human-derived subcellular fractions (microsomes, cytosol), whole cells (hepatocytes) and recombinant enzymes (CYP, UGTs) of documented quality are routinely used to generate human-based metabolites. The availability of highly-specific monoclonal inhibitory CYP antibodies and selective chemical inhibitors used in combination with human hepatic subcellular systems facilitates phenotyping studies that lead to the identification of enzymes involved in metabolic clearance (Mei et al. 1999, 2002). Consequently, by the start of human studies, a reasonable scientific foundation can be available for rational design of clinical pharmacology programs. These data along with information from clinical drug metabolism studies may provide the rationale for the conduct of specific drug-drug interaction studies and the characterization of the pharmacokinetics in special populations. For example, *in vitro* phenotyping studies may implicate a particular CYP isozyme (e.g., 3A4 or 2D6) as a major contributor to the metabolism of an NCE. Early clinical drug metabolism studies showing that elimination of the drug proceeds primarily via these oxidative pathways justifies the early evaluation of co-administration of clinically significant CYP inhibitors (e.g., ketoconazole or quinidine) in drug-drug interaction (DDI) studies. A clinical drug metabolism study suggesting a low risk of DDIs may justify a minimal set of clinical pharmacology studies, while an unfavorable DDI profile could lead to project termination, depending on the risk benefit associated with the therapeutic indication. The benefit of reaching the latter decision before the initiation of large-scale clinical trials is obvious. Conversely, establishing that glucuronidation or renal excretion were quantitatively most important could lead to clinical studies assessing the effect on drug clearance of co-administration of valproic acid (a UGT inhibitor) or of renal impairment (Lin and Wong 2002).

While solid directional data on clearance mechanism(s) is obtained from preclinical animal and *in vitro* studies, an *in vivo* clinical drug metabolism study is needed for definitive characterization of human clearance pathways. This definitive data is usually obtained from a human ADME study conducted with radiolabeled drug. However, evaluation of drug metabolism during early clinical studies (e.g., first-in-human, FIH) conducted with unlabeled material can provide a valuable opportunity to explore human drug disposition. Information regarding circulating levels of key metabolites (major or active), metabolic pathways, and in certain instances, insight into the elimination pathways of an NCE may be obtained from these experiments.

Administration of a radiolabeled drug candidate to human subjects affords a unique opportunity to determine quantitatively the *in vivo* disposition and metabolism of the molecule. When mass balance is achieved, the clearance mechanisms of an NCE can be fully elucidated through characterization of the excretion profile of parent drug and associated metabolites. Routes of clearance determined through the course of a study may validate previous insights made on the basis of *in vitro* human data, pre-clinical interspecies extrapolations, or early clinical metabolism studies conducted without radiolabel. Alternatively, results from the radiolabel study may highlight unforeseen ADME knowledge gaps requiring additional research efforts to support advancement of a potential drug. Efficacy- and safety-related concerns are also addressed in the context of the radiolabel human ADME study, as metabolites present in circulation are identified and quantified in order to evaluate their possible contribution to pharmacological or toxicological effects (in accordance with regulatory guidance). Given the relative ease with which radiolabeled molecules and their metabolites are identified and quantified amidst complex endogenous background components, radioisotopes are an essential tool in the assessment of the *in vivo* fate of drug candidates.

Clinical Drug Metabolism with Non-Radiolabeled Drug

Qualitative Approaches

In the absence of quantitative tools (i.e., radiolabeled material or synthetic standards), useful information regarding *in vivo* metabolic pathways of an NCE can be obtained via qualitative means. Exploratory analysis of human urine or plasma may reveal important details concerning the biotransformation of an investigational drug. Generally, *in vitro* human data provide a framework for conduct of exploratory investigations of urinary or plasma. However, there are cases where *in vitro* data is of limited value due to slow metabolite formation rates and in these instances the detection of key *in vivo* human metabolites may still be feasible. Piperaquine (PQ) is an antimalarial agent initially synthesized in the 1960s. In combination with dihydroartemisinin, use of PQ in malaria treatment recently increased due to its efficacy and tolerability (Davis et al. 2005). Despite PQ's lengthy clinical use, little was known about the biotransformation of this drug in humans. Complicating the study of PQ biotransformation was the low turnover rate in standard *in vitro* systems, resulting in limited formation of metabolites. Following oral administration of PQ (960 mg) to human volunteers, five oxidative metabolites were detected in urine at quantities sufficient to permit structural elucidation by liquid chromatography-mass spectrometry (LC-MS)/MS and NMR analysis (Tarning et al. 2006). Information derived from early studies using unlabeled drug can also identify differences in biotransformation profiles between humans and pre-clinical species. Analysis of urine samples collected from subjects receiving a 1000 mg oral dose of indinavir, an HIV protease inhibitor, revealed the formation of several prominent oxidative metabolites including a novel quaternary *N*-glucuronide (Balani et al. 1995). While good agreement was observed across species (rat, dog, monkey, and human) for oxidative metabolites, the quaternary *N*-glucuronide was observed only in human and non-human primates (Balani et al. 1996; Lin et al. 1996).

When measurement of biliary secretion of parent drug or metabolites is warranted, bile can be collected from either the patients undergoing certain surgical procedures (e.g., cholecystectomy, temporary bile shunts, and nasobiliary drainage) or in healthy subjects using either duodenal perfusion or oroentric tubes (Ghibellini et al. 2006). A recent study applied oroentric tubes to collect bile for the evaluation of metabolites of piperacillin (2 g IV dose) in normal volunteers (Ghibellini et al. 2007). Piperacillin was excreted predominantly into urine, while its metabolites desethylpiperacillin and desethylpiperacillin-glucuronide were excreted predominantly in bile. The glucuronide conjugate of desethylpiperacillin was a novel metabolite not previously described, potentially as a result of hydrolysis by intestinal β-glucuronidases. The bile collection method used involves the oral insertion of a customized multiluminal oroentric tube that is modified for the aspiration of gastric and duodenal contents (Ghibellini et al. 2004). A small balloon is inflated on the distal end of the tube to prevent the loss of biliary secretions into the lower GI tract, which facilitates quantitative bile collections. In addition, administration of cholecystokinin-8 to stimulate gall-bladder contraction enables complete recovery of biliary secretions (Ghibellini et al. 2004). This technique, also used to study biliary disposition of [^{14}C]muraglitazar and metabolites (Wang et al. 2006) and demonstrate low biliary excretion of [^{14}C]apixaban (Raghavan et al. 2009), may provide a less invasive method of bile collection from human volunteers for purposes of clinical drug metabolism studies.

While either duodenal perfusion or oroentric tubes are less invasive than older methods of bile collection and have facilitated bile sampling from human volunteers for purposes of clinical drug metabolism studies, a novel minimally invasive technique utilizing a diagnostic device (Entero-Test™) has recently been reported (Guiney et al. 2011). The device is composed of highly absorbent nylon string encapsulated by a dissolvable gelatin capsule. Once swallowed, the distal end of the string, which is weighed, passes into the duodenum. Bile excretion is stimulated and, following an appropriate period of time, the string is withdrawn via the mouth and the sample is extracted. Metabolites observed following administration of simvastatin using the Entero-Test™ device were consistent with metabolites described in previous *in vitro* and *in vivo* (intubated) experiments. Additionally, a new direct glucuronide conjugate of parent drug was discovered in this study. The technique has been used in subsequent studies coupled with NMR to assess the major metabolic pathways of a novel compound, GSK1325756 (Bloomer et al. 2013). Data showed that the major metabolite excreted in bile was the direct glucuronide conjugate, with only a minor contribution from oxidative metabolism. Human disposition of [^{14}C]GSK1322322 was also evaluated using this technique (Mamaril-Fishman et al. 2014). In this study, the authors observed an *N*-glucuronide as the major metabolite in bile, which was largely absent in feces, suggesting this metabolite was not stable in the GI tract.

Semiquantitative Plasma Analysis for Metabolite Exposure Determination

Regulatory FDA and EMA guidance establish expectations for safety assessment of either human-specific metabolites or "disproportionate" metabolites achieving higher exposures in humans at steady-state than in preclinical toxicology studies (see section "Impact of FDA Guidance for Industry *Safety*

Testing of Drug Metabolites on Clinical Drug Metabolism Studies"). Failure to identify such metabolites early could delay development timelines overall given a potential need to perform additional safety studies to determine the safety profile for the metabolite(s) of concern at established exposures. Common industry practice, therefore, involves semiquantitative analysis of plasma samples generated during first-in-human (FIH) clinical testing from single ascending dose (SAD) and/or multiple ascending dose (MAD) studies to identify human-specific or disproportionate metabolites as soon as feasible. Valuable semiquantitative exposure data is gained by pooling plasma from individual subjects in proportion to sampling time (Hamilton et al. 1981; Riad et al. 1991; Hop et al. 1998) to create a single sample where levels of each component reflect their relative AUC exposures when analyzed, typically by LC-MS. Methodologies have been described (Ma and Chowdhury 2011) in which plasma pools similarly prepared from FIH-enabling (GLP) toxicology studies in rodent and non-rodent species can be analyzed and compared to clinical samples to assess whether exposures in toxicology species are sufficient to qualify metabolite coverage as adequate or insufficient per the regulatory guidance (Figure 20.2). Should insufficient coverage be observed for a metabolite, toxicology studies for that metabolite could be contemplated at an earlier stage. Approaches generally involve either using a normalized matrix (combined human and animal plasma) with appropriate internal standard (Gao et al. 2010), or a calibrated mass spectrometry response factor to account for ionization differences between parent and metabolite(s) if mass spectrometry serves as the analytical platform (Yu et al. 2007; Wright et al. 2009).

Validation of the semiquantitative approach investigating metabolite exposure ratios (i.e., coverage) between preclinical species and human has been demonstrated with SCH-A and its circulating oxidative deamination metabolite, M18, in rabbits (Ma et al. 2010). A validated LC-MS/MS method was first used to quantify SCH-A and M18 employing a standard, quantitative bioanalytical method using authentic standards and calibration curves for each analyte. Exposure multiples for M18 determined at doses of 30, 100, and 300 mg/kg (relative to a 100 mg human dose) were 2.55, 12.4, and 16.6, respectively. Samples pooled using a normalized matrix approach and analyzed by high-resolution MS (HRMS) using the semiquantitative method revealed exposure multiples of 2.70, 12.0, and 16.0, respectively, which were in good agreement (within 10%) compared to the validated bioanalytical method. SCH-A exposure multiples determined by the same two approaches also exhibited good agreement. A second example evaluated SCH-B and its circulating oxidative metabolite, M7, in dogs (Ma et al. 2010). Exposure multiples for M7 determined at doses of 10 and 20 mg/kg (relative to a 100 mg human dose) were 0.703 and 2.36, respectively, using a validated bioanalytical method. Like the standard method, the semiquantitative HRMS pooling approach established sufficient coverage at the higher dose only, with exposure multiples determined to be 0.671 and 2.41 at 10 and 20 mg/kg doses, respectively (within 15% of the values obtained using the fully quantitative method). These examples demonstrate that exposure multiples may be determined using early clinical SAD/MAD samples and multi-dose pre-FIH toxicokinetic samples from preclinical safety species. Accurate evaluation of exposure multiples can be obtained for identified metabolites early in clinical development without the need for synthesized standards and validated assays.

While semiquantitative methods can address metabolite coverage questions for specific metabolites, there may be circumstances where they do not fully inform on the need to perform additional safety studies. As described previously, regulatory guidance provides a threshold (10% of total drug-related material in circulation) below which further evaluation may be unnecessary, even if a metabolite lacks coverage in preclinical safety species. Semiquantitative approaches may identify such a metabolite; however, all circulating drug-related metabolites and parent drug must also be accounted for in order to establish whether the 10% threshold has been exceeded. Though HRMS applications can greatly enhance the likelihood of capturing many drug-related species (Tiller et al. 2008b; Ma and Chowdhury 2011), use of radioisotopes provides a definitive advantage in assuring all drug-related material is characterized and quantified.

With the advent of more sensitive and selective LC/MS systems, earlier clinical metabolism studies utilizing microdosing may be feasible. An investigation comparing plasma metabolites detected following oral nicardipine administration at doses of 20 mg (clinical dose) or 100 µg (microdose) using a randomized cross-over design revealed similar results at both dose levels (Yamane et al. 2009). Based on mass transitions specific to 9 metabolites determined from *in vitro* experiments, 7 metabolites were

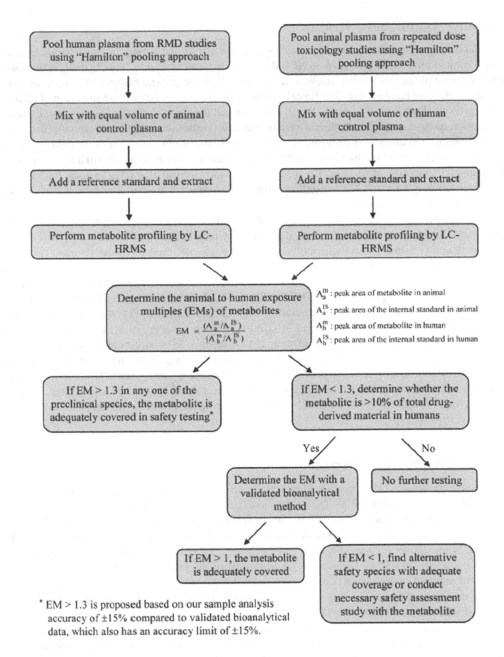

FIGURE 20.2 A schematic diagram for work procedures and proposed decision tree for assessing human metabolite coverage in preclinical safety testing.

observed in plasma collected following the 20 mg dose while 6 metabolites were detected in plasma following the 100 µg dose. One metabolite, with the lowest abundance following administration of the clinical dose, was not observed after microdosing. Moreover, the kinetic profiles of the metabolites detected at both dose levels were comparable as well (based on peak area ratios). As with other qualitative approaches, the mass transitions of putative metabolites must be known *a priori*, unless an HRMS approach is utilized. Nevertheless, as technology continues to improve, this approach may continue to be informative to address specific questions pertaining to clinical drug metabolism prior to the conduct of Phase I experiments.

Quantitative Approaches—Plasma

The availability of synthetic standards of key metabolites allows for a more quantitative understanding of the human biotransformation of an NCE during early clinical studies. Timely data on the role of circulating metabolites can be instrumental in understanding the pharmacological response of a new agent, since active metabolites can significantly impact the intensity, duration, and spectrum of pharmacological activity (Fura 2006). In early clinical development, often the challenge is the lack of definitive data on which to base selection of relevant metabolite(s) to synthesize and measure. *In vitro* data using human-derived tissue, qualitative or semiquantitative metabolite ID from preclinical or clinical studies, or *a priori* knowledge as to the likelihood of pharmacological activity all may inform a decision to synthesize a given metabolite. In addition, the complexity of biotransformation often impacts the ease with which a decision may be made. Circumstances where only a limited number of metabolites are formed make this approach more feasible.

In the case of AMG 487, an investigational CXCR3 inhibitor, analysis of *in vitro* human microsomal and hepatocyte incubations showed that only three primary metabolites were formed: a pyridyl *N*-oxide (M1—major) and two minor metabolites (*O*-deethylated AMG 487 and the *O*-deethylated AMG 487 *N*-oxide). Evaluation of synthetic M1 demonstrated similar potency for CXCR3 inhibition as parent. Quantitation of M1 in human plasma samples collected from FIH studies showed this metabolite circulated at levels 2- to 6-fold greater than AMG 487 (Floren et al. 2003). These data highlighted the need to evaluate both AMG 487 and M1 concentrations to understand the PK/PD of parent, and to ensure the selection of appropriate doses in preclinical safety testing for coverage of M1 concentrations across preclinical species. The latter posed a considerable challenge since M1 concentrations were considerably lower in the species used for safety testing than in humans. Predicting plasma metabolite concentrations based on *in vitro* data is not straightforward. This is because plasma metabolite levels are not only a function of a metabolite's formation rate, but are also determined by its elimination rate, sequential metabolism (i.e., the availability of the metabolite to blood from the site of formation), and its volume of distribution (Houston 1981).

Quantitative Approaches—Excreta

Quantitation of parent and/or metabolites in excreta (urine, bile, feces) provides useful information about the routes of elimination of an NCE. This information can be helpful in designing key clinical experiments (e.g., drug-drug interaction trials or studies in special populations). The contribution of metabolism to the overall elimination of a drug can often be inferred by measuring the excretion of parent drug in the urine. High recovery of parent drug in urine indicates that renal excretion, rather than metabolism and/or biliary secretion pathways (or others), will dominate the elimination of an NCE. The urinary recoveries of atenolol, many cephalosporin antibiotics, hydrochlorothiazide, and lisinopril are >90%, suggesting that biotransformation of these agents plays only a minor role while renal excretion is dominant in their elimination (Benet et al. 1995).

Efforts to determine mass balance of an NCE solely on the basis of parent drug recovery in excreta would be expected to yield incomplete recovery for most drug candidates. Therefore, measuring both parent drug and metabolite(s) in excreta provides considerably more insight as to the elimination routes of an NCE. In the optimal case of quantitative mass balance, a more detailed description of the elimination pathways emerges. This was the case with acetaminophen. Following a 1000 mg oral dose of acetaminophen, essentially complete (100%) recovery was obtained by measurement of the acetaminophen, Phase I oxidative metabolites, and Phase II conjugates (glucuronide, sulfate, and glutathione conjugates) excreted in urine over a 24-hour period (Slattery et al. 1987). In the case of this drug, the complete accounting of the dose was aided by the historical understanding of the major metabolites of this compound and their excretion profile. Unfortunately, quantification of drug-related material using cold assay techniques rarely results in complete recovery; however, important information can still be obtained from early clinical studies. In Phase 1 studies of maribavir, a novel anti-viral agent, less than 2% of the dose was excreted in urine as parent drug, while 30%–40% of the dose was recovered as the corresponding *N*-dealkylated metabolite (Wang et al. 2003). *In vitro*-based phenotyping demonstrated that formation of this *N*-dealkylated metabolite was mediated almost exclusively by CYP3A4 (Koszalka et al. 2002). Despite the incomplete recovery of material in this study, it was clear that CYP3A4-mediated biotransformation contributed significantly to the overall elimination of the drug. Although the exact extent to which the elimination of maribavir was dependent on CYP3A4 could not be determined from these data, prioritization of CYP3A4-oriented drug-drug interaction studies may be warranted based on these data and the intended patient population.

Classically, urinary excretion of parent drug and metabolites has formed the basis of phenotyping humans for polymorphic CYP enzymes. For example, urinary ratios of 4-hydroxydebrisoquine to debrisoquine or dextrorphan to dextromethorphan are often used as a means of determining CYP2D6 phenotype (Chladek et al. 2000; Christensen et al. 2003). In the case of atomoxetine, a blocker of presynaptic norepinephrine transporter, the 4-hydroxyatomoxetine metabolite was shown to result from CYP2D6-mediated biotransformation (Ring et al. 2002). A 90 mg oral dose of atomoxetine was administered to "extensive" and "poor" CYP2D6 metabolizers (EMs and PMs, respectively). In EMs, approximately 60% of the oral dose was recovered in urine over 24 hours as either parent, *N*-desmethylatomoxetine, 4-hydroxyatomoxetine, or the glucuronide conjugate of 4-hydroxyatomoxetine (Mullen et al. 2005). The majority of the dose was recovered as 4-hydroxyatomoxetine (1.2%) and the corresponding glucuronide conjugate (59%), suggesting that oxidative metabolism of atomoxetine to 4-hydroxyatomoxetine was a key elimination pathway for this drug. In PMs, the total recovery was much lower (11%) and the pattern of metabolites recovered was different, as a greater degree of *N*-desmethylatomoxetin formation and excretion of unchanged parent drug was reported (Mullen et al. 2005). The impact of CYP2D6 phenotype on the biotransformation of atomoxetin was confirmed subsequently in a radiolabel mass balance study (Sauer et al. 2003). It is important to note that low recovery of parent and known metabolites may not provide a comprehensive view regarding the disposition of an NCE. Low recovery may be due to incomplete absorption of the compound following oral administration, incomplete understanding of the elimination routes in humans, or drug-related material being excreted in another matrix.

Quantitative Approaches—Fluorine NMR

Fluorine (^{19}F) NMR provides an alternate means for metabolite quantitation without the prerequisite of synthetic reference standards or radiolabeled material. ^{19}F NMR shares some attributes of radiochemical analysis because the method is highly selective for drug-related material due to the low background of endogenous fluorine, and the NMR signal is directly proportional to the number of fluorine nuclei in a molecule (Martino et al. 2005). The large range of chemical shifts and the high sensitivity of the fluorine nuclei to its environment allows for the differentiation of the various chemical species within a biological sample, often without prior chromatographic separation (Bernadou et al. 1985; Martino et al. 2005). Depending on the sample matrix, only limited sample work up is generally required. Exceptions are matrices prone to macromolecular binding (e.g., plasma) and micellar substructures (e.g., bile), which can obscure the NMR signal (Martino et al. 2005). The key limitations of ^{19}F NMR compared to LC-MS/MS and radiochemical techniques are related to access to equipment, lower sensitivity, and increased sample volume. Nevertheless, this technique is very powerful in selected instances for studying clinical drug metabolism.

Using ^{19}F NMR analysis, a total of 8 metabolites were detected in human urine following oral administration of 150 and 800 mg flurbiprofen (Wade et al. 1990). Base hydrolysis abolished the major putative metabolite peaks while increasing those corresponding to parent drug and another metabolite, suggesting that these were acyl glucuronide conjugates. Further characterization of the second metabolite led to its assignment as the glucuronide of 4-hydroxyflurbiprofen. Another case demonstrated the utility of LC-^{19}F/^{1}H NMR-MS to identify a novel metabolite of the experimental reverse transcriptase inhibitor, BW935U83, in human urine (Shockcor et al. 2000). Analysis of urine samples collected following oral administration of a 1000 mg dose detected parent drug, a known glucuronide conjugate, and a second unknown metabolite. This latter metabolite was not detected using LC-MS/MS or ^{1}H NMR methods due to background interference from endogenous components. Subsequent structural characterization using LC-^{19}F/^{1}H NMR coupled with tandem MS analysis identified this metabolite as 3-fluoro-ribolactone, a metabolite believed to be derived from the CYP-mediated cleavage of the nucleoside-sugar bond of the parent molecule (Shockcor et al. 2000). In the presence of a known concentration of standard (e.g., trifluoromethylbenzoic acid, fluoroacetate, trifluoroacetic acid, etc.) quantitation of the ^{19}F signal is also possible (Martino et al. 2005).

Several reports have demonstrated good concordance between ^{14}C and ^{19}F NMR mass balance approaches in non-clinical species (Monteagudo et al. 2007; Mutlib et al. 2012; Hu et al. 2015). A mass balance study of an experimental HIV-1 integrase inhibitor conducted in rats demonstrated comparable total recoveries determined by standard radiometric and ^{19}F NMR methods (Monteagudo et al. 2007). A good correlation was also observed for the recovery in urine and bile of individual metabolite components (e.g., parent, the glucuronide conjugate, and an *N*-demethylated metabolite). The utility of this approach has also been demonstrated in the clinical setting with GSK1325756 (Bloomer et al. 2013). Analysis of human bile using ^{19}F NMR following preparative HPLC was able to demonstrate that an *O*-glucuronide metabolite (M11) was the major metabolite in bile, representing 80% of the drug related material within the sample collected. Additionally, minor metabolites (2%–5%) and unchanged drug (6%) constituted the remainder of the drug related material. The limit of quantitation of the method was 1% of drug related material. Overall, provided the fluorine substituent is metabolically stable within the molecule of interest, ^{19}F NMR represents a useful technique for the quantification of drug metabolites without reference standards or radiolabel. For additional information on this technique the reader is referred to an excellent review describing ^{19}F NMR application to drug disposition (Martino et al. 2005).

Radiolabel Human ADME Study—Background

Exploratory analyses of clinical samples from standard, non-radiolabel Phase I dose escalation studies can provide valuable information about metabolite exposure in certain instances, where *in vivo* metabolism closely follows *in vitro* prediction and is not overly complicated (see section "Clinical Drug Metabolism with Non-Radiolabeled Drug"). In cases where metabolism is not completely understood or may be more extensive *in vivo* than observed *in vitro*, the obvious concern centers around which metabolites are potentially missed in the absence of a detection method specific for exogenous drug-related material. Scenarios involving complex metabolic pathways or unknown clearance mechanisms highlight the value of radiolabel when dosed *in vivo*—radioisotopes can be used to identify and quantify *all* drug-related material without the need for metabolite standards and standard curves. These benefits are brought about by the fact that the decay of a radioactive isotope and the ability to detect and quantitate radiolabeled material is independent of molecular structure. Quantitation of the radioisotope requires only a simple measurement of disintegrations per minute (dpm) by liquid scintillation counting (LSC) and the specific activity of the radiolabel dose, which is known at the outset of the study. Furthermore, given the very low background of naturally-occurring radioisotopes *in vivo*, unchanged drug and its metabolites are readily distinguished from components of the complicated and diverse biological matrices in which they reside.

Drug candidates are most commonly labeled with low-energy radioisotopes of carbon (Carbon-14, ^{14}C) or hydrogen (Tritium, ^{3}H) to enable characterization of their *in vivo* ADME properties in humans (Dain et al. 1994; Roffey et al. 2007), as well as preclinical species (Marathe et al. 2004; Roffey et al. 2007). Between these two radioisotopes, ^{14}C is generally preferred due to its relatively high degree of chemical stability and detection efficiency by standard LSC when compared to ^{3}H. A potential advantage of ^{3}H is the relative ease with which it may be incorporated into an investigational drug; however, the possibility of isotope exchange with water must be carefully investigated through additional experimental efforts (Shaffer and Langer 2007). Whether ^{14}C or ^{3}H is utilized as an isotopic label, specific attention must be paid to placement of the label within the molecule. Incorporation of the label at a position of chemical or metabolic instability that results in the formation of a very low molecular weight entity (i.e., tritiated water, HTO) or volatile entity (i.e., ^{14}CO$_2$) may easily confound interpretation of results or lead to poor radiolabel recovery. At a minimum, it is prudent to utilize *in vitro* cross-species metabolic stability data together with chemical stability information and chemical synthesis feasibility assessments to optimize placement of the radiolabel.

The dosing of radioisotopes to humans is done with the proper oversight with regard to the safety of the study participants. Guidance on the appropriate conduct of studies involving the administration of radiolabeled drugs to humans is set forth by 21 CFR § 361.1, which mandates protocol review by both an FDA-approved Radioactive Drug Research Committee (comprised of a physician specializing in nuclear medicine, a specialist in radiation dosimetry and/or safety, and at least three other medical experts) and an Institutional Review Board. Radiolabel studies are most frequently conducted in healthy volunteers; however, those where narrow therapeutic index agents (i.e., anticancer agents) are administered are generally conducted in patients (Beumer et al. 2006). The amount of radioactivity given to subjects in a single dose must be as low as feasible to achieve study objectives without exceeding 3 rem exposure for whole body, active blood-forming organs, lens of the eye, and gonads; and 5 rem exposure for all other organs. Annually, these limits increase to 5 and 15 rem, respectively, for sponsors planning multiple-dose administration (which is less common than single-dose studies). Exposure to radioactivity in human is estimated by means of a dosimetry experiment using pre-clinical models, most often rat (Dain et al. 1994). In a dosimetry experiment, radioactivity exposure is measured for each tissue type either by direct quantitation in dissected organs (Potchoiba et al. 1998) or whole-body autoradioluminography imaging techniques (Sonada et al. 1983; Potchoiba et al. 1995, 1998; Solon and Kraus 2002; Potchoiba and Nocerini 2004). A survey of major pharmaceutical companies (*circa* 1994) revealed that these guidelines translate to radioisotope doses ranging from 10 to 300 μCi for ^{14}C (100 μCi most commonly) and 50 to 1000 μCi for ^{3}H (Dain et al. 1994). Recently, another survey of industry practices pertaining to conduct of clinical drug metabolism studies (*circa* 2008–2012) was conducted and confirmed these same isotopes are still commonly utilized as other aspects of ADME study design may continue to evolve (Slatter et al. 2014). Administration of a radiolabel dose was most often by the oral route, since the intended clinical route of dosing is oral for most small molecule drugs. Examples of intravenous (IV) (Harrison et al. 1993; Nave et al. 1994; Cocquyt et al. 1999; Vree et al. 1999; Johnson et al. 2003; Hoffmann et al. 2007) and dermal (Weichers et al. 1990) administration are also present in the literature.

Though the data generated from a radiolabel human ADME study are key to understanding human disposition and metabolism of a drug candidate *in vivo*, the investments required to synthesize radiolabeled material and to perform the requisite dosimetry analysis are not trivial. Therefore, the timing of the radiolabel ADME study with respect to development stage may vary depending on the need to address scientific questions early (Phase 1) or the philosophy that the conduct of the study can be performed later (Phase 2). Purely from a scientific perspective, earlier would be ideal in order to utilize ADME data to design the development plan prospectively in terms of clinical DDI studies and metabolite monitoring strategies for toxicology and clinical studies. However, resource limitations or lower confidence in a high risk (i.e., unvalidated) therapeutic target may dictate a later human ADME study (Rohatagi et al. 2004). Naturally, the decision to collect *in vivo* human ADME data later in Phase II carries with it a risk that unexpected findings may arise, resulting in program delays or termination of the candidate after more costly proof-of-concept clinical trials.

Key Deliverables of the Radiolabel Human ADME Study and Examples

Radiolabel human ADME studies provide insight into the disposition and metabolism of a drug candidate in three primary ways: (1) determination of mass balance of the drug and drug-related material; (2) characterization of routes of elimination and clearance mechanisms of the drug; and (3) identification and quantitation of drug metabolites in circulatory and excretory matrices. Each element of the study is discussed in detail in this section with specific examples to highlight both typical findings and unexpected outcomes at the conclusion of the study. Details and recommendations regarding the design and conduct of the studies, with specifics about sample work-up and analysis, are reviewed elsewhere (Rohatagi et al. 2004; Beumer et al. 2006).

Mass Balance

The most straightforward human ADME deliverable is the determination of mass balance. Careful characterization of the dose administered to each subject measured against the total recovery of radioactivity in excretory matrices from each subject determines this outcome. If total recovery approaches or exceeds 85%–90% of dose, the consensus in the ADME discipline would be that mass balance is complete (Sunzel 2004; Rohatagi et al. 2004; Beumer et al. 2006). Celecoxib (Celebrex®), a well-known cyclooxygenase-2 inhibitor, was administered to eight healthy volunteers at a 300 mg dose containing approximately 100 μCi of ^{14}C-labeled drug (Paulson et al. 2000). Total recovery of dose was an acceptable 85%, with 27% excreted in urine and 58% excreted in feces. Profiling of these matrices revealed metabolism as the major clearance route with only three major metabolites. In the case of valdecoxib (Bextra®), a closely related analog with similar pharmacology, a 50 mg dose containing 100 μCi of ^{14}C-labeled drug was administered as a single dose to eight volunteers, and 94% recovery was achieved (76% in urine and 18% in feces). Valdecoxib exhibited more extensive metabolism than celecoxib, with more than 10 metabolites observed; nonetheless, complete recovery was achieved. Therefore, in the absence of other factors, the degree of metabolism is not necessarily a determinant of recovery (note: for valdecoxib the majority of radioactivity in the form of metabolites was excreted in urine). Together, celecoxib and valdecoxib are representative of a large number of human ^{14}C mass balance studies with successful recoveries (Roffey et al. 2007).

Potential reasons for lower recovery in a human radiolabel ADME study include limitations brought about by the excretion profile of the investigational drug and the pharmacology related to the drug and its target. Imatinib (Gleevec®), a tyrosine kinase inhibitor effective in the treatment of certain cancers, was administered at a 200 mg dose (free-base equivalent) containing 32 μCi of ^{14}C drug (Gschwind et al. 2005). Recovery of radiolabeled dose hit a plateau by day 7, and continued collections through day 11 resulted in little additional radioisotope retrieval. At the end of the study, approximately 68% of drug-related material was found in feces and approximately 13% in urine, with total recovery lower than the consensus 85% goal. Investigators hypothesized that recovery was limited by a slow terminal elimination half-life in feces estimated at 3 weeks. A likely driving force behind the prolonged fecal elimination was the concurrent observation that the terminal elimination half-life of radioactivity in plasma was 57 hours, suggesting that excretion would continue via the fecal route for a protracted period. This is consistent with data tabulated from a review of radiolabeled ADME studies that demonstrated an inverse relationship between plasma half-life and recovery of total dose (Roffey et al. 2007). It was shown that compounds exhibiting radioactivity plasma half-lives of <50 hours achieved mass balance (defined as >85% recovery) about 80% of the time, meaning those compounds with radioactivity half-lives in plasma exceeding 50 hours (like imatinib) were much less likely to achieve full recovery.

Aside from technical challenges associated with recovery in the fecal matrix (e.g., inter-subject variability in time course of excretion, high sample mass, sample consistency, etc.), additional reasons cited for low mass balance recoveries were tissue sequestration, phospholipid affinity, and subject compliance. Alendronate (Fosamax®), a bisphosphonate inhibitor of osteoclast-mediated bone resorption used in the treatment of osteoporosis, provides a good example of tissue sequestration limiting recovery of a radiolabeled dose as a result of pharmacology (Cocquyt et al. 1999). Clinically relevant alendronate doses given in animal models revealed unsaturable uptake in bone tissue, the site of action, with estimated elimination half-lives of more than 200 days in rats and 1000 days in dogs (Lin et al. 1991). In these species, approximately half of the administered dose was excreted unchanged in urine. In human, a pharmacokinetic study at a 30 mg/kg IV dose (7.5 mg/day × 4 consecutive days; unlabeled drug) revealed prolonged urinary excretion similar to preclinical species with detectable drug 18 months after dosing (Khan et al. 1997). A follow-on clinical investigation was subsequently carried out in the context of a ^{14}C-ADME study (performed in oncology patients), where a 10 mg IV dose containing 26 μCi ^{14}C-labeled alendronate was administered to 12 patients (Cocquyt et al. 1999). Observations from the earlier pharmacokinetic study were confirmed, as 47% of the radiolabeled dose was recovered in urine within 3 days and negligible dose was excreted in feces. Incomplete recovery was attributed to a high degree of distribution to bone. By way of comparison to alendronate, tigecycline (Tygacil®), a first-in-class glycylcycline antibiotic, distributed extensively to bone in rats after a single IV dose (Tombs 1999). A human tigecycline ADME study was subsequently conducted with a radiolabeled dose (50 μCi IV) administered to six study subjects who had been dosed previously with non-labeled compound to reach steady-state (Hoffmann et al. 2007). In this case, recovery was considered complete (excluding two subjects who had incomplete fecal sample collection), with 92% of total dose excreted predominantly in feces and more sparingly in urine. These findings demonstrate that, in contrast to alendronate, saturable tissue distribution of tigecycline may be overcome by dosing to steady-state prior to administration of the labeled dose in order to improve mass balance recovery.

Molecules that form covalent bonds with their therapeutic target, or other proteins non-specifically, may represent a challenge in terms of definitive mass balance. As a class, thiol-containing angiotensin-converting enzyme (ACE) inhibitors generally exhibit lower recoveries than other non-thiol compounds. The free thiol present in this group of ACE inhibitors binds to the zinc atom at the active site of the enzyme and is important with respect to mechanism of action. However, free thiols also react with sulfur-containing moieties present in other proteins and small molecules, which serves as the basis for concern in terms of recovery of drug-related material. With no requirement for bioactivation processes, the entire dose is available to form disulfide linkages or react with endogenous molecules in other ways (i.e., nucleophilic addition reactions). The investigational drug gemopatrilat, a more recent entry to the thiol-containing ACE inhibitor class, was dosed orally to humans at a dose of 50 mg containing 112 µCi of ^{14}C-labeled drug (Wait et al. 2006). A sustained presence of total radioactivity was observed in plasma (half-life of 85 hours), and only 77% of the administered dose was recovered. Investigators specified that approximately half of the drug-derived radioactivity in circulation was bound via disulfide bonds to protein, as determined by extraction recovery experiments in the presence and absence of reducing equivalents. This was likely the main cause for low recovery of gemopatrilat and was also suspected to limit recovery of omapatrilat (Iyer et al. 2001) and captopril (Capoten®) (Kripalani et al. 1980). In contrast to free thiol-containing pharmaceutical agents, compounds that require metabolic bioactivation to generate thiol-containing metabolites that bind to proteins in circulation (or in tissues) tend to exhibit much higher recoveries. Clopidogrel (Plavix®) is a thienopyridine compound that antagonizes platelet aggregation by means of binding to the platelet P2Y$_{12}$ receptor via disulfide linkage (Savi et al. 2000). Unlike gemopatrilat, clopidogrel requires cytochrome P450 (CYP)-mediated biotransformation to convert the thienopyridine moiety to one exhibiting a free thiol—the active form of the drug (see Figure 20.3). [^{14}C]Clopidogrel human ADME studies were conducted in six healthy volunteers at a dose of 75 mg containing 76 µCi radiolabeled drug (Lins et al. 1999). Despite the established on-mechanism covalent binding to P2Y$_{12}$ receptor (and presumably other circulatory components), mass balance was achieved at a level of 92% of dose, excreted almost equally in urine and feces. Elimination half-life in plasma was a prolonged 338 hours. Prasugrel (Effient®), an irreversible P2Y$_{12}$ inhibitor very similar in nature to clopidogrel, is also essentially a pro-drug that requires both hydrolysis and CYP activity to transform it into a free thiol (Rehmel et al. 2006; Farid et al. 2007). In a study utilizing [^{14}C] prasugrel administered as an oral dose of 15 mg (containing 100 µCi radioactivity), 95% mass balance was achieved with the majority of recovery occurring in urine. Like clopidogrel, a substantial fraction of radioactivity in plasma was covalently bound to protein and the terminal radioactivity half-life in plasma was >180 hours.

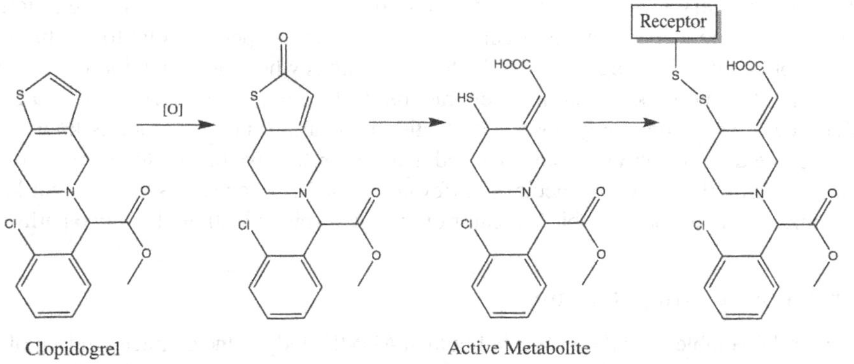

FIGURE 20.3 Metabolism of Clopidogrel to form a thiol-containing active metabolite.

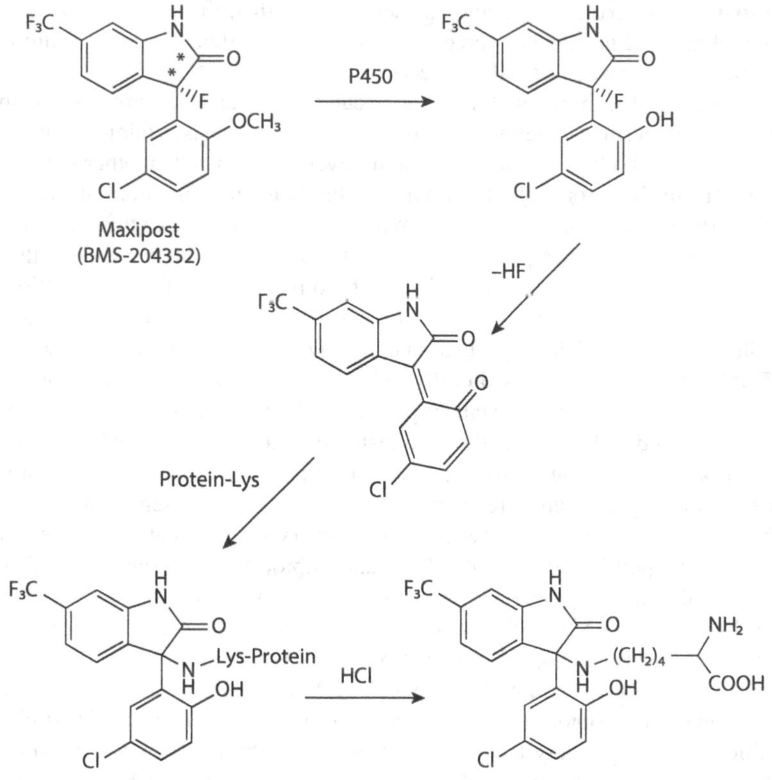

FIGURE 20.4 Metabolism of Maxipost to form a quinone methide metabolite that binds to protein macromolecules.

Aside from thiol-containing compounds, the investigational drug maxipost (BMS-204352) for treatment of ischemic stroke serves as an example of metabolic activation involving covalent bond formation to plasma proteins via a mechanism other than disulfide bond formation. CYP-mediated *O*-demethylation of maxipost forms a phenol that undergoes subsequent CYP-mediated bioactivation to generate a quinone methide, which was shown to bind covalently to macromolecules (Zhang et al. 2003), as depicted in Figure 20.4. IV dosing of maxipost (10 mg) containing 50 μCi ^{14}C-labeled drug resulted in 97% recovery over 14 days (37% in urine and 60% in feces) (Zhang et al. 2005). In this case, significant covalent binding to plasma protein (particularly at later time points) coincided with a terminal plasma half-life in excess of 250 hours, which together did not limit radioactivity excretion to the extent it would cause low mass balance recovery. Overall, compounds that initially contain a protein-reactive functional group (e.g., thiol) tend to stand a poor chance of achieving mass balance, perhaps due to the high fraction of dose available for covalent binding. Conversely, for compounds where bioactivation is a prerequisite for covalent binding, it is more likely that a lower fraction of dose is cleared exclusively via bioactivation and complete recovery is commonly observed. Additional examples of compounds known to undergo bioactivation (and exhibit toxicity) are summarized in a comprehensive review focusing on mass balance outcomes in pre-clinical and human species (Roffey et al. 2007). A consensus view is that low recovery in a mass balance study is not a reliable indicator of an *in vivo* bioactivation clearance pathway.

Characterization of Drug Clearance

A second major deliverable from the radiolabel human ADME study is the characterization of drug clearance. This assessment mainly involves the quantitative determination of whether the administered dose is primarily excreted unchanged, or whether the majority of dose is excreted in the form of metabolites. When metabolism is a primary clearance route, the identity of the metabolites is expected to provide insight into the classes of enzymes responsible. A thorough example of the characterization of metabolic clearance in the design and conduct of a radiolabel human ADME study can be seen with the investigational drug traxoprodil, a potential treatment for the prevention of neuronal death associated with brain injury (Johnson et al. 2003). Typical of CNS drugs, traxoprodil contains a tertiary basic amine as part of a lipophilic scaffold—a common feature in CYP2D6 substrates. In light of this and the inter-subject variability in pharmacokinetic behavior observed during early Phase 1 clinical trials, the investigators chose to examine the role of CYP2D6 in the metabolic clearance of traxoprodil *in vitro* and *in vivo*, enrolling both PM and EM CYP2D6 phenotypes in a ^{14}C ADME study. *In vitro* data showed a relatively low microsomal K_m of 1.7 μM (V_{max} of 0.66 nmol/nmol/min), and confirmation of a major contribution to *in vitro* metabolism by CYP2D6 was made on the basis of correlation analyses, inhibition of microsomal turnover by quinidine, and traxoprodil metabolism by recombinant enzyme. *In vivo* data generated from a single IV infusion of a 50 mg (100 μCi) dose revealed lower mass balance recovery in EM subjects when compared to PM subjects (61% and 89%, respectively), with the majority of drug-related material excreted in urine. Metabolite profiling in urine from PM subjects revealed predominantly parent drug and its direct glucuronide conjugate (M6), while EM subjects displayed only low levels of unchanged parent drug accompanied by two major metabolites (M7 and M14) formed via CYP-mediated oxidation and subsequent Phase II metabolic processes (as shown in Figure 20.5). Plasma and fecal matrices further demonstrated an abundance of Phase I metabolites (and their conjugates) in EMs, while metabolites in PMs arose mainly from Phase II conjugation of traxoprodil itself. Quantitative recovery of individual metabolites as a percentage of dose in EM and PM subjects is summarized in Table 20.1. With regard to persistence of drug in circulation, traxoprodil had a 3-hour half-life in EM subjects and a much longer 27-hour half-life in PM subjects. Interestingly, in EMs, plasma half-life of total radioactivity was estimated to be >140 hours, which by comparison to other previously mentioned examples, may partly explain the low recovery in these subjects. Overall, the results of the *in vivo* study highlighted the role of metabolism in the clearance of traxoprodil, most importantly contributions by CYP2D6 as a key enzyme in the metabolic pathway.

A heavy reliance on any single clearance pathway increases the risk of a pharmacokinetic DDI (Ito et al. 2005). The traxoprodil example further serves to demonstrate the added value of the ^{14}C-ADME study where, in the absence of a specific clinical DDI study, insight may be gained into the potential for a meaningful DDI. As a comparison of the PM and EM data indicated, reduced capacity for CYP2D6-mediated metabolism was directly linked to increased traxoprodil exposure in circulation for the PM subjects (Johnson et al. 2003). Therefore, co-administered agents with a more potent CYP2D6

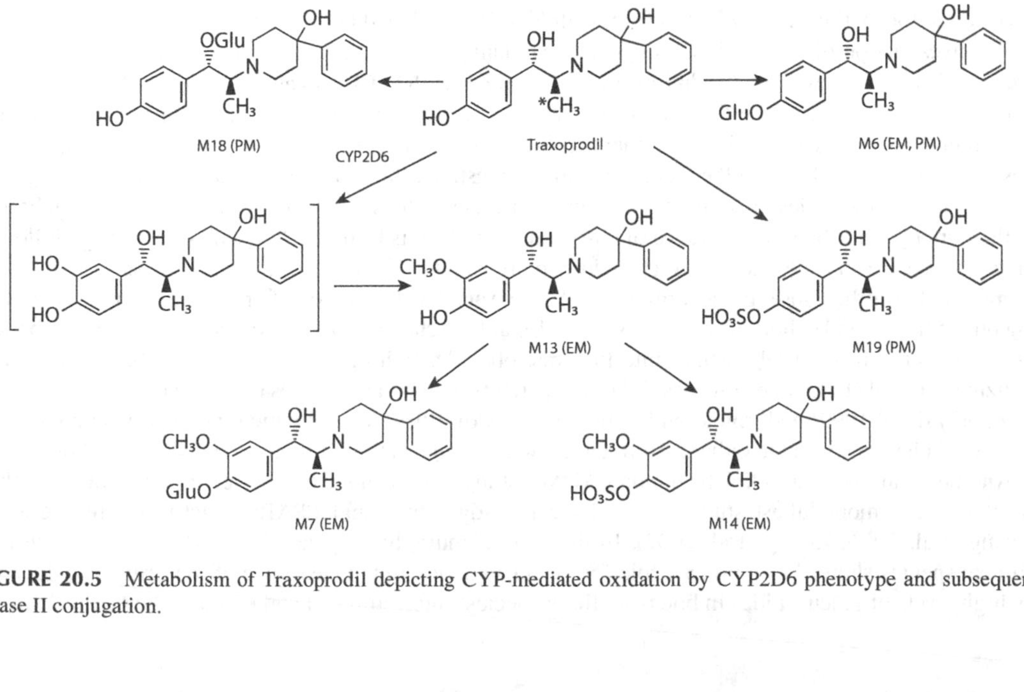

FIGURE 20.5 Metabolism of Traxoprodil depicting CYP-mediated oxidation by CYP2D6 phenotype and subsequent Phase II conjugation.

TABLE 20.1

Mean Recovery of Traxoprodil Metabolites in CYP2D6 Extensive Metabolizer (EM) and Poor Metabolizer (PM) Subjects.

	Mean Recovery (% Administered Dose)	
Component	EM Subjects (n = 4)	PM Subjects (n = 2)
M6	0.68	25
M7	8.8	ND
M13	2.8	ND
M14	39	ND
M18	ND	1.4
M19	ND	12
Traxoprodil	7.1	50

Source: Johnson, K. et al., *Drug Metab. Dispos.*, 31, 76–87, 2003.
ND = Not detected

interaction (with respect to K_m) may be expected to affect traxoprodil exposure similarly. Such data are very valuable in the development process as they are an important factor in assessing the clinical utility of a compound with regard to the kinds of therapeutic agents likely to be co-administered. In the case of traxoprodil and at least one other investigational agent (Colizza et al. 2007), enrollment of a special population in the radiolabel study (CYP2D6 PMs) allowed for a quantitative assessment of the role of a specific enzyme and its potential for pharmacokinetic DDI in human.

Biliary excretion and its contribution to clearance is directly measurable in radiolabel ADME studies in pre-clinical species due to the availability of bile duct cannulated animals. In human, this information is far more challenging to obtain, leaving investigators to infer human biliary clearance on the basis of cross-species extrapolation and/or characterization of drug-related material in feces collected during a standard radiolabel human ADME study. While this method is potentially simplified when dosing occurs through the IV route, most compounds are dosed orally where it is impossible to distinguish unabsorbed dose in feces from that excreted unchanged in bile or that secreted in the intestine. Recent advances in medical technology involving the use of oroentric or modified nasogastric tubes (Ghibellini et al. 2006), however, have led to a non-surgical method of obtaining bile from healthy subjects participating in radiolabel studies (see section "Clinical Drug Metabolism with Non-Radiolabeled Drug"). Such a technique was applied to the investigation of montelukast (Singulair®) (Balani et al. 1997). Two cohorts were enrolled in a ^{14}C radiolabel study; one was orally administered a 102 mg dose (84 µCi) and another was orally administered a 55 mg dose (122 µCi). The first cohort was studied in accordance with a "typical" protocol, while the second underwent bile collection for either a 2–8-hour interval post-dose (fasted) or a 6–12-hour interval post-dose (fed). Results from the second cohort demonstrated little biliary excretion of parent drug with much more significant levels of oxidative montelukast metabolites in bile, thereby confirming metabolism as the primary contributor to clearance of absorbed dose. Results from the "typical" study design followed in the first cohort showed trace recovery of dose in urine and 86% recovery in feces, consistent with biliary excretion of absorbed dose (in the form of metabolites) and fecal excretion of unabsorbed drug. By collecting bile in the second cohort, investigators were also able to characterize biliary metabolites in the absence of any influence from metabolism by intestinal microbes. Though similar data may have been obtained by utilizing surgical cholecystectomy candidates or patients with biliary T-tubes (as in the case of atorvastatin (Lipitor®) [Pool 1999] and irinotecan [Slatter et al. 2000]), these special patient populations may present additional challenges due to either enrollment difficulty or the nature of their pre-existing conditions.

Another example of a radiolabel human ADME study that included bile collection utilizing a method similar to the montelukast study involved the investigational dual PPARα/γ activator, muraglitazar (Wang et al. 2006; Zhang et al. 2007). In the case of muraglitazar, radiolabel ADME studies in pre-clinical species showed a significant role for glucuronidation in the clearance of the drug, as evidenced by high levels of glucuronides in bile from these species. Interestingly, fecal extracts showed little in the way of glucuronides, presumably as a result of gluronidase activity present in gut microbes or chemical instability. Of particular interest was acyl glucuronide formation at the carboxylic acid moiety, which was readily detected in bile but proved elusive in the fecal matrix. Investigators sought confirmation of *in vivo* acyl glucuronide formation in humans, choosing to sample bile during the course of a [^{14}C] muraglitazar study. A single 20 mg (103 µCi) oral dose was administered to study participants, with collection of bile, urine, feces, and plasma. Feces was determined to be the major route of elimination of drug-related material (>90%), with urine playing only a very minor role (<5%). Total recovery of radiolabeled dose was approximately 94% in both bile-sampled subjects and those with conventional collection. Human bile contained a substantial fraction of administered dose (40%), and many of these components were found to be acyl glucuronides. These data confirmed a role for glucuronidation in the clearance of muraglitazar that may otherwise have gone underestimated if fecal elimination had been relied upon solely, as feces contained either low or undetectable levels of these metabolites.

Identification of Circulating Metabolites

The third major deliverable derived from radiolabel human ADME data is the identification and quantitation of drug metabolites in circulatory and excretory matrices. As mentioned in the previous section, the identity of metabolites present in any matrix provides essential information about the biotransformation pathways involved in the clearance of an NCE. However, circulating metabolites in plasma (or blood) generally receive a higher degree of attention as they contribute to systemic exposure. If active, metabolites in circulation may help drive the intended pharmacological effect, or cause toxicity by exaggeration of on-target pharmacology. Conversely, toxicity may be the result of unintended off-target pharmacology or chemical toxicity. FDA and EMA guidance focusing specifically on metabolite-related toxicity (described in detail in section "Evolving Regulatory Environment and Clinical Drug Metabolism") sets forth the expectation that any metabolite in circulation at exposures exceeding 10% total drug-related material must be independently evaluated for toxicity *unless* coverage can be verified in pre-clinical toxicology studies. The value of radiolabel in this regard is that contributions of each metabolite to circulating radioactivity can be quantitatively assessed cross-species to distinguish any metabolites in human that are not adequately covered in pre-clinical toxicology studies. Upon confirmation of structural identity, metabolites can be synthesized, if necessary, and tested in accordance with regulatory guidance. CP-122,721, an investigational neurokinin-1 (NK1) receptor antagonist evaluated for the treatment of various neurological conditions, was administered to healthy volunteers as part of a radiolabel human ADME study (Colizza et al. 2007). A 30 mg (100 µCi) [^{14}C]CP-122,721 dose was extensively metabolized, with recovery of radiolabeled drug primarily in urine (>70%) in the form of several oxidative metabolites. One of these, a carboxylic acid cleavage product (5-trifluoromethoxy salicylic acid) formed via *O*-demethylation, *N*-dealkylation, and subsequent oxidation, was only a minor component accounting for <5% of the administered dose. A potentially unimportant metabolite at first glance, investigators determined that this low-level excretory component was present in circulation as a major contributor to circulating radioactivity (>50% in EM subjects and 29% in PM subjects), far exceeding parent drug levels. Complete mass-spectral and NMR characterization definitively established the identity of this important metabolite, which was subsequently confirmed with synthetic standard. Though inactive in terms of NK1 antagonism, off-target toxicity associated with this metabolite could not be excluded since it was not observed in pre-clinical toxicology species (Kamel et al. 2006). In the case of CP-122,721, the radiolabel human ADME study led to the discovery of a significant human-specific metabolite due to its systemic exposure in circulation. Such a finding would likely require further evaluation according to current FDA and EMA guidance.

Current and Emerging Technologies Applied in Clinical Drug Metabolism Studies

Current practice for the quantification of unlabeled analytes and the structure elucidation of metabolites employs the use of liquid chromatography (LC) coupled with atmospheric pressure ionization (API) tandem mass spectrometry (MS/MS), collectively abbreviated LC-API/MS/MS. Where radioisotopes are assayed, in-line radiochemical flow detectors are readily integrated into these analytical systems to aid in metabolite identification efforts. Ultra-high-performance liquid chromatography (UPLC) is the primary front-end LC separation technology used for analysis of small molecules, particularly metabolite identification applications. Better peak resolution and shorter analysis times (via higher pressures) are achieved relative to the more classical high-performance liquid chromatography (HPLC) variant. The most widely-employed API technique for drug-like analytes is electrospray ionization (ESI), since it is well-suited for ionization of a diverse array of molecules in the liquid state as they exit the LC system and enter the ion source of the MS instrument. In addition to ESI, atmospheric pressure chemical ionization (APCI) is important for certain analytes (most notably steroids), where ionization occurs by chemical reaction in the gas phase. Tandem MS experiments following ion formation can be performed in a variety of ways, as advances in technology relating to ion optics continue to introduce powerful new MS instruments to the ADME laboratory. A versatile and nearly ubiquitous platform is the triple quadrupole mass spectrometer (TQMS), which is both an exemplary quantitative instrument and a metabolite identification platform. The use of TQMS for metabolite identification, however, has diminished in recent years giving way to linear ion trap instruments, like the Q-Trap and LTQ, which are ideal for metabolite identification applications given their MS^3 and MS^n and capabilities, respectively. Finally, quadrupole time-of-flight (QTOF) and Orbitrap instruments bring high-resolution MS capabilities to bear when more definitive elemental composition data describing metabolites and their fragment ions are required, or for some semiquantitative full-scan methods discussed previously (see section "Semiquantitative Plasma Analysis for Metabolite Exposure Determination"). High resolution instruments are also routinely utilized to more selectively distinguish drug-related material from biological background by means of mass-defect filtering techniques (Zhu et al. 2006, 2007; Zhang et al. 2007; Ruan et al. 2008; Tiller et al. 2008a), which makes them a platform of choice for metabolite identification in FIH exploratory experiments as well as later-stage definitive studies. More detailed reviews of these technologies, and others associated with drug metabolism studies have been published recently (Papac and Shahrokh 2001; Kamel and Prakash 2006; Prakash et al. 2007). Overall, LC-API/MS/MS technology encompasses a variety of instrument platforms and experimental approaches that may be viewed as complimentary to one another. The specialized ADME analytical laboratory is best served if all these tools are available and applied according to the needs of the challenge at-hand.

Despite the availability of numerous MS platforms ranging from unit mass to high-resolution, the ability to unequivocally identify metabolites using MS technology is ultimately limited by the nature of the metabolite and the extent to which its tandem MS (or MS^n) fragments are informative with respect to structure. Definitive structure elucidation often requires nuclear magnetic resonance (NMR) spectroscopy for correct assignment of stereochemical or isomeric configurations, which are rarely readily apparent on the basis of MS data alone. ^1H and ^{13}C nuclei are among the more common targets for NMR experiments, which by virtue of either homonuclear or heteronuclear design are well-suited to establish bond connectivity and molecular structure if adequate sample is available. Particularly in cases where metabolites are of high interest, either due to their relative abundance or potential for toxicity, definitive structure assignment is critical and underlies the importance of close alignment between ADME scientists and the NMR spectroscopist. For additional discussion, the reader is directed to (refer to NMR-focused chapter).

When the use of radiolabel is employed in clinical ADME studies, quantitation of drug-related material in biological matrices is most commonly performed by standard LSC techniques. Using traditional LSC methodologies, detection and quantification of radioisotope is a function of radioactive decay (disintegrations), and robust measurements require a reasonable quantity of material (doses in the μCi range) and/or sufficiently long counting times in order to accurately determine disintegrations per minute. Though history has proven this approach to be widely successful, continued efforts to reduce the levels of radioactivity dosed to humans (and to minimize radioactive waste) have recently led to the utilization of a technology platform new to the ADME field. With its roots in carbon dating and varied earth science applications, accelerator mass spectrometry (AMS) directly measures $^{14}C/^{12}C$ radioisotope ratios at the atomic level with no dependence on isotope decay for detection (Lappin and Garner 2005; Vogel 2005). Biological samples are oxidized completely to CO_2, which may be analyzed directly or subsequently reduced to solid carbon prior to being subjected to ionization by a cesium sputter source, mass selection, collision at high voltage to break down carbon hydride isobars (e.g., $^{12}CH_2$, ^{13}CH), and detection. Using AMS, samples containing approximately 1 mg of carbon can be reliably assayed for ^{14}C at attomole (10^{-18}) levels with good accuracy and precision. At such low isotope levels, LSC detection would not be a viable option, since decay of ^{14}C nuclei would occur less frequently than 1 per hour (Vogel 2005). This enhanced sensitivity relative to conventional radiometric detection has allowed for administration of ^{14}C doses on the order of 100 nCi in pre-clinical and human radiolabel ADME studies, which is far below doses used in conventional ADME experiments (Lappin and Garner 2005). The benefit of lower, "trace" level doses are that they are similar to the naturally occurring ^{14}C levels in human (Lappin and Garner 2005) and generally do not require dosimetry calculations (Turteltaub and Vogel 2000). Therefore, these truly minimal radiolabel doses facilitate earlier timing for definitive ADME studies in human, if desired. Sub-μCi doses may also enable administration of radiolabeled drug candidates that are highly potent, those exhibiting significant tissue retention or long half-life, or those prone to radiolytic degradation. In addition to ^{14}C, AMS has also been adapted to measure trace quantities of other radioisotopes like ^{3}H (Chiarappa-Zucca et al. 2002; Vogel and Love 2005), making it a versatile technology for many biopharmaceutical and toxicological applications.

AMS validation studies and applications in ADME and toxicology experiments have been described in the literature regularly in the past several years. A comparison of conventional LSC analysis and AMS detection of [^{14}C]fluconazole (Diflucan®) and [^{14}C]fluticasone (Flonase®) in circulatory, urinary, and fecal matrices from human and rat revealed good agreement between the two approaches (Garner et al. 2000). In one experiment, samples analyzed by LSC required nearly 12,000-fold dilution prior to AMS analysis, where a similar result was achieved. AMS was subsequently used in a clinical study to establish a 94% mass balance recovery of an investigational farnesyl transferase inhibitor, R115777, administered at a dose of 50 mg containing only 34 nCi of radioactivity (Garner et al. 2002). Profiles of drug and human metabolites (reconstructed from LC fractions) were also obtained in urine, feces, and plasma. Similar success was observed with ixabepilone (Ixempra®), a microtubule stabilizing agent, which achieved a recovery of 77% dose after administration of only 80 nCi of radiolabel (70 mg) (Beumer et al. 2007). In this example, AMS was selected due to the high radiolytic degradation observed at specific activities required for the administration of a 100 uCi dose. Investigators measured total plasma ^{14}C pharmacokinetics by AMS and pharmacokinetics of ixabepilone by LC-MS/MS to establish a major contribution to circulating ^{14}C. Subsequently, LC-AMS was used to produce a quantitative profile of metabolites circulating in plasma as well as metabolites present in excreta (Comezoglu et al. 2009).

In a recent study conducted to determine the ADME profile of cerlapirdine, only low doses of radioactivity were acceptable based on dosimetry calculations as a result of prolonged retention in pigmented tissues (Tse et al. 2014). In this case, a dose of 200 nCi was administered alongside approximately 5 mg of unlabeled material. The results achieved similar outcomes to more traditional ADME studies (i.e., good recovery, determination of excretion routes, and profiling of metabolites); however, compromises due to low levels of radioactivity were required. For instance, plasma samples were pooled across time points as well as subjects, resulting in the loss of the metabolite time course data and inter subject variability information. The authors suggest that good outcomes were achieved in this study due to the uncomplicated biotransformation pathways for this compound (i.e., two major metabolites).

Utility of AMS detection applied in a circumstance where radioactivity dose was limited by low clearance was demonstrated in an ADME study with vismodegib (Graham et al. 2011). In addition to long plasma half-life precluding the administration of high levels of radioactivity due to dosimetry constraints (radioactive dose was 1000 nCi), low levels of radioactivity were expected to be excreted over long periods of time resulting in dilution of the radioactive signal and limiting the likelihood of good recovery. Notably, however, recovery from urine and feces was good (>85%) over a 56-day period. LC-AMS was also used to generate the profile of vismodegib metabolites. In another example, AMS was used for quantitation of radioactivity following the administration of the peptide drug, [^{14}C]etelcalcetide (Subramanian et al. 2016). A dose of 10 mg (710 nCi) was administered to patients with chronic kidney disease undergoing dialysis. Blood, dialysate, urine, and feces were collected for 176 days. An estimated 67% of the radioactivity was recovered, with the bulk (60%) recovered in dialysis. AMS enabled the measurement of low levels of radioactivity in high volumes of dialysate.

AMS was also successfully utilized in the determination of nelfinavir (Viracept®) bioavailability in humans (Sarapa et al. 2005), and for the quantitation of *in vivo* DNA adduct formation in human colon tissue after administration of tamoxifen (Nolvadex®) (Brown et al. 2007). DNA adducts were also observed in rodents using AMS technology after the dosing of various halogenated hydrocarbons (Watanabe et al. 2007). For additional information about AMS applications in drug metabolism, the reader is directed to (refer to AMS-focused chapter).

Looking forward, both regulatory drivers (FDA and EMA guidance on *Safety Testing of Metabolites*) and technology developments (LC-MS/MS and AMS) continue to provide added impetus for early human ADME studies through implementation of microdosing strategies. While drug metabolism scientists working within this environment recognize the need for high quality, progressive science, and push for rigorous characterization of NCEs on the registration pathway, caveats remain to the general application of microdosing in clinical drug metabolism studies. Firstly, administration of microdose quantities of an NCE may only provide insight into pharmacokinetic behavior and metabolism characteristics of a molecule that are relevant at very low (i.e., non-pharmacological) doses. Without a complete understanding of whether clearance processes are linear or non-linear across a wide dose range, there are risks associated with heavy reliance on microdose data in early development. Studies have been conducted to evaluate dose-linearity between microdoses and more pharmacologically relevant doses (Sandhu et al. 2004; Balani et al. 2006; Lappin et al. 2006; Vlaming et al. 2015), and for many compounds dose linearity has been demonstrated. However, each novel NCE presents a unique challenge whereby prediction of linear pharmacokinetics over a wide dose range (microdose to pharmacological dose) may be difficult. Secondly, AMS instrumentation and enabling technology is not widely available commercially, and a robust LC (or other) interface remains an active area of research to simplify sample work-flows and improve throughput. A combustion interface using an elemental analyzer was recently described, capable of enabling AMS analysis of 70 samples daily (van Duijn et al. 2014). In routine practice, however, AMS analyses remain cumbersome due to the need for fraction collection, graphitization, and other technical steps involved in sample processing. Off-site or CRO-based collaborations may require sample shipment.

Whether or not microdoses will routinely provide sufficient metabolite quantities for more definitive metabolite characterization by standard LC-MS/MS techniques or NMR is also unclear. What remains certain is that clinical drug metabolism studies provide key information about the disposition of potential drug molecules that may impact the evaluation of their safety and efficacy. Earlier characterization of human ADME properties, perhaps even in the context of exploratory IND (eIND) filings, may ultimately become routine for compounds or programs where this information forms the basis of critical success factors.

REFERENCES

Baillie, T. A., M. N. Cayen, H. Fouda et al. 2002. Drug metabolites in safety testing. *Toxicology & Applied Pharmacology* 182 (3):188–196.

Balani, S. K., B. H. Arison, L. Mathai et al. 1995. Metabolites of L-735,524, a potent HIV-1 protease inhibitor, in human urine. *Drug Metabolism & Disposition* 23 (2):266–270.

Balani, S. K., E. J. Woolf, V. L. Hoagland et al. 1996. Disposition of indinavir, a potent HIV-1 protease inhibitor, after an oral dose in humans. *Drug Metabolism & Disposition* 24 (12):1389–1394.

Balani, S. K., N. V. Nagaraja, M. G. Qian et al. 2006. Evaluation of microdosing to assess pharmacokinetic linearity in rats using liquid chromatography-tandem mass spectrometry. *Drug Metabolism & Disposition* 34 (3):384–388.

Balani, S. K., X. Xu, V. Pratha et al. 1997. Metabolic profiles of montelukast sodium (Singulair), a potent cysteinyl leukotriene1 receptor antagonist, in human plasma and bile. *Drug Metabolism & Disposition* 25 (11):1282–1287.

Benet, L.Z., S. Oie, and J.B. Schwartz. 1995. Design and optimization of dosage regimens; pharmacokinetic data. In *The Pharmacological Basis of Therapeutics*, edited by J. G. Hardman, L. E. Limbird, P. B. Molinoff, R. W. Ruddon, and A. Goodman Gillman. New York: McGraw-Hill.

Bernadou, J., R. Martino, M.C. Malet-Martino, A. Lopez, and J.P. Armand. 1985. Fluorine-19 NMR: A technique for metabolism and disposition studies of fluorinated drugs. *Trends in Pharmacological Sciences* 6 (3):103–105.

Beumer, J. H., J. H. Beijnen, and J. H. Schellens. 2006. Mass balance studies, with a focus on anticancer drugs. *Clinical Pharmacokinetics* 45 (1):33–58.

Beumer, J. H., R. C. Garner, M. B. Cohen et al. 2007. Human mass balance study of the novel anticancer agent ixabepilone using accelerator mass spectrometry. *Investigational New Drugs* 25 (4):327–334.

Bloomer, J. C., M. Nash, A. Webb et al. 2013. Assessment of potential drug interactions by characterization of human drug metabolism pathways using non-invasive bile sampling. *British Journal of Clinical Pharmacology* 75 (2):488–496.

Brown, K., E. M. Tompkins, D. J. Boocock et al. 2007. Tamoxifen forms DNA adducts in human colon after administration of a single [14C]-labeled therapeutic dose. *Cancer Research* 67 (14):6995–7002.

Chiarappa-Zucca, M. L., K. H. Dingley, M. L. Roberts, C. A. Velsko, and A. H. Love. 2002. Sample preparation for quantitation of tritium by accelerator mass spectrometry. *Analytical Chemistry* 74 (24):6285–6290.

Chladek, J., G. Zimova, M. Beranek, and J. Martinkova. 2000. *In-vivo* indices of CYP2D6 activity: Comparison of dextromethorphan metabolic ratios in 4-h urine and 3-h plasma. *European Journal of Clinical Pharmacology* 56 (9–10):651–657.

Christensen, M., K. Andersson, P. Dalen et al. 2003. The Karolinska cocktail for phenotyping of five human cytochrome P450 enzymes. *Clinical Pharmacology & Therapeutics* 73 (6):517–528.

Cocquyt, V., W. F. Kline, B. J. Gertz et al. 1999. Pharmacokinetics of intravenous alendronate. *Journal of Clinical Pharmacology* 39 (4):385–393.

Colizza, K., M. Awad, and A. Kamel. 2007. Metabolism, pharmacokinetics, and excretion of the substance P receptor antagonist CP-122,721 in humans: Structural characterization of the novel major circulating metabolite 5-trifluoromethoxy salicylic acid by high-performance liquid chromatography-tandem mass spectrometry and NMR spectroscopy. *Drug Metabolism & Disposition* 35 (6):884–897.

Comezoglu, S. N., V. T. Ly, D. Zhang et al. 2009. Biotransformation profiling of [(14)C]ixabepilone in human plasma, urine and feces samples using accelerator mass spectrometry (AMS). *Drug Metabolism & Pharmacokinetics* 24 (6):511–522.

Dain, J. G., J. M. Collins, and W. T. Robinson. 1994. A regulatory and industrial perspective of the use of carbon-14 and tritium isotopes in human ADME studies. *Pharmaceutical Research* 11 (6):925-928.

Davis, T. M., T. Y. Hung, I. K. Sim, H. A. Karunajeewa, and K. F. Ilett. 2005. Piperaquine: A resurgent antimalarial drug. *Drugs* 65 (1):75–87.

Espina, R., L. Yu, J. Wang et al. 2009. Nuclear magnetic resonance spectroscopy as a quantitative tool to determine the concentrations of biologically produced metabolites: Implications in metabolites in safety testing. *Chemical Research in Toxicology* 22 (2):299–310.

Farid, N. A., R. L. Smith, T. A. Gillespie et al. 2007. The disposition of prasugrel, a novel thienopyridine, in humans. *Drug Metabolism & Disposition* 35 (7):1096–1104.

Floren, L.C., K. Berry, G.R. Tonn et al. 2003. T0906487 (T487), a novel CXCR3 antagonist: First time in human study of safety and pharmacokinetics. *Paper Read at 6th Annual World Congress of Inflammation*, at Vancouver, BC.

Fura, A. 2006. Role of pharmacologically active metabolites in drug discovery and development. *Drug Discovery Today* 11 (3–4):133–142.

Gao, H., and R. S. Obach. 2011. Addressing MIST (Metabolites in Safety Testing): Bioanalytical approaches to address metabolite exposures in humans and animals. *Current Drug Metabolism* 12 (6):578–586.

Gao, H., S. Deng, and R. S. Obach. 2010. A simple liquid chromatography-tandem mass spectrometry method to determine relative plasma exposures of drug metabolites across species for metabolite safety assessments. *Drug Metabolism & Disposition* 38 (12):2147–2156.

Garner, R. C., I. Goris, A. A. Laenen et al. 2002. Evaluation of accelerator mass spectrometry in a human mass balance and pharmacokinetic study-experience with 14C-labeled (R)-6-[amino(4- chlorophenyl)(1-methyl-1H-imidazol-5-yl)methyl]-4-(3-chlorophenyl)-1-methyl-2(1H)-quinolinone (R115777), a farnesyl transferase inhibitor. *Drug Metabolism & Disposition* 30 (7):823–830.

Garner, R. C., J. Barker, C. Flavell et al. 2000. A validation study comparing accelerator MS and liquid scintillation counting for analysis of 14C-labelled drugs in plasma, urine and faecal extracts. *Journal of Pharmaceutical & Biomedical Analysis* 24 (2):197–209.

Ghibellini, G., A. S. Bridges, C. N. Generaux, and K. L. Brouwer. 2007. *In vitro* and *in vivo* determination of piperacillin metabolism in humans. *Drug Metabolism & Disposition* 35 (3):345–349.

Ghibellini, G., B. M. Johnson, R. J. Kowalsky, W. D. Heizer, and K. L. Brouwer. 2004. A novel method for the determination of biliary clearance in humans. *AAPS Journal* 6 (4):e33.

Ghibellini, G., E. M. Leslie, and K. L. Brouwer. 2006. Methods to evaluate biliary excretion of drugs in humans: An updated review. *Molecular Pharmaceutics* 3 (3):198–211.

Graham, R. A., B. L. Lum, G. Morrison et al. 2011. A single dose mass balance study of the Hedgehog pathway inhibitor vismodegib (GDC-0449) in humans using accelerator mass spectrometry. *Drug Metabolism & Disposition* 39 (8):1460–1467.

Gschwind, H. P., U. Pfaar, F. Waldmeier et al. 2005. Metabolism and disposition of imatinib mesylate in healthy volunteers. *Drug Metabolism & Disposition* 33 (10):1503–1512.

Guiney, W. J., C. Beaumont, S. R. Thomas et al. 2011. Use of Entero-Test, a simple approach for non-invasive clinical evaluation of the biliary disposition of drugs. *British Journal of Clinical Pharmacology* 72 (1):133–142.

Hamilton, R. A., W. R. Garnett, and D. J. Kline. 1981. Determination of mean valproic acid serum level by assay of a single pooled sample. *Clinical Pharmacology & Therapeutics* 29 (3):408–413.

Harrison, M. P., S. J. Haworth, S. R. Moss, D. M. Wilkinson, and A. Featherstone. 1993. The disposition and metabolic fate of 14C-meropenem in man. *Xenobiotica* 23 (11):1311–1323.

Hochman, J. H., N. Pudvah, J. Qiu et al. 2004. Interactions of human P-glycoprotein with simvastatin, simvastatin acid, and atorvastatin. *Pharmaceutical Research* 21 (9):1686–1691.

Hoffmann, M., W. DeMaio, R. A. Jordan et al. 2007. Metabolism, excretion, and pharmacokinetics of [14C] tigecycline, a first-in-class glycylcycline antibiotic, after intravenous infusion to healthy male subjects. *Drug Metabolism & Disposition* 35 (9):1543–1553.

Hop, C. E., Z. Wang, Q. Chen, and G. Kwei. 1998. Plasma-pooling methods to increase throughput for *in vivo* pharmacokinetic screening. *Journal of Pharmaceutical Sciences* 87 (7):901–903.

Houston, J. B. 1981. Drug metabolite kinetics. *Pharmacology & Therapeutics* 15 (3):521–552.

Hu, H., N. Huang, P. Yi et al. 2015. Utilizing 19F NMR to investigate drug disposition early in drug discovery. *Xenobiotica* 45 (12):1081–1091.

Ito, K., D. Hallifax, R. S. Obach, and J. B. Houston. 2005. Impact of parallel pathways of drug elimination and multiple cytochrome P450 involvement on drug-drug interactions: CYP2D6 paradigm. *Drug Metabolism & Disposition* 33 (6):837–844.

Iyer, R. A., J. Mitroka, B. Malhotra et al. 2001. Metabolism of [(14)C]omapatrilat, a sulfhydryl-containing vasopeptidase inhibitor in humans. *Drug Metabolism & Disposition* 29 (1):60–69.

Johnson, K., A. Shah, S. Jaw-Tsai, J. Baxter, and C. Prakash. 2003. Metabolism, pharmacokinetics, and excretion of a highly selective N-methyl-D-aspartate receptor antagonist, traxoprodil, in human cytochrome P450 2D6 extensive and poor metabolizers. *Drug Metabolism & Disposition* 31 (1):76–87.

Kamel, A., and C. Prakash. 2006. High performance liquid chromatography/atmospheric pressure ionization/ tandem mass spectrometry (HPLC/API/MS/MS) in drug metabolism and toxicology. *Current Drug Metabolism* 7 (8):837–852.

Kamel, A., J. Davis, M. J. Potchoiba, and C. Prakash. 2006. Metabolism, pharmacokinetics and excretion of a potent tachykinin NK1 receptor antagonist (CP-122,721) in rat: Characterization of a novel oxidative pathway. *Xenobiotica* 36 (2–3):235–258.

Khan, S. A., J. A. Kanis, S. Vasikaran et al. 1997. Elimination and biochemical responses to intravenous alendronate in postmenopausal osteoporosis. *Journal of Bone & Mineral Research* 12 (10):1700–1707.

Koszalka, G. W., N. W. Johnson, S. S. Good et al. 2002. Preclinical and toxicology studies of 1263W94, a potent and selective inhibitor of human cytomegalovirus replication. *Antimicrobial Agents & Chemotherapy* 46 (8):2373–2380.

Kripalani, K. J., D. N. McKinstry, S. M. Singhvi, D. A. Willard, R. A. Vukovich, and B. H. Migdalof. 1980. Disposition of captopril in normal subjects. *Clinical Pharmacology & Therapeutics* 27 (5):636–641.

Lappin, G., and R. C. Garner. 2005. The use of accelerator mass spectrometry to obtain early human ADME/ PK data. *Expert Opinion On Drug Metabolism & Toxicology* 1 (1):23–31.

Lappin, G., W. Kuhnz, R. Jochemsen et al. 2006. Use of microdosing to predict pharmacokinetics at the therapeutic dose: Experience with 5 drugs.[see comment]. *Clinical Pharmacology & Therapeutics* 80 (3):203–215.

Lin, J. H., and B. K. Wong. 2002. Complexities of glucuronidation affecting *in vitro in vivo* extrapolation. *Current Drug Metabolism* 3 (6):623–646.

Lin, J. H., D. E. Duggan, I. W. Chen, and R. L. Ellsworth. 1991. Physiological disposition of alendronate, a potent anti-osteolytic bisphosphonate, in laboratory animals. *Drug Metabolism & Disposition* 19 (5):926–932.

Lin, J. H., M. Chiba, S. K. Balani et al. 1996. Species differences in the pharmacokinetics and metabolism of indinavir, a potent human immunodeficiency virus protease inhibitor. *Drug Metabolism & Disposition* 24 (10):1111–1120.

Lins, R., J. Broekhuysen, J. Necciari, and X. Deroubaix. 1999. Pharmacokinetic profile of 14C-labeled clopidogrel. *Seminars in Thrombosis and Hemostasis* 25 (Suppl. 2):29–33.

Ma, S., and S. K. Chowdhury. 2011. Analytical strategies for assessment of human metabolites in preclinical safety testing. *Analytical Chemistry* 83 (13):5028–5036.

Ma, S., Z. Li, K. J. Lee, and S. K. Chowdhury. 2010. Determination of exposure multiples of human metabolites for MIST assessment in preclinical safety species without using reference standards or radiolabeled compounds. *Chemical Research in Toxicology* 23 (12):1871–1873.

Mamaril-Fishman, D., J. Zhu, M. Lin et al. 2014. Investigation of metabolism and disposition of GSK1322322, a peptidase deformylase inhibitor, in healthy humans using the entero-test for biliary sampling. *Drug Metabolism & Disposition* 42 (8):1314–1325.

Marathe, P. H., W. C. Shyu, and W. G. Humphreys. 2004. The use of radiolabeled compounds for ADME studies in discovery and exploratory development. *Current Pharmaceutical Design* 10 (24):2991–3008.

Martin, I. J., S. E. Hill, J. A. Baker, S. V. Deshmukh, and E. F. Mulrooney. 2016. A pharmacokinetic modeling approach to predict the contribution of active metabolites to human efficacious dose. *Drug Metabolism & Disposition* 44 (8):1435–1440.

Martino, R., V. Gilard, F. Desmoulin, and M. Malet-Martino. 2005. Fluorine-19 or phosphorus-31 NMR spectroscopy: A suitable analytical technique for quantitative *in vitro* metabolic studies of fluorinated or phosphorylated drugs. *Journal of Pharmaceutical & Biomedical Analysis* 38 (5):871–891.

Mei, Q., C. Tang, C. Assang et al. 1999. Role of a potent inhibitory monoclonal antibody to cytochrome P-450 3A4 in assessment of human drug metabolism. *Journal of Pharmacology & Experimental Therapeutics* 291 (2):749–759.

Mei, Q., C. Tang, Y. Lin, T. H. Rushmore, and M. Shou. 2002. Inhibition kinetics of monoclonal antibodies against cytochromes P450. *Drug Metabolism & Disposition* 30 (6):701–708.

Monteagudo, E., S. Pesci, M. Taliani et al. 2007. Studies of metabolism and disposition of potent human immunodeficiency virus (HIV) integrase inhibitors using 19F-NMR spectroscopy. *Xenobiotica* 37 (9):1000–1012.

Mullen, J. H., R. L. Shugert, G. D. Ponsler et al. 2005. Simultaneous quantification of atomoxetine as well as its primary oxidative and O-glucuronide metabolites in human plasma and urine using liquid chromatography tandem mass spectrometry (LC/MS/MS). *Journal of Pharmaceutical & Biomedical Analysis* 38 (4):720–733.

Mutlib, A., R. Espina, J. Atherton et al. 2012. Alternate strategies to obtain mass balance without the use of radiolabeled compounds: Application of quantitative fluorine (19F) nuclear magnetic resonance (NMR) spectroscopy in metabolism studies. *Chemical Research in Toxicology* 25 (3):572–583.

Nave, R., T.D. Bethke, S.P. van Marle, and K. Zech. 1994. Pharmacokinetics of [14C]Ciclesonide after oral and intravenous administration to healthy subjects. *Clinical Pharmacokinetics* 43 (7):479–486.

Papac, D. I., and Z. Shahrokh. 2001. Mass spectrometry innovations in drug discovery and development. *Pharmaceutical Research* 18 (2):131–145.

Paulson, S. K., J. D. Hribar, N. W. Liu et al. 2000. Metabolism and excretion of [(14)C]celecoxib in healthy male volunteers. *Drug Metabolism & Disposition* 28 (3):308–314.

Pool, W.F. 1999. Clinical drug metabolism studies. In *Handbook of Drug Metabolism*, edited by T. F. Woolf. New York: Marcel Dekker.

Potchoiba, M. J., and M. R. Nocerini. 2004. Utility of whole-body autoradioluminography in drug discovery for the quantification of tritium-labeled drug candidates. *Drug Metabolism & Disposition* 32 (10):1190–1198.

Potchoiba, M. J., M. West, and M. R. Nocerini. 1998. Quantitative comparison of autoradioluminographic and radiometric tissue distribution studies using carbon-14 labeled xenobiotics. *Drug Metabolism & Disposition* 26 (3):272–277.

Potchoiba, M. J., T. G. Tensfeldt, M. R. Nocerini, and B. M. Silber. 1995. A novel quantitative method for determining the biodistribution of radiolabeled xenobiotics using whole-body cryosectioning and autoradioluminography. *Journal of Pharmacology & Experimental Therapeutics* 272 (2):953–962.

Powley, M. W., C. B. Frederick, F. D. Sistare, and J. J. DeGeorge. 2009. Safety assessment of drug metabolites: Implications of regulatory guidance and potential application of genetically engineered mouse models that express human P450s. *Chemical Research in Toxicology* 22 (2):257–262.

Prakash, C., C. L. Shaffer, and A. Nedderman. 2007. Analytical strategies for identifying drug metabolites. *Mass Spectrometry Reviews* 26 (3):340–369.

Prueksaritanont, T., J. H. Lin, and T. A. Baillie. 2006. Complicating factors in safety testing of drug metabolites: Kinetic differences between generated and preformed metabolites. *Toxicology & Applied Pharmacology* 217 (2):143–152.

Raghavan, N., C. E. Frost, Z. Yu et al. 2009. Apixaban metabolism and pharmacokinetics after oral administration to humans. *Drug Metabolism & Disposition* 37 (1):74–81.

Rehmel, J. L., J. A. Eckstein, N. A. Farid et al. 2006. Interactions of two major metabolites of prasugrel, a thienopyridine antiplatelet agent, with the cytochromes P450. *Drug Metabolism & Disposition* 34 (4):600–607.

Riad, L. E., K. K. Chan, and R. J. Sawchuk. 1991. Determination of the relative formation and elimination clearance of two major carbamazepine metabolites in humans: A comparison between traditional and pooled sample analysis. *Pharmaceutical Research* 8 (4):541–543.

Ring, B. J., J. S. Gillespie, J. A. Eckstein, and S. A. Wrighton. 2002. Identification of the human cytochromes P450 responsible for atomoxetine metabolism. *Drug Metabolism & Disposition* 30 (3):319–323.

Roffey, S. J., R. S. Obach, J. I. Gedge, and D. A. Smith. 2007. What is the objective of the mass balance study? A retrospective analysis of data in animal and human excretion studies employing radiolabeled drugs. *Drug Metabolism Reviews* 39 (1):17–43.

Rohatagi, S., Y. Wang, and D. Argenti. 2004. Mass balance studies. *Pharmacokinetics in Drug Development* 1:121–148.

Ruan, Q., S. Peterman, M. A. Szewc et al. 2008. An integrated method for metabolite detection and identification using a linear ion trap/Orbitrap mass spectrometer and multiple data processing techniques: Application to indinavir metabolite detection. *Journal of Mass Spectrometry* 43 (2):251–261.

Sandhu, P., J. S. Vogel, M. J. Rose et al. 2004. Evaluation of microdosing strategies for studies in preclinical drug development: Demonstration of linear pharmacokinetics in dogs of a nucleoside analog over a 50-fold dose range. *Drug Metabolism & Disposition* 32 (11):1254–1259.

Sarapa, N., P. H. Hsyu, G. Lappin, and R. C. Garner. 2005. The application of accelerator mass spectrometry to absolute bioavailability studies in humans: Simultaneous administration of an intravenous microdose of 14C-nelfinavir mesylate solution and oral nelfinavir to healthy volunteers. *Journal of Clinical Pharmacology* 45 (10):1198–1205.

Sauer, J. M., G. D. Ponsler, E. L. Mattiuz et al. 2003. Disposition and metabolic fate of atomoxetine hydrochloride: The role of CYP2D6 in human disposition and metabolism. *Drug Metabolism & Disposition* 31 (1):98–107.

Savi, P., J. M. Pereillo, M. F. Uzabiaga et al. 2000. Identification and biological activity of the active metabolite of clopidogrel. *Thrombosis & Haemostasis* 84 (5):891–896.

Shaffer, C. L., and C. S. Langer. 2007. Metabolism of a 14C/3H-labeled GABAA receptor partial agonist in rat, dog and human liver microsomes: Evaluation of a dual-radiolabel strategy. *Journal of Pharmaceutical & Biomedical Analysis* 43 (4):1195–1205.

Shockcor, J. P., S. E. Unger, P. Savina, J. K. Nicholson, and J. C. Lindon. 2000. Application of directly coupled LC-NMR-MS to the structural elucidation of metabolites of the HIV-1 reverse-transcriptase inhibitor BW935U83. *Journal of Chromatography. B, Biomedical Sciences & Applications* 748 (1):269–279.

Slatter, J. G., L. J. Schaaf, J. P. Sams et al. 2000. Pharmacokinetics, metabolism, and excretion of irinotecan (CPT-11) following I.V. infusion of [(14)C]CPT-11 in cancer patients. *Drug Metabolism & Disposition* 28 (4):423–4233.

Slatter, J.G., N. Agrawal, S. Chowdhury et al. 2014. Current industry practices in the *in vivo* assessment of human drug metabolism: A survey by the drug metabolism and clinical pharmacology leadership groups of the IQ consortium. *Clinical Pharmacology & Therapeutics* 95 (Supplement 1):S64.

Slattery, J. T., J. M. Wilson, T. F. Kalhorn, and S. D. Nelson. 1987. Dose-dependent pharmacokinetics of acetaminophen: Evidence of glutathione depletion in humans. *Clinical Pharmacology & Therapeutics* 41 (4):413–418.

Smith, D. A., and R. S. Obach. 2006. Metabolites and safety: What are the concerns, and how should we address them? *Chemical Research in Toxicology* 19 (12):1570–1579.

Solon, E.G., and L. Kraus. 2002. Quantitative whole-body autoradiography in the pharmaceutical industry: Survey results on study design, methods, and regulatory compliance. *Journal of Pharmacological and Toxicological Methods* 46:73–81.

Sonada, M., M. Takana, J. Miyahara, and H. KAto. 1983. Computed radiography utilising scanning laser stimulated luminescence. *Radiology* 148:833–838.

Subramanian, R., X. Zhu, M. B. Hock et al. 2016. Pharmacokinetics, biotransformation, and excretion of [14C]Etelcalcetide (AMG 416) following a single microtracer intravenous dose in patients with chronic kidney disease on hemodialysis. *Clinical Pharmacokinetics* 56 (2):179–192.

Sunzel, M. 2004. In *New Drug Development, Regulatory Paradigms for Clinical Pharmacology and Biopharmaceutics*, edited by C. G. Sahajwalla. New York: Marcel Decker.

Tarning, J., Y. Bergqvist, N. P. Day et al. 2006. Characterization of human urinary metabolites of the antimalarial piperaquine. *Drug Metabolism & Disposition* 34 (12):2011–2019.

Tiller, P. R., S. Yu, J. Castro-Perez, K. L. Fillgrove, and T. A. Baillie. 2008a. High-throughput, accurate mass liquid chromatography/tandem mass spectrometry on a quadrupole time-of-flight system as a "first-line" approach for metabolite identification studies. *Rapid Communications in Mass Spectrometry* 22 (7):1053–1061.

Tiller, P. R., S. Yu, K. P. Bateman et al. 2008b. Fractional mass filtering as a means to assess circulating metabolites in early human clinical studies. *Rapid Communications in Mass Spectrometry* 22 (22):3510–3516.

Tombs, N.I. 1999. Tissue distribution of Gar-936, a broad-spectrum antibiotic, in male rats. *Abstracts Interscience Conference on Antimicrobial Agents and Chemotherapy* 39:302.

Tse, S., L. Leung, S. Raje, M. Seymour, Y. Shishikura, and R. S. Obach. 2014. Disposition and metabolic profiling of [(14)C]cerlapirdine using accelerator mass spectrometry. *Drug Metabolism & Disposition* 42 (12):2023–2032.

Turteltaub, K. W., and J. S. Vogel. 2000. Bioanalytical applications of accelerator mass spectrometry for pharmaceutical research. *Current Pharmaceutical Design* 6 (10):991–1007.

van Duijn, E., H. Sandman, D. Grossouw, J. A. Mocking, L. Coulier, and W. H. Vaes. 2014. Automated combustion accelerator mass spectrometry for the analysis of biomedical samples in the low attomole range. *Analytical Chemistry* 86 (15):7635–7641.

Vishwanathan, K., K. Babalola, J. Wang et al. 2009. Obtaining exposures of metabolites in preclinical species through plasma pooling and quantitative NMR: Addressing metabolites in safety testing (MIST) guidance without using radiolabeled compounds and chemically synthesized metabolite standards. *Chemical Research in Toxicology* 22 (2):311–322.

Vlaming, M. L., E. van Duijn, M. R. Dillingh et al. 2015. Microdosing of a carbon-14 labeled protein in healthy volunteers accurately predicts its pharmacokinetics at therapeutic dosages. *Clinical Pharmacology & Therapeutics* 98 (2):196–204.

Vogel, J. S., and A. H. Love. 2005. Quantitating isotopic molecular labels with accelerator mass spectrometry. *Methods in Enzymology* 402:402–422.

Vogel, JS. 2005. Accelerator mass spectrometry for quantitative *in vivo* tracing. *BioTechniques* 38:S25–S29.

Vree, T. B., J. Waitzinger, A. Hammermaier, and S. Radhofer-Welte. 1999. Absolute bioavailability, pharmacokinetics, renal and biliary clearance of distigmine after a single oral dose in comparison to i.v. administration of 14C-distigmine-bromide in healthy volunteers. *International Journal of Clinical Pharmacology & Therapeutics* 37 (8):393–403.

Wade, K. E., I. D. Wilson, J. A. Troke, and J. K. Nicholson. 1990. 19F and 1H magnetic resonance strategies for metabolic studies on fluorinated xenobiotics: Application to flurbiprofen [2-(2-fluoro-4-biphenylyl) propionic acid]. *Journal of Pharmaceutical & Biomedical Analysis* 8 (5):401–410.

Wait, J. C., N. Vaccharajani, J. Mitroka et al. 2006. Metabolism of [14C]gemopatrilat after oral administration to rats, dogs, and humans. *Drug Metabolism & Disposition* 34 (6):961–970.

Wang, L. H., R. W. Peck, Y. Yin, J. Allanson, R. Wiggs, and M. B. Wire. 2003. Phase I safety and pharmacokinetic trials of 1263W94, a novel oral anti-human cytomegalovirus agent, in healthy and human immunodeficiency virus-infected subjects. *Antimicrobial Agents & Chemotherapy* 47 (4):1334–1342.

Wang, L., D. Zhang, A. Swaminathan et al. 2006. Glucuronidation as a major metabolic clearance pathway of 14c-labeled muraglitazar in humans: Metabolic profiles in subjects with or without bile collection. *Drug Metabolism & Disposition* 34 (3):427–439.

Watanabe, K., R. G. Liberman, P. L. Skipper, S. R. Tannenbaum, and F. P. Guengerich. 2007. Analysis of DNA adducts formed *in vivo* in rats and mice from 1,2-dibromoethane, 1,2-dichloroethane, dibromomethane, and dichloromethane using HPLC/accelerator mass spectrometry and relevance to risk estimates. *Chemical Research in Toxicology* 20 (11):1594–600.

Weichers, J.W., R.E. Herder, B.F.H. Drenth, and R.A. de Zeeuw. 1990. Percutaneous absorption, disposition, metabolism, and excretion of 14C-labelled Cyoctol in humans after a single dermal application. *International Journal of Pharmaceutics* 65 (1–2):77–84.

Wright, P., Z. Miao, and B. Shilliday. 2009. Metabolite quantitation: Detector technology and MIST implications. *Bioanalysis* 1 (4):831–845.

Yamane, N., T. Takami, Z. Tozuka, Y. Sugiyama, A. Yamazaki, and Y. Kumagai. 2009. Microdose clinical trial: Quantitative determination of nicardipine and prediction of metabolites in human plasma. *Drug Metabolism and Pharmacokinetics* 24 (4):389–403.

Yu, C., C. L. Chen, F. L. Gorycki, and T. G. Neiss. 2007. A rapid method for quantitatively estimating metabolites in human plasma in the absence of synthetic standards using a combination of liquid chromatography/mass spectrometry and radiometric detection. *Rapid Communications in Mass Spectrometry* 21 (4): 497–502.

Zhang, D., L. Wang, N. Raghavan et al. 2007. Comparative metabolism of radiolabeled muraglitazar in animals and humans by quantitative and qualitative metabolite profiling. *Drug Metabolism & Disposition* 35 (1):150–67.

Zhang, D., M. Ogan, R. Gedamke et al. 2003. Protein covalent binding of maxipost through a cytochrome P450-mediated ortho-quinone methide intermediate in rats. *Drug Metabolism & Disposition* 31 (7):837–845.

Zhang, D., P. T. Cheng, and H. Zhang. 2007. Mass defect filtering on high resolution LC/MS data as a methodology for detecting metabolites with unpredictable structures: Identification of oxazole-ring opened metabolites of muraglitazar. *Drug Metabolism Letters* 1 (4):287–292.

Zhang, D., R. Krishna, L. Wang et al. 2005. Metabolism, pharmacokinetics, and protein covalent binding of radiolabeled MaxiPost (BMS-204352) in humans. *Drug Metabolism & Disposition* 33 (1):83–93.

Zhu, M., L. Ma, D. Zhang et al. 2006. Detection and characterization of metabolites in biological matrices using mass defect filtering of liquid chromatography/high resolution mass spectrometry data. *Drug Metabolism & Disposition* 34 (10):1722–1733.

Zhu, M., L. Ma, H. Zhang, and W. G. Humphreys. 2007. Detection and structural characterization of glutathione-trapped reactive metabolites using liquid chromatography-high-resolution mass spectrometry and mass defect filtering. *Analytical Chemistry* 79 (21):8333–8341.

21

Managing Metabolic Activation Issues in Drug Discovery

Sanjeev Kumar, Kaushik Mitra, and Thomas A. Baillie

CONTENTS

Overview: Relevance of Metabolic Activation in Drug Safety and Toxicity

Adverse safety findings occur at both preclinical and clinical stages of drug candidate evaluation, where they contribute significantly to attrition in the overall drug development process. As such, considerable efforts are devoted by the pharmaceutical industry to understand the underlying mechanisms of toxicity with a view to being able to predict *a priori*, those structural and biological characteristics of a new chemical entity that are likely to elicit a toxic response, and to incorporate these considerations into drug design activities [1–5]. While it is apparent that molecular mechanisms of drug-induced toxicity are numerous, it is now generally accepted that the metabolism of chemically stable drug candidates to highly reactive, electrophilic intermediates represents one risk factor for serious adverse reactions, notably those involving the metabolically active organ systems such as liver, skin, and hematological systems with drug-induced liver injury (DILI) being the most prevalent and of greatest concern. The underlying hypothesis for these adverse effects is that the covalent modification of proteins by reactive metabolites can either cause direct toxicity by negatively impacting critical protein function or convert these endogenous proteins into *haptens* that, in susceptible individuals, can trigger an immune-mediated response that is manifest as an "idiosyncratic toxicity [6–8]." These idiosyncratic toxicities generally are not detected during preclinical safety evaluation, have a low clinical incidence (1 in 10000 or more), and may only become apparent during large scale clinical trials when a significant resource investment has already been made in the drug candidate or, even worse, after a compound has been introduced onto the market, thus posing a significant patient hazard as well as economic loss for the sponsor company.

Based on these observations, screening strategies were implemented by many companies in the early 2000s to detect reactive metabolite formation from new chemical entities, either through appropriate *in vitro* incubations supplemented with nucleophilic "trapping agents" or by the characterization of glutathione (GSH) adducts or *N*-acetylcysteine conjugates in animals dosed *in vivo* with the experimental compound [9]. While these studies provide data largely of a qualitative nature and afford an insight into the molecular structure of the reactive intermediates in question, quantitative information on the metabolic activation process generally requires the synthesis of a radiolabeled analog of the drug candidate to assess metabolism-dependent covalent binding to cellular proteins [10]. Collectively, these approaches form the basis of "avoidance" strategies in drug discovery whose goal is not only to eliminate from consideration those molecules that undergo appreciable metabolic activation, but also to develop an appreciation of the structural motifs that typically are associated with bioactivation for intervention by medicinal chemists. In addition, a substantial body of information has accumulated over the years on so-called "structural alerts" for bioactivation and their prevalence in both experimental agents and approved drugs that exhibit various types of toxicity [11]. For example, functional groups such as anilines, precursors of quinones and related electrophiles, hydrazines, thiophenes, furans, terminal olefins and alkynes, and nitroaromatics frequently undergo metabolism to reactive species that have been implicated in the toxicity of their respective parent molecules [12,13]. Mechanistic studies with representative examples of compounds containing these functional groups have yielded a wealth of information on the underlying biochemical processes leading to metabolic activation and on the identities of the reactive metabolites themselves. Substituted thiophenes, for example, have received much attention in this regard in view of the presence of this heterocycle in several approved drugs [14]; in some cases (e.g., tienilic acid), oxidation of the thiophene ring is associated with liver toxicity, which led to removal of the compound from the market [15], while in others (e.g., prasugrel), the product of thiophene ring oxidation actually is responsible for the pharmacological activity of the drug through thiolation of the P_2Y_{12} purinoreceptor on the surface of blood platelets [16,17]. The latter example serves to illustrate one of the core complexities of the metabolic activation phenomenon, namely that reactive intermediates are not always toxic to the host cell, and the specific determinants of a toxic *versus* non-toxic response to individual reactive species are poorly understood. In general, it appears that covalent binding of reactive drug metabolites to critical cellular macromolecules, when combined with certain host-specific genetic, environmental, and/or disease factors, can render certain individuals more susceptible to drug-induced idiosyncratic toxicity [18]. Since it is not possible to identify these individual-specific factors during preclinical safety testing and map their relationship to drug-induced idiosyncratic toxicity, our ability to predict the potential for these toxicities remains limited. Consequently, efforts to avoid, or at least minimize, exposure to reactive intermediates represent a reasonable approach towards reducing the potential for toxicity during drug development [2–5], although it is acknowledged that toxicological triggers and mechanisms can be numerous and, in many cases, may not involve metabolic activation of the drug candidate.

Over the past decade, considerable progress has been made in addressing the limitations of the avoidance strategy and further refining the process of managing metabolic activation issues in drug discovery. These efforts stemmed from the observation that the extent of drug bioactivation and/or covalent binding of drug-related material to liver proteins alone did not differentiate effectively between hepatotoxic and non-hepatotoxic drugs and other factors likely contributed to hepatotoxicity risk [19,20]. Thus, it was proposed that using bioactivation alone to assess toxicity risk could lead to discontinuation of development of potentially safe and effective drug candidates or to the implementation of lead optimization efforts that are not truly warranted. The ensuing work over the past 5–10 years has focused on integrating bioactivation risk with other drug candidate attributes, such as total daily dose and fractional clearance to reactive species that together determine *daily total body burden* of reactive species. Additional indices that have been considered include mitochondrial and cellular effects of drug candidates in metabolically competent cell systems as key indicators of cell health, as well as other risk factors for drug-induced liver injury (DILI) such as the effects on bile salt homeostasis *via* inhibition of bile salt export pump (BSEP). Collectively, these integrative approaches aim to enhance the predictive power of broader preclinical assessment of toxicity risk that includes bioactivation as one contributing factor [21–28]. With the limited amount of literature available on this topic at the present time, it is encouraging to note that integrative approaches that take into account the multifactorial nature of drug toxicity and integrate bioactivation risk into a broader context do appear to perform better in differentiating between high *versus* low toxicity risk compounds [25]. It should be acknowledged, however, that much still remains to be learned about the multiplicity of factors that combine to cause tissue injury, and this probably will require the adoption of systems pharmacology/toxicology approaches employing contemporary toxicogenomics and associated bioinformatics tools [29], toxicity biomarkers [30,31], and novel, more physiologically relevant *in vitro* systems, such as organoids and/or microfluidic "organs-on-chips," to assess these effects [32].

In contrast to the more complex relationship between metabolic activation and idiosyncratic or target organ toxicities, there are other important drug attributes that can be more directly impacted by chemically reactive metabolites. The role of electrophilic metabolites in genotoxicity and carcinogenesis is well established for structural motifs such as polycyclic aromatic hydrocarbons and aromatic amines [33,34]. For example, a number of quinone and/or quinone methide reactive intermediates derived from estrogens and the "anti-estrogen" tamoxifen have been shown to bind to DNA bases and induce DNA damage [35,36]. Similarly, there are numerous examples where cytochrome P450-mediated formation of reactive metabolites and their subsequent irreversible binding to the apoprotein and/or prosthetic heme leads to suicide inactivation of the enzyme, which is manifested as time-dependent or mechanism-based P450 inhibition [37,38]. This suicide inactivation of P450 enzymes has been responsible for many serious drug-drug interactions, notably those involving the CYP3A4 enzyme, and have even led to market withdrawals (e.g., mibefradil). Thus, reducing the formation of chemically reactive metabolites can often provide a direct and rational approach for minimizing such adverse drug properties during pharmaceutical lead optimization.

Progress in assessing the role of metabolic activation as a causative factor in drug toxicity has been greatly facilitated by the strides that have been made in recent years in the analytical techniques employed for the detection, identification, and quantitative assessments of reactive metabolites, notably those based on the use liquid chromatography-tandem mass spectrometry (LC-MS/MS) [39]. Adducts to GSH and other low molecular weight nucleophiles provide indirect evidence of the structures of electrophilic intermediates, a critical piece of information for medicinal chemists involved in the rational design of drug candidates that are refractory to metabolic activation. Developments in the field of proteomics mass spectrometry can now provide information on the identities of covalent drug-protein adducts. While still challenging from an analytical standpoint, this field of research is evolving rapidly and promises to provide insights into the macromolecular targets of reactive intermediates and potential epitopes on proteins that may be involved in triggering an immune response through activation of T-cells [40].

In the following sections of this chapter, we elaborate on aspects of reactive metabolite formation in the context of pharmaceutical research and development. Specifically, we address topics related to minimizing the metabolic activation potential of new chemical entities, approaches to evaluate risk associated with bioactivation, and the impact of reactive metabolite formation on decision-making in the drug discovery process.

Minimizing Metabolic Activation in Drug Discovery

Several qualitative and quantitative tools are available for the assessment and remediation of the propensity of drug candidates to form reactive intermediates. The qualitative assessment identifies the reactive metabolite(s) in question, with particular attention to the sub-structural motif that is involved in bioactivation. This information guides the introduction of appropriate structural modifications to block the undesired metabolic pathway(s). A quantitative assessment serves a dual purpose; firstly, it allows appropriate comparisons to be drawn among different candidates as improvements are made in structure; and secondly, it allows an absolute assessment of risk in terms of body burden of reactive species.

TABLE 21.1

Summary of Available Methods to Assess and Minimize the Potential for Metabolic Activation During Drug Discovery

Methods	Purpose	Timing	Resource
In silico			
Chemical structural alerts (Qualitative)	Information on potential risk based on structural analogy to known offenders	Early	Low
In silico analysis of structure and toxicity risk (Qualitative/Quantitative)	Identifies compounds with known alerts	Early	Low
Experimental			
Metabolism studies (Qualitative/Quantitative)	Identification of putative reactive intermediates from *in vitro* or *in vivo* studies as trapped products	Early to late	Medium
Acyl glucuronide half-life (Quantitative)	Stability of an acyl glucuronide to hydrolyze to parent molecule or undergo rearrangement to ring opened products	Early to late	Low
Protein/amino acid adduct identification (Quantitative)	Identification of the conjugate of the drug to a peptide/amino acid residue following digestion of the adducted protein	Mid to late	High
Covalent binding (Quantitative)	Measurement of the amount of drug-related material covalently bound to protein under defined experimental conditions	Mid	High
Quantitative trapping assays (Quantitative)	Estimate of the amount of putative reactive intermediate formed under defined experimental conditions using radioactive or fluorescent labeled trapping agents	Early to late	Medium
Toxicogenomics (Qualitative)	Analysis of the transcriptome, proteome and metabolome from *in vitro* or *in vivo* drug-exposed tissues to assess risk relative to a standard validated set of DILI-causing drugs	Mid to late	High

In order to provide meaningful and actionable information in a timely manner, industrial drug metabolism scientists utilize one or more of the available tools in a fit-for-purpose manner depending upon the stage of the discovery process and the question being addressed. Table 21.1 above lists the tools that scientists have at their disposal, along with the resource implications, achievable throughput, nature of the output they provide, and the timing of the analysis in a typical drug discovery project.

The following sections discuss the merits and limitations of each of these tools in detail.

Chemical Structural Alerts

Certain chemical substructures are particularly prone to forming reactive electrophilic metabolites capable of covalently binding to cellular macromolecules. Examples of these, as noted above, include anilines, hydrazines, nitroarenes, α,β-unsaturated carbonyls, thiophenes, terminal alkenes, or alkynes. Circumstantial evidence in the literature links bioactivation of these functional groups to various forms of toxicity observed with certain drugs (e.g., ticlodipine, tienilic acid and zileuton for thiophene; carbutamide, procainamide, and tocainide for aniline; phenelzine, hydralazine, dihydralazine, and isoniazid for hydrazine; chloramphenicol, tolcapone, flutamide, and metronidazole for nitroaromatics, etc.) [11,41–43]. In some cases, replacement of the offending substructure with a metabolically benign functional group has indeed led to a safer and less toxic second-generation agent, lending support to the idea that formation of reactive metabolites was a key feature in the toxicity of the original agent. For example, the antidiabetic agent, carbutamide, was withdrawn from the market due to severe bone marrow toxicity; however, replacement of the aniline moiety of carbutamide with a toluene substituent led to the discovery of tolbutamide, which is devoid of this toxicity. Similarly, the antiarrhythmics, procainamide and tocainide, both contain an aniline substructure and cause bone marrow aplasia and lupus syndrome, while a closely related congener, flecainide, lacks the aniline motif and is devoid of these toxicities. This subject has been reviewed in depth in several articles [11,42–44]. It should be noted that, as a result of medicinal chemistry efforts to access novel chemical space in support of drug discovery programs, new structural alerts are being recognized on an ongoing basis and require continued vigilance from drug metabolism scientists. For example, it has been reported that boronic acid-containing structures such as those found in the proteasome inhibitors bortezomib and ixazomib can become bioactivated to chemically reactive imine amide derivatives [45]. Also, while the potential for metabolic activation of the carboxylic acid moiety through conversion to the corresponding acyl glucuronide has been recognized for many years [46], recent studies have pointed to a potential role for coenzyme A [47,48] and GSH-linked thioesters [49] as reactive metabolites of carboxylic acids, and even the intermediate acyl adenylate that is the immediate precursor of the acyl-CoA could serve as an intracellular electrophile [50,51]. Other examples of such recently discovered structural alerts include the thiazolidinedione, pyrazinone, isoxazole, and piperazine functionalities, as well as *N*-substituted piperidines and ureas [52–56]. It should be borne in mind, however, that the mere presence of a structural alert does not necessarily mean that a given molecule will undergo metabolism to a reactive intermediate since the functional group in question may not be accessible to drug metabolizing enzymes—this needs to be determined on a case-by-case basis through appropriate experimentation. Thus, strict avoidance of structural alerts in drug design is an overly conservative approach that could severely limit the exploration of the full chemical space for structure-activity relationships (SAR) in the discovery of optimal drug candidates. Instead, it is recommended that the analysis of structural alerts should be performed in conjunction with appropriate and timely experimental investigation in order to assess the risk associated with the molecule in question. Such experiments may involve metabolite identification studies *in vitro* and analysis of elimination routes of the drug candidate *in vivo*. The exact nature of these experiments and their timing varies across pharmaceutical companies, but it is generally accepted that assessment of the perceived risk associated with a structural alert should be performed early in the lead optimization phase.

In Silico Assessment of Toxicity Risk

In silico analysis of toxicity risk encompasses a range of predictive, integrative and visualization tools that may utilize prior knowledge as well as empirical or mechanistic modeling (e.g., Quantitative Structure Activity Relationships [QSAR]; molecular docking). Sophisticated software applications such as TIBCO® Spotfire can be valuable to visualize and correlate multi-parametric data. In the future, one could imagine the construction of a user-friendly interface where a large number of compounds with clinical DILI or genetic toxicity can be associated with known bioactivation mechanisms, physicochemical properties, specific structural motifs, drug elimination pathways, dose levels, population distributions and genetic descriptors.

Relatively mature *in silico* tools are available for assessing the risk of genetic toxicity such that general recommendations of their use are included in regulatory guidelines. The recent ICH M7 regulatory guideline recommends that the genetic toxicity risk assessment should be performed using two QSAR prediction methodologies complementing each other: a statistical- and an expert rule-based method [57,58]. The application of two orthogonal models increases sensitivity and coverage. DEREK Nexus (The Deductive Estimation of Risk from Existing Knowledge, an expert rule-based system) and Sarah Nexus (a statistical system), when analyzed against several public and proprietary databases, displayed 70%–85% agreement. In addition, when agreements were achieved between the two methods, accuracy of mutagenicity predictions was found to be as high as 90% [59]. Software such as DEREK can be used to differentiate a potentially genotoxic aromatic amine from a benign one; such applications are useful in early drug discovery when more resource-intensive evaluations (such as the Ames assay) of many non-optimized leads may not be warranted. It is not fully understood why aromatic amines differing only in the position of a methyl group or a ring nitrogen, often contrary to electronic principles, can show contrasting mutagenic properties. Molecular modeling approaches can be applied to gain insight into such unanticipated mechanisms. For example, activation of amines by CYP1A2 has been extensively studied to delineate whether $Ar-NH_2$ to $Ar-NH-OH$ conversion occurs *via* a radical or an anionic pathway. Such mechanistic information can provide useful hints regarding the electronics of the drug molecule and potentially help in the design of safer drug candidates [60–62]. In an Amgen AKT program suffering from bioactivation issues involving an aminothiazole scaffold, Gaussian calculations were used to measure the relative energies of epoxidation, the suspected offending metabolic pathway. Coupled with metabolite identification and covalent binding studies, such analysis helped guide appropriate SAR efforts to yield a molecule lacking bioactivation liability [63]. Furthermore, the accuracy of *in silico* tools for prediction of drug metabolism such as Metasite™ (Molecular Discovery Ltd., Pinner, Middlesex, UK) and Meteor Nexus™ (Lhasa Ltd., Leeds, UK) is also steadily improving and these tools can be used in conjunction with the above described molecular modeling or genetic toxicity assessment software to assess toxicity risks with potential metabolites of drug candidates at early stages of drug discovery.

Newer advanced system-based approaches such as the one exemplified by the DILIsym® group (Research Triangle Park, NC, USA) strive to assess the risk of a more complex toxicity endpoint, namely DILI, during drug discovery and development. The DILIsym® software encompasses a mechanistic computational model of DILI the structure of which includes key liver cells (e.g., hepatocytes, Kupffer cells), intracellular biochemical systems (e.g., mitochondrial dysfunction), and whole-body dynamics (drug distribution and metabolism) and allows *in vitro* to *in vivo* extrapolation as well as preclinical to clinical translation of DILI risk based on prior knowledge. In addition to representing physiological data for preclinical species and humans, DILIsym® also includes indices of inter-individual variability. Using a simulated human population, DILIsym® successfully differentiated clinical outcomes between the hepatotoxic agent, tolcapone, and its structurally-related but non-hepatotoxic analog, entacapone. In a simulated population receiving recommended clinical doses of the two drugs, serum alanine transaminase (ALT) >3 times the upper limit of normal (ULN) were observed in 2.2% of the population for tolcapone, while no simulated patients on entacapone experienced serum ALT >3 times ULN [64]. As these software tools become more data rich, it is envisioned that they will provide enhanced predictive power for a larger selection of molecules and add to the arsenal of available predictive tools.

Liquid Chromatography-Mass Spectrometry (LC-MS) Based Identification of Chemically-Reactive Metabolites via "Trapping" Studies

LC-MS based approaches likely represent the single most important tool for assessing bioactivation liabilities in a drug discovery setting. An early intervention entails incubation of a number of drug candidates with appropriately cofactor-fortified liver preparations (e.g., hepatocytes, microsomes, or S9) from selected preclinical species and humans. The reactive electrophilic species formed from drug candidates generally do not exhibit sufficient stability to be detected as such and, therefore, they need to be captured following adduction with small nucleophiles that are included as "traps" in the incubation. Some exceptions are reactive species such as acyl glucuronides or CoA thioesters and, rarely, some epoxides that may exhibit sufficient stability under the analytical conditions being employed, allowing their direct detection. The underlying assumption of the "trapping" approach is that the reactive species that are trapped by surrogate small molecule trapping agents will also covalently bind to biological macromolecules. The tripeptide glutathione (γ-glutamylcysteinylglycine, GSH) is the most common trapping agent used in such applications, where its cysteinyl thiol nucleophilic center reacts covalently with the electrophilic intermediate, such as the aromatic epoxide **1** shown in Figure 21.1. As an extension of this approach, other thiols, such as *N*-acetylcysteine, cysteine, and 2-mercaptoethanol, have also been used in such studies [39,65]. Interestingly, cysteine has been shown to react *via* both its thiol and amine functional groups to trap bifunctional electrophiles. For example, the enedial intermediate **2** from the furan-containing compound, ipomeanine, is trapped by cysteine to form a cyclic adduct (Figure 21.1) [66]. It is to be noted that these thiol derivatives are "soft" nucleophiles and react readily with "soft" electrophiles (e.g., quinones, epoxides; Figure 21.1), but they are not efficient at trapping "hard" electrophiles such as iminium ions and other reactive species such as electrophilic carbonyls (e.g., aldehydes and activated ketones). These latter reactive intermediates are more efficiently trapped by the non-thiol hard nucleophiles such as cyanide, semicarbazide, methoxyamine, and DNA bases.

Cyanide has been used to trap "hard" electrophiles such as iminium ions resulting from metabolic activation of compounds such as *S*-nicotine (intermediate **3** in Figure 21.2a) and other alicyclic tertiary amines [67]. For compounds suspected to yield aldehydes as reactive intermediates, the most commonly used trapping agents include semicarbazide and methoxyamine. For example, furan-containing compounds undergo oxidative ring opening to form aldehyde intermediates (represented by compound **4**, Figure 21.2b), which can be trapped by methoxyamine and semicarbazide [44,68]. An interesting product from

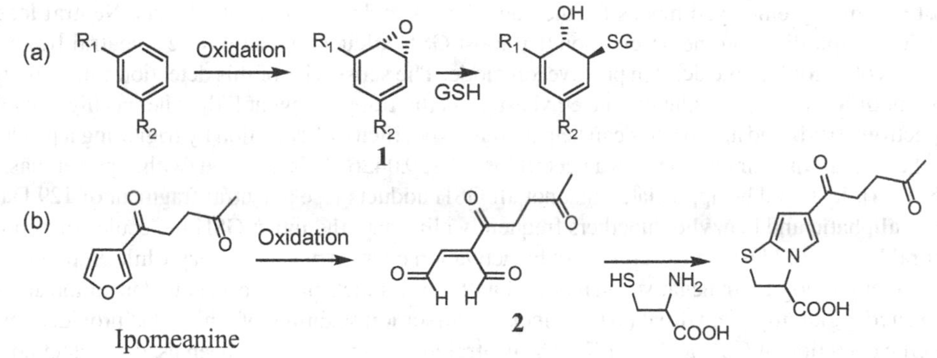

FIGURE 21.1 Thiol nucleophiles as trapping agents. (a) Trapping of an aromatic epoxide with glutathione, (b) Bifunctional trapping of an enedial by cysteine.

semicarbazide trapping of the furan-derived intermediate **5** of pulegone is the tetrahydrocinnoline derivative **6**, supposedly arising from condensation of one molecule of semicarbazide with the γ-ketoenal intermediate **7** of furan ring metabolism (Figure 21.2c) [69].

The LC-MS analysis of adducts of drug candidates with trapping agents typically involves two steps. In the first step, the molecular mass of the adduct is determined from the *m/z* value of its molecular ion and, in the second, a product ion spectrum is generated by collision-induced dissociation (CID) of the parent ion to determine the sub-structural motif(s) involved in bioactivation. Advances in mass spectrometry and separation technologies over the last decade have provided drug metabolism scientists with extremely sensitive and reliable tools for detection of small amounts of metabolites in complex biological matrices. In the positive ionization mode, neutral fragment loss and precursor ion scans are

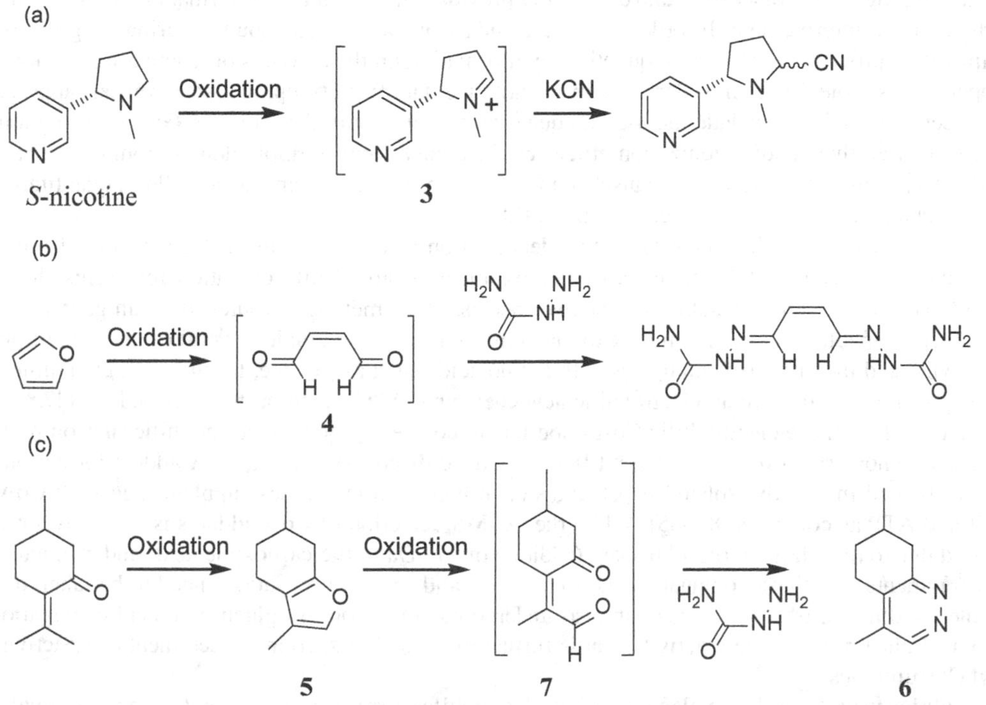

FIGURE 21.2 Reactive intermediate capture by the use of nucleophilic trapping agents; cyanide for an iminium ion (a) and semicarbazide for 1,4-dicarbonyls (b) and (c).

the most commonly employed modes for the detection of molecular ions of adducts. Neutral loss scan methodology capitalizes on the observation that most GSH adducts typically lose a neutral fragment of 129 Da (loss of pyroglutamic acid) in positive ion mode. The sensitivity of this detection can be increased by using modified GSH (e.g., glutathione ethyl ester) as the trapping agent [70], whereas high-resolution mass spectrometry-based approaches can help increase specificity of detection by triggering a product ion scan of the relevant precursor ion when a neutral loss of 129.0426 Da is detected (within preset mass error windows) [71]. It should be appreciated that not all GSH adducts lose a neutral fragment of 129 Da upon CID (e.g., aliphatic and benzylic thioethers frequently eliminate the intact GSH molecule corresponding to a neutral loss of 307 Da), and awareness of bioactivation chemistry is necessary while employing these screening methodologies. In negative ion mode, glutathione adducts produce an abundant anion at m/z 272 (deprotonated γ-glutamyl-dehydroalanyl-glycine), precursor ion scanning of which that provides sensitive and specific detection of GSH adducts [72]. The neutral loss scans also have been used to detect non-thiol adducts of drug candidates; for example, a high-throughput method that employs the neutral loss of 27 Da to detect cyanide adducts of a series of compounds forming iminium ions has been reported [73].

In addition to the above "older" methods, high-resolution mass spectrometry-based approaches capitalize on the similarity of the mass between the parent molecule and its metabolites, and on the fact that most xenobiotics exhibit negative mass-defects relative to endogenous materials; thus, by defining preset filter windows, ions that fall outside the mass defect range can be filtered out and compound-of-interest-related ions selected over those from the matrix to further increase the specificity, speed and throughput of detection [74–76].

Another commonly used approach for the identification of molecular ion(s) of adducts is a knowledge-based search for the expected masses from full scan MS data. Rule-based algorithms are available within the LC-MS software to generate exhaustive lists of masses of expected metabolites, the detection of which can be used to trigger further CID scans to provide structural information [77]. Variations of these methods include the use of equimolar mixtures of naturally occurring and stable-isotope-labeled GSH (which incorporates [$^{13}C_2,^{15}N$]glycine) as a trapping agent in microsomal incubations, such that the resulting adducts are readily detectable *via* the "isotopic signature" with enhanced specificity [78–80].

The trapping assays discussed above generally provide only qualitative information on the formation of the reactive intermediate. In order to make comparisons across compounds during drug discovery optimization process, some level of quantitative information on the amounts of reactive species formed/ trapped is desirable. In order to derive semi-quantitative data from trapping assays, various approaches have been reported that include the use of a quaternary ammonium derivative of GSH carrying a fixed positive charge that reduces ionization efficiency differences across thiol adducts from different drug candidates, or use of a fluorescent dansylated GSH as the trapping agent, which allows quantitation of the adduct amounts *via* fluorescence detection [81,82].

The discussion above has focused on the identification of reactive intermediates formed from drug candidates *via* (usually P450-mediated) oxidative metabolism. While oxidation represents the most prolific pathway for the generation of reactive species, other metabolic routes also can generate reactive species capable of covalent binding to macromolecules. For example, several drugs containing the carboxylic acid moiety form conjugates with amino acids such as glycine, taurine, and glutamine, and this is presumed to involve an electrophilic acyl coenzyme A (CoA) thioester intermediate [47,83–85]. The potential for these electrophilic CoA thioesters to covalently modify nucleophilic sites on proteins has been demonstrated *in vivo* in the rat [83]. In a drug discovery setting, CoA adduct formation can be investigated in freshly isolated hepatocytes or in hepatic microsomes supplemented with CoASH, Mg^{2+} and ATP as cofactors [83–85]. While the LC-MS detection of CoA adducts is relatively straightforward due to their large molecular mass (addition of 749 Da to the carboxylic acid) and characteristic CID fragmentation, these conjugates tend to be labile and special precautions need to be taken during sample handling. Carboxylic acids can also undergo bioactivation *via* glucuronic acid conjugation to form acyl glucuronides, the reactivity that is further discussed in section "Assessment of Reactivity of Acyl Glucuronides."

In addition to proteins, low molecular weight electrophiles formed from xenobiotics can also covalently bind to DNA, with the potential consequences of mutagenicity and carcinogenicity. DNA modifications generally are detected as adducts to individual bases following digestion of the adducted DNA strands. Several selective estrogen receptor modulators (SERMs) are known to form such adducts. For example, guanine adducts of tamoxifen that are postulated to be formed *via* transient carbocation, quinone or quinone methide intermediates have been observed in endometrial tissues from patients taking the drug [86]. Chemically prepared quinone methides of desmethyl arzoxifene and acolbifene have been shown to form adducts *in vitro* when incubated with deoxynucleosides [87,88]. In drug discovery, drug candidates sometimes test positive in early mutagenicity testing in a metabolism-dependent manner (Ames bacterial mutagenicity assay in the presence of liver S9 fractions). In such instances, follow-up metabolism studies can be conducted using DNA bases (e.g., guanine) as trapping agents to identify the biotransformation step(s) responsible for the generation of the DNA-damaging electrophile(s) in concert with mutagenicity assay results and an SAR developed to alleviate the liability. In addition, metabolism studies can be used proactively to eliminate potentially problematic pathways and help lower risk to the pipeline. In a recent Merck Research Laboratories (MRL) drug discovery program, the aminoisoxazole compound **8** (Figure 21.3) represented a promising lead. The hydrolysis product diaminoisoxazole **9** and *N-O* cleaved derivative of the parent **10** were found to be prominent metabolites. This observation led to the deduction that, although not detected (perhaps due to lack of LC retention), the *N-O* cleaved aniline **11** is a likely metabolite. Compound **11** was synthesized and assessed for mutagenicity in the Ames assay, along with compounds **8** and **9**. While compounds **8** and **9** were negative, compound **11** was found to be Ames positive, demonstrating that the release of the aniline, coupled with the cleavage of the isoxazole ring, generated a mutagenic moiety. Subsequent SAR studies led to a follow-up molecule that lacked the potential to form this mutagenic metabolite. Note that compound **11** was not experimentally observed as a metabolite of candidate **8**, but its presence was anticipated *via* mechanistic understanding of the available metabolism data. Thus, insight into the biotransformation route allowed proactive assessment of mutagenicity risk at a very early stage.

Another area where trapping studies can be helpful is to design out P450 time-dependent inhibition (TDI) during lead optimization where one or more reactive species formed from metabolism of the drug candidate bind to P450 heme or apoprotein and result in irreversible inactivation of the enzyme. Compound **12** was found to be a very potent time-dependent inhibitor of CYP3A4. In order to identify the potential reactive metabolite responsible for the observed TDI, compound **12** was incubated at a high concentration (50 µM) with 200 pmol of recombinant human CYP3A4 supplemented with GSH (5 mM), and the supernatant concentrated to allow detection of small amounts of adduct(s). LC-MS analysis of this sample identified compound **13** as a glutathione adduct. The proposed mechanism to form adduct **13** involves hydroxylation of one of the urea nitrogens as the first step. Subsequent flow of electrons from the second urea nitrogen releases the hydroxylamine moiety **14** as a good leaving group and produces a highly reactive isocyanate derivative **15**. Intermediate **15** is trapped by GSH to form product **13** (Figure 21.4). It was hypothesized that the isocyanate **15** is responsible for the observed TDI. In addition, the aromatic hydroxylamine may be further oxidized to the corresponding nitroso derivative **16** that can also play a role in CYP TDI *via* coordination to the heme iron. The conclusion that urea bioactivation is the causal step for CYP3A4 TDI was supported by subsequent SAR studies, where follow-up compounds lacking the urea function were devoid of any enzyme inhibition. This example illustrates the value of fit-for-purpose studies and application of knowledge of bioactivation mechanisms to solve important lead optimization challenges.

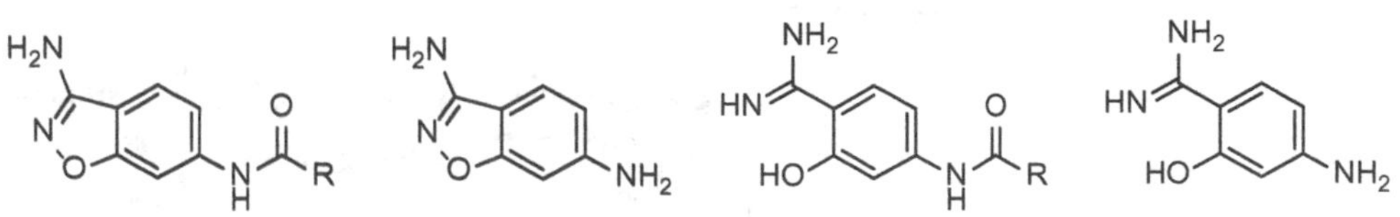

FIGURE 21.3 Structures of drug candidate **8** and its known/proposed metabolites.

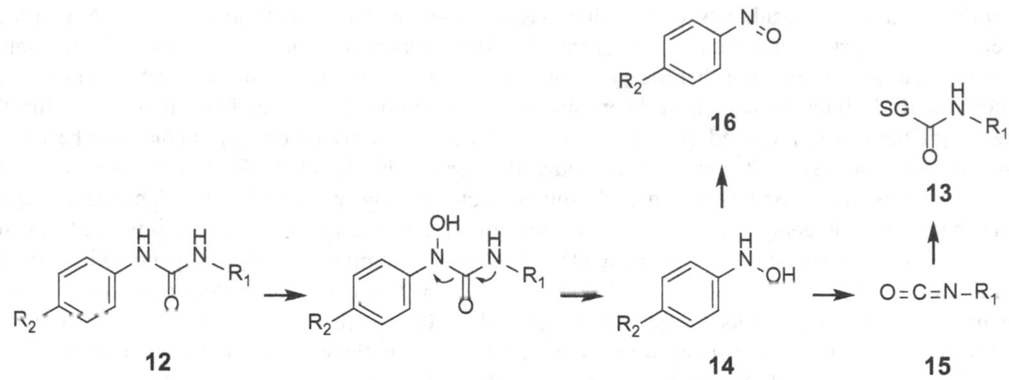

FIGURE 21.4 Bioactivation of a urea functionality as a proposed mechanism of CYP3A4 TDI.

Assessment of Reactivity of Acyl Glucuronides

Acyl glucuronidation represents a common elimination pathway of carboxylic acid-containing drugs. While acyl glucuronides can react with nucleophiles, they are sufficiently stable to allow their synthesis, isolation and characterization. The reactivity of acyl glucuronides can involve two mechanisms: firstly, transacylation (Figure 21.5a) where the sugar moiety of the acyl glucuronide **17** is replaced by a

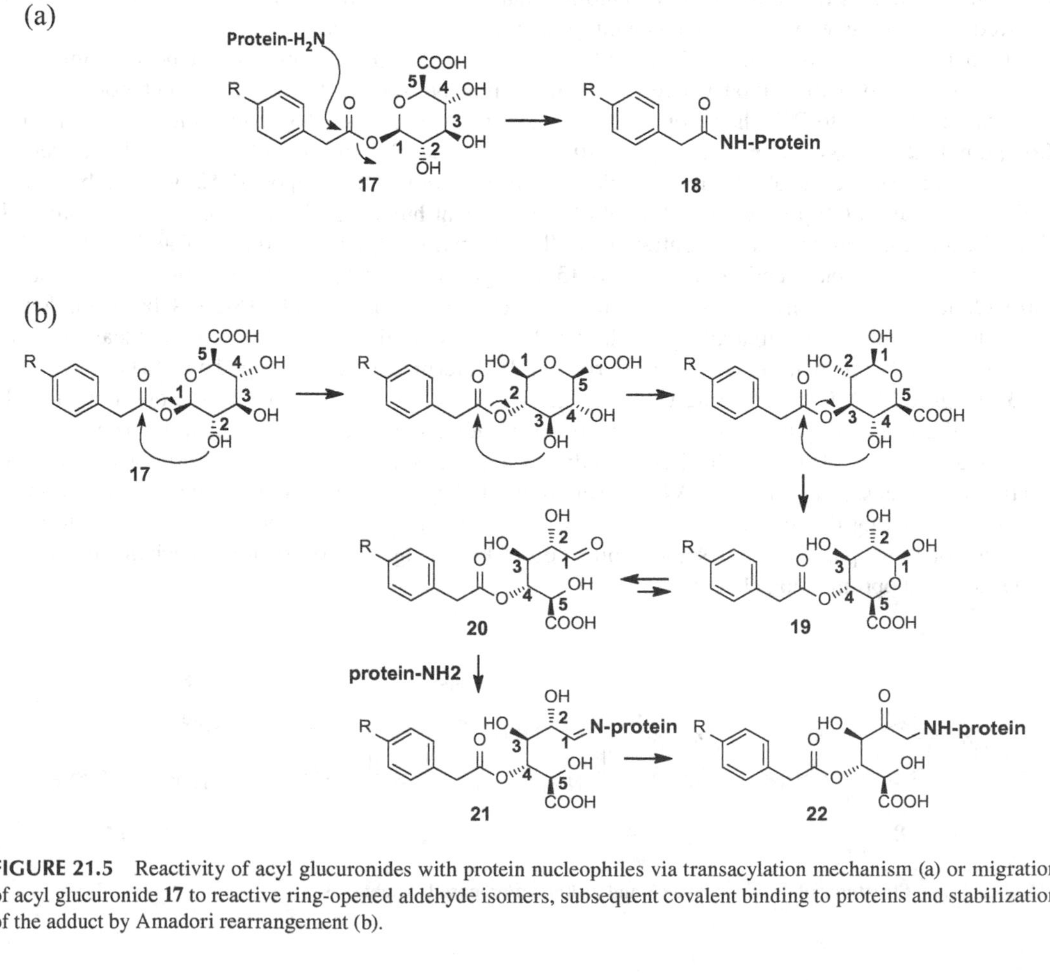

(a)

(b)

FIGURE 21.5 Reactivity of acyl glucuronides with protein nucleophiles via transacylation mechanism (a) or migration of acyl glucuronide **17** to reactive ring-opened aldehyde isomers, subsequent covalent binding to proteins and stabilization of the adduct by Amadori rearrangement (b).

protein to produce amide **18**, and secondly, acyl migration within the glucuronide conjugate **17** to form hemiacetal intermediates (e.g., **19**) that exist in equilibrium with ring-opened aldehyde isomers (e.g., **20**) (Figure 21.5b). These aldehyde species can react with proteins to form imines (e.g., **21**) that are then stabilized *via* Amadori rearrangement to an amine **22** [48]. The potential of such transacylation and acyl migration processes is thought to be dependent on the electrophilicity of the carbonyl group of the glucuronide.

A measure of the stability, or the half-life, of the acyl glucuronide and its ability to undergo acyl migration to yield isomeric conjugates can be used to estimate its potential for reacting with protein residues. A typical experiment would entail the preparation of an authentic standard of the acyl glucuronide and determination of its half-life in aqueous buffer in the absence of any protein. Acyl glucuronides generated biosynthetically *in vitro* or *in vivo* have also been used in cases where preparation of the pure synthetic standard is complex. In an analysis of 21 molecules spanning the spectrum of DILI risk, the cut-off value of the acyl glucuronide half-life, which separated safe drugs from those withdrawn from market, was calculated to be 3.6 hours [46]. It is important to recognize that the panel of drugs included in this analysis ranged in dose 10–4000 mg and had multiple mechanisms of bioactivation, including the formation of reactive CoA intermediates that are known to form protein adducts that could also contribute to liver toxicity. It is nonetheless noteworthy that the acyl glucuronide half-life did appear to correlate with the potential for liver toxicity, supporting the approach of measuring the acyl glucuronide reactivity as a tool for de-risking carboxylic acid containing drug candidates for potential DILI liabilities.

Detection and Identification of Drug-Protein Adducts

The most direct approach to assessing the bioactivation potential of a drug candidate is the identification and quantification of the adduct(s) formed between the chemically-reactive species and protein or DNA, the macromolecules considered most relevant to toxicological consequences of bioactivation. However, the throughput and speed of currently available technologies for this purpose is not adequate for a fast-paced drug discovery setting, and hence such an approach is not commonly used. However, methodologies are available to help understand protein adduction mechanisms in cases where traditional trapping studies do not provide actionable data. As in the case of GSH conjugates, the structures of drug-protein adducts reveal the identities of the reactive intermediates from which they were derived. As an example, radiolabeled compound **23** (Figure 21.6) irreversibly modified liver and kidney proteins in the rat *in vivo* in a dose- and time-dependent manner. Following nonspecific proteolytic digestion of liver and kidney proteins with pronase, a single major amino acid adduct was obtained. From LC-MS and NMR data, this adduct **25** was found to be the product of a novel metabolic activation pathway, where the azetidine moiety underwent oxidative ring opening to afford an α,β-unsaturated aldehyde **24**, with subsequent conjugation to the ε-amino group of a lysine residue. Further digestion studies of rat liver homogenates led to the identification of the adducted peptide, which was further deduced to originate from covalent labeling of acyl-CoA synthetase-1 (ACSL1) [89].

Other examples of recent work in this area include a study on the suite of proteins in the human liver that become adducted upon exposure to the reactive metabolite of acetaminophen *in vitro*, showing that four mitochondrial oxidative stress related proteins (GATM, PARK7, PRDX6, and VDAC2) are targets [90], and an investigation into the identities of protein adducts in patients given the antiretroviral drug abacavir that revealed the formation of novel intramolecular cross-linked adducts to human serum albumin resulting from its reaction with an electrophilic α,β-unsaturated aldehyde metabolite of the drug [91].

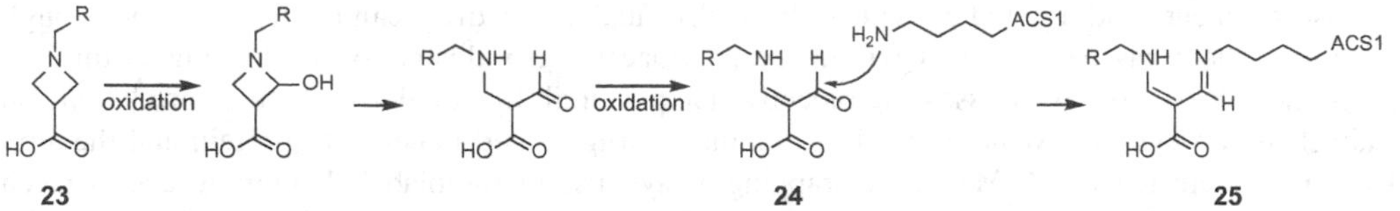

FIGURE 21.6   Protein adducts of compound **23** formed via oxidative opening of the azetidine ring.

Similarly, characterization of the protein adducts from isoniazid [92], a widely-used anti-tubercular agent that causes liver injury, has provided evidence in support of a revised theory of the mechanism by which this drug undergoes bioactivation [93].

Application of Covalent Binding Studies in Drug Discovery

The above LC-MS based approaches aimed at evaluating the potential for bioactivation risk currently provide, at best, qualitative or semi-quantitative information, and are not likely to be applicable universally for studying all types of reactive intermediates. The current "gold standard" approach for reliably quantifying the extent of drug-protein adduction remains the traditional covalent binding studies that are conducted with radiolabeled analogs of drug candidates. The requirement for synthesis of a radiolabeled analog of the drug candidate makes these studies low-throughput, costly and not amenable to the rapid screening strategies desired in a drug discovery setting. Thus, covalent binding studies generally are conducted as a second step in the lead optimization process following synthesis of radiolabeled analogs of a limited number of more mature lead candidates. The usual approach involves measuring the extent of covalent binding of drug-related material to animal and human liver microsomal protein or hepatocytes *in vitro*, and to liver and plasma proteins from animals *in vivo* [10,94]. The covalent binding data (expressed as pmol equiv/mg protein) obtained from these assays are indicative of the propensity of the drug candidate to form reactive species that are capable of covalent adduction to proteins under both *in vitro* and *in vivo* conditions. The data generated in hepatocytes and *in vivo* are considered more meaningful since they utilize a more complete biological system with all relevant metabolic pathways and native protective mechanisms (e.g., GSH conjugation, quinone reductases). In particular, studies in human hepatocytes, in principle, provide data in a system that is most relevant to the clinical situation. Studies *in vivo* allow factors such as dose, systemic exposure, blood-to-liver partitioning, and plasma protein binding to be taken into account. Furthermore, the key to correct interpretation of the covalent binding data is the qualitative and quantitative understanding of bioactivation routes of the drug in animals and humans. This information can serve to "bridge" the preclinical data to man and help project potential exposure of humans to chemically reactive metabolites after administration of the drug candidate at a clinically relevant dose. These covalent binding studies, albeit somewhat crude in terms of their relevance to predicting toxicological outcomes, afford a means during drug discovery to differentiate lead candidates in terms of their potential to generate reactive species in animal safety testing and eventually in humans. Over the past 10–15 years, this approach has been utilized frequently across the pharmaceutical industry to measure and minimize the potential for metabolic activation in drug candidates [2,54,65,95].

An example of the utility of covalent binding studies is illustrated by compound **26** from a recent drug discovery program at MRL, which demonstrated high levels of protein adduction (~800 pmol-eq/mg protein) in human hepatocytes. Traditional trapping studies failed to identify the structural moiety that was subject to bioactivation and responsible for the observed binding to protein. From pronase-catalyzed digestion of the adducted proteins, sulfide product **27** was identified (Figure 21.7). The obligate precursor of product **27** is hypothesized to be the carbon-centered radical intermediate **28**, formed by opening of the cyclopropyl ring of **26** by a mechanism reminiscent of single electron oxidation of cyclopropyl amines. Based on this hypothesis, follow-up molecule **29** was designed and was found to be practically devoid of covalent binding (10 pmol-eq/mg) (Figure 21.7) (MRL, unpublished data).

Higher-Throughput Surrogate Assays for Quantifying the Potential for Bioactivation

Because covalent binding studies with radiolabeled analogs of drug candidates are low-throughput and costly, there has been interest within the pharmaceutical industry to develop higher-throughput approaches for quantitatively assessing bioactivation potential. In situations where a correlation can be established between the extent of covalent binding of drug-related material to protein and the amount of adduct(s) detected in LC-MS based trapping assays, use of radiolabeled trapping agents (such as [^{3}H]GSH, [^{35}S]GSH, [^{35}S]β-mercaptoethanol and K^{14}CN) have been explored. The resulting radioactive adducts can then be separated from excess trapping agent by appropriate extraction procedures and

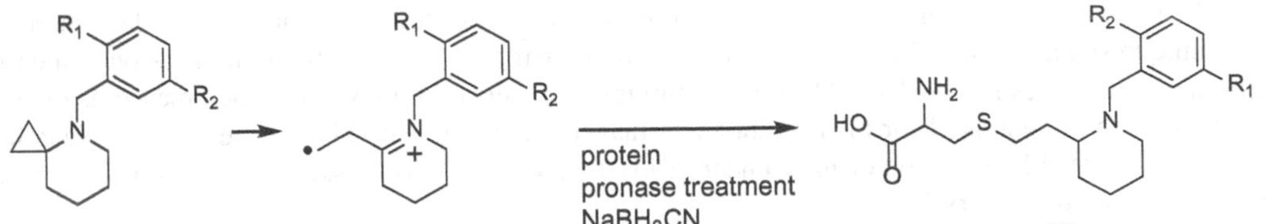

FIGURE 21.7 Proposed mechanism of bioactivation of cyclopropane derivative **26** and formation of cysteine adduct **27**, identification of which led to the design of compound **29** that was resistant to metabolic activation.

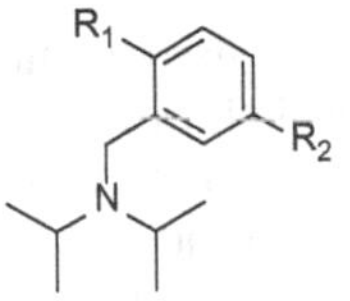

quantified using plate-based radioactivity detection methods. This assay format is easily amenable to automation, thus dramatically increasing the speed and throughput of data generation. It was shown that a series of compounds that were bioactivated to electrophilic iminium intermediates, when subjected to microsomal incubations fortified with $K^{14}CN$, produced radiolabeled cyanide adducts the amounts of which correlated reasonably well with the covalent binding of these analogs to protein [96]. Similarly, a series of compounds that formed reactive intermediates that could be scavenged by GSH, when subjected to microsomal incubations fortified with $[^{35}S]\beta$-mercaptoethanol, produced labeled thiol adducts the amounts of which afforded a reasonable correlation with the corresponding covalent binding values [97]. Similarly, Masubuchi et al. [98] demonstrated a good correlation between the amount of GSH conjugates formed (using both unlabeled and $[^{35}S]GSH$) from a set of 10 model compounds with the extent of covalent binding of radiolabeled drug-related material to human and rat liver microsomal protein, and to rat liver protein *in vivo* when systemic exposure (plasma AUC) and plasma free fraction were taken into account. A key consideration for the successful utilization of trapping assays for reactive intermediate screening is the judicious selection of the trapping agent(s) based on a sound understanding of the mechanism of bioactivation/covalent binding and the nature of the resulting chemically-reactive species (e.g., hard *versus* soft electrophiles). Such studies can help increase the speed, efficiency and throughput, and lower the overall cost of bioactivation studies by significantly reducing the number of radiolabeled drug candidates that need to be synthesized for this purpose.

Approaches to Assess Oxidative and Electrophilic Cellular Stress Resulting from Drug Bioactivation

As discussed at the outset, a fundamental gap in our knowledge in assessing toxicity risk associated with bioactivation is that only some, and not all, reactive metabolites have been implicated in drug toxicity. In recent years, efforts have been initiated within the pharmaceutical industry to assess chemical mechanisms of bioactivation in combination with the potential downstream effects on cellular health in the hope of differentiating problematic forms of bioactivation from those that may be relatively benign. Assessment of these downstream effects has included endpoints ranging from simpler readouts, such as gross cytotoxicity and effects on mitochondrial function, to more ambitious toxicogenomic, proteomic, and metabolomic assessments that aim to identify broad changes in the biological system in response to xenobiotic and reactive metabolite assault. These latter analyses are based on the hypothesis that a foreign compound and its bioactivated products would modulate the transcriptome, proteome, or metabolome with a specific signature that could be correlated to toxicological outcome or a lack thereof. Such a unique signature may then serve as a predictive biomarker of a downstream toxicity outcome for future drug candidates [31,99–101]. The current limited experience in integrating such measures of cellular stress with the potential for bioactivation to enhance the predictive value of these assessments for toxicity is discussed later in this chapter under "Bioactivation, Toxicity Risk, and Decision-Making in the Pharmaceutical Industry."

Challenges in Interpreting Bioactivation Risk

As discussed above, a variety of approaches are used within the pharmaceutical industry to assess the risk of formation of chemically reactive metabolites from drug candidates. In addition to the fundamental challenge of assessing relevance of specific bioactivation pathways to potential toxicity, there remain significant difficulties in generating and interpreting human relevant data from these studies that can be used objectively to assess risk with individual drug candidates. The LC-MS based trapping studies aimed at evaluating the potential for bioactivation currently provide, at best, qualitative or semi-quantitative information, and are not applicable universally for trapping all types of reactive intermediates. While these studies can be useful to understand structural features of drug candidates that lead to reactive metabolites, it should be recognized that they represent a somewhat artificial system that lacks the full physiological complement of various dispositional and detoxifying pathways, and no direct link to potential toxicity risk can, or should, be drawn from readouts in these systems. In spite of substantial debate and clarification of this point over the past few years [2,24–26,65,102], detection of GSH conjugates or downstream products thereof *in vitro* or *in vivo* is still frequently mistaken by drug discovery teams to represent a marker of toxicity. It should be noted that these thiol products reflect the operation of a *detoxification* pathway for the reactive species and, when detected, indicate that detoxification machinery is functioning to serve its intended purpose. The risk, however, is that this detoxification pathway potentially can be overwhelmed in the setting of high doses or certain patient or disease specific situations and lead to toxicity.

Assessment of inhibition of P450 enzymes in a time-dependent manner is considered an additional approach/filter to assess the potential formation of reactive species during drug discovery where irreversible time-dependent inhibition of the enzyme suggests formation of a reactive species that inactivates P450 by binding to prosthetic heme or apoprotein. However, in most companies, this time-dependent P450 inhibition assessment is limited to CYP3A due to the prevalent role of this enzyme in drug metabolism and its resulting high importance for drug interaction risk. However, there are multiple examples where the reactive species formed by enzymes other than CYP3A have led to time-dependent inhibition of a different enzyme and also resulted in toxicity (e.g., tienilic acid [98]).

As discussed previously, covalent binding studies that assess irreversible binding of radioactivity to microsomal or hepatocyte protein *in vitro* or total liver protein *in vivo* following incubation or administration of the radiolabeled drug candidate provide the most reliable quantitative data on its bioactivation potential. The following sections discuss some key points that should be considered while generating and interpreting appropriate covalent binding data and assessing its relevance for humans.

Acceptable Levels of Covalent Binding

There has been much debate within the pharmaceutical industry as to what constitutes an acceptable level of covalent binding for a drug candidate. Considering the limitations of our understanding of the biochemical mechanisms by which some reactive intermediates may cause toxicities, a simple answer to this question remains elusive. Originally, it was proposed by scientists at MRL that a value of 50 pmol eq/mg protein (under well-defined experimental conditions [10]) be used as an upper-end target for advancing drug candidates into development. This target was based on the crude observation that the extent of covalent binding of a number of known hepatotoxins (e.g., acetaminophen, bromobenzene, furosemide, and 4-ipomeanol) in animal liver, under conditions where liver necrosis was evident, is of the order of ~1 nmol equiv/mg protein. Thus, the 50 pmol equiv/mg protein value provides an ~20-fold "safety margin" over the levels of binding that have been associated with frank hepatic necrosis with some hepatotoxic agents. It should be emphasized that the 50 pmol equiv/mg protein figure was never intended to be a rigid threshold for covalent binding, but rather was proposed as a target value above which other considerations would need to be taken into account before progressing a particular drug candidate. Subsequent to the MRL publication on this subject, other pharmaceutical companies, such as Glaxo SmithKline [26] and AstraZeneca [23], have developed their own protocols for assessing covalent binding, which typically involve upper target values higher than 50 pmol equiv/mg protein.

Covalent Binding in Relation to Drug Exposure

An additional point of discussion relates to the assay conditions under which the extent of covalent binding is measured, including considerations such as the concentration of the drug candidate in incubations with liver preparations *in vitro* and the dose, formulation, bioavailability, and systemic exposure in studies *in vivo*. Since the extent of bioactivation of a drug candidate is expected to depend upon the pathways and kinetics of its metabolism, which, in turn, could be modulated by its absorption, systemic exposure, and tissue (liver) partitioning, it would appear reasonable that these factors be taken into account while designing covalent binding studies to cover bounds of intended clinical exposure.

Low Metabolic Turnover

For a substantial fraction of drug candidates, the extent of metabolic turnover during the typical incubation time period (1–2 hours) in traditional *in vitro* systems used for covalent binding studies (liver microsomes, hepatocytes) is low because a key goal of many drug discovery programs is to decrease rates of metabolism and thereby extend elimination half-life in order to achieve once-a-day dosing regimen. The low metabolic turnover, in turn, presents challenges in fully assessing the bioactivation potential of lead candidates and makes identification of the bioactivation pathways more difficult. This also results in a reduced level of confidence in understanding qualitative and quantitative species differences in various metabolic pathways (including those involved in bioactivation) across species, leading to a less robust "bridging" of preclinical data to the human situation [65]. The newer engineered liver systems and organoids that incorporate co-culture of hepatocytes with other liver cell types in a 3D format offer considerable promise in providing more physiologically-relevant preparations with a significantly prolonged viability for fully assessing the bioactivation potential of compounds that are not significantly turned over in traditional liver preparations [103].

Relationship Between Overall Metabolic Clearance and Bioactivation

Typically, the metabolic pathway(s) that lead to the generation of reactive metabolites represent only one component of the overall clearance of the drug candidate. Since different drug candidates display variable rates of metabolism and clearance in various *in vitro* and *in vivo* assay systems, it is important to understand the fraction of the metabolism that occurs *via* the bioactivation pathway in order to appropriately benchmark different molecules and assess total body burden of reactive species for risk-assessment [25].

Inter-species Differences in Metabolism

While qualitative species-differences in the metabolism of xenobiotics across mammalian species are relatively uncommon, differences in the quantitative contribution of various metabolic pathways to drug disposition, including those involved in the formation of chemically reactive metabolites, are the rule rather than the exception [104]. Thus, it is important to understand the disposition of the drug candidate(s) and gain a mechanistic view of the pathways involved in bioactivation and covalent binding for accurate assessment of the relevance of covalent binding data generated in animals to humans. In this regard, efforts to understand mechanisms of metabolic activation can be of value in rationalizing foreign compound-mediated toxicities that are species-specific. Such understanding can, in turn, provide

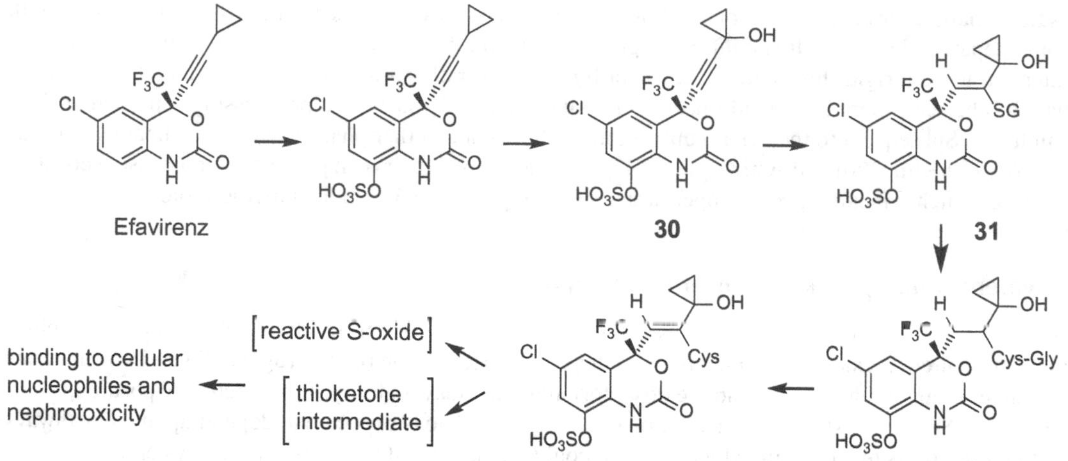

FIGURE 21.8 Proposed mechanism for the rat-specific metabolic activation of efavirenz and its role in nephrotoxicity in the rat. (Adapted from references Mutlib, A.E. et al., *Drug Metab. Dispos.*, 27, 1319–1333, 1999; Mutlib, A.E. et al., *Toxicol. Appl. Pharmacol.*, 169, 102–113, 2000.)

a framework for assessing the risk of certain toxicities in humans that may be mediated through metabolic activation. An elegant illustration of this point is provided by studies with the non-nucleoside HIV reverse transcriptase inhibitor, efavirenz, which causes renal tubular epithelial cell necrosis in rats but not in cynomolgus monkeys or humans at equivalent or greater systemic exposures [105,106]. The sulfate conjugate of hydroxylated efavirenz is metabolized to a cyclopropanol metabolite **30** *via* oxidation at the methine position of the cyclopropane moiety that is linked to an alkyne functionality (Figure 21.8); this cyclopropanol metabolite likely serves as a substrate for a *rat-specific* glutathione-*S*-transferase(s) and results in the addition of GSH to the alkyne moiety of efavirenz in rats to form metabolite **31**. Interestingly, this pathway is not seen in other species. The GSH conjugate **31** is processed further in the rat kidney to a cysteinylglycine conjugate via γ-glutamyltranspeptidase-catalyzed removal of the glutamic acid residue, and the cysteinylglycine conjugate is either excreted in urine or is involved in further bioactivation events that eventually lead to nephrotoxicity in the rat. Strong evidence for this hypothesis was obtained when decreases in the formation of the cysteinylglycine conjugate, either by suppressing the formation of the cyclopropanol metabolite or by inhibiting γ-glutamyltranspeptidase activity, led to reductions in the incidence and severity of nephrotoxicity.

Another striking example of differences in biotransformation across (and within) species was published recently by Taub et al. [107] who reported on the sex-, species-, and tissue-specific metabolic activation in male CD-1 mouse kidney of empagliflozin, an SGLT2 inhibitor for the treatment of Type 2 diabetes (Figure 21.9a). In an effort to account for the formation of renal tumors only in male animals in a 2-year mouse carcinogenicity study, but not in female mice or in male or female rats, it was shown through *in vitro* studies that empagliflozin undergoes oxidative metabolism in mouse renal microsomes to yield an unstable hemiacetal species **32**. This intermediate, generated only in preparations from male animals, degrades spontaneously to yield 4-hydroxycrotonaldehyde (Figure 21.9a), a reactive, cytotoxic α,β-unsaturated aldehyde that was trapped by GSH and characterized by LC-MS/MS techniques. Since glucuronidation is the prevalent pathway of empagliflozin metabolism in humans, and oxidation is minor, it was concluded that renal toxicity due to the formation of 4-hydroxycrotonaldehyde from empagliflozin would not be expected in humans. A further example of species differences in bioactivation is found in a report by Hadi et al. [108] who studied the metabolism and toxicity of 3′-hydroxyacetanilide (AMAP, Figure 21.9b), the alleged non-hepatotoxic regioisomer of acetaminophen (APAP, Figure 21.9c). Both compounds had been found to undergo CYP-dependent oxidation to reactive quinoid species (APBQ and NAPQI, respectively), yet only APAP was believed to be toxic. However, the early toxicology studies with AMAP had been carried out in mice and hamsters, and when the compound was re-evaluated in precision-cut liver slices from rat and human, it proved to be equally or more toxic than APAP.

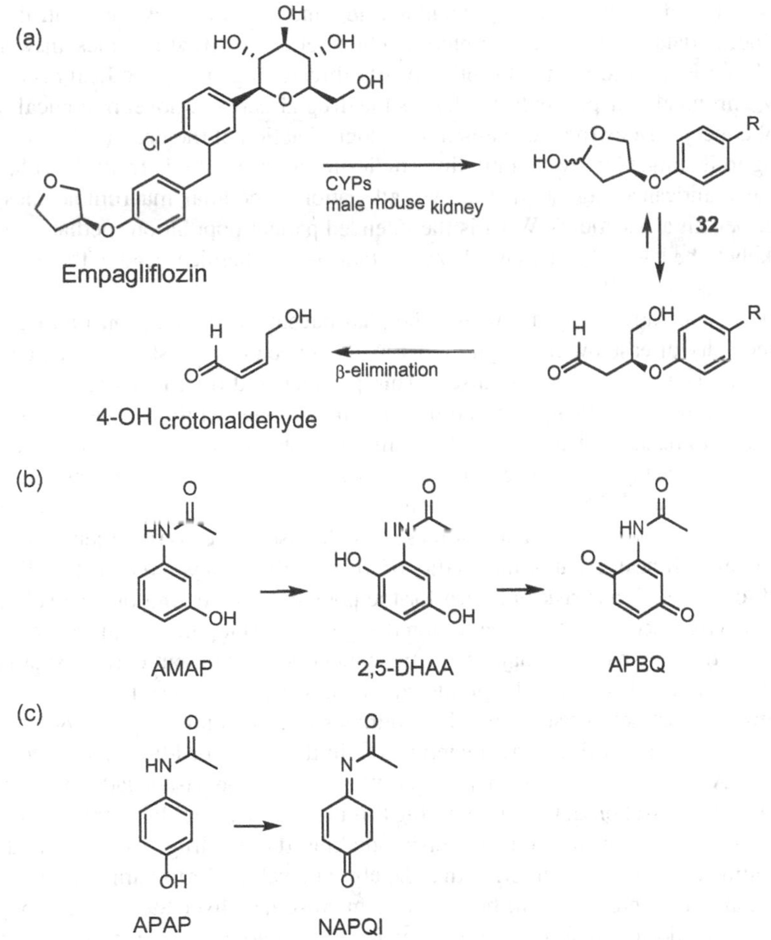

FIGURE 21.9 Metabolic activation pathways of (a) empagliflozin, (b) AMAP, and (c) APAP.

This species difference in AMAP toxicity appears to be related to species differences in exposure to the reactive metabolites APBQ and NAPQI, a conclusion that was supported by a subsequent *in silico* analysis of the potential of these two agents to cause liver injury in mice [109]. These examples clearly illustrate the value of understanding bioactivation mechanisms and their relationship to toxicity findings in preclinical species in order to assess risk in humans.

The points above on practical limitations of the covalent binding data support the notion that rigid "cut-off" values for the extent of covalent binding to protein for decision-making in drug discovery are inappropriate and should be avoided. The extent of bioactivation and covalent binding should be interpreted in light of knowledge of the overall metabolic turnover of the compounds and systemic exposure to drug-related material in relation to the target clinical exposure, and species-differences in metabolism should be taken into account when extrapolating covalent binding risk to humans.

Bioactivation, Toxicity Risk, and Decision-Making in Pharmaceutical Industry

As noted above, a framework for addressing metabolic activation issues in drug discovery was first proposed by Evans et al. [10] and broadly adopted at MRL [2,10,65]. Due to the imprecise relationship of metabolic activation with toxicity and the fact that this attribute is only one aspect of the overall risk/benefit assessment for advancing a particular lead candidate into development, it was advocated that covalent binding data should be interpreted in a broader context that includes answers to questions such as: Is the drug intended to treat a disabling or life-threatening unmet medical need? Will the drug be used acutely, chronically or prophylactically? Is the drug aimed at a novel biological target awaiting clinical proof of concept? Does the mechanism of biological action of the drug involve bioactivation and covalent binding to its target? (Covalent binding studies for antimicrobials from the β-lactam class and for many cytotoxic anticancer agents that act *via* alkylation of cellular macromolecules would not be relevant for risk/benefit assessment). What is the intended patient population (pediatric, elderly)? Is the clinical dose likely to be low (≤10 mg/day)? How tractable is the chemical lead with respect to modification at the site of bioactivation?

The heightened focus in recent years within the pharmaceutical industry on finding targeted medicines for rare specialty diseases with a high unmet medical need (e.g., cystic fibrosis, Duchenne's muscular dystrophy, etc. [110]) as well as on discovering personalized treatments for smaller segments of the overall disease population, brings an additional point of consideration. These so-called *precision medicines* are likely to be administered to only small segments of the patient population of a few thousand people. Given the average incidence of idiosyncratic toxicity of 1 in 10,000 patients, such precision medicines may never be administered to a large enough population to pose a significant population hazard. Furthermore, since patients with many of these rare diseases have no treatment options and face an inevitable decline in their health status and quality of life over time, they and their families are generally more motivated to accept higher risk in return for the potential for slowing or reversal of their disease progression. In such instances, it may appear rational to pursue development of drug candidates that have the potential to positively impact the majority of the patient population but carry a small risk for a rare idiosyncratic adverse event that cannot be predicted with any degree of certainty.

These mitigating factors notwithstanding, there remains a substantial body of evidence that suggests that chemically reactive metabolites play a central role in the direct or idiosyncratic toxicity observed with certain drugs. As such, there have been multiple attempts over the past decade to enhance the predictive value of metabolic activation data by integrating this drug property with other risk factors to improve overall toxicity risk-assessment and aid in decision-making during drug discovery and development. These efforts stemmed from the observation that the absolute values for the amount of covalent binding of drug-related material to protein from human liver microsomes, liver S9 and hepatocytes following *in vitro* incubations could not differentiate a set of nine hepatotoxic and nine non-hepatotoxic agents [19,20]. However, when total daily dose and the fractional clearance to chemically reactive metabolites that covalently bind to protein were used to estimate the *total daily body burden* of reactive species, there was an improvement in parsing hepatotoxic and non-hepatotoxic compounds. Furthermore, human hepatocytes appeared somewhat better at making this differentiation relative to liver microsomes and S9 fractions, which lack the full complement of metabolic and detoxification pathways [19,20]. A similar conclusion was reached independently by Usui et al. who compared a set of twelve compounds known to cause drug-induced liver injury with twelve other compounds that are considered safe [111]. Covalent binding of drug-related radioactivity to protein was measured following incubation of test compounds with liver microsomes in the presence or absence of additional cofactors such as UDPGA and GSH, as well as in human hepatocytes. A significant amount of overlap was observed in all *in vitro* systems in the covalent binding values of compounds known to cause DILI and those that do not. However, increasing differentiation between hepatotoxic and non-hepatotoxic drugs was achieved when covalent binding values were multiplied by the C_{max} or total daily dose, with the latter being the best discriminator [111]. Nakayama et al. [21] extended this type of analysis to the covalent binding in human liver microsomes, hepatocytes and rat liver in *vivo* of a larger set of 42 marketed drugs in which other types of idiosyncratic toxicity, such as neutropenia, agranulocytosis, and Steven Johnson Syndrome, in addition to serious liver injury, were considered. When covalent binding in human hepatocytes was plotted against the recommended daily dose of each drug, the 42 agents could be parsed into 3 zones denoted as "safe," "toxic" (defined as those withdrawn from market or with a black box warning for idiosyncratic toxicity), and those with a warning for idiosyncratic toxicity in their label [21]. This "zone classification system" represented an important advance in that it allowed for the identification of compounds with low *versus* high risk of causing liver toxicity, although many compounds fell between these two extremes and could not be accurately classified. Additional variations of integrating the recommended daily dose in risk assessment have utilized other measures of assessing metabolic activation such as GSH adduct formation and time-dependent P450 inhibition, in addition to covalent binding [27,112]. All of these analyses are consistent with the notion that *daily total body burden* of reactive species, which is determined by the fractional metabolism to reactive species and the total daily dose, is an important determinant of the toxicity risk posed by metabolic activation. In one analysis [24], it was suggested that the total body burden of reactive metabolites should not exceed 1 mg/day, while in another, a more liberal value of <10mg/day was proposed as a safe upper limit [113]. Of course, these upper target values are largely empirical in nature, but nevertheless provide a useful guide for benchmarking activities. It should be noted that a significant limitation of this approach is that there is often a substantial amount of uncertainty in the estimates of the clinical dose of drug candidates early in development, thus complicating estimates of the body burden of reactive metabolite based on the fractional clearance through the bioactivation pathway.

Clearly, many factors beyond daily dose come into play in the decision to advance into development a new chemical entity that is subject to some degree of metabolic activation, such as the expected risk/benefit ratio of the intended therapy. A case in point is the family of "first generation" tyrosine kinase inhibitors (TKIs) for indications in oncology; erlotinib, gefatinib, lapatinib, and dasatinib all are high-dose TKIs that undergo CYP-mediated metabolism to reactive quinoid species that are believed to play a role in drug-induced liver injury [114,115]. Given the life-threatening nature of the disease for which these drugs are intended, a higher degree of risk for toxicity may be tolerated, but it is interesting to note that newer TKIs, such as the family of EGFR inhibitors being developed for the treatment of non-small cell lung carcinoma, are low-dose compounds that are devoid of metabolic activation liabilities, but which are designed to covalently modify their molecular target (EGFR with activating mutations and deletions) in a highly selective fashion [116]. While the long-term safety of these "second generation" agents, e.g., afatinib and osimertinib, remains to be established, preliminary indications are promising.

In all of the above retrospective studies, while it appears possible to differentiate drugs at the extreme ends of the risk profile using covalent binding data and recommended daily dose or total body burden of reactive metabolites (e.g., <10 mg *versus* several hundred to >1000 mg daily dose), there remains a significant grey area of risk in the middle zone. This limitation is significant given that the majority of drug candidates are likely to fall into this daily dose range of 10 to low hundreds of mg and, as noted above, the fact that there is often a significant amount of uncertainty in the prediction of pharmacokinetic profile and optimal clinical dose at the discovery stage, especially for agents targeting novel biological mechanisms.

There has been increasing recognition in recent years that the gap in being able to precisely link metabolic activation and dose (or total body burden of reactive species) to potential toxicity risk is likely due to two broad reasons: (1) toxicity is multifactorial in nature and other mechanisms of cellular stress, in combination with metabolic activation, lead to toxicity outcomes for certain drugs, and (2) the nature of the macromolecular targets modified and the ensuing cellular insult may be a key determinant of toxicological outcomes or lack thereof. Thus, the missing piece in the armamentarium of approaches to assess toxicity risk related to metabolic activation may be the assays to assess these additional mechanisms that could lead to cellular stress and the tools to evaluate/measure this cellular stress in metabolism-competent human relevant systems. Such a broader approach would also need to be complemented with integrative data handling and interpretation for a multifactorial hazard assessment. To this end, Thompson et al. [24] proposed a multi-pronged approach that included evaluation of the inhibitory potential of drugs against the bile-salt export pump (BSEP) and multidrug resistance-associated protein 2 (Mrp2) as potential mechanisms for cellular stress *via* effects on hepato-biliary homeostasis, in addition to assessment of total daily burden of reactive species based on covalent binding *in vitro* to human hepatocyte protein as a fraction of overall metabolism and recommended daily dose. Further, CYP3A-dependent and metabolism-independent cytotoxicity in THLE cells (SV40 T-antigen-immortalized human liver epithelial cells) and cytotoxicity in HepG2 cells, cultured in glucose *versus* galactose containing media to evaluate potential for mitochondrial injury, were included as markers for cellular insult. The data output from each readout was digitized to 0 (no concern) or 1 (concern) based on specific cut-off values for various assays and composite risk scores were calculated. When the aggregate *in vitro* panel scores were plotted against total daily body burden of covalent binding for a set of 36 agents, of which 27 are known to have severe or marked concern and 9 with low concern for idiosyncratic toxicity, 4 different risk zones in an *integrated in vitro hazard matrix* could be identified. The compounds were segregated into low *versus* high reactive metabolite burden (using a cut-off of 1 mg/day daily predicted covalent binding) and low *versus* high *in vitro* panel score (using a cut-off score of 1.5 out of a possible 4). The zone with low reactive metabolite burden and a low *in vitro* panel score contained only low concern compounds, whereas the other zones contained all 27 compounds known to exhibit severe or marked concern for idiosyncratic toxicity, with a small number (2 out of 7) of low concern agents. Overall, this approach allowed differentiation between drugs known to cause idiosyncratic toxicity *versus* those that are considered safe with 100% sensitivity and 78% specificity [24]. This work again highlighted the importance of the "body burden" of reactive metabolites and suggested that agents that produced less than 1 mg/day of reactive species in humans tended to have a low risk of hepatotoxicity, particularly in the absence of other *in vitro* indices of liver injury. Application of this methodology to a retrospective analysis of the hepatotoxic properties of three endothelin receptor antagonists, namely sitaxentan, bosentan, and ambrisentan, correctly rank-ordered these agents and suggested that multiple mechanisms contribute to the rare, but potentially severe, liver injury caused by sitaxentan in humans [117]. Other variations on this approach have been published recently where slightly different measures of metabolic activation burden (e.g., GSH adduction formation, CYP3A time-dependent inhibition), systemic exposure (e.g., dose, C_{max}), and cellular and mitochondrial stress in different cell systems have been used to differentiate between agents that have high risk of causing idiosyncratic drug toxicity from those that do not [28,118]. On the other hand, a simple empirical approach termed "Rule of Two" proposed by the scientists at the FDA argues that compounds with log P $\geq$ 3 and dose $\geq$ 100 mg carry a greater risk for hepatotoxicity; this analysis is consistent with the notion that greater lipophilicity can impact cellular partitioning, metabolism profile (including bioactivation pathways) and general off-target promiscuous binding to cellular macromolecules [119,120]. A deeper mechanistic analysis of the data presented in this argument would provide critical insights for further validation. All of the above studies have further emphasized the multifactorial nature of drug-induced toxicities and serve to reinforce the concept that metabolic activation and covalent binding alone do not necessarily translate to a high potential for adverse reactions to a new chemical entity. Many of these approaches that account for multiple drug attributes in addition to bioactivation potential do appear to result in improved risk classification for marketed drugs and could find use in drug discovery to enrich for compounds that have a lower overall risk for causing idiosyncratic drug toxicity. It should be noted, however, that these methods are likely not suitable in their present form for assessing absolute risk of idiosyncratic toxicity with individual compounds and in making definitive decisions on advancing or terminating development of drug candidates. Since the drug discovery process is a complex multidimensional endeavor that requires concurrent optimization of many molecular attributes, it often results in compounds that appear attractive from an efficacy perspective and promise to address an important medical need but have other potential risks (e.g., metabolic activation and risk of idiosyncratic toxicity) that need to be understood with each individual candidate before making major investment decisions. The fact that the above multifactorial risk-assessment approaches, as yet, lack the precision to assess this risk with individual compounds is perhaps the reason that such methods have not been adopted universally across the pharmaceutical industry. This is especially true for small or mid-size companies where there is greater competition for limited resources, a culture of higher tolerance for risks that cannot be easily predicted or mitigated, and an urgency to progress projects and portfolio to ensure continued investor interest.

The limitations of the current integrative approaches to toxicity risk assessment are likely due to the *in vitro* models and the relatively crude readouts (cytotoxicity) that have been used thus far to assess cellular insult. Significant developments have occurred in the past 5 years in both areas that promise to enhance the reliability of these multifactorial toxicity risk assessments in the future. In terms of improved cellular systems, there has been an explosion in the number of available 3D liver or hepatic organoid models that are based on co-cultures of human hepatocytes with other liver cell types. Some examples of these systems include Hepatopac® (micropatterned co-culture of hepatocytes with fibroblasts; Ascendance Biotechnology, Medford, MA, USA), Hμrel® (co-culture of hepatocytes with non-parenchymal stromal cells; Hμrel Corporation, North Brunswick, NJ, USA), ExVive3D® (multiple cell types including hepatocytes, stellate, and endothelial cells cultured in a spatially controlled manner using NovoGen Bioprinting platform™; Organovo Holdings, Inc., San Diego, CA, USA), LiverChip® (microfluidic flow-through co-culture; CN Bio Innovations Ltd., Hertfordshire, UK), and many others. These models provide an improved microphysiological environment for hepatocytes and create a cellular phenotype that is claimed to be closer to the *in vivo* situation. Furthermore, many of these systems have extended viability that allows their use for several weeks at a time, with stable expression of drug metabolizing enzymes and transporters. As a result, these systems should allow assessment of cellular drug effects after multiple dosing in the presence of normal processes of detoxification and bioactivation to more closely simulate the clinical situation. With advances in stem cell technologies, it is also now possible to obtain iPSC-derived hepatocytes from patients [121] who may have experienced toxicity; these cells, when cultured in the improved 3D configurations described above, may also allow incorporation of patient-specific factors into assessment of toxicity risk. In addition to these improved *in vitro* models, there has also been substantial progress over the past few years in developing novel *human relevant* animal models that can be used to assess toxicity risk due to chemically reactive metabolites. These include genetically-engineered and chimeric animals that express single, multiple, or the entire complement of human drug metabolizing enzymes and transporters [122]. The chimeric mouse models that have the majority of their liver populated with human hepatocytes on an immune-deficient background are particularly attractive for assessing the risk of hepatotoxicity since they have been shown to quantitatively recapitulate human metabolic pathways of many drugs [123,124]. Early studies to investigate the utility of these mice for parent drug- or metabolism-dependent liver toxicity show substantial promise and warrant further study with additional hepatotoxic agents [124,125]. Future development of these chimeric models also promises to incorporate engraftment of the human immune system along with human hepatocytes in the liver, which could, in theory, allow assessment of hepatotoxicity that has an immune component in response to an insult from chemically-reactive metabolites [126].

As for the improved end-points to assess cellular stress that eventually leads to toxicological outcomes, perhaps it is the toxicogenomic, proteomic, and metabolomic approaches that hold the greatest promise due to their broad potential to provide insights into perturbation of various biological networks in response to drug exposure as a prelude to toxicity [31,101,127–130]. These analyses can help recognize early patterns of change across a broad range of biological networks in response to toxicants and identify potential trigger mechanisms and biomarkers that precede full manifestation of toxicity. There have been initial successes with the utilization of these approaches to identify signatures as predictive markers that may provide a link to toxicity. However, much more work needs to be done to assess whether such changes in response to drug exposure in more physiological and metabolically-competent *in vitro* and *in vivo* models described above can help address the central question in assessing the risk of toxicity with metabolic activation as to why only some, and not all, chemically-reactive metabolites lead to drug toxicity.

In summary, it has been well understood for many years that metabolic activation is an important risk factor in causing direct or indirect immune-mediated idiosyncratic toxicity for some drugs, while in other cases it appears to be relatively benign. The challenge during drug discovery is to be able to differentiate these two types of metabolic activation to allow accurate projection of risk for decision-making. However, our current state of biological understanding and the available tools are not adequate to allow this differentiation, with the exception that dose and total body burden of reactive metabolites appear to be important determinants of toxicity risk. As a result, recent approaches for assessing toxicity risk with metabolic activation have evolved to include other risk factors and readouts such as dose/exposure, daily body burden of reactive species, BSEP inhibition, and measures of cellular stress or cytotoxicity in various cell systems to take into account the multifactorial nature of drug toxicity and integrate all of these readouts into composite risk scores. These approaches do appear to result in incrementally improved toxicity risk classification for marketed drugs. However, in spite of the progress made in recent years, it should be acknowledged that our scientific approach to addressing this issue remains rather rudimentary, both in terms of the quality of assay systems and readouts that are employed for human risk assessment, and in our understanding of the biological mechanisms that result in toxic insult following exposure to chemically-reactive metabolites. For these reasons, different pharmaceutical companies appear to have adopted different strategies on this issue over the past few years depending upon the availability of resources and their tolerance for risk. These strategies range from routinely optimizing for a reduced potential for metabolic activation to not evaluating bioactivation at all and simply relying on routine animal toxicology studies to capture the potential for direct toxicities. Assessing the risk of idiosyncratic toxicities that appear to be immunologically mediated represents the greatest challenge of all, and we are only beginning to understand the complex molecular events by which reactive drug metabolites can trigger an adverse reaction through activation of the immune system [18]. Over the past 5 years, exciting breakthroughs have begun to occur in developing significantly improved *in vitro* and *in vivo* liver models that appear to be closer to native human tissue and are able to quantitatively recapitulate human drug metabolism pathways. These models, when combined with more robust measures of cellular stress based on broader toxicogenomic, proteomic, and/or metabolomic signatures in response to exposure to parent drug and metabolite (both stable and chemically-reactive), provide a potentially promising path to a new more scientific approach to assessing the role of metabolic activation in drug toxicity and minimizing this risk in humans.

REFERENCES

1. Stachulski, A.V. et al., The generation, detection, and effects of reactive drug metabolites. *Med Res Rev*, 2013. **33**(5): 985–1080.
2. Kumar, S. et al., Approaches for minimizing metabolic activation of new drug candidates in drug discovery. *Handb Exp Pharmacol*, 2010. **196**: 511–44.
3. Leung, L., A.S. Kalgutkar, and R.S. Obach, Metabolic activation in drug-induced liver injury. *Drug Metab Rev*, 2012. **44**(1): 18–33.
4. Dalvie, D., A.S. Kalgutkar, and W. Chen, Practical approaches to resolving reactive metabolite liabilities in early discovery. *Drug Metab Rev*, 2015. **47**(1): 56–70.
5. Kalgutkar, A.S. and D. Dalvie, Predicting toxicities of reactive metabolite-positive drug candidates. *Annu Rev Pharmacol Toxicol*, 2015. **55**: 35–54.
6. Uetrecht, J. and D.J. Naisbitt, Idiosyncratic adverse drug reactions: Current concepts. *Pharmacol Rev*, 2013. **65**(2): 779–808.
7. Johnston, A. and J. Uetrecht, Current understanding of the mechanisms of idiosyncratic drug-induced agranulocytosis. *Expert Opin Drug Metab Toxicol*, 2015. **11**(2): 243–257.
8. Ikeda, T., Idiosyncratic drug hepatotoxicity: Strategy for prevention and proposed mechanism. *Curr Med Chem*, 2015. **22**(4):528–537.
9. Baillie, T.A., Future of toxicology-metabolic activation and drug design: Challenges and opportunities in chemical toxicology. *Chem Res Toxicol*, 2006. **19**(7): 889–893.
10. Evans, D.C. et al., Drug-protein adducts: An industry perspective on minimizing the potential for drug bioactivation in drug discovery and development. *Chem Res Toxicol*, 2004. **17**(1): 3–16.
11. Stepan, A.F. et al., Structural alert/reactive metabolite concept as applied in medicinal chemistry to mitigate the risk of idiosyncratic drug toxicity: A perspective based on the critical examination of trends in the top 200 drugs marketed in the United States. *Chem Res Toxicol*, 2011. **24**(9): 1345–1410.
12. Eno, M.R. and M.D. Cameron, Gauging reactive metabolites in drug-induced toxicity. *Curr Med Chem*, 2015. **22**(4): 465–489.
13. Kalgutkar, A.S., Should the incorporation of structural alerts be restricted in drug design? An analysis of structure-toxicity trends with aniline-based drugs. *Curr Med Chem*, 2015. **22**(4): 438–464.
14. Gramec, D., L. Peterlin Masic, and M. Sollner Dolenc, Bioactivation potential of thiophene-containing drugs. *Chem Res Toxicol*, 2014. **27**(8): 1344–1358.
15. Zuniga, F.I. et al., Idiosyncratic reactions and metabolism of sulfur-containing drugs. *Expert Opin Drug Metab Toxicol*, 2012. **8**(4): 467–485.
16. Dansette, P.M. et al., Formation and fate of a sulfenic acid intermediate in the metabolic activation of the antithrombotic prodrug prasugrel. *Chem Res Toxicol*, 2010. **23**(7): 1268–1274.
17. Dansette, P.M. et al., Metabolic activation of prasugrel: Nature of the two competitive pathways resulting in the opening of its thiophene ring. *Chem Res Toxicol*, 2012. **25**(5): 1058–1065.
18. Meng, X. et al., Immunological mechanisms of drug hypersensitivity. *Curr Pharm Des*, 2016. **22**(45): 6734–6747.

19. Bauman, J.N. et al., Can *in vitro* metabolism-dependent covalent binding data distinguish hepatotoxic from nonhepatotoxic drugs? An analysis using human hepatocytes and liver S-9 fraction. *Chem Res Toxicol*, 2009. **22**(2): 332–340.
20. Obach, R.S. et al., Can *in vitro* metabolism-dependent covalent binding data in liver microsomes distinguish hepatotoxic from nonhepatotoxic drugs? An analysis of 18 drugs with consideration of intrinsic clearance and daily dose. *Chem Res Toxicol*, 2008. **21**(9): 1814–1822.
21. Nakayama, S. et al., A zone classification system for risk assessment of idiosyncratic drug toxicity using daily dose and covalent binding. *Drug Metab Dispos*, 2009. **37**(9): 1970–1977.
22. Nakayama, S. et al., Combination of GSH trapping and time-dependent inhibition assays as a predictive method of drugs generating highly reactive metabolites. *Drug Metab Dispos*, 2011. **39**(7): 1247–1254.
23. Thompson, R.A. et al., Risk assessment and mitigation strategies for reactive metabolites in drug discovery and development. *Chem Biol Interact*, 2011. **192**(1–2): 65–71.
24. Thompson, R.A. ct al., *In vitro* approach to assess the potential for risk of idiosyncratic adverse reactions caused by candidate drugs. *Chem Res Toxicol*, 2012. **25**(8): 1616–1632.
25. Thompson, R.A. et al., Reactive metabolites: Current and emerging risk and hazard assessments. *Chem Res Toxicol*, 2016. **29**(4): 505–533.
26. Reese, M. et al., An integrated reactive metabolite evaluation approach to assess and reduce safety risk during drug discovery and development. *Chem Biol Interact*, 2011. **192**(1–2): 60–64.
27. Sakatis, M.Z. et al., Preclinical strategy to reduce clinical hepatotoxicity using *in vitro* bioactivation data for >200 compounds. *Chem Res Toxicol*, 2012. **25**(10): 2067–2082.
28. Schadt, S. et al., Minimizing DILI risk in drug discovery-A screening tool for drug candidates. *Toxicol In Vitro*, 2015. **30**(1 Pt B):429–437.
29. Stamper, B.D., Transcriptional profiling of reactive metabolites for elucidating toxicological mechanisms: A case study of quinoneimine-forming agents. *Drug Metab Rev*, 2015. **47**(1): 45–55.
30. Pelkonen, O. et al., Reactive metabolites in early drug development: Predictive *in vitro* tools. *Curr Med Chem*, 2015. **22**(4): 538–550.
31. Qin, S. et al., Identification of organ-enriched protein biomarkers of acute liver injury by targeted quantitative proteomics of blood in acetaminophen- and carbon-tetrachloride-treated mouse models and acetaminophen overdose patients. *J Proteome Res*, 2016. **15**(10): 3724–3740.
32. Bhatia, S.N. and D.E. Ingber, Microfluidic organs-on-chips. *Nat Biotechnol*, 2014. **32**(8): 760–772.
33. Miller, J.A., Brief history of chemical carcinogenesis. *Cancer Lett*, 1994. **83**(1–2): 9–14.
34. Miller, J.A., The metabolism of xenobiotics to reactive electrophiles in chemical carcinogenesis and mutagenesis: A collaboration with Elizabeth Cavert Miller and our associates. *Drug Metab Rev*, 1998. **30**(4): 645–674.
35. Bolton, J.L. et al., Role of quinones in toxicology. *Chem Res Toxicol*, 2000. **13**(3): 135–160.
36. Liu, X. et al., Antiestrogenic and DNA damaging effects induced by tamoxifen and toremifene metabolites. *Chem Res Toxicol*, 2003. **16**(7): 832–837.
37. Kalgutkar, A.S., R.S. Obach, and T.S. Maurer, Mechanism-based inactivation of cytochrome P450 enzymes: Chemical mechanisms, structure-activity relationships and relationship to clinical drug-drug interactions and idiosyncratic adverse drug reactions. *Curr Drug Metab*, 2007. **8**(5): 407–447.
38. Orr, S.T. et al., Mechanism-based inactivation (MBI) of cytochrome P450 enzymes: Structure-activity relationships and discovery strategies to mitigate drug-drug interaction risks. *J Med Chem*, 2012. **55**(11): 4896–4933.
39. Grillo, M.P., Detecting reactive drug metabolites for reducing the potential for drug toxicity. *Expert Opin Drug Metab Toxicol*, 2015. **11**(8): 1281–1302.
40. Monks, T.J. and S.S. Lau, Reactive intermediates: Molecular and MS-based approaches to assess the functional significance of chemical-protein adducts. *Toxicol Pathol*, 2013. **41**(2): 315–321.
41. Boelsterli, U.A. et al., Bioactivation and hepatotoxicity of nitroaromatic drugs. *Curr Drug Metab*, 2006. **7**(7): 715–727.
42. Kalgutkar, A.S. and J.R. Soglia, Minimising the potential for metabolic activation in drug discovery. *Expert Opin Drug Metab Toxicol*, 2005. **1**(1): 91–142.
43. Kalgutkar, A.S. et al., A comprehensive listing of bioactivation pathways of organic functional groups. *Curr Drug Metab*, 2005. **6**(3): 161–225.
44. Dalvie, D.K. et al., Biotransformation reactions of five-membered aromatic heterocyclic rings. *Chem Res Toxicol*, 2002. **15**(3): 269–299.

45. Li, A.C. et al., Boronic acid-containing proteasome inhibitors: Alert to potential pharmaceutical bioactivation. *Chem Res Toxicol*, 2013. **26**(4): 608–615.

46. Sawamura, R. et al., Predictability of idiosyncratic drug toxicity risk for carboxylic acid-containing drugs based on the chemical stability of acyl glucuronide. *Drug Metab Dispos*, 2010. **38**(10): 1857–1864.

47. Darnell, M. and L. Weidolf, Metabolism of xenobiotic carboxylic acids: Focus on coenzyme A conjugation, reactivity, and interference with lipid metabolism. *Chem Res Toxicol*, 2013. **26**(8): 1139–1155.

48. Lassila, T. et al., Toxicity of carboxylic acid-containing drugs: The role of acyl migration and CoA conjugation investigated. *Chem Res Toxicol*, 2015. **28**(12): 2292–2303.

49. Grillo, M.P., Drug-S-acyl-glutathione thioesters: Synthesis, bioanalytical properties, chemical reactivity, biological formation and degradation. *Curr Drug Metab*, 2011. **12**(3): 229–244.

50. Grillo, M.P., M. Tadano Lohr, and J.C. Wait, Metabolic activation of mefenamic acid leading to mefenamyl-S-acyl-glutathione adduct formation *in vitro* and *in vivo* in rat. *Drug Metab Dispos*, 2012. **40**(8): 1515–1526.

51. Horng, H. and L.Z. Benet, Characterization of the acyl-adenylate linked metabolite of mefenamic Acid. *Chem Res Toxicol*, 2013. **26**(3): 465–476.

52. Kassahun, K. et al., Studies on the metabolism of troglitazone to reactive intermediates *in vitro* and *in vivo*. Evidence for novel biotransformation pathways involving quinone methide formation and thiazolidinedione ring scission. *Chem Res Toxicol*, 2001. **14**(1): 62–70.

53. Singh, R. et al., Metabolic activation of a pyrazinone-containing thrombin inhibitor. Evidence for novel biotransformation involving pyrazinone ring oxidation, rearrangement, and covalent binding to proteins. *Chem Res Toxicol*, 2003. **16**(2): 198–207.

54. Doss, G.A. et al., Metabolic activation of a 1,3-disubstituted piperazine derivative: Evidence for a novel ring contraction to an imidazoline. *Chem Res Toxicol*, 2005. **18**(2): 271–276.

55. Yin, W. et al., Conversion of the 2,2,6,6-tetramethylpiperidine moiety to a 2,2-dimethylpyrrolidine by cytochrome P450: Evidence for a mechanism involving nitroxide radicals and heme iron. *Biochemistry*, 2004. **43**(18): 5455–5466.

56. Yu, J. et al., Elucidation of a novel bioactivation pathway of a 3,4-unsubstituted isoxazole in human liver microsomes: formation of a glutathione adduct of a cyanoacrolein derivative after isoxazole ring opening. *Drug Metab Dispos*, 2011. **39**(2): 302–311.

57. Amberg, A. et al., Principles and procedures for implementation of ICH M7 recommended (Q)SAR analyses. *Regul Toxicol Pharmacol*, 2016. **77**: 13–24.

58. Pavan, M. et al., The consultancy activity on *in silico* models for genotoxic prediction of pharmaceutical impurities. *Methods Mol Biol*, 2016. **1425**: 511–529.

59. Barber, C. et al., Establishing best practise in the application of expert review of mutagenicity under ICH M7. *Regul Toxicol Pharmacol*, 2015. **73**(1): 367–377.

60. Shamovsky, I. et al., Explanation for main features of structure-genotoxicity relationships of aromatic amines by theoretical studies of their activation pathways in CYP1A2. *J Am Chem Soc*, 2011. **133**(40): 16168–16185.

61. Shamovsky, I. et al., Theoretical studies of chemical reactivity of metabolically activated forms of aromatic amines toward DNA. *Chem Res Toxicol*, 2012. **25**(10): 2236–2252.

62. Ripa, L. et al., Theoretical studies of the mechanism of N-hydroxylation of primary aromatic amines by cytochrome P450 1A2: Radicaloid or anionic? *Chem Res Toxicol*, 2014. **27**(2): 265–278.

63. Subramanian, R. et al., Cytochrome P450-mediated epoxidation of 2-aminothiazole-based AKT inhibitors: Identification of novel GSH adducts and reduction of metabolic activation through structural changes guided by *in silico* and *in vitro* screening. *Chem Res Toxicol*, 2010. **23**(3): 653–663.

64. Longo, D.M. et al., Elucidating differences in the hepatotoxic potential of tolcapone and entacapone with DILIsym((R)), a mechanistic model of drug-induced liver injury. *CPT Pharmacom Syst Pharmacol*, 2016. **5**(1): 31–39.

65. Kumar, S. et al., Minimizing metabolic activation during pharmaceutical lead optimization: Progress, knowledge gaps and future directions. *Curr Opin Drug Discov Devel*, 2008. **11**(1): 43–52.

66. Chen, L.J., E.F. DeRose, and L.T. Burka, Metabolism of furans *in vitro*: Ipomeanine and 4-ipomeanol. *Chem Res Toxicol*, 2006. **19**(10): 1320–1329.

67. Kalgutkar, A.S. et al., On the diversity of oxidative bioactivation reactions on nitrogen-containing xenobiotics. *Curr Drug Metab*, 2002. **3**(4): 379–424.

68. Peterson, L.A., Electrophilic intermediates produced by bioactivation of furan. *Drug Metab Rev*, 2006. **38**(4): 615–626.

69. Khojasteh-Bakht, S.C. et al., Metabolism of (R)-(+)-pulegone and (R)-(+)-menthofuran by human liver cytochrome P-450s: Evidence for formation of a furan epoxide. *Drug Metab Dispos*, 1999. **27**(5): 574–580.

70. Soglia, J.R. et al., The development of a higher throughput reactive intermediate screening assay incorporating micro-bore liquid chromatography-micro-electrospray ionization-tandem mass spectrometry and glutathione ethyl ester as an *in vitro* conjugating agent. *J Pharm Biomed Anal*, 2004. **36**(1): 105–116.

71. Castro-Perez, J. et al., A high-throughput liquid chromatography/tandem mass spectrometry method for screening glutathione conjugates using exact mass neutral loss acquisition. *Rapid Commun Mass Spectrom*, 2005. **19**(6): 798–804.

72. Dieckhaus, C.M. et al., Negative ion tandem mass spectrometry for the detection of glutathione conjugates. *Chem Res Toxicol*, 2005. **18**(4): 630–638.

73. Argoti, D. et al., Cyanide trapping of iminium ion reactive intermediates followed by detection and structure identification using liquid chromatography-tandem mass spectrometry (LC-MS/MS). *Chem Res Toxicol*, 2005. **18**(10): 1537–1544.

74. Ruan, Q. et al., An integrated method for metabolite detection and identification using a linear ion trap/ Orbitrap mass spectrometer and multiple data processing techniques: Application to indinavir metabolite detection. *J Mass Spectrom*, 2008. **43**(2): 251–261.

75. Bateman, K.P. et al., MSE with mass defect filtering for *in vitro* and *in vivo* metabolite identification. *Rapid Commun Mass Spectrom*, 2007. **21**(9): 1485–1496.

76. Wen, B. and M. Zhu, Applications of mass spectrometry in drug metabolism: 50 years of progress. *Drug Metab Rev*, 2015. **47**(1): 71–87.

77. Ma, S. and S.K. Chowdhury, Application of LC-high-resolution MS with "intelligent" data mining tools for screening reactive drug metabolites. *Bioanalysis*, 2012. **4**(5): 501–510.

78. Mutlib, A. et al., Application of stable isotope labeled glutathione and rapid scanning mass spectrometers in detecting and characterizing reactive metabolites. *Rapid Commun Mass Spectrom*, 2005. **19**(23): 3482–3492.

79. Yan, Z. and G.W. Caldwell, Stable-isotope trapping and high-throughput screenings of reactive metabolites using the isotope MS signature. *Anal Chem*, 2004. **76**(23): 6835–6847.

80. Yan, Z. et al., Rapid detection and characterization of minor reactive metabolites using stable-isotope trapping in combination with tandem mass spectrometry. *Rapid Commun Mass Spectrom*, 2005. **19**(22): 3322–3330.

81. Gan, J. et al., Dansyl glutathione as a trapping agent for the quantitative estimation and identification of reactive metabolites. *Chem Res Toxicol*, 2005. **18**(5): 896–903.

82. Soglia, J.R. et al., A semiquantitative method for the determination of reactive metabolite conjugate levels *in vitro* utilizing liquid chromatography-tandem mass spectrometry and novel quaternary ammonium glutathione analogues. *Chem Res Toxicol*, 2006. **19**(3): 480–490.

83. Li, C. et al., Covalent binding of 2-phenylpropionyl-S-acyl-CoA thioester to tissue proteins *in vitro*. *Drug Metab Dispos*, 2003. **31**(6): 727–730.

84. Olsen, J. et al., *In vitro* and *in vivo* studies on acyl-coenzyme A-dependent bioactivation of zomepirac in rats. *Chem Res Toxicol*, 2005. **18**(11): 1729–1736.

85. Olsen, J. et al., Studies on the metabolism of tolmetin to the chemically reactive acyl-coenzyme A thioester intermediate in rats. *Drug Metab Dispos*, 2007. **35**(5): 758–764.

86. Shibutani, S. et al., Identification of tamoxifen-DNA adducts in the endometrium of women treated with tamoxifen. *Carcinogenesis*, 2000. **21**(8): 1461–1467.

87. Liu, H. et al., Bioactivation of the selective estrogen receptor modulator desmethylated arzoxifene to quinoids: 4'-fluoro substitution prevents quinoid formation. *Chem Res Toxicol*, 2005. **18**(2): 162–473.

88. Liu, J. et al., Bioactivation of the selective estrogen receptor modulator acolbifene to quinone methides. *Chem Res Toxicol*, 2005. **18**(2): 174–182.

89. Aloysius, H. et al., Metabolic activation and major protein target of a 1-benzyl-3-carboxyazetidine sphingosine-1-phosphate-1 receptor agonist. *Chem Res Toxicol*, 2012. **25**(7): 1412–1422.

90. Bruderer, R. et al., Extending the limits of quantitative proteome profiling with data-independent acquisition and application to acetaminophen-treated three-dimensional liver microtissues. *Mol Cell Proteomics*, 2015. **14**(5): 1400–1410.

91. Meng, X. et al., Abacavir forms novel cross-linking abacavir protein adducts in patients. *Chem Res Toxicol*, 2014. **27**(4): 524–535.

92. Koen, Y.M. et al., Protein targets of isoniazid-reactive metabolites in mouse liver *in vivo*. *Chem Res Toxicol*, 2016. **29**(6): 1064–1072.

93. Metushi, I., J. Uetrecht, and E. Phillips, Mechanism of isoniazid-induced hepatotoxicity: Then and now. *Br J Clin Pharmacol*, 2016. **81**(6): 1030–1036.

94. Day, S.H. et al., A semi-automated method for measuring the potential for protein covalent binding in drug discovery. *J Pharmacol Toxicol Methods*, 2005. **52**(2): 278–285.

95. Tang, C. et al., Bioactivation of 2,3-diaminopyridine-containing bradykinin B1 receptor antagonists: Irreversible binding to liver microsomal proteins and formation of glutathione conjugates. *Chem Res Toxicol*, 2005. **18**(6): 934–945.

96. Meneses-Lorente, G. et al., A quantitative high-throughput trapping assay as a measurement of potential for bioactivation. *Anal Biochem*, 2006. **351**(2): 266–272.

97. Samuel, K. et al., Addressing the metabolic activation potential of new leads in drug discovery: A case study using ion trap mass spectrometry and tritium labeling techniques. *J Mass Spectrom*, 2003. **38**(2): 211–221.

98. Masubuchi, N., C. Makino, and N. Murayama, Prediction of *in vivo* potential for metabolic activation of drugs into chemically reactive intermediate: correlation of *in vitro* and *in vivo* generation of reactive intermediates and *in vitro* glutathione conjugate formation in rats and humans. *Chem Res Toxicol*, 2007. **20**(3): 455–464.

99. Laifenfeld, D. et al., Utilization of causal reasoning of hepatic gene expression in rats to identify molecular pathways of idiosyncratic drug-induced liver injury. *Toxicol Sci*, 2014. **137**(1): 234–48.

100. Leone, A. et al., Oxidative stress/reactive metabolite gene expression signature in rat liver detects idiosyncratic hepatotoxicants. *Toxicol Appl Pharmacol*, 2014. **275**(3): 189–197.

101. Qin, C. et al., Toxicogenomics in drug development: A match made in heaven? *Expert Opin Drug Metab Toxicol*, 2016. **12**(8): 847–849.

102. Park, B.K. et al., Managing the challenge of chemically reactive metabolites in drug development. *Nat Rev Drug Discov*, 2011. **10**(4): 292–306.

103. Hutzler, J.M., B.J. Ring, and S.R. Anderson, low-turnover drug molecules: A current challenge for drug metabolism scientists. *Drug Metab Dispos*, 2015. **43**(12): 1917–1928.

104. Baillie, T.A. and A.E. Rettie, Role of biotransformation in drug-induced toxicity: Influence of intra- and inter-species differences in drug metabolism. *Drug Metab Pharmacokinet*, 2011. **26**(1): 15–29.

105. Mutlib, A.E. et al., Identification and characterization of efavirenz metabolites by liquid chromatography/mass spectrometry and high field NMR: Species differences in the metabolism of efavirenz. *Drug Metab Dispos*, 1999. **27**(11): 1319–1333.

106. Mutlib, A.E. et al., The species-dependent metabolism of efavirenz produces a nephrotoxic glutathione conjugate in rats. *Toxicol Appl Pharmacol*, 2000. **169**(1): 102–113.

107. Taub, M.E. et al., Sex-, species-, and tissue-specific metabolism of empagliflozin in male mouse kidney forms an unstable hemiacetal metabolite (M466/2) that degrades to 4-hydroxycrotonaldehyde, a reactive and cytotoxic species. *Chem Res Toxicol*, 2015. **28**(1): 103–115.

108. Hadi, M. et al., AMAP, the alleged non-toxic isomer of acetaminophen, is toxic in rat and human liver. *Arch Toxicol*, 2013. **87**(1): 155–65.

109. Howell, B.A., S.Q. Siler, and P.B. Watkins, Use of a systems model of drug-induced liver injury (DILIsym((R))) to elucidate the mechanistic differences between acetaminophen and its less-toxic isomer, AMAP, in mice. *Toxicol Lett*, 2014. **226**(2): 163–172.

110. Ashley, E.A., Towards precision medicine. *Nat Rev Genet*, 2016. **17**(9): 507–522.

111. Usui, T. et al., Evaluation of the potential for drug-induced liver injury based on *in vitro* covalent binding to human liver proteins. *Drug Metab Dispos*, 2009. **37**(12): 2383–2392.

112. Gan, J. et al., *In vitro* screening of 50 highly prescribed drugs for thiol adduct formation-Comparison of potential for drug-induced toxicity and extent of adduct formation. *Chem Res Toxicol*, 2009. **22**(4): 690–698.

113. Dahal, U.P., R.S. Obach, and A.M. Gilbert, benchmarking *in vitro* covalent binding burden as a tool to assess potential toxicity caused by nonspecific covalent binding of covalent drugs. *Chem Res Toxicol*, 2013. **26**(11): 1739–1745.

114. Hardy, K.D. et al., Studies on the role of metabolic activation in tyrosine kinase nhibitor-dependent hepatotoxicity: Induction of CYP3A4 enhances the cytotoxicity of lapatinib in HepaRG cells. *Drug Metab Dispos*, 2014. **42**(1): 162–171.

115. Teo, Y.L., H.K. Ho, and A. Chan, Formation of reactive metabolites and management of tyrosine kinase inhibitor-induced hepatotoxicity: A literature review. *Expert Opin Drug Metab Toxicol*, 2015. **11**(2): 231–242.

116. Baillie, T.A., Targeted covalent inhibitors for drug design. *Angew Chem Int Ed Engl*, 2016. **55**: 13408–13421.

117. Kenna, J.G. et al., Multiple compound-related adverse properties contribute to liver injury caused by endothelin receptor antagonists. *J Pharmacol Exp Ther*, 2015. **352**(2): 281–290.

118. Shah, F. et al., Setting clinical exposure levels of concern for drug-induced liver injury (DILI) using mechanistic *in vitro* assays. *Toxicol Sci*, 2015. **147**(2): 500–514.

119. Chen, M., J. Borlak, and W. Tong, High lipophilicity and high daily dose of oral medications are associated with significant risk for drug-induced liver injury. *Hepatology*, 2013. **58**(1): 388–396.

120. Chen, M. et al., A testing strategy to predict risk for drug-induced liver injury in humans using high-content screen assays and the "rule-of-two" model. *Arch Toxicol*, 2014. **88**(7): 1439–1449.

121. Roy-Chowdhury, N. et al., Hepatocyte-like cells derived from induced pluripotent stem cells. *Hepatol Int*, 2016. **11**(1): 54–69.

122. Scheer, N. and I.D. Wilson, A comparison between genetically humanized and chimeric liver humanized mouse models for studies in drug metabolism and toxicity. *Drug Discov Today*, 2016. **21**(2): 250–263.

123. Bateman, T.J. et al., Application of chimeric mice with humanized liver for study of human-specific drug metabolism. *Drug Metab Dispos*, 2014. **42**(6): 1055–1065.

124. Xu, D. and G. Peltz, Can humanized mice predict drug "Behavior" in humans? *Annu Rev Pharmacol Toxicol*, 2016. **56**: 323–338.

125. Xu, D. et al., Humanized thymidine kinase-NOG mice can be used to identify drugs that cause animal-specific hepatotoxicity: A case study with furosemide. *J Pharmacol Exp Ther*, 2015. **354**(1): 73–78.

126. Strick-Marchand, H. et al., A novel mouse model for stable engraftment of a human immune system and human hepatocytes. *PLoS One*, 2015. **10**(3): e0119820.

127. Choucha Snouber, L. et al., Metabolomics-on-a-chip of hepatotoxicity induced by anticancer drug flutamide and its active metabolite hydroxyflutamide using HepG2/C3a microfluidic biochips. *Toxicol Sci*, 2013. **132**(1): 8–20.

128. Eun, J.W. et al., Characteristic molecular and proteomic signatures of drug-induced liver injury in a rat model. *J Appl Toxicol*, 2015. **35**(2): 152–164.

129. Hu, Z. et al., Quantitative liver-specific protein fingerprint in blood: A signature for hepatotoxicity. *Theranostics*, 2014. **4**(2): 215–228.

130. Rodrigues, R.M. et al., Toxicogenomics-based prediction of acetaminophen-induced liver injury using human hepatic cell systems. *Toxicol Lett*, 2016. **240**(1): 50–9.

22

Kinetic Differences between Generated and Preformed Metabolites: A Dilemma in Risk Assessment

Thomayant Prueksaritanont and Jiunn H. Lin

CONTENTS

Introduction

During the drug development process, monitoring plasma profiles of parent drug and its metabolites in the nonclinical toxicology studies are required to ensure adequate systemic exposure to characterize organ toxicity and to cover the expected plasma profiles in clinical studies. In some cases, however, significant qualitative or quantitative differences in metabolite profiles occur between the test animal species and humans because of species differences in drug metabolism. Concerns have arisen regarding potential inadequacy of the animal toxicology studies with only parent drugs. In the past few years, the issue of drug metabolites in safety testing and the role of metabolites as potential mediators of the toxicity of new drug products have gained increased attention by both pharmaceutical companies and regulatory agencies [1–4]. After much debate, the Food and Drug Administration (FDA) issued the *Guidance for Industry on Safety Testing of Drug Metabolites* in February 2008, which outlined recommendations on when and how to characterize and evaluate the safety of "disproportionate" metabolites of small molecule drug products [5]. Metabolites are defined as disproportionate if they present only in humans or present at higher plasma concentrations in humans than in the animals used in nonclinical studies. In cases where a relevant animal species that forms the metabolites at adequate exposure cannot be identified, a bridging study will be required to evaluate safety of the specific metabolite by dosing preformed metabolite(s) in animals. The risk assessment of drug metabolites is considered to be part of an investigational new drug (IND) application and recommended to be completed before beginning large-scale clinical trials prior to new drug application (NDA) in the United States.

The main objective of this chapter is to examine the kinetic differences between preformed and generated metabolites and highlight potential complications associated with the approaches in risk assessment of drug metabolites by dosing preformed metabolites. We hope to convey that considerations to conduct the metabolite testing be based on knowledge and understanding of the kinetic behavior of a metabolite generated *in vivo* versus those given exogenously, and that this chapter would promote continued discussions on finding alternatives/approaches to the proposed nonclinical testing of drug metabolites to better ensure the clinical safety of new therapeutic agents.

Theoretical Considerations

From a pharmacokinetic viewpoint, in order to achieve the goals set forth by FDA Guidance, two key assumptions have to be met: (i) the kinetic behavior, with respect to the relationship between systemic exposure and tissue distribution, of a preformed (synthesized) metabolite administered exogenously is the same as that of the metabolite formed *in vivo* following administration of the parent compound and (ii) the kinetics of a preformed metabolite in an animal species selected for nonclinical testing reflect those of the corresponding metabolite formed *in vivo* in humans following administration of its parent. While these two assumptions may be valid for many drug metabolites, there are cases that the assumptions may not be valid, so that the results of toxicity testing of a drug metabolite can be misleading or fail to characterize the true toxicological contribution of the metabolite when formed from the parent.

The processes of absorption, distribution, metabolism, and excretion (ADME) of a compound are known to be influenced by (i) the specific characteristics of the compound, including its physicochemical properties and ability to interact with transporters, drug-metabolizing enzymes, and binding proteins, and (ii) physiological factors, which govern the exposure of the compound to those proteins, such as distribution, tissue localization, and organ blood flow [6,7]. While the pharmacokinetics of a preformed metabolite, measured as systemic or tissue concentrations as a function of time, will depend largely on the ADME properties of the synthesized metabolite per se, the kinetics of a metabolite generated *in vivo* also are influenced by the ADME properties of the parent compound, in addition to its own [6,8]. Therefore, differences between the kinetic behavior of a preformed metabolite and the metabolite generated from the parent drug could arise because of intrinsic differences between the parent and its metabolite in physicochemical properties and/or the nature of their interactions with transporters, drug-metabolizing enzymes, and/or binding proteins. Moreover, the kinetics of a preformed metabolite in an animal species selected for nonclinical testing may not be the same as those of a metabolite formed *in vivo*, either in that animal species or humans, following administration of the parent, due to species differences in the interaction of a compound with transporters, enzymes, or plasma/tissue-binding proteins, and intrinsic activities or distribution across organs [9].

There are many physicochemical and biological factors that may contribute to the kinetic differences between preformed and generated metabolites [10,11]. This chapter focuses mainly on three major factors, namely physicochemical properties, drug transporters, and drug-metabolizing enzymes. In addition, species differences in transporters and drug-metabolizing enzymes and the interplay between transporter and metabolizing enzyme are also discussed.

Physicochemical Factors

Lipophilicity is generally considered as a key determinant of permeability across tissue membranes, and consequently in determining the extent of drug absorption, distribution to tissues (particularly brain), and elimination processes such as hepatic transport and renal reabsorption [10]. Uptake of lipophilic compounds across the basolateral membrane usually is very efficient as compared with that of hydrophilic molecules. Since metabolites are generally more polar than their parent compounds, they commonly experience much greater diffusional barriers to tissues [11,12]. Consequently, the distribution of a preformed metabolite to organs and tissues may be more limited than when the metabolite is formed *in vivo*; thus, it may restrict potential toxicities to somewhat limited tissues, as compared with that generated from the parent. Additionally, because of the larger permeability barrier to transverse out of cells, the metabolite, once formed *in vivo*, also has a greater potential to accumulate inside the cells. If the site of metabolite formation is tissue specific, the difference in polarity between a metabolite and its parent could lead to differences in tissue-specific distribution or retention between the generated versus preformed metabolite and, hence, in their tissue-specific toxicity profiles.

Other physicochemical properties that may impact the disposition of a compound include chemical stability [13]. If a metabolite is less stable chemically than its parent, administration of the preformed metabolite may lead to more limited distribution of the metabolite than is the case when the parent is dosed. The distribution of a metabolite formed *in vivo* is expected to be dependent on the tissue distribution of both the parent drug and the metabolizing enzymes responsible for the parent-to-metabolite conversion. Furthermore, there are cases when the generated metabolite, because of its instability, leads to regeneration of the precursor within the body ("futile cycling"). Many conjugated metabolites (e.g., glucuronides) can be hydrolyzed back to their corresponding aglycones either chemically or, more commonly, via the action of β-glucuronidase enzymes [14–16]. In such cases, the exposure ratio between a metabolite and its parent in the systemic circulation and/or in a given organ following administration of a preformed metabolite may differ appreciably from that following administration of the parent, depending on the interconversion rate and the efficiency of competing pathways. Additionally, if the locus of formation of a labile metabolite differs from that at which it causes toxicity, the tissue distribution (and hence toxic effects) of the preformed metabolite would be anticipated to be quite distinct from those of the corresponding metabolite generated endogenously. For example, hydroxylamine metabolites of certain carcinogenic aromatic amines are themselves carcinogenic. However, when given as the parent aromatic amines, the hydroxylamine metabolites are subject to efficient hepatic glucuronidation and subsequent "transport" from the liver to the kidney in the form of labile N-glucuronide conjugates. Upon exposure of these conjugates to the acidic urinary pH in the bladder, reactive intermediates are generated causing bladder-specific tumors [17]. It is very likely that the toxicity profiles would be quite different when the parent aromatic amines or N-glucuronides of hydroxylamine are given.

Transporter Factors

The results of a large number of *in vivo* and *in vitro* studies indicate that transporters represent an important determinant of drug disposition [10]. Drug transporters generally can be separated into two major classes—uptake and efflux transporters. Several of these transporters have been demonstrated to possess substrate specificities and are known to localize in different tissues/organs [18]. For example, the ABC-B family (P-glycoprotein, P-gp, and its relatives) mediates ATP-driven efflux transport of cationic and neutral xenobiotics [19], while the ABC-C family (the multidrug resistance associated proteins, MRPs) is ATP-driven drug pumps that handle anionic compounds [20,21]. Both are highly expressed in brain and several peripheral tissues, particularly excretory organs. A family of polyspecific uptake transporters, the organic anion transporting polypeptides, or OATPs [22], which also are prominent in excretory organs and barrier epithelia, handle somewhat large hydrophobic organic anions. Human OATP1B1, OATP1B3, and rat Oatp1b2, which are known to be expressed exclusively in liver, have been shown to be responsible for the selective liver uptake of pravastatin [23,24]. The organic cation and anion transporters, OCTs and OATs, respectively, accommodate relatively small molecular weight molecules and exhibit tissue-specific expression [25,26]. In humans, OCT1 is expressed ubiquitously with relatively robust expression in the liver, and OCT2 is highly expressed in the kidney [27]. In rodents, Oct1 is expressed in both the liver and kidney, whereas Oct2 is expressed mainly in the kidney. Recently, the high levels of Oct1/2 in kidney have been reported to be responsible for selective tissue retention of tetraethylammonium (TEA) in mouse kidney (kidney/plasma ratio ~80) [28], while that of Oct1 has been shown to be associated with high intra-hepatic concentrations of metformin, resulting in a known potentially lethal side effect, lactic acidosis [29]. Similarly, OAT1 and OAT3 are known to be expressed exclusively in kidney tissue. Indeed, OAT1-mediated renal uptake has been implicated as a contributing factor in the intracellular accumulation of adefovir and cidofovir, leading to the nephrotoxicity of these agents [30]. Conceivably, differences in tissue-selective exposure or accumulation between a metabolite formed *in vivo* versus given exogenously would ensue if the metabolite and its parent are substrates of different uptake transporters, which exhibit tissue selectivity. Similarly, there may be differences in excretory profiles or tissue localization/exposure between preformed and generated metabolites when the metabolite and its parent are substrates of different excretory transporters, which are in different tissues.

It is noteworthy that transporter-mediated drug disposition reflects the dynamic interplay between uptake and efflux transporters within any given epithelial cell, where the translocation of drugs across membranes may be impeded or facilitated by the presence of transporters on apical or basolateral membranes [31,32]. Therefore, for many drugs, the combined and sometimes complementary actions of transporters expressed within specific membrane domains of epithelial cells determine the extent and direction of drug movement across organs such as the liver, kidney, and brain. It is to be expected that differences between a metabolite and its parent in their interactions with uptake and efflux transporters would lead to differences in disposition between a preformed metabolite and a metabolite generated *in vivo*.

Compounding this issue further is the question of species differences in the expression level, functional activity, and tissue distribution of transporters. Recent data have revealed that rat liver contains much more (~10-fold) Mrp2 protein resulting in a much higher capacity for the biliary excretion of organic anions in rats than in humans or other preclinical species [32]. Species differences between rat and human OATs also have been reported; hOAT1 accepts cimetidine as a substrate, whereas rOat1 does not interact with cimetidine [33–35]. These differences have been associated with species differences in the renal elimination of cimetidine, as well as a number of organic anions and cations [34]. Similarly, OCTs expressed in the kidney differ between rodents and humans. Both Oct1 (Slc22a1) and Oct2 (Slc22a2) are involved in the renal uptake of organic cations on the basolateral membrane of the proximal tubules in rodents, whereas OCT2, but not OCT1, is abundant in the human kidney [36]. As a result of species differences in drug and metabolite-transporter interactions, it is conceivable that the disposition of a preformed metabolite in animals may differ substantially from that of the corresponding metabolite formed *in vivo* in humans following administration of its parent.

Metabolizing Enzyme Factors

Drug-metabolizing enzymes have been shown to exhibit heterogeneity in distribution within an organ. An enrichment of cytochromes (CYPs), glutathione-S-transferases (GSTs), carboxylesterases, and UDP-glucuronyltransferases (UGTs) was demonstrated in the perihepatic venous region of the liver, while sulfotransferases (SULTs) were found predominantly in the periportal region [11,37–39]. This zonal distribution of enzymes has been proposed, both on theoretical and experimental grounds, to represent one determinant of metabolite disposition, resulting in differences in the fate of a preformed metabolite entering the liver from the circulation relative to that of the same metabolite formed within the liver. In-depth reviews of this topic with specific examples are provided in Pang et al. [11] and Abu-Zahra and Pang [38].

In theory, differences in the disposition between a preformed versus an *in vivo* generated metabolite, especially with respect to formation of downstream metabolites, may result from differences in tissue distribution or exposure between the preformed and generated metabolite (as a consequence of the aforementioned physicochemical and/or transporter factors). This potential difference in the formation of downstream metabolites could be complicated further by the fact that some drug-metabolizing enzymes, as is the case with transporters, exhibit tissue-specific expression. Although most CYPs are found in the liver, some CYPs are expressed preferentially in extrahepatic tissues, which may lead to unique extrahepatic metabolites and tissue-specific consequences in terms of cellular toxicity and organ pathology. Among those in the CYP2 gene family, CYP2A6, 2B6, 2C18, and 2J2 are expressed preferentially in extrahepatic tissues, including epithelial tissues at the environmental interface such as skin, nasal, respiratory, and digestive systems [40,41]. Similarly, UGT1A8 and UGT1A10 are expressed exclusively in gastrointestinal tissues, each with a unique distribution pattern [42,43]. SULT1A1 is the major adult liver SULT1A subfamily member, whereas SULT1A3 is barely detectable in the adult human liver but is highly expressed in jejunum and intestine [44]. In the brain, the cellular and regional distribution of drug-metabolizing enzymes is known to be heterogeneous, with the blood–brain interfaces bearing special drug-metabolic capacities; MAO-B and class III alcohol dehydrogenase (ADH) appear to be highly expressed and active at the blood–CSF barrier in rat and human choroid plexuses [45].

Additionally, species differences in drug-metabolizing enzyme activities are well recognized and the reader is referred to reviews on this topic [9]. These differences may lead to the formation of species-selective metabolites, and consequently to species-selective toxicity. An increase in CYP-mediated hydroxylation, low esterase activity, and relatively high aldehyde dehydrogenase activity in rats relative to humans have been linked to the characteristic toxic effects of felbamate in humans, which are not seen in rats [46]. Also, as is the case for the drug transporters, several enzymes are known to exhibit species differences in tissue distribution, including acylases (N-acetyl-L-cysteine-deacetylating enzyme) and GSTs [47,48]. In rats, e.g., a cysteinylglycine adduct formed by renal γ-glutamyltranspeptidase-mediated cleavage of a GSH adduct of efavirenz (generated by a species-specific GST) was demonstrated to be associated with nephrotoxicity. This kidney toxicity was observed only in rats, and not in cynomulgus monkeys or humans [49]. Moreover, some drug-metabolizing enzymes have been shown to exhibit species differences in intracellular distribution. In guinea pig, as in humans, the liver ciprofibroyl-CoA hydrolase is localized in the mitochondrial and soluble fractions of cells, while in rats, the enzyme has a microsomal localization [50]. In principle, these differences could contribute to tissue-selective exposure and species differences in toxicity profiles between the preformed and generated metabolite.

Interplay Between Membrane Permeability/Transporters and Drug-Metabolizing Enzymes

As will be evident from the above discussion, the disposition of a compound is dependent on a number of factors, including membrane permeability, drug transporters, and drug-metabolizing enzymes. These factors work either in concert with or competitively against each other, and it is reasonable to expect that differences in the interplay between a metabolite and its parent with these systems would lead to differences in the disposition of a preformed metabolite relative to its counterpart generated *in vivo*. Using computer modeling, Miyauchi and coworkers [51] demonstrated that when there is no diffusional barrier for the metabolite, differences in the extraction ratio between the preformed and generated metabolite are dependent on enzyme activity and could be as large as fivefold. In cases where a diffusional barrier exists for the metabolite, a much higher hepatic extraction ratio (up to 10-fold) is observed for the endogenously generated metabolite relative to the exogenously dosed preformed metabolite [51]. Recent studies [7,52] also have demonstrated the importance of the interplay of uptake and efflux transporters with metabolic enzymes in drug disposition as the access of drug molecules to the enzymes is controlled by drug transporters. Both transporter activities and localization of enzymes in the liver influenced the mean hepatic residence time of a metabolite formed *in vivo* [53]. In the case of CPT-11, the interplay between esterases, UGTs, β-glucuronidases, and the efflux transporter MRP2, has been implicated in the localization of its active metabolite, SN-38, in the intestinal tract, leading to diarrhea, the dose-limiting toxicity of CPT-11 [54,55]. SN-38 is formed by esterases from CPT-11, deactivated by UGTs, excreted via MRP2- and/or P-gp-mediated biliary excretion, and deconjugated by β-glucuronidases in the intestinal lumen.

The interplay discussed above also has been shown to impact the metabolic pattern and extraction ratio of compounds given orally. Thus, luminal administration of phenol yielded phenol glucuronide as the primary metabolite, while following vascular administration, sulfation represented the primary metabolic pathway of phenol [56]. A much greater overall extraction also was obtained following luminal than following vascular administration [56]. This was attributed to a greater and/or more prolonged exposure of the perorally administered phenol to the apically placed UGTs. Phenol required more time to diffuse across the lipid-rich barrier of the ER to access the active site of the UGTs, as compared with the readily accessible cytosolic SULTs, whereas the phenol glucuronide, being more polar and much larger than its aglycone, experienced a greater diffusional barrier to its efflux from the ER lumen. A similar route-of-administration-dependent metabolism, resulting from a dynamic interplay between UGTs and efflux transporters, has been reported for morphine and its glucuronide metabolite [57]. A logical extension of these observations is that the route of administration may have a significant effect on the toxicity profile of a drug metabolite, such that the findings from a study in which the preformed metabolite is dosed may not reflect those of a study in which the metabolite is generated from the parent.

Specific Examples

In the section that follows, examples are provided to illustrate the differences in the disposition kinetics of a preformed metabolite versus the same metabolite generated *in vivo* from the parent, either within a given animal species or between animals and humans. Where applicable, the consequences of these differences in disposition, either pharmacological or toxicological, are highlighted.

Acetaminophen and Phenacetin

Quantitative differences in the sequential metabolism of a preformed metabolite and its counterpart generated by metabolism are best exemplified by the case of acetaminophen. Both phenacetin and acetaminophen (the O-de-ethylated metabolite of phenacetin) distribute equally and rapidly from blood to hepatocytes; i.e., there is little, if any, diffusional barrier in the process [58]. Using the rat isolated liver perfusion technique, Pang and Gillette [59] demonstrated that the hepatic extraction ratio (the fraction of dose metabolized by the liver during each passage) of [14C]acetaminophen derived from [14C] phenacetin was lower than that of preformed [3H]acetaminophen when given exogenously (0.50 vs. 0.68). These results suggest that the hepatic exposure to acetaminophen formed *in vivo* would be higher than that when preformed acetaminophen is given exogenously, assuming an equimolar molar dose of the two species. This lower extraction ratio of generated [14C]acetaminophen was proposed to be due to the uneven distribution of the corresponding enzyme systems responsible for the metabolism of phenacetin (CYPs) and acetaminophen (UGTs and SULTs). The CYP-mediated O-deethylation of phenacetin occurred predominantly in the centrilobular region, while a sequential metabolic step, sulfate conjugation, occurred predominantly in the periportal region [58,60]. This hypothesis is consistent with computer simulations under various patterns of enzyme distribution and membrane permeability [51,60]. It is noteworthy that acetaminophen undergoes oxidative metabolism to a product, namely N-acetyl-pbenzoquinone imine (NAPQI), that is toxic to the liver [61,62]. Therefore, the hepatic exposure to the hepatotoxic intermediate, and consequently hepatotoxicity, would conceivably be significantly greater, as a result of greater hepatic exposure to acetaminophen, in animals dosed with acetaminophen than in animals given an equimolar amount of phenacetin itself.

Enalaprilat and Enalapril

Unlike the acetaminophen/phenacetin pair, differential effects of a diffusional barrier on generated and preformed metabolite kinetics have been reported to be important factors in the disposition of enalaprilat, an ACE inhibitor employed for the treatment of hypertension. In animals and humans, enalapril, an inactive prodrug, is hydrolyzed completely by carboxylesterases to its polar dicarboxylic acid metabolite, enalaprilat [63,64]. Studies in the perfused rat liver with simultaneous delivery of [14C] enalapril and its active metabolite, [3H]enalaprilat, revealed a marked difference in the biliary recovery of the generated [14C]enalaprilat (18% dose) and the preformed [3H]enalaprilat (5% dose). A higher hepatic exposure (>3-fold) of enalaprilat was obtained when the compound was generated from the parent drug than when given as the preformed metabolite [63]. In a subsequent study using a perfused rat liver preparation, these authors showed that the biliary clearance of generated [14C]enalaprilat was 15-fold higher than the biliary clearance of the preformed [3H]enalaprilat [65]. Similarly, a significant difference in the urinary clearance for the generated versus preformed enalaprilat was reported in studies using the isolated perfused rat kidney [66]. Collectively, these results suggest that a diffusional barrier for enalaprilat served to limit entry of the preformed enalaprilat into hepatocytes or renal epithelium cells, thereby decreasing biliary or urinary excretion. This differential diffusional barrier between enalapril and enalaprilat is consistent with differences in their physical properties; under physiological pH, the dicarboxylic acid metabolite is present in ionized form, which is very polar in nature. Both compounds also differ in their ability to interact with OATP1, a drug transporter; thus, enalapril, but not enalaprilat, has been shown to be taken up by rat Oatp1a1 and human OATP1B1 and OATP1B3 in the liver [67,68].

Dopamine and L-Dopa

In addition to the liver, a profound difference in tissue-specific distribution and retention between a preformed metabolite and the metabolite generated from the parent drug also may occur as a result of the presence of a diffusional barrier or specific influx transporters in extrahepatic tissues, as illustrated by the penetration of dopamine into the central nervous system (CNS). Many transport systems, which play an important role in the uptake of water-soluble nutrients from the blood circulation into the brain, are known to be present at the blood–brain barrier (BBB) [69]. The large neutral amino acid carrier (LAT) mediates the uptake of phenylalanine and other neutral amino acids from the circulation into the brain. L-dopa, used for the treatment of Parkinson's disease, is a neutral amino acid analog that traverses the BBB via the LAT into the brain, where it is decarboxylated to the pharmacologically active metabolite, dopamine [70]. Since dopamine is not a substrate for the LAT and is highly water soluble, it does not cross the BBB. When given exogenously, dopamine has no therapeutic effect in the treatment of Parkinson's disease.

Nucleotides, Nucleosides, and Nucleoside Prodrugs

Similar to L-dopa, an active uptake system (adenosine nucleoside transporter) is involved in the uptake of nucleosides into various tissues where they are converted to the corresponding pharmacologically active nucleotides. Since nucleotides are not substrates for adenosine nucleoside transporter and are very water soluble, they usually do not cross cell membranes by passive diffusion. Consequently, the tissue exposure of nucleotides would be expected to be much higher when given as nucleosides than when dosed exogenously as the preformed metabolites (nucleotides). Indeed, following oral administration of MRL111, a nucleoside analog, in rats, mice, dogs, and monkeys, the AUC of the active triphosphate metabolite in the liver was ~25- to 30-fold higher than the plasma AUC of the parent nucleoside (data on file, Merck Research Laboratories). In rat hepatocyte studies, MRL111 showed time- and temperature-dependent uptake, consistent with the involvement of equilibrative transport into hepatocytes, commonly mediated by nucleoside transporters [71].

Tenofovir, a dianion at physiological pH, belongs to a class of nucleotide analogs that exhibit prolonged intracellular half-lives [72]. The long intracellular half-life of tenofovir is a result of rapid metabolism within the cell to the nucleotide diphosphate, the active metabolite. The low cellular permeability of the nucleotide metabolite limits its efflux from cells. The amidate prodrug GS 7340 was designed to overcome the permeability limitations of tenofovir by masking the dianion with a neutral promoiety and increasing the plasma stability of the prodrug relative to its intracellular stability. *In vivo* administration of GS 7340 to dogs resulted in an enhanced distribution to lymphatic tissue compared with tenofovir; concentrations of tenofovir in peripheral blood mononuclear cells (PBMCs) versus plasma were much higher (>10-fold) following GS 7340 than following tenofovir [73]. Consistent with this finding, GS 7340 also was found to distribute widely to lymphatic tissues [73]. This expanded distribution and the higher intracellular levels of tenofovir after administration of GS 7340 than after tenofovir raises the possibility of safety issues that may not be observed with tenofovir itself.

Statin Acids and Lactones

HMG-CoA reductase inhibitors, or "statins," which target HMG-CoA reductase, the rate-limiting enzyme in cholesterol biosynthesis, are used widely for the treatment of hypercholesterolemia and hypertriglyceridemia. Except for simvastatin and lovastatin, which are administered in the inactive lactone forms, all currently available statins are administered as the pharmacologically active™-hydroxy acids. The statin lactones are hydrolyzed to their open acids chemically or enzymatically by esterases or paraoxonases [16]. The major physicochemical difference between the lactone and acid form for each statin is that the lactone has a higher partition coefficient (log P) or lipophilicity (log D), compared with the acid [74,75]. The acid versus lactone forms of statins, including atorvastatin, lovastatin, and simvastatin, also have differential activities toward several transporters, including P-gp [76,77].

Simvastatin is not a P-gp substrate, whereas the acid form of both simvastatin and atorvastatin exhibit a moderate level of P-gp-mediated transport [76]. Therefore, it is possible that the superior membrane permeability of the statin lactone (due to increased lipophilicity) and its inability to interact with P-gp may allow ready access of the lactone form to tissues. Indeed, the acid form of simvastatin accumulated in muscle and brain to a greater degree (2–3-fold) when given to dogs as the lactone than as the open acid, even though plasma levels of the open acid were comparable in each case (data on file, Merck Research Laboratories). In an earlier dog study, the disposition of simvastatin lactone also was found to be more hepatoselective than that of simvastatin acid; thus, simvastatin lactone exhibited a higher hepatic extraction ratio than simvastatin acid (93% vs. 80%), resulting in a lower systemic burden of prodrug and active drug after administration of simvastatin lactone versus simvastatin acid [78]. Evidently, treatment with simvastatin lactone is more selective with respect to inhibition of hepatic versus extrahepatic HMG-CoA reductase. This was substantiated further by the finding that plasma levels of active drug equivalents, after administration of simvastatin acid and lactone to dogs at doses that produced a similar degree of cholesterol lowering, are approximately 10-fold higher when simvastatin acid is given [78]. Hence, the safety or toxicity profile of simvastatin acid in dogs may be different when the open acid is given exogenously as compared with when it is formed *in vivo* from the lactone.

Interestingly, the above observation was found to be species specific. As shown in an earlier study [78], the half-life of simvastatin in rodent plasma is approximately four minutes due to very rapid hydrolysis of the lactone, while essentially no hydrolysis occurs in human or dog plasma. Consistent with this observation, the oral bioavailability of the lactone was essentially zero when simvastatin was dosed to rodents [78]. Studies on the disposition and metabolism of simvastatin lactone and open acid in rodents revealed that the systemic levels of the acid form, active or total HMG-CoA inhibitory activity, and total radioactivity following administration of simvastatin acid were similar to those observed following dosing with simvastatin lactone in the same species and gender (data on file, Merck Research Laboratories). Tissue distribution patterns of radioactivity following a dose of [14C] simvastatin acid to rats also were similar to those found after [14C]simvastatin lactone was given [78]. Thus, the safety or toxicity profile of preformed and metabolically generated simvastatin acid in rodents would be expected to be similar. However, this is not likely to be the case in dogs, and possibly also in humans.

Morphine and Its Glucuronides

In mammals, morphine, a potent analgesic, is metabolized mainly by glucuronidation to yield morphine-3-glucuronide (M3G) and morphine-6-glucuronide (M6G). Because of their greater polarity relative to the parent aglycone, these conjugates are subject to significant diffusional barriers. Studies using the isolated perfused rat liver demonstrated that the hepatic disposition of the pharmacologically inactive metabolite M3G is indeed membrane permeability-rate limited; the biliary excretion and extraction ratio of hepatically generated M3G is much more efficient (>10-fold) than that of M3G given exogenously [79,80]. Additionally, using a loading wash-out design and a physiologically based pharmacokinetic model, the volume of distribution of hepatically generated M3G was found to be approximately 50 times the intracellular space of the rat liver, suggesting that the generated M3G accumulates within hepatocytes, consistent with its poor membrane permeability [81].

Unlike M3G, M6G is an opioid agonist that plays a role in the clinical effects of morphine. M6G has been shown to exhibit much lower BBB permeability than morphine, as supported by studies showing lower brain penetration with M6G than morphine [82]. Also consistent with the limited membrane permeability, plasma M6G, unlike morphine, was below detection limits after intracerebroventricular injection of M6G, and the apparent elimination clearance of M6G from the cerebrospinal fluid was 10 times lower than that of morphine after central administration of morphine to rats [83]. Using a brain slice uptake method, the same authors showed that morphine was distributed in the brain parenchyma cells, whereas M6G was in the extracellular fluid. It has been suggested recently that morphine is a substrate for P-gp [84], but M6G may be a substrate for an active uptake transporter and MRP [80,85].

This difference may account for the differential brain distribution between morphine and M6G, given that P-gp is expressed mainly in the cerebral capillary endothelium, whereas MRP is expressed predominantly elsewhere in the brain [86].

To complicate the matter further, brain UGT(s) is capable of catalyzing the conjugation of morphine [87] and exhibits a regioselectivity toward morphine that is different from the liver enzyme. M6G is the primary metabolite in brain, whereas M3G is the major conjugate in liver [88]. Additionally, human kidney preferentially forms M3G (M3G/M6G ratio ~20) relative to human liver (M3G/M6G ratio ~5) [89]. Furthermore, the metabolism of morphine also differs markedly between animal species, and between animals and humans [89,90]. Whereas in human and guinea pig liver microsomes fortified with UDPGA, both the M3G and M6G are generated, with M3G being the major product, in rat and mouse liver microsomes, morphine forms almost exclusively M3G (M3G/M6G ratio ~90). Consequently, the distribution of the two isomeric glucuronides to various brain regions or tissues following administration of preformed M6G or M3G may be different in animals and humans.

Acyl Glucuronides and Aglycones

Acyl glucuronides are a unique class of electrophilic metabolites, capable of hydrolysis to reform the parent aglycone and of intramolecular rearrangement. Both intra- and extrahepatic exposure to acyl glucuronides depends not only on the efficiency of competing glucuronidation and hydrolysis processes in the liver, but also on the efficiency of the hepatic membrane transport systems. Sallustio et al. [91] used the isolated perfused liver preparation to examine the hepatic disposition of the fibrate hypolipidemic agent gemfibrozil and its acyl glucuronide metabolite, 1-O-gemfibrozil-β-D-glucuronide (GG). Unlike observations with morphine, acetaminophen or 4-nitrophenol and their respective ether glucuronide conjugates [79,92], the hepatic extraction ratio of gemfibrozil was found to be lower than that of GG (0.09 vs. 0.65, respectively), consistent with its lower unbound fraction in perfusate (0.004), compared with that of GG (0.018). The fraction of gemfibrozil excreted in bile as the glucuronide conjugate also was lower (0.35 vs. 0.53, respectively) after administration of gemfibrozil than after GG. The relatively lower biliary excretion of the hepatically generated GG was attributed to the more efficient sinusoidal efflux into perfusate. On the basis of the finding of high concentration gradients (>40) for GG between the liver and perfusate and between bile and the liver [93], it was also suggested that the movement of GG from perfusate into bile is a two-step concentrative process involving carrier-mediated systems at both the sinusoidal and canalicular membranes of hepatocytes, possibly via OATP2 and MRP2, respectively [14,91]. Similarly, naproxen acyl glucuronide was excreted in bile in much higher quantities (~25% vs. 4% of the dose) following administration of naproxen acyl glucuronide than after dosing with naproxen [94]. In addition, rearranged isomers of naproxen acyl glucuronide were not observed following naproxen administration, whereas they were detected in significant levels in bile (3% of the dose) after naproxen acyl glucuronide administration [96].

Acyl glucuronides are intrinsically reactive; following rearrangement, positional isomers can react with amino acids of macromolecules to form protein adducts, potentially contributing to hepatotoxicity. Dipeptidylpeptidase IV, UGTs, and tubulin have been identified as intra-hepatic targets of adduct formation by acyl glucuronides [91,97]. The concentrative effect of carrier-mediated hepatic membrane transport observed following dosing with preformed acyl glucuronides, together with the detection of their rearranged isomers, suggests that significantly higher intra-hepatic protein adduct formation would follow, even in the absence of detectable plasma acyl glucuronide concentrations, after administration of the preformed acyl glucuronides than after the corresponding aglycones. Thus, it may be anticipated that the toxicity profile obtained following administration of preformed acyl glucuronides could be different from (in this case more toxic) that following the respective aglycones, even with comparable systemic exposure of the glucuronides. Consistent with this hypothesis, increased covalent naproxen-protein adducts in the liver were observed following perfusion of naproxen acyl glucuronide, as compared with perfusion with naproxen (0.34%–0.20% of the doses, respectively) in an isolated rat liver perfusion system [94]. Similar findings also have been reported with diflunisal and diflunisal acyl glucuronide [96].

Conclusions and Perspectives

Risk assessment of drug metabolites is a complex issue that has been discussed extensively by pharmaceutical, academic, and regulatory scientists [1–4,97]. As aforementioned, the kinetic behavior of a preformed metabolite given exogenously may differ significantly from that of the corresponding metabolite generated endogenously from the parent compound in animals or humans. In some cases, this complication may be overcome by administering high doses of preformed metabolites to generate sufficient systemic and tissue exposure. However, for hydrophilic metabolites, it may not readily be overcome by giving high doses of preformed metabolites because of poor passive permeability and/or interactions with specialized transporters and/or drug-metabolizing enzymes. Additionally, potential differences in physiological factors such as tissue-selective distribution and species differences in transporters and/or metabolizing enzymes could contribute to differences in tissue- and species-specific toxicities depending on the compound administered (preformed metabolite vs. metabolite generated from the parent drug). It is, therefore, important to better understand the kinetic behavior of a metabolite generated *in vivo* versus that given exogenously before conducting the so-called bridging study to evaluate the safety of the drug metabolite.

Over the past few decades, considerable progress has been made in the generation of transgenic animal models for drug metabolism studies [98]. Significant qualitative or quantitative differences in metabolite profiles between the test animal species and humans could theoretically be addressed by these animal models. To date, at least six mouse models expressing human CYP1A1, CYP1A2, CYP2D6, CYP2E1, and CYP3A4 have been generated and characterized [98–100]. The usefulness of these mouse models is, however, still limited because of variable expression levels and erroneous localization of CYP enzymes. More recently, transgenic mouse models expressing human CYP3A4 in a tissue-specific expression manner (particularly liver vs. intestine) have been established and initial characterization showed promising results [101]. Additionally, a chimeric mouse model with approximately 80% replacement by humanized liver has been reported to express functionally active, although not quantitatively as compared to, results obtained with human livers, human drug-metabolizing enzymes, and transporters [102]. Conceivably, in the next decade humanized mouse lines expressing selected drug transporters and metabolizing enzymes in specific tissues could be available for use in risk assessment of drug metabolites that are disproportionately higher in humans than in animal species used for toxicity studies.

ACKNOWLEDGMENTS

The authors would like to thank Dr. Thomas A. Baillie of the Department of Global Drug Metabolism and Pharmacokinetics, Merck Research Laboratories, for his careful review and valuable suggestions.

REFERENCES

1. Baillie TA, Cayen MN, Fouda H, Gerson RJ, Green JD, Grossman SJ, Klunk LJ, LeBlanc B, Perkins DC, Shipley LA. Drug metabolites in safety testing. *Toxicol Appl Pharmacol* 2002; 182:188–196.
2. Smith DA, Obach RS. Seeing through the MIST: Abundance versus percentage. *Drug MetabDispos* 2005; 33:1409–1417.
3. Davis-Bruno KL, Atrakchi A. A regulatory perspective on issues and approaches in characterizing human metabolites. *Chem Res Toxicol* 2006; 19:1561–1563.
4. Prueksaritanont T, Lin JH, Baillie TA. Complicating factors in safety testing of drug metabolites: Kinetic differences between generated and preformed metabolites. *Toxicol Appl Pharmacol* 2006; 217:143–152.
5. US Food and Drug Administration. *Guidance to Industry Safety Testing of Drug Metabolites Revision 1* 2016. Available at: www.fda.gov/cder/guidance (accessed February 2019).
6. Rowland M, Tozer TN. *Clinical Pharmacokinetics: Concepts and Applications*. 3rd ed. New York: Lee & Febiger, 1995.
7. Liu LC, Pang KS. The roles of transporters and enzymes in hepatic drug processing. *DrugMetab Dispos* 2005; 33:1–9.

8. Houston JB. Drug metabolite kinetics. *Pharmacol Ther* 1982; 15:521–552.

9. Lin JH. Species similarities and differences in pharmacokinetics. *Drug Metab Dispos* 1995; 23:1008–1021.

10. Lin JH. Tissue distribution and pharmacodynamics: A complicated relationship. *Curr DrugMetab* 2006; 7:39–65.

11. Pang KS, Xin X, St Pierre MV. Determinants of metabolite disposition. *Annu Rev Pharmacol Toxicol* 1992; 32:623–669.

12. Evans AM. Membrane transport as a determinant of the hepatic elimination of drugs and metabolites. *Clin Exp Pharmacol Physiol* 1996; 23:970–974.

13. Dell D. Labile metabolites. *Chromatographia* 2004; 59(suppl):S139–S148.

14. Sallustio BC, Fairchild BA, Shanahan K, Evans AM, Nation RL. Disposition of gemfibrozil and gemfibrozil acyl glucuronide in the rat isolated perfused liver. *Drug Metab Dispos* 1996; 24:984–989.

15. Tan E, Lu T, Pang KS. Futile cycling of estrone sulfate and estrone in the recirculating perfused rat liver preparation. *J Pharmacol Exp Ther* 2001; 297:423–436.

16. Prueksaritanont T, Subramanian R, Fang X, Ma B, Qiu Y, Lin JH, Pearson PG, Baillie TA. Glucuronidation of statins in animals and humans: A novel mechanism of statin lactonization. *Drug Metab Dispos* 2002; 30:505–512.

17. Kadlubar FF, Unruh LE, Flammang TJ, Sparks D, Mitchum RK, Mulder GJ. Alteration of urinary levels of the carcinogen, N-hydroxy-2-naphthylamine, and its N-glucuronide in the rat by control of urinary pH, inhibition of metabolic sulfation, and changes in biliary excretion. *Chem Biol Interact* 1981; 33:129–147.

18. Maher JM, Slitt AL, Cherrington NJ, Cheng X, Klaassen CD. Tissue distribution and hepatic and renal ontogeny of the multidrug resistance-associated protein (MRP) family in mice. *Drug Metab Dispos* 2005; 33:947–955.

19. Schinkel AH, Jonker JW. Mammalian drug efflux transporters of the ATP binding cassette(ABC) family: An overview. *Adv Drug Deliv Rev* 2003; 55:3–29.

20. Kruh GD, Belinsky MG. The MRP family of drug efflux pumps. *Oncogene* 2003; 22:7537–7552.

21. Haimeur A, Conseil G, Deeley RG, Cole SPC. The MRP-related and BCRP/ABCG2 multidrug resistance proteins: Biology, substrate specificity and regulation. *Curr Drug Metab* 2004; 5:21–53.

22. Hagenbuch B, Meier PJ. The superfamily of organic anion transporting polypeptides. *Biochim Biophys Acta* 2003; 1609:1–18.

23. Yamazaki M, Tokui T, Ishigami M, Sugiyama Y. Tissue-selective uptake of pravastatin in rats: Contribution of a specific carrier-mediated uptake system. *Biopharm Drug Dispos* 1996; 17:775–789.

24. Hirano M, Maeda K, Shitara Y, Sugiyama Y. Contribution of OATP2 (OATP1B1) andOATP8 (OATP1B3) to the hepatic uptake of pitavastatin in humans. *J Pharmacol Exp Ther* 2004; 311:139–146.

25. Koepsell H, Endou H. The SLC22 drug transporter family. *Pflugers Arch* 2004; 447:666–676.

26. You GF. The role of organic ion transporters in drug disposition: An update. *Curr Drug Metab* 2004; 5:55–62.

27. Ito S, Alcorn J. Xenobiotic transporter expression and function in the human mammary gland. *Adv Drug Deliv Rev* 2003; 55:653–665.

28. Jonker JW, Wagenaar E, Mol CA, Buitelaar M, Koepsell H, Smit JW, Schinkel AH. Deficiency in the organic cation transporters 1 and 2 (Oct1/Oct2 [Slc22a1/Slc22a2]) in mice abolishes renal secretion of organic cations. *Mol Cell Biol* 2001; 23:7902–7908.

29. Wang DS, Kusuhara H, Kato Y, Jonker JW, Schinkel AH, Sugiyama Y. Involvement of organic cation transporter 1 in the lactic acidosis caused by metformin. *Mol Pharmacol* 2003; 63:844–848.

30. Ho ES, Lin DC, Mendel DB, Cihlar T. Cytotoxicity of antiviral nucleotides adefovir and cidofovir is induced by the expression of human renal organic anion transporter 1. *J Am Soc Nephrol* 2000; 11:383–393.

31. Kusuhara H, Sugiyama Y. Role of transporters in the tissue-selective distribution and elimination of drugs: Transporters in the liver, small intestine, brain and kidney. *J Control Release* 2002; 78:43–54.

32. Zamek-Gliszczynski MJ, Hoffmaster KA, Nezasa K, Tallman MN, Brouwer KLR. Integration of hepatic drug transporters and phase II metabolizing enzymes: Mechanisms of hepatic excretion of sulfate, glucuronide, and glutathione metabolites. *Eur J Pharm Sci* 2006; 27:447–486.

33. Nagata Y, Kusuhara H, Endou H, Sugiyama Y. Expression and functional characterization of rat organic anion transporter 3 (rOat3) in the choroid plexus. *Mol Pharmacol* 2002; 61:982–988.

34. Tahara H, Kusuhara H, Endou H, Koepsell H, Imaoka T, Fuse E, Sugiyama Y. A species difference in the transport activities of H-2 receptor antagonists by rat and human renal organic anion and cation transporters. *J Pharmacol Exp Ther* 2005; 315:337–345.

35. Tahara H, Shono M, Kusuhara H, Kinoshita H, Fuse E, Takadate A, Otagiri M, Sugiyama Y. Molecular cloning and functional analyses of OAT1 and OAT3 from cynomolgus monkey kidney. *Pharm Res* 2005; 22:647–660.

36. Wright SH, Dantzler WH. Molecular and cellular physiology of renal organic cation and an ion transport. *Physiol Rev* 2004; 84:987–1049.

37. Tirona RG, Pang KS. Sequestered endoplasmic reticulum space for sequential metabolism of salicylamide—Coupling of hydroxylation and glucuronidation. *Drug Metab Dispos* 1996; 24:821–833.

38. Abu-Zahra TN, Pang KS. Effect of zonal transport and metabolism on hepatic removal: Enalapril hydrolysis in zonal, isolated rat hepatocytes *in vitro* and correlation with perfusion data. *Drug Metab Dispos* 2000; 28:807–813.

39. Schwab AJ, Tao L, Kang M, Meng L, Pang KS. Moment analysis of metabolic heterogeneity: Conjugation of benzoate with glycine in rat liver studied by multiple indicator dilution technique. *J Pharmacol Exp Ther* 2003; 305:279–289.

40. Ding XX, Kaminsky LS. Human extrahepatic cytochromes P450: Function in xenobiotic metabolism and tissue-selective chemical toxicity in the respiratory and gastrointestinal tracts. *Annu Rev Pharmacol Toxicol* 2003; 43:149–173.

41. Du LP, Hoffman SMG, Keeney DS. Epidermal CYP2 family cytochromes P450. *Toxicol Appl Pharmacol* 2004; 195:278–287.

42. Gregory PA, Lewinsky RH, Gardner-Stephen DA, Mackenzie PI. Regulation of UDP glucuronosyl transferases in the gastrointestinal tract. *Toxicol Appl Pharmacol* 2004; 199:354–363.

43. Kiang TKL, Ensom MHH, Chang TKH. UDP-glucuronosyltransferases and clinical drug-drug interactions. *Pharmacol Ther* 2005; 106:97–132.

44. Gamage N, Barnett A, Hempel N, Duggleby RG, Windmill KF, Martin JL, McManus ME. Human sulfotransferases and their role in chemical metabolism. *Toxicol Sci* 2006; 90:5–22.

45. Strazielle N, Khuth ST, Ghersi-Egea JF. Detoxification systems, passive and specific transport for drugs at the blood-CSF barrier in normal and pathological situations. *Adv Drug Deliv Rev* 2004; 56:1717–1740.

46. Dieckhaus CM, Miller TA, Sofia RD, Macdonald TL. A mechanistic approach to understanding species differences in felbamate bioactivation: Relevance to drug-induced idiosyncratic reactions. *Drug Metab Dispos* 2000; 28:814–822.

47. Urrea R, Bronfman M. Species differences in the intracellular distribution of ciprofibroyl-CoA hydrolase. Implications for peroxisome proliferation. *FEBS Lett* 1996; 389:219–223.

48. Their R, Wiebel FA, Hinkel A, Burger A, Brüning T, Morgenroth K, Senge T, Wilhelm M, Schulz TG. Species differences in the glutathione transferase GSTT1-1 activity towards the model substrates methyl chloride and dichloromethane in liver and kidney. *Arch Toxicol* 1998; 72:622–629.

49. Mutlib AE, Chen H, Nemeth GA, Markwalder JA, Seitz SP, Gan LS, Christ DD. Identification and characterization of efavirenz metabolites by liquid chromatography/mass spectrometry and high field NMR: Species differences in the metabolism of efavirenz. *Drug Metab Dispos* 1999; 27:1319–1333.

50. Yamauchi A, Ueda N, Hanafusa S, Yamashita E, Kihara M, Naito, S. Tissue distribution of and species differences in deacetylation of N-acetyl-L-cysteine and immunohistochemical localization of acylase I in the primate kidney. *J Pharm Pharmacol* 2002; 54:205–212.

51. Miyauchi S, Sugiyama Y, Sato H, Sawada Y, Iga T, Hanano M. Effects of a diffusional barrier to a metabolite across hepatocytes on its kinetics in "enzyme-distributed" model a computer aided simulation study. *J Pharmacokinet Biopharm* 1987; 15:399–421.

52. Benet LZ, Cummins CL, Wu CY. Unmasking the dynamic interplay between efflux transporters and metabolic enzymes. *Int J Pharm* 2004; 277:3–9.

53. Schwab AJ, Pang KS. The multiple indicator-dilution method for the study of enzyme heterogeneity in liver: Theoretical basis. *Drug Metab Dispos* 1999; 27:746–755.

54. Mathijssen RHJ, van Alphen RJ, Verweij J, Loos WJ, Nooter K, Stoter G, Sparreboom A. Clinical pharmacokinetics and metabolism of irinotecan (CPT-11). *Clin Cancer Res* 2001; 7:2182–2194.

55. Ma MK, McLeod HL. Lessons learned from the irinotecan metabolic pathway. *Curr MedChem* 2003; 10:41–49.

56. Kothare PA, Zimmerman CL. Intestinal metabolism: The role of enzyme localization in phenol metabolite kinetics. *Drug Metab Dispos* 2002; 30:586–594.

57. Doherty MM, Pang KS. Route-dependent metabolism of morphine in the vascularly perfused rat small intestine preparation. *Pharm Res* 2000; 17:291–298.

58. Pang KS, Waller L, Horning MG, Chan KK. Metabolite kinetics-formation of acetaminophen from dueterated and non-dueterated phenacetin and acetanilide on acetaminophen sulfation kinetics in the perfused-rat liver preparation. *J Pharmacol Exp Ther* 1982; 222:14–19.

59. Pang KS, Gillette JR. Kinetics of metabolite formation and elimination in the perfused rat liver preparation: Differences between elimination of preformed acetaminophen and acetaminophen formed from phenacetin. *J Pharmacol Exp Ther* 1978; 207:178–194.

60. Pang KS, Terrell A. Conjugation kinetics of acetaminophen by the perfused rat-liver preparation. *Biochem Pharmacol* 1981; 30:1959–1965.

61. James LP, Mayeux PR, Hinson JA. Acetaminophen-induced hepatotoxicity. *Drug Metab Dispos* 2003; 31:1499–1506.

62. Bender RP, Lindsey RH, Burden DA, Osheroff, N. N-acetyl-p-benzoquinone imine, the toxic metabolite of acetaminophen, is a topoisomerase II poison. *Biochemistry* 2004; 43:3731–3739.

63. Pang KS, Cherry WF, Terrell JA, Ulm EH. Disposition of enalapril and its diacid metabolite, enalaprilat, in a perfused rat liver preparation. Presence of a diffusional barrier into hepatocytes. *Drug Metab Dispos* 1984; 12:309–313.

64. Pang KS, Baker F, Cherry WF, Goresky CA. Esterases for enalapril hydrolysis are concentrated in the perihepatic venous region of the rat-liver. *J Pharmacol Exp Ther* 1991; 257:294–301.

65. de Lannoy IAM, Baker F, Pang KS. Formed and preformed metabolite excretion clearances in liver, a metabolite formation organ: Studies on enalapril and enalaprilat in the single-pass and recirculating perfused rat liver. *J Pharmacokint Biopharm* 1993; 21:395–422.

66. de Lannoy IAM, Nespeca R, Pang KS. Renal handling of enalapril and enalprilat: Studies in the isolated red blood cell-perfused rat kidney. *J Pharmacol Exp Ther* 1989; 251:1211–1222.

67. Pang KS, Wang PJ, Chung AYK, Wolkoff AW. The modified dipeptide, enalapril, an angiotensin-converting enzyme inhibitor, is transported by the rat liver organic anion transport protein. *Hepatology* 1998; 28:1341–1346.

68. Liu LC, Cui YH, Chung AY, Shitara Y, Sugiyama Y, Keppler D, Pang KS. Vectorial transport of enalapril by Oatp1a1/Mrp2 and OATP1B1 and OATP1B3/MRP2 in rat and human livers. *J Pharmacol Exp Ther* 2006; 318:395–402.

69. Pardridge WM. Recent advances in blood-brain barrier transport. *Annu Rev Pharmacol Toxicol* 1988; 28:25–39.

70. Nutt JG, Woodward WR, Hammerstad JP, Carter MN, Anderson JL. The "on-off" phenomenon in Parkinson's disease. Relation to levodopa absorption and transport. *N Engl J Med* 1984; 310:483–488.

71. Pastor-Anglada M, Cano-Soldado P, Molina-Arcas M, Pilar Lostaob M, Larra´yozb I, Martı´nez-Picadoc J, Casado FJ. Cell entry and export of nucleoside analogues. *Virus Res* 2005; 107:151–164.

72. Pauwels R, Baba M, Balzarini J, Herdewijn P, Desmyter J, Robins MJ, Zou R, Madej D, deClercq, E. Investigations on the anti-HIV activity of 2′,3′-dideoxyadenosine analogs with modification in either the pentose or purine moiety—Potent and selective anti-HIV activity of 2,6-diaminopurine 2′,3′-dideoxyriboside. *Biochem Pharmacol* 1988; 37, 1317–1325.

73. Lee WA, He GX, Eisenberg E, Cihlar T, Swaminathan S, Mulato A, Cundy KC. Selective intracellular activation of a novel prodrug of the human immunodeficiency virus reverse transcriptase inhibitor tenofovir leads to preferential distribution and accumulation in lymphatic tissue. *Antimicrob Agents Chemother* 2005; 49:1898–1906.

74. Serajuddin AT, Ranadive SA, Mahoney EM. Relative lipophilicities, solubilities, and structure-pharmacological considerations of 3-hydroxy-3-methylglutaryl-coenzyme A (HMG-CoA) reductase inhibitors pravastatin, lovastatin, mevastatin, and simvastatin. *J Pharm Sci* 1991; 80:830–834.

75. Ishigami M, Honda T, Takasaki W, Ikeda T, Komai T, Ito K, Sugiyama Y. A comparison of the effects of 3-hydroxy-3-methylglutaryl-coenzyme A (HMG-CoA) reductase inhibitors on the CYP3A4-dependent oxidation of mexazolam *in vitro*. *Drug Metab Dispos* 2001; 29:282–288.

76. Hochman JH, Pudvah NT, Qiu Y, Yamazaki M, Tang C, Lin JH, Prueksaritanont T. Interactions of human P-glycoprotein with simvastatin, simvastatin acid, and atorvastatin. *Pharm Res* 2004; 21:1688–1693.

77. Chen C, Mireles RJ, Campbell SD, Lin J, Mills JB, Xu JJ, Smolarek TA. Differential interaction of 3-hydroxy-3-methylglutaryl-coenzyme A reductase inhibitors with ABCB1, ABCC2, and OATP1B1. *Drug Metab Dispos* 2005; 33:537–546.

78. Vickers S, Duncan CA, Chen, I.-W, Rosegay A, Duggan DE. Metabolic disposition studies of simvastatin, a cholesterol-lowering prodrug. *Drug Metab Dispos* 1990; 18:138–145.

79. Evans AM, Shanahan K. Biliary excretion of hepatically-generated and pre-formed morphine3-glucuronide (M-3-G) in the isolated perfused rat liver: Evidence for a diffusional barrier. *Clin Exp Pharmacol Physiol* 1993; 10(suppl 1):S22.

80. Doherty MM, Poon IM, Tsang C, Pang KS. Transport is not rate-limiting in morphine glucuronidation in the single-pass perfused rat liver preparation. *J Pharmacol Exp Ther* 2006; 317:890–900.

81. Evans AM, O'Brien J, Nation RL. Application of a loading wash-out method for investigating the hepatocellular efflux of a hepatically-generated metabolite morphine-3-glucuronide. *J Pharm Pharmacol* 1999; 51:1289–1297.

82. Wu DF, Kang YS, Bickel U, Pardridge WM. Blood-brain barrier permeability to morphine-6glucuronide is markedly reduced compared with morphine. *Drug Metab Dispos* 1997; 25:768–771.

83. Okura T, Saito M, Nakanishi M, Komiyama N, Fujii A, Yamada S, Kimura R. Different distribution of morphine and morphine-6 b-glucuronide after intracerebroventricular injection in rats. *Br J Pharmacol* 2003; 140:211–217.

84. Cisternino S, Rousselle C, Debray M, and Scherrmann JM. *In situ* transport of vinblastine and selected P-glycoprotein substrates: Implications for drug-drug interactions at the mouse blood brain barrier. *Pharm Res* 2004; 21:1382–1389.

85. Bourasset F, Cisternino S, Temsamani J, Scherrmann, JM. Evidence for an active transport of morphine-6-beta-D-glucuronide but not P-glycoprotein-mediated at the blood-brain barrier. *J Neurochem* 2003; 86:1564–1567.

86. Regina A, Koman A, Piciotti M, El Hafny B, Center MS, Bergmann R, Couraud PO, Roux F. Mrp1 multidrug resistance-associated protein and P-glycoprotein expression in rat brain microvessel endothelial cells. *J Neurochem* 1998; 71:705–715.

87. Wahlstro¨m A, Winblad B, Bixo M, Rane A. Human brain metabolism of morphine and naloxone. *Pain* 1998; 35:121–127.

88. Nagano W, Yamada H, Oguri K. Characteristic glucuronidation pattern of physiologic concentration of morphine in rat brain. *Life Sci* 2000; 67:2453–2464.

89. Coughtrie MWH, Ask B, Rane A, Burchell B, Hume R. The enantioselective glucuronidation of morphine in rats and humans. *Biochem Pharmacol* 1989; 19:3273–3280.

90. Kuo CK, Hanioka N, Hoshikawa Y, Oguri K, Yoshimura H. Species difference of site selective glucuronidation of morphine. *J Pharmacobiodyn* 1991; 14:187–193.

91. Sallustio BC, Sabordo L, Evans AM, Nation RL. Hepatic disposition of electrophilic acylglucuronide conjugates. *Curr Drug Metab* 2000; 1:163–180.

92. Watari N, Iwai M, Kaneniwa N. Pharmacokinetic study of the fate of acetaminophen and its conjugates in rats. *J Pharmacokinet Biopharm* 1983; 11:245–272.

93. Sabordo L, Sallustio BC, Evans AM, Nation RL. Hepatic disposition of the acyl glucuronide1O-gemfibrozil-b-D-glucuronide: Effects of dibromosulfophthalein on membrane transport and aglycone formation. *J Pharmacol Exp Ther* 1999; 288:414–420.

94. Lo A, Addison RS, Hooper WD, Dickinson RG. Disposition of naproxen, naproxen acylglucuronide and its rearrangement isomers in the isolated perfused rat liver. *Xenobiotica* 2001; 31:309–319.

95. Wang M, Gorrell MD, McCaughan GW, Dickinson RG. Dipeptidyl peptidase IV is a target for covalent adduct formation with the acyl glucuronide metabolite of the anti-inflammatory drug zomepirac. *Life Sci* 2001; 68:785–797.

96. Wang M, Dickinson RG. Disposition and covalent binding of diflunisal and diflunisal acylglucuronide in the isolated perfused rat liver. *Drug Metab Dispos* 1998; 26:98–104.

97. Naito S, Furuta S, Yoshida T, Kitada M, Fueki O, Unno T, Ohno Y et al. Current opinion: Safety evaluation of drug metabolites in development of pharmaceuticals. *J Toxicol Sci* 2007; 32:329–341.

98. Gonzalez FJ, Yu A-M. Cytochrome P450 and xenobiotic receptor humanized mice. *Annu Rev Pharmacol Toxicol* 2006; 46:41–64.

99. Gonzalez FJ. CYP3A4 and pregnane X receptor humanized mice. *J Biochem Mol Toxicol* 2007; 21:158–162.

100. Dragin N, Uno S, Wang B, Dalton TP, Nebert DW. Generation of humanized hCYP1A1_1A2_Cyp1a1/1a2 (–/–) mouse line. *Biochem Biophys Res Commun* 2007; 359:635–642.

101. Van Herwaarden AE, Wagenaar E, van der Kruijssen CMM, van Waterschoot RAB, Smit JW, Song JY, van der Valk MA et al. Knockout of cytochrome P450 3A yields new mouse models for understanding xenobiotic metabolism. *J Clin Invest* 2007; 117:3583–3592.
102. Okumura H, Katoh M, Sawada T, Nakajima M, Soeno Y, Yabuuchi H, Ikeda T, Tateno C, Yoshizato K, Yokoi T. Humanization of excretory pathway in chimeric mice with humanized liver. *Toxicol Sci* 2007; 97:533–538.

23

Numerical Approaches to Drug Metabolism Kinetics and Pharmacokinetics

Ken Korzekwa and Swati Nagar

CONTENTS

Introduction

In 1979, Cleland proposed that all kinetic analyses should be conducted using appropriate regression methods [1]. This allows for statistical analyses of kinetic parameters. Knowledge of errors in statistical parameters allows for the selection of the correct kinetic model (e.g., competitive versus noncompetitive inhibition). In reality, the computational capabilities to perform these analyses were not readily available at the time and it was several years before nonlinear least-squares were routinely used. A similar situation exists today. With the emergence of user-friendly computational software, e.g., Mathematica (Wolfram Research, Inc., Mathematica, Version 10.4, Champaign, IL [2016]) and Matlab (The MathWorks, Inc., Natick, Massachusetts, United States), enzyme kinetics, pharmacokinetics (PK), and any other quantitative modeling effort can be approached using numerical methods. We will loosely define numerical methods as methods to solve series of ordinary differential equations (partial differential equations will not be discussed here). As discussed below, numerical methods are particularly useful for analysis of complex kinetic schemes. This was discussed by Segel [2], but sufficient computational capabilities were not routinely available at that time.

Complex enzyme kinetics can arise from several factors. These include multiple binding sites, multiprotein interactions, non-specific substrate–enzyme interactions, and experimental design considerations. Of particular importance to this chapter, absorption, distribution, metabolism, and excretion (ADME) processes are necessarily driven by non-specific interactions. As opposed to most biochemical processes that are designed to accomplish a single biochemical task, the systems that distribute, metabolize, and eliminate foreign compounds must contend with the diversity of these compounds. For example, most hydrophobic compounds can be metabolized by the Cytochrome P450 (CYP) enzymes. In humans, most of these metabolic transformations are catalyzed by a very small number of enzymes (4–6) [3]. Thus drug metabolizing enzymes, drug transporters, and some ADME-specific receptors have broader ligand selectivity than most other enzymes, transporters, and receptors.

Similar to ADME enzymes and transporters, membrane partitioning and passive permeability across a cellular membrane is driven to a large extent by non-specific interactions. Membrane partitioning has a large impact on the volume of distribution of a drug, and membrane permeability determines the rate and extent of drug absorption and organ distribution. Primary determinants of membrane partitioning and permeability include the hydrophobicity and ionization state of a compound [4]. The specific orientation of various functional groups is less important than bulk compound properties.

In pharmacokinetic compartmental modeling, concentration as a function of time profiles, C(t), are commonly described by multi-exponential functions. These functions are derived from ordinary differential equations (ODEs) and numerical solutions directly from the ODEs are common. The advantage of using numerical methods instead of integrated equations is that the complexities of physiologic processes (e.g., enzyme, transporter, and membrane kinetics) can be directly incorporated into PK models. For example, physiologically-based pharmacokinetic (PBPK) models use numerical methods for their solutions [5–7]. Similarly, pharmacodynamic (PD) models can be built and readily solved by numerical approaches.

This chapter details the use of numerical methods in simple and complex enzyme kinetics, compartmental- and physiologically-based PK models, and PK-PD. The flexibility allowed by the numerical method to incorporate various mechanistic complexities into a model and to combine various enzyme kinetics, PK, and PD models will be discussed. Model development and validation with rigorous statistical analyses will be included and examples of several modeling exercises will be provided.

Michaelis–Menten Kinetics

Assumptions and Limitations

The Michaelis–Menten (MM) equation is the best-known model to describe saturable enzyme kinetics [8]. The model for MM kinetics is shown in Scheme 23.1. Scheme 23.1 can be used to derive Eq. 23.1, with the assumptions that there is insignificant substrate depletion as well as insignificant reverse reaction (the initial rate assumption) and that there is a rapid equilibrium (i.e., the rate of ES dissociation to E and S is much faster than its conversion to E and P). Briggs and Haldane revised the derivation by assuming that the rate of change of the concentration of the ES complex is zero (the steady-state assumption) with no assumption about rapid equilibrium or the rate of reverse reaction [9].

$$v = \frac{V_{max}[S]}{K_m + [S]} \tag{23.1}$$

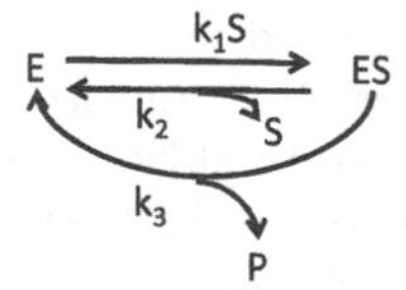

SCHEME 23.1 Scheme for Michaelis–Menten enzyme kinetics. E: enzyme, S: substrate, ES: enzyme-substrate complex, P: product, k_1: second order binding constant, k_2: first-order debinding constant, k_3: first-order rate constant for product formation.

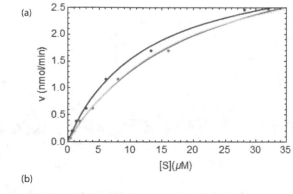

(a)

(b)

Parameter	Simulated	Eq.1 with S	Eq. 1 with Ŝ	Numerical
Km (uM)	10	20.4	12.5	12.7
Vmax (nmol/min)	3	4.0	3.5	3.5

FIGURE 23.1 MM kinetics with substrate depletion. (a) Velocity versus [S] profiles are depicted. Black closed circles: velocity versus [S] data. Light-gray closed circles: velocity versus [Ŝ] data. Model fits are shown with solid lines for Eq. 23.1 with [S] (solid gray), Eq. 23.1 with [Ŝ] (solid black), and the numerical method (dashed gray). (b) True (simulated) and model estimates of K_m and V_{max} are listed with the three methods.

In Eq. 23.1, v is the initial velocity of the reaction, [S] is the substrate concentration, V_{max} is the maximal velocity, and K_m is the substrate concentration yielding half-maximal velocity. K_m is also called the Michaelis–Menten constant, or the Michaelis constant. Eq. 23.1 is the rate equation based on ODEs for each species in Scheme 23.1. The derivation of Eq. 23.1 along with detailed discussions on the underlying assumptions and interpretation of K_m are covered by Segel [2].

Use of the steady-state rate equation for MM kinetics is sometimes limited by the underlying assumptions. Thus, Eq. 23.1 will hold if substrate depletion is minimal over the duration of an experiment. Experiments are recommended to be designed such that there is less than 10% substrate depletion [10]. However, in scenarios such as novel substrates being tested or unknown enzyme levels, significant substrate depletion may occur. If this occurs, the logarithmic mean of substrate concentration ($\hat{S} = (S_0 - S_t)/Ln S_0/S_t$ instead of S) can be used to correctly calculate K_m with Eq. 23.1 [11]. Figure 23.1 shows the impact of substrate depletion on kinetic parameters estimated with Eq. 23.1 using either $\hat{S}$ or S, as well as with numerical methods. As can be seen in Figure 23.1, use of Eq. 23.1 with substrate depletion results in inaccurate kinetic parameters. Use of either $\hat{S}$ or the numerical method gives better and virtually identical estimates.

Another assumption key to the derivation of Eq. 23.1 with the Briggs–Haldane approach is the steady-state assumption. It is assumed that the rate of formation of the ES complex is equal to its rate of consumption, such that the net rate of change of [ES] with time is zero. Practically, the steady-state assumption is valid at high ratios of $S_0/[E]_t$ (S_0: substrate concentration at time zero, E_t: total enzyme concentration) and when binding and debinding are rapid relative to other steps. Thus, when assays are performed at high substrate concentrations relative to low concentrations of enzyme and when equilibrium can be achieved, Eq. 23.1 is valid. Another experimental issue that can invalidate the assumptions of the MM equation is enzyme instability. If the enzyme system is inherently unstable, equilibrium cannot be achieved, and the steady-state assumption is invalid.

Advantages of the Numerical Method

As stated above, the steady-state rate equation for MM kinetics is valid under certain simplifying assumptions. In contrast, no such assumptions are necessary when working directly with ODEs and numerical methods. Figure 23.2 shows an example of analyses of an unstable enzyme that displays hyperbolic saturation kinetics using Eq. 23.1 and the numerical solution. For a solution directly from the ODEs, an additional rate constant for first-order enzyme loss (k_4) is included in the model. Significant

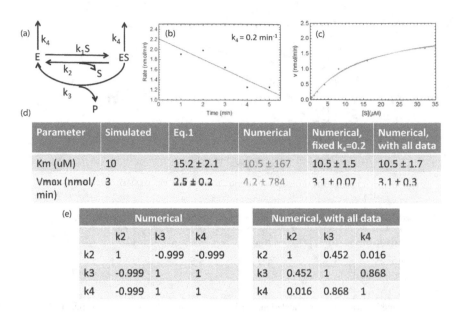

FIGURE 23.2 MM kinetics with non-specific enzyme loss. (a) Scheme for MM kinetics with non-specific enzyme loss, where k_4 is the first-order rate constant for enzyme loss. (b) Plot of product formation rate versus time. A linear fit to the data estimates k_4 to be 0.2 min^{-1}. (c) Velocity versus [S] profiles are depicted. Black closed circles: velocity versus [S] data. Solid lines are model fits with Eq. 23.1 (solid) or the numerical method (dashed). (d) True (simulated) and model estimates of K_m and V_{max} are listed with Eq. 23.1, and the numerical method using either velocity-[S] data alone, with k_4 fixed at 0.2 min^{-1} based on data in Figure 23.2b, or simultaneous use of velocity-[S] and velocity-time data. (e) Correlation matrices for model fitting for the numerical method using either velocity-[S] data alone (left) or simultaneous use of velocity-[S] and velocity-time data (right).

loss of enzyme during an experiment can cause significant changes in estimated parameters. As shown in Figure 23.2, parameters resulting from Eq. 23.1 are inaccurate. Also, the numerical method cannot be used to solve for k_4 using only velocity-[S] data. Enzyme loss still results in a hyperbolic saturation curve, and k_2, k_3, and k_4 become highly correlated. Highly correlated parameters will result in very large parameter errors and this can be directly observed from the correlation matrix (Figure 23.2e). Additional data are required, and an easy solution is to use the preliminary data collected from a time linearity study. The velocity-[S] data and time linearity (velocity-time) data can be simultaneously used in the numerical method to provide accurate parameter estimates including k_4, as shown in Figure 23.2d. Another option is to conduct a preincubation–time velocity study to characterize the rate of enzyme loss. The enzyme loss rate constant can then be fixed to solve for K_m and V_{max}.

Another practical advantage of numerical methods is that experimental events can be incorporated into the model. For example, while not recommended, if one spills coffee into their CYP incubation, and (1) the coffee is tepid (37°C), (2) caffeine is not an inhibitor (not CYP2E1), and (3) the change in volume is known, a dilution step can be incorporated into the model and kinetic parameters can be estimated. A more serious and relevant example is provided below in section "TDI Modeling with a Dilution Step: An Example."

Non-Michaelis–Menten Kinetics

Often, atypical or non-MM kinetics are observed with deviation from hyperbolic velocity-[S] relationships (e.g., sigmoidal curves, biphasic curves, partial inhibition curves, etc.). Mechanistically, multiple binding sites on a protein or multiple ligand molecules binding to the same binding site will often lead to atypical kinetics. Non-MM enzyme kinetics have been reported for CYPs, uridine diphospho-glucuronosyltransferases (UGTs), sulfotransferases (SULTs), and transporters [12–14]. In ADME, the CYP superfamily of enzymes plays an important role in drug oxidation and has been the most well studied system [15]. We will use CYP kinetics to exemplify numerical approaches to solve non-MM kinetics in this section.

Background on CYPs and CYP Kinetics

The CYP superfamily includes numerous functional isozymes in humans, but a relatively small number of enzymes—CYPs 1A2, 2A6, 2B6, 2C8, 2C9, 2C19, 2D6, 2E1, and 3A4/5—are responsible for most of the CYP mediated oxidations. Of these, CYPs 2C9, 2D6, and 3A4 mediate over 90% of human drug oxidations [3]. CYPs are understood to be versatile with respect to ligand selectivity, and many drug molecules are substrates for the same CYP enzyme. Crystal structures support the conclusion that the active sites of some CYPs are very flexible, particularly those involved in the metabolism of xenobiotics [16]. These non-specific binding interactions between CYPs and ligands can result in some unusual binding and metabolism kinetics. In general, non-hyperbolic saturation kinetics and noncompetitive inhibition kinetics are sometimes observed for CYPs. This appears to occur when more than one substrate can simultaneously occupy the active site (or multiple regions within the active site). Simultaneous substrate binding to the CYP active site can have a marked impact on the observed enzyme kinetics as well as interpretation of kinetic data [17]. Knowledge of the catalytic cycle of CYP-mediated oxidation is important in order to understand the resultant complex enzyme kinetics. The present discussion focuses on MM and non-MM CYP enzyme kinetic models.

One Substrate Binding Profiles (ESS)

When a single substrate binds a CYP binding site in a 2:1 ratio, an ESS complex is formed (Scheme 23.2). The result can be non-hyperbolic saturation kinetics. Scheme 23.2a and b depict two possibilities: two substrate molecules bind to the CYP active site in an indistinguishable manner, with the same product resulting from both ES and ESS (Scheme 23.2a), and two substrate molecules bind to two independent binding sites within the CYP active site with potentially different products or product ratios from each binding event (Scheme 23.2b). When a single product is formed in a reaction, Scheme 23.2a and b will fit the data equally well. However, when more than one product is formed, Scheme 23.2b can be used to vary product ratios.

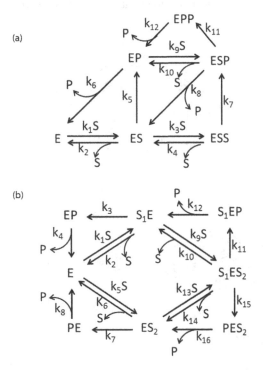

SCHEME 23.2 Schemes for multi-binding (ESS) non-MM enzyme kinetics. (a) Two substrate molecules bind to the CYP active site in an indistinguishable manner, with the same product resulting from ES and ESS. (b) Two substrate molecules bind to two independent binding sites within the CYP active site, possibly resulting in different products or product ratios from each binding event.

In the event of [ESS] formation, saturation profiles can exhibit hyperbolic, sigmoidal, biphasic, or substrate inhibition characteristics. Hyperbolic saturation kinetics can be observed when the kinetic characteristics of the two binding events are similar. Sigmoidal saturation kinetics can be observed if (A) the second substrate molecule binds with a lower K_m than the first substrate molecule, (B) if the second substrate molecule is metabolized faster than the first, or (C) a combination of both. Biphasic kinetics is observed when the second binding event has a higher K_m and a higher V_{max} than the first event. Finally, substrate inhibition is observed when the second binding event has a lower V_{max} than the first event.

Multi-substrate Binding Profiles (ESB)

Analogous to ESS kinetics, different substrates can simultaneously bind to the CYPs. Figure 23.3a depicts ESB formation, where B is a substrate, inhibitor, or activator. Multi-substrate interactions are most apparent during competitive inhibition experiments, generally used to predict drug interactions. Profiles that can be observed include complete inhibition, partial inhibition, activation, or a combination of activation followed by inhibition. The profiles are generally hyperbolic in nature (Figure 23.3b) and are determined by the two binding events (ES and ESB formation) and product formation from these species. Multi-substrate binding profiles can be further complicated when S and B can bind twice forming ESS and EBB in addition to ESB. When this occurs the velocity profiles can be quite complicated. For example, one can observe activation occurring at low [B] and inhibition at high [B]. These models can be easily constructed with ODEs without the need for explicit derivation of rate equations.

Numerical Solutions to Multi-substrate Kinetics

A fit of an ESB scheme (Figure 23.3a) to data using the numerical method is shown in Figure 23.3b and c and the Mathematica program to solve the ODEs is given on next page. For this kinetic scheme, the fit using the numerical method will be identical to the fit to a standard multi-site binding equation:

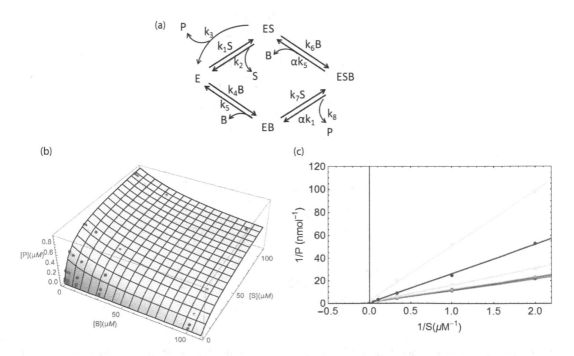

FIGURE 23.3 Multi-binding (ESB) enzyme kinetics. (a) Scheme for ESB formation upon multi-binding kinetics. B denotes a substrate, an inhibitor, or an activator. (b) A 3D plot of product formation versus [S] and [B]. (c) A double reciprocal plot of the data. Data and the numerical solution in Mathematica are provided below.

$$\frac{v}{E_t} = \frac{k_3\left(\dfrac{S}{K_S}\right) + k_8\left(\dfrac{S\,B}{\alpha K_S K_B}\right)}{1 + \left(\dfrac{S}{K_S}\right) + \left(\dfrac{S\,B}{\alpha K_S K_B}\right)} \tag{23.2}$$

where E_t is total enzyme concentration, $K_S = k_2/k_1$, $K_B = k_5/k_4$, and α is the constant that defines the effect of B on S binding to E and the effect of S on B binding to E.

ESB Kinetics

This program fits an ESB model

```
ClearAll["Global`*"];
```

Data {[B],[S],[P]} for a 20 minute incubation

```
data = {{0.0001, 0.5, 0.0446732}, {0.0001, 1, 0.0846008}, {0.0001, 3, 0.221733},
    {0.0001, 10, 0.491599}, {0.0001, 30, 0.750456}, {0.0001, 100, 0.867364},
    {1, 0.5, 0.0422905}, {1, 1, 0.0841401}, {1, 3, 0.220819}, {1, 10, 0.455583},
    {1, 30, 0.703897}, {1, 100, 0.945641}, {3, 0.5, 0.0395237}, {3, 1, 0.0751188},
    {3, 3, 0.217412}, {3, 10, 0.419241}, {3, 30, 0.742473}, {3, 100, 0.884652},
    {10, 0.5, 0.0312889}, {10, 1, 0.0608708}, {10, 3, 0.158427}, {10, 10, 0.398627},
    {10, 30, 0.61712}, {10, 100, 0.78687}, {30, 0.5, 0.0188269}, {30, 1, 0.0379214},
    {30, 3, 0.103891}, {30, 10, 0.250932}, {30, 30, 0.476263}, {30, 100, 0.655345},
    {100, 0.5, 0.00893282}, {100, 1, 0.0192194}, {100, 3, 0.0556214},
    {100, 10, 0.148711}, {100, 30, 0.294211}, {100, 100, 0.488861}};

Et = 0.005;
```

For a 10 uM Kd, k1=k4=10^4/M,sec

```
k1 = 60;
k2init = 600;
k3init = 10;
k4 = 60;
k5init = 1200;
k6init = 2;
ainit = 5;

ClearAll[k2, k3, k5, k6, a, B0, S0, fit, modelSB];

modelSB[k2_?NumericQ, k3_?NumericQ, k5_?NumericQ,
    k6_?NumericQ, a_?NumericQ, B0_?NumericQ, S0_?NumericQ] :=
  (modelSB[k2, k3, k5, k6, a, B0, S0] = P[20] /. First[NDSolve[{
        Eu'[t] == -k1 Eu[t] S[t] + k2 ES[t] + k3 ES[t] - k4 Eu[t] Bu[t] + k5 EB[t],
        ES'[t] == k1 Eu[t] S[t] - (k2 + k3 + k4 Bu[t]) ES[t] + a k5 ESB[t],
        EB'[t] == - (k5) EB[t] + k4 Eu[t] Bu[t] - k1 EB[t] S[t] + a k2 ESB[t] + k6 ESB[t],
        ESB'[t] == - (a k5 + a k2 + k6) ESB[t] + k4 ES[t] Bu[t] + k1 EB[t] S[t],
        S'[t] == -k1 Eu[t] S[t] + k2 ES[t] - k1 EB[t] S[t] + a k2 ESB[t],
        P'[t] == k3 ES[t] + k6 ESB[t],
        Bu'[t] == -k4 Eu[t] Bu[t] + k5 EB[t] - k4 ES[t] Bu[t] + a k5 ESB[t],
        S[0] == S0,
        Eu[0] == Et,
        ES[0] == 0,
        EB[0] == 0,
        ESB[0] == 0,
        P[0] == 0,
        Bu[0] == B0},
        {Eu, ES, EB, ESB, S, P, Bu},
        {t, 0, 60}, MaxSteps -> 100 000, PrecisionGoal -> ∞]]);

fit = NonlinearModelFit[data, modelSB[k2, k3, k5, k6, a, B0, S0],
    {{k2, k2init}, {k3, k3init}, {k5, k5init}, {k6, k6init}, {a, ainit}},
    {B0, S0}, Weights -> (1 / #3 &)];
```

```
fit["ParameterTable"]
```

	Estimate	Standard Error	t-Statistic	P-Value
k2	586.646	21.7664	26.9519	4.44409×10^{-23}
k3	9.93914	0.143304	69.3568	1.42287×10^{-35}
k5	961.471	102.796	9.35316	1.54379×10^{-10}
k6	3.26305	0.554121	5.88869	1.68494×10^{-6}
a	4.8681	0.777182	6.26378	5.8057×10^{-7}

```
fit["RSquared"]
```

0.998545

```
fit["AICc"]
```

-157.971

```
TableForm[fit["CorrelationMatrix"]]
```

1.	0.732713	0.469158	-0.229942	-0.466942
0.732713	1.	0.0268296	0.0291053	-0.537506
0.469158	0.0268296	1.	-0.859675	-0.0169071
-0.229942	0.0291053	-0.859675	1.	-0.14265
-0.466942	-0.537506	-0.0169071	-0.14265	1.

This will be true for any model provided that the assumptions used to derive the rate equations are valid. When one or more of these assumptions cannot be made (e.g., steady-state, initial rates, or rapid-equilibrium kinetics), the numerical method will provide better results. Also, to any of these models, any mechanistic insights to the model can be incorporated by addition or modification of the ODEs. For example, an enzyme loss pathway can be added to any model with the addition of a single rate constant.

An important consideration for any enzymatic rate model is the range of the experimental concentrations relative to the binding constants. If a significant amount of saturation of a binding site is not achieved experimentally, it will not be possible to solve for either the binding constant K or the velocity from that species (V). Only the ratio of the two parameters (V/K) can be estimated. This can be accomplished by fixing either K (both binding and debinding constants) or V and solving for the other. The absolute values of K and V are meaningless and only V/K, the clearance at sub-saturating concentrations, has value.

Time-Dependent Inactivation

Overlapping drug metabolism pathways are the most common mechanism for drug-drug interactions (DDIs). One of the most difficult DDIs to predict with preclinical data is the time-dependent inhibition (TDI) of the CYPs. Unanticipated DDIs can have two important consequences. First, if a DDI is under predicted, unsafe drug candidates will be advanced into the clinic. Second, over prediction of DDIs can prevent or delay useful drugs from reaching the market.

Since TDIs result in a loss of enzyme over time [18–22], the *in vivo* impact of TDI is more difficult to assess than competitive inhibitors. Whereas the DDI potential of a competitive inhibitor can be predicted from free drug concentration at the active site and a binding constant (at least in theory), the DDI potential of a TDI will depend on the affinity (K_I), inactivation rate (k_{inact}), and rate of enzyme regeneration (k_{deg}) [22,23]. When the substrate and inhibitor display normal hyperbolic binding kinetics and the inhibitor displays simple irreversible inactivation, TDIs can be identified by an IC_{50} shift upon preincubation with the compound in the presence of NADPH [20]. However, prediction of *in vivo* DDIs requires an accurate assessment of K_I, k_{inact}, and k_{deg}.

If the substrate and inhibitor display normal hyperbolic binding kinetics and the inhibitor displays simple irreversible inhibition, the binding constant (K_I) and inactivation rate constant (k_{inact}) can be determined through a replot method [18]. To determine binding and rate constants, enzyme activity is measured at several inhibitor concentrations and several preincubation times. The log of percent remaining activity versus time is plotted (PRA plot), and the slope for each inhibitor concentration gives the observed rate constant (k_{obs}) for enzyme loss. Fitting a hyperbola to a plot of k_{obs} versus inhibitor concentration gives the apparent binding constant for the inhibitor (K_I) and the k_{cat} for inactivation (k_{inact}). Although this is the current method to determine TDI parameters, it has provided limited success in predicting clinical outcomes [24–27]. A recent survey of 17 PhRMA (Pharmaceutical Research and Manufacturers of America) member companies provides a number of reservations on the current use of TDI methodology [23].

The standard replot method described above requires a number of assumptions, including Michaelis–Menten kinetics, initial rates, steady-state, and irreversible steps. As described above, CYP kinetics are often complex and therefore the numerical method provides significant advantages over the replot method [28,29].

TDI with MM Kinetics

It has been shown previously that the replot method suffers from propagation of errors [28]. Since the numerical method considers all data simultaneously, propagation of errors does not occur. Figure 23.4 shows the results of 500 simulations for MM TDI (Scheme 22.3a) in which random error was introduced to the data and the parameters estimated by the replot and numerical methods were determined. As can be seen in Figure 23.4, the numerical method has ~8 × less error in K_I values than the replot method. The k_{inact} values are similar, because the plateau is better defined with experimental data. In fact, we accurately determine both K_I and k_{inact} using a 6 × 2 experimental protocol (equivalent to an IC_{50} shift assay). This suggests that when simple MM kinetics are involved, better parameters can be generated with less experimental data.

A complicating factor for TDI experiments is the nonspecific loss of enzyme over time (Scheme 23.3b). This enzyme loss is observed as a decrease in activity over time in the absence of inhibitor. The replot method generally uses the [I] = 0 data as the control against which the remaining data are normalized.

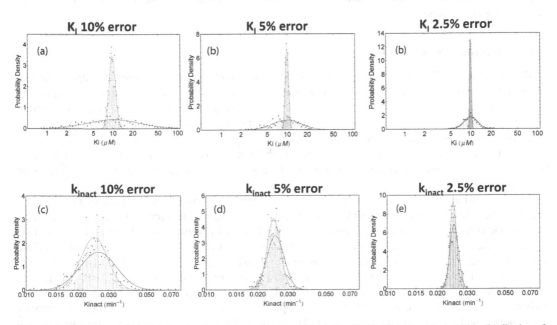

FIGURE 23.4 Comparison of the replot and numerical methods for TDI with MM kinetics. Probability distribution of K_I (a–c) and k_{inact} (d–f) estimates is depicted for the numerical (dark gray) and standard replot (light gray) methods, from simulated MM data at 10% (a, d), 5% (b, e), and 2.5% (c, f) error. Distribution is shown for 500 runs at each condition. (Reproduced with permission Nagar, S. et al., *Drug Metab. Dispos.*, 42, 1575–1586, 2014.)

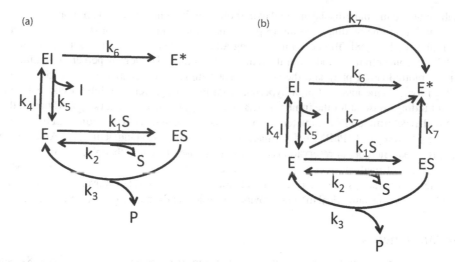

SCHEME 23.3   Scheme for TDI with MM kinetics. (a) TDI with MM kinetics, and (b) TDI with MM kinetics and non-specific enzyme loss. Non-specific enzyme loss is modeled with k_7, a first-order rate constant.

This treatment accounts for nonspecific enzyme loss, but propagates error. Nonspecific enzyme loss must be explicitly modeled with a first order rate constant in the numerical method. The schemes for MM TDI kinetics without or with nonspecific enzyme loss are depicted in Scheme 23.3a and b, respectively. In our experience, nonspecific enzyme loss typically follows first-order kinetics. The first-order rate constant (k_7 in Scheme 23.3b) is easily parameterized by the numerical method, and its inclusion does not hinder model optimization. It should be noted, however, that enzyme loss may occur from specific enzyme species (e.g., enzyme protection by ligand binding). If additional experimental data are available, this can be easily incorporated into the model. In the absence of such data, enzyme loss adds uncertainty to the parameterized values of k_{inact}.

TDI with Non-MM Kinetics

As discussed above, CYP kinetics are often non-MM due to multiple binding events. Complex kinetics are observed with TDI experiments as well, and more complex models provide additional parameters that are required to describe CYP TDI kinetics. An irreversible inhibitor can bind twice to form an EII complex or can bind simultaneously with a substrate to form an ESI complex. In these cases, sufficient experimental data points are needed in order to provide estimates of multi-binding kinetic parameters [29]. Scheme 23.4 depicts TDI models with formation of either an EII (Scheme 23.4a) or an ESI (Scheme 23.4b) complex. A number of *in vitro* TDI experiments modeled with EII kinetics have been previously reported [29].

In addition to multi-substrate/inhibitor kinetics, other complexities have been reported for TDI kinetics. These include partial, quasi-irreversible intermediate, and sequential metabolism TDI (Scheme 23.5). Partial inactivation (Scheme 23.5a) occurs when a TDI binds irreversibly to a CYP apoprotein. This binding causes a decrease but not a complete loss in activity [30,31]. Quasi-irreversible intermediate kinetics (Scheme 23.5b) result from the formation of a metabolic intermediate complex (MIC) with the heme. The first complex is reversible, but is converted to an irreversible complex by further reduction of the enzyme [32]. When a TDI is a product of a prior metabolic step, sequential metabolism kinetics (Scheme 23.5c) should be used. Each of these complexities results in nonlinear PRA plots. For partial inactivation, the log (percent remaining activity) time curves are concave upward, with the curve at each [I] approaching the same asymptote [28]. The PRA curves for quasi-irreversible intermediate formation are also concave upward, but increasing [I] results in parallel biphasic curves. Many amine-containing drugs that form MICs require an initial de-alkylation reaction prior to forming the nitroso TDI [33].

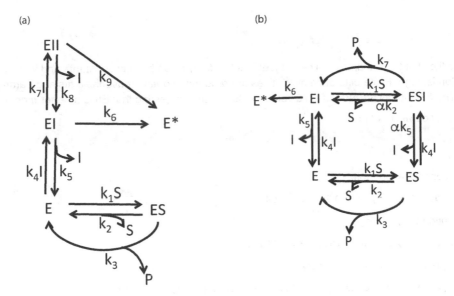

SCHEME 23.4 Schemes for TDI with non-MM multi-binding kinetics. (a) TDI with formation of EII complex. (b) TDI with formation of ESI complex.

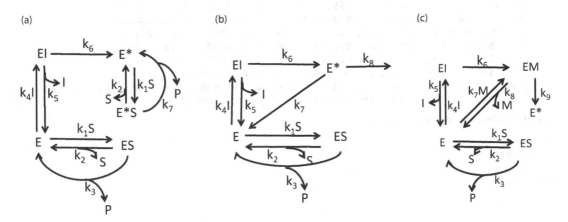

SCHEME 23.5 Schemes for TDI with non-MM complex kinetics. (a) TDI with partial inactivation. (b) TDI with quasi-irreversible intermediate formation. (c) TDI with sequential metabolism to form the inactivator.

The result is a short lag time prior to inactivation. Often, the appropriate kinetic model can be identified from the shape of the PRA plot. However, model selection should always be based on objective statistical criteria as discussed below.

TDI Modeling with a Dilution Step: An Example

In vitro TDI experiments are often conducted with a dilution step after the primary incubation with inactivator, in order to minimize competitive inhibition during the secondary incubation (addition of substrate). While a dilution step is not necessary when using the numerical method to obtain kinetic parameters, if conducted as part of the experiment it can be easily incorporated into the modeling procedure. An example of substrate addition for the secondary incubation with dilution for an EII model is presented in a Mathematica file below.

EII versus MM Time Dependent Inhibition.

EII is a difficult fit for this dataset. The dataset has two fairly close binding constants and velocities, and correlation is high. Finite difference derivatives are required to obtain reasonable fits and parameter errors. The MM fit has an AICc of -276 versus -286 for EII, suggesting that EII is a better model.

```
ClearAll["Global`*"];
```

```
Et = 0.1;
S0 = 100;
```

Inhibitor concentration table

```
IOt = {0.01, 2., 4., 8., 16., 32., 64.};
```

Preincubation time Table

```
tSt = {0.01, 1., 2., 5., 10., 15., 30.};
```

Data {[I], preincubation time, product}

```
data = {{0.01, 0.01, 0.119}, {0.01, 1., 0.117}, {0.01, 2., 0.121},
    {0.01, 5., 0.106}, {0.01, 10., 0.118}, {0.01, 15., 0.113}, {0.01, 30., 0.112},
    {2., 0.01, 0.113}, {2., 1., 0.117}, {2., 2., 0.107}, {2., 5., 0.105},
    {2., 10., 0.103}, {2., 15., 0.0943}, {2., 30., 0.0791}, {4., 0.01, 0.116},
    {4., 1., 0.11}, {4., 2., 0.107}, {4., 5., 0.104}, {4., 10., 0.0908},
    {4., 15., 0.077}, {4., 30., 0.0595}, {8., 0.01, 0.102}, {8., 1., 0.11},
    {8., 2., 0.0982}, {8., 5., 0.0903}, {8., 10., 0.0778}, {8., 15., 0.0659},
    {8., 30., 0.0406}, {16., 0.01, 0.106}, {16., 1., 0.112}, {16., 2., 0.0982},
    {16., 5., 0.0878}, {16., 10., 0.0714}, {16., 15., 0.0532}, {16., 30., 0.0254},
    {32., 0.01, 0.105}, {32., 1., 0.0992}, {32., 2., 0.0942}, {32., 5., 0.0763},
    {32., 10., 0.0599}, {32., 15., 0.0417}, {32., 30., 0.0151},
    {64., 0.01, 0.109}, {64., 1., 0.0949}, {64., 2., 0.0839}, {64., 5., 0.0672},
    {64., 10., 0.0472}, {64., 15., 0.0333}, {64., 30., 0.00927}}};
```

Fixed parameters and initial values.

```
k1 = 270.;
k2 = 2700.;
k3init = 5;
k4 = 270.;
k5init = 2000.;
k6init = 0.1;
k7 = 270.;
k8init = 6000.;
k9init = 0.1;
```

Build the EII model solving for k3,k5,k6,k8,k9. 20-fold dilution at time tS (WhenEvent).

```
ClearAll[k3, k5, k6, k8, k9, I0, tS, model1, fit]
model1[k3_?NumericQ, k5_?NumericQ, k6_?NumericQ,
    k8_?NumericQ, k9_?NumericQ, I0_?NumericQ, tS_?NumericQ] :=
  (model[k3, k5, k6, k8, k9, I0, tS] = P[tS + 5.] /. First[NDSolve[{
          Eu'[t] == -k1 Eu[t] S[t] + k2 ES[t] + k3 ES[t] - k4 Eu[t] Iu[t] + k5 EI[t],
          ES'[t] == k1 Eu[t] S[t] - (k2 + k3) ES[t],
          EI'[t] == k4 Eu[t] Iu[t] - (k5 + k6) EI[t] - k7 EI[t] Iu[t] + k8 EII[t],
          EII'[t] == k7 EI[t] Iu[t] - (k8 + k9) EII[t],
          E2'[t] == k6 EI[t] + k9 EII[t],
          S'[t] == -k1 Eu[t] S[t] + k2 ES[t],
          P'[t] == k3 ES[t],
          Iu'[t] == -k4 Eu[t] Iu[t] + k5 EI[t] - k7 EI[t] Iu[t] + (k8 + k9) EII[t],
          S[0] == 0,
          Eu[0] == Et,
          ES[0] == 0,
          EI[0] == 0,
          EII[0] == 0,
          P[0] == 0,
          Iu[0] == I0,
          E2[0] == 0,
          WhenEvent[t == tS, {S[t] -> S0, Eu[t] -> Eu[t] / 20,
            ES[t] -> ES[t] / 20, EI[t] -> EI[t] / 20, EII[t] -> EII[t] / 20,
            E2[t] -> E2[t] / 20, P[t] -> P[t] / 20, Iu[t] -> Iu[t] / 20}]},
        {Eu, ES, EI, EII, E2, S, P, Iu}, {t, 0, 40}, MaxSteps -> 100 000,
        PrecisionGoal -> Infinity]]);
```

Fit model to the data.

```
fit = NonlinearModelFit[data, model1[k3, k5, k6, k8, k9, I0, tS],
    {{k3, k3init}, {k5, k5init}, {k6, k6init}, {k8, k8init}, {k9, k9init}},
    {I0, tS}, PrecisionGoal -> 14, MaxIterations -> 10 000, Weights -> (1 / #3 &),
    Gradient -> {"FiniteDifference", "DifferenceOrder" -> 4}];
```

```
fit["ParameterTable"]
```

	Estimate	Standard Error	t-Statistic	P-Value
k3	4.98723	0.0420906	118.488	9.17862×10^{-57}
k5	872.769	195.298	4.46891	0.0000544516
k6	0.0271077	0.00581118	4.66475	0.0000289267
k8	6700.83	2164.01	3.09649	0.0034029
k9	0.0987243	0.00843509	11.704	4.19898×10^{-15}

```
fit["RSquared"]
```

0.998538

```
fit["AICc"]
```

-286.464

```
TableForm[fit["CorrelationMatrix"]]
```

```
1.            -0.566078    -0.314617    -0.184851    -0.13472
-0.566078      1.           0.774696     0.376033     0.342735
-0.314617      0.774696     1.           0.785268     0.660531
-0.184851      0.376033     0.785268     1.           0.934945
-0.13472       0.342735     0.660531     0.934945     1.
```

Build the MM model solving for k3,k5,k6. 20-fold dilution at time tS.

```
ClearAll[k3, k5, k6, IO, tS, model1, fit]
model2[k3_?NumericQ, k5_?NumericQ, k6_?NumericQ, IO_?NumericQ, tS_?NumericQ] :=
   (model[k3, k5, k6, IO, tS] = P[tS + 5.] /. First[NDSolve[{
           Eu'[t] == -k1 Eu[t] S[t] + k2 ES[t] + k3 ES[t] - k4 Eu[t] Iu[t] + k5 EI[t],
           ES'[t] == k1 Eu[t] S[t] - (k2 + k3) ES[t],
           EI'[t] == k4 Eu[t] Iu[t] - (k5 + k6) EI[t],
           E2'[t] == k6 EI[t],
           S'[t] == -k1 Eu[t] S[t] + k2 ES[t],
           P'[t] == k3 ES[t],
           Iu'[t] == -k4 Eu[t] Iu[t] + k5 EI[t],
           S[0] == 0,
           Eu[0] == Et,
           ES[0] == 0,
           EI[0] == 0,
           P[0] == 0,
           Iu[0] == IO,
           E2[0] == 0,
           WhenEvent[t == tS, {S[t] -> S0, Eu[t] -> Eu[t] / 20, ES[t] -> ES[t] / 20, EI[t] ->
               EI[t] / 20, E2[t] -> E2[t] / 20, P[t] -> P[t] / 20, Iu[t] -> Iu[t] / 20}]},
           {Eu, ES, EI, E2, S, P, Iu}, {t, 0, 40}, MaxSteps -> 100 000,
           PrecisionGoal -> Infinity]]);
```

Fit model to the data.

```
fit = NonlinearModelFit[data, model2[k3, k5, k6, IO, tS],
   {{k3, k3init}, {k5, k5init}, {k6, k6init}}, {IO, tS},
   PrecisionGoal -> 14, MaxIterations -> 10000, Weights -> (1 / #3 &),
   Gradient -> {"FiniteDifference", "DifferenceOrder" -> 4}];
```

```
fit["ParameterTable"]
```

	Estimate	Standard Error	t-Statistic	P-Value
k3	4.89581	0.0390745	125.294	6.00003×10^{-60}
k5	4217.94	421.371	10.0101	3.94215×10^{-13}
k6	0.100092	0.00450939	22.1963	3.23358×10^{-26}

```
fit["RSquared"]
```

0.998012

```
fit["AICc"]
```

-276.48

```
TableForm[fit["CorrelationMatrix"]]
```

```
1.          -0.293048    -0.0201307
-0.293048    1.           0.87315
-0.0201307   0.87315      1.
```

Incorporating Numerical Enzyme Models in Pharmacokinetic Models

Analogous to enzyme kinetics, compartmental PK models can utilize either integrated C(t) equations or directly use the ODEs. Fitting ODEs to PK data provide identical results as fitting the integrated C(t) equations, provided that identical weighting schemes are used. Numerical methods in compartmental PK modeling are commonly utilized in commercial software packages. The principal advantage of working with ODEs is that numerical enzyme kinetic models can seamlessly be incorporated into PK models. When clearance is modeled directly from the central compartment in a compartmental PK model, the ODEs of the enzyme kinetic model can be directly linked to central compartment concentrations.

If the clearance organ is not part of the central compartment, i.e. the drug is permeability rate limited, or if the drug is a transporter substrate, the organ may need to be modeled explicitly. These models are usually referred to as hybrid PBPK models. In this case, the enzyme kinetics ODEs can be linked to intracellular organ concentrations [34].

Practical Aspects of Numerical Approaches to Drug Metabolism Kinetics

There are several steps that can help in the construction and parameterization of kinetic models for drug metabolism.

1. First and foremost, it is useful to plot the data in an appropriate format to determine the best starting model. Eadie-Hofstee plots are useful to analyze saturation kinetics. For inhibition kinetics, a double reciprocal or Dixon plot, and for TDI, a PRA plot should be used. For enzyme inhibition kinetics, most multi-substrate/inhibitor interactions result in mixed inhibition kinetics (i.e., changes in both the slope and intercept of a double reciprocal plot) or in activation. For saturation kinetics, ESS models can result in sigmoidal, biphasic, of substrate inhibition kinetics. For TDI models, curvature in the PRA plots will determine if quasi-irreversible intermediate, partial inactivation, or sequential metabolism models should be used. Although more difficult to detect, non-hyperbolic spacing of the different lines of a PRA plot indicates that an EII model should be used.

2. For any enzyme-ligand species in an enzyme kinetic model, at least one on- or off-rate must be assumed or measured (e.g., by a surface plasmon resonance assay). For most models, experimental on- and off-rates are not available, nor are they required to build a useful model. For most CYP oxidations, measured on-rates are much faster than rates of substrate oxidation. Since on-rates of 80–490 and 270 μM^{-1}, min^{-1} have been reported for the binding of ketoconazole [35] and podophyllotoxin [32], respectively, we use a value of 270 μM^{-1}, min^{-1}. The maximum rate of substrate metabolism by a CYP is ~1 min^{-1} and K_m values are usually in the μM range. Therefore, on- and off-rates are much faster than oxidation rates and the K_m is similar to the binding constant (rapid equilibrium assumption). During model parameterization, on-rates are assumed, and off-rates are parameterized, to determine the binding constant (k_{off}/k_{on}). In the absence of experimental rate constants, the absolute values of the rate constants are not meaningful since one rate constant was assumed. The rapid equilibrium assumption may not be valid for reactions with very low K_m values. For a 10 nM K_m, an on-rate of 270 μM^{-1}, min^{-1} will result in an off-rate of 2.7 μM^{-1}, min^{-1}, in the range of many CYP oxidation rates. In this case, the K_m (or effective K_m for complex schemes) will be determined by both the dissociation rate constant and the catalytic rate constant. It is noteworthy that for complex schemes, net rate constants are useful to describe fluxes through enzyme species [36].

3. Correlation matrices should be generated and analyzed (see Figure 23.2). Highly correlated parameters must be identified since the fitted values of these parameters have no information content. This situation generally requires that one or more of the parameters must be fixed. Depending on the reason for the modeling exercise, this may or may not change the interpretation of the results. For example, a substrate saturation dataset that does not approach saturation cannot be used to define K_m or V_{max}, and the parameters will be highly correlated. However, V_{max}/K_m will be meaningful, and if the relevant substrate concentrations *in vivo* do not approach the K_m, V_{max}/K_m will define the intrinsic clearance for the process ($V_{max}/K_m \times S$ = rate of metabolism). Correlation is particularly common when circular pathways exist (e.g., Scheme 23.4b). Also, greater error in the experimental data will tend to mask highly correlated variables and can cause independent parameters to appear correlated.

4. Any model should be fit to a dataset using the appropriate weighting scheme. Generally, 1/Y weighting is used to account for increasing errors with increasing values of Y. If the residuals are increasing with increasing Y and random for the logarithm of Y, 1/Y weighting is appropriate.

Model selection should be based on statistical analyses. The goodness of fit for a given dataset and a given model can be determined by any error-based function such as RMSE, SSE, R^2, etc. When selecting between multiple models objective selection criteria such as AICc or BICc should be used. AICcs can essentially compare models for the same dataset. We should point out that using AICc to compare models when a parameter has been fixed in one model and is optimized in another is not appropriate. Finally, residual plots are useful to highlight model deficiencies.

5. Simulation is a powerful tool. When many parameters are being optimized, simulations can be used to search for starting estimates. Also, after a model has been constructed, simulated datasets can be generated with and without random error to explore the covariance between parameters. When conducting sensitivity analyses, simulations can be conducted over a range of selected parameters and the impact on the other parameters and overall model fit can be determined.

Summary

Numerical methods provide a flexible and powerful approach to model drug metabolism processes. Rate and integrated equations remain useful and provide clear and useful relationships for model components. However, experimental and model complexities may preclude their derivation and use without simplifying assumptions. ODEs can be easily written for most time-dependent biological processes in drug metabolism and pharmacokinetics. Current computational software packages allow for the solution of complex systems directly from the ODEs.

Both MM and non-MM enzyme kinetic models can be parameterized with the numerical method without the need for simplifying assumptions. When events occur within an experiment (e.g., dilution in a TDI experiment), these events can be readily incorporated into the models. Finally, the ODEs for enzyme kinetic models can be seamlessly added to PK models including compartmental, PBPK, and hybrid models. With the availability of user-friendly interfaces, robust optimizers, and improved quality and quantity of experimental data, we expect that numerical approaches will become the standard modeling approach in drug metabolism science.

ACKNOWLEDGMENTS

The authors acknowledge funding from National Institutes of General Medical Sciences (NIGMS), Grants R01 GM114369, and R01 GM104178.

REFERENCES

1. Cleland WW (1979) Statistical analysis of enzyme kinetic data. *Methods Enzymol* 63:103–138.
2. Segel IH (1975) *Enzyme Kinetics*. John Wiley & Sons, New York.
3. August JT, Li AP, Anders MW, Murad F, and Coyle JT (1997) *Drug-drug Interactions: Scientific and Regulatory Perspectives*. San Diego: Academic Press.
4. Balaz S (2009) Modeling kinetics of subcellular disposition of chemicals. *Chem Rev* 109:1793–899. doi:10.1021/cr030440j.
5. Rodgers T, Leahy D, and Rowland M (2005) Physiologically based pharmacokinetic modeling 1: Predicting the tissue distribution of moderate-to-strong bases. *J Pharm Sci* 94:1259–1276. doi:10.1002/jps.20322.
6. Rodgers T and Rowland M (2006) Physiologically based pharmacokinetic modelling 2: Predicting the tissue distribution of acids, very weak bases, neutrals and zwitterions. *J Pharm Sci* 95:1238–1257. doi:10.1002/jps.20502.
7. Peyret T, Poulin P, and Krishnan K (2010) A unified algorithm for predicting partition coefficients for PBPK modeling of drugs and environmental chemicals. *Toxicol Appl Pharmacol* 249:197–207. doi:10.1016/j.taap.2010.09.010.

8. Michaelis L, Menten ML, Johnson KA, and Goody RS (2011) The original Michaelis constant: Translation of the 1913 Michaelis–Menten paper. *Biochemistry* 50:8264–8269. doi:10.1021/bi201284u.

9. Briggs GE and Haldane JBS (1925) A note on the kinetics of enzyme action. *Biochem J* 19:338.

10. Seibert E and Tracy TS (2014) Fundamentals of enzyme kinetics. *Methods Mol Biol* 1113:9–22. doi:10.1007/978-1-62703-758-7_2.

11. Tweedie DJ (2014) Case study 7. Compiled aha moments in enzyme kinetics: Authors' experiences. *Methods Mol Biol* 1113:513–519. doi:10.1007/978-1-62703-758-7_24.

12. Hutzler JM and Tracy TS (2002) Atypical kinetic profiles in drug metabolism reactions. *Drug Metab Dispos* 30:355–362.

13. Wu B (2011) Substrate inhibition kinetics in drug metabolism reactions. *Drug Metab Rev* 43:440–456. doi:10.3109/03602532.2011.615320.

14. Subramanian M and Tracy TS (2010) Allosteric enzyme-and transporter-based interactions. K. Sandy Pang, A. David Rodrigues, Raimund M. Peter (Eds.), In: *Enzyme-and Transporter-Based Drug-Drug Interactions*. Springer, New York, pp. 497–515.

15. Ortiz de Montellano PR (2005) *Cytochrome P450: Structure, Mechanism, and Biochemistry*. Springer, New York.

16. Li H and Poulos TL (2004) Crystallization of cytochromes P450 and substrate-enzyme interactions. *Curr Top Med Chem* 4:1789–1802.

17. Korzekwa K (2014) Enzyme kinetics of oxidative metabolism: Cytochromes p450. *Methods Mol Biol* 1113:149–66. doi:10.1007/978-1-62703-758-7_8.

18. Silverman RB (1995) [10] Mechanism-based enzyme inactivators. *Meth Enzymol* 249:240–283.

19. Ortiz de Montellano PR and Correia M (1995) Inhibition of cytochrome P450 enzymes. P.R. Ortiz de Montellano (Ed.) In: *Cytochrome P450*. Plenum Press, New York, pp. 305–364.

20. Obach RS, Walsky RL, and Venkatakrishnan K (2007) Mechanism-based inactivation of human cytochrome p450 enzymes and the prediction of drug-drug interactions. *Drug Metab Dispos* 35:246–255. doi:10.1124/dmd.106.012633.

21. Grime KH, Bird J, Ferguson D, and Riley RJ (2009) Mechanism-based inhibition of cytochrome P450 enzymes: An evaluation of early decision making *in vitro* approaches and drug-drug interaction prediction methods. *Eur J Pharm Sci* 36:175–191. doi:10.1016/j.ejps.2008.10.002.

22. Mohutsky M and Hall SD (2014) Irreversible enzyme inhibition kinetics and drug-drug interactions. *Methods Mol Biol* 1113:57–91. doi:10.1007/978-1-62703-758-7_5.

23. Grimm SW, Einolf HJ, Hall SD, He K, Lim HK, Ling KH, Lu C et al. (2009) The conduct of *in vitro* studies to address time-dependent inhibition of drug-metabolizing enzymes: A perspective of the pharmaceutical research and manufacturers of America. *Drug Metab Dispos* 37:1355–1370. doi:10.1124/dmd.109.026716.

24. Obach RS (2011) Predicting clearance in humans from *in vitro* data. *Curr Top Med Chem* 11:334–339. doi:10.2174/156802611794480873.

25. Fahmi OA, Hurst S, Plowchalk D, Cook J, Guo F, Youdim K, Dickins M, Phipps A, Darekar A, Hyland R, and Obach RS (2009) Comparison of different algorithms for predicting clinical drug-drug interactions, based on the use of CYP3A4 *in vitro* data: Predictions of compounds as precipitants of interaction. *Drug Metab Dispos* 37:1658–166. doi:10.1124/dmd.108.026252.

26. Wang YH (2010) Confidence assessment of the Simcyp time-based approach and a static mathematical model in predicting clinical drug-drug interactions for mechanism-based CYP3A inhibitors. *Drug Metab Dispos* 38:1094–1104. doi:10.1124/dmd.110.032177.

27. Yan Z and Caldwell GW (2012) The current status of time dependent CYP inhibition assay and in silico drug-drug interaction predictions. *Curr Top Med Chem* 12:1291–1297. doi:10.2174/156802612800672871.

28. Nagar S, Jones JP, and Korzekwa K (2014) A numerical method for analysis of *in vitro* time-dependent inhibition data. Part 1. Theoretical considerations. *Drug Metab Dispos* 42:1575–1586. doi:10.1124/dmd.114.058289.

29. Korzekwa K, Tweedie D, Argikar UA, Whitcher-Johnstone A, Bell L, Bickford S, and Nagar S (2014) A numerical method for analysis of *in vitro* time-dependent inhibition data. Part 2. Application to experimental data. *Drug Metab Dispos* 42:1587–1595. doi:10.1124/dmd.114.058297.

30. Chun J, Kent UM, Moss RM, Sayre LM, and Hollenberg PF (2000) Mechanism-based inactivation of cytochromes P450 2B1 and P450 2B6 by 2-phenyl-2-(1-piperidinyl)propane. *Drug Metab Dispos* 28:905–911.

31. Hollenberg PF, Kent UM, and Bumpus NN (2008) Mechanism-based inactivation of human cytochromes p450s: Experimental characterization, reactive intermediates, and clinical implications. *Chem Res Toxicol* 21:189–205. doi:10.1021/tx7002504.

32. Barnaba C, Yadav J, Nagar S, Korzekwa K, and Jones JP (2016) Mechanism-based inhibition of CYP3A4 by podophyllotoxin: Aging of an intermediate is important for in *vitro/in vivo* correlations. *Mol Pharm* 13:2833–2843.

33. Hanson KL, VandenBrink BM, Babu KN, Allen KE, Nelson WL, and Kunze KL (2010) Sequential metabolism of secondary alkyl amines to metabolic-intermediate complexes: Opposing roles for the secondary hydroxylamine and primary amine metabolites of desipramine, (s)-fluoxetine, and N-desmethyldiltiazem. *Drug Metab Dispos* 38:963–972. doi:10.1124/dmd.110.032391.

34. Pang KS and Chow EC (2012) Commentary: Theoretical predictions of flow effects on intestinal and systemic availability in physiologically based pharmacokinetic intestine models: The traditional model, segregated flow model, and QGut model. *Drug Metab Dispos* 40:1869–1877. doi:10.1124/dmd.112.045872.

35. Pearson JT, Hill JJ, Swank J, Isoherranen N, Kunze KL, and Atkins WM (2006) Surface plasmon resonance analysis of antifungal azoles binding to CYP3A4 with kinetic resolution of multiple binding orientations. *Biochemistry* 45:6341–6353. doi:10.1021/bi0600042.

36. Cleland WW (1975) Partition analysis and the concept of net rate constants as tools in enzyme kinetics. *Biochemistry* 14:3220–3224. doi:10.1021/bi00685a029.

24

Active Metabolites in Drug Development

Sylvie E. Kandel and Jed N. Lampe

CONTENTS

Introduction

Many currently marketed drugs produce metabolites that are pharmacologically active, enhancing efficacy or toxicity, or exhibiting a completely different type of pharmacological profile. Aberra Fura has suggested that approximately 22% of the top 50 drugs prescribed in the US in 2003 produced metabolites that significantly affected their pharmacodynamics (PD), pharmacokinetics (PK), or both [1]. In our own assessment of the literature for the top 100 prescribed drugs reported for 2013–2014, we found that ~39% produce at least one active metabolite. Given the importance of active metabolites in drug safety and efficacy, extending the patent life of a drug or becoming drug leads in their own right, it is important to identify active metabolites early in the drug development process.

It is in this context that we wish to distinguish between the terms *active metabolite* and *prodrug*, where the former refers to a pharmacologically *active metabolic product* from an *active parent drug*, and the latter refers to an *active metabolic product* produced from an *inactive parent drug*. For simplicity, we will limit our discussion to active metabolites as defined above.

It has been known for some time that metabolites can affect the efficacy or toxicity of a parent drug [2]. However, until recently [3] there has not been concerted efforts to identify active metabolites early in the drug discovery and development process. In addition to regulatory guidance that has focused on identification of all significant human metabolites, there is a growing appreciation of how active metabolites can influence safety and efficacy through dispositional effects—i.e., distribution, pharmacokinetics, and elimination, as well as pharmacodynamics (Figure 24.1). While not all active metabolites contribute substantially to the safety or efficacy of any particular drug, their study is worthwhile in at least two additional aspects. Firstly, understanding their receptor specificity and how they elicit their effect often contributes to an understanding of the mechanism of action of the parent drug. Secondly, in situations where a parent drug may fail in late stage clinical trials, due to toxicity, PK, or other concerns, the active metabolite has the potential to serve as an effective back-up candidate.

Active metabolite identification often occurs in various phases of the drug discovery and development process. In early drug discovery, identification of active metabolites can be useful in order to identify leads with improved absorption, distribution, metabolism, excretion (ADME), and PD properties over the parent drug. In the clinical phase of the drug development cycle, identification of active metabolites with plasma half-lives longer than the parent can potentially increase the therapeutic advantage of a drug by allowing for a significant decrease in dose, thereby decreasing the risk for toxic off-target side effects. Thus, in order to have a comprehensive understanding of mechanism of action and disposition of any new drug candidate, one must first elucidate the role of potentially active metabolites.

Active metabolites can be roughly grouped into three main categories based on their pharmacological and/or toxicological properties. Category 1 represents metabolites that illicit a pharmacological response similar to the parent drug. The effect from the active metabolite may be similar, greater, or less than the parent drug, but is likely to involve the same or a closely related receptor. Category 2 are metabolites whose spectrum of pharmacological activity is entirely different than that of the parent drug. In this case, the metabolite either has opposing activity at the same receptor as the parent drug or targets an entirely different receptor. Category 3 is comprised of toxic active metabolites. This includes both reactive metabolites and metabolites that exhibit their toxicity directly.

Therefore, production of active metabolites must be considered in any new drug development program due to their potential impact on pharmacodynamics, pharmacokinetics, toxicity, and prospect as new drug leads.

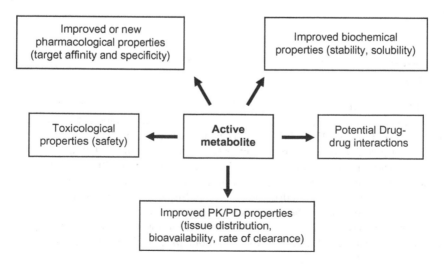

FIGURE 24.1 Importance of active metabolites in drug development.

How Are Active Metabolites Formed?

Active metabolites are formed from the typical biotransformation reactions that have been described in detail in other chapters of this volume. These include Phase I oxidation/reduction reactions and, in certain cases, Phase II conjugation reactions. Although the Phase I reactions that produce active metabolites are mediated primarily by cytochrome P450 enzymes, they can occasionally be catalyzed by non-CYP enzymes [2], such as FMOs [4–7], esterases, peroxidases, or reductases [2,8]. Examples of active metabolites formed from the top 100 prescribed drugs for 2013–2014 can be found in Table 24.1.

In order for a metabolite to become "active," the chemical change imparted to the parent drug must be such that it does not eliminate the biological activity of the drug. These modifications typically result in a change in receptor specificity or affinity. Therefore, they tend to be either minor modifications of the drug in the region of receptor binding, such as heteroatom dealkylation or oxidation, or modifications in a region of the drug that is not critical for receptor binding, but may enhance the molecule's pharmacokinetic properties. This, of course, is to be distinguished from the usual occurrence where an oxidative modification either interferes with receptor binding or leads to a significant alteration of physiochemical properties, thereby leading to decreased pharmacodynamic and/or pharmacokinetic performance.

Next, we will examine some examples of active metabolites, each chosen because they reinforce one or more of the general conclusions that can be made regarding active metabolite formation. For a more complete list of active metabolites that are formed from common drugs, the reader is directed to the excellent review by Obach [9].

Examples of Phase I Active Metabolites

Given the chemical versatility of oxidation reactions performed by cytochromes P450 and other Phase I enzymes [2,10], it is perhaps not surprising that drug oxidation can lead to the production of active metabolites. The variety of oxidative cytochrome P450 reactions reported include, but are not limited to: aliphatic and aromatic hydroxylations, epoxidations, *N*- and *O*-dealkylations, heteroatom oxidations, and even reductions [2,10]. There are examples from the literature of each type of reaction generating active metabolites from the respective parent drug. Here, we will provide a limited set of examples of drugs producing active metabolites through Phase I oxidative metabolism in order to illustrate some of the principles outlined above.

Aliphatic or Aromatic Hydroxylation

The addition of an alcohol to a drug at a position not critical for target binding may increase the metabolic stability and/or effect its intrinsic pharmacological activity. An example of this is one of the active metabolites of the selective estrogen-receptor modulator tamoxifen, 4-hydroxytamoxifen (Figure 24.2) [6,11–15]. 4-Hydroxytamoxifen is a major tamoxifen metabolite produced by CYP2D6 [14]. It has been reported to exhibit equivalent or greater potency than the parent drug and is thought to significantly contribute to the pharmacological activity of tamoxifen *in vivo* [16–18]. As confirmation of this, reduced efficacy was observed in CYP2D6 poor metabolizer patients or those taking drugs acting as CYP2D6 competitive inhibitors [19,20]. Here, confidence of assigning pharmacological activity to the metabolite was greatly increased by knowledge of the particular CYP metabolic pathway involved in tamoxifen oxidation. However, the case of tamoxifen activity is somewhat more complicated as at least one other metabolite is also responsible for its *in vivo* effect (described below).

In some instances, the active metabolite may not have a higher affinity for the target receptor, but it may still substantially contribute to the pharmacological effect due to altered PK. Such is the case with the anxiolytic agent buspirone and its active metabolite, 6-hydroxybuspirone [21,22]. Buspirone is rapidly converted to 6-hydroxybuspirone and its metabolite circulates at much higher effective concentrations, and for longer duration, than the parent compound resulting in an increased contribution to the biological activity of the drug.

Another example of hydroxyl metabolites contributing significantly to the efficacy of a drug are the active metabolites of the HMG-CoA reductase inhibitor, atorvastatin [23,24]. Atorvastatin is predominantly metabolized by CYP3A4 to form active 2-hydroxy and 4-hydroxy metabolites (Figure 24.3), in addition to

TABLE 24.1

Representative Drugs and Their Active Metabolites as Defined by Therapeutic Indication, Pharmacological Activity, Biotransformation, and Category

Drug	Therapeutic Indications	Pharmacological Activity	Biotransformation	Active Metabolite(s)	Active Metabolite Category: Potency to Parent Drug
Aripiprazole	Antipsychotic	Partial dopamine 2 and serotonin 1A receptor agonist	Dehydrogenation (P450)	Dehydroaripiprazole [160]	Cat. 1: equal potency for dopamine 2 receptor
Atomoxetine	Attention-deficit hyperactivity disorder	Norepinephrine (NRI) and serotonine (SRI) transporter inhibitor	Hydroxylation (P450)	4-Hydroxyatomoxetine [161]	Cat. 1: equal potency as NRI and greater potency as SRI
Buprenorphine	Acute and chronic pain, opioid addiction	Mixed partial agonist opioid receptor modulator	N-Dealkylation (P450) Glucuronidation (UGT)	Norbuprenorphine [162] Buprenorphine-3-glucuronide [163] Norbuprenorphine-3-glucuronide [163]	Cat. 1(/2): greater potency Cat. 1(/2): lower potency Cat. 1(/2): lower potency
Dabigatran etexilate (a dabigatran pro-drug)	Anticoagulant	Direct thrombin inhibitor	Glucuronidation (UGT) following ester hydrolysis	Dabigatran-O-acylglucuronide [164]	Cat. 1: equal potency to dabigatran
Dutasteride	Benign prostatic hyperplasia	5α-Reductase inhibitor	Hydroxylation (P450)	6-Hydroxydutasteride [165] 4'-Hydroxydutasteride [165] 1,2-Hydroxydutasteride [165]	Cat. 1: equal potency Cat. 1: lower potency Cat. 1: lower potency
Eletriptan	Migraine headaches	Serotonin receptor agonist	N-Demethylation (P450)	N-Desmethyl eletriptan [166]	Cat. 1: equal potency
Ezetemibe	Dyslipidemia	Niemann-Pick C1 like-1 inhibition	Glucuronidation (UGT)	Ezetimibe-glucuronide [167]	Cat. 1: greater potency
Febuxostat	Chronic gout and hyperuricemia	Xanthine oxidase inhibitor	Hydroxylation (P450)	Febuxostat 67M-1, 67M-2 and 67-M4 metabolites [168]	Cat. 1: equal potency
Lisdexamfetamine (a dextroamphetamine pro-drug)	Attention deficit hyperactivity disorder and binge eating disorder	Trace amine-associated receptor 1 agonist and vesicular monoamine transporter 2 inhibitor	Hydroxylation (P450 and DBH) following cleavage	4-Hydroxyamphetamine [169, 70] 4-Hydroxynorephedrine [169, 170]	Cat. 1: equal potency Cat. 1: lower potency
Lurasidone	Antipsychotic	Dopamine 2 and serotonin 2A receptor antagonist	Hydroxylation (P450)	Exo-hydroxylurasidone [171] Endo-hydroxylurasidone [171]	Cat. 1: equal potency Cat. 1: equal potency

(Continued)

TABLE 24.1 (Continued)

Representative Drugs and Their Active Metabolites as Defined by Therapeutic Indication, Pharmacological Activity, Biotransformation, and Category

Drug	Therapeutic Indications	Pharmacological Activity	Biotransformation	Active Metabolite(s)	Active Metabolite Category: Potency to Parent Drug
Mometasone furoate	Inflammation	Potent agonist of progesterone receptor	Oxidation (P450)	6β-Hydroxymometasone furoate [45] 9,11-Epoxymometasone furoate [45]	Cat 1: lower potency Cat 1: lower potency (chemically reactive)
Nebivolol	Hypertension	Vasodilatory β₁-adrenoreceptor antagonist	Hydroxylation (P450)	4-Hydroxynebivolol [172,173]	Cat 1: equal potency
Norethindrone acetate (a norethindrone pro-drug)	Hormonal contraceptive	Progestogen	Reduction (5α-steroid reductase) following hydrolysis	5α-Dehydronorethindrone [174,175]	Cat 2: - Anti-progestational/contragestational effect - Not aromatizable; a potential aromatase inhibitor for breast cancer
Oxycodone	Severe and acute pain	μ-Opioid receptor agonist	N-Demethylation (P450) O-Demethylation (P450) N- and O-demethylation (P450)	Noroxycodone [176] Oxymorphone [176] Noroxymorphone [176]	Cat 1: lower potency Cat 1: higher potency Cat 1: higher potency
Quetiapine fumarate	Antipsychotic	Dopamine, serotonin and adrenergic receptor antagonist	N-Dealkylation (P450)	N-Desalkyl quetiapine [177,178]	Cat 1: greater potency (activity mediator)
Ritonavir	HIV/AIDS treatment	HIV-1 protease inhibitor (use in combinatorial therapy)	Hydroxylation (P450)	Ritonavir M2 metabolite (isopropylthiazole hydroxylation) [179]	Cat 1: equal potency
Rivastigmine	Mild/moderate dementia	Carbamate-type inhibitor of acetylcholinesterase	Esterase hydrolysis	NAP 226-90 [180]	Cat 1: lower potency
Rosuvastatin	Dyslipidemia	3-Hydroxy-3-ethylglutaryl coenzyme A (HMG-CoA) reductase inhibitor	N-Demethylation (P450)	N-Desmethyl rosuvastatin [181]	Cat 1: lower potency

(Continued)

TABLE 24.1 (*Continued*)

Representative Drugs and Their Active Metabolites as Defined by Therapeutic Indication, Pharmacological Activity, Biotransformation, and Category

Drug	Therapeutic Indications	Pharmacological Activity	Biotransformation	Active Metabolite(s)	Active Metabolite Category: Potency to Parent Drug
Saxagliptin	Type 2 diabete	Dipeptidyl peptidase-4 inhibitor	Hydroxylation (P450)	5-Hydroxysaxagliptin [182,187]	Cat 1: lower potency
Sildenafil	Erectile dysfunction and pulmonary arterial hypertension	cGMP-specific phosphodiesterase type 5 inhibitor	N-Demethylation (P450)	N-Desmethyl sildenafil (UK-1C3 320) [184,185]	Cat 1: lower potency
Simvastatin	Dyslipidemia	3-Hydroxy-3-ethylglutaryl coenzyme A (HMG-CoA) reductase inhibitor	Hydroxylation (P450) with hydrolysis to the β-hydroxy acid form	6′-Hydroxysimvastatin hydroxy acid [186]	Cat 1: lower potency
Solifenacin	Overactive bladder	Cholinergic receptor antagonist	Hydroxylation (P450)	4R-Hydroxysolifenacin [187]	Cat 1: lower potency

Source: Valotis, A., and Hogger, P., *Respir. Res.*, 5, 7, 2004; Huang, P. et al., *J. Pharmacol. Exp. Ther.*, 297, 688–695, 2001; Sauer, J.M. et al., *Clin. Pharmacokinet.*, 44, 571–590, 2005; Molden, E. et al., *Ther. Drug. Monit.*, 28, 744–749, 2006; Lalovic, B. et al., *Clin. Pharmacol. Ther.*, 79, 461–479, 2006; Briciu, C. et al., *Clujul. Med.*, 88, 208–213, 2015; Prisant, L.M., *J. Clin. Pharmacol.*, 48, 225–239, 2008; Caccia, S. et al., *Neuropsychiatr. Dis. Treat.*, 8, 155–168, 2012; Wenger, G.R., and Rutledge, C.O., *J. Pharmacol. Exp. Ther.*, 189, 725–732, 1974; Hutson, P.H. et al., *Neuropharmacology*, 87, 41–50, 2014; Love, B.L. et al., *Pharmacotherapy*, 30, 594–608, 2010; Hawes, B.E. et al., *Mol. Pharmacol.*, 71, 19–29, 2007; Evans, D.C. et al., *Drug Metab. Dispos.*, 31, 861–869, 2003; Wu, C., and Kapoor, A., *Expert Opin. Pharmacother.*, 14, 1399–1408, 2013; Ebner, T. et al., *Drug Metab. Dispos.*, 38, 1567–1575, 2010; Kennedy, J.S. et al., *J. Clin. Psychopharmacol.*, 19, 513–521, 1999; Denissen, J.F. et al., *Drug Metab. Dispos.*, 25, 489–501, 1997; Brown, S.M. et al., *Anesthesiology*, 115, 1251–1260; Bakken, G.V. et al., *Drug Metab. Dispos.*, 40, 1778–1784, 2012; Jensen, N.H. et al., *Neuropsychopharmacology*, 33, 2303–2312, 2008; Yamamoto, T. et al., *Eur. J. Endocrinol.*, 130, 634–640, 1994; Perez-Palacios, G. et al., *J. Steroid Biochem. Mol. Biol.*, 41, 479–485, 1992; Doroshyenko, O., and Fuhr, U., *Clin Pharmacokinet.*, 48, 281–302, 2009; Vickers, S. et al., *Drug Metab. Dispos.*, 18, 138–145, 1990; Hyland, R. et al., *Br. J. Clin. Pharmacol.*, 51, 239–248, 2001. Walker, D.K. et al., *Xenobiotica*, 29, 297–310, 1999; Su, H. et al., *Drug Metab. Dispos.*, 40, 1345–1356, 2012; Fura, A. et al., *Drug Metab. Dispos.*, 37, 1164–1171, 2009; Olsson, A.G. et al., *Cardiovasc. Drug. Rev.*, 20, 303–328, 2002.

Note: See main chapter text for definition of the individual categories.

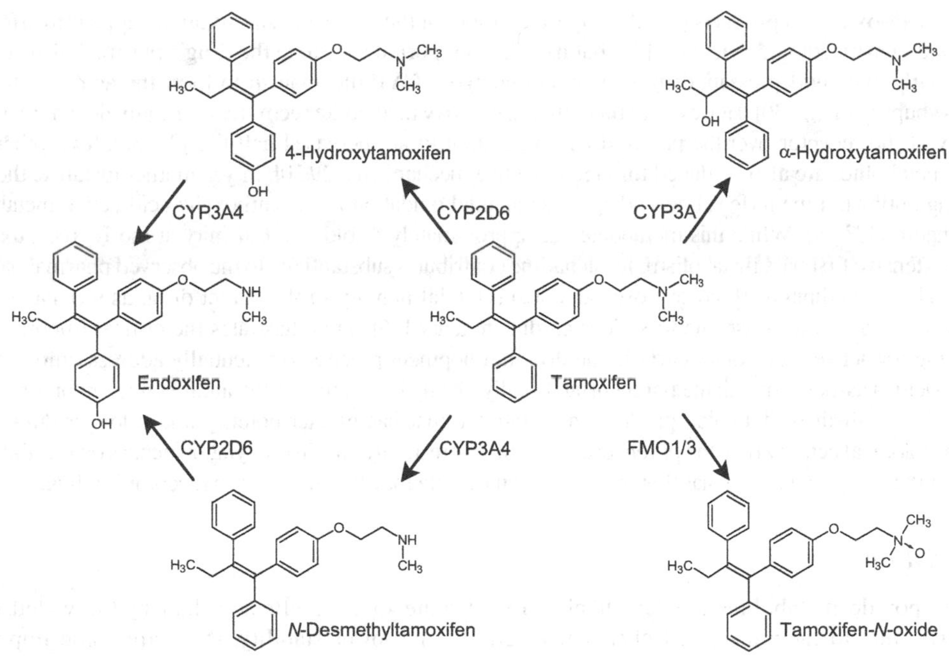

FIGURE 24.2 Tamoxifen and its active metabolites.

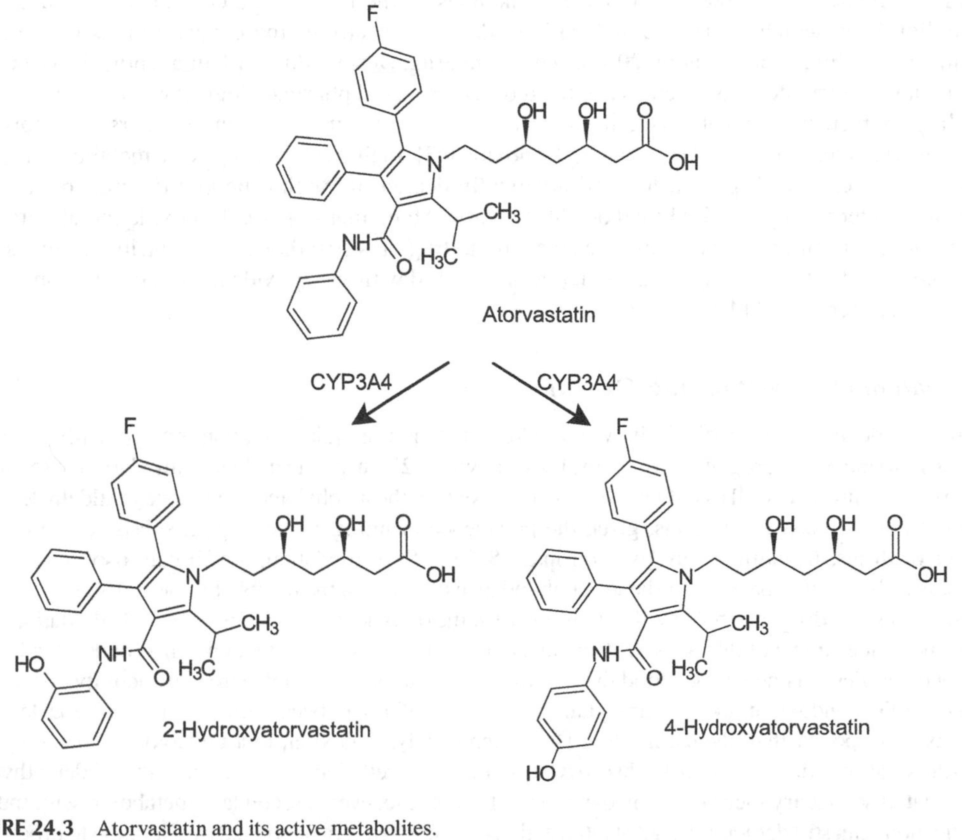

FIGURE 24.3 Atorvastatin and its active metabolites.

several beta-oxidation products [25–27]. Hydroxylations at the 2 and 4 positions do not appear to effect the observed pharmacological activity [27] but have been reported to extend the drug's plasma half-life [28].

Similarly, the antidepressant drug bupropion undergoes CYP metabolism to form the active metabolite hydroxybupropion [29,30]. However, in this case the hydroxy metabolite seems to have equivalent or increased activity at the receptor over the parent drug, in addition to an increased half-life [30–32]. Two other, less active metabolites are also produced through reductive mechanisms [29,30]. In yet another instance, the non-sedating antihistamine terfenadine undergoes sequential oxidation to the carboxylic acid active metabolite, fexofenadine [33,34]. While this metabolite has approximately 4-fold lower affinity at the H_1 receptor [35], due to extensive first pass metabolism, fexofenadine contributes substantially to the observed pharmacological effect. This serendipitous discovery overcame a substantial liability of the parent drug, as terfenadine was withdrawn from clinical use due to serious cardiac toxicity [36]. This illustrates the critical importance of screening for active metabolites early in the drug development process to potentially address unforeseen *in vivo* toxicities associated with the parent drug. Finally, the hydroxylation of the androgen receptor antagonist flutamide to 2-hydroxyflutamide produces a metabolite that has greater potency and a longer duration of pharmacological activity than the parent drug [37,38]. Interestingly, this hydroxylation occurs on the alkyl side chain of the drug, suggesting that this region of the molecule may be important in receptor binding.

Epoxidation

While epoxide metabolites are less likely to contribute to drug efficacy than hydroxylated ones, primarily due to their increased chemical reactivity and lower stability, there are some important examples of epoxides as active metabolites [39]. Probably the most well-known is the epoxide formed from carbamazepine, carbamazepine-10,11-epoxide [40]. Carbamazepine, a drug used clinically to treat epileptic seizures since the late 1950s, is oxidized by CYP3A isoforms to produce the carbamazepine-10,11-epoxide [40]. While the epoxide metabolite has comparable affinity for the intended receptor, the voltage gated sodium channels in the brain, it quickly undergoes hydrolysis to the diol form, which is inactive [41]. This leads to lower circulating concentrations of the active epoxide metabolite, approximately 20% of the parent drug. Despite this, carbamazepine-10,11-epoxide is thought to contribute to as much as one third of the observed pharmacological response *in vivo* [42]. The drug mometasone furoate, used in the treatment of inflammatory skin disorders, also forms an active epoxide metabolite, mometasone-9,11-epoxide [43]. In this case, the epoxide metabolite is a very short-lived species, with plasma levels dramatically decreasing with time and the metabolite being difficult to detect using standard methods [44]. While the mometasone-9,11-epoxide metabolite has a somewhat lower affinity to the receptor as the parent drug, it is still thought to contribute significantly to the biological activity of the drug. Toxicities associated with the epoxide metabolite of mometasone have not been reported [44,45].

Heteroatom Dealkylation and Oxidation

Heteroatom dealkylation, particularly *N*- and *O*-dealkylation, is quite common, energetically favorable, reactions carried out on drugs by cytochrome P450 enzymes [2]. These can include dealkylation of secondary and tertiary amines, as well as C-O bond cleavage to obtain the alcohol and the ketone or aldehyde. These are an important class of reactions, given the prevalence of nitrogen and oxygen substituents in a large number of drugs, including many psychotropics. Sulfur (*S*)-dealkylation, which can also occur, is less commonly observed in part due to the lower abundance of sulfur substituents present in drugs.

In most cases, a drug metabolite will retain at least some of its activity after an *N*- or *O*-dealkylation event. One important example of this is the *N*-demethylated metabolite of tamoxifen, known as endoxifen [15]. As mentioned earlier, it is now understood that the majority of tamoxifen's antiestrogenic activity comes from the metabolites endoxifen and 4-hydroxytamoxifen. Endoxifen has been demonstrated to be at least 100 times as more potent than the parent drug [16]. Interestingly, tamoxifen first undergoes *N*-demethylation (or hydroxylation), then followed by hydroxylation (or *N*-demethylation) to produce the *N*-demethylated, hydroxylated secondary metabolite, endoxifen [18]. In this case, even a secondary metabolite with multiple modifications can still demonstrate substantial activity. Tamoxifen is metabolized by CYP2D6 to produce the

4-hydroxy metabolite (see above), whereas CYP3A4 is thought to be responsible for producing the observed *N*-demethylation event (Figure 24.2). Therefore, the circulating levels of endoxifen can be considerably impacted by CYP2D6 polymorphisms. Indeed, it has been observed that CYP2D6 poor metabolizers have worse clinical outcomes in response to tamoxifen therapy than do CYP2D6 extensive metabolizers [46].

In the case of the analgesic codeine, *O*-demethylation, performed primarily by CYP2D6, produces morphine (Figure 24.4) [47,48]. Morphine has a 600-fold higher affinity for the μ-opioid receptor

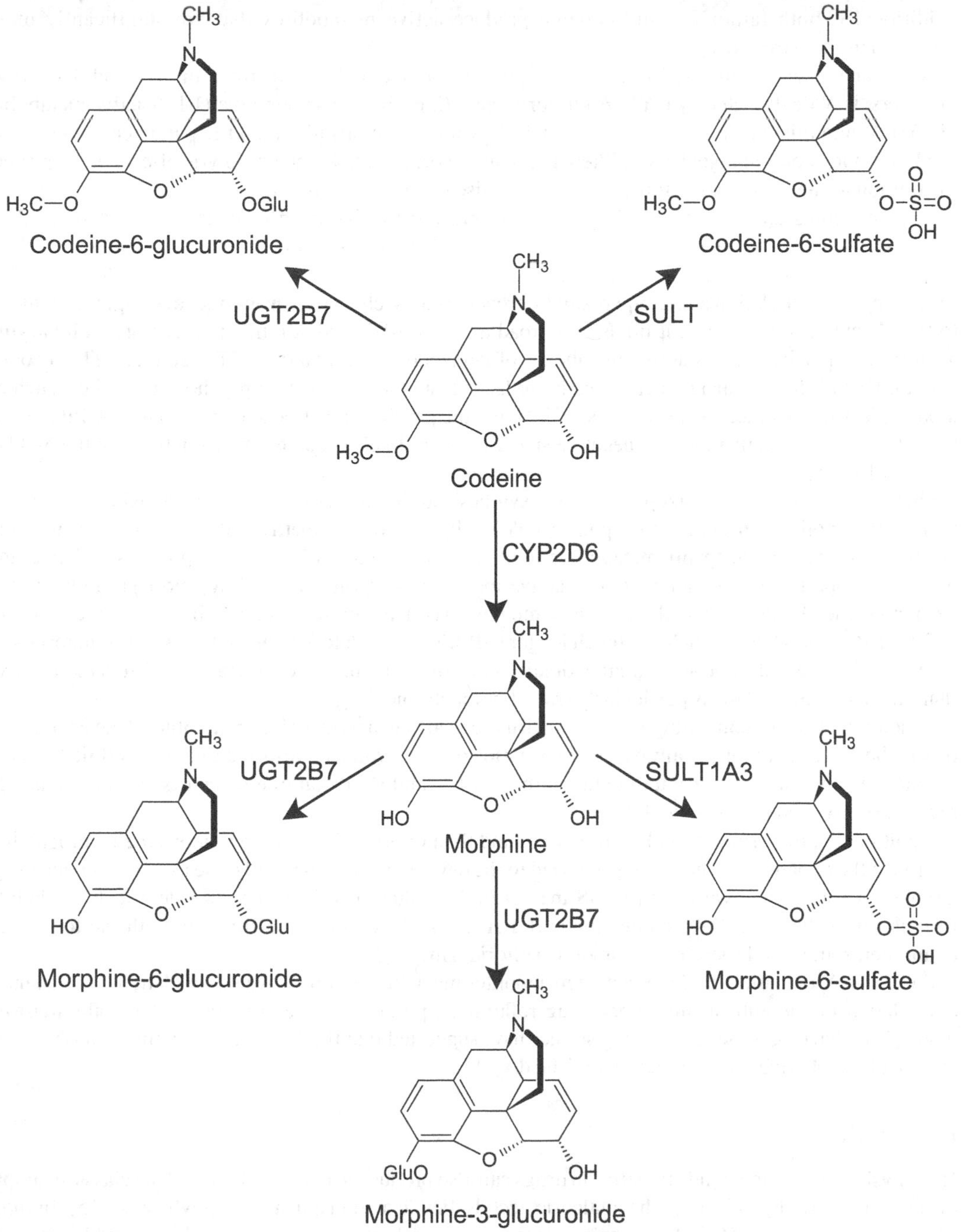

FIGURE 24.4 Metabolism of codeine to morphine and its active metabolites.

than codeine [49–51]. Additionally, the metabolite exhibits a longer half-life than the parent drug, contributing to a 40-fold greater total exposure level [52]. However, N-demethylation to norcodeine produces an inactive metabolite. Since activation of the drug is also CYP2D6 dependent, there is a large degree of interindividual variability in the analgesic response. This discrepancy has led to tragic consequences, such as the case of a new mother who was an ultra-rapid CYP2D6 metabolizer and had been prescribed a standard dose of codeine [53]. Morphine quickly accumulated in her breast milk and caused the overdose of her newborn infant. This again underscores the fact that CYP genotype can have a significant impact on the type and amount of active metabolite produced. Additionally, both tamoxifen and codeine produce active metabolites that are significantly more potent than the parent drug.

Buspirone, a serotonin 5-HT type 1A receptor partial agonist used to treat anxiety and depressive disorders, is N-dealkylated by CYP3A4 to form the 1-(2-pyrimidyl)-piperazine (1-PP) active metabolite [54,55]. While this metabolite binds to the 5-HT$_{1A}$ with a lower affinity than the parent compound, it is a α2-adrenoreceptor antagonist and likely plays an important role in the anxiolytic effects of buspirone, in addition to the 6-hydroxybuspirone metabolite discussed above [56–58].

The antidepressant serotonin 5-HT$_{2A}$ receptor antagonist nefazodone is extensively metabolized by CYP3A4 to the metabolites hydroxynefazodone, triazoledione, and m-chlorophenylpiperazine (mCPP) [59,60]. While hydroxynefazodone and triazoledione display similar activity to nefazodone, m-CPP, formed by N-dealkylation at the piperazinyl nitrogen, is a psychoactive drug in its own right. Belonging to the phenylpiperazine class, it binds to a broad array of 5-HT and adrenergic receptors with varying affinities. In particular, this active metabolite of nefazodone is a potent 5-HT$_{1A}$ and a 5-HT$_{2C}$ agonist [61,62]. Due to these disparate activities, it produces a number of negative psychotropic effects such as anxiety, loss of appetite, and headaches [63]. While the psychedelic effects attributed to m-CPP are due to 5-HT$_{2A}$ receptor activation, the negative side effects are likely mediated by its actions on the 5-HT$_{2C}$ receptor [64,65].

One of the first benzodiazepines to be synthesized in the 1950s, chlordiazepoxide, undergoes N-demethylation to produce the pharmacologically active desmethyl (desmethyldiazepam) and desmethylhydroxy (oxazepam) metabolites [66,67]. Indeed, much of chlordiazepoxide's sedative and hypnotic properties can be attributed to active metabolites of the parent drug, most prominently the desmethyl metabolite. While the parent compound has a medium to long half-life (on the order of 5–30 hr), desmethyldiazepam has a much longer half-life, from 36 to 200 hr [68]. It is again important to note here that multiple, and sequential, oxidations of a drug can produce a metabolite that is more active than the parent drug. This is particularly true of psychotropic drugs.

Oxidation of sulfur containing moieties in drugs can also generate active metabolites. One example of this is the S-oxidation of the antipsychotic, thioridazine, to produce mesoridazine [69]. While both the parent drug and the active metabolite target the D2, D3, and D4 dopamine receptors, mesoridazine has higher affinity than thioridazine [68,70].

Additionally, mesoridazine is less protein bound than thioridazine, thereby increasing its probability to bind at the dopamine receptor [71]. This led to the development of mesoridazine as a stand-alone drug, although it was withdrawn from the US market in 2004 due to serious cardiac side effects, including irregular heart beat and QT-prolongation [72]. Further oxidation of the sulfur atom to the sulfone leads to another, somewhat less active metabolite, sulforidazine [73].

Similarly, N-oxidation produces active metabolites much in the same way as S-oxidation. For instance, N-oxidation of the anti-inflammatory drug roflumilast produces the active metabolite roflumilast-N-oxide [74]. Pharmacokinetic modeling studies have suggested that the N-oxide metabolite contributes up to 93% of the pharmacological activity of the drug [9].

Hydrolysis

Hydrolysis of esters and amide moieties in drugs can also produce active metabolites. One classic example of this is the ester hydrolysis of the analgesic acetylsalicylic acid (aspirin) to salicylic acid [75]. In most individuals, more than 50% of the aspirin dose is converted into salicylic acid, which provides most of the pharmacological effect observed with this drug. Another example is the hydrolysis of cefotaxime, which generates the active metabolite desacetyl cefotaxime. This is the major metabolite, accounting for 15%–25% of the administered dose of the parent drug and is thought to provide a significant contribution to the drug's activity [76]. Esterification, in fact, has been a primary method to convert an existing drug into a prodrug to alter its PK or toxicity profile.

Reduction

While reduction can be cytochrome P450-mediated, it is more commonly performed by reductases. For example, the electron transfer partner of cytochrome P450 enzymes, cytochrome P450 reductase (CPR) is responsible for reduction of a number of drugs and plays a role in active metabolite formation for several of them. One such instance is acetoheximide, where the carbonyl is reduced to a hydroxyl group [77]. The resulting metabolite, hydroxyhexamide, has been demonstrated to decrease plasma glucose and increase circulating insulin levels in rats. Interestingly, both the (*R*) and (*S*) enantiomers of the metabolite were found to be biologically active. Cytochrome P450 reductase is also known to reductively activate several antineoplastic agents, such as anthracycline antibiotic adriamycin [78]. Similarly, CPR reduces mitomycin C to produce the active metabolite that is responsible for DNA alkylation [79]. The antipsychotic agent haloperidol, used in the treatment of schizophrenia, also undergoes a reversible reduction mediated by CPR to form an active metabolite [80]. While this metabolite is less active than the parent compound, it demonstrates increased stability and may be responsible for the long terminal half-life of the drug *in vivo*. In the case of dolasetron, a serotonin receptor antagonist, reduction of the carbonyl on the parent drug produces the active metabolite hydrodolasetron, which is thought to be responsible for the majority of the antiemetic activity of the drug [81]. Dolasetron is substantially metabolized *in vivo* to produce the alcohol metabolite leading to higher circulating concentrations of the metabolite over the parent drug. This, in conjunction with the fact that the metabolite has between 20- and 60-fold greater affinity for the serotonin receptor than the parent compound [82], supports the conclusion that the entire *in vivo* efficacy of the drug is due to production of the hydrodolasetron metabolite. The antidepressant and smoking cessation adjuvant bupropion produces several active metabolites, including the reduced form of the drug, dihydrobupropion [83]. While it's unclear how much of the observed pharmacological effect is directly due to dihydrobupropion versus the parent drug, in part because the mechanism of action has yet to be completely elucidated, its reported circulating concentration is in the micromolar range suggesting that it may make a substantial contribution [84].

Other reductases are also responsible for producing active metabolites, such as the activation of idarubicin to idarubicinol by aldo-keto reductase [85]. Idarubicinol has been previously determined to be equipotent to the parent drug, idarubicin. Also, glutathione reductase is thought to catalyze the reduction of the anti-alcoholic drug disulfiram to the active metabolite diethyldithio carbamate [86,87].

Phase II Active Metabolites

In addition to oxidation, dealkylation, and reduction, active metabolites can also be generated through Phase II conjugation reactions. While this is a less common pathway for active metabolite production, it is important for a number of drugs from different classes. In most circumstances, conjugation of a drug at a site of receptor interaction has the effect of diminishing or blocking the interaction entirely. However, in some cases it can enhance the interaction and prolong the circulating half-life of the drug. Also, depending on the stability of the conjugate, the original parent drug species may be regenerated through enterohepatic cycling, providing another pathway for extending the effects of the parent compound.

Glucuronidation

After oxidation, glucuronidation is second most common metabolic fate for a drug. Glucuronidation is an enzymatic process mediated by UDP-glucuronosyltransferases (UGTs) that conjugates a glucuronide moiety to an O or N and, occasionally, S heteroatom functional group. This often occurs after the parent drug has undergone oxidation, as discussed above, and generally produces a more hydrophilic species that is more readily excreted. However, the more hydrophobic drug conjugates that are excreted into the bile are susceptible to hydrolysis by β-glucuronidase enzymes present in the intestine. The hydrolyzed drug may then be reabsorbed into the intestine, leading to enterohepatic cycling [88].

Perhaps the most famous example of an active glucuronide drug conjugate is the glucuronidation of the opiate analgesic morphine to produce morphine-6-glucuronide (M6G) via the enzyme UGT2B7 (Figure 24.4) [89,90]. While almost 10% of the given dose is converted into this Phase II conjugate, its circulating concentration is estimated to be equivalent to the parent drug primarily due to its longer half-life [91]. In *in vitro* receptor activation studies, the M6G conjugate demonstrated equivalent potency in activating the μ–opioid receptor when compared with the parent drug [92]. Interestingly, there is some data to suggest that the M6G conjugate is more likely to enter the brain due to a conformational switch that increases the lipophilicity while reducing hydration, which may account for some of its activity [93]. However, the possible involvement of a specific transporter cannot be ruled out, as this has proven to be a convenient way for glucuronide conjugates to enter cells.

An additional example of an active glucuronide metabolite is the *O*-glucuronide conjugate of the anticoagulant factor Xa inhibitor, darexaban. Darexaban-*O*-glucuronide is a major pharmacologically active metabolite that is present in plasma after oral administration of darexaban [94–96]. Previous studies have implicated UGT1A9 as the predominant isoform involved in the production of darexaban-*O*-glucuronide, suggesting that mutant alleles in this particular gene may be partially responsible for different clinical responses observed with the drug [94].

Sulfation

Another Phase II modification, that of the addition of a sulfate group mediated by sulfotransferases, can also result in the production of active metabolites. Sulfotransferases are a class of conjugation enzymes that utilize the co-factor 3′-phosphoadenosine-5′-phosphosulfate (PAPS) to attach a sulfate group to either an alcohol or amine functional group on the drug of interest [97]. These functional groups are either generated or exposed by Phase I oxidative enzymes, such as the cytochrome P450 family. As in the case of glucuronidation, sulfation typically abolishes the pharmacological activity of a drug. However, it has been known for some time that sulfation is an important step in the bioactivation of certain procarcinogens, such as aromatic amines and benzylic alcohols. Additionally, there is significant inter-individual genetic variability associated with sulfotranferase expression and function, leading to variation in enzymatic activity. In addition to producing active glucuronide metabolites, both morphine and codeine undergo sulfation at the C6 position to produce active metabolites [98,99]. For its part, morphine-6-sulfate has been found to be a 30-fold more potent analgesic than morphine at the μ–opiate receptors following intracerebroventricular administration [98,100]. Codeine-6-sulfate also has analgesic activity, but it is only 1/10th as potent as the parent compound. Additionally, it has the ability to induce seizures in a rodent model when given at doses below full analgesic activity, limiting its utility as a potential drug candidate [98]. Therefore, while morphine-6-sulfate has potent analgesic properties similar to the morpine-6-glucuronide conjugate, codeine-6-sulfate is unlikely to be therapeutically useful due to its toxicity component.

The antihypertensive vasodilator and hair growth agent minoxidil is also modified by sulfotransferases to produce the active metabolite minoxidil sulfate [101]. Minoxidil sulfate is produced mainly by SULT1A1 and is thought to be responsible for most of the pharmacological activity associated with the drug [101]. In regard to the promotion of hair growth, the principle indication for current use of the drug, a number of studies have shown that the amount of sulfotransferase activity in treated hair follicles can accurately predict the hair growth response, demonstrating the importance of the sulfated metabolite [102,103].

Acetylation

Acetylation is a common metabolic mechanism for the elimination of drugs and other xenobiotics, particularly those containing primary amines. This includes primary aromatic amines, hydrazines, hydrazides, sulfonamides, and primary aliphatic amines. This reaction involves the transfer of the acetyl group from acetyl-CoA to the parent drug or Phase I drug metabolite by hepatic *N*-acetyltransferases

(NATs). Again, as seen with glucuronidation and with glutathionylation (below), this reaction typically terminates the biological activity of the drug under most circumstances, with a few exceptions. One of these is the antiarrhythmic drug procainamide, which undergoes acetylation to produce *N*-acetylprocainamide [104]. The circulating half-life of *N*-acetylprocainamide is significantly longer than procainamide (upwards of 15 hr), and it is substantially less protein bound than the parent drug. Since NATs are known to exhibit a high degree of genetic variation, studies have been conducted to understand what role this plays in the pharmacological response to the drug [105]. The results of one such study indicated that the NAT2* (fast acetylator) genotype was more positively correlated with clinical drug response than other NAT genotypes occurring in the population examined.

Glutathionylation

Glutathionylation, or attachment of the tri-peptide glutathione (GSH) to a drug substrate, is often mediated by glutathione-*S*-transferase (GST) enzymes [106]. Given that this is such a significant modification of the parent drug, often leading to changes in the compound's electrostatics and sterics, it rarely gives rise to active metabolites. An exception to this is the GSH-conjugated metabolite of the antiplatelet aggregator $P2Y_{12}$ antagonist, clopidogrel. Clopidogrel is bioactivated to its pharmacologically active metabolite initially by hepatic cytochrome P450 enzymes, predominantly CYP2C19 through two sequential oxidation steps [107–110]. In the first step, clopidogrel is mono-oxygenated to yield 2-oxo-clopidogrel, which is pharmacologically inactive. In the second step, 2-oxo-clopidogrel is further oxidized to yield an unstable sulfenic acid intermediate. Reduction of the sulfenic acid by GSH leads to opening of the thiolactone ring to yield a glutathione conjugate. While it is not currently known if this GSH conjugate is active in itself, it provides the substrate for a thiol-disulfide exchange to occur to produce the penultimate active metabolite that then forms a disulfide bridge with the platelet $P2Y_{12}$ ADP receptor.

On occasion, GSH adduction can lead to a decomposition of the parent drug to produce an active metabolite. An example of this occurs with the immunosuppressive agent, azathioprine. Azathioprine is glutathionylated by hepatic GST enzymes to produce 1-methyl-4-nitro-5-(*N*-acetyl-*S*-cysteinyl)imidazole adduct and 6-mercaptopurine [111,112]. Classic studies by Elion's lab and others demonstrated that the majority of the immunosuppressive activity of azathioprine was indeed due to the 6-mercaptopurine metabolite [113–115].

Sub-Classes of Active Metabolites

Drugs That Form Multiple Active Metabolites Contributing to the Pharmacological Effect (Category 1)

As noted above, there are many cases in which a drug will produce multiple active metabolites. This is especially true for drugs that have high affinity for their particular receptor(s) and undergo extensive Phase I metabolism. Tamoxifen is a case in point, where at least three metabolites are known to contribute to the pharmacological effect. These include 4-hydroxytamoxifen, *N*-desmethyltamoxifen, and endoxifen (Figure 24.2). While their individual receptor affinities may vary greatly, from 500 nM for *N*-desmethyltamoxifen to 3 nM for 4-hydroxytamoxifen and endoxifen, together they are responsible for the majority of the pharmacological activity associated with the drug. As Obach points out [9], it is interesting to note that tamoxifen had been in clinical use for a number of years before it was discovered that much of its biological activity was due to active metabolites. This underscores the need for identification of all active, or potentially active, metabolites for a particular drug early in the development process.

Another example of a drug that forms multiple active metabolites responsible for much of the observed pharmacological activity is codeine (Figure 24.4). As in the case with tamoxifen, through metabolism of the parent drug (to morphine) and further metabolism of the active metabolite (to morphine-6-glucuronide), a more potent and longer lasting effect is observed than would otherwise be achieved with the parent compound alone [116,117]. This is particularly interesting, and unusual, in that the observed effects are due to both Phase I and Phase II metabolites.

In the case of the benzodiazepine sedative chlordiazepoxide, at least four different metabolites are thought to contribute to its activity at the benzodiazepine receptor, including: norchlordiazepoxide, demoxepam, desmethyldiazepam, and oxazepam [68]. In particular, the half-life of desmethyldiazepam has been determined to be between 36 and 200 hr dramatically extending the action of the drug [118]. The half-life of the parent drug has been reported to significantly increase in the elderly, which may suggest altered metabolism in this population and/or decreased efficiency in clearing the active metabolites [119].

As noted earlier, another psychotropic drug, the antipsychotic thioridazine produces at least two known metabolites that are pharmacologically active, mesoridazine and sulforidazine. As with the examples noted above, these metabolites have greater affinity for the target receptor than the parent drug [120]. In contrast to the others, these metabolites are unique in that the oxidation occurs on the sulfur atom, which leads to decreased protein binding and greater bioavailability

The phenomenon of multiple active metabolites being produced from a single parent drug seems to occur more often with psychotropic agents than with other drug classes. This may have more to do with the nature of the types of receptors and their interaction with a particular drug than the actual drugs themselves. Additionally, due to the fact that many of the drugs in this class are cytochrome P450 CYP2D6 substrates, the effect of genetic polymorphisms in certain individuals can be an important determinant of efficacy.

Drugs That Form Metabolites with Pharmacological Activity Significantly Different from the Parent Drug (Category 2)

Under certain circumstances, active metabolites may take on an altered activity profile when compared with the parent drug. This occurs with clomipramine, a tricyclic antidepressant used clinically for over fifty years. Oxidation of clomipramine produces three hydroxylated active metabolites: 8-hydroxyclomipramine, norclomipramine, and 8-hydroxynorclomipramine. While clomipramine and 8-hydroxyclomipramine are potent serotonin reuptake inhibitors, norclomipramine and 8-hydroxynorclomipramine are more effective at inhibiting uptake at the norepinephrine receptor [121–123]. A similar pattern occurs with another tricyclic antidepressant, amitriptyline, which is *N*-demethylated to produce nortriptyline, which has been approved as a drug in its own right, and then further metabolized to 10-hydroxynortriptyline. Studies have demonstrated that while amitriptyline is more active at the serotonin transporter than the norepinephrine transporter, both nortriptyline and 10-hydroxynortriptyline are more active at the norepinephrine transporter than the serotonin transporter [124]. Since the highly polymorphic CYP2D6 enzyme is primarily responsible for metabolism of both amitriptyline and nortriptyline, inter-individual genetic variability can impact the clinical response.

In the case of the angiotensin II receptor antagonist losartan, the cytochrome P450 isoforms CYP3A4 and CYP2C9 oxidize the parent drug to produce an aldehyde metabolite that has angiotensin II receptor-independent anti-inflammatory and anti-aggregatory properties [125]. Additionally, losartan can be further metabolized to produce the 5-carboxylic acid metabolite, designated as EXP3174. Approximately 14% of the oral dose is transformed into this metabolite, which exhibits a long half-life, 6–8 hr, and functions as a noncompetitive antagonist at the AT_1 receptor, contributing to some of the pharmacological effects observed with losartan. EXP3174 has been shown to be 10–40 times more potent in blocking AT_1 receptors than losartan itself [125].

Drugs That Form Toxic Metabolites (Category 3)

Generation of active metabolites may not always lead to a beneficial pharmacological effect. In some cases, the metabolites themselves may be toxic. One of the oldest and best known examples of this is generation of the reactive metabolite *N*-acetyl-*p*-benzoquinone imine (NAPQI) from the analgesic acetaminophen [126–128]. Under normal conditions, acetaminophen is metabolized to produce the glucuronide conjugate, ~55% of total, (as catalyzed by UGT1A1 and UGT1A6), the sulfate conjugate, ~25% (as catalyzed by SULT1A1), and the reactive NAPQI (~15%; produced predominantly by CYP2E1) [126]. Under normal circumstances, the electrophilic NAPQI reacts with excess cellular glutathione and is detoxified in this fashion. However, under conditions when the glucuronide and sulfate conjugation systems are overwhelmed, as occurs in the case of a clinical overdose, cellular glutathione is depleted and toxicity results from formation of protein adducts with the NAPQI conjugate and increased oxidative stress [129]. This, in turn, can lead to cellular necrosis and hepatotoxicity. The bioactivation of acetaminophen is a prototypical example of metabolic activation of a drug to a reactive species. Furthermore, the metabolism of drugs to reactive intermediates, followed by covalent binding to cellular components, is generally considered to be the basis for many of the idiosyncratic toxicities caused by some drugs [130,131]. Examples of this are numerous and beyond the scope of this chapter, but many excellent reviews exist on the subject [132–134].

Establishing the Presence of an Active Metabolite

Over the past thirty years, metabolic profiling and identification have been accelerated to the forefront of the drug development process [135]. This is due, at least in part, for the need to select the most relevant animal model that recapitulates human drug metabolite exposure. It also provides an opportunity to identify and characterize active metabolites early in drug development and before a final candidate molecule is selected [136].

In any active metabolite identification program, there are several questions that first need to be addressed before accessing the overall impact of the active metabolite on the drug development process. Is the active metabolite a major metabolite? In many cases, it may not be. This may pose a particular challenge for bioanalytical identification and production scale-up for further testing.

Understanding the metabolic disposition, PK, and toxicity of metabolites can simultaneously help limit the liability of prospective drug candidates and provide an opportunity for structure guided lead discovery and optimization. This is now a recommended part of any new drug development program [3].

Despite the difficulties involved in identification of active metabolites, there are certain unique structural and functional characteristics generally shared by most active metabolites that may aid in their identification. Firstly, in most cases the active metabolite bears a large structural similarity to the parent drug compound. Secondly, compounds that are extensively metabolized by Phase I enzymes are more likely to generate active metabolites that those that primarily undergo Phase II metabolism, as noted above. An exception to this is when oxidation occurs on a functional group that is important for the drug's structure-activity relationship. In these cases, it is unlikely that an active metabolite will be formed (at least one with similar activity to the parent drug).

In addition to their identification, due to their importance as potential drug leads or toxicants, active metabolites need to be identified and characterized as to their intrinsic potency, bioavailability, pharmacokinetics, distribution, and clearance. These fundamental physiochemical properties may differ dramatically from the parent drug. Many times this may pose a challenge, due to the limited amount of metabolite formed, its inherent instability, or the difficulty involved in synthesizing it.

Experimental clues from pre-clinical and phase I clinical studies can be useful in indicating the presence of an active metabolite (Figure 24.5) [1]. Once all of the metabolites of a particular drug have been identified, a good knowledge of the SAR combined with a substantial amount of chemical and biological intuition, can be instrumental in identifying putative active metabolites even before animal studies have begun. As noted above, many active metabolites structurally resemble the parent drug, so these types of metabolites would be the first under consideration in trying to identify an active metabolite.

After animal studies have begun, much more data can be brought to bear to identify active metabolites of the drug being examined. Often, a pharmacological response significantly greater than predicted by PK modeling or *in vitro* bioassay data may suggest the involvement of an active metabolite. This is perhaps particularly notable when testing an analog series where only one compound is producing an active metabolite. Similarly, if a drug that has been predicted to have a short half-life tends to exhibit a sustained effect *in vivo*, it also may suggest the involvement of an active metabolite. As mentioned above, drugs that are extensively metabolized by Phase I enzymes are more likely to produce active metabolites than those that are metabolized via other pathways. For a sub-set of these drugs that experience

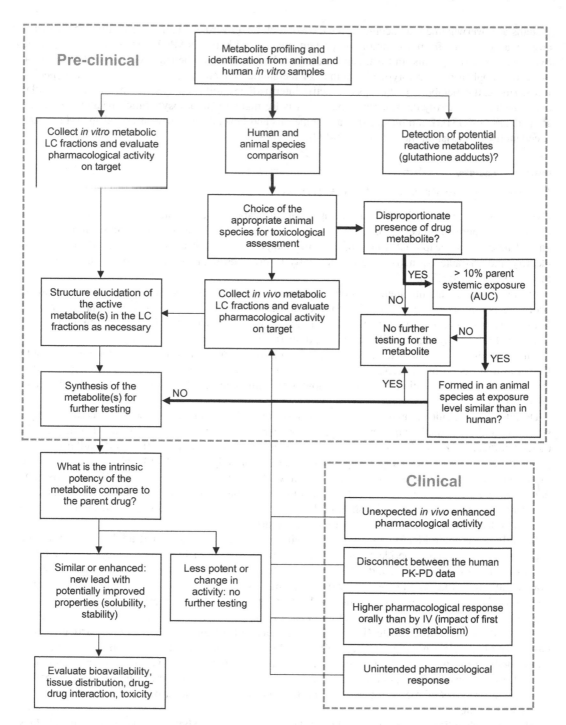

FIGURE 24.5   Flow-chart diagram for the identification and characterization of active metabolites in the drug development process.

significant first pass metabolism, the circulating metabolite concentration normally is higher when the drug is administered orally versus intravenously. Therefore, if increased pharmacodynamic activity is observed when the drug is given orally versus intravenously, this might suggest the involvement of active metabolites in the pharmacological response. Likewise, when compounds or drugs that are known to stimulate or induce Phase I metabolism are given concurrently and are observed to *increase* the pharmacological activity of a drug candidate instead of *decreasing* it, it is possible an active metabolite might be involved. This would also be the case if a particular drug candidate demonstrated increased activity in a cohort of patients who are extensive metabolizers of the drug. Conversely, if the specific metabolic pathway is known, cytochrome P450 isoform selective inhibitors can be used to probe for active metabolites by blocking metabolite formation when dosed simultaneously. In this instance, one would expect to observe a decrease in the pharmacodynamic response. Additionally, if the metabolic pathway is known, PD/PK and metabolic data can be examined to determine if there are genetic outliers in the drug response, due to poor or extensive metabolizers of the drug, which may suggest the involvement of an active metabolite. This is likely to be more common with drugs that are predominantly metabolized by a single pathway. Unintended pharmacological or toxic responses may also be indicative of an active metabolite, particularly when the metabolite is acting on a different biological target than the parent drug. Finally, any other factors that may affect metabolism, such as age, gender, diet, drug-drug interactions, or specific pathology, that lead to a difference in drug response may point to the involvement of an active metabolite.

Methods to Characterize and Quantify Active Metabolites

Metabolite characterization is often hampered by either lack of a sufficient quantity of material for characterization and/or a robust separation procedure. Historically, high performance/ultra-high performance liquid chromatography coupled mass spectrometry (HPLC/UHPLC-MS) has been the workhorse technique for metabolite identification and separation. However, over the past few years nuclear magnetic resonance (NMR) combined with novel biomimetic methods have given us new tools with increased potential for characterization of active metabolites.

While significant challenges still remain to identify all of the important metabolites of a candidate drug, HPLC-MS and now more commonly UHPLC-MS, remain the primary methods of metabolite structural elucidation and quantification [137]. They are typically employed in the pre-clinical phase of drug development after the drug candidate has been incubated in the presence of animal and human liver microsomes (HLMs) or hepatocytes, or dosed in a model animal species. Parent drug and metabolites are extracted from supernatant, cell media, or body fluids (in the case of animal dosing) and quantified using authentic metabolic standards (when available).

Alternatively, metabolism of a radiolabeled drug candidate can be evaluated using a HPLC coupled with a radiometric detector and a mass spectrometer, by splitting the LC-eluent between the two detectors, for a more comprehensive understanding of the drug's disposition [138]. However, the cost and difficultly of synthesis of the radiolabeled drug may be prohibitive during the early pre-clinical stages.

Cost-effective approaches to identifying and characterizing active metabolites can be employed even during early stages of drug development. One such approach involves standard HPLC/UHPLC-MS identification of the metabolite combined with a diverter valve that allows half of the eluent to be collected with an automated fraction collector for off-line bioactivity studies at the target receptor [1,9]. In this way, the LC-MS chromatogram can be compared to the target receptor bioactivity profile in order to generate an "activitygram" that relates the LC-MS peak to some specific pharmacological activity of the drug in question. While the quantity of metabolite isolated by this approach is necessarily limited, once the active metabolite has been identified production scale-up may be accomplished by using either a bioreactor [139,140] or biomimetic [141,142] approach. A similar method was successfully employed to detect binding of active metabolites of tamoxifen using a fluorescence-based displacement assay [143–145]. Using this method, 15 active metabolites were identified, including five primary and ten secondary metabolites, and six with an unknown order of metabolism [144].

In vitro bioreactors can be set up in most laboratories that are routinely performing drug metabolism studies [146]. Typically, these consist of: (1) mg to gram quantities of lead drug compound, (2) a metabolite generation system (either recombinant CYP enzymes, such as Supersomes™, yeast microsomes, *E. coli* expressed enzyme, HLMs, or hepatocytes—in general, if the CYP generating the metabolite is known, a recombinant system is preferred over HLMs or hepatocytes due to its superior metabolite generating capacity), and (3) a preparative HPLC system (most analytical HPLC systems can be converted into a preparative HPLC system simply by adding a semi-preparative or preparative column and adjusting the flow rate) [9]. This type of analytical characterization is also amenable to a high-throughput format using a 96-well microtiter plate, as previously described [143]. In this system, drug-metabolite mixtures are first separated and collected into fractions into 96-well plates. The fractions may then be assayed for activity in a receptor binding assay.

More recently, methods have been developed to incorporate a flow-based approach for generating and characterizing metabolites using an analytical-based chip method, aka the "liver-on-a-chip" [147,148]. This is a micro-fabricated device that contains hepatic cells expressing drug metabolizing enzymes in line with an analytical capture system; typically HPLC-MS, but newer modalities could also incorporate NMR. This has the advantage that a metabolite may be generated and analyzed using a single system with minimal user involvement. These types of approaches are preferred for metabolites that are intractable using traditional synthetic techniques.

An alternative to production of active metabolites by an *in vitro* bioreactor system is the recent development of biomimetic systems to generate metabolites [141]. These systems utilize a diverse array of organometallic catalysts and oxidants arranged in a microtiter plate format to perform oxidative chemistry on the drug of interest. Metabolite production involves a three-step method involving screening, optimization, and reaction scale-up. Since the biomimetic chemistry uses organic solvents, the reactions can be conducted with a much higher concentration of drug than a microsomal reaction, increasing the yields of the active metabolite [141]. Additionally, the biomimetic system is generally more amenable to scale-up than a comparative HLM system. However, since the system uses a non-biological catalyst it may not always be able to generate the metabolite of interest in sufficient quantity or with the proper stereochemistry. Depending on the efficiency of the reaction and the amount of metabolite needed for downstream applications, the biomimetic system may be more (or less) cost-effective than bioreactor metabolite generation.

Once the metabolite has been successfully purified and concentrated for bioactivity assays, the problem of concentration determination remains. Mutlib and colleagues have described a clever solution to this problem using a quantitative NMR (qNMR) approach [149–151]. Since ^{1}H NMR can provide a direct measurement of the absolute number of ^{1}H in a drug metabolite, and since the absolute number of ^{1}H is proportional to the absolute number of metabolite molecules in solution, the total concentration of metabolite may be determined by obtaining a quantitative ^{1}H NMR spectrum using the aSICCO (artificial Signal Insertion for Calculation of Concentration Observed) method [149] in combination with a known internal standard, typically maleic acid [149,152]. An added advantage of this method is that, since NMR is a non-destructive technique, the sample can be used in downstream applications such as *in vitro* and *in vivo* bioassays [150].

Full structural and functional characterization of the metabolite also allows for the possibility of late stage lead diversification [153]. A variety of related structural analogues is necessary for a complete understanding of the structure activity relationships (SAR) and mechanism of action of a drug. However, this can be an expensive and time-consuming undertaking. Since metabolism introduces chemical "handles," via functional groups such as hydroxyl groups or epoxides into a variety of locations on the drug of interest, these can be exploited in a semi-synthetic fashion to quickly generate new drug analogues. Combined with a recombinant enzyme method to scale up production of any metabolite, this can be a powerful tool for drug discovery and development. An instructive example of this technique was recently published by Obach and colleagues where they utilized generated deoxyfluorinated metabolites of midazolam, celecoxib, ramelteon, and risperidone that demonstrated increased metabolic stability [153]. In the same fashion, Bright and colleagues used a microbial cytochrome P450 biotransformation system combined with Suzuki–Miyaura coupling reactions to introduce fluorine at particular metabolic "hotspots" to increase the metabolic half-life of certain compounds [154].

Another advancement that has taken place in recent years has been the improved implementation of computational techniques to identify and predict drug metabolites [155]. With the increasing sophistication and availability of software to reliably predict sites of metabolism on new drug entities, this opens the possibility of predicting *a priori* potential active metabolites. In this regard, the use of principal component analysis (PCA) and pattern recognition techniques to obtain a new SAR for potential active metabolites can help to guide medicinal chemistry design of new drugs [156–158].

Conclusions

Forty years ago, Drayer et al. produced a list of approximately 50 drugs that were recognized to have active metabolites [159]. Since that time, the number of drugs with known active metabolites has expanded dramatically, along with our knowledge of how to identify and characterize them. Given the recent advancements in NMR, LC-MS, and separation technologies, the prospects are bright for future identification of as yet unknown active metabolites of existing and future drugs. As such, it is critical that active metabolite identification and characterization be included in any drug discovery and development program. Knowledge of the PD and PK properties of each active metabolite will provide enhanced opportunities for new drug leads and second-generation drug candidates.

Just as important, in some cases, active metabolites may lead to toxicities that need to be addressed early in the drug development cycle.

A vital challenge moving forward is to identify the *in vivo* pharmacology of critical active metabolites in a cost effective and expeditious manner. As analytical sensitivity and in line analysis techniques improve, this is quickly becoming an achievable goal.

REFERENCES

1. Fura, A. (2006) Role of pharmacologically active metabolites in drug discovery and development. *Drug Discov Today* **11**, 133–142.
2. Ortiz de Montellano, P. R. (2005) *Cytochrome P450: Structure, Mechanism, and Biochemistry*, 3rd. ed., Kluwer Academic/Plenum Publishers, New York.
3. Baillie, T. A., Cayen, M. N., Fouda, H., Gerson, R. J., Green, J. D., Grossman, S. J., Klunk, L. J., LeBlanc, B., Perkins, D. G., and Shipley, L. A. (2002) Drug metabolites in safety testing. *Toxicol Appl Pharmacol* **182**, 188–196.
4. Foster, A. B., Griggs, L. J., Jarman, M., van Maanen, J. M., and Schulten, H. R. (1980) Metabolism of tamoxifen by rat liver microsomes: Formation of the *N*-oxide, a new metabolite. *Biochem Pharmacol* **29**, 1977–1979.
5. McCague, R. and Seago, A. (1986) Aspects of metabolism of tamoxifen by rat liver microsomes. Identification of a new metabolite: E-1-[4-(2-dimethylaminoethoxy)-phenyl]-1, 2-diphenyl-1-buten-3-ol *N*-oxide. *Biochem Pharmacol* **35**, 827–834.
6. Mani, C., Hodgson, E., and Kupfer, D. (1993) Metabolism of the antimammary cancer antiestrogenic agent tamoxifen. II. Flavin-containing monooxygenase-mediated *N*-oxidation. *Drug Metab Dispos* **21**, 657–661.
7. Parte, P. and Kupfer, D. (2005) Oxidation of tamoxifen by human flavin-containing monooxygenase (FMO) 1 and FMO3 to tamoxifen-*N*-oxide and its novel reduction back to tamoxifen by human cytochromes P450 and hemoglobin. *Drug Metab Dispos* **33**, 1446–1452.
8. Hartyanszky, I., Kalasz, H., Adeghate, E., Gulyas, Z., Hasan, M. Y., Tekes, K., Adem, A., and Sotonyi, P. (2012) Active metabolites resulting from decarboxylation, reduction and ester hydrolysis of parent drugs. *Curr Drug Metab* **13**, 835–862.
9. Obach, R. S. (2013) Pharmacologically active drug metabolites: Impact on drug discovery and pharmacotherapy. *Pharmacol Rev* **65**, 578–640.
10. Guengerich, F. P. (2001) Common and uncommon cytochrome P450 reactions related to metabolism and chemical toxicity. *Chem Res Toxicol* **14**, 611–650.
11. Fabian, C., Tilzer, L., and Sternson, L. (1981) Comparative binding affinities of tamoxifen, 4-hydroxytamoxifen, and desmethyltamoxifen for estrogen receptors isolated from human breast carcinoma: Correlation with blood levels in patients with metastatic breast cancer. *Biopharm Drug Dispos* **2**, 381–390.
12. Ruenitz, P. C., Bagley, J. R., and Pape, C. W. (1984) Some chemical and biochemical aspects of liver microsomal metabolism of tamoxifen. *Drug Metab Dispos* **12**, 478–483.
13. Katzenellenbogen, B. S., Norman, M. J., Eckert, R. L., Peltz, S. W., and Mangel, W. F. (1984) Bioactivities, estrogen receptor interactions, and plasminogen activator-inducing activities of tamoxifen and hydroxy-tamoxifen isomers in MCF-7 human breast cancer cells. *Cancer Res* **44**, 112–119.

14. Crewe, H. K., Ellis, S. W., Lennard, M. S., and Tucker, G. T. (1997) Variable contribution of cytochromes P450 2D6, 2C9 and 3A4 to the 4-hydroxylation of tamoxifen by human liver microsomes. *Biochem Pharmacol* **53**, 171–178.

15. Desta, Z., Ward, B. A., Soukhova, N. V., and Flockhart, D. A. (2004) Comprehensive evaluation of tamoxifen sequential biotransformation by the human cytochrome P450 system *in vitro*: Prominent roles for CYP3A and CYP2D6. *J Pharmacol Exp Ther* **310**, 1062–1075.

16. Furr, B. J. and Jordan, V. C. (1984) The pharmacology and clinical uses of tamoxifen. *Pharmacol Ther* **25**, 127–205.

17. Johnson, M. D., Westley, B. R., and May, F. E. (1989) Oestrogenic activity of tamoxifen and its metabolites on gene regulation and cell proliferation in MCF-7 breast cancer cells. *Br J Cancer* **59**, 727–738.

18. Johnson, M. D., Zuo, H., Lee, K. H., Trebley, J. P., Rae, J. M., Weatherman, R. V., Desta, Z., Flockhart, D. A., and Skaar, T. C. (2004) Pharmacological characterization of 4-hydroxy-*N*-desmethyl tamoxifen, a novel active metabolite of tamoxifen. *Breast Cancer Res Treat* **85**, 151–159.

19. Jin, Y., Desta, Z., Stearns, V., Ward, B., Ho, H., Lee, K. H., Skaar, T. et al. (2005) CYP2D6 genotype, antidepressant use, and tamoxifen metabolism during adjuvant breast cancer treatment. *J Natl Cancer Inst* **97**, 30–39.

20. Goetz, M. P., Rae, J. M., Suman, V. J., Safgren, S. L., Ames, M. M., Visscher, D. W., Reynolds, C. et al. (2005) Pharmacogenetics of tamoxifen biotransformation is associated with clinical outcomes of efficacy and hot flashes. *J Clin Oncol* **23**, 9312–9318.

21. Dockens, R. C., Salazar, D. E., Fulmor, I. E., Wehling, M., Arnold, M. E., and Croop, R. (2006) Pharmacokinetics of a newly identified active metabolite of buspirone after administration of buspirone over its therapeutic dose range. *J Clin Pharmacol* **46**, 1308–1312.

22. Wong, H., Dockens, R. C., Pajor, L., Yeola, S., Grace, J. E., Jr., Stark, A. D., Taub, R. A., Yocca, F. D., Zaczek, R. C., and Li, Y. W. (2007) 6-Hydroxybuspirone is a major active metabolite of buspirone: Assessment of pharmacokinetics and 5-hydroxytryptamine1A receptor occupancy in rats. *Drug Metab Dispos* **35**, 1387–1392.

23. Kantola, T., Kivisto, K. T., and Neuvonen, P. J. (1998) Effect of itraconazole on the pharmacokinetics of atorvastatin. *Clin Pharmacol Ther* **64**, 58–65.

24. Park, J. E., Kim, K. B., Bae, S. K., Moon, B. S., Liu, K. H., and Shin, J. G. (2008) Contribution of cytochrome P450 3A4 and 3A5 to the metabolism of atorvastatin. *Xenobiotica* **38**, 1240–1251.

25. Lennernas, H. (2003) Clinical pharmacokinetics of atorvastatin. *Clin Pharmacokinet* **42**, 1141–1160.

26. Lins, R. L., Matthys, K. E., Verpooten, G. A., Peeters, P. C., Dratwa, M., Stolear, J. C., and Lameire, N. H. (2003) Pharmacokinetics of atorvastatin and its metabolites after single and multiple dosing in hypercholesterolaemic haemodialysis patients. *Nephrol Dial Transplant* **18**, 967–976.

27. Jacobsen, W., Kuhn, B., Soldner, A., Kirchner, G., Sewing, K. F., Kollman, P. A., Benet, L. Z., and Christians, U. (2000) Lactonization is the critical first step in the disposition of the 3-hydroxy-3-methylglutaryl-CoA reductase inhibitor atorvastatin. *Drug Metab Dispos* **28**, 1369–1378.

28. Mason, R. P., Walter, M. F., Day, C. A., and Jacob, R. F. (2006) Active metabolite of atorvastatin inhibits membrane cholesterol domain formation by an antioxidant mechanism. *J Biol Chem* **281**, 9337–9345.

29. Hesse, L. M., Venkatakrishnan, K., Court, M. H., von Moltke, L. L., Duan, S. X., Shader, R. I., and Greenblatt, D. J. (2000) CYP2B6 mediates the *in vitro* hydroxylation of bupropion: Potential drug interactions with other antidepressants. *Drug Metab Dispos* **28**, 1176–1183.

30. Damaj, M. I., Carroll, F. I., Eaton, J. B., Navarro, H. A., Blough, B. E., Mirza, S., Lukas, R. J., and Martin, B. R. (2004) Enantioselective effects of hydroxy metabolites of bupropion on behavior and on function of monoamine transporters and nicotinic receptors. *Mol Pharmacol* **66**, 675–682.

31. Butz, R. F., Welch, R. M., and Findlay, J. W. (1982) Relationship between bupropion disposition and dopamine uptake inhibition in rats and mice. *J Pharmacol Exp Ther* **221**, 676–685.

32. Martin, P., Massol, J., Colin, J. N., Lacomblez, L., and Puech, A. J. (1990) Antidepressant profile of bupropion and three metabolites in mice. *Pharmacopsychiatry* **23**, 187–194.

33. Lalonde, R. L., Lessard, D., and Gaudreault, J. (1996) Population pharmacokinetics of terfenadine. *Pharm Res* **13**, 832–838.

34. Chen, C. (2007) Some pharmacokinetic aspects of the lipophilic terfenadine and zwitterionic fexofenadine in humans. *Drugs R D* **8**, 301–314.

35. Gillard, M. and Chatelain, P. (2006) Changes in pH differently affect the binding properties of histamine H1 receptor antagonists. *Eur J Pharmacol* **530**, 205–214.

36. Woosley, R. L., Chen, Y., Freiman, J. P., and Gillis, R. A. (1993) Mechanism of the cardiotoxic actions of terfenadine. *JAMA* **269**, 1532–1536.
37. Marugo, M., Bernasconi, D., Miglietta, L., Fazzuoli, L., Ravera, F., Cassulo, S., and Giordano, G. (1992) Effects of dihydrotestosterone and hydroxyflutamide on androgen receptors in cultured human breast cancer cells (EVSA-T). *J Steroid Biochem Mol Biol* **42**, 547–554.
38. Shet, M. S., McPhaul, M., Fisher, C. W., Stallings, N. R., and Estabrook, R. W. (1997) Metabolism of the antiandrogenic drug (Flutamide) by human CYP1A2. *Drug Metab Dispos* **25**, 1298–1303.
39. Tekes, K., Kalasz, H., Hasan, M. Y., Adeghate, E., Darvas, F., Ram, N., and Adem, A. (2011) Aliphatic and aromatic oxidations, epoxidation and *S*-oxidation of prodrugs that yield active drug metabolites. *Curr Med Chem* **18**, 4885–4900.
40. Kerr, B. M., Thummel, K. E., Wurden, C. J., Klein, S. M., Kroetz, D. L., Gonzalez, F. J., and Levy, R. H. (1994) Human liver carbamazepine metabolism. Role of CYP3A4 and CYP2C8 in 10,11-epoxide formation. *Biochem Pharmacol* **47**, 1969–1979.
41. McLean, M. J. and Macdonald, R. L. (1986) Carbamazepine and 10,11-epoxycarbamazepine produce use- and voltage-dependent limitation of rapidly firing action potentials of mouse central neurons in cell culture. *J Pharmacol Exp Ther* **238**, 727–738.
42. Johannessen, S. I., Gerna, M., Bakke, J., Strandjord, R. E., and Morselli, P. L. (1976) CSF concentrations and serum protein binding of carbamazepine and carbamazepine-10,11-epoxide in epileptic patients. *Br J Clin Pharmacol* **3**, 575–582.
43. Sahasranaman, S., Issar, M., and Hochhaus, G. (2006) Metabolism of mometasone furoate and biological activity of the metabolites. *Drug Metab Dispos* **34**, 225–233.
44. Valotis, A., Neukam, K., Elert, O., and Hogger, P. (2004) Human receptor kinetics, tissue binding affinity, and stability of mometasone furoate. *J Pharm Sci* **93**, 1337–1350.
45. Valotis, A. and Hogger, P. (2004) Significant receptor affinities of metabolites and a degradation product of mometasone furoate. *Respir Res* **5**, 7.
46. Schroth, W., Goetz, M. P., Hamann, U., Fasching, P. A., Schmidt, M., Winter, S., Fritz, P. et al. (2009) Association between CYP2D6 polymorphisms and outcomes among women with early stage breast cancer treated with tamoxifen. *JAMA* **302**, 1429–1436.
47. Otton, S. V., Schadel, M., Cheung, S. W., Kaplan, H. L., Busto, U. E., and Sellers, E. M. (1993) CYP2D6 phenotype determines the metabolic conversion of hydrocodone to hydromorphone. *Clin Pharmacol Ther* **54**, 463–472.
48. Kirchheiner, J., Schmidt, H., Tzvetkov, M., Keulen, J. T., Lotsch, J., Roots, I., and Brockmoller, J. (2007) Pharmacokinetics of codeine and its metabolite morphine in ultra-rapid metabolizers due to CYP2D6 duplication. *Pharmacogenomics J* **7**, 257–265.
49. Volpe, D. A., McMahon Tobin, G. A., Mellon, R. D., Katki, A. G., Parker, R. J., Colatsky, T., Kropp, T. J., and Verbois, S. L. (2011) Uniform assessment and ranking of opioid mu receptor binding constants for selected opioid drugs. *Regul Toxicol Pharmacol* **59**, 385–390.
50. Caraco, Y., Sheller, J., and Wood, A. J. (1996) Pharmacogenetic determination of the effects of codeine and prediction of drug interactions. *J Pharmacol Exp Ther* **278**, 1165–1174.
51. Caraco, Y., Tateishi, T., Guengerich, F. P., and Wood, A. J. (1996) Microsomal codeine *N*-demethylation: Cosegregation with cytochrome P4503A4 activity. *Drug Metab Dispos* **24**, 761–764.
52. Quiding, H., Anderson, P., Bondesson, U., Boreus, L. O., and Hynning, P. A. (1986) Plasma concentrations of codeine and its metabolite, morphine, after single and repeated oral administration. *Eur J Clin Pharmacol* **30**, 673–677.
53. Madadi, P., Koren, G., Cairns, J., Chitayat, D., Gaedigk, A., Leeder, J. S., Teitelbaum, R., Karaskov, T., and Aleksa, K. (2007) Safety of codeine during breastfeeding: Fatal morphine poisoning in the breastfed neonate of a mother prescribed codeine. *Can Fam Physician* **53**, 33–35.
54. Goa, K. L. and Ward, A. (1986) Buspirone. A preliminary review of its pharmacological properties and therapeutic efficacy as an anxiolytic. *Drugs* **32**, 114–129.
55. Blier, P., Bergeron, R., and de Montigny, C. (1997) Selective activation of postsynaptic 5-HT1A receptors induces rapid antidepressant response. *Neuropsychopharmacology* **16**, 333–338.
56. Zhu, M., Zhao, W., Jimenez, H., Zhang, D., Yeola, S., Dai, R., Vachharajani, N., and Mitroka, J. (2005) Cytochrome P450 3A-mediated metabolism of buspirone in human liver microsomes. *Drug Metab Dispos* **33**, 500–507.
57. Kivisto, K. T., Lamberg, T. S., Kantola, T., and Neuvonen, P. J. (1997) Plasma buspirone concentrations are greatly increased by erythromycin and itraconazole. *Clin Pharmacol Ther* **62**, 348–354.

58. Caccia, S., Conti, I., Vigano, G., and Garattini, S. (1986) 1-(2-Pyrimidinyl)-piperazine as active metabolite of buspirone in man and rat. *Pharmacology* **33**, 46–51.

59. Rotzinger, S. and Baker, G. B. (2002) Human CYP3A4 and the metabolism of nefazodone and hydroxynefazodone by human liver microsomes and heterologously expressed enzymes. *Eur Neuropsychopharmacol* **12**, 91–100.

60. Mayol, R. F., Cole, C. A., Luke, G. M., Colson, K. L., and Kerns, E. H. (1994) Characterization of the metabolites of the antidepressant drug nefazodone in human urine and plasma. *Drug Metab Dispos* **22**, 304–311.

61. Fiorella, D., Rabin, R. A., and Winter, J. C. (1995) The role of the 5-HT2A and 5-HT2C receptors in the stimulus effects of m-chlorophenylpiperazine. *Psychopharmacology (Berl)* **119**, 222–230.

62. Conn, P. J. and Sanders-Bush, E. (1987) Relative efficacies of piperazines at the phosphoinositide hydrolysis-linked serotonergic (5-HT-2 and 5-HT-1c) receptors. *J Pharmacol Exp Ther* **242**, 552–557.

63. Ghaziuddin, N., Welch, K., and Greden, J. (2003) Central serotonergic effects of m-chlorophenylpiperazine (mCPP) among normal control adolescents. *Neuropsychopharmacology* **28**, 133–139.

64. Kennett, G. A., Whitton, P., Shah, K., and Curzon, G. (1989) Anxiogenic-like effects of mCPP and TFMPP in animal models are opposed by 5-HT1C receptor antagonists. *Eur J Pharmacol* **164**, 445–454.

65. Kennett, G. A. and Curzon, G. (1988) Evidence that mCPP may have behavioural effects mediated by central 5-HT1C receptors. *Br J Pharmacol* **94**, 137–147.

66. Mizuno, K., Katoh, M., Okumura, H., Nakagawa, N., Negishi, T., Hashizume, T., Nakajima, M., and Yokoi, T. (2009) Metabolic activation of benzodiazepines by CYP3A4. *Drug Metab Dispos* **37**, 345–351.

67. Greenblatt, D. J., Shader, R. I., MacLeod, S. M., Sellers, E. M., Franke, K., and Giles, H. G. (1978) Absorption of oral and intramuscular chlordiazepoxide. *Eur J Clin Pharmacol* **13**, 267–274.

68. Richelson, E., Nelson, A., and Neeper, R. (1991) Binding of benzodiazepines and some major metabolites at their sites in normal human frontal cortex *in vitro*. *J Pharmacol Exp Ther* **256**, 897–901.

69. Chakraborty, B. S., Hawes, E. M., McKay, G., Hubbard, J. W., Korchinski, E. D., Midha, K. K., Choc, M. G., and Robinson, W. T. (1988) S-oxidation of thioridazine to psychoactive metabolites: An oral dose-proportionality study in healthy volunteers. *Drug Metabol Drug Interact* **6**, 425–437.

70. Roth, B. L., Tandra, S., Burgess, L. H., Sibley, D. R., and Meltzer, H. Y. (1995) D4 dopamine receptor binding affinity does not distinguish between typical and atypical antipsychotic drugs. *Psychopharmacology (Berl)* **120**, 365–368.

71. Dinovo, E. C., Pollak, H., and Gottschalk, L. A. (1984) Partitioning of thioridazine and mesoridazine in human blood fractions. *Methods Find Exp Clin Pharmacol* **6**, 143–146.

72. Mackin, P. (2008) Cardiac side effects of psychiatric drugs. *Hum Psychopharmacol* **23 Suppl 1**, 3–14.

73. Niedzwiecki, D. M., Mailman, R. B., and Cubeddu, L. X. (1984) Greater potency of mesoridazine and sulforidazine compared with the parent compound, thioridazine, on striatal dopamine autoreceptors. *J Pharmacol Exp Ther* **228**, 636–639.

74. Milara, J., Armengot, M., Banuls, P., Tenor, H., Beume, R., Artigues, E., and Cortijo, J. (2012) Roflumilast N-oxide, a PDE4 inhibitor, improves cilia motility and ciliated human bronchial epithelial cells compromised by cigarette smoke *in vitro*. *Br J Pharmacol* **166**, 2243–2262.

75. Davison, C. (1971) Salicylate metabolism in man. *Ann N Y Acad Sci* **179**, 249–268.

76. Hansen, B. G. and Sogaard, P. (1985) Population analysis of susceptibility to cefotaxime and desacetyl-cefotaxime in Staphylococcus and Enterobacteriaceae. *Acta Pathol Microbiol Immunol Scand B* **93**, 243–247.

77. Imamura, Y., Sanai, K., Seri, K., and Akita, H. (2001) Hypoglycemic effect of S(-)-hydroxyhexamide, a major metabolite of acetohexamide, and its enantiomer R(+)-hydroxyhexamide. *Life Sci* **69**, 1947–1955.

78. Bartoszek, A. (2002) Metabolic activation of adriamycin by NADPH-cytochrome P450 reductase; overview of its biological and biochemical effects. *Acta Biochim Pol* **49**, 323–331.

79. Bligh, H. F., Bartoszek, A., Robson, C. N., Hickson, I. D., Kasper, C. B., Beggs, J. D., and Wolf, C. R. (1990) Activation of mitomycin C by NADPH: Cytochrome P-450 reductase. *Cancer Res* **50**, 7789–7792.

80. Chang, W. H. (1992) Reduced haloperidol: A factor in determining the therapeutic benefit of haloperidol treatment? *Psychopharmacology (Berl)* **106**, 289–296.

81. Keung, A. C., Landriault, H., Lefebvre, M., Gossard, D., Dempsey, E. E., Juneau, M., Dimmitt, D., Castles, M., Roberts, L., and Spenard, J. (1997) Pharmacokinetics and safety of single intravenous and oral doses of dolasetron mesylate in healthy women. *Biopharm Drug Dispos* **18**, 361–369.

82. Gregory, R. E. and Ettinger, D. S. (1998) 5-HT3 receptor antagonists for the prevention of chemotherapy-induced nausea and vomiting. A comparison of their pharmacology and clinical efficacy. *Drugs* **55**, 173–189.

83. Warner, C. and Shoaib, M. (2005) How does bupropion work as a smoking cessation aid? *Addict Biol* **10**, 219–231.

84. Golden, R. N., De Vane, C. L., Laizure, S. C., Rudorfer, M. V., Sherer, M. A., and Potter, W. Z. (1988) Bupropion in depression. II. The role of metabolites in clinical outcome. *Arch Gen Psychiatry* **45**, 145–149.

85. Zhong, L., Shen, H., Huang, C., Jing, H., and Cao, D. (2011) AKR1B10 induces cell resistance to daunorubicin and idarubicin by reducing C13 ketonic group. *Toxicol Appl Pharmacol* **255**, 40–47.

86. Stromme, J. H. and Eldjarn, L. (1966) Distribution and chemical forms of diethyldithiocarbamate and tetraethylthiuram disulphide (disculfiram) in mice in relation to radioprotection. *Biochem Pharmacol* **15**, 287–297.

87. Stromme, J. H. (1963) Effects of diethyldithiocarbamate and disulfiram on glucose metabolism and glutathione content of human erythrocytes. *Biochem Pharmacol* **12**, 705–715.

88. Roberts, M. S., Magnusson, B. M., Burczynski, F. J., and Weiss, M. (2002) Enterohepatic circulation: Physiological, pharmacokinetic and clinical implications. *Clin Pharmacokinet* **41**, 751–790.

89. Kilpatrick, G. J. and Smith, T. W. (2005) Morphine-6-glucuronide: Actions and mechanisms. *Med Res Rev* **25**, 521–544.

90. Mulder, G. J. (1992) Pharmacological effects of drug conjugates: Is morphine 6-glucuronide an exception? *Trends Pharmacol Sci* **13**, 302–304.

91. van Dorp, E. L., Romberg, R., Sarton, E., Bovill, J. G., and Dahan, A. (2006) Morphine-6-glucuronide: Morphine's successor for postoperative pain relief? *Anesth Analg* **102**, 1789–1797.

92. Lotsch, J., Stockmann, A., Kobal, G., Brune, K., Waibel, R., Schmidt, N., and Geisslinger, G. (1996) Pharmacokinetics of morphine and its glucuronides after intravenous infusion of morphine and morphine-6-glucuronide in healthy volunteers. *Clin Pharmacol Ther* **60**, 316–325.

93. Gaillard, P., Carrupt, P. A., Testa, B., and Boudon, A. (1994) Molecular lipophilicity potential, a tool in 3D QSAR: Method and applications. *J Comput Aided Mol Des* **8**, 83–96.

94. Shiraga, T., Yajima, K., Teragaki, T., Suzuki, K., Hashimoto, T., Iwatsubo, T., Miyashita, A., and Usui, T. (2012) Identification of enzymes responsible for the *N*-oxidation of darexaban glucuronide, the pharmacologically active metabolite of darexaban, and the glucuronidation of darexaban *N*-oxides in human liver microsomes. *Biol Pharm Bull* **35**, 413–421.

95. Hashimoto, T., Suzuki, K., Kihara, Y., Iwatsubo, T., Miyashita, A., Heeringa, M., Onkels, H. et al. (2013) Absorption, metabolism and excretion of darexaban (YM150), a new direct factor Xa inhibitor in humans. *Xenobiotica* **43**, 534–547.

96. Iwatsuki, Y., Sato, T., Moritani, Y., Shigenaga, T., Suzuki, M., Kawasaki, T., Funatsu, T., and Kaku, S. (2011) Biochemical and pharmacological profile of darexaban, an oral direct factor Xa inhibitor. *Eur J Pharmacol* **673**, 49–55.

97. Negishi, M., Pedersen, L. G., Petrotchenko, E., Shevtsov, S., Gorokhov, A., Kakuta, Y., and Pedersen, L. C. (2001) Structure and function of sulfotransferases. *Arch Biochem Biophys* **390**, 149–157.

98. Zuckerman, A., Bolan, E., de Paulis, T., Schmidt, D., Spector, S., and Pasternak, G. W. (1999) Pharmacological characterization of morphine-6-sulfate and codeine-6-sulfate. *Brain Res* **842**, 1–5.

99. Kurogi, K., Chepak, A., Hanrahan, M. T., Liu, M. Y., Sakakibara, Y., Suiko, M., and Liu, M. C. (2014) Sulfation of opioid drugs by human cytosolic sulfotransferases: Metabolic labeling study and enzymatic analysis. *Eur J Pharm Sci* **62**, 40–48.

100. Brown, C. E., Roerig, S. C., Burger, V. T., Cody, R. B., Jr., and Fujimoto, J. M. (1985) Analgesic potencies of morphine 3- and 6-sulfates after intracerebroventricular administration in mice: Relationship to structural characteristics defined by mass spectrometry and nuclear magnetic resonance. *J Pharm Sci* **74**, 821–824.

101. Anderson, R. J., Kudlacek, P. E., and Clemens, D. L. (1998) Sulfation of minoxidil by multiple human cytosolic sulfotransferases. *Chem Biol Interact* **109**, 53–67.

102. Goren, A., Shapiro, J., Roberts, J., McCoy, J., Desai, N., Zarrab, Z., Pietrzak, A., and Lotti, T. (2015) Clinical utility and validity of minoxidil response testing in androgenetic alopecia. *Dermatol Ther* **28**, 13–16.

103. Roberts, J., Desai, N., McCoy, J., and Goren, A. (2014) Sulfotransferase activity in plucked hair follicles predicts response to topical minoxidil in the treatment of female androgenetic alopecia. *Dermatol Ther* **27**, 252–254.

104. Connolly, S. J. and Kates, R. E. (1982) Clinical pharmacokinetics of *N*-acetylprocainamide. *Clin Pharmacokinet* **7**, 206–220.

105. Okumura, K., Kita, T., Chikazawa, S., Komada, F., Iwakawa, S., and Tanigawara, Y. (1997) Genotyping of *N*-acetylation polymorphism and correlation with procainamide metabolism. *Clin Pharmacol Ther* **61**, 509–517.

106. Mahajan, S., and Atkins, W. M. (2005) The chemistry and biology of inhibitors and pro-drugs targeted to glutathione S-transferases. *Cell Mol Life Sci* **62**, 1221–1233.

107. Dansette, P. M., Rosi, J., Bertho, G., and Mansuy, D. (2012) Cytochromes P450 catalyze both steps of the major pathway of clopidogrel bioactivation, whereas paraoxonase catalyzes the formation of a minor thiol metabolite isomer. *Chem Res Toxicol* **25**, 348–356.

108. Dansette, P. M., Libraire, J., Bertho, G., and Mansuy, D. (2009) Metabolic oxidative cleavage of thioesters: Evidence for the formation of sulfenic acid intermediates in the bioactivation of the antithrombotic prodrugs ticlopidine and clopidogrel. *Chem Res Toxicol* **22**, 369–373.

109. Dansette, P. M., Levent, D., Hessani, A., and Mansuy, D. (2015) Bioactivation of clopidogrel and prasugrel: Factors determining the stereochemistry of the thiol metabolite double bond. *Chem Res Toxicol* **28**, 1338–1345.

110. Dansette, P. M., Levent, D., Hessani, A., Bertho, G., and Mansuy, D. (2013) Thiolactone sulfoxides as new reactive metabolites acting as bis-electrophiles: Implication in clopidogrel and prasugrel bioactivation. *Chem Res Toxicol* **26**, 794–802.

111. de Miranda, P., Beacham, L. M., 3rd, Creagh, T. H., and Elion, G. B. (1975) The metabolic disposition of 14C-azathioprine in the dog. *J Pharmacol Exp Ther* **195**, 50–57.

112. De, M. P., Beacham, L. M., 3rd, Creagh, T. H., and Elion, G. B. (1973) The metabolic fate of the methylnitroimidazole moiety of azathioprine in the rat. *J Pharmacol Exp Ther* **187**, 588–601.

113. Chalmers, A. H. (1974) Studies on the mechanism of formation of 5-mercapto-1-methyl-4-nitroimidazole, a metabolite of the immunosuppressive drug azathioprine. *Biochem Pharmacol* **23**, 1891–1901.

114. Elion, G. B. (1967) Symposium on immunosuppressive drugs. Biochemistry and pharmacology of purine analogues. *Fed Proc* **26**, 898–904.

115. Elion, G. B., Rideout, J. L., de Miranda, P., Collins, P., and Bauer, D. J. (1975) Biological activities of some purine arabinosides. *Ann N Y Acad Sci* **255**, 468–480.

116. Skarke, C., Darimont, J., Schmidt, H., Geisslinger, G., and Lotsch, J. (2003) Analgesic effects of morphine and morphine-6-glucuronide in a transcutaneous electrical pain model in healthy volunteers. *Clin Pharmacol Ther* **73**, 107–121.

117. Murthy, B. R., Pollack, G. M., and Brouwer, K. L. (2002) Contribution of morphine-6-glucuronide to antinociception following intravenous administration of morphine to healthy volunteers. *J Clin Pharmacol* **42**, 569–576.

118. Martinez, M. N. and Jackson, A. J. (1991) Suitability of various noninfinity area under the plasma concentration-time curve (AUC) estimates for use in bioequivalence determinations: Relationship to AUC from zero to time infinity (AUC0-INF). *Pharm Res* **8**, 512–517.

119. Vozeh, S. (1981) Pharmacokinetic of benzodiazepines in old age. *Schweiz Med Wochenschr* **111**, 1789–1793.

120. Richtand, N. M., Welge, J. A., Logue, A. D., Keck, P. E., Jr., Strakowski, S. M., and McNamara, R. K. (2007) Dopamine and serotonin receptor binding and antipsychotic efficacy. *Neuropsychopharmacology* **32**, 1715–1726.

121. Tatsumi, M., Groshan, K., Blakely, R. D., and Richelson, E. (1997) Pharmacological profile of antidepressants and related compounds at human monoamine transporters. *Eur J Pharmacol* **340**, 249–258.

122. Banger, M., Hermes, B., Hartter, S., and Hiemke, C. (1997) Monitoring serum concentrations of clomipramine and metabolites: Fluorescence polarization immunoassay versus high performance liquid chromatography. *Pharmacopsychiatry* **30**, 128–132.

123. Agnel, M., Esnaud, H., Langer, S. Z., and Graham, D. (1996) Pharmacological characterization of the cloned human 5-hydroxytryptamine transporter. *Biochem Pharmacol* **51**, 1145–1151.

124. Owens, M. J., Morgan, W. N., Plott, S. J., and Nemeroff, C. B. (1997) Neurotransmitter receptor and transporter binding profile of antidepressants and their metabolites. *J Pharmacol Exp Ther* **283**, 1305–1322.

125. Le, M. T., Vanderheyden, P. M., Szaszak, M., Hunyady, L., Kersemans, V., and Vauquelin, G. (2003) Peptide and nonpeptide antagonist interaction with constitutively active human AT1 receptors. *Biochem Pharmacol* **65**, 1329–1338.

126. Hinson, J. A., Roberts, D. W., and James, L. P. (2010) Mechanisms of acetaminophen-induced liver necrosis. *Handb Exp Pharmacol* **196**, 369–405.

127. Dahlin, D. C., Miwa, G. T., Lu, A. Y., and Nelson, S. D. (1984) N-acetyl-p-benzoquinone imine: A cytochrome P-450-mediated oxidation product of acetaminophen. *Proc Natl Acad Sci USA* **81**, 1327–1331.

128. Dahlin, D. C. and Nelson, S. D. (1982) Synthesis, decomposition kinetics, and preliminary toxicological studies of pure N-acetyl-p-benzoquinone imine, a proposed toxic metabolite of acetaminophen. *J Med Chem* **25**, 885–886.

129. Du, K., Ramachandran, A., and Jaeschke, H. (2016) Oxidative stress during acetaminophen hepatotoxicity: Sources, pathophysiological role and therapeutic potential. *Redox Biol* **10**, 148–156.

130. Park, B. K., Laverty, H., Srivastava, A., Antoine, D. J., Naisbitt, D., and Williams, D. P. (2011) Drug bioactivation and protein adduct formation in the pathogenesis of drug-induced toxicity. *Chem Biol Interact* **192**, 30–36.

131. Lammert, C., Bjornsson, E., Niklasson, A., and Chalasani, N. (2010) Oral medications with significant hepatic metabolism at higher risk for hepatic adverse events. *Hepatology* **51**, 615–620.

132. Baillie, T. A. (2015) The contributions of Sidney D. Nelson to drug metabolism research. *Drug Metab Rev* **47**, 4–11.

133. Kalgutkar, A. S. and Dalvie, D. (2015) Predicting toxicities of reactive metabolite-positive drug candidates. *Annu Rev Pharmacol Toxicol* **55**, 35–54.

134. Grillo, M. P. (2015) Detecting reactive drug metabolites for reducing the potential for drug toxicity. *Expert Opin Drug Metab Toxicol* **11**, 1281–1302.

135. Wienkers, L. C. and Heath, T. G. (2005) Predicting *in vivo* drug interactions from *in vitro* drug discovery data. *Nat Rev Drug Discov* **4**, 825–833.

136. Kerns, E. H. and Di, L. (2003) Pharmaceutical profiling in drug discovery. *Drug Discov Today* **8**, 316–323.

137. Prakash, C., Shaffer, C. L., and Nedderman, A. (2007) Analytical strategies for identifying drug metabolites. *Mass Spectrom Rev* **26**, 340–369.

138. Penner, N., Xu, L., and Prakash, C. (2012) Radiolabeled absorption, distribution, metabolism, and excretion studies in drug development: Why, when, and how? *Chem Res Toxicol* **25**, 513–531.

139. Lampe, J. N., Fernandez, C., Nath, A., and Atkins, W. M. (2008) Nile Red is a fluorescent allosteric substrate of cytochrome P450 3A4. *Biochemistry* **47**, 509–516.

140. Rushmore, T. H., Reider, P. J., Slaughter, D., Assang, C., and Shou, M. (2000) Bioreactor systems in drug metabolism: Synthesis of cytochrome P450-generated metabolites. *Metab Eng* **2**, 115–125.

141. Bernadou, J. and Meunier, B. (2004) Biomimetic chemical catalysts in the oxidative activation of drugs. *Adv Synth Catal* **346**, 171–184.

142. Rocha, B. A., de Oliveira, A. R., Pazin, M., Dorta, D. J., Rodrigues, A. P., Berretta, A. A., Peti, A. P. et al. (2014) Jacobsen catalyst as a cytochrome P450 biomimetic model for the metabolism of monensin A. *Biomed Res Int* **2014**, 152102.

143. Kool, J., Ramautar, R., van Liempd, S. M., Beckman, J., de Kanter, F. J., Meerman, J. H., Schenk, T., Irth, H., Commandeur, J. N., and Vermeulen, N. P. (2006) Rapid on-line profiling of estrogen receptor binding metabolites of tamoxifen. *J Med Chem* **49**, 3287–3292.

144. van Liempd, S. M., Kool, J., Niessen, W. M., van Elswijk, D. E., Irth, H., and Vermeulen, N. P. (2006) On-line formation, separation, and estrogen receptor affinity screening of cytochrome P450-derived metabolites of selective estrogen receptor modulators. *Drug Metab Dispos* **34**, 1640–1649.

145. Oosterkamp, A. J., Villaverde Herraiz, M. T., Irth, H., Tjaden, U. R., and van der Greef, J. (1996) Reversed-phase liquid chromatography coupled on-line to receptor affinity detection based on the human estrogen receptor. *Anal Chem* **68**, 1201–1206.

146. Martinez, C. A. and Rupashinghe, S. G. (2013) Cytochrome P450 bioreactors in the pharmaceutical industry: Challenges and opportunities. *Curr Top Med Chem* **13**, 1470–1490.

147. Novik, E., Maguire, T. J., Chao, P., Cheng, K. C., and Yarmush, M. L. (2010) A microfluidic hepatic coculture platform for cell-based drug metabolism studies. *Biochem Pharmacol* **79**, 1036–1044.

148. Chang, S. Y., Weber, E. J., Ness, K. V., Eaton, D. L., and Kelly, E. J. (2016) Liver and kidney on chips: Microphysiological models to understand transporter function. *Clin Pharmacol Ther* **100**, 464–478.

149. Walker, G. S., Ryder, T. F., Sharma, R., Smith, E. B., and Freund, A. (2011) Validation of isolated metabolites from drug metabolism studies as analytical standards by quantitative NMR. *Drug Metab Dispos* **39**, 433–440.

150. Walker, G. S., Bauman, J. N., Ryder, T. F., Smith, E. B., Spracklin, D. K., and Obach, R. S. (2014) Biosynthesis of drug metabolites and quantitation using NMR spectroscopy for use in pharmacologic and drug metabolism studies. *Drug Metab Dispos* **42**, 1627–1639.

151. Mutlib, A., Espina, R., Vishwanathan, K., Babalola, K., Chen, Z., Dehnhardt, C., Venkatesan, A. et al. (2011) Application of quantitative NMR in pharmacological evaluation of biologically generated metabolites: Implications in drug discovery. *Drug Metab Dispos* **39**, 106–116.

152. Espina, R., Yu, L., Wang, J., Tong, Z., Vashishtha, S., Talaat, R., Scatina, J., and Mutlib, A. (2009) Nuclear magnetic resonance spectroscopy as a quantitative tool to determine the concentrations of biologically produced metabolites: Implications in metabolites in safety testing. *Chem Res Toxicol* **22**, 299–310.

153. Obach, R. S., Walker, G. S., and Brodney, M. A. (2016) Biosynthesis of fluorinated analogs of drugs using human cytochrome P450 enzymes followed by deoxyfluorination and quantitative nuclear magnetic resonance spectroscopy to improve metabolic stability. *Drug Metab Dispos* **44**, 634–646.

154. Bright, T. V., Dalton, F., Elder, V. L., Murphy, C. D., O'Connor, N. K., and Sandford, G. (2013) A convenient chemical-microbial method for developing fluorinated pharmaceuticals. *Org Biomol Chem* **11**, 1135–1142.

155. Kirchmair, J., Goller, A. H., Lang, D., Kunze, J., Testa, B., Wilson, I. D., Glen, R. C., and Schneider, G. (2015) Predicting drug metabolism: Experiment and/or computation? *Nat Rev Drug Discov* **14**, 387–404.

156. Bajorath, J. (2016) Computational chemistry and computer-aided drug discovery: Part II. *Future Med Chem* **8**, 1799–1800.

157. Bajorath, J. (2016) Computational chemistry and computer-aided drug discovery: Part 1. *Future Med Chem* **8**, 1705–1706.

158. Nassar, A. E. and Talaat, R. E. (2004) Strategies for dealing with metabolite elucidation in drug discovery and development. *Drug Discov Today* **9**, 317–327.

159. Drayer, D. E. (1976) Pharmacologically active drug metabolites: Therapeutic and toxic activities, plasma and urine data in man, accumulation in renal failure. *Clin Pharmacokinet* **1**, 426–443.

160. Huang, P., Kehner, G. B., Cowan, A., and Liu-Chen, L. Y. (2001) Comparison of pharmacological activities of buprenorphine and norbuprenorphine: Norbuprenorphine is a potent opioid agonist. *J Pharmacol Exp Ther* **297**, 688–695.

161. Sauer, J. M., Ring, B. J., and Witcher, J. W. (2005) Clinical pharmacokinetics of atomoxetine. *Clin Pharmacokinet* **44**, 571–590.

162. Molden, E., Lunde, H., Lunder, N., and Refsum, H. (2006) Pharmacokinetic variability of aripiprazole and the active metabolite dehydroaripiprazole in psychiatric patients. *Ther Drug Monit* **28**, 744–749.

163. Lalovic, B., Kharasch, E., Hoffer, C., Risler, L., Liu-Chen, L. Y., and Shen, D. D. (2006) Pharmacokinetics and pharmacodynamics of oral oxycodone in healthy human subjects: Role of circulating active metabolites. *Clin Pharmacol Ther* **79**, 461–479.

164. Briciu, C., Neag, M., Muntean, D., Bocsan, C., Buzoianu, A., Antonescu, O., Gheldiu, A. M., Achim, M., Popa, A., and Vlase, L. (2015) Phenotypic differences in nebivolol metabolism and bioavailability in healthy volunteers. *Clujul Med* **88**, 208–213.

165. Prisant, L. M. (2008) Nebivolol: Pharmacologic profile of an ultraselective, vasodilatory beta1-blocker. *J Clin Pharmacol* **48**, 225–239.

166. Caccia, S., Pasina, L., and Nobili, A. (2012) Critical appraisal of lurasidone in the management of schizophrenia. *Neuropsychiatr Dis Treat* **8**, 155–168.

167. Wenger, G. R. and Rutledge, C. O. (1974) A comparison of the effects of amphetamine and its metabolites, p-hydroxyamphetamine and p-hydroxynorephedrine, on uptake, release and catabolism of 3H-norepinephrine in cerebral cortex of rat brain. *J Pharmacol Exp Ther* **189**, 725–732.

168. Hutson, P. H., Pennick, M., and Secker, R. (2014) Preclinical pharmacokinetics, pharmacology and toxicology of lisdexamfetamine: A novel d-amphetamine pro-drug. *Neuropharmacology* **87**, 41–50.

169. Love, B. L., Barrons, R., Veverka, A., and Snider, K. M. (2010) Urate-lowering therapy for gout: Focus on febuxostat. *Pharmacotherapy* **30**, 594–608.

170. Hawes, B. E., O'Neill K, A., Yao, X., Crona, J. H., Davis, H. R., Jr., Graziano, M. P., and Altmann, S. W. (2007) *In vivo* responsiveness to ezetimibe correlates with niemann-pick C1 like-1 (NPC1L1) binding affinity: Comparison of multiple species NPC1L1 orthologs. *Mol Pharmacol* **71**, 19–29.

171. Evans, D. C., O'Connor, D., Lake, B. G., Evers, R., Allen, C., and Hargreaves, R. (2003) Eletriptan metabolism by human hepatic CYP450 enzymes and transport by human P-glycoprotein. *Drug Metab Dispos* **31**, 861–869.

172. Wu, C. and Kapoor, A. (2013) Dutasteride for the treatment of benign prostatic hyperplasia. *Expert Opin Pharmacother* **14**, 1399–1408.

173. Ebner, T., Wagner, K., and Wienen, W. (2010) Dabigatran acylglucuronide, the major human metabolite of dabigatran: *In vitro* formation, stability, and pharmacological activity. *Drug Metab Dispos* **38**, 1567–1575.

174. Kennedy, J. S., Polinsky, R. J., Johnson, B., Loosen, P., Enz, A., Laplanche, R., Schmidt, D., Mancione, L. C., Parris, W. C., and Ebert, M. H. (1999) Preferential cerebrospinal fluid acetylcholinesterase inhibition by rivastigmine in humans. *J Clin Psychopharmacol* **19**, 513–521.

175. Denissen, J. F., Grabowski, B. A., Johnson, M. K., Buko, A. M., Kempf, D. J., Thomas, S. B., and Surber, B. W. (1997) Metabolism and disposition of the HIV-1 protease inhibitor ritonavir (ABT-538) in rats, dogs, and humans. *Drug Metab Dispos* **25**, 489–501.

176. Brown, S. M., Holtzman, M., Kim, T., and Kharasch, E. D. (2011) Buprenorphine metabolites, buprenorphine-3-glucuronide and norbuprenorphine-3-glucuronide, are biologically active. *Anesthesiology* **115**, 1251–1260.

177. Bakken, G. V., Molden, E., Knutsen, K., Lunder, N., and Hermann, M. (2012) Metabolism of the active metabolite of quetiapine, N-desalkylquetiapine *in vitro*. *Drug Metab Dispos* **40**, 1778–1784.

178. Jensen, N. H., Rodriguiz, R. M., Caron, M. G., Wetsel, W. C., Rothman, R. B., and Roth, B. L. (2008) N-desalkylquetiapine, a potent norepinephrine reuptake inhibitor and partial 5-HT1A agonist, as a putative mediator of quetiapine's antidepressant activity. *Neuropsychopharmacology* **33**, 2303–2312.

179. Yamamoto, T., Tamura, T., Kitawaki, J., Osawa, Y., and Okada, H. (1994) Suicide inactivation of aromatase in human placenta and uterine leiomyoma by 5 alpha-dihydronorethindrone, a metabolite of norethindrone, and its effect on steroid-producing enzymes. *Eur J Endocrinol* **130**, 634–640.

180. Perez-Palacios, G., Cerbon, M. A., Pasapera, A. M., Castro, J. I., Enriquez, J., Vilchis, F., Garcia, G. A., Morali, G., and Lemus, A. E. (1992) Mechanisms of hormonal and antihormonal action of contraceptive progestins at the molecular level. *J Steroid Biochem Mol Biol* **41**, 479–485.

181. Doroshyenko, O. and Fuhr, U. (2009) Clinical pharmacokinetics and pharmacodynamics of solifenacin. *Clin Pharmacokinet* **48**, 281–302.

182. Vickers, S., Duncan, C. A., Chen, I. W., Rosegay, A., and Duggan, D. E. (1990) Metabolic disposition studies on simvastatin, a cholesterol-lowering prodrug. *Drug Metab Dispos* **18**, 138–145.

183. Hyland, R., Roe, E. G., Jones, B. C., and Smith, D. A. (2001) Identification of the cytochrome P450 enzymes involved in the N-demethylation of sildenafil. *Br J Clin Pharmacol* **51**, 239–248.

184. Walker, D. K., Ackland, M. J., James, G. C., Muirhead, G. J., Rance, D. J., Wastall, P., and Wright, P. A. (1999) Pharmacokinetics and metabolism of sildenafil in mouse, rat, rabbit, dog and man. *Xenobiotica* **29**, 297–310.

185. Su, H., Boulton, D. W., Barros, A., Jr., Wang, L., Cao, K., Bonacorsi, S. J., Jr., Iyer, R. A., Humphreys, W. G., and Christopher, L. J. (2012) Characterization of the *in vitro* and *in vivo* metabolism and disposition and cytochrome P450 inhibition/induction profile of saxagliptin in human. *Drug Metab Dispos* **40**, 1345–1356.

186. Fura, A., Khanna, A., Vyas, V., Koplowitz, B., Chang, S. Y., Caporuscio, C., Boulton, D. W. et al. (2009) Pharmacokinetics of the dipeptidyl peptidase 4 inhibitor saxagliptin in rats, dogs, and monkeys and clinical projections. *Drug Metab Dispos* **37**, 1164–1171.

187. Olsson, A. G., McTaggart, F., and Raza, A. (2002) Rosuvastatin: A highly effective new HMG-CoA reductase inhibitor. *Cardiovasc Drug Rev* **20**, 303–328.

25

ADME of Antibody Drug Conjugates

Jiajie Yu, Cinthia Pastuskovas, and Brooke M. Rock

CONTENTS

Introduction: Understanding ADME Properties of ADCs

Antibody drug conjugates (ADCs) represent a relatively new therapeutic modality, mainly focused towards the treatment of cancer. ADCs are monoclonal antibodies with covalently bound cytotoxic drugs. In general terms the ADC is designed to bind to antigens that are overly expressed on cancer cells, but minimally expressed on healthy cells. The targeted delivery and use of highly potent cytotoxic carries the hope of killing the cancer cells with minimal systemic toxicities. The concept of ADCs was first validated in the clinic with gemtuzumab ozogamicin, a conjugate of an anti-CD33 antibody and the cytotoxic agent calicheamicin, and was approved for bone cancer by the FDA in 2000. The product was recently withdrawn from the market after raised safety concerns and its failure to demonstrate benefit to patients. In 2011, Brentuximab vedotin (Adcetris™) was approved for Hodgkin's disease and anaplastic large cell lymphoma. Later that year, ado-trastuzumab emtansine (Kadcyla™) was approved for metastatic HER2 positive breast cancer [1,2].

In general, ADCs are comprised of an IgG antibody conjugated to a drug via a linker. Two distinct classes of linkers are available: cleavable, and non-cleavable. Most cleavable linkers ADCs release the drug from the antibody following internalization of the ADC into the endo-lysosomal pathway where protease recognition, disulfide reduction, or a change in pH leads to linker-drug cleavage [3–5]. Highly potent drugs including monomethyl auristatin E, pyrrolobenzodiazepines, and the maytansinoids often employ cleavable linkers [6–8]. Release of highly potent drugs from cleavable linkers lead to bystander activity, as the released drugs can cross cell membranes of target and non-target cells [5]. Both the ADC itself or the released drug of a cleavable-linker based ADC can contribute to toxicity [9].

ADCs with non-cleavable linkers internalize into cells followed by antibody catabolism in lysosomes to generate amino acid-linker-drug [10–12]. Amino acid-linker-drug catabolites containing maytansine, such as Lysine-MCC-DM1, are transported from the lysosome to the cytoplasm by the lysosomal transporter SLC46A3 [13]. Once the catabolite reaches the cytoplasm the catabolite inhibits tubulin polymerization, which leads to cell death. Lysine-MCC-DM1, the catabolite of non-cleavable linker ADC Ab-MCC-DM1, is significantly less potent in cell-based assays than DM1 itself [14]. Non-cleavable linker ADC potency is derived solely from internalization and production of the catabolite as non-cleavable linker-ADC catabolites do not readily enter cells and therefore do not exhibit bystander activity [5]. The poor cell membrane permeability and lack of metabolism suggest that non-cleavable linker ADC toxicity is primarily due to the ADC, in contrast to cleavable linker ADCs where both the released drug and the ADC itself can mediate the toxicity (Figure 25.1).

The majority of ADCs currently in clinical trials are conjugated to antibody native lysines or cysteines, which generate heterogeneous drug antibody ratio (DAR) profiles [15]. Purified fractions of cleavable monomethyl auristatin E (MMAE) conjugates with different DARs demonstrated that ADC half-life and therapeutic index inversely correlated with DAR [16]. Much of the current focus of ADC optimization is directed toward the generation of homogeneous site-specific ADCs using different techniques such as engineered cysteines, non-natural amino acids, enzymes, or reagents to bridge native disulfides in an attempt to improve therapeutic index [17–23]. Junutula et al. demonstrated that the pharmacokinetic profile and therapeutic index of a site-specific cysteine antibody drug conjugate was superior to a heterogeneous ADC [20].

The promise of ADCs is still rapidly evolving with many ADC drug candidates in preclinical and clinical development stages across the industry. The development of this emerging class of bio-therapeutics has been challenging particular in regard to appropriate bioanalytical techniques, biodistribution studies, and development of PK-PD modeling to inform both safety and efficacy; an overview of these challenges and successes is discussed through the remainder of this chapter.

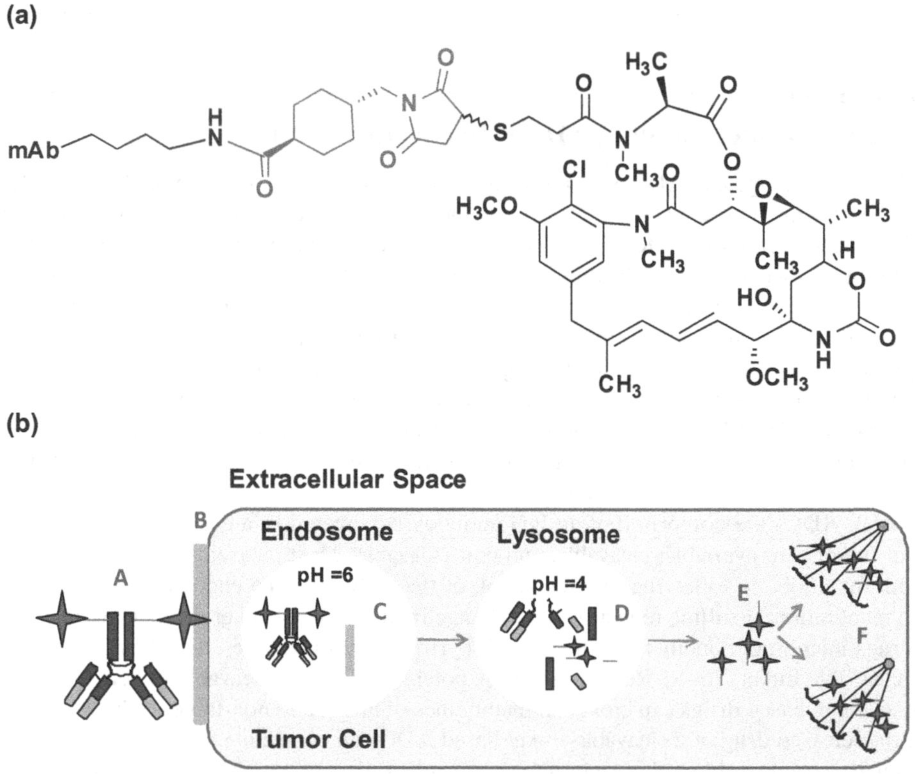

FIGURE 25.1   (a) General structure of non-cleavable antibody maytansiod conjugate. (b) Mechanism of ADC activity where (A) localization of ADC to the tumor cell, (B) binding of ADC to specific antigen, (C) internalization into the endosome release the antigen from ADC, (D) catabolism of ADC in the lysosome, (E) release of Lys-MCC-DM1 into the cytoplasm, and (F) binding of Lys-MCC-DM1to tubulin resulting in cell cycle arrest and apoptosis.

Biodistribution Studies and Analytical Techniques
for Characterization of ADCs

Understanding the kinetics of distribution of ADCs to normal and disease tissues is critical for interpreting the safety and efficacy. Over the past few decades, strategies to accomplish this pre-clinically have been established in the setting of drug discovery and development and have proven instrumental in providing valuable information regarding the mechanism of action, identification of off-target tissues, and kinetics of distribution to tumor relative to normal tissues, as well as providing insight into mechanisms of clearance.

The biodistribution of an ADC is driven by both the biological and biophysical features of the antibody and the small molecule, respectively [24]. In cancer therapy, the antigen binding domain of the antibody is designed to target an epitope uniquely expressed by the tumor, or otherwise with a low expression in healthy tissues, to enable efficient delivery of the conjugated cytotoxic molecule intracellularly following antibody internalization [25,26]. If working properly, systemic exposure to the cytotoxic molecule is minimized. However, the therapeutic window of an ADC can be impacted by partial or full de-conjugation of the linker-drug from the ADC regardless of the linkage type, cleavable and non-cleavable [27–29], poor antibody internalization, and binding of the ADC to normal tissues.

ADC tissue distribution is driven by the targeting properties of the antibody and as such its distribution is led through the lymphatic system resulting in substantial ADC concentrations in the blood and highly vascularized tissues at earlier time points: liver, lungs, heart, and kidneys. As these early concentrations are dependent on blood extravasation through the tissues, concentrations are expected to decrease over time in parallel with the blood kinetic profiles. These observations have demonstrated to be consistent among data reported with different ADCs containing a variety of linkers and cytotoxic drugs [30–34]. However, conjugation of the antibody to the cytotoxic drug, by conventional and/or engineered strategies can impact the properties of the antibody including its overall charge, hydrophobicity, and polarity, which in turn may change the expected ADC tissue distribution. Changes of the antibody molecular charge can have an impact on the antibody distribution phase and clearance (e.g., increases in molecular charge can lead to a faster distribution phase and, therefore, faster clearance relative to those antibodies with lower charge [35]). On the other hand, lowering binding affinity for FcRn can shorten systemic circulation of the antibody and increase catabolism in liver and spleen [36]. Therefore, tissue distribution studies in preclinical models are specifically designed to compare the tissue disposition of the ADC relative to that of the unconjugated antibody.

Methodologies to assess ADC biodistribution have been developed from both the small and large molecule fields to provide information on the distribution and fate of the ADC when in an *in vivo* system. The modalities utilized to evaluate ADC tissue distribution in preclinical models have involved *ex vivo* and *in vivo* methodologies such as the traditional cut and count and autoradiography (i.e., whole-body autoradiography) and micro-positron emission tomography (micro-PET) and single photon emission computed tomography (SPECT), respectively. These approaches require the use of radioactive isotopes to label either the antibody and/or the cytotoxic component of the ADC. Among the most common radioactive probes to label the antibody portion of the ADC are ^{125}I and ^{111}In, where the latter is attached to the antibody via a chelator (tetraxetan [DOTA] or pentetic acid [DTPA]). Based on the physicochemical properties of the radioactive probes, ^{125}I allows measurements of the antibody binding to the cell surface while metal ions such as ^{111}In are retained and accumulate within the cell upon internalization [37,38] ADC distribution can be effectively characterized by using either of these probes independently [30,39,40] or as a mixture to demonstrate ADC distribution to normal tissues relative to antigen and as proof-of-concept of receptor internalization in non-binding species, for the study of antigen-independent distribution, or in xenograft models by comparing tumor uptake of the conjugated versus unconjugated mAb [32,41].

One of these antibody candidates for an ADC was developed against STEAP1, a cell surface antigen overexpressed in prostate cancer with limited expression in normal tissues. Distribution in rats showed no substantial changes in tissue uptake between the unconjugated and conjugated antibody, except a trend for hepatic uptake of the conjugated most likely due to the metabolism of the small molecule (Boswell et al., 2011).

Mandler et al. (2004) provides a good example of the characterization of ADC distribution relative to unconjugated antibody in xenograft models, where tumor specific uptake between Herceptin and H-GA, an ADC consisting of Herceptin conjugated to geldanamycin (GA) was evaluated. In this study, both unconjugated Herceptin and Herceptin in the ADC were labeled with ^{111}In and ^{125}I in order to identify tumor associated internalized and bound fractions, respectively. Data revealed similar tumor uptake suggesting that Herceptin targeting properties were not affected by the linkage chemistry to geldanamycin (GA) (Figure 25.2).

Micro-PET imaging from antibodies labeled with positron zirconium-89 (^{89}Zr) have also been studied in preclinical and clinical settings to obtain non-invasive, real-time data about ADC distribution and tumor targeting. Importantly, the tracking of 89Zr-antibody has been used as a tool to assess antibody internalization and target expression to predict patient response to the ADC version of the antibody [42–45].

Other modalities pertain to non-invasive methodologies, such as fluorescence molecular tomography (FMT), which uses the near infrared (NIR) spectral region (600–900 nm) where the biologic component of the ADC is labeled with a fluorescent dye. Although at the cost of losing resolution, gains such as avoiding the labor-intensive requirements implied on the synthesis of the radiolabeled compounds and the use of a large number of animals have proven to be of advantage. In addition, the ability of assessing multiple fluorophores simultaneously due to the wide spectra has been consider a plus. Examples of this modality used in the context of ADC whole-body biodistribution are reported by Giddabasappa et al. [46], using IRDye 800 CW and fluorophore VivoTag 680XL (VT680), demonstrating no significant differences in biodistribution, PK, or tumor targeting between naked antibody and ADC. A trend to higher tumor accumulation of the signal in the antibody group was hypothesized to be due to the ADC-induced tumor growth inhibition or cell killing. Liver accumulation of the signal in both antibody and ADC groups was attributed to the metabolism of VT680 (Figure 25.3).

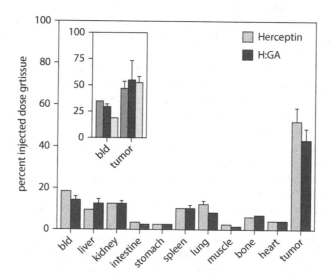

FIGURE 25.2 Tissue distribution of 111In-Herceptin and 111In-Herceptin-GA at 4 days after IV administration in xenografts bearing mice. Tumor uptake between naked and conjugated antibody did not show significant differences (p = 0.077). Inset depict kinetics in blood relative to tumor at 1, 2, and 4 days of 111In-Herceptin-GA administration. (From Mandler, R. et al., *Cancer Res.*, 64, 1460–1467.)

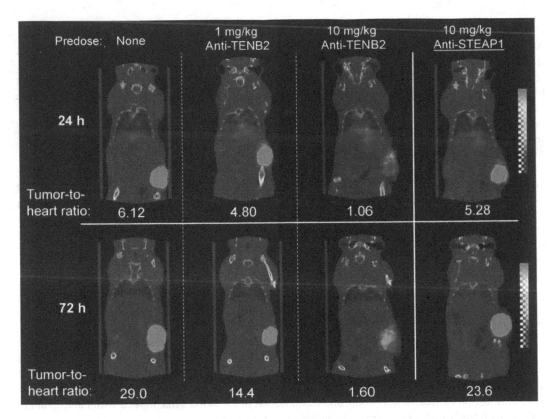

FIGURE 25.3 SPECT/CT fusion images of xenograft bearing mice showing the impact of pre-treatment with 0, 1, or 10 mg/kg of anti-TENB2 or 10 mg/kg of STEAP antibody (control antibody), 24 hrs prior to the intravenous administration of 111In-anti-TENB2-MMAE (3 mg/kg) at 24 or 72 hrs. Pre-treatment with another anti-prostate cancer antibody did not impact tumor uptake of anti-TENB2. Tumor-to-heart ratio increased over time, depicting the increase of anti-TENB2 ADC associated signal in tumor against the decrease in blood and highly perfused organs, i.e., heart. (From Boswell, K.A. et al., *Breast*, 21, 701–706, 2012.)

Relevance of Target Expression in Healthy and Pathological Tissues

Together with the stability of the linker in circulation and the unchanged targeting properties of the mAb due to conjugation, target expression is of particular consideration when selecting an antibody as a candidate for the design of an ADC. Due to the potency of the cytotoxic drug, even low expression of the target in normal tissues may limit the ADC therapeutic window [47]. In order to reduce ADC binding to healthy tissues and to enhance uptake by tumors, it appears possible to pre-block antibody binding to non-target tissues by pre-dosing with unconjugated antibody. This approach has been successfully implemented by radio-immunotherapy in preclinical and clinical studies [48–50], in which saturation of the non-target sites was achieved by pre-dosing of the unconjugated antibody. Hence, identification of target expression in normal tissues does not necessarily prevent achievement of a reasonable therapeutic window. In a case study with an anti-TENB2 antibody directed against another prostate cancer antigen, TENB2, and candidate antibody for an ADC, Boswell et al. 2013 identified normal tissue expression of TENB2. Thus, an unconjugated anti-TENB2 dose-escalation study in mice bearing tumors was performed to select the optimal pre-dose level based on the ability of the antibody to saturate specific binding in normal tissues without hampering 111In-TENB2 ADC tumor uptake and subsequent efficacy (Boswell et al. 2012a). These results are depicted by SPECT/CT (Figure 25.3).

Complementing Biodistribution with ADC Catabolism

ADCs can be catabolized in a variety of ways, depending on their antibody, linker and drug components, thereby releasing distinct species that can contribute to both efficacy and toxicity. Novel technologies are increasingly being applied to better characterize the catabolic fate of the ADC and therefore complement biodistribution data conventionally referred to as "total." Concomitantly, bioanalytical methods, such as immunoassays or LC-MS, have been applied to investigate the concentrations of an ADC as intact, products of catabolism, or identification of relevant metabolites in different biological matrices. Multiple review articles have addressed the complexities of ADC analyte mixtures and the need for multiple and diverse analytical techniques used for characterization.

Studies to characterize the ADME properties of an ADC typically use radioactivity labels such as ^{14}C and ^{3}H on the cytotoxic drug. Case studies of this type where biodistribution is complemented with ADC metabolism and excretion are described by Pastuskovas et al. (2005) and Shen et al. (2012). In the first case, the study was aimed to characterize the tissue distribution, metabolism and route of elimination of Herceptin-Val-Cit-[^{14}C]MMAE after intravenous administration in rats. Tissue distribution was assessed by quantitative whole-body autoradiography showing that ADC followed a distribution similar to that of an antibody in a non-binding species. Persistence of radioactivity in rapidly dividing cells tissues, such as the thymus by day 7, was associated to the cytotoxic drug (Figure 25.4). Overall, tissue distribution data reinforced the understanding of the antibody as the driver of ADC distribution in tissues. These data were complemented with characterization of the ADC biotransformation and it postulated feces as the main route of elimination of the free drug (Figure 25.5).

In addition, Shen et al. (2012) investigated trastuzumab-MCC-[^{3}H]DM1 distribution, metabolism and excretion in rats after intravenous administration. Tissue distribution was evaluated by cut and count and results demonstrated, as shown before, that the ADC distributed non-specifically to highly vascularized tissues, with no evidence of accumulation or retention. These data were complemented by evidences of DM1 elimination by fecal/biliary route and identification of catabolites that agreed with those found in patients with Her2-positive cancer receiving the ADC as treatment.

Diversified bioanalytical assays and considerate biodistribution studies will continue to expand the understanding of ADCs, and the potential to increase therapeutic window to ultimately treat disease as well as inform more accurate PK-PD modeling.

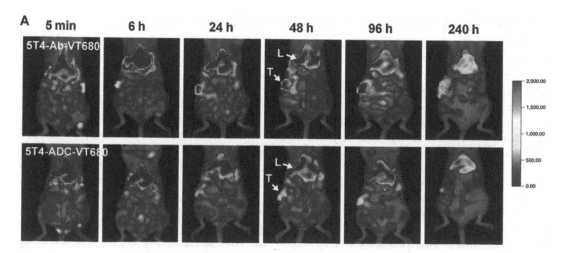

FIGURE 25.4 Whole-body FMT images depicting Tumor targeting and clearance of 5T4-Ab-VT680 and 5T4-ADC-VT680 at different time points after intravenous administration in tumor bearing mice. Arrows show the location of tumor (T) and liver (L). (From Giddabasappa et al., 2016.)

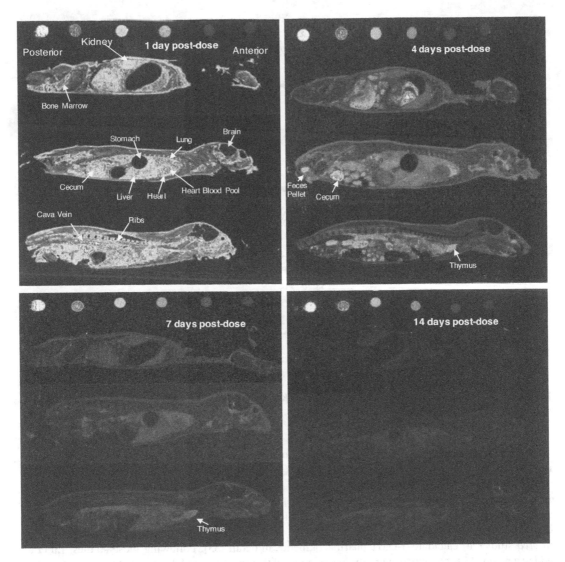

FIGURE 25.5 Representative sagittal autoradiograms at different sectioning levels of a rat showing the distribution of Herceptin-Val-Cit-[^{14}C] MMAE at different time points post-administration of a single dose of the ADC. Heat map depicts radioactivity concentrations. (From Pastuskovas, C.V. et al., *Cancer Res.*, 65, 1195–1196, 2005.)

Utilizing PK-PD Modeling to Inform Efficacy of ADCs

Due to the multi-components of the ADC and its complex disposition at organ and cellular levels, a quantitative understanding and evaluation of the ADC PK-PD relationship are needed in the early stages of development to optimize the ADC design, assess target feasibility, and guide translational studies.

Early attempts of developing PK-PD models for ADCs started with the semi-mechanistic modeling approaches. For example, Jumbe et al. developed a PK-PD model for trastuzumab-DM1 (T-DM1) [51]. In this study, the conventional two-compartment model was used to describe T-DM1 PK and a transit tumor killing model was used to model the efficacy. PK and PD models were sequentially fitted to various mice studies. The final model was used to evaluate the optimal dosing regimen in the clinical study. A similar approach has been used to study the clinically efficacious concentration for an anti-5T4 ADC [52]. Population modeling combining the two-compartment PK model with a transit PD model was also utilized to analyze patient platelet profile in the clinical development [53].

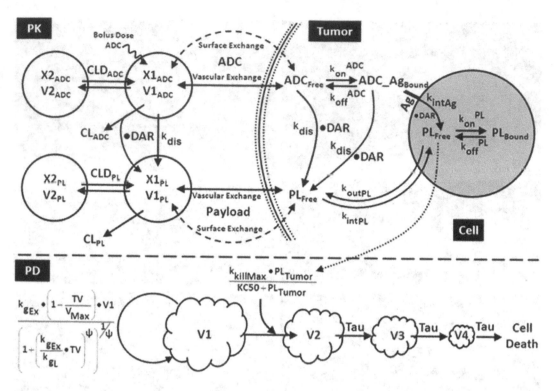

FIGURE 25.6   Model structure diagram of the multiscale PK-PD model developed for predicting ADC clinical outcomes using preclinical measurements.

Chudasama et al. developed a semi-mechanistic population model focused solely on pharmacokinetics to characterize T-DM1 deconjugation [54]. In this model, the pharmacokinetics of individual ADC species with different DAR values were described using the two-compartment model and individual ADC species were connected with first-order deconjugation rates (Figure 25.6). The model was used to explain why T-DM1 had shorter terminal half-life than Trastuzumab™ in clinical studies. Bender et al. later on extended this approach and measured individual DAR moieties in preclinical *in vitro* and *in vivo* studies to elucidate T-DM1 pharmacokinetics in detail [55]. Following these studies, Lu et al. added a payload PK compartment to the existing model that the final model was able to characterize total ADC, conjugated ADC and free payload PK of an anti-CD79b-MMAE ADC in the preclinical study [56]. Sukumanran et al. correlated the clearance of individual DAR moieties with its DAR values and investigated the impact of conjugation-site dependent payload deconjugation on PK and the tumor killing efficacy [57]. The same group also applied the similar modeling approach for predicting human PK of an anti-STEAP1-vc-MMAE ADC [58].

More mechanistic models were also developed with increasing model complexity. Shah et al. developed a multiscale model by modeling ADC and free payload physiological disposition separately [59]. In this study, the ADC and free payload disposition were modeled at tissue and cellular levels (Figure 25.7). While the two-compartment model was used to fit the plasma PK of both ADC and free payload, a published tumor disposition model [60,61] was adapted to describe ADC and free payload transport between plasma and tumor. At the tumor cellular level, the ADC binding to antigen, bound ADC internalization, free payload transport, and free payload binding with cellular target were also considered. The total tumor payload concentration was linked to a transit tumor killing model for modeling efficacy. The final PK-PD model was used to predict clinical progression free survival rates and complete response rates for Brentuximab-vedotin as well as the tumor concentration of ADC and free payload for the anti-5T4 ADC [59,62]. Later on, the same model was used to predict clinical responses of Inotuzumab ozogamicin [63]. Additional efforts have been made to integrate more cellular disposition mechanisms into the model [64].

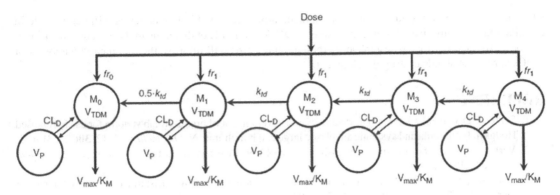

FIGURE 25.7 Model structure diagram a semi-mechanistic with the consideration of individual ADC species with different DAR values.

The target-mediated drug disposition (TMDD) model, which has been frequently used for characterizing antibody non-linear PK [65], was also being adapted to describe PK of ADCs. Gibiansky et al. applied the TMDD modeling approach to individual DAR species of the ADC [66]. In this study, payload deconjugation was assumed to occur only in the central compartment. Individual DAR species were assumed to have same distribution parameters and target binding kinetics, while the non-specific clearance and payload deconjugation rate of individual DAR species were allowed to be different. The general TMDD model has also been simplified with quassi-equilibrium, quassi-steady-state and Michaelis–Menten approximations in order to improve the parameter identifiability and estimation precision.

Whole-body physiologically based pharmacokinetic (PBPK) models have been frequently used to characterize tissue specific toxicity and PD at the site of action for both small molecule and monoclonal antibodies [67,68]. Developing whole-body PBPK model for ADC is more complicated since the disposition of intact ADC, free antibody and free freeload all would need to be considered. While it is challenging, Cilliers et al. developed a multiscale PBPK model to describe ADC disposition at tissue and cellular levels. In this study, a published PBPK model was combined with the aforementioned tumor disposition model and *in vivo* biodistribution studies were performed to validate model. The model was used to study the tumor penetration of the T-DM1 ADC and suggested that when free payload is potent enough, lowing the DAR of the ADC or co-administration of a monoclonal antibody that competes the same target with the ADC may improve the ADC tumor penetration hence potentially improve the efficacy [69]. Interestingly, a minimal PBPK model with reduced model complexity that describe both ADC and free payload PK was also developed based on the commercially available software Simcyp® to assess DDI risks of the free payload [70].

Overall, PK-PD modeling of ADCs is still a relatively new field and requires understanding of both monoclonal antibodies and small molecular payloads physiological disposition. It is unlikely that a one-size-fits-all modeling strategy would be developed. The choice of model needs to be determined based on the purpose of the study, data availability, and understanding of the physiology. The "right" model could be very helpful for optimizing ADC design, evaluating target, identifying key issues, and guiding the preclinical and clinical developments.

Conclusions

Antibody-drug conjugates are targeted therapeutic conjugates that employ antibodies for its specificity and long half-life, and small molecules for their cytotoxic effect. Even though ADCs have been investigated for decades, there are numerous knowledge gaps in understanding the relationship between selective delivery and toxicity. For example, the optimum difference in the expression of target required between the tumor and normal tissues for a better therapeutic index of an ADC is unknown.

Utilizing biodistribution studies along with implementing accurate PK-PD modeling will begin to aid in establishing a quantitative relationship between ADC dose and PK of different analytes in plasma, tumor, and other tissues. Ultimately, establishing these relationships will improve the therapeutic outcomes of ADCs across the stages of drug development.

REFERENCES

1. Senter, P.D. and E.L. Sievers, The discovery and development of brentuximab vedotin for use in relapsed Hodgkin lymphoma and systemic anaplastic large cell lymphoma. *Nat Biotechnol*, 2012. **30**(7): 631–637.
2. Verma, S. et al., Trastuzumab emtansine for HER2-positive advanced breast cancer. *N Engl J Med*, 2012. **367**(19): 1783–1791.
3. Doronina, S.O. et al., Development of potent monoclonal antibody auristatin conjugates for cancer therapy. *Nat Biotechnol*, 2003. **21**(7): 778–784.
4. Hamann, P.R. et al., Gemtuzumab ozogamicin, a potent and selective anti-CD33 antibody-calicheamicin conjugate for treatment of acute myeloid leukemia. *Bioconjug Chem*, 2002. **13**(1): 47–58.
5. Kovtun, Y.V. et al., Antibody-drug conjugates designed to eradicate tumors with homogeneous and heterogeneous expression of the target antigen. *Cancer Res*, 2006. **66**(6): 3214–3221.
6. Kung Sutherland, M.S. et al., SGN-CD33A: A novel CD33-targeting antibody-drug conjugate using a pyrrolobenzodiazepine dimer is active in models of drug-resistant AML. *Blood*, 2013. **122**(8): 1455–1463.
7. Li, D. et al., DCDT2980S, an anti-CD22-monomethyl auristatin E antibody-drug conjugate, is a potential treatment for non-Hodgkin lymphoma. *Mol Cancer Ther*, 2013. **12**(7): 1255–1265.
8. Widdison, W.C. et al., Semisynthetic maytansine analogues for the targeted treatment of cancer. *J Med Chem*, 2006. **49**(14): 4392–4408.
9. Polakis, P., Antibody drug conjugates for cancer therapy. *Pharmacol Rev*, 2016. **68**(1): 3–19.
10. Doronina, S.O. et al., Enhanced activity of monomethylauristatin F through monoclonal antibody delivery: Effects of linker technology on efficacy and toxicity. *Bioconjug Chem*, 2006. **17**(1): 114–124.
11. Erickson, H.K. et al., Antibody-maytansinoid conjugates are activated in targeted cancer cells by lysosomal degradation and linker-dependent intracellular processing. *Cancer Res*, 2006. **66**(8): 4426–4433.
12. Rock, B.M. et al., Intracellular catabolism of an antibody drug conjugate with a noncleavable linker. *Drug Metab Dispos*, 2015. **43**(9): 1341–1344.
13. Hamblett, K.J. et al., SLC46A3 is required to transport catabolites of noncleavable antibody maytansine conjugates from the lysosome to the cytoplasm. *Cancer Res*, 2015. **75**(24): 5329–5340.
14. Junttila, T.T. et al., Trastuzumab-DM1 (T-DM1) retains all the mechanisms of action of trastuzumab and efficiently inhibits growth of lapatinib insensitive breast cancer. *Breast Cancer Res Treat*, 2011. **128**(2): 347–356.
15. Sassoon, I. and V. Blanc, Antibody-drug conjugate (ADC) clinical pipeline: A review. *Methods Mol Biol*, 2013. **1045**: 1–27.
16. Hamblett, K.J. et al., Effects of drug loading on the antitumor activity of a monoclonal antibody drug conjugate. *Clin Cancer Res*, 2004. **10**(20): 7063–7070.
17. Badescu, G. et al., Bridging disulfides for stable and defined antibody drug conjugates. *Bioconjug Chem*, 2014. **25**(6): 1124–1136.
18. Drake, P.M. et al., Aldehyde tag coupled with HIPS chemistry enables the production of ADCs conjugated site-specifically to different antibody regions with distinct *in vivo* efficacy and PK outcomes. *Bioconjug Chem*, 2014. **25**(7): 1331–1341.
19. Jeffrey, S.C. et al., A potent anti-CD70 antibody-drug conjugate combining a dimeric pyrrolobenzodiazepine drug with site-specific conjugation technology. *Bioconjug Chem*, 2013. **24**(7): 1256–1263.
20. Junutula, J.R. et al., Site-specific conjugation of a cytotoxic drug to an antibody improves the therapeutic index. *Nat Biotechnol*, 2008. **26**(8): 925–932.
21. Panowksi, S. et al., Site-specific antibody drug conjugates for cancer therapy. *MAbs*, 2014. **6**(1): 34–45.
22. Tian, F. et al., A general approach to site-specific antibody drug conjugates. *Proc Natl Acad Sci USA*, 2014. **111**(5): 1766–1771.

23. Zimmerman, E.S. et al., Production of site-specific antibody-drug conjugates using optimized non-natural amino acids in a cell-free expression system. *Bioconjug Chem*, 2014. **25**(2): 351–361.

24. Schmidt, M.M. and K.D. Wittrup, A modeling analysis of the effects of molecular size and binding affinity on tumor targeting. *Mol Cancer Ther*, 2009. **8**(10): 2861–2871.

25. Garnett, M.R. et al., Altered cellular metabolism following traumatic brain injury: A magnetic resonance spectroscopy study. *J Neurotrauma*, 2001. **18**(3): 231–240.

26. Chari, R.V., Targeted delivery of chemotherapeutics: Tumor-activated prodrug therapy. *Adv Drug Deliv Rev*, 1998. **31**(1–2): 89–104.

27. Sanderson, R.J. et al., *In vivo* drug-linker stability of an anti-CD30 dipeptide-linked auristatin immunoconjugate. *Clin Cancer Res*, 2005. **11**(2 Pt 1): 843–852.

28. Ducry, L. and B. Stump, Antibody-drug conjugates: Linking cytotoxic payloads to monoclonal antibodies. *Bioconjug Chem*, 2010. **21**(1): 5–13.

29. Erickson, H.K. et al., Tumor delivery and *in vivo* processing of disulfide-linked and thioether-linked antibody-maytansinoid conjugates. *Bioconjug Chem*, 2010. **21**(1): 84–92.

30. Pastuskovas, C.V. et al., Tissue distribution, metabolism, and excretion of the antibody-drug conjugate Herceptin-monomethyl auristatin E in rats. *Cancer Res*, 2005. **65**(9 Supplement): 1195–1196.

31. Shen, B.Q. et al., Catabolic fate and pharmacokinetic characterization of trastuzumab emtansine (T-DM1): An emphasis on preclinical and clinical catabolism. *Curr Drug Metab*, 2012. **13**(7): 901–910.

32. Boswell, C.A. et al., An integrated approach to identify normal tissue expression of targets for antibody-drug conjugates: Case study of TENB2. *Br J Pharmacol*, 2013. **168**(2): 445–457.

33. Boswell, C.A. et al., Differential effects of predosing on tumor and tissue uptake of an 111In-labeled anti-TENB2 antibody-drug conjugate. *J Nucl Med*, 2012a. **53**(9): 1454–1461.

34. Han, T.H. and B. Zhao, Absorption, distribution, metabolism, and excretion considerations for the development of antibody-drug conjugates. *Drug Metab Dispos*, 2014. **42**(11): 1914–1920.

35. Li, B. et al., Framework selection can influence pharmacokinetics of a humanized therapeutic antibody through differences in molecule charge. *MAbs*, 2014. **6**(5): 1255–1264.

36. Yip, V. et al., Quantitative cumulative biodistribution of antibodies in mice: Effect of modulating binding affinity to the neonatal Fc receptor. *MAbs*, 2014. **6**(3): 689–696.

37. Naruki, Y. et al., Differential cellular catabolism of 111In, 90Y and 125I radiolabeled T101 anti-CD5 monoclonal antibody. *Int J Rad Appl Instrum B*, 1990. **17**(2): 201–207.

38. Kobayashi, H. et al., Pharmacokinetics of 111In- and 125I-labeled antiTac single-chain Fv recombinant immunotoxin. *J Nucl Med*, 2000. **41**(4): 755–762.

39. Boswell, C.A. et al., Impact of drug conjugation on pharmacokinetics and tissue distribution of anti-STEAP1 antibody-drug conjugates in rats. *Bioconjug Chem*, 2011. **22**(10): 1994–2004.

40. Boswell, K.A. et al., Disease burden and treatment outcomes in second-line therapy of patients with estrogen receptor-positive (ER+) advanced breast cancer: A review of the literature. *Breast*, 2012b. **21**(6): 701–706.

41. Mandler, R. et al., Herceptin-geldanamycin immunoconjugates: Pharmacokinetics, biodistribution, and enhanced antitumor activity. *Cancer Res*, 2004. **64**(4): 1460–1467.

42. Doran, M.G. et al., Annotating STEAP1 regulation in prostate cancer with 89Zr immuno-PET. *J Nucl Med*, 2014. **55**(12): 2045–2049. doi:10.2967/jnumed.114.145185.

43. Gebhart, G. et al., Molecular imaging as a tool to investigate heterogeneity of advanced HER2-positive breast cancer and to predict patient outcome under trastuzumab emtansine (T-DM1): The ZEPHIR trial. *Ann Oncol*, 2016. **27**(4): 619–624. doi:10.1093/annonc/mdv577.

44. Weekes, C.D. et al., A phase I study of the human monoclonal anti-NRP1 antibody MNRP1685A in patients with advanced solid tumors. *Invest New Drugs*, 2014. **32**(4): 653–660. doi:10.1007/s10637-014-0071-z.

45. ter Weele, E.J. et al., Imaging the distribution of an antibody-drug conjugate constituent targeting mesothelin with 89Zr and IRDye 800CW in mice bearing human pancreatic tumor xenografts. *Oncotarget*. 2015. **6**(39): 42081–42090. doi:10.18632/oncotarget.5877..

46. Giddabasappa, A. et al., Biodistribution and targeting of anti-5T4 antibody-drug conjugate using fluorescence molecular tomography. *Mol Cancer Ther*, 2016. **15**(10): 2530–2540.

47. Tijink, B.M. et al., A phase I dose escalation study with anti-CD44v6 bivatuzumab mertansine in patients with incurable squamous cell carcinoma of the head and neck or esophagus. *Clin Cancer Res*, 2006. **12**(20 Pt 1): 6064–6072.

48. Buchsbaum, D.J. et al., Therapy with unlabeled and 131I-labeled pan-B-cell monoclonal antibodies in nude mice bearing Raji Burkitt's lymphoma xenografts. *Cancer Res*, 1992. **52**(23): 6476–6481.

49. Blumenthal, R.D. et al., Tumor-specific dose scheduling of bimodal radioimmunotherapy and chemotherapy. *Anticancer Res*, 2003. **23**(6C): 4613–4619.

50. Kletting, P. et al., Potential of optimal preloading in anti-CD20 antibody radioimmunotherapy: an investigation based on pharmacokinetic modeling. *Cancer Biother Radiopharm*, 2010. **25**(3): 279–287. doi:10.1089/cbr.2009.0746.

51. Jumbe, N.L. et al., Modeling the efficacy of trastuzumab-DM1, an antibody drug conjugate, in mice. *J Pharmacokinet Pharmacodyn*, 2010. **37**(3): 221–242.

52. Haddish-Berhane, N. et al., On translation of antibody drug conjugates efficacy from mouse experimental tumors to the clinic: A PK/PD approach. *J Pharmacokinet Pharmacodyn*, 2013. **40**(5): 557–571.

53. Bender, B.C. et al., A population pharmacokinetic/pharmacodynamic model of thrombocytopenia characterizing the effect of trastuzumab emtansine (T-DM1) on platelet counts in patients with HER2-positive metastatic breast cancer. *Cancer Chemother Pharmacol*, 2012. **70**(4): 591–601.

54. Chudasama, V.L. et al., Semi-mechanistic population pharmacokinetic model of multivalent trastuzumab emtansine in patients with metastatic breast cancer. *Clin Pharmacol Ther*, 2012. **92**(4): 520–527.

55. Bender, B. et al., A mechanistic pharmacokinetic model elucidating the disposition of trastuzumab emtansine (T-DM1), an antibody–drug conjugate (ADC) for treatment of metastatic breast cancer. *AAPS J*, 2014. **16**(5): 994–1008.

56. Lu, D. et al., Semi-mechanistic multiple-analyte pharmacokinetic model for an antibody-drug-conjugate in cynomolgus monkeys. *Pharm Res*, 2015. **32**(6): 1907–1919.

57. Sukumaran, S. et al., Mechanism-based pharmacokinetic/pharmacodynamic model for THIOMAB™ drug conjugates. *Pharm Res*, 2015. **32**(6): 1884–1893.

58. Sukumaran, S. et al., Development and translational application of an integrated, mechanistic model of antibody-drug conjugate pharmacokinetics. *AAPS J*, 2016: 1–11.

59. Shah, D.K., N. Haddish-Berhane, and A. Betts, Bench to bedside translation of antibody drug conjugates using a multiscale mechanistic PK/PD model: A case study with brentuximab-vedotin. *J Pharmacokinet Pharmacodyn*, 2012. **39**(6): 643–659.

60. Thurber, G.M., M.M. Schmidt, and K.D. Wittrup, Factors determining antibody distribution in tumors. *Trends Pharmacol Sci*, 2008. **29**(2): 57–61.

61. Thurber, G.M., S.C. Zajic, and K.D. Wittrup, Theoretic criteria for antibody penetration into solid tumors and micrometastases. *J Nucl Med*, 2007. **48**(6): 995–999.

62. Shah, D.K. et al., A priori prediction of tumor payload concentrations: Preclinical case study with an Auristatin-based anti-5T4 antibody-drug conjugate. *AAPS J*, 2014. **16**(3): 452–463.

63. Betts, A.M. et al., Preclinical to clinical translation of antibody-drug conjugates using PK/PD modeling: A retrospective analysis of inotuzumab ozogamicin. *AAPS J*, 2016. **18**(5): 1101–1116.

64. Singh, A.P. et al., Evolution of antibody-drug conjugate tumor disposition model to predict preclinical tumor pharmacokinetics of trastuzumab-emtansine (T-DM1). *AAPS J*, 2016. **18**(4): 861–875.

65. Dua, P., E. Hawkins, and P.H. van der Graaf, A tutorial on target-mediated drug disposition (TMDD) models. *Pharmacometrics Syst Pharmacol*, 2015. **4**(6): 324–337.

66. Gibiansky, L. and E. Gibiansky, Target-mediated drug disposition model and its approximations for antibody–drug conjugates. *J Pharmacokinet Pharmacodyn*, 2014. **41**(1): 35–47.

67. Lipscomb, J.C. et al., Physiologically-Based Pharmacokinetic (PBPK) Models in Toxicity Testing and Risk Assessment, in *New Technologies for Toxicity Testing*, M. Balls, R.D. Combes, and N. Bhogal, (Eds.). 2012, Springer: New York. pp. 76–95.

68. Shah, D.K. and A.M. Betts, Towards a platform PBPK model to characterize the plasma and tissue disposition of monoclonal antibodies in preclinical species and human. *J Pharmacokinet Pharmacodyn*, 2012. **39**(1): 67–86.

69. Cilliers, C. et al., Multiscale modeling of antibody-drug conjugates: Connecting tissue and cellular distribution to whole animal pharmacokinetics and potential implications for efficacy. *AAPS J*, 2016. **18**(5): 1117–1130.

70. Chen, Y. et al., Physiologically based pharmacokinetic modeling as a tool to predict drug interactions for antibody-drug conjugates. *Clin Pharmacokinet*, 2015. **54**(1): 81–93.

26

Managing Reactive Metabolites in Drug Discovery and Development

Amit S. Kalgutkar

CONTENTS

Introduction

The biotransformation of relatively innocuous chemicals to electrophilic reactive metabolites (RMs), commonly referred to as bioactivation, is viewed as an unfavorable feature in drug candidates given the propensity of RMs to covalently modify of DNA resulting in genotoxicity (Dobo et al., 2009) and/or inactivate cytochrome P450 (CYP) isoform(s) leading to clinical drug–drug interactions (DDIs) (Orr et al., 2012). In addition, it is now widely accepted that the generation of an RM is an obligatory step in the pathogenesis of some idiosyncratic adverse drug reactions (IADRs) (Guengerich and MacDonald, 2007; Li and Uetrecht, 2010; Uetrecht, 2008). IADRs can manifest as rare and sometimes life-threatening reactions (e.g., drug-induced liver injury [DILI], skin rashes, and blood dyscracias) in drug-treated patients that cannot be explained by the primary pharmacology of the drug. For instance, nefazodone is used to treat depression but can cause DILI (Kalgutkar et al., 2005a). Many IADRs are immune mediated and occur in very low frequency (1 in 10,000 or 1 in 100,000) in a small subset of patients either acutely or as a delayed response. IADRs, by definition, are difficult to reproduce in the human population and there are few, if any, generally applicable animal models for examining these toxicities in preclinical discovery/development (Uetrecht, 2006). Consequently, these reactions are often not detected until the drug has gained broad exposure in a large patient population. Amongst all IADRs, DILI remains a leading cause of acute hepatic failure and a major reason for withdrawal of marketed therapeutic agents (Leise et al., 2014).

The underlying mechanisms of IADRs remain unclear. However, it is believed that the vast majority are caused by immunogenic conjugates formed via the covalent interaction of an RM with cellular proteins resulting in direct cellular dysfunction or an immune response via the formation of a hapten (Uetrecht and Naisbitt, 2013). The observations that certain IADRs (e.g., hypersensitivity associated with the antiretroviral agent abacavir) are linked to specific human leukocyte antigen (HLA) genes provide compelling evidence for the immune-mediated component of these toxicities (Ogese et al., 2016). As such, the link between RM formation and drug toxicity was first demonstrated in studies on the hepatotoxic anti-inflammatory agent acetaminophen. Mechanistic studies, which established the CYP-mediated oxidation of the *p*-hydroxyacetanilide moiety in acetaminophen to a reactive quinone-imine species, which can cause hepatotoxicity via depletion of endogenous glutathione (GSH) pools and/or covalent binding to hepatic proteins, have served as a gold standard for drug toxicity assessment over the decades (Park et al., 2005).

Screening for Reactive Metabolites in Preclinical Discovery

Predicting the IADR potential of new drug candidates is practically difficult, if not impossible. Under the basic premise that a drug candidate devoid of RM formation could mitigate IADR risks, proto-cols have been implemented by pharmaceutical companies to evaluate RM formation potential of new chemical entities (NCEs) with the goal of minimizing or eliminating the liability by rational structural modifications on the NCE (Argikar et al., 2011; Kalgutkar and Dalvie, 2015; Park et al., 2011; Prakash et al., 2008; Stachulski et al., 2013; Thompson et al., 2012, 2016). Tactics to evaluate the generation of RMs via oxidative metabolism of NCEs has been previously reviewed (Evans et al., 2004); incubation of the radiolabeled (^{14}C or ^{3}H-labeled) NCE with NADPH-supplemented human liver microsomes and/or human hepatocytes followed by quantification of the amount of un-extractable radioactivity (presumably due to covalent binding of the electrophilic RM to hepatic proteins) constitute prototypic methods. Lack of availability of radiolabeled material particularly in early preclinical discovery, however, precludes routine application of this method for screening vast numbers of NCEs. A more convenient solution, which is also flexible to a high-throughput screening format, is the implementation of assays in which nucleophilic trapping reagents are included in NADPH-supplemented liver microsomal incubations with NCEs, and the trapped electrophiles (RM-nucleophile adducts) are detected using liquid chromatography tandem mass spectrometry (LC/MSMS) (Argoti et al., 2005; Ma and Subramanian, 2006). Soft elec-trophiles (e.g., epoxides, quinones, quinone-imines, quinone-methides, etc.) generated via the oxidative bioactivation of phenyl, phenolic, amino-, and alkylphenolic substituents can be trapped with nucleo-philes of comparable softness (e.g., GSH or cysteine) in RM screens. In contrast, hard nucleophiles such as cyanide and amines (e.g., semicarbazide or methoxylamine) are frequently utilized to trap hard elec-trophiles (e.g., iminiums and aldehydes) that result from the oxidative bioactivation of cyclic (or acylic) amines and primary alcohols (Kalgutkar, 2005b, 2017). In some instances, soft sulfydryl nucleophiles (e.g., GSH and cysteine) have also been utilized to trap aldehydes to yield cyclized thiazolidine adducts (Inoue et al., 2015; Lenz et al., 2014).

Excluding Toxicophores in Drug Design

Besides the implementation of RM screens, exclusion of certain functional groups (referred to as structural alerts or toxicophores) that are either intrinsically electrophilic or are known to undergo enzyme-catalyzed bioactivation to RMs is a standard *modus operandi* in modern medicinal chemistry. The categorization of functional groups as toxicophores (Kalgutkar et al., 2005b) has originated from numerous mechanistic studies on pathways leading to RM formation with drugs associated with idio-syncratic toxicity (associated with a black box warning (BBW) or recalled from commercial use). Out of 68 drugs recalled or associated with a BBW for idiosyncratic toxicity, 55 (80.8%) contained one or more toxicophores, and evidence for RM formation (characterization of stable adducts with nucleo-philes and/or covalent binding to target organ tissue (e.g., liver microsomes)) is available for 36 out of the 55 drugs (65%) (Stepan et al., 2011). In this meta-analysis, the aniline/anilide motif emerged as a prominent toxicophore, which was present in more than half of the toxic drugs (Kalgutkar, 2015; Stepan et al., 2011). Amongst all known toxicophores, the aniline/anilide motif is perhaps most notorious for its association with mutagenicity, direct organ toxicity, methemoglobinemia, and immunogenic allergenic toxicity (Shamovsky et al., 2012). Bioactivation pathways of the aniline/ anilide motif leading to RMs have been previously reviewed (Kalgutkar, 2015).

A persuasive argument for chemotype driven toxicity also becomes evident from structure-activity relationship (SAR) studies, wherein absence of RM liability is consistent with the improved safety profile of successor drugs (Kalgutkar, 2011; Kalgutkar and Didiuk, 2009; Stepan et al., 2011). For instance, the high incidence of agranulocytosis and hepatotoxicity noted with clozapine use in the clinic is rarely encountered with the structural analogs quetiapine and loxapine. *In vitro*, clozapine undergoes oxidative bioactivation on its dibenzodiazepine ring via the action of myeloperoxidase (MPO) enzyme to afford a reactive iminium ion **1**, which covalently binds to target tissue (e.g., human neutrophils) and GSH to yield adduct **2** (Figure 26.1) (Gardner et al., 1998; Liu and Uetrecht, 1995). Proteins covalently modified with clozapine have been detected in neutrophils of patients being treated with the drug, which reaffirms the relevance of the *in vitro* studies (Gardner et al., 1998). In the case of quetiapine and loxapine, the bridging nitrogen atom is replaced with a sulfur or oxygen atom (Figure 26.1). Consequently, these drugs cannot form a reactive iminium species (Uetrecht et al., 1997). Although anecdotal for the most part, such structure-toxicity relationships suggest that avoiding toxicophores in drug design would yield small molecule therapeutics potentially devoid of IADRs.

There are several shortcomings on the application of the toxicophore concept in drug design. First and perhaps most importantly, there is no clear distinction as to when a particular functional motif is viewed as a toxicophore. This is because toxicophores are divided into a simple binary categorization; ones that form RMs versus all other functional groups. The vast majority of marketed medicinal agents possess a phenyl ring, which is a toxicophore. Oxidative metabolism of the phenyl ring to the corresponding phenol metabolite by CYP enzymes proceeds through a reactive epoxide intermediate, which can be trapped with GSH (Kalgutkar et al., 2005b; Stepan et al., 2011). It is essentially impossible to remove simple aryl rings from the collection of organic functional groups in drug design, and mankind would be deprived of myriad useful drugs if compounds containing a phenyl ring were suspended from development because a phenyl ring is considered to be a toxicophore.

Second, since the categorization of toxicophores is knowledge-based, it is not possible to avoid as yet unknown structures that can form RMs. For example, the mechanism for RM formation with the anticonvulsant felbamate, which is associated with aplastic anemia and hepatotoxicity, involves the formation of the electrophilic α,β-unsaturated aldehyde 2-phenylpropenal (**3**) via an atypical bioactivation pathway

IADRs: agranulocytosis, hepatotoxicity

(Quetiapine, loxapine are not associated with the IADRs noted with clozapine)

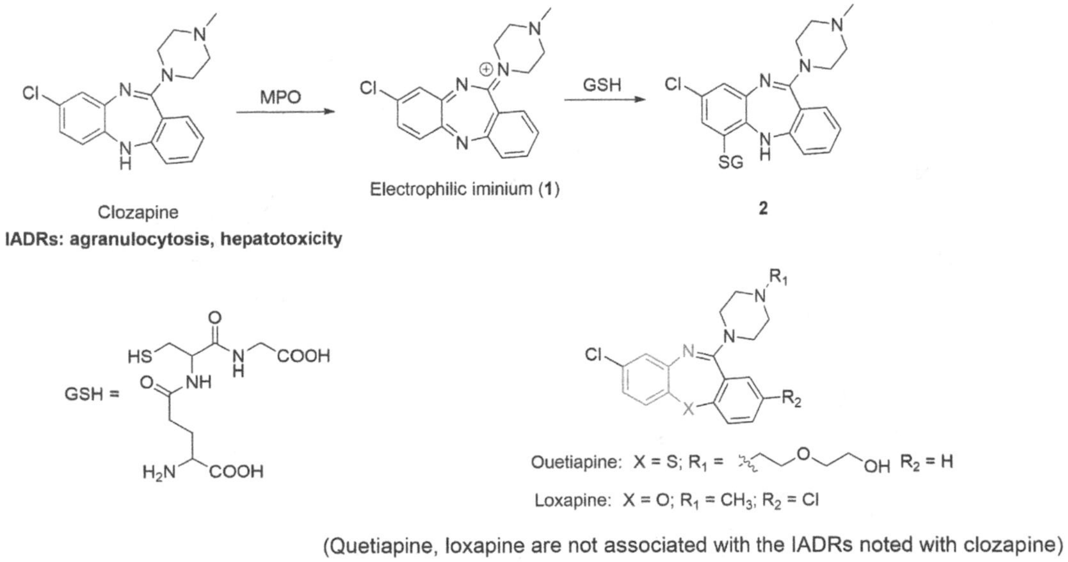

FIGURE 26.1 Structure-toxicity relationships for dibenzodiazepine class of antipsychotic agents—Clozapine versus loxapine and quetiapine.

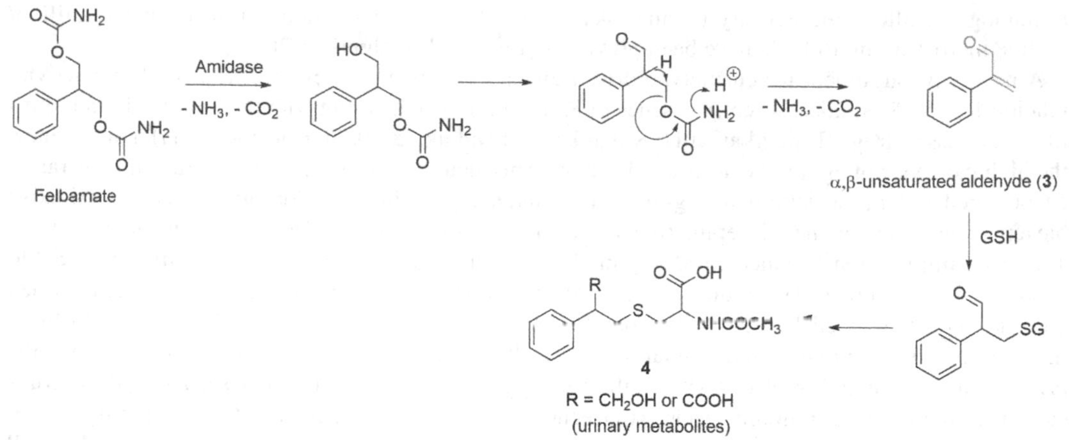

FIGURE 26.2 Bioactivation of the anticonvulsant felbamate to a reactive α,β-unsaturated aldehyde **3**.

shown in Figure 26.2 (Dieckhaus et al., 2002). Evidence for the occurrence of this pathway *in vivo* has been demonstrated via the characterization of urinary mercapturic acid conjugates (e.g., adduct **4**) following felbamate administration to humans (Thompson et al., 1999). As seen in Figure 26.2, felbamate is devoid of prototypic toxicophores. The enzyme(s) responsible for felbamate bioactivation in humans remain to be characterized.

Finally, not all toxicophores will be necessarily bioactivated to RMs. The selective direct factor Xa inhibitors and anticoagulants apixaban and rivaroxaban (Figure 26.3) contain toxicophores (*p*-methoxyaniline and *bis*-anilide motifs in apixaban; chlorothiophene and *bis*-anilide motifs in rivaroxaban). Human mass balance studies using ^{14}C radiolabeled apixaban and rivaroxaban reveal that the toxicophores in apixaban and rivaroxaban are not prone to metabolism, thus negating the possibility of RM formation (Weinz et al., 2009; Zhang et al., 2009). In the case of rivaroxaban, the pendant chlorothiophene motif is essential for pharmacology and cannot be replaced. The aniline toxicophore is also

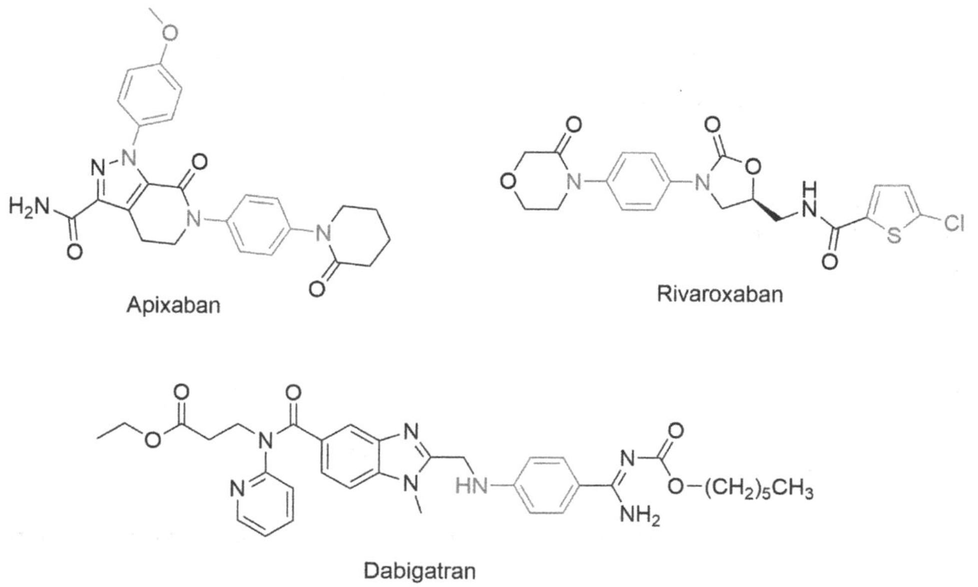

FIGURE 26.3 Anticoagulants apixaban, rivaroxaban, and dabigatran possess toxicophores but do not form RMs.

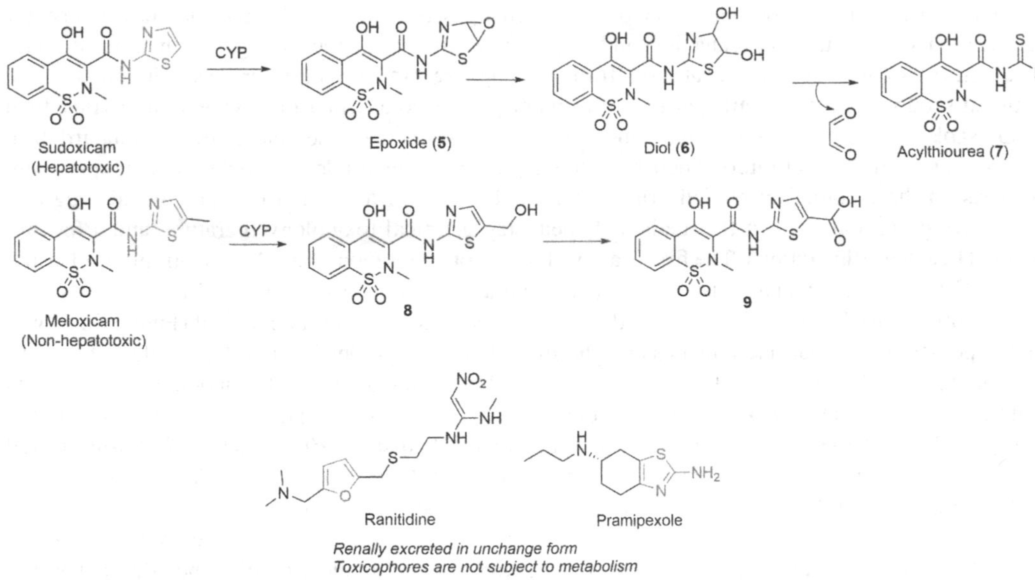

FIGURE 26.4 Examples of drugs that contain toxicophores but do not form RMs.

present in the oral direct thrombin inhibitor dabigatran (see Figure 26.3). However, dabigatran is not subject to oxidative metabolism by CYP enzymes in humans (Stangier, 2008).

The likelihood of RM formation will depend on the binding pose of the NCE in the catalytic active site of the metabolizing enzyme (e.g., CYP) and subsequent positioning of the toxicophore towards the catalytic center to yield an RM. Thus, it is entirely possible that metabolism could potentially occur at a region distinct from the toxicophore and lead to non-reactive products as metabolites. For instance, the 2-aminothiazole toxicophore is present in the enol-carboxamide class of non-steroidal anti-inflammatory drugs sudoxicam and meloxicam, but only sudoxicam is oxidized by CYP enzyme(s) to the reactive acylthiourea intermediate **7** via the epoxide and diol intermediate **5** and **6**, respectively (Figure 26.4). The acylthiourea **7** appears to be responsible for sudoxicam hepatoxicity (Obach et al., 2008a). Although introduction of a methyl group at the C-5 position on the thiazole ring in meloxicam is the only structural difference, the change dramatically alters the metabolic profile. Oxidation of the *C*-5 methyl group to the alcohol **8** and carboxylic acid **9** metabolites constitutes the major metabolic fate of meloxicam in humans (Figure 26.4) (Davies and Skjodt, 1999). Additionally, elimination mechanisms other than metabolism could be a principal mitigating factor with regards to bioactivation. For example, ranitidine and pramipexole (Figure 26.4) are primarily eliminated by urinary excretion in unchanged parent form (Bell et al., 1980; Diao et al., 2010) and no evidence for bioactivation to RMs has been deciphered on the furan and 2-aminothiazole toxicophores present in these drugs. It is noteworthy to point out that ranitidine and pramipexole are marketed agents for the treatment of peptic ulcers and Parkinson's disease, and are generally devoid of IADRs.

Elimination of RM Liability in Preclinical Drug Discovery

While toxicophores must be used with caution particularly at the chemical lead optimization stage, it is pivotal to experimentally determine their susceptibility to form RMs. For RM-positive compounds, the structure of the reactive species (usually inferred from the characterization of a stable adduct(s) with nucleophiles), the biochemical pathway(s) and the enzyme(s) responsible for their generation must be determined. The information can then be used, as appropriate, for structural modifications aimed at eliminating the liability. In practice, however, eliminating or reducing RM formation in a lead chemical series is not trivial; medicinal chemistry solutions to eliminate RM formation could result in a detrimental effect on primary pharmacology (e.g., changes in subtype selectivity for target receptor or enzyme, agonist/antagonist behavior) and/or pharmacokinetic attributes (e.g., attenuation of aqueous solubility or passive cell permeability). If the toxicophore can be readily replaced with an alternate functional group without a significant loss of primary pharmacology/pharmacokinetic properties, then it is advisable to do so and thereby avoid the need for additional risk assessment beyond standard drug safety packages and further internal debate on this topic for the remainder of the development program.

Reports on the metabolism-guided drug design to abolish RM formation in a preclinical drug discovery setting are abundant in the medicinal chemistry/chemical toxicology literature, and a few are discussed below as illustrations. The first example focuses on pyrazinone-based corticotrophin-releasing factor-1 (CRF$_1$) receptor antagonists and potential antidepressant/anti-anxiolytic drugs (Hartz et al., 2009a, 2009b, 2010; Zhuo et al., 2010). In the course of SAR studies, pyrazinone **10** (Figure 26.5) was found to possess good pharmacokinetics and pharmacodynamics properties in rodent models of anxiety (Hartz et al., 2009a). However, extensive oxidative metabolism including the formation of GSH adducts was noted in subsequent *in vivo* disposition studies on **10** in bile duct-cannulated rats (Hartz et al., 2009b; Zhuo et al., 2010). A major component of the elimination mechanism of **10** in rats (~40% of drug-related material recovered in rat bile) comprised of conjugation with GSH, consistent with RM formation *in vivo* (Zhuo et al., 2010). Two distinct bioactivation mechanisms (both mediated by CYP enzyme(s)) were elucidated from subsequent *in vitro* studies on **10** using NADPH-supplemented liver microsomes (Figure 26.5): (a) oxidation on the chloropyrazinone ring to yield an electrophilic epoxide **11** that was trapped with GSH to generate stable adduct **12** and (b) *O*-dealkylation of the difluoromethylphenoxy moiety to afford phenol **13**, followed by a two-electron oxidation to generate a reactive quinone-imine species **14**, which reacted with GSH in a 1,4-Michael fashion to yield adduct **15**. This bioactivation pathway is analogous to the one described with the 2,6-dichloro-4-hydroxyaniline analogs and non-steroidal anti-inflammatory drugs diclofenac and lumiracoxib (Li et al., 2008; Tang et al., 1999). On the basis of this information, medicinal chemistry strategies were initiated with the goal of eliminating the bioactivation liability in **10**. Quinone-imine formation was eliminated by replacing the 2,6-dichloroaniline motif with a bioisosteric pyridyl group, whereas epoxide formation on the 5-chloropyrazinone ring was attenuated by replacing the chlorine atom with the more strongly electron-withdrawing cyano group. Out of this exercise emerged **16** (Figure 26.5) with sufficiently diminished RM formation both rat and human liver microsomes (Hartz et al., 2009b). Consistent with the *in vitro* finding, <2%–4% of GSH conjugates were recovered in rat bile following *in vivo* administration of **16**. Compound **16** also retained all of the primary pharmacology and pharmacokinetic properties of the lead compound **10** (Hartz et al., 2009b, 2010). As such, replacement of the phenyl ring with a pyridyl group is frequently utilized in

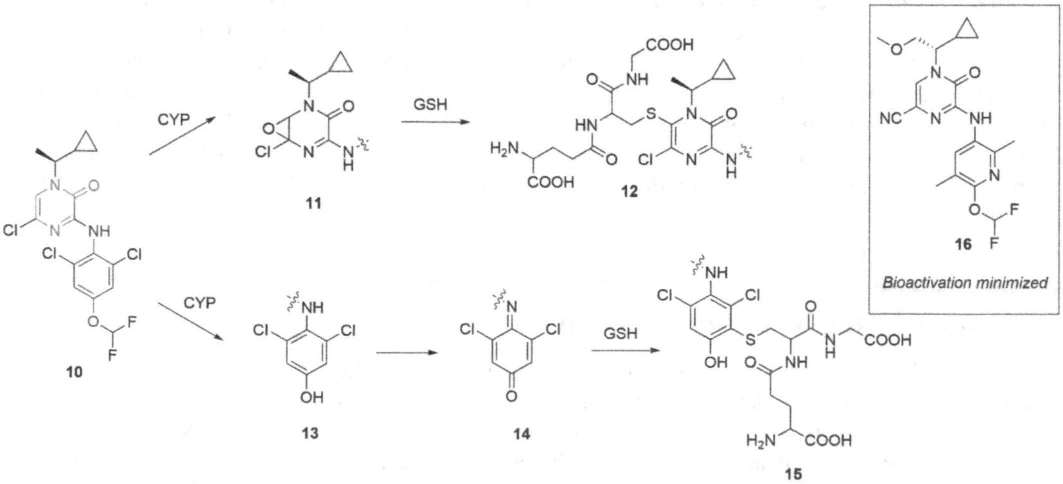

FIGURE 26.5 Metabolism-guided efforts in reducing RM formation with a pyrazinone-based corticotropin-releasing factor-1 receptor antagonist **10**.

medicinal chemistry to attenuate the formation of reactive quinonoid species derived from oxidation of electron-rich aromatic systems (e.g., aminophenols, catechols, etc.) (Kalgutkar et al., 2010).

The second illustration depicts strategies towards eliminating bioactivation of the electron rich 4-hydroxyaniline motif in the antimalarial agent amodiaquine **17** (Figure 26.6) (Maggs et al., 1987, 1998; O'Neill et al., 1994, 2003, 2009a; Tingle et al., 1995). Several cases of hepatotoxicity and agranulocytosis have been noted with the clinical use of **17**, and the detection of IgG antibodies in patients exposed to **17** is consistent with immune-mediated hypersensitivity reactions (Neftel et al., 1986; Schulthess et al., 1983). The immune-mediated toxicity is thought to arise from the bioactivation of the 4-hydroxyaniline motif in **17** to a reactive quinone-imine species **18**, which can covalently bind to cellular proteins or GSH (Figure 26.6). Exchanging the C'-4-phenolic OH group with a fluorine atom results in **19** that does not undergo the obligatory two-electron oxidation process to the electrophilic quinone-imine species (Figure 26.6) (O'Neill et al., 1994; Tingle et al., 1995). In addition, isomerization of the 3' and 4' substituents in **17** affords analogs **20** and **21** (Figure 26.6), which do not form RMs (judged from the lack of formation of GSH conjugates) (O'Neill et al., 2003, 2009a). Compound **21**, in particular, was identified as a candidate for further development based on potent activity versus chloroquine-sensitive and resistant parasites, moderate to excellent oral bioavailability, low toxicity in *in vitro* studies and an acceptable safety profile (Davis et al., 2009; O'Neill et al., 2009a, 2009b).

The third example pertains to the discovery efforts on taranabant (**23**, Figure 26.6), a selective and potent inhibitor of the cannabinoid-1 receptor, which has been studied in phase III clinical trials for the treatment of obesity. The lead compound **22** (Figure 26.6) revealed a high level of covalent binding to human liver microsomes in a NADPH-dependent fashion, consistent with CYP-mediated formation of RM(s). Elucidation of the structure of the GSH conjugate obtained in subsequent trapping studies in liver microsomes suggested that the RM was an epoxide intermediate derived from a CYP-mediated oxidation of the electron-rich phenoxy ring (Hagmann, 2008). Replacement of the

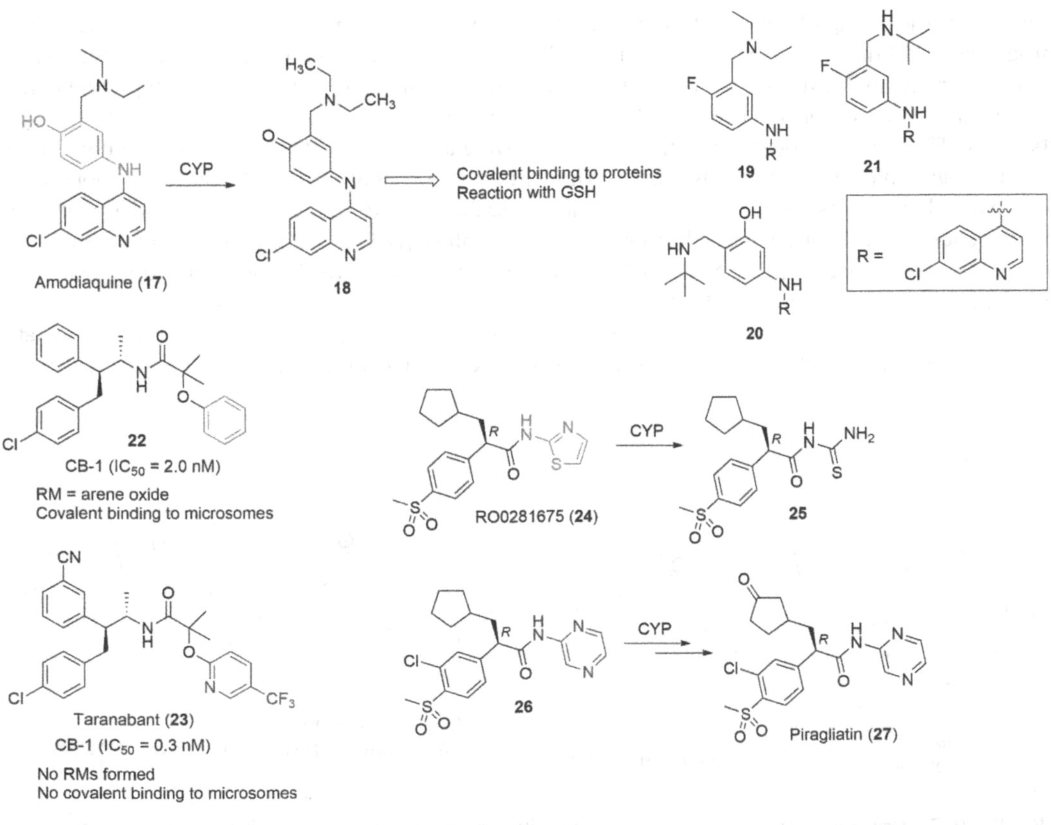

FIGURE 26.6 Case studies on elimination of bioactivation liability in lead chemical series.

phenoxy ring in **22** with a trifuoromethylpyridyl ring afforded **23**, which was devoid of RM formation, while retaining potency and selectivity against the cannabinoid-1 receptor.

The final example revolves around the discovery of the first glucokinase activator, piragliatin (**27**,
Figure 26.6), which has demonstrated efficacy (e.g., lowering of pre- and postprandial glucose levels,
improvements in insulin secretory profile) in phase II clinical trials in patients with type 2 diabetes (Sarabu
et al., 2012). The prototype candidate RO0281675 (**24**, Figure 26.6) was withdrawn from phase I clinical
studies due to its narrow safety margin in preclinical toxicology studies. RO0281675 caused reversible
hepatic lipidosis in chronic toxicology studies in rats and dogs, which was believed to occur via the metabolism of the 2-aminothiazole motif to the reactive thiourea metabolite (**25**). The hypothesis was further
substantiated on the basis of two observations: (a) the thiourea derivative **25** was formed as a metabolite
upon incubating **24** in NADPH-supplemented liver microsomes from preclinical species and humans, and
(b) five day toxicity studies in rats with an authentic standard of **25** led to hepatic lipidosis in a manner
similar to that noted with **24**. Subsequent SAR studies seeking thiazole ring replacements led to the identification of a pyrazine-based lead analog **26** (Figure 26.6). *In vitro* metabolite identification on **26** revealed
several oxidative metabolites on the cyclopentyl ring, which were synthesized and shown to possess pharmacological activity comparable to **26**. Additional profiling of *in vitro* and *in vivo* safety and efficacy of
the oxidative metabolites led to the selection of piragliatin (**27**) as the clinical candidate. Subchronic and
chronic toxicology studies with **27** in rats and dogs revealed no evidence of hepatic lipidosis. Furthermore,
27 is relatively less lipophilic than **26** (clog P of **26** = 2.69 vs. clog P of **27** = 0.47) and exhibits superior oral
absorption (lower plasma clearance leading to increased oral absorption) in preclinical species and humans.

Critical Evaluation of the Toxicophore Concept as Utilized in Medicinal Chemistry

Potentially alleviating IADR risks by eliminating RM formation may represent a viable starting point in
drug design, but there is a growing concern that the perceived safety risks associated with incorporation
of a toxicophore and RM-positive compounds may be over accentuated. First of all, it is important to note
that the lack of a toxicophore and/or RM formation in a drug candidate does not serve as a warranty of
its safety. There is no evidence that the idiosyncratic DILI associated with the recalled thrombin inhibitor ximelagatran (Figure 26.7) is associated with RM formation and, as such, the drug does not contain
any toxicophores in its chemical structure (Testa et al., 2007). Likewise, there are no toxicophores and
no evidence for RM formation with drugs such as pemoline (DILI), chlormezanone (toxic epidermal
necrolysis), and isoxicam (toxic epidermal necrolysis) (Figure 26.7), which have been withdrawn due to
idiosyncratic toxicity (Stepan et al., 2011).

Several marketed blockbuster drugs also contain toxicophores and form RMs, but are rarely associated
with idiosyncratic toxicity. Out of 108 structurally distinct and most prescribed small molecule drugs in

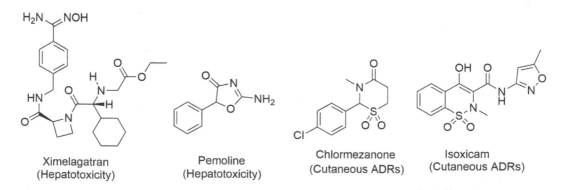

Ximelagatran
(Hepatotoxicity)

Pemoline
(Hepatotoxicity)

Chlormezanone
(Cutaneous ADRs)

Isoxicam
(Cutaneous ADRs)

FIGURE 26.7 Drugs associated with idiosyncratic toxicity that do not contain toxicophores and are devoid of RM
formation.

2009, 58 (53%) contained toxicophores and evidence for RM formation was provided in 24 out of the 58 (41%) cases (Stepan et al., 2011). Likewise, 13 out of the 15 small molecule drugs, which constituted the most sold drugs in 2009, were found to contain toxicophores in their structures. *In vitro* and/or *in vivo* experimental evidence for RM formation has been presented for 10 out of the 13 drugs (Stepan et al., 2011). The toxicophores are fairly diverse in nature and include aniline/anilide, thiophene, olefin, and quinone precursors found in the toxic drugs. Atorvastatin, clopidogrel, and duloxetine (Figure 26.8) are perhaps the most provocative illustrations of marketed blockbuster agents that contain toxicophores and are prone to RM formation. In the case of atorvastatin, monohydroxylation(s) on the acetanilide toxicophore by CYP3A4 yields the pharmacologically active *ortho-* and *para*-hydroxyacetanilide metabolites (Lannernas, 2003), which can be further oxidized to reactive quinone-imine species in a manner similar to that noted for the anti-inflammatory agent acetaminophen. The observation that atorvastatin covalently binds to human liver microsomes in a NADPH-dependent fashion partially validates the bioactivation hypothesis (Nakayama et al., 2009). It is interesting to note that atorvastatin was ranked number one in terms of dispensed prescriptions and total sales for 2009. The P2Y$_{12}$ purinoreceptor antagonist and clot-buster agent clopidogrel contains the thiophene ring toxicophore, which is metabolized by CYP enzyme(s) to a pharmacologically active RM (speculated to be an electrophilic sulfenic acid **28**), which forms a covalent disulfide linkage with a cysteinyl residue on the P2Y$_{12}$ receptor in platelets, leading to inhibition of platelet aggregation (Dansette et al., 2009, 2012; Savi et al., 1994, 2006). Similar to clopidogrel, the anti-depressant duloxetine possesses a pendant thiophene ring, which can be potentially oxidized by CYP to reactive species. Incubation of duloxetine in NADPH- and GSH-supplemented human liver microsomes has indicated the presence of several GSH conjugates (e.g., compound **30**) derived from adduction of the sulfhydryl nucleophile to arene oxide intermediates (e.g., compound **29**) on the naphthalene ring (Wu et al., 2010). The thiophene ring in duloxetine does not appear to be prone to oxidative bioactivation. Overall, the analysis by Stepan et al. (2011) reveals that the percentage of toxicophore- and/or

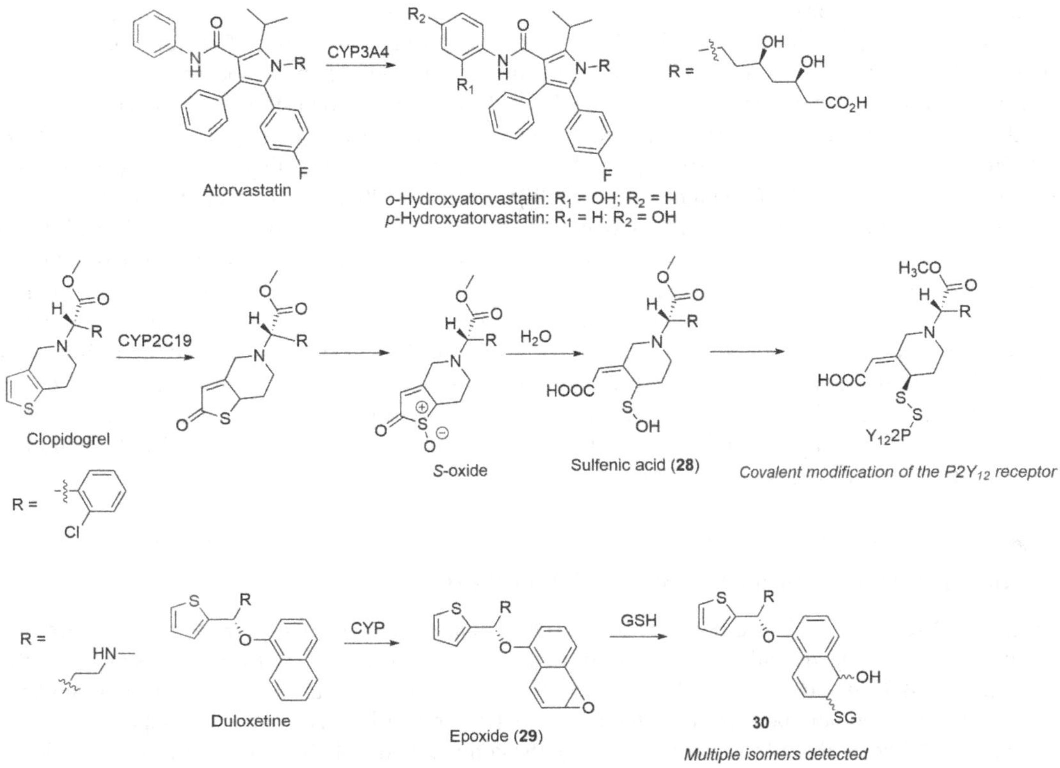

FIGURE 26.8 Bioactivation of blockbuster marketed drugs atorvastatin, clopidogrel, and duloxetine.

RM-positive compounds in the most prescribed or total sales drug category is largely similar to that noted for drugs recalled or associated with a BBW for idiosyncratic toxicity. These observations also imply that the toxicophore concept and RM screening tools in preclinical drug discovery may be too rigorous and in its current form could halt the progression of novel and much-needed medicines.

Total Daily Dose as a Mitigating Factor for IADRs

Influence of the administered total daily dose on IADRs has been a topic of discussion across several reviews (Boelsterli, 2003; Dalvie et al., 2015; Kalgutkar and Dalvie, 2015; Lammert et al., 2008; Stepan et al., 2011; Uetrecht, 2000). Comparison of the daily dosing regimen of drugs associated with idiosyncratic toxicity versus drugs rarely associated with this liability indicates that high dose drugs (>100 mg) tend to be the ones that most frequently lead to IADRs, while low dose drugs (<50 mg) are rarely problematic in this regard (whether or not these agents are prone to RM formation) (Stepan et al., 2011). Among US prescription medicines, a statistically significant relationship has also been noted between daily dose of oral medicines and reports of liver failure ($p = 0.009$), liver transplantation ($p < 0.001$), and death caused by DILI ($p = 0.004$). Of 598 eligible Swedish DILI cases, 9% belonged to the ≤10 mg/day group, 14.2% to the 11–49 mg/day group, and 77% of cases were caused by medications given at dose ≥50 mg/day (Lammert et al., 2008).

The meta-analysis by Stepan et al. (2011) indicates that the vast majority of toxicophore- and/or RM-positive drugs in the top 200 list (prescription/sales) are low total daily dose drugs. Thus, olanzapine (Figure 26.9), which is not associated with a significant incidence of agranulocytosis, forms a reactive iminium metabolite analogous to the one observed with clozapine (Gardner et al., 1998). A key difference between the two drugs is the total daily dose; clozapine is dosed at >300 mg/day, while the maximum recommended daily dose of olanzapine is 10 mg/day. Likewise, the tricyclic antidepressants amineptine and tianeptine (Figure 26.9) form reactive arene oxide species but only amineptine is hepatotoxic (Fromenty and Pessayre 1995; Genève et al., 1987; Stepan et al., 2011). The improved tolerance of tianeptine in the clinic has been speculated to arise from the ~5–6-fold lower recommended dose (daily doses of amineptine and tianeptine are 200 and 37.5 mg, respectively) (Stepan et al., 2011). A similar argument has been made for DILI differences between the three thiazolidinedione (TZD) derivatives and anti-diabetic agents troglitazone, pioglitazone, and rosiglitazone (Figure 26.9). All three agents are prone to bioactivation on the TZD ring framework yielding reactive species *in vitro* (Alvarez-Sanchez et al., 2006; Baughman et al., 2005; He et al., 2004; Kassahun et al., 2001). However, pioglitazone and rosiglitazone are not associated with idiosyncratic DILI noted in the clinical use of troglitazone. A plausible explanation is the lower total daily doses of pioglitazone and rosiglitazone relative to troglitazone (troglitazone, 200–600 mg; pioglitazone, 30 mg; rosiglitazone, 8 mg). Finally, in the case of clopidogrel, the majority (>70%) of its daily dose of 75 mg is undergoes rapid ester hydrolysis by carboxylesterases to yield an inactive carboxylic acid metabolite (~ 80%–85% of circulating metabolites) (Farid et al., 2010). This observation implies that only a small percentage of the parent drug (20 mg or less) is theoretically available for conversion to the pharmacologically active RM. Indeed, covalent binding to platelets accounts for only 2% of radiolabeled clopidogrel in human mass balance studies (Plavix® package insert).

Competing Detoxication Pathways of Metabolism

In vitro RM screens (conducted in GSH- and NADPH-supplemented human liver microsomes) are only capable of inspecting oxidative bioactivation mediated by CYP enzymes. In some instances, CYP-dependent RM formation may be observed in microsomes, but *in vivo*, the compound may undergo a distinctly different and perhaps more facile metabolic fate that by-passes and/or competes with RM formation (Dalvie et al., 2015). The more diverse the competing metabolic routes for a NCE, the lesser the fraction metabolized via the bioactivation pathway leading to RM. This phenomenon is illustrated further with the anti-depressant paroxetine and the selective estrogen receptor modulator raloxifene,

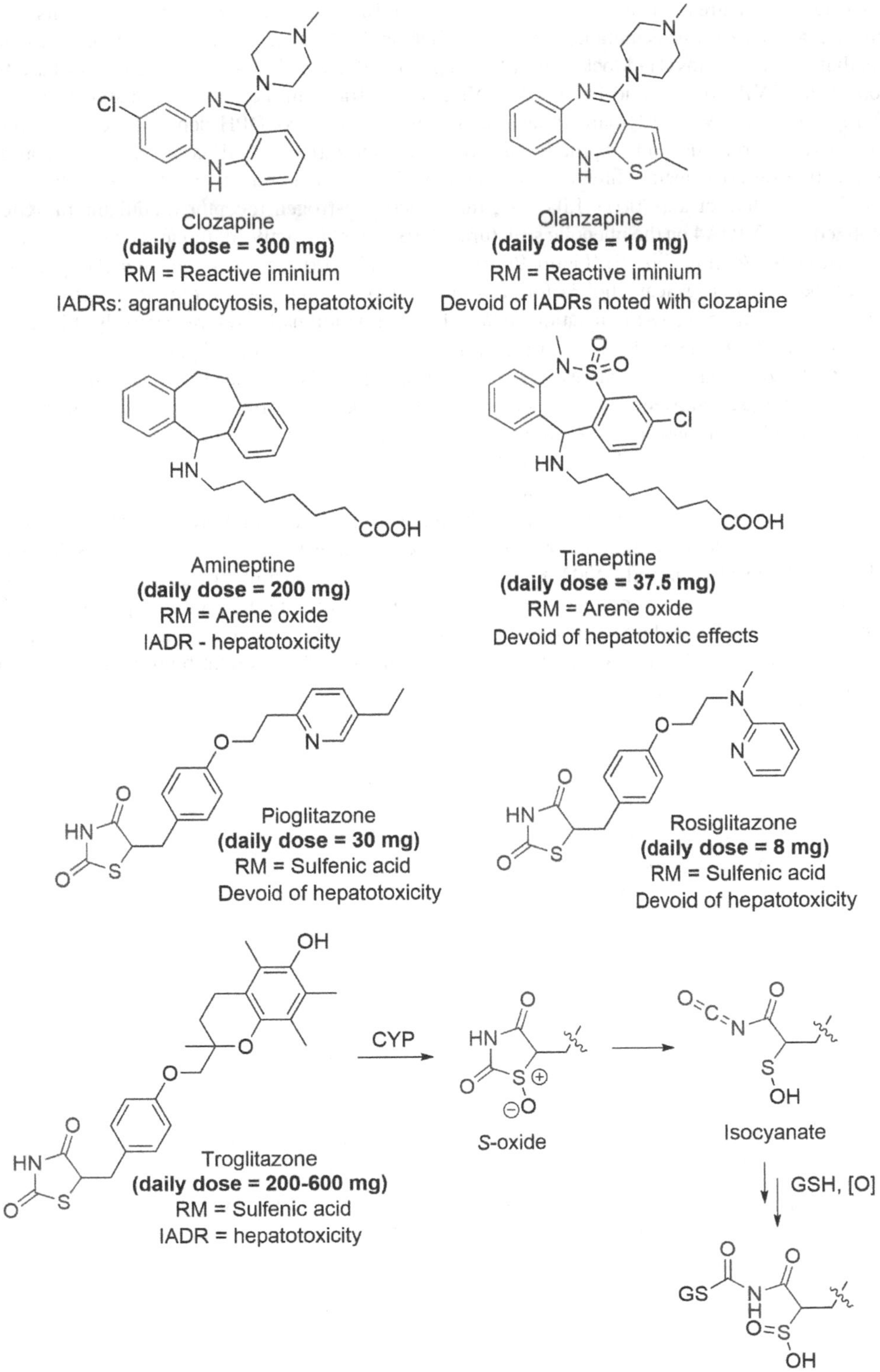

FIGURE 26.9 Impact of low total daily dose on IADR potential of drugs that contain toxicophores and/or form RMs.

marketed agents that are rarely associated with IADRs, and are part of the "most-prescribed" list of medications in 2009. Paroxetine is metabolized by CYP2D6 on the 1,3-benzdioxole toxicophore to a catechol intermediate **31** in humans (Haddock et al., 1989); a process that also leads to the mechanism-based inactivation of the CYP isozyme and DDIs with CYP2D6 substrates in the clinic (Venkatakrishnan et al., 2005). *In vitro* studies with [³H]-paroxetine have demonstrated the NADPH-dependent covalent binding to human liver microsomal and S9 proteins, and the characterization of GSH conjugates (e.g., compound **33**) of reactive quinone metabolites (e.g., compound **32**) obtained from two-electron oxidation of **31** (Figure 26.10) (Zhao et al., 2007). Likewise, the selective estrogen receptor modulator raloxifene is metabolized by CYP3A4 on the phenolic structural alerts to yield reactive quinone species **34** that can be trapped with GSH (compound **35**) (Figure 26.10) (Chen et al., 2002). However *in vivo*, the quinone precursors of these two drugs (catechol **31** for paroxetine and parent compound raloxifene) are principally metabolized via competing *O*-methylation and/or glucuronidation pathways, respectively (Figure 26.10) (Zhao et al., 2007; Dalvie et al., 2008). In fact, the principal metabolites of paroxetine in humans are the *O*-methylated guaiacol derivatives of paroxetine (compounds **36** and **37**), obtained via catechol-*O*-methyl transferase-catalyzed methylation of **31** (Haddock et al., 1989). In the case of raloxifene, Dalvie et al. (2008) demonstrated the influence of the competing glucuronidation pathway on covalent binding of raloxifene-related RMs to human liver microsomes. The studies revealed that preincubation of raloxifene with uridine 5-diphosphoglucuronic acid-fortified human intestinal microsomes reduces the amount of [¹⁴C]-raloxifene that is covalently bound to liver microsomal proteins. Thus, efficient and extensive raloxifene glucuronidation (compounds **38**–**40**) by intestinal uridine glucuronosyltransferase UGT 1A10 and 1A8 (Kemp et al., 2002; Kishi et al., 2016) probably limits the amount of drug undergoing bioactivation to the corresponding quinones in the liver. Overall, it is tempting to speculate that in the modern drug discovery paradigm, paroxetine and raloxifene would unlikely be considered as candidates for clinical development because of the high degree of microsomal covalent binding and GSH adduct formation (Obach et al., 2008b).

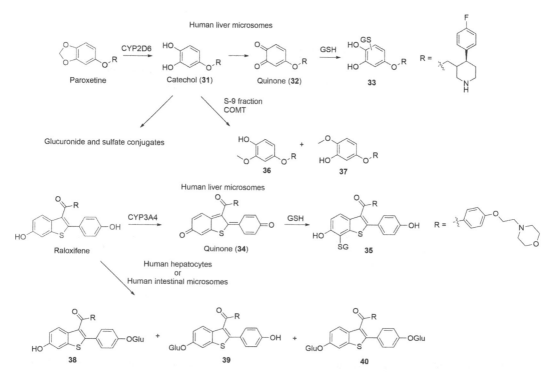

FIGURE 26.10 Impact of competing detoxication pathways on RM formation and protein covalent binding as illustrated with paroxetine and raloxifene.

These observations point out the importance for detailed follow-up studies in fully integrated *in vitro* biological matrices (e.g., hepatocytes and/or liver S-9 fractions) from both human and animal species to minimize false positives generated in preliminary RM screens (Dalvie et al., 2009). Establishing a clear understanding of the *in vivo* clearance mechanisms in animals and how that relates to RM formation *in vitro* matrices would lead to data-driven decision making with regards to compound selection. Consequently, the improved safety of low total daily dose drugs could potentially arise from a marked reduction in the total body burden to RM exposure via efficient detoxication processes involving scavenging by the endogenous GSH pool and/or competing metabolic pathways, such that the RMs are unlikely to exceed the safety threshold needed for toxicity.

Managing RM Liability of Drug Candidates in Preclinical Discovery

The mere presence of toxicophores cannot in itself predict the type, severity or incidence of IADRs associated with drug candidates. Likewise, RM screening tools (exogenous trapping with nucleophiles and/or protein covalent binding in human liver microsomes) are not intended to predict toxicity but rather detect the formation of RMs, some of which may carry a toxic liability. Experiments that unambiguously define a 1:1 relationship between RM formation (e.g., the *in vitro* and *in vivo* characterization of GSH conjugates) and toxicity in humans are extremely rare. Although GSH adducts and/or downstream mercapturic acid metabolites that are measured *in vivo* represent short-term exposure to RMs, protein adducts reflect the internal exposure of cells to RMs *in vivo*, which is more relevant for risk assessment purposes. Whether covalent binding measures *in vivo* is likely to be more informative of the *in vivo* safety risk than covalent binding studies *in vitro*, remains to be established. This is because of a paucity of data on absolute levels of *in vivo* covalent binding that could lead to a toxic outcome versus levels of binding that are safe. At the present time, there is no consensus on a preclinical discovery strategy to investigate safety hazard and risk posed by RM formation for a particular drug candidate in humans. Ultimately, only studies in humans can currently be used to unearth mechanisms of serious IADRs, and determine "cause and effect" with respect to RM formation in humans and clinical outcome. While reducing exposure to RM is viewed as a pragmatic approach to minimize IADR risks during drug development, these strategies should not rely solely on structural alert/RM information, as overall metabolic fate and other considerations (e.g., toxicity arising from the parent compound itself via inhibition of critical hepatobiliary transport proteins) provide additional valuable information that can be used in a "weight of evidence" approach for risk assessment and management. Recent advances in risk assessment methodologies, such as the estimate of total daily body burden of covalent binding in hepatocytes or by zone classification taking the clinical dose into consideration, are positive steps towards quantitative prediction of IADR risks with drug candidates (Bauman et al., 2009; Schadt et al., 2015; Thompson et al., 2012, 2016). Given this general trend on low daily dose as a key factor in reducing IADR risks, optimization of lead compounds in drug discovery programs should focus on improving intrinsic pharmacologic potency and optimizing pharmacokinetics (e.g., reducing metabolic clearance) as a means of decreasing the projected clinically efficacious plasma concentrations (and hence the dose) and the associated "body burden" of parent drug and its metabolites (Smith and Obach, 2009).

With respect to optimization of oxidative metabolic clearance (i.e., reduction in CYP mediated metabolism) of NCEs, it is necessary to emphasize that a correlation has been established between DILI and drugs undergoing high hepatic metabolism (Lammert et al., 2010). Out of ~ 207 most widely prescribed oral medications in the United States, 12 drugs with no reported hepatic metabolism had no reports of liver failure, liver transplantation, or fatal DILI. In contrast, drugs significantly metabolized in the liver (>50% hepatic metabolism, $n = 149$) had significantly higher frequency of alanine aminotransferase >3 times the upper limit of normal (35% vs. 11%, $p = 0.001$), liver failure (28% vs. 9%, $p = 0.004$), and fatal DILI (23% vs. 4%, $p = 0.001$). When the relationship between DILI and combination of hepatic metabolism and daily dose was examined, compounds with both significant hepatic metabolism and daily dose >50 mg ($n = 50$) were significantly more hepatotoxic than compounds belonging to other groups. Compared with medications without biliary excretion, compounds with biliary excretion ($n = 50$) had significantly higher frequency of jaundice (74% vs. 40%, $p = 0.0001$).

Yu et al. (2014) extended the findings of Lammert et al. (2010) by collecting known CYP-mediated metabolism data for 254 orally administered drugs in the Liver Toxicity Knowledge Base Benchmark Dataset with a known daily dose and applied logistic regression to identify trends between oxidative metabolism and DILI. These authors found that drugs oxidatively metabolized by CYP enzymes have a higher likelihood of causing DILI (odds ratio, 3.99; 95% confidence interval, 2.07–7.67; $p < 0.0001$) in a dose-dependent manner. These findings have been recently broadened by Weng et al. (2015) using 975 oral drugs used worldwide that have a Defined Daily Dose (DDD) designated in the World Health Organization's Anatomical Therapeutic Chemical classification system and whose IADR potential and metabolism data are available in the Micromedex Drugdex® compendium. Of the 975 drugs examined, 49% ($n = 478$) have the potential to induce at least one type of idiosyncratic DILI (e.g., acute liver failure, significant ALT/AST elevation, hepatitis, jaundice, and/or fatal DILI). A higher DDD (≥100 mg) was found to be associated with all types of IADRs, and extensive liver metabolism ($\geq50\%$) was associated with a subset of IADRs including hepatitis, jaundice, and fatal DILI. As was the case in the analysis of Stepan et al. (2011), lipophilicity (e.g., log P) did not correlate with IADR incidence or severity.

Against this backdrop, it is noteworthy to point out that several marketed drugs generate RMs, cause idiosyncratic toxicity, and carry a BBW for adverse reactions (Kalgutkar and Dalvie, 2015). Such drugs remain on the market and are widely prescribed because of favorable benefit-risk considerations. Lapatinib (Figure 26.11) is one such example that illustrates the weight of unmet medical need over the risk of hepatotoxicity. Lapatinib is used in combination with capecitabine for treatment of advanced or metastatic breast cancer and is associated with several cases of hepatotoxicity (some resulting in fatalities). Not only is the drug bioactivated to a quinoneimine **41** resulting in covalent interactions with GSH (compound **42**) and CYP3A4 isozyme (Teng et al., 2010; Hardy et al., 2014; Towles et al., 2016), its recommended daily dose is 1.25–1.5 g. What these observations suggest is that the level of risk (e.g., idiosyncratic toxicity, DDI due to CYP inhibition, etc.) that would deemed acceptable for drug candidates intended to treat major unmet medical need, life-threatening diseases, and/or orphan diseases is significantly higher relative to treatment of chronic non-debilitating conditions where alternate treatment options are already available. This also raises a philosophical question for debate regarding medicinal chemistry investments in removing structural alert(s) such the aniline motif, which is widely utilized in kinase inhibitor programs in oncology and is challenging to mimic by isosteric replacement. The risk-benefit argument also applies to unprecedented pharmacologic targets or molecules that carry a significant risk with regards to predicted human pharmacokinetics, where the primary goal is to first demonstrate early sign of efficacy in the clinic and/or adequate human pharmacokinetics. For such programs, RM-positive molecules can be progressed into first-in-human studies as probes to address

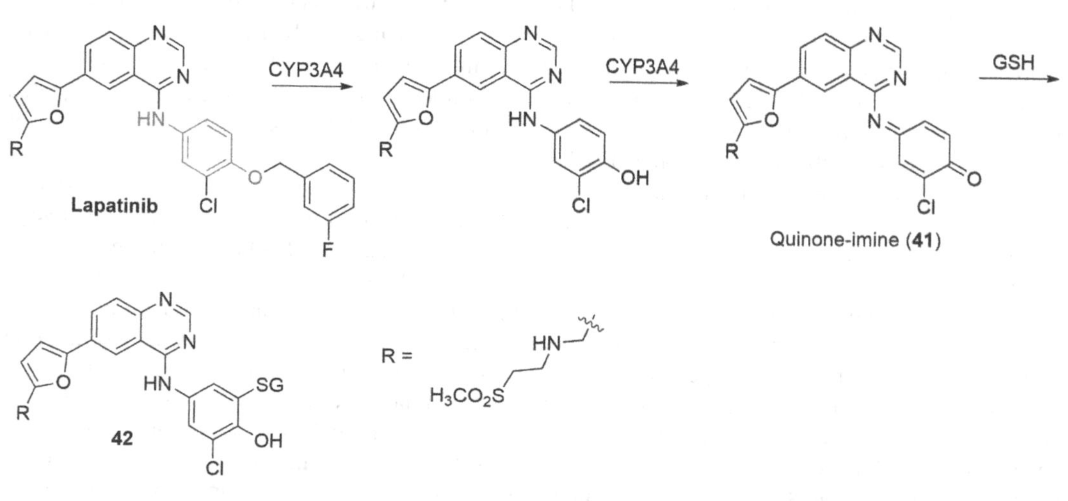

FIGURE 26.11 Bioactivation of the tyrosine kinase inhibitor lapatinib by CYP3A to an RM.

pharmacokinetics and proof-of-mechanism provided they are deemed safe in standard preclinical toxicology studies. While proof-of-mechanism is being obtained, additional efforts can be invested in the identification of back-up molecules that are devoid of RM formation.

REFERENCES

Alvarez-Sanchez, R., Montavon, F., Hartung, T., and Pahler, A. "Thiazolidinedione Bioactivation: A Comparison of the Bioactivation Potentials of Troglitazone, Rosiglitazone, and Pioglitazone Using Stable Isotope-Labeled Analogues and Liquid Chromatography Tandem Mass Spectrometry." *Chemical Research in Toxicology* 19 no. 8 (2006):1106–1116.

Argikar, U. A., Mangold, J. B., and Harriman, S. P. "Strategies and Chemical Design Approaches to Reduce the Potential for Formation of Reactive Metabolic Species." *Current Topics in Medicinal Chemistry* 11 no. 4 (2011):419–449.

Argoti, D., Liang, L., Conteh, A. et al. "Cyanide Trapping of Iminium Ion Reactive Intermediates Followed by Detection and Structure Identification Using Liquid Chromatography-tandem Mass Spectrometry (LC-MS/MS)." *Chemical Research in Toxicology* 18 no. 10 (2005):1537–1544.

Baughman, T. M., Graham, R. A., Wells-Knecht, K., Silver, I. S., Tyler, L. O., Wells-Knecht, M., and Zhao, Z. "Metabolic Activation of Pioglitazone Identified from Rat and Human Liver Microsomes and Freshly Isolated Hepatocytes." *Drug Metabolism and Disposition* 33 no. 6 (2005):733–738.

Bauman, J. S., Kelly, J. M., Tripathy, S. et al. "Can *In Vitro* Metabolism-Dependent Covalent Binding Data Distinguish Hepatotoxic From Nonhepatotoxic drugs? An Analysis Using Human Hepatocytes and Liver S-9 Fraction." *Chemical Research in Toxicology* 22 no. 2 (2009):332–340.

Bell, J. A., Dallas, F. A., Jenner, W. N., and Martin, L. E. "The metabolism of Ranitidine in Animals and Man." *Biochemical Society Transactions* 8 no. 1 (1980):93.

Boelsterli, U. A. "Disease-Related Determinants of Susceptibility to Drug-Induced Idiosyncratic Hepatotoxicity." *Current Opinion in Drug Discovery and Development* 6 no. 1 (2003):81–91.

Chen, Q., Ngui, J. S., Doss, G. A. et al. "Cytochrome P450 3A4-Mediated Bioactivation of Raloxifene: Irreversible Enzyme Inhibition and Thiol Adduct Formation." *Chemical Research in Toxicology* 15 no. 7 (2002):907–914.

Dalvie, D., Kalgutkar, A. S., and Chen, W. "Practical Approaches to Resolving Reactive Metabolite Liabilities in Early Discovery." *Drug Metabolism Reviews* 47 no. 1 (2015):56–70.

Dalvie, D., Kang, P., Zientek, M., Xiang, C., Zhou, S., and Obach, R. S. "Effect of Intestinal Glucuronidation in Limiting Hepatic Exposure and Bioactivation of Raloxifene in Humans and Rats." *Chemical Research in Toxicology* 21 no. 12 (2008):2260–2271.

Dalvie, D., Obach, R. S., Kang, P. et al. "Assessment of Three Human *In Vitro* Systems in the Generation of Major Human Excretory and Circulating Metabolites." *Chemical Research in Toxicology* 22 no. 2 (2009):357–368.

Dansette, P. M., Libraire, J., Bertho, G., and Mansuy, D. "Metabolic Oxidative Cleavage of Thioesters: Evidence for the Formation of Sulfenic Acid Intermediates in the Bioactivation of the Antithrombotic Prodrugs Ticlopidine and Clopidogrel." *Chemical Research in Toxicology* 22 no. 2 (2009):369–373.

Dansette, P. M., Rosi, J., Bertho, G., and Mansuy, D. "Cytochromes P450 Catalyze Both Steps of the Major Pathway of Clopidogrel Bioactivation, Whereas Paraoxonase Catalyzes the Formation of a Minor Thiol Metabolite Isomer." *Chemical Research in Toxicology* 25 no. 2 (2012):348–356.

Davies, N. M. and Skjodt, N. M. "Clinical Pharmacokinetics of Meloxicam. A Cyclo-Oxygenase-2 Preferential Nonsteroidal Anti-Inflammatory Drug." *Clinical Pharmacokinetics* 36 no. 2 (1999):115–126.

Davis, C. B., Bambal, R., Moorthy, G. S. et al. "Comparative Preclinical Drug Metabolism and Pharmacokinetic Evaluation of Novel 4-Aminoquinoline Anti-Malarials." *Journal of Pharmaceutical Sciences* 98 no. 1 (2009):362–377.

Diao, L., Shu, Y., and Polli, J. E. "Uptake of Pramipexole by Human Organic Cation Transporters." *Molecular Pharmaceutics* 7 no. 4 (2010):1342–1347.

Dieckhaus, C. M., Thompson, C. D., Roller, S. G., and Macdonald, T. L. "Mechanisms of Idiosyncratic Drug Reactions: The Case of Felbamate." *Chemico-Biological Interactions* 142 no. 1–2 (2002):99–117.

Dobo, K. L., Obach, R. S., Luffer-Atlas, D., and Bercu, J. P. "A Strategy for the Risk Assessment of Human Genotoxic Metabolites." *Chemical Research in Toxicology* 22 no. 2 (2009):348–356.

Evans, D. C., Watt, A. P., Nicoll-Griffith, D. A., and Baillie, T. A. "Drug-Protein Adducts: An Industry Perspective on Minimizing the Potential for Drug Bioactivation in Drug Discovery and Development." *Chemical Research in Toxicology* 17 no. 1 (2004):3–16.

Farid, N. A., Kurihara, A., and Wrighton, S. A. "Metabolism and Disposition of the Thienopyridine Antiplatelet Drugs Ticlopidine, Clopidogrel, and Prasugrel in Humans." *Journal of Clinical Pharmacology* 50 no. 2 (2010):126–142.

Fromenty, B. and Pessayre, D. "Inhibition of Mitochondrial Beta-Oxidation as a Mechanism of Hepatotoxicity." *Pharmacology and Therapeutics* 67 no. 1 (1995):101–154.

Gardner, I., Leeder, J. S., Chin, T., Zahid, N., and Uetrecht, J. P. "A Comparison of the Covalent Binding of Clozapine and Olanzapine to Human Neutrophils *in Vitro* and *in Vivo*." *Molecular Pharmacology* 53 no. 6 (1998):999–1008.

Genève, J., Degott, C., Letteron, P. et al. "Metabolic Activation of the Tricyclic Antidepressant Amineptine—II Protective Role of Glutathione Against *In Vitro* and *In Vivo* Covalent Binding." *Biochemical Pharmacology* 36 no. 3 (1987):331–337.

Guengerich F. P. and MacDonald, J. S. "Applying Mechanisms of Chemical Toxicity to Predict Drug Safety." *Chemical Research in Toxicology* 20 no. 3 (2007):344–369.

Haddock, R. E., Johnson, A. M., Langley, P. F. et al. "Metabolic Pathways of Paroxetine in Animals and Man and the Comparative Pharmacological Properties of the Metabolites." *Acta Psychiatrica Scandinavica Supplement* 350 (1989):24–26.

Hagmann, W. K. "The Discovery of Taranabant, a Selective Cannabinoid-1 Receptor Inverse Agonist for the Treatment of Obesity." *Archiv der Pharmazie (Weinheim)* 341 no. 7 (2008):405–411.

Hardy, K. D., Wahlin, M. D., Papageorgiou, I., Unadkat, J. D., Rettie, A. E., and Nelson, S. D. "Studies on the Role of Metabolic Activation in Tyrosine Kinase Inhibitor-Dependent Hepatotoxicity: Induction of CYP3A4 Enhances the Cytotoxicity of Lapatinib in HepaRG Cells." *Drug Metabolism and Disposition* 42 no. 1 (2014):162–171.

Hartz, R. A., Ahuja, V. T., Rafalski, M. et al. "*In Vitro* Intrinsic Clearance-Based Optimization of N3-Phenylpyrazinones as Corticotropin-Releasing Factor-1 (CRF1) Receptor Antagonists." *Journal of Medicinal Chemistry* 52 no. 14 (2009a): 4161–4172.

Hartz, R. A., Ahuja, V. T., Schmitz, W. D. et al. "Synthesis and Structure-activity Relationships of N3-Pyridylpyrazinones as Corticotropin-Releasing Factor-1 (CRF-1) Receptor Antagonists." *Bioorganic Medicinal Chemistry letters* 20 no. 6 (2010):1890–1894.

Hartz, R. A., Ahuja, V. T., Zhuo, X. et al. "A Strategy to Minimize Reactive Metabolite Formation: Discovery of (S)-4-(1-Cyclopropyl-2-methoxyethyl)-6-[6-(difluoromethoxy)-2,5-dimethylpyridin-3-ylamino]-5-oxo-4,5-dihydropyrazine-2-carbonitrile as a Potent, Orally Bioavailable Corticotropin-Releasing Factor-1 Receptor Antagonist." *Journal of Medicinal Chemistry* 52 no. 23 (2009b):7653–7668.

He, K., Talaat, R. E., Pool, W. F. et al. "Metabolic Activation of Troglitazone: Identification of a Reactive Metabolite and Mechanisms Involved." *Drug Metabolism and Disposition* 32 no. 6 (2004):639–646.

Inoue, K., Fukuda, K., Yoshimura, T., and Kusano, K. "Comparison of the Reactivity of Trapping Agents Towards Electrophiles: Cysteine Derivatives can be Bifunctional Trapping Reagents." *Chemical Research in Toxicology* 28 no. 8 (2015):1546–1555.

Kalgutkar, A. S. "Handling Reactive Metabolite Positives in Drug Discovery: What has Retrospective Structure-toxicity Analyses Taught Us?" *Chemico-Biological Interactions* 192 no. 1–2 (2011):46–55.

Kalgutkar, A. S. "Liabilities Associated with the Formation of 'Hard' Electrophiles in Reactive Metabolite Trapping Screens." *Chemical Research in Toxicology* 30 no. 1 (2017):220–238.

Kalgutkar, A. S. "Should the Incorporation of Structural Alerts be Restricted in Drug Design? An Analysis of Structure-Toxicity Trends with Aniline-based Drugs." *Current Medicinal Chemistry* 22 no. 4 (2015):438–464.

Kalgutkar, A. S. and Dalvie, D. "Predicting Toxicities of Reactive Metabolite-Positive Drug Candidates." *Annual Reviews in Pharmacology and Toxicology* 55 (2015):35–54.

Kalgutkar, A. S. and Didiuk, M. T. "Structural Alerts, Reactive Metabolites, and Protein Covalent Binding: How Reliable are These Attributes as Predictors of Drug Toxicity." *Chemistry and Biodiversity* 6 no. 11 (2009):2115–2137.

Kalgutkar, A. S., Gardner, I., Obach, R. S. et al. "A Comprehensive Listing of Bioactivation Pathways of Organic Functional Groups." *Current Drug Metabolism* 6 no. 3 (2005b):161–225.

Kalgutkar, A. S., Griffith, D. A., Ryder, T. et al. "Discovery Tactics to Mitigate Toxicity Risks Due to Reactive Metabolite Formation with 2-(2-Hydroxyaryl)-5-(trifluoromethyl)pyrido[4,3-d]pyrimidin-4(3H)-one Derivatives, Potent Calcium-Sensing Receptor Antagonists and Clinical Candidate(s) for the Treatment of Osteoporosis." *Chemical Research in Toxicology* 23 no. 6 (2010):1115–1126.

Kalgutkar, A. S., Vaz, A. D., Lame, M. E. et al. "Bioactivation of the Nontricyclic Antidepressant Nefazodone to a Reactive Quinone-Imine Species in Human Liver Microsomes and Recombinant Cytochrome P4503A4." *Drug Metabolism and Disposition* 33 no. 2 (2005a):243–253.

Kassahun, K., Pearson, P. G., Tang, W. et al. "Studies on the Metabolism of Troglitazone to Reactive Intermediates *In Vitro* and *In Vivo*. Evidence for Novel Biotransformation Pathways Involving Quinone Methide Formation and Thiazolidinedione Ring Scission." *Chemical Research in Toxicology* 14 no. 1 (2001):62–70.

Kemp, D. C., Fan, P. W., and Stevens, J. C. "Characterization of Raloxifene Glucuronidation *In Vitro*: Contribution of Intestinal Metabolism to Presystemic Clearance." *Drug Metabolism and Disposition* 30 no. 6 (2002):694–700.

Kishi, N., Takasuka, A., Kokawa, Y. et al. "Raloxifene Glucuronidation in Liver and Intestinal Microsomes of Humans and Monkeys: Contribution of UGT1A1, UGT1A8 and UGT1A9." *Xenobiotica* 46 no. 4 (2016):289–295.

Lammert, C., Bjornsson, E., Niklasson, A., and Chalasani, N. "Oral Medications with Significant Hepatic Metabolism at Higher Risk for Hepatic Adverse Events." *Hepatology* 51 no. 2 (2010):615–620.

Lammert, C., Einarsson, S., Saha, C., Niklasson, A., Bjornsson, E., and Chalasani, N. "Relationship Between Daily Dose of Oral Medications and Idiosyncratic Drug-Induced Liver Injury: Search for Signals." *Hepatology* 47 no. 6 (2008):2003–2009.

Leise, M. D., Poterucha, J. J., and Talwalkar, J. A. "Drug-Induced Liver Injury." *Mayo Clinic Proceedings* 89 no. 1 (2014):95–106.

Lannernas, H. "Clinical Pharmacokinetics of Atorvastatin." *Clinical Pharmacokinetics* 42 no. 13 (2003):1141–1160.

Lenz, E. M., Martin, S., Schmidt, R. et al. "Reactive Metabolite Trapping Screens and Potential Pitfalls: Bioactivation of a Homomorpholine and Formation of an Unstable Thiazolidine Adducts." *Chemical Research in Toxicology* 27 no. 6 (2014):968–980.

Li, J. and Uetrecht, J. P. "The Danger Hypothesis Applied to Idiosyncratic Drug Reactions." *Handbook in Experimental Pharmacology* 196 (2010):493–509.

Li, Y., Slatter, J. G., Zhang, Z. et al. "*In Vitro* Metabolic Activation of Lumiracoxib in Rat and Human Liver Preparations." *Drug Metabolism and Disposition*, 36 no. 2 (2008):469–473.

Liu, Z. C. and Uetrecht, J. P. "Clozapine is Oxidized by Activated Human Neutrophils to a Reactive Nitrenium Ion that Irreversibly Binds to the Cells." *Journal of Pharmacology and Experimental Therapeutics* 275 no. 3 (1995):1476–1483.

Ma, S. and Subramanian, R. "Detecting and Characterizing Reactive Metabolites by Liquid Chromatography/tandem Mass Spectrometry." *Journal of Mass Spectrometry* 41 no. 9 (2006) 1121–1139.

Maggs, J. L., Colbert, J., Winstanley, P. A., Orme, M. L., and Park, B. K. "Irreversible Binding of Amodiaquine to Human Liver Microsomes: Chemical and Metabolic Factors." *British Journal of Clinical Pharmacology* 23 (1987):649.

Maggs, J. L., Tingle, M. D., Kitteringham, N. R., and Park, B. K. "Drug–Protein Conjugates. 14. Mechanisms of Formation of Protein-Arylating Intermediates from Amodiaquine, a Myelotoxin and Hepatotoxin in Man." *Biochemical Pharmacology* 37 no. 2 (1988):303–311.

Nakayama, S., Atsumi, R., Takakusa, H. et al. "A Zone Classification System for Risk Assessment of Idiosyncratic Drug Toxicity Using Daily Dose and Covalent Binding. *Drug Metabolism and Disposition* 37 no. 9 (2009):1970–1977.

Neftel, K. A., Woodtly, W., Schmid, M., Frick, P. G., and Fehr, J. "Amodiaquine Induced Agranulocytosis and Liver Damage." *British Medical Journal* 292 no. 6552 (1986):721–723.

O'Neill, P. M., Mukhtar, A., Stocks, P. A. et al. "Isoquine and Related Amodiaquine Analogues: A New Generation of Improved 4-Aminoquinoline Antimalarials." *Journal of Medicinal Chemistry* 46 no. 23 (2003):4933–4945.

O'Neill, P. M., Park, B. K., Shone, A. E. et al. "Candidate Selection and Preclinical Evaluation of N-tert-Butyl Isoquine (GSK369796), an Affordable and Effective 4-Aminoquinoline Antimalarial for the 21st Century." *Journal of Medicinal Chemistry*, 52 no. 5 (2009b):1408–1415.

O'Neill, P. M., Shone, A. E., Stanford, D. et al. "Synthesis, Antimalarial Activity, and Preclinical Pharmacology of a Novel Series of 4′-Fluoro and 4′-Chloro Analogues of Amodiaquine. Identification of a Suitable "Back-up" Compound for N-tert-Butyl Isoquine." *Journal of Medicinal Chemistry* 52 no.7 (2009a):1828–1844.

O'Neill, P.M., Harrison, A. C., Storr, R. C., Hawley, S. R., Ward, S. A., and Park, B. K. "The Effect of Fluorine Substitution on the Metabolism and Antimalarial Activity of Amodiaquine." *Journal of Medicinal Chemistry* 37 no. 9 (1994):1362–1370.

Obach, R. S., Kalgutkar, A. S., Ryder, T. F., and Walker, G. S. "*In Vitro* Metabolism and Covalent Binding of Enol-carboxamide Derivatives and Anti-inflammatory Agents Sudoxicam and Meloxicam: Insights into the Hepatotoxicity of Sudoxicam." *Chemical Research in Toxicology* 21 no. 9 (2008a):1890–1899.

Obach, R. S., Kalgutkar, A. S., Soglia, J. R., and Zhao, S. X. "Can *in Vitro* Metabolism-Dependent Covalent Binding Data in Liver Microsomes Distinguish Hepatotoxic from Nonhepatotoxic Drugs? An Analysis of 18 Drugs with Consideration of Intrinsic Clearance and Daily Dose." *Chemical Research in Toxicology* 21 no. 9 (2008b):1814–1822.

Ogese, M. O., Ahmed, S., Alfirevic, A. et al. "New Approaches to Investigate Drug-Induced Hypersensitivity." *Chemical Research in Toxicology* 30 no. 1 (2016):239–259.

Orr, S. T., Ripp, S. L., Ballard, T. E. et al. "Mechanism-Based Inactivation (MBI) of Cytochrome P450 Enzymes: Structure-Activity Relationships and Discovery Strategies to Mitigate Drug-Drug Interaction Risks. *Journal of Medicinal Chemistry* 55 no. 11 (2012):4896–4933.

Park, B. K., Boobis, A., Clarke, S. et al. "Managing the Challenge of Chemically Reactive Metabolites in Drug Development." *Nature Reviews in Drug Discovery and Development* 10 no. 4 (2011):292–306.

Park, B. K., Kitteringham, N. R., Maggs, J. L., Pirmohamed, M., and Williams, D. P. "The Role of Metabolic Activation in Drug-Induced Hepatotoxicity." *Annual Review of Pharmacology and Toxicology* 45 (2005):177–202.

Prakash, C., Sharma, R., Gleave, M., and Nedderman, A. "*In Vitro* Screening Techniques for Reactive Metabolites for Minimizing Bioactivation Potential in Drug Discovery." *Current Drug Metabolism* 9 no. 9 (2008):952–964.

Sarabu, R., Bizzarro, F. T., Corbett, W. L. et al. "Discovery of Piragliatin—First Glucokinase Activator Studied in Type 2 Diabetic Patients." *Journal of Medicinal Chemistry* 55 no. 16 (2012):7021–7036.

Savi, P., Comalbert, J., Gaich, C. et al. "The Antiaggregating activity of Clopidogrel is Due to a Metabolic Activation by the Hepatic Cytochrome P450-1A." *Thrombosis and Haemostasis* 72 no. 2 (1994):313–317.

Savi, P., Zachayus, J. L., Delesque-Touchard, N. et al. "The Active Metabolite of Clopidogrel Disrupts P2Y12 Receptor Oligomers and Partitions Them Out of Lipid Rafts. *Proceedings of the National Academy of Sciences USA* 103 no. 29 (2006):11069–11074.

Schadt, S., Simon, S., Kustermann, S. et al. "Minimizing DILI Risk in Drug Discovery—A Screening Tool for Drug Candidates." *Toxicology In Vitro* 30 no. 1 Pt B (2015):429–437.

Schulthess, H. K., von Felten, A., Gmur, J., and Neftel, K. "Amodiaquine-Induced Agranulocytosis During Suppressive Treatment of Malaria–Demonstration of an Amodiaquine-Dependent Granulocytotoxic Antibody." *Schweizer Medizinische Wochenschr* 113 no. 50 1983:1912–1913.

Shamovsky, I., Ripa, L., Blomberg, N. et al. "Theoretical Studies of Chemical Reactivity of Metabolically Activated Forms of Aromatic Amines Towards DNA." *Chemical Research in Toxicology* 25 no. 10 (2012):2236–2252.

Smith, D. A. and Obach, R. S. "Metabolites in Safety Testing (MIST): Considerations of Mechanisms of Toxicity with Dose, Abundance, and Duration of Treatment." *Chemical Research in Toxicology* 22 no. 2 (2009):267–279.

Stachulski, A. V., Baillie, T. A., Park, B. K. et al. "The Generation, Detection, and Effects of Reactive Drug Metabolites." *Medicinal Research Reviews* 33 no. 5 (2013):985–1080.

Stangier, J. 2008. "Clinical Pharmacokinetics and Pharmacodynamics of the Oral Direct Thrombin Inhibitor Dabigatran Etexilate." *Clinical Pharmacokinetics* 47 no. 5 (2008):285–295.

Stepan, A. F., Walker, D. P., Bauman, J. et al. "Structural Alert/Reactive Metabolite Concept as Applied in Medicinal Chemistry to Mitigate Risk of Idiosyncratic Drug Toxicity: A Perspective Based on the Critical Examination of Trends in the Top 200 Drugs Marketed in the United States." *Chemical Research in Toxicology* 24 no. 9 (2011):1345–1410.

Tang, W., Stearns, R. A., Wang, R. W., Chiu, S. H., and Baillie, T. A. "Roles of Human Hepatic Cytochrome P450s 2C9 and 3A4 in the Metabolic Activation of Diclofenac." *Chemical Research in Toxicology* 12 no. 2 (1999):192–199.

Teng, W. C., Oh, J. W., New, L. S. et al. "Mechanism-Based Inactivation of Cytochrome P450 3A4 by Lapatinib." *Molecular Pharmacology* 78 no. 4 (2010):693–703.

Testa, L., Bhindi, R., Agostoni, P., Abbate, A., Zoccai, G. G., and van Gaal, W. J. "The Direct Thrombin Inhibitor Ximelagatran/Melagatran: A Systematic Review on Clinical Applications and an Evidence Based Assessment of Risk Benefit Profile." *Expert Opinion on Drug Safety* 6 no. 4 (2007):397–406.

Thompson, C. D., Barthen, M. T., Hopper, D. W. et al. "Quantification in Patient Urine Samples of Felbamate and Three Metabolites: Acid Carbamate and Two Mercapturic Acids." *Epilepsia* 40 no. 6 (1999):769–776.

Thompson, R. A., Isin, E. M., Li, Y. et al. "*In Vitro* Approach to Assess the Potential for Risk of Idiosyncratic Adverse Reactions Caused by Candidate Drugs." *Chemical Research in Toxicology* 25 no. 8 (2012):1616–1632.

Thompson, R. A., Isin, E. M., Ogese, M. O., Mettetal, J. T., and Williams, D. P. "Reactive Metabolites: Current and Emerging Risk and Hazard Assessments." *Chemical Research in Toxicology* 29 no. 4 (2016):505–533.

Tingle, M. D., Jewell, H., Maggs, J. L., O'Neill, P. M., and Park, B. K. "The Bioactivation of Amodiaquine by Human Polymorphonuclear Leucocytes *In Vitro*: Chemical Mechanisms and the Effects of Fluorine Substitution." *Biochemical Pharmacology* 50 no. 7 (1995):1113–1119.

Towles, J. K., Clark, R. N., Wahlin, M. D., Uttamsingh, V., Rettie, A. E., and Jackson, K. D. "Cytochrome P450 3A4 and CYP3A5-Catalyzed Bioactivation of Lapatinib." *Drug Metabolism and Disposition* 44 no. 10 (2016):1584–1597.

Uetrecht, J. "Evaluation of Which Reactive Metabolite, If Any, is Responsible for a Specific Idiosyncratic Reaction." *Drug Metabolism Reviews* 38 no. 4 (2006):745–753.

Uetrecht, J. and Naisbitt, D. J. "Idiosyncratic Adverse Drug Reactions: Current Concepts." *Pharmacology Reviews* 65 no. 2 (2013):779–808.

Uetrecht, J. P. "Idiosyncratic Drug Reactions: Past, Present, and Future." *Chemical Research in Toxicology* 21 no. 1 (2008):84–92.

Uetrecht, J. P. "Is It Possible to More Accurately Predict Which Drug Candidates Will Cause Idiosyncratic Drug Reactions?" *Current Drug Metabolism* 1 no. 2 (2000):133–141.

Uetrecht, J., Zahid, N., Tehim, A., Fu, J. M., and Rakhit, S. "Structural Features Associated with Reactive Metabolite Formation in Clozapine Analogues." *Chemico-Biological Interactions* 104 no. 2–3 (1997):117–129.

Venkatakrishnan, K. and Obach, R. S. "*In Vitro-in Vivo* Extrapolation of CYP2D6 Inactivation by Paroxetine: Prediction of Nonstationary Pharmacokinetics and Drug Interaction Magnitude." *Drug Metabolism and Disposition* 33 no. 6 (2005):845–852.

Weinz, C., Schwarz, T., Kubiza, D., Mueck, W., and Lang, D. "Metabolism and Excretion of Rivaroxaban, an Oral, Direct Factor Xa Inhibitor, in Rats, Dogs, and Humans." *Drug Metabolism and Disposition* 37 no. 5 (2009):1056–1064.

Weng, Z., Wang, K., Li, H., and Shi, Q. "A Comprehensive Study of the Association Between Drug Hepatotoxicity and Daily Dose, Liver Metabolism, and Lipophilicity Using 975 Oral Medications." *Oncotarget* 10 no. 6 (2015):17031–17038.

Wu, G., Vashishtha, S. C., and Erve, J. C. "Characterization of Glutathione Conjugates of Duloxetine by Mass Spectrometry and Evaluation of In Silico Approaches to Rationalize the Site of Conjugation for Thiophene Containing Drugs." *Chemical Research in Toxicology* 23 no. 8 (2010):1393–1404.

Yu, K., Geng, X., Chen, M. et al. "High Daily Dose and Being a Substrate of Cytochrome P450 Enzymes are Two Important Predictors of Drug-Induced Liver Injury." *Drug Metabolism and Disposition* 42 no. 4 (2014):744–750.

Zhang, D., He, K., Raghavan, N. et al. "Comparative Metabolism of 14C-Labeled Apixaban in Mice, Rats, Rabbits, Dogs and Humans." *Drug Metabolism and Disposition* 37 no. 8 (2009):1738–1748.

Zhao, S. X., Dalvie, D. K., Kelly, J. M. et al. "NADPH-Dependent Covalent Binding of [3H]Paroxetine to Human Liver Microsomes and S-9 Fractions: Identification of an Electrophilic Quinone Metabolite of Paroxetine." *Chemical Research in Toxicology*. 20 no. 11 (2007):1649–1657.

Zhuo, X., Hartz, R. A., Bronson, J. J. et al. "Comparative Biotransformation of Pyrazinone-containing Corticotropin-Releasing Factor Receptor-1 Antagonists: Minimizing the Reactive Metabolite Formation." *Drug Metabolism and Disposition* 38 no. 1 (2010):5–15.

27

Applications of ^{14}C Accelerator Mass Spectrometry in Drug Development

Raju Subramanian and Mark Seymour

CONTENTS

Introduction

Accelerator mass spectrometry (AMS) is an ultra-sensitive technique for quantitative analysis of low abundance isotopes that has found utility in very-low-level tracer (commonly referred to as microtracer) analysis in biological samples using, almost exclusively, ^{14}C (the radioactive isotope of carbon; natural isotopic abundance $\sim 10^{-12}\%$). AMS was developed in the second half of the twentieth century and has been widely applied for radiocarbon dating in fields such as archaeology, wherein the ^{14}C-content in organic matter within ancient artifacts is measured to determine their age [1]. Since the 1990s, AMS as a radiotracer technique has been applied in biomedical research to measure ultra-low concentrations of ^{14}C in a wide range of biological samples. AMS sensitivity is unmatched because the technique measures the mass to charge ratio of atoms and typically an absolute count of approximately 1000 ^{14}C atoms in a sample provides an adequate signal-to-noise ratio for a valid measurement. An overview of biomedical AMS methodology is provided in the next section. This atom level measurement yields a method capable

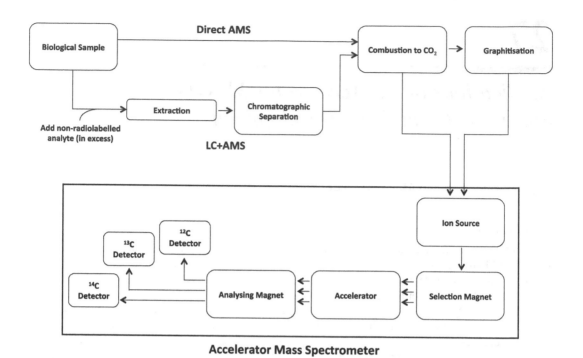

FIGURE 27.1 Biomedical accelerator mass spectrometry modes of operation. Biological samples may be analyzed intact (Direct AMS), to determine total ^{14}C following analyte extraction and/or chromatographic separation (LC+AMS), to quantify specific analyte(s). The modes of operation are explained in the text. (Adapted with permission from Seymour, M.A., *J Labelled Comp. Radiopharm.*, 59, 640–647, 2016.)

of quantifying ^{14}C concentrations in the range of 10^{-16} to 10^{-18} g/mL. At a practical level this equates to lower limits of quantification (LLOQs) for total ^{14}C measurements in biological samples (direct AMS; see Figure 27.1) 300–1000-fold lower than those typically obtained using liquid scintillation counting [2,3]. Despite impressive and on-going improvements in "conventional" liquid chromatography-tandem mass spectrometry (LC-MS/MS), the sensitivity of LC+AMS remains orders of magnitude lower, with LLOQs routinely in the sub-pg/mL range for the quantification of a specific small molecule analyte using LC+AMS [4].

AMS is now an established bioanalytical technique in pharmaceutical development and has two major advantages [5]. Firstly, prior to AMS analysis, each sample irrespective of the biomatrix origin is converted to one single ultimate analyte—initially carbon dioxide, which in most cases is then reduced to solid carbon (graphite). The analyte response is based on carbon atom counting; therefore, it is constant and unaffected by sample type—ionization is not compound specific and is unaffected by matrix components. Secondly, AMS measures the ^{14}C amount in each biomatrix that was introduced with the dosing and is independent of the total mass of analyte present.

AMS has found a wide range of applications in drug development [2–9] and examples from select categories are presented in later sections. These applications include, but are not limited to:

- Intravenous (IV) and extravascular pharmacokinetics (PK): Determination of fundamental PK parameters; absolute bioavailability following single dose and at steady-state following repeat doses.
- PK following low absorption routes of delivery: Ocular, dermal, intranasal.
- Disposition (absorption, distribution, metabolism and excretion; ADME) characterization in healthy subjects and vulnerable populations: These include studies where human dosimetry is dose limiting; where a drug is eliminated slowly or rapidly; where the ^{14}C-labeled compound

is unstable due to radiolysis; or where the radioactive dosed is limited by the study population; for, e.g., pediatric studies, studies in cancer patients, etc.

- Early read on metabolite safety liability in humans: Adding a microtracer to early clinical studies provides assurance that no human-disproportionate metabolites, which are not covered by existing safety toxicology data, will be uncovered late in development.
- Specimen limited analysis: Pediatric PK and disposition; PK at the target site of action—for example, peripheral blood mononuclear cells, cerebrospinal fluid, biopsy tissues.
- Drug-drug interactions.
- Drug polymorphisms.
- Tracing endogenous compound PK/turnover.

In this chapter, the utility of these applications in the context of pharmaceutical development is discussed: what information can AMS provide, and how can it be integrated with other techniques to add real value?

Analytical Methodology

An overview of biomedical AMS modes of operation is presented in Figure 27.1. The core concept of ^{14}C-AMS detection [10] and the considerations for bioanalytical method development and validation have been described recently [2,11]. Two types of workflows are followed. In the "direct AMS" mode, the total ^{14}C content is determined by AMS in the intact biological sample. Alternately, in the "LC+AMS" mode, the biological sample is prepared for and then fractionated via liquid chromatographic separation (HPLC or UPLC). The ^{14}C content in each fraction is then determined by AMS. LC+AMS can be sub-divided into bioanalytical and profiling modes. In the former, one or more fractions containing specific analyte(s) is analyzed; in the latter, all fractions across the chromatographic run are analyzed. In all modes, a common sample preparation process is used whereby the sample is combusted to convert all the carbon in the sample to carbon dioxide. The CO_2 is then either reduced to elemental carbon (graphitized) and loaded into the ion source or introduced directly into the ion source of the AMS instrument.

A carbon carrier (diluent) is typically added to each sample when the amount of natural carbon in the sample is small or highly variable [12,13]. An example of sample preparation for AMS is as follows [14]:

- ^{14}C-depleted carbon carrier (sodium benzoate) is added as necessary during sample preparation to achieve approximately 2 mg of carbon.
- Dialysate (25 to 500 µL), 10-fold diluted urine (100 µL), plasma or 10-fold diluted plasma (60 µL), blood (20 µL), and lyophilized feces (2 to 4 mg) were directly analyzed by AMS.
- Each sample was prepared in quartz sample tubes, which were heat-sealed under vacuum and then heated for 2 hours at 900°C to oxidize all carbon in the sample to CO_2.
- The CO_2 was then cryogenically transferred and sealed into an evacuated glass tube containing reducing agent (TiH_2 and Zn), with cobalt powder as catalyst.
- Samples were heated for 4 hours at 500°C, then for 6 hours at 550°C, reducing CO_2 to solid carbon (graphite).
- The resultant graphite/cobalt mixture was pressed into aluminum cathodes.
- The prepared cathodes were placed in the ion source of a 250 kV single-stage AMS (National Electrostatics Corp., Middleton, WI).
- In the ion source, a Cs^+ ion beam was focused onto the surface of the pressed graphite, producing carbon ions, These are passed through a selection magnet that sequentially pulses the three isotopes of carbon (^{14}C, ^{13}C, and ^{12}C) into the accelerator, where the ions are accelerated to a sufficiently high kinetic energy to allow separation in a detecting mass spectrometer. The three isotopes are quantified in separate detectors, and the instrument reports the results as isotope ratios (e.g., ^{14}C: ^{12}C, and ^{13}C: ^{12}C; Figure 27.1).

All carbon from biological sources contains background levels of ^{14}C measurable by AMS. Therefore, in order to quantify ^{14}C arising from exogenously administered ^{14}C-labeled compounds, background ^{14}C:^{12}C ratios must be measured in relevant background material, e.g., predose samples, and subtracted from the ratios determined for post dose sample.

The sample processing to prepare the aluminum cathode for each sample is time and labor intensive—it takes a 1–3 days to prepare a batch of up to 134 cathodes [15], although experienced analysts can easily sustain a production rate of two or more batches of samples ready for analysis per working day. Several groups have recently introduced automated combustion AMS methods, wherein the CO_2 formed from initial combustion of the sample is infused directly into the ion source of the AMS [16–19]. In the most advanced automated method [17], a solid sample formed by placing the biomedical sample in a tin foil cup and evaporated to dryness is introduced to an elemental analyzer and then combusted to CO_2. The liberated CO_2 is mixed with a helium stream and infused to AMS. This method requires only ~50 µg (e.g., equivalent to as little as 2 µL of plasma). Most importantly, this method allows for automated sample introduction to AMS and enables a significantly faster overall analysis cycle time (including sample preparation and AMS analysis) for individual samples. Maximum throughput for the automated CO_2 analysis system is currently at approximately 90 samples per day and set to increase to 160/day (W Vaes, TNO, personal communication). It is also likely to provide the basis of a practical on-line interface between liquid chromatography and AMS.

Dosing Paradigms in AMS Studies

The disposition and pharmacokinetics of an administered compound is driven by the total mass dose. As described above, AMS detects the ^{14}C in each sample and this ^{14}C tracer is introduced with the intravenous or extravascular dose. A "microtracer" ^{14}C amount of <1 µCi, at the time of dose administration, is added to the non-radiolabeled dose. The typical dose combinations used in AMS studies are listed in Table 27.1.

The mass of non-radiolabeled dose in the total mass administered is selected to meet the aims of the study. The non-radiolabeled dose could be a macrodose (>100 µg), in designs defined herein as "macrodose with microtracer" studies. Two dosing paradigms are possible here—the ^{14}C tracer and the non-radiolabeled dose are administered at the same time via the same route, for example in a human ADME study, or the ^{14}C tracer is administered separately and via different routes, for example in an absolute bioavailability study. Applications with these two designs are provided in section "Macrodose with Microtracer Studies." Alternately, the non-radiolabeled dose could be a microdose (≤100 µg)

TABLE 27.1

Typical Doses for AMS Tracer Studies

Dose Paradigm	^{14}C Tracer Radioactivity (µCi)	Mass (mg)	Mass of Non-Radiolabeled Dose (mg)	Total Mass Administered (mg)
Macrodose with microtracer[a]	0.2–1	0.0014[c]–0.1	10–100[d]	10–100
Macrodose with microtracer— concomitant dosing[b]	0.2–1	0.0014[c]–0.1	10–100[d]	10–100
Microdose with microtracer	0.2–1	0.0014[c]–0.1	NA	0.0014–0.1[e]

NA = not applicable

[a] ^{14}C tracer dose and non-radiolabeled dose are typically co-formulated and administered as a single dose.

[b] ^{14}C tracer dose and non-radiolabeled dose administered separately, e.g., by different dose routes.

[c] Based on maximum theoretical specific radioactivity for incorporation of a single ^{14}C atom into molecule with molecular weight = 450 g/mol.

[d] Typical values; actual dose depends on study type and therapeutic dose.

[e] Maximum = 100 µg (30 nmol for protein); must not exceed 1/100th of dose calculated to give pharmacological effect.

defined herein as "microdose with microtracer" studies, and examples of applications using this design are provided in section "Microdose with Microtracer Studies." There is confusion over the use of the "microdose" terminology in the literature, where it is incorrectly used when a microtracer radiodose is co-administered with a macrodose as well as when the total dose (radiolabeled + non-radiolabeled) is below 100 µg [8]. The use of "microtracer" distinguishes these two scenarios.

Macrodose with Microtracer Studies

The sensitivity of ^{14}C AMS detection is ideal for a whole range of PK and disposition studies—by adding a microtracer amount of ^{14}C label (Table 27.1) to the administered dose, either by the same or a different dose route, the total ^{14}C and the LC-fractionated ^{14}C of the administered compound and the ^{14}C-label related analytes of interest (metabolites, additions to endogenous biomarkers) can be followed in circulating and excreted biofluids and tissues. A study design with a ^{14}C microtracer delivers several advantages [7] over conventional macrotracer designs: enabling tissue dosimetry animal studies are not needed; the low level of radioactivity means there are no radiological protection concerns once the tracer has been administered; and the ^{14}C microtracer dose enables determination of routes of excretion and biotransformation pathways in any clinical study. Where the microtracer and macrodose are administered by different dose routes, there are additional advantages over stable-isotope or two-way non-radiolabeled cross-over designs—the microtracer dose is too small to perturb the kinetics of the extravascular dose; intravenous formulation is simplified; the plasma compartment mixing of the microtracer and macro non-radiolabeled doses ensure equal clearance for the two doses; and lastly, the microtracer study delivers in a single arm what used to require two tests with a cross-over design and in between wash-out periods wherein the individuals serve as their own control and thereby improves the statistical power of the study.

Concomitant Dosing

An area of biomedical AMS that has gained considerable traction within the pharmaceutical development industry is that of concomitant clinical dosing, whereby an isotopically labeled intravenous dose of test compound and a non-labeled extravascular dose of the same compound are co-administered to the same human subject. The AMS technique is particularly well suited to this type of study because it measures the ^{14}C-label, not the compound it is attached to, facilitating discrimination between compound arising from the two different dose routes. Furthermore, the sensitivity of AMS means that the intravenous dose can be extremely small in mass terms, ensuring that it does not affect the pharmacokinetics of the extravascular dose and minimizing the galenic and regulatory hurdles that are often cited as reasons for not carrying out intravenous studies during the development of drugs intended for extravascular administration in the clinic. The intravenous dose itself is typically below the threshold for a microdose (Table 27.1). However, because the extravascular dose is given at a pharmacologically relevant dose, the total dose exceeds the microdose definition.

Although the current regulatory guidelines make allowance for sponsors to scientifically justify to not include absolute bioavailability data in their regulatory submission [20], the feasibility of using the AMS-enabled approach to generate the required intravenous data means the regulatory authorities are less likely to accept of rationale in the future. Additionally, from the drug developer's point of view, the fundamental pharmacokinetic information generated, including clearance and volume of distribution, can be invaluable aids to decision making during the development process.

The principle of the concomitant dosing study design is that the intravenous dose is delivered, usually as a short infusion (typically 15–30 minutes), to coincide with the maximum systemic concentrations arising from the extravascular dose (i.e., at time to maximum concentration; t_{max}). Concentrations of the test compound arising from each of the dose routes are measured in samples collected from the same subject during a single study period. Consequently, the intravenous and extravascular pharmacokinetics can both be determined under identical conditions. This is scientifically superior to the traditional cross-over study design, in which subjects receive separate intravenous and extravascular doses, with a washout period in between. The cross-over study design adds an additional source of variability due to day-to day fluctuations and also engenders the potential for errors due to dose-dependent kinetics if the drug exposures resulting from the two doses are not closely matched. This can be difficult to achieve, since by definition, the bioavailability is unknown. Furthermore, the intravenous dose level for a cross-over study is likely to be orders of magnitude higher than for a microtracer study, which can dramatically increase the resource (time, money and establishment) required to develop a suitable intravenous formulation.

A schematic of the concomitant dosing study design is shown in Figure 27.2. The underlying principle in this approach is that the isotopic label attached to the test compound administered intravenously enables it to be differentiated analytically from the non-labeled form of the same compound administered by a different dosing route (most often oral, but the methodology is applicable to any extravascular route) present in the same sample. The earliest studies with this approach used ^{13}C-labeled analogues, for example, the determination of the intravenous PK and absolute bioavailability of *N*-acetylprocainamide was published by Strong et al. in 1975 [21]. There are some advantages to using a stable, non-radioactive isotope, such as ^{13}C, including not requiring the designated facilities or regulatory approvals necessary to handle radioactivity and the ability to quantify both labeled and non-labeled analyte using "conventional" analytical techniques (invariably LC-MS/MS). On the other hand, the use of a single analytical platform implies that the lower limits of quantification for both analytes are the same. This limits how far the labeled tracer dose can be lowered, increasing the proportion of total circulating compound concentration that originates from the intravenous dose (and thereby the likelihood that it will influence the pharmacokinetics being measured), and potentially the time and cost of developing a suitable clinical formulation for the intravenous dose. Furthermore, because of the relatively high natural abundance of stable isotopes (for ^{13}C that is 1.1%), the potential for isotopic interference between the assays must be assessed. It should also be noted that, in many cases, the LC-MS/MS assay for the non-labeled analyte will use a stable-labeled internal standard (IS). The labeled form used for the intravenous dose has to be distinct from the IS and the isotopic interference issue is complicated further.

A key consideration in the decision on which isotope to use is analytical sensitivity and the concentration range expected for a given mass of drug given intravenously. The latter depends on the volume of distribution and clearance of the compound in humans, the very parameters that the study is designed to determine and, therefore, are unknown at the study design stage. If, based on estimates from *in vitro* and/or preclinical studies, the expected systemic concentrations are below the LLOQ of the bioanalytical method to be used for the non-labeled (extravascular) analyte, the options are either to increase the intravenous dose or to use an alternative analytical platform, such as AMS, with adequate sensitivity.

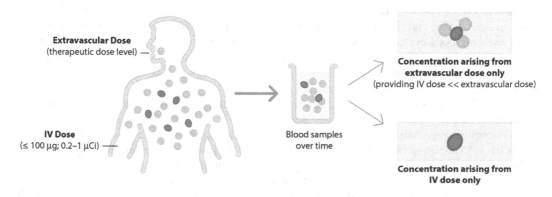

FIGURE 27.2 Intravenous ^{14}C microtracer study design. Non-radiolabeled test compound (●) light gray is administered, at a pharmacologically relevant dose, *via* an extravascular route. Subsequently, at the expected T_{max} of the extravascular dose, an intravenous microtracer dose (●) dark gray of the ^{14}C-labeled compound is administered to the same subject. Plasma, containing compound arising from both dose routes, is obtained at timed intervals after dosing. Concentrations of the non-radiolabeled compound, arising from the extravascular dose, are measured using a conventional bioanalytical method; plasma concentrations of ^{14}C-labeled compound, arising from the intravenous dose, are determined using LC+AMS. Figure kindly provided by Xceleron Inc and reproduced with permission.

The issue with increasing the intravenous dose is that this also increases the proportion of total circulating compound it contributes, raising the likelihood that it will affect the kinetics being measured. In practice, it is recommended that the expected concentrations arising from the intravenous dose should be ≤1% of those arising from the extravascular dose.

As discussed above, the sensitivity of AMS depends on the amount of ^{14}C administered, rather than the total mass of compound, in other words the specific radioactivity of the dose. Assuming substitution with a single radionuclide atom, the theoretical maximum achievable specific radioactivity for ^{14}C is 62.4 mCi/mmol; this equates to 125 µCi/mg for a "typical" small molecule drug with a molecular weight of 500 Da. In practice, commercially available radiolabeled compounds are typically synthesized at a specific activity of around ~100 µCi/mg. Assuming a total radioactivity dose of 1 µCi, the theoretical minimum mass dose is therefore just 10 ng. The maximum radioactivity dose depends on the local legal and regulatory framework and, therefore, varies geographically; this amount of radioactivity can generally be administered to human subjects without specific regulatory approval. In practice, the challenges involved in preparing and administering such an extremely small quantity means that doses are generally between 1 and 10 µg.

Xu et al. [22] note that, because both labeled and non-labeled compounds can be measured simultaneously with LC-MS/MS, using a stable label is more cost effective than using ^{14}C, but point out that for compounds with high volumes of distribution and/or poor LC-MS/MS response the use of ^{14}C with LC+AMS detection would be indicated. Lappin [8] suggests that, given a typical lower limit of quantification (LLOQ) for LC-MS/MS of 10–100 pg/mL, a compound with a volume of distribution of 100 L or greater would need to be administered at a dose of more than 100 µg for the resulting circulating concentrations to be high enough to enable adequate definition of the pharmacokinetic profile. Interestingly, Lappin's calculations are based on being able to follow the disposition of the compound for a little more than three half-lives, whereas it is more usually held that a minimum of five or six half-lives is required. A typical LLOQ for an LC+AMS assay in human plasma, assuming a dose of 1 µCi (37 kBq)/10 µg, is around 0.15 pg/mL. With a volume of distribution of 100 L, the expected circulating concentration at time zero (C_0) is 0.1 µg/L or 100 pg/mL. Thus, the LC+AMS assay would easily be capable of quantifying concentrations after three half-lives (i.e., 12.5 pg/mL), and indeed after six half-lives (1.6 pg/mL) and beyond. It would also have adequate sensitivity for a compound with a much higher volume of distribution. In their paper, Xu and co-authors present a decision tree to assist decision making on whether to choose whether to use ^{14}C- or a stable label. A similar decision tree, shown in Figure 27.3 [23], builds on this by introducing an assessment of the relative predicted concentrations arising from the intravenous and extravascular doses.

The first decision box in Figure 27.3 relates to the fact that a range of additional analyses are facilitated by the presence of the ^{14}C in the microtracer. These include:

- **Measurement of total ^{14}C in plasma and/or excreta by direct AMS:** This can yield information on the extent of systemic metabolism and, by comparison with similar data for the extravascular dose route, to help assess the extent of first-pass metabolism [8, 24–28].
- **Collection of human bile samples:** These samples can be analyzed for total ^{14}C, for radiolabeled metabolites and/or parent compound. Although only semi-quantitative, because the fraction of total bile recovered is unknown and variable, the technique can provide valuable insight if an understanding of biliary excretion in human is important for the development of the compound, [29,30].
- **Collection and analysis of other tissues:** Although clinical collection of tissues is limited by ethical and technical considerations, if samples can be obtained in the presence of the ^{14}C-tracer facilitates quantitative analysis due to the universal applicability of AMS [31–34].

Another key feature of the concomitant dosing study design is that the intravenous microtracer dose is administered to coincide with maximum circulating concentration arising from the extravascular dose, again in order to ensure that the pharmacokinetics is always driven by the extravascular dose. Ideally, the intravenous dose is given as a short infusion (typically 15–30 min), timed to end at the expected t_{max} for the extravascular dose, as this mirrors the absorption phase of the extravascular dose. Additionally, calculation of the area under the plasma concentration curve (AUC) for a constant infusion is based entirely on observed data, whereas for a bolus dose concentration at time zero (C_0) must be estimated by

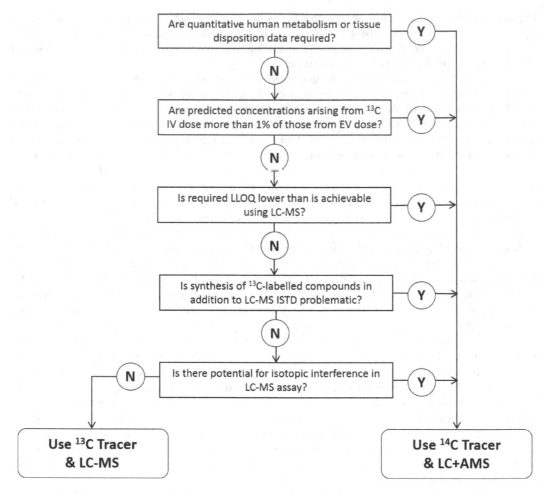

FIGURE 27.3 Decision tree for selection of isotope label for concomitant microtracer studies. (From English, S. et al., *What's the Best Way to Measure Absolute Bioavailability?* Land O'Lakes Bioanalytical Meeting 2014, Madison, WI, 2014.)

back extrapolation and this can introduce error into the calculation. However, if necessary, for example for a test compound that binds extensively to the infusion apparatus, administering the microtracer dose as a bolus at t_{max} is acceptable. Several examples of macrodose with concomitant microtracer dosing are among the examples discussed in section "Examples of Macrodose with Microtracer Studies."

Examples of Macrodose with Microtracer Studies

There are numerous literature examples available in the application categories presented in the introduction section [32,33,35–48]; recent select examples addressing PK and disposition questions utilizing macrodose with microtracer amounts are presented below. Additional examples employing IV microtracers are summarized in a recent review [8].

Etelcalcetide

Etelcalcetide is an intravenous calcimimetic approved for treatment of secondary hyperthyroidism in chronic kidney disease (CKD) patients on hemodialysis [49–52]. Etelcalcetide is a 1048 Da novel synthetic peptide composed of a linear chain of seven D-amino acids (referred to as the "D-amino acid backbone") and an L-cysteine linked to the D-cysteine by a disulfide bond. The PK, biotransformation, and excretion in CKD patients on hemodialysis was characterized following a single intravenous dose of [¹⁴C]etelcalcetide (10 mg; 710 nCi) [14]. Blood, urine, feces (from each discharge), dialysate (entire amounts from each hemodialysis session), and vomit from each emesis session were collected for up to approximately 180 days to characterize the PK, mass balance, and biotransformation product profiles of etelcalcetide. Blood was also collected from arterial and venous lines during the first hemodialysis session following dose administration. The hemodialyzer apparatus (dialysis cartridge and lead lines) were saved from each session to assess non-specific binding.

Higher amounts of radioactivity typical for a conventional human ADME study were considered in the study design phase for dosing but were not pursued. A microtracer study was compelling for several reasons. The PK and disposition needed to be characterized in a vulnerable clinical population. If a conventional dose (such as ~100 µCi) was administered, there were concerns in controlling radioactivity contamination should a hospitalization be required—one patient in the study required hospitalization and the microtracer dosing obviated the need for contamination controls. The duration of the study was uncertain at the time of study design due to significant differences in PK of the molecule in healthy subjects versus CKD patients [53,54]—the study was initiated with a 40 day collection period and was extended to almost 180 days to achieve the mass balance objective. Lastly, it was important to determine the ¹⁴C excretion in all matrices and in particular in dialysate, which would have required the ultrasensitivity of AMS detection to determine the total ¹⁴C in dialysate collections past the initial few hemodialysis sessions. AMS sensitivity was remarkable—¹⁴C concentrations of ~6.7 fCi/g of ¹⁴C (~0.06 ng-equivalents of etelcalcetide/g) were quantified in a ~0.35 g dialysate sample prepared from ~150 kg of dialysate collected on study day 176.

The PK of total ¹⁴C and etelcalcetide (determined with an LC-MS/MS method) in systemic circulation and during the first hemodialysis session following the IV dose is shown in Figure 27.4, panels A and B,

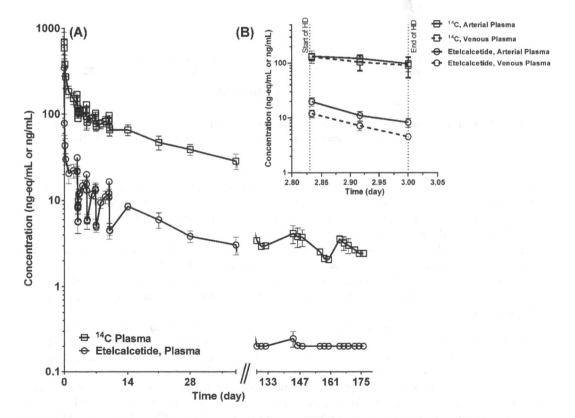

FIGURE 27.4 Total ¹⁴C and etelcalcetide plasma pharmacokinetics following a single intravenous dose in systemic circulation (panel A) and during the first hemodialysis period post dose (panel B). The total ¹⁴C and etelcalcetide concentrations were determined by AMS and LC-MS/MS, respectively. HD = hemodialysis. (Adapted with permission from Subramanian, R. et al., *Clin. Pharmacokinet.*, 56, 179–192, 2017.)

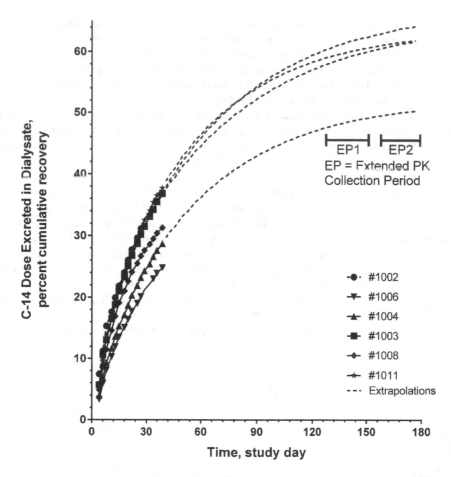

FIGURE 27.5   Cumulative recovery of [^{14}C]etelcalcetide dose in the dialysate following administration of a single intravenous dose. (Adapted with permission from Subramanian, R. et al., *Clin. Pharmacokinet.*, 56, 179–192, 2017.)

respectively. The PK for the measured analytes was characterized outside and during hemodialysis periods. The mean total ^{14}C elimination half-life was similar for dialysate (~40 days) and plasma (~36 days).

The cumulative excretion in dialysate following the microtracer dose administration is shown in Figure 27.5. Mass balance data showed that hemodialysis (approximately 60% of the administered dose; 89% of the recovered dose) was the predominant clearance and elimination pathway for etelcalcetide. A small proportion of the dose was excreted in urine and feces (each <5% of the administered dose). Radioactivity was below the limit of quantification even of AMS in the sole vomit sample and only trace levels of ^{14}C (0.005% of administered dose) were recovered in extracts from the dialyzer cartridge used in the first session.

LC+AMS and LC-HRMS chromatograms from pooled plasma, urine, and dialysate samples were acquired in the study. LC+AMS chromatograms from plasma and dialysate are shown in Figure 27.6. LC-HRMS chromatograms were acquired with a parallel LC set up to identify the etelcalcetide related components. In plasma from the first interdialytic period after dosing, intact etelcalcetide accounted for approximately 17% of radioactivity in plasma AUC pool [55]. Serum albumin peptide conjugate (SAPC) formed via a covalent disulfide exchange of the L-cysteine in etelcalcetide with the free thiol cysteine in serum albumin was the most abundant biotransformation product (73%) in the plasma AUC pool. The dialysate profile consisted of all components in plasma except the SAPC as anticipated; SAPC is not removed from dialysate because its molecular weight (~67 kDa) is well above the dialyzer cut off (~10 kDa).

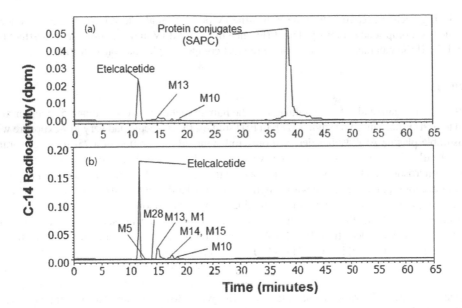

FIGURE 27.6 LC+AMS chromatograms. (a) AUC pooled plasma from the 1st interdialytic period. LC separation was performed on non-extracted diluted plasma. (b) Dialysate from first hemodialysis session (panel B) following the IV dose. Identities of metabolites and SAPC are explained in the reference. (Adapted with permission from Subramanian, R. et al., *Clin. Pharmacokinet.*, 56, 179–192, 2017.)

Overall, the cumulative dataset from this study also enabled a drug disposition model that provided a quantitative approach to describe the biotransformation, distribution, and elimination of etelcalcetide, a unique synthetic D-amino acid peptide, in the relevant patient population [56].

Pomaglumetad Methionil (LY2140023)

Pomaglumetad methionil (LY2140023) is the methionine prodrug of LY404039, a novel metabotropic glutamate 2/3 receptor agonist currently in clinical development for the treatment of schizophrenia [27]. LY2140023 is actively absorbed in the gastrointestinal (GI) tract with uptake mediated by human peptide transporter 1 (PEPT1), and during the GI epithelium transit, the prodrug undergoes complete or partial hydrolysis by the esterases. If the GI hydrolysis is incomplete, a significant fraction of the prodrug could enter systemic circulation and be taken up in tissue sites that express PEPT1 or PEPT2. The relative contribution of these intestinal and systemic processes is not predicted—in part because the plasma esterase activity is high in nonclinical species.

The absolute bioavailability of the prodrug (LY2140023) and the extent of conversion to the active form (LY404039) were estimated at presystemic and systemic sites in a two-period clinical study using a microtracer approach with AMS detection. In period 1, subjects received a single oral dose of the prodrug (80 mg) immediately followed by a 2-hour IV infusion of the [^{14}C]-labeled prodrug (100 μg; 100 nCi). In period 2, subjects received a single oral dose of the prodrug (80 mg) immediately followed by a 2-hour IV infusion of the [^{14}C]-labeled active form (100 μg; 100 nCi). The duration of the infusion was chosen so that the oral and IV plasma concentrations peaked at similar times. The plasma concentrations of the non-radiolabeled prodrug and the active form were determined by LC-MS/MS and ^{14}C concentrations of the prodrug and the active form were determined by LC+AMS.

PK results showed the prodrug mean absolute oral bioavailability was 68%, and the prodrug fraction reaching systemic circulation is completely converted to the active form. The simultaneous oral and IV dosing approach enabled by the AMS sensitivity to estimate absolute oral bioavailability minimized the intrasubject variability and also mitigated issues that may arise due to non-linear kinetics with the traditional study design to determine absolute bioavailability [8,57]. In the traditional study design, the IV and oral dosing occur in separate time periods—the IV dose is usually lower due to safety concerns or limits in the test compound solubility. The difference in the total IV and oral doses could affect the test compound PK if the clearance is dependent on the test compound plasma concentration [57].

Lu AF09535

Lu AF09535 is a negative allosteric modulator of the human metabotropic glutamate 5 receptor and was advanced to first-in-human (FIH) studies [28]. In FIH studies, the molecule had very low exposure with the first measurable plasma AUC values detected only following administration of a 75-mg single oral dose. For this molecule, the human *in vivo* clearance was predicted to be low, because the intrinsic clearance in human liver microsome and hepatocyte was low as did the *in vitro* and *in vivo* clearances in the nonclinical species rat, mouse, and dog, along with a high oral bioavailability (60%–70%). Various *in vitro-in vivo* extrapolation approaches, including allometric scaling, also predicted low clearance in human.

The mechanism(s) behind the low human exposure of this molecule was elucidated with a microtracer clinical study with AMS detection. [14C]Lu AF09535 (263 nCi) was coadministered with the highest non-radiolabeled dose (75 mg) in the FIH study. Plasma, urine, and feces were collected and analyzed in the study. Of the administered 14C dose, 80% was recovered in the first 96 hours. Comparison of plasma total 14C PK profile obtained by direct AMS analysis and the Lu AF09535 PK obtained by LC-MS/MS analysis (Figure 27.7) showed that total 14C AUC was 22-fold higher than the intact drug AUC. LC+AMS analysis revealed that the test compound was fully absorbed, and the low exposure was caused by extensive first pass metabolism. AUC pooled plasma LC+AMS and parallel LC-MS/MS revealed that circulating radioactivity was predominantly composed of a multiple oxidative (mono, di, and tri-hydroxy) metabolites; intact test compound was not detected. Additional *in vitro* experiments revealed the aldehyde oxidase (AO) catalyzed the formation of the primary monohydroxy metabolite. Overall, the poor initial prediction of human PK was attributed to difficulty of scaling AO-mediated clearance determined from *in vitro* methods to an *in vivo* setting.

Vismodegib

Vismodegib is an oral small molecule inhibitor of the hedgehog signaling pathway and is approved for the treatment of basal cell carcinoma. Vismodegib exhibited a long elimination half-life (terminal half-life of ~12 days after a single 150 mg dose) and unique nonlinear plasma pharmacokinetics in cancer

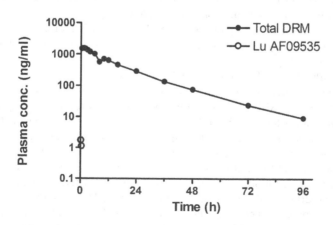

FIGURE 27.7 Plasma pharmacokinetic profile following a single [14C]Lu AF09535 (75 mg; 263 nCi) oral dose in humans. Total DRM = total 14C concentration determined by direct AMS; Lu AF09535 = intact test compound concentration determined by LC-MS/MS. (Reproduced with permission from Jensen, K.G. et al., *Drug Metab. Dispos.*, 45, 68–75, 2017.)

patients and healthy subjects [24,58]. Vismodegib steady-state concentrations were achieved much faster (within 7 days) than expected (~50 days) and the accumulation was 5-fold lower than expected. Also, nonlinearity with respect to dose was observed—an increase in dose from 150 to 270 mg or 540 mg did not result in an increase in steady-state concentration. Furthermore, vismodegib binds to plasma α-1-acid glycoprotein (AAG) and serum albumin with a 10-fold higher affinity binding to AAG. Thus, two separate nonlinear processes were hypothesized to contribute to the observed nonlinearity—solubility limited absorption and high affinity saturable plasma protein binding. A microtracer approach with AMS detection was used to characterize the human ADME and to understand the mechanisms contributing to the nonlinear PK in two clinical studies with female human subjects of non-child-bearing potential.

In the human ADME study [58], [^{14}C]Vismodegib (150 mg; 1 µCi) was administered to subjects; blood, urine, and feces were collected for 56 days. Intact vismodegib in plasma was determined with a LC-MS/MS method. Total ^{14}C in all biomatrices was determined by direct AMS, and ^{14}C metabolite profiles were obtained by LC+AMS analysis. Results revealed that vismodegib was slowly eliminated by a combination of metabolism and excretion of intact drug through feces. Vismodegib was the most dominate component in a plasma AUC pool (98%).

The systemic clearance and absolute bioavailability of vismodegib following single and repeat dosing was determined in a separate clinical study [24]. In the first study group, subjects received a single oral dose of vismodegib (150 mg) followed by a single IV dose of [^{14}C]vismodegib (10 µg; 500 nCi) at 2 hours post the oral dose to match the time to maximum concentration following the oral dose. In the second study group, subjects received repeat oral doses of vismodegib (150 mg) once a day for 7 days; subjects then received a single IV dose of [^{14}C]vismodegib (10 µg; 500 nCi) at 2 hours post day 7 dose. Plasma PK of non-radiolabeled and radiolabeled vismodegib were characterized following the first and last microtracer doses, with plasma concentrations determined by LC-MS/MS and LC+AMS respectively. Vismodegib protein binding was also measured in plasma obtained after single and repeat doses. Results revealed an elimination limited plasma PK following single and repeat doses. The PK profiles following oral (vismodegib) and IV ([^{14}C]vismodegib) administration were parallel in both study groups—the terminal half-life was similar at approximately 12 days after single dose and at approximately 10 days at steady-state after repeating oral dosing. The IV clearance and the volume of distribution at steady-state after repeating oral doses were 81% and 63% higher, respectively, compared to their values after single oral dose. This change in the fundamental PK parameters was explained by the 2.4-fold increase in fraction unbound of vismodegib after repeat dosing, likely due to saturable plasma protein binding. The absolute bioavailability following single dose was moderate (~32%) and following repeat dosing decreased by 77%. This decrease in vismodegib bioavailability was also inferred to be due to poor intestinal solubility and slow drug absorption; it was not due to metabolic enzyme induction. Finally, the increase in clearance and decrease in bioavailability observed in this study explained the 5-fold lower than expected accumulation of vismodegib with continuous repeat dosing.

Recombinant Placental Alkaline Phosphatase

Human recombinant placental alkaline phosphatase (hRESCAP), a recombinant protein (dimer molecular weight ~110 kDa), is being investigated for treatment of chronic inflammatory diseases. A two phase hRESCAP microtracer study was performed to characterize the PK at four doses starting with a microdose leading up to the target therapeutic dose [59]. In the first phase, three healthy human male volunteers were administered a single intravenous microdose with microtracer amount of [^{14}C]hRESCAP (53 µg; ~16 nCi). In the second phase, three healthy volunteers were administered a single intravenous macrodose with microtracer amount of [^{14}C]hRESCAP at three dose levels—a low (~0.4 mg; ~17 nCi), a mid (~1.2 mg; ~17 nCi), and a high (~5.3 mg; ~16 nCi) dose with each cohort dosed 1 week apart. Blood was collected at predose and regular time points and processed to plasma; the total ^{14}C plasma concentrations were determined by automated direct AMS method [17]. A non-compartmental analysis of the time -^{14}C concentration data, assuming the dosed hRESCAP was intact, showed the hRESCAP PK was linear from the microdose to the therapeutic doses of the protein in healthy volunteers. This study is the first published example of the application of the ^{14}C-AMS microtracer dose to a biological therapeutic.

Saxagliptin and Dapagliflozin

Saxagliptin (Onglyza™) is a dipeptidyl peptidase-4 inhibitor and dapagliflozin is a sodium glucose co-transporter-2 inhibitor. Both compounds have been developed for the treatment of type 2 diabetes mellitus. A concomitant dosing macrodose with microtracer approach was used to determine the absolute oral bioavailability of both compounds [26].

In the saxagliptin cohort, eight healthy male subjects each received a single oral dose of non-labeled saxagliptin (5 mg) followed by an IV microtracer dose of [14C]saxagliptin (40 μg; <270 nCi; 5 mL of solution infused over 15 min, beginning 1 hour after the oral dose). In the dapagliflozin cohort, seven subjects each received a single oral dose of dapagliflozin (10 mg), followed after 1 hour by a single intravenous dose of [14C]-dapagliflozin (80 μg; ~200 nCi; 0.32 mL of solution infused over 1 min).

Plasma concentrations of radiolabeled saxagliptin and dapagliflozin arising from the 14C-microtracer doses were quantified using separate LC+AMS methods. The saxagliptin assay utilized a standard curve, generated using standards prepared at known concentrations of [14C]saxagliptin [60], whereas the dapagliflozin method used a recovery standard methodology that relies on the absolute 14C-quantitation provided by AMS and measurement of the analyte extraction efficiency for each individual sample using UV detection [11,15]. Both assays were validated for accuracy, precision, and selectivity using scientifically justified, technology-based validation procedures. The LLOQs of the saxagliptin and dapagliflozin assays were 1.91 and 9.074 pg/mL, respectively, at the specific radioactivities dosed.

Plasma concentrations of saxagliptin and dapagliflozin arising from the non-radiolabeled oral doses were determined using separate validated LC-MS/MS assays. The LLOQs were 0.1 ng/mL for saxagliptin and 1 ng/mL for dapagliflozin, i.e., more than 50- and 100-fold higher than the values for the corresponding LC+AMS assays.

The half-life values for the intravenous and oral doses were similar—saxagliptin, 7.5 hours from the IV data versus 5.7 hours from the oral data; dapagliflozin, 12.2 hours from the IV data versus 13.7 hours from the oral data—and the terminal (elimination) phases of the plasma concentration-time for each dose route were parallel. The observed half-life differences for saxagliptin were attributed to differences in the sampling schemes used for the two dose routes: when the same time points were used for half-life determination, the two values for saxagliptin were virtually identical. These results confirmed the disposition of extravascular macrodose and concomitantly-administered microtracer dose were same for both compounds.

The concomitant microtracer approach allowed an accurate and precise determination of absolute bioavailability at therapeutically relevant concentrations using a single-period study design—the mean absolute oral bioavailability for saxagliptin and dapagliflozin was 50% and 78%, respectively. Furthermore, the approach required less time and resources than traditional study designs. The data generated were successfully used in the regulatory submissions for saxagliptin and dapagliflozin.

Microdose with Microtracer Studies

According to the International Council for Harmonization of Technical Requirements for Pharmaceuticals for Human Use (ICH) guidance [61], a microdose is a sub-pharmacologic dose of a compound at the time of intravenous or extravascular dose administration. In a single dose setting, it is 1/100th of the known or anticipated active dose or 100 μg total adult dose, whichever is smaller. In a repeat dose setting, up to 500 μg can be administered in ≤5 dose administrations. The sensitivity of 14C AMS detection is ideal in microdose studies—by adding a microtracer amount of 14C label (as stated above, typically <1 μCi achieved with 1–100 μg of 14C-labeled compound) the goals of microdose studies are achieved. Although use of conventional LC-MS/MS methods is possible and cheaper, it would require an ultrasensitive analytical method [4,6,22,62].

In a pure microdose study, the sub-therapeutic dose is administered without any additional non-tracer dose, i.e., a concomitant dosing microtracer study is *not* microdosing, despite the fact that the microdosing guidelines are invoked in order to avoid having to carry out route-specific toxicological testing for the tracer dose. Furthermore, microdosing does not necessarily involve the use of a microtracer: if sufficient sensitivity is available using conventional bioanalytical platforms these may be used and, indeed, despite the association of biomedical AMS with microdosing from its earliest days, over recent years more microdose studies appear to have been supported by LC-MS/MS than by LC+AMS (personal communications) Nevertheless, as already discussed, the inherent sensitivity of AMS means it is an invaluable tool whenever dose is restricted (e.g., for a very potent drug), or the required LLOQ is unachievable using MS-based assays.

Because the dose administered is, by definition, below the level where any pharmacological effects are expected, microdosing is not intended to provide efficacy or safety data. Rather it is a way of obtaining human clinical pharmacokinetic data at the earliest possible opportunity, with the minimum amount of enabling pre-clinical effort. Originally conceived by some as a paradigm-shifting advance that would completely replace the traditional iterative process of repeating a more extensive suite of Phase 1 clinical studies on successive development candidates, microdosing has established itself more as a niche application. Thus, it is used mainly in situations where a specific question needs to be answered; for example, when the actual human PK of a lead candidate is significantly different to that predicted from pre-clinical data and not compatible with the clinical requirements. Microdosing can be used to screen several potential back-ups quickly, with very specific go-no-go criteria specified.

Three main issues seem to have prevented the wider adoption of microdosing in drug development:

- The inevitable questions about how well sub-pharmacologic dose predicts the PK of the therapeutic dose;
- The apparent unreliability, high cost and lack of routine availability of AMS;
- The practical issues around the implementation of microdosing within a highly-regulated industry that can significantly reduce the time and cost advantage of the approach.

The question of predictivity has dogged microdosing since it was first conceived and, on the face of it, it seems reasonable to ask whether the pharmacokinetics measured will be relevant to the clinical situation when, by definition, the drug candidate is administered at a level at least two orders of magnitude below the expected therapeutic dose. After all, many drugs are known to exhibit non-dose-linear pharmacokinetics, due to saturation of absorption or elimination pathways or through an effect (inhibition or induction) of the enzymes that mediate their disposition.

Three large research projects have been run to try to generate experimental evidence to inform the debate—the CREAM (Consortium for Resourcing and Evaluating AMS Microdosing) trial [63], EUMAPP (European Union Microdose AMS Partnership Programme) [36,37], and NEDO-MD (New Energy and Industrial Technology Development Organization Microdosing Project) [64]. These studies investigated marketed pharmaceuticals and drug candidates withdrawn during clinical development, chosen as representative of types of compounds for which the PK at a microdose might not be expected to predict PK at the therapeutic dose level (e.g., midazolam, which is subject to extensive first pass metabolism) or for which the human data provided by microdosing could be particularly helpful during development (e.g., phenobarbital, which has very low clearance that is difficult to predict from pre-clinical data). There has been some criticism of the fact that these programs did not test compounds more representative of the types of chemistries that are seen in more modern drugs. Nevertheless, in most cases, the results showed good correlation between the PK at a microdose and the therapeutic doses. Where there were discrepancies, generally, these could be explained from a knowledge of the properties of the compound, and often other parameters for the same compound were well predicted [65]. For example, the clearance of the anti-arrhythmia drug propafenone was under-predicted by the microdose [37], due to saturation of metabolism by CYP2D6 at the therapeutic dose. However, the plasma half-life was dose-proportional within a factor of two, the threshold used to determine whether an observed difference was significant.

The NEDO-MD project is interesting because it was not focused solely on AMS. In fact, most of the clinical microdosing carried out as part of the project was supported analytically using sensitive LC-MS/MS. However, the broader range of endpoints available using of ^{14}C-microtracers supported by AMS-detection is fully acknowledged. The NEDO-MD collaborators have also published some interesting work looking at ways in which *in vitro* data might be used to assess the dose-proportionality of novel compounds in a quantitative mathematical fashion. For example, the relationship between dose-normalized clinical AUC values at least two doses and dose/Km (termed the linearity index, LIN) for P-gp (a membrane transporter that mediates the efflux of oral drugs in the gastrointestinal tract) and CYP3A4 (a drug-metabolizing enzyme that is an important determinant of first-pass metabolism) was analyzed for 38 compounds. Substrates with a P-gp LIN above 0.77 L or a CYP3A4 LIN above 2.8 L exhibited non-linear PK. The authors present a decision tree for predicting non-linear PK based on LIN and F_aF_g (product of the fraction absorbed and the fraction escaping intestinal metabolism), which correctly predicted linearity or non-linearity for 24/29 drugs [66].

A review published in 2013 [9] found that overall, for those compounds where data had been reported both for a microdose and a pharmacologically relevant dose (including the results from CREAM, EUMAPP, and NEDO-MD), 100% of the twelve intravenous microdoses identified accurately predicted the therapeutic dose pharmacokinetics. The figure was lower for the oral dose route, presumably reflecting the influence of saturable uptake processes. However, at 80% (20 out of a total of 25 administrations identified), extravascular microdosing is still significantly better at predicting the human PK of a therapeutic dose than the best achievable using modeling techniques (45%, according to a review published on behalf of PhRMA in 2011[67]).

One of the reasons that ^{14}C-microdosing has not been adopted wholesale by the pharmaceutical industry appears to be a reluctance to commit to the changes in organizational thinking necessary to fully realize the potential time and resource savings. For example, the Chemistry, Manufacturing and Controls (CMC) section of the 2006 US FDA guidance document on Exploratory IND studies [68] states that "although in each phase of a clinical investigational program sufficient information should be submitted to ensure the proper identification, strength, quality, purity, and potency of the investigational candidate, the amount of information that will provide that assurance will vary with the phase of the investigation, the proposed duration of the investigation, the dosage form, and the amount of information already available." However, many drug development companies, particularly the larger ones, have internal policies that do not allow deviation from the CMC requirements that apply to the later stages of clinical development. As a consequence, the time taken to screen 3–5 candidate compounds using a microdosing approach can be increased significantly, to the point where there is little advantage compared to the traditional iterative Phase 1 approach.

Examples of Microdose with Microtracer Studies

There are numerous examples available in the literature [9,37,63,69–75]. A select example is presented below.

AR-709

AR-709 is an anti-infective that was being developed to treat lung infections. The developer needed answers to two key questions: does the active compound reach the target tissues in the lung and, if so, is its oral bioavailability sufficient to make it viable as an orally-administered drug?

The study was carried out in healthy male volunteers with a two-part study design [34]. In part A, four subjects each received two single, microdoses of [^{14}C]AR-709 (100 µg, ~200 nCi) 7 days apart: the first was administered IV, the second orally. The data were used to calculate oral bioavailability. In part B, a separate group of 15 subjects each received a single IV microdose (100 µg, ~200 nCi). In addition to blood, bronchial mucosa biopsy (BM), and bronchoalveolar lavage (BAL) samples were collected. BAL was collected by introducing a saline solution into the lungs and removing it with a syringe. The aspirated liquid contained fluid (epithelial lining fluid; ELF) and cellular (alveolar macrophages; AM) components from the respiratory regions of the lungs. A single set of lung samples was collected from each subject, with five subjects being sampled at each of 3-time points after dosing, in a composite design.

Plasma concentrations of total ^{14}C radioactivity and [^{14}C]AR-709 were determined using direct AMS and LC+AMS, respectively (Figure 27.8). Based on these data, the absolute oral bioavailability was calculated to be just 2.5%.

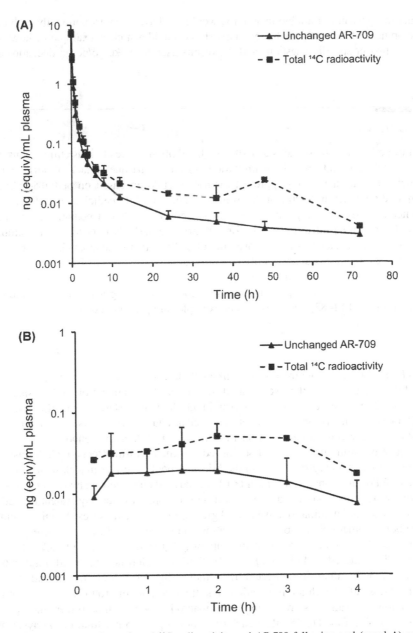

FIGURE 27.8 Plasma concentrations of total ¹⁴C radioactivity and AR-709 following oral (panel A) and intravenous administration (panel B) of a microdose of [¹⁴C]AR-709 (100 μg; 7.4 kBq). Note the difference in both x- and y-scales for the two panels. (Reproduced with permission from Lappin, G. et al., *Eur. J. Clin. Pharmacol.*, 69, 1673–1682, 2013.)

Tissue to plasma concentration ratios from Part B, calculated from total ¹⁴C measurements made using direct AMS, showed that there was a time-dependent concentration of radioactivity in ELF, AM, and BM, indicating that AR-709 and/or its metabolites had reached the intended site of action, i.e., the alveoli of the lung. Subsequently, AM extracts from were profiled using LC+AMS to determine the number and relative amounts of ¹⁴C-labeled metabolites present. The majority of the radioactivity was associated with unchanged AR-709.

The conclusion from this study was that AR-709 reached the target tissues. However, due to its very low oral bioavailability, use of the drug would have been restricted to hospitals and, in view of its relatively narrow spectrum of antibiotic activity, would not have been economically viable. Therefore, further development of AR-709 was halted. This study provides a clear example of how microdosing can be used to answer specific questions and the results used to make go/no-go decisions during drug development.

Pediatric Studies

The conduct of pediatric trials remains a challenge. In addition to the obvious ethical constraints, there are significant technical and procedural limitations in large part due to lack of sufficiently sensitive analytical methods. The medicines approved for use in children based on pediatric clinical studies remains minor, at approximately 20% of the overall number of adult medicines listed in the Physician's Desk Reference [76]. Evolving regulations have increased the number of pediatric clinical studies and improved the number of new drugs available for pediatric use in the last decade—for example, approximately 40% of new molecular entities approved in 2002–2008 also include labeling language for use in children [77,78]. A microtracer approach offers a promising alternative [76,79,80]—the exquisite sensitivity of AMS detection allows for facile analysis of the limited bio fluid volumes (blood, ~20 μL; urine ~100 μL). Pediatric studies with approximately four molecules using a microtracer study design are reported in literature [31,81–83]; two most recent examples are presented below.

Ursodiol

Ursodiol is a bile acid used in the treatment of infant cholestasis. Cholestasis is a condition caused by a reduction of bile acid flow from the liver to small intestine. The treatment of cholestasis is designed to minimize adverse consequences of elevated bilirubin. Orally administered ursodial is effective in treatment of cholestasis in term and preterm neonates, as well as adults. Ursodiol is an endogenous secondary bile acid and is a bacterial metabolism product of the primary bile acid chenodeoxycholic acid formed in the small intestine. Administration of ursodiol reduces the harmful effects of cholestasis by displacing the more cytotoxic primary bile acids in the bile acid pool. The pharmacokinetics of ursodiol was studied in infants following a single microtracer (≤10 nCi) dose administration in two groups of neonates [82]. The radioactivity exposure from this microtracer dose was approximately equivalent to 1/8th of a chest X-ray and was considered nominal relative to background radiation exposures. The five infants in group A, with three born prematurely at 36 weeks gestation and two born at full term, were given three consecutive oral microdoses with microtracer amounts of [14C]ursodiol—8 ng (1.0 nCi), 26 ng (3.3 nCi), and 80 ng (10 nCi) separated by 48 hours. Blood (0.25 mL at each timepoint; 6 mL total in 6 days; <4% of infant's total blood volume) was collected by an indwelling catheter at predose and at 7-time points in 24 hours post dose after each administration. The three infants in group B, all born prematurely at 36 weeks gestation, were administered a single oral macrodose with a microtracer amount of [14C]ursodiol (40 mg/kg; 10 nCi). Blood (0.25 mL at each timepoint; up to 1.5 mL total in 14 days) was collected by a heel stick or an indwelling catheter at predose and at 4-time points in 24 hours post dose after each dose. Serum was collected following clotting of each blood sample, and the total [14C]ursodiol-derived radioactivity from each serum sample was determined by direct AMS. Serum LC+AMS analysis was not performed in this study but was planned for a future date. A total of 115 total [14C]ursodiol derived radioactivity concentration time data points were available and quantifiable by AMS. Assuming the total radioactivity represents the intact ursodiol, a PK model describing ursodiol concentrations was developed using nonlinear mixed-effects modeling.

Acetaminophen

Acetaminophen (Paracetomol) is routinely used as an analgesic and antipyretic in children. A microtracer study was conducted in ten infants aged 0.1–83.1 months. These infants were administered a single oral [14C]acetaminophen dose of (3.3 nCi/kg) in addition to intravenous therapeutic doses of acetaminophen

(15 mg/kg every 6 hours). Blood samples (0.5 mL) were collected via an indwelling catheter at 7-time points and processed to plasma. [¹⁴C]Acetaminophen and the primary metabolites (acetaminophen glucuronide; acetaminophen-4-sulfate) were determined by automated LC+AMS [17] and intact acetaminophen (non-radiolabeled) was determined with an immunoassay. Results showed concentrations of [¹⁴C] acetaminophen were in the same range as previously reported in neonates and children. The average [¹⁴C]acetaminophen and the metabolite maximal concentrations in these infants were also similar to those reported in a previous microdose with microtracer study in adults[72]. The concentration of [¹⁴C] acetaminophen-4-sulfate in a 4-day old neonate was much higher than in a 2.4 year infant, in line with developmental changes of acetaminophen metabolism. A follow-up study with 50 additional patients is planned to study the developmental changes in acetaminophen disposition further.

Regulatory Acceptance

In general, the regulatory authorities are very accepting of AMS as a suitable methodology for use in drug development; many of the examples described in this chapter are from approved drugs. In its landmark 2004 publication *Challenge and Opportunity on the Critical Path to New Medical Products*, the US FDA called on the scientists engaged in developing new medicines to develop a "new product development toolkit—containing powerful new scientific and technical methods such as animal or computer-based predictive models, biomarkers for safety and effectiveness, and new clinical evaluation techniques." The use of ¹⁴C-AMS to enable the early and efficient collection of clinical DMPK data is surely part of the response to that. Subsequently, regulatory authorities around the globe have introduced procedures to facilitate microdosing [68,84]. Almost 25% of the 27 novel drugs approved by the FDA in 2013 included some AMS-generated data as part of the supporting dossier [3], and the authors have personal experience of regulatory agencies requesting absolute bioavailability data so late in the development process that using the concomitant dosing ¹⁴C-microtracer approach is the only feasible option. LC+AMS has also become accepted as a valid, quantitative bioanalytical tool, albeit not generally applied to regulated bioanalysis as defined by bodies such as the European Bioanalytical Forum [85].

Although, on an intellectual level and based on their publications, the regulatory agencies accept AMS as a valid technique. It is noted that individual assessors are not necessarily as well versed in the nuances of the different applications. For example, in 2011, having submitted data from a macrodose with microtracer AME study to the EMEA in support of a marketing application, one multinational pharmaceutical company was surprised to receive the suggestion that they would have to repeat the study on the basis of the rapporteur's concerns about the applicability of "microdose" data. Of course, it was easy enough for the company to respond to that question to say that the total mass dose administered level was in the pharmacologically relevant range, and it is to be hoped that, the same question would not now arise. However, this experience does highlight the need to be aware of the tendency for the non-initiated to assume that any AMS-enabled study *must* be a microdose.

Future Perspective

Smaller, cheaper AMS instruments and adoption of CO_2 detection by AMS will continue to increase versus the currently more prevalent graphitization technique. This will bring benefits in flexibility and cost reduction, e.g., LC+AMS method development and possibly improve throughput. The biggest effect is likely to be the development of a practical LC-AMS interface—current "moving wire set-ups" are not practical [16]. Adoption of a consensus on LC+AMS validation will also help in adoption of LC+AMS as a mainstream tool to address PK questions. The development of alternative technologies for the quantification of ¹⁴C is also likely. At one time, intracavity optogalvanic spectroscopy seemed promising in this area [86], but other researchers have not been able to reproduce the inventor's findings [87]. Now, ring down cavity laser detection seems to be the front runner, offering a potentially lower-cost ¹⁴C detector with a similar sensitivity to AMS [85] and an approach that eliminates many of the shortcomings of an accelerator-based system and would supplement the use of AMS in biomedical research.

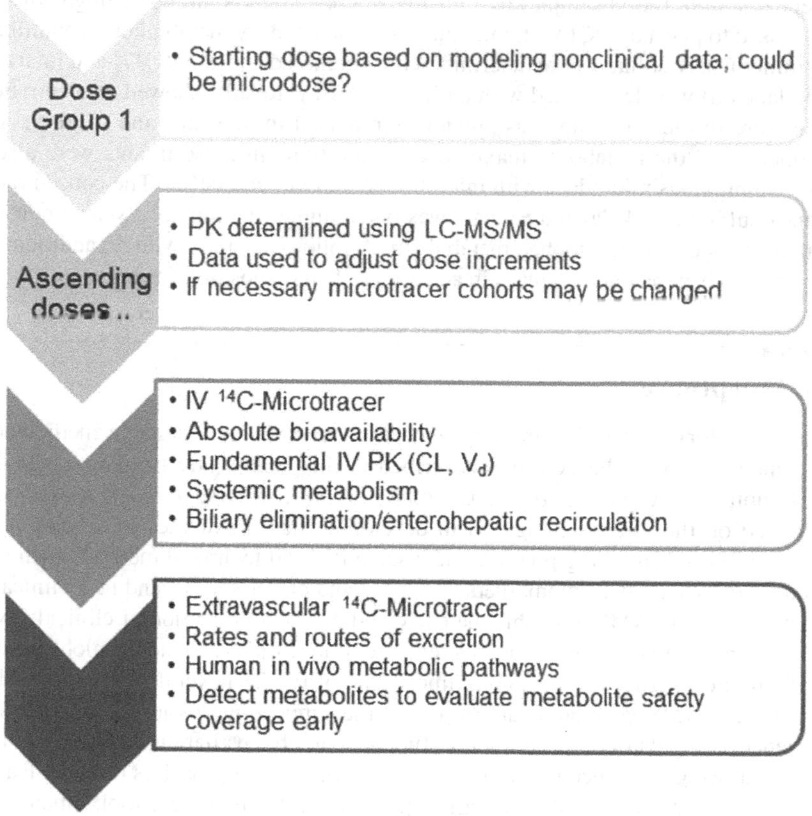

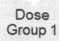

Dose Group 1
- Starting dose based on modeling nonclinical data; could be microdose?

Ascending doses ..
- PK determined using LC-MS/MS
- Data used to adjust dose increments
- If necessary microtracer cohorts may be changed

- IV ^{14}C-Microtracer
- Absolute bioavailability
- Fundamental IV PK (CL, V_d)
- Systemic metabolism
- Biliary elimination/enterohepatic recirculation

- Extravascular ^{14}C-Microtracer
- Rates and routes of excretion
- Human in vivo metabolic pathways
- Detect metabolites to evaluate metabolite safety coverage early

FIGURE 27.9   Microtracer enhanced FIH study design. (Adapted with permission from Seymour, M.A., *J. Labelled Comp. Radiopharm.*, 59, 640–647, 2016.)

A judicious incorporation of ^{14}C-labeled microtracer dose(s) can significantly enhance the quality and quantity of data obtained from the FIH study [5]. A generic microtracer-enhanced FIH study design is presented in Figure 27.9. Dosing cohorts suitable for inclusion of microtracer doses are preselected based on the planned-dose escalation strategy and the predicted therapeutic dose level. However, the clinical protocol is written to allow flexibility in these selections based on data emerging from earlier cohorts as the study progresses. The IV ^{14}C microtracer cohort is designed to generate fundamental PK parameters and absolute bioavailability data and is executed as part of the main study, without compromising its original objectives but generating significant additional data, for example on biotransformation. Inclusion of the second ^{14}C dose, administered by the extravascular (therapeutic) dose route, again as part of the main study, requires no additional effort or cost for radiosynthesis and in most cases, formulation. However, it is possible to design the extravascular ^{14}C microtracer cohort to meet the requirements for a definitive human mass balance study, suitable for submission as part of a marketing application. In such cases, it is recommended that the extravascular microtracer cohort is dosed in parallel to the main study, to allow co-formulation of the ^{14}C compound and non-radiolabeled drug and optimization of the sample collection regimen.

Whether as part of a FIH study or another "routine" clinical trial, the microtracer approach with AMS detection at a therapeutic dose is now a mature technique, and administration of macrotracer levels of radioactivity (typically ~100 µCi) in a separate clinical study is no longer necessary.

REFERENCES

1. Vogel JS, Turteltaub KW, Finkel R, Nelson DE. Accelerator mass spectrometry. *Analytical Chemistry.* 1995;67(11):353A–359A.
2. Dueker SR, Lohstroh PN, Giacomo JA, Vuong LT, Keck BD, Vogel JS. Early human ADME using microdose and microtracer: Bioanalytical considerations. *Bioanalysis.* 2010;2(3):441–454.
3. Young GC, Seymour M. Application of 14C-Accelerator MS in pharmaceutical development. *Bioanalysis.* 2015;7(5):513–517.
4. Burt T, John C, Ruckle J, Vuong L. Phase-0/microdosing studies using AMS, PET, and LC-MS/MS: A range of study methodologies and conduct considerations. Accelerating development of novel pharmaceuticals through safe testing in humans—A practical guide. *Expert Opinion on Drug Delivery.* 2017;14(5):657–672.
5. Seymour MA. Adding value through accelerator mass spectrometry-enabled first in human studies. *Journal of Labelled Compounds & Radiopharmaceuticals.* 2016;59(14):640–647.
6. Burt T, Yoshida K, Lappin G, Vuong L, John C, de Wildt SN, et al. Microdosing and other phase 0 clinical trials: Facilitating translation in drug development. *Clinical Translational Science.* 2016;9(2):74–88.
7. Dueker SR, Lohstroh PN, Giacomo JA, Vuong LT, Keck BD, Vogel JS. Quantifying exploratory low dose compounds in humans with AMS. *Advanced Drug Delivery Reviews.* 2011;63(7):518–531.
8. Lappin G. Approaches to intravenous clinical pharmacokinetics: Recent developments with isotopic microtracers. *Journal of Clinical Pharmacology.* 2016;56(1):11–23.
9. Lappin G, Noveck R, Burt T. Microdosing and drug development: Past, present and future. *Expert Opinion on Drug Metabolism & Toxicology.* 2013;9(7):817–834.
10. Vogel JS, Giacomo JA, Schulze-König T, Keck BD, Lohstroh P, Dueker SR. AMS best practices for accuracy and precision in bioanalytical ^{14}C measurements. *Bioanalysis.* 2010;2(3):455–468.
11. Lappin G, Seymour M, Young G, Higton D, Hill HM. An AMS method to determine analyte recovery from pharmacokinetic studies with concomitant extravascular and intravenous administration. *Bioanalysis.* 2011;3(4):407–410.
12. Vogel J, Love AH. Quantitating isotopic molecular labels with accelerator mass spectrometry. In: Burlingame AL, editor. *Methods in enzymology.* New York: Academic Press; 2005.
13. Vogel JS. Accelerator mass spectrometry for quantitative *in vivo* tracing. *Biotechniques.* 2005; 38(Suppl6):25–29.
14. Subramanian R, Zhu X, Hock MB, Sloey BJ, Wu B, Wilson SF et al. Pharmacokinetics, biotransformation, and excretion of [14C]Etelcalcetide (AMG 416) following a single microtracer intravenous dose in patients with chronic kidney disease on hemodialysis. *Clinical Pharmacokinetics.* 2017;56(2):179–192.
15. Lappin G, Seymour M, Young G, Higton D, Hill HM. AMS method validation for quantitation in pharmacokinetic studies with concomitant extravascular and intravenous administration. *Bioanalysis.* 2011;3(4):393–405.
16. Ognibene TJ, Thomas AT, Daley PF, Bench G, Turteltaub KW. An interface for the direct coupling of small liquid samples to AMS. *Nuclear Instruments and Methods in Physics Research Section B.* 2015;361:173–177.
17. van Duijn E, Sandman H, Grossouw D, Mocking JA, Coulier L, Vaes WH. Automated combustion accelerator mass spectrometry for the analysis of biomedical samples in the low attomole range. *Analytical Chemistry.* 2014;86(15):7635–7641.
18. Thomas AT, Stewart BJ, Ognibene TJ, Turteltaub KW, Bench G. Directly coupled high-performance liquid chromatography-accelerator mass spectrometry measurement of chemically modified protein and peptides. *Analytical Chemistry.* 2013;85(7):3644–3650.
19. Flarakos J, Liberman RG, Tannenbaum SR, Skipper PL. Integration of continuous-flow accelerator mass spectrometry with chromatography and mass-selective detection. *Analytical Chemistry.* 2008;80(13):5079–5085.
20. Australian Government Department of Health Therapeutic Goods Administration, Guidance 15: Biopharmaceutic Studies July 2014.
21. Strong JM, Dutcher JS, Lee WK, Atkinson AJ, Jr. Absolute bioavailability in man of N-acetylprocainamide determined by a novel stable isotope method. *Clinical Pharmacology and Therapeutics.* 1975; 18(5 Pt 1):613–622.

22. Xu XS, Jiang H, Christopher LJ, Shen JX, Zeng J, Arnold ME. Sensitivity-based analytical approaches to support human absolute bioavailability studies. *Bioanalysis.* 2014;6(4):497–504.

23. English S, Croft M, Lin JL, Pankratz T, Seymour MA, Yamashita J. What's the best way to measure absolute bioavailability? *Land O'Lakes Bioanalytical Meeting* 2014; Madison, WI.

24. Graham RA, Hop CE, Borin MT, Lum BL, Colburn D, Chang I et al. Single and multiple dose intravenous and oral pharmacokinetics of the hedgehog pathway inhibitor vismodegib in healthy female subjects. *British Journal of Clinical Pharmacology.* 2012;74(5):7887–96.

25. Lappin G, Seymour M, Gross G, Jørgensen M, Kall M, Kværnø L. Meeting the regulatory requirements in MIST: Human metabolism data early in phase-1 using accelerator-MS combined with a tiered bioanalytical approach in metabolite quantification. *Bioanalysis.* 2012;4(4):407–416.

26. Boulton DW, Kasichayanula S, Keung CF, Arnold ME, Christopher LJ, Xu XS et al. Simultaneous oral therapeutic and intravenous (1)(4)C-microdoses to determine the absolute oral bioavailability of saxagliptin and dapagliflozin. *British Journal of Clinical Pharmacology.* 2013;75(3):763–768.

27. Annes WF, Long A, Witcher JW, Ayan-Oshodi MA, Knadler MP, Zhang W et al. Relative contributions of presystemic and systemic peptidases to oral exposure of a novel metabotropic glutamate 2/3 receptor agonist (LY404039) after oral administration of prodrug pomaglumetad methionil (LY2140023). *Journal of Pharmaceutical Sciences.* 2015;104(1):207–214.

28. Jensen KG, Jacobsen AM, Bundgaard C, Nilausen DO, Thale Z, Chandrasena G et al. Lack of exposure in a first-in-man study due to aldehyde oxidase metabolism: Investigated by use of 14C-microdose, humanized mice, monkey pharmacokinetics, and *in vitro* methods. *Drug Metabolism.* 2017;45(1):68–75.

29. Guiney WJ, Beaumont C, Thomas SR, Robertson DC, McHugh SM, Koch A et al. Use of Entero-Test, a simple approach for non-invasive clinical evaluation of the biliary disposition of drugs. *British Journal of Clinical Pharmacology.* 2011;72(1):133–142.

30. Bloomer JC, Nash M, Webb A, Miller BE, Lazaar AL, Beaumont C et al. Assessment of potential drug interactions by characterization of human drug metabolism pathways using non-invasive bile sampling. *British Journal of Clinical Pharmacology.* 2013;75(2):488–496.

31. Gunnarsson M, Leide-Svegborn S, Stenstrom K, Skog G, Nilsson LE, Hellborg R et al. No radiation protection reasons for restrictions on ^{14}C urea breath tests in children. *The Bristish Journal of Radiology.* 2002;75(900):982–986.

32. Brown K, Tompkins EM, Boocock DJ, Martin EA, Farmer PB, Turteltaub KW et al. Tamoxifen forms DNA adducts in human colon after administration of a single [14C]-labeled therapeutic dose. *Cancer Research.* 2007;67(14):6995–7002.

33. Chen J, Garner RC, Lee LS, Seymour M, Fuchs EJ, Hubbard WC et al. Accelerator mass spectrometry measurement of intracellular concentrations of active drug metabolites in human target cells *in vivo*. *Clinical Pharmacology and Therapeutics.* 2010;88(6):796–800.

34. Lappin G, Boyce MJ, Matzow T, Lociuro S, Seymour M, Warrington SJ. A microdose study of ^{14}C-AR-709 in healthy men: Pharmacokinetics, absolute bioavailability and concentrations in key compartments of the lung. *European Journal of Clinical Pharmacology.* 2013;69(9):1673–1682.

35. Sarapa N, Hsyu PH, Lappin G, Garner RC. The application of accelerator mass spectrometry to absolute bioavailability studies in humans: Simultaneous administration of an intravenous microdose of ^{14}C-nelfinavir mesylate solution and oral nelfinavir to healthy volunteers. *Journal of Clinical Pharmacology.* 2005;45(10):1198–1205.

36. Lappin G, Shishikura Y, Jochemsen R, Weaver RJ, Gesson C, Houston B et al. Pharmacokinetics of fexofenadine: Evaluation of a microdose and assessment of absolute oral bioavailability. *European Journal of Pharmaceutical Sciences: Official Journal of the European Federation for Pharmaceutical Sciences.* 2010;40(2):125–131.

37. Lappin G, Shishikura Y, Jochemsen R, Weaver RJ, Gesson C, Houston JB et al. Comparative pharmacokinetics between a microdose and therapeutic dose for clarithromycin, sumatriptan, propafenone, paracetamol (acetaminophen), and phenobarbital in human volunteers. *European Journal of Pharmaceutical Sciences.* 2011;43:141–150.

38. Ross AB, Vuong le T, Ruckle J, Synal HA, Schulze-Konig T, Wertz K et al. Lycopene bioavailability and metabolism in humans: An accelerator mass spectrometry study. *The American Journal of Clinical Nutrition.* 2011;93(6):1263–1273.

39. Chen J, Flexner C, Liberman RG, Skipper PL, Louissaint NA, Tannenbaum SR et al. Biphasic elimination of tenofovir diphosphate and nonlinear pharmacokinetics of zidovudine triphosphate in a microdosing study. *Journal of Acquired Immune Deficiency Syndromes*. 2012;61(5):593–599.

40. Denton CL, Minthorn E, Carson SW, Young GC, Richards-Peterson LE, Botbyl J et al. Concomitant oral and intravenous pharmacokinetics of dabrafenib, a BRAF inhibitor, in patients with BRAF V600 mutation-positive solid tumors. *Journal of Clinical Pharmacology*. 2013;53(9):955–961.

41. Hoffmann E, Wald J, Lavu S, Roberts J, Beaumont C, Haddad J et al. Pharmacokinetics and tolerability of SRT2104, a first-in-class small molecule activator of SIRT1, after single and repeated oral administration in man. *British Journal of Clinical Pharmacology*. 2013;75(1):186–196.

42. Schwab D, Portron A, Backholer Z, Lausecker B, Kawashima K. A novel double-tracer technique to characterize absorption, distribution, metabolism and excretion (ADME) of [14C]tofogliflozin after oral administration and concomitant intravenous microdose administration of [13C]tofogliflozin in humans. *Clinical Pharmacokinetics*. 2013;52(6):463–473.

43. Leonowens C, Pendry C, Bauman J, Young GC, Ho M, Henriquez F et al. Concomitant oral and intravenous pharmacokinetics of trametinib, a MEK inhibitor, in subjects with solid tumours. *British Journal of Clinical Pharmacology*. 2014;78(3):524–532.

44. Tse S, Leung L, Raje S, Seymour M, Shishikura Y, Obach RS. Disposition and metabolic profiling of [^{14}C]Cerlapirdine utilizing accelerator mass spectrometry (AMS). *Drug Metabolism and Disposition: The Biological Fate of Chemicals*. 2014;42(12):2023–2032.

45. Devineni D, Murphy J, Wang SS, Stieltjes H, Rothenberg P, Scheers E et al. Absolute oral bioavailability and pharmacokinetics of canagliflozin: A microdose study in healthy participants. *Clinical Pharmacology in Drug Development*. 2015;4(4):295–304.

46. Negash K, Andonian C, Felgate C, Chen C, Goljer I, Squillaci B et al. The metabolism and disposition of GSK2140944 in healthy human subjects. *Xenobiotica; the Fate of Foreign Compounds in Biological Systems*. 2016;46(8):683–702.

47. Suri A, Pusalkar S, Li Y, Prakash S. Absorption, Distribution, and excretion of the investigational agent orteronel (TAK-700) in healthy male subjects: A phase 1, open-label, single-dose study. *Clinical Pharmacology in Drug Development*. 2016;5(3):108–107.

48. Hickey MJ, Allen PH, Kingston LP, Wilkinson DJ. The synthesis of [(14) C]AZD5122. Incorporation of an IV (14) C-microtracer dose into a first in human study to determine the absolute oral bioavailability of AZD5122. *Journal of Labelled Compounds & Radiopharmaceuticals*. 2016;59(6):245–249.

49. Bell G, Huang S, Martin KJ, Block GA. A randomized, double-blind, phase 2 study evaluating the safety and efficacy of AMG 416 for the treatment of secondary hyperparathyroidism in hemodialysis patients. *Current Medical Research and Opinion*. 2015;31(5):943–952.

50. Bushinsky DA, Block GA, Martin KJ, Bell G, Huang S, Sun Y et al. Treatment of secondary hyperparathyroidism: Results of a phase 2 trial evaluating an intravenous peptide agonist of the calcium-sensing receptor. *American Journal of Nephrology*. 2015;42(5):379–388.

51. Block GA, Bushinsky DA, Cheng S, Cunningham J, Dehmel B, Drueke TB et al. Effect of etelcalcetide versus cinacalcet on serum parathyroid hormone in patients receiving hemodialysis with secondary hyperparathyroidism: A randomized clinical trial. *JAMA*. 2017;317(2):156–164.

52. Block GA, Bushinsky DA, Cunningham J, Drueke TB, Ketteler M, Kewalramani R et al. Effect of etelcalcetide versus placebo on serum parathyroid hormone in patients receiving hemodialysis with secondary hyperparathyroidism: Two randomized clinical trials. *JAMA*. 2017;317(2):146–155.

53. Martin KJ, Bell G, Pickthorn K, Huang S, Vick A, Hodsman P et al. Velcalcetide (AMG 416), a novel peptide agonist of the calcium-sensing receptor, reduces serum parathyroid hormone and FGF23 levels in healthy male subjects. *Nephrology, Dialysis, Transplantation: Official Publication of the European Dialysis and Transplant Association—European Renal Association*. 2014;29(2):385–392.

54. Martin KJ, Pickthorn K, Huang S, Block GA, Vick A, Mount PF et al. AMG 416 (velcalcetide) is a novel peptide for the treatment of secondary hyperparathyroidism in a single-dose study in hemodialysis patients. *Kidney International*. 2014;85(1):191–197.

55. Hamilton RA, Garnett WR, Kline BJ. Determination of mean valproic acid serum level by assay of a single pooled sample. *Clinical Pharmacology and Therapeutics*. 1981;29(3):408–413.

56. Wu L, Melhem M, Subramanian R, Wu B. Drug disposition model of radiolabeled etelcalcetide in patients with chronic kidney disease and secondary hyperparathyroidism on hemodialysis. *Journal of Pharmacokinetics and Pharmacodynamics.* 2017;44(1):43–53.

57. Lappin G, Rowland M, Garner RC. The use of isotopes in the determination of absolute bioavailability of drugs in humans. *Expert Opinion on Drug Metabolism & Toxicology.* 2006;2(3):419–427.

58. Graham RA, Lum BL, Morrison G, Chang I, Jorga K, Dean B et al. A single dose mass balance study of the hedgehog pathway inhibitor vismodegib (GDC-0449) in humans using accelerator mass spectrometry. *Drug Metabolism and Sisposition: The Biological Fate of Chemicals.* 2011;39(8):1460–1467.

59. Vlaming MLH, van Duijn E, Dillingh MR, Brands R, Windhorst AD, Hendrikse NH et al. Microdosing of a carbon-14 labeled protein in healthy volunteers accurately predicts its pharmacokinetics at therapeutic dosages. *Clinical Pharmacology and Therapeutics.* 2015;98(2):196–204.

60. Xu W, Dueker SR, Christopher LJ, Lohstroh PN, Keung CF, Cao K et al. Overcoming bioanalytical challenges in an Onglyza intravenous [14C]microdose absolute bioavailability study with accelerator MS. *Bioanalysis.* 2012;4(15):1855–1870.

61. ICH M3 R2. *Guidance on Nonclinical Safety Studies for the Conduct of Human Clinical Trials and Marketing Authorization for Pharmaceuticals.* 2009; Last Accessed February 17, 2019.

62. Sun L, Li H, Willson K, Breidinger S, Rizk ML, Wenning L et al. Ultrasensitive liquid chromatography-tandem mass spectrometric methodologies for quantification of five HIV-1 integrase inhibitors in plasma for a microdose clinical trial. *Analytical Chemistry.* 2012;84(20):8614–8621.

63. Lappin G, Kuhnz W, Jochemsen R, Kneer J, Chaudhary A, Oosterhuis B et al. Use of microdosing to predict pharmacokinetics at the therapeutic dose: Experience with 5 drugs. *Clinical Pharmacology and Therapeutics.* 2006;80(3):203–215.

64. Yamashita S. Impact of NEDO project on microdosing clinical studies: Toward the eIND study in Japan. *Drug Metabolism and Pharmacokinetics.* 2011;26(6):549–550.

65. Bosgra S, Vlaming MLH, Vaes WHJ. To apply microdosing or not? Recommendations to single out compounds with non-linear pharmacokinetics. *Clinical Pharmacokinetics.* 2016;55(1):1–15.

66. Tachibana T, Kato M, Sugiyama Y. Prediction of nonlinear intestinal absorption of CYP3A4 and P-glycoprotein substrates from their *in vitro* Km values. *Pharmaceutical Research.* 2012;29(3):651–668.

67. Ring BJ, Chien JY, Adkison KK, Jones HM, Rowland M, Jones RD et al. PhRMA CPCDC initiative on predictive models of human pharmacokinetics, part 3: Comparative assessement of prediction methods of human clearance. *Journal of Pharmaceutical Sciences.* 2011;100(10):4090–4110.

68. Center for Drug Evaluation and Research (CDER; Food and Drug Administration). Guidance for Industry, Investigators, and Reviewers—Exploratory Investigational New Drug Studies. 2006; Last Accessed February 17, 2019.

69. Knutson CG, Skipper PL, Liberman RG, Tannenbaum SR, Marnett LJ. Monitoring *in vivo* metabolism and elimination of the endogenous DNA adduct, M1dG {3-(2-deoxy-beta-D-erythro-pentofuranosyl) pyrimido[1,2-alpha]purin-10(3H)-one}, by accelerator mass spectrometry. *Chemical Research in Toxicology.* 2008;21(6):1290–1294.

70. Zhou XJ, Garner RC, Nicholson S, Kissling CJ, Mayers D. Microdose pharmacokinetics of IDX899 and IDX989, candidate HIV-1 non-nucleoside reverse transcriptase inhibitors, following oral and intravenous administration in healthy male subjects. *Journal of Clinical Pharmacology.* 2009;49(12):1408–1416.

71. Vuong LT, Ruckle JL, Blood AB, Reid MJ, Wasnich RD, Synal H-A et al. Use of accelerator mass spectrometry to measure the pharmacokinetics and peripheral blood mononuclear cell concentrations of zidovudine. *Journal of Pharmaceutical Sciences.* 2008;97(7):2833–2843.

72. Tozuka Z, Kusuhara H, Nozawa K, Hamabe Y, Ikushima I, Ikeda T et al. Microdose study of 14C-acetaminophen with accelerator mass spectrometry to examine pharmacokinetics of parent drug and metabolites in healthy subjects. *Clinical Pharmacology and Therapeutics.* 2010;88(6):824–830.

73. Dueker SR, Vuong le T, Lohstroh PN, Giacomo JA, Vogel JS. Quantifying exploratory low dose compounds in humans with AMS. *Advanced Drug Delivery Reviews.* 2011;63(7):518–531.

74. Duchateau G, Cochrane B, Windebank S, Herudzinska J, Sanghera D, Burian A et al. Absolute oral bioavailability and metabolic turnover of beta-sitosterol in healthy subjects. *Drug Metabolism and Disposition: The Biological Fate of Chemicals.* 2012;40(10):2026–2030.

75. Madeen E, Corley RA, Crowell S, Turteltaub K, Ognibene T, Malfatti M et al. Human *in Vivo* pharmacokinetics of [(14)C]Dibenzo[def, p]chrysene by accelerator mass spectrometry following oral microdosing. *Chemical Research in Toxicology.* 2015;28(1):126–134.

76. Vuong LT, Blood AB, Vogel JS, Anderson ME, Goldstein B. Applications of accelerator MS in pediatric drug evaluation. *Bioanalysis*. 2012;4(15):1871–1882.
77. Sachs AN, Avant D, Lee CS, Rodriguez W, Murphy MD. Pediatric information in drug product labeling. *JAMA*. 2012;307(18):1914–1915.
78. Turner MA, Catapano M, Hirschfeld S, Giaquinto C, Global Research in P. Paediatric drug development: The impact of evolving regulations. *Advanced Drug Delivery Reviews*. 2014;73:2–13.
79. Roth-Cline M, Nelson RM. Microdosing studies in children: A US regulatory perspective. *Clinical Pharmacology and Therapeutics*. 2015;98(3):232–233.
80. Turner MA, Mooij MG, Vaes WH, Windhorst AD, Hendrikse NH, Knibbe CA et al. Pediatric microdose and microtracer studies using ^{14}C in Europe. *Clinical Pharmacology and Therapeutics*. 2015;98(3):234–237.
81. Mooij MG, Van Duijn E, Knibbe CA, Windhorst AD, Hendrikse NH, Vaes WH et al. Pediatric microdose study of [14C] paracetamol to study drug metabolism using accelerator mass spectrometry: Proof of concept. *Clinical Pharmacokinetics*. 2014;53:1045–1051.
82. Gordi T, Baillie R, Vuong le T, Abidi S, Dueker S, Vasquez H et al. Pharmacokinetic analysis of ^{14}C-ursodiol in newborn infants using accelerator mass spectrometry. *Journal of Clinical Pharmacology*. 2014;54(9):1031–1037.
83. Aklamati EK, Mulenga M, Dueker SR, Buchholz BA, Peerson JM, Kafwembe E et al. Accelerator mass spectrometry can be used to assess vitamin A metabolism quantitatively in boys in a community setting. *Journal of Nutrition*. 2010;140:1588–1594.
84. ICH Topic M3 (R2) (CPMP/ICH/286/95) Non-Clinical Safety Studies for the Conduct of Human Clinical Trials and Marketing Authorization for Pharmaceuticals. 2008 & 2009; Last Accessed February 17, 2019.
85. Higton D, Young G, Timmerman P, Abbott R, Knutsson M, Svensson LD. European bioanalysis forum recommendation: Scientific validation of quantification by accelerator mass spectrometry. *Bioanalysis*. 2012;4:2669–2679.
86. Murnick DE, Dogru O, Ilkmen E. Intracavity optogalvanic spectroscopy. An analytical technique for ^{14}C analysis with subattomole sensitivity. *Analytical Chemistry*. 2008;80(13):4820–4824.
87. Persson A, Salehpour M. Intracavity optogalvanic spectroscopy: Is there any evidence of a radiocarbon signal? *Nuclear Instruments and Methods in Physics Research Section B: Beam Interactions with Materials and Atoms*. 2015;361:8–12.

Index

Note: Page numbers in italic and bold refer to figures and tables, respectively.